T0338392

HANDBOOK OF APPLIED DOG BEHAVIOR AND TRAINING

Volume Three

Procedures and Protocols

HANDBOOK OF
APPLIED DOG BEHAVIOR AND TRAINING

Volume Three

Procedures and Protocols

Steven R. Lindsay

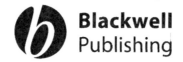
Blackwell
Publishing

Steven R. Lindsay, MA, is a dog behavior consultant and trainer who lives in Newtown Square, Pennsylvania, where he provides a variety of behavioral training and counseling services. In addition to his long career in working with companion dogs, he previously evaluated and trained military working dogs as a member of the U.S. Army Biosensor Research Team (Superdog Program).

©2005 Blackwell Publishing

Blackwell Publishing Professional
2121 State Avenue, Ames, Iowa 50014, USA

Orders: 1-800-862-6657
Office: 1-515-292-0140
Fax: 1-515-292-3348
Web site: www.blackwellprofessional.com

Blackwell Publishing Ltd
9600 Garsington Road, Oxford OX4 2DQ, UK
Tel.: +44 (0)1865 776868

Blackwell Publishing Asia
550 Swanston Street, Carlton, Victoria 3053, Australia
Tel.: +61 (0)3 8359 1011

Cover image: "Puppies in Snow," by Katsushika Hokusai (1760-1849), Japanese Edo period. Courtesy of the Freer Gallery of Art, Smithsonian Institution, Washington, D.C.

First edition, 2005

Printed and bound in Malaysia by Vivar Printing Sdn Bhd

The Library of Congress has catalogued Volume One as follows:
Lindsay, Steven R.
Handbook of applied dog behavior and training / Steven R. Lindsay; foreword by Victoria Lea Voith.— 1st ed.
  p. cm.
  Contents: v. 1. Adaption and learning
  ISBN 978-0-8138-0738-6

  1. Dogs—Behavior. 2. Dogs—Training. I. Title.

SF433.1.56 1999
636.7'0887—dc21

                                                                      99-052013

Contents

9   *Biobehavioral Monitoring and Electronic Control of Behavior*

Preface

A unifying focus of the *Handbook of Applied Dog Behavior and Training* has been to collect and organize a coherent and integrated body of scientific knowledge with practical and theoretical relevance for understanding and controlling dog behavior—especially problem behavior. The information has been collected from diverse areas of scientific research, including canine evolution and domestication, ethology, behavioral ontogeny, neurobiology, cognition and emotion, and learning. The process of assembling and organizing the information contained in this work bears a resemblance to what E. O. Wilson (1998) has referred to as *consilience*, that is, an inventive linking together of facts and theory from different scientific disciplines to produce a framework of explanation and novel hypotheses. This eclectic process of tying together data-based theoretical accounts and experimental findings from diverse fields not only reveals a significant interdisciplinary order and unity between them, it also produces an astonishing diversity of new ideas and possibilities for taking a fresh look at the organization and disorganization of dog behavior.

The selection of topics covered in Volume 3, *Procedures and Protocols*, has been largely based on criteria of practical relevance and value for dog behavior specialists providing professional behavior therapy, counseling, and training services. Various themes introduced in Volumes 1 and 2 are revisited and expanded upon, especially with regard to significant social, biological, and behavioral influences that impact the etiology of behavior problems and their treatment. Although Volume 3 can stand alone for reference purposes, fully appreciating the finer details and distinctions referred to in the text requires that readers be familiar with the contents of Volumes 1 and 2. There is extensive cross-referencing to these previous volumes, especially when a topic covered requires additional background information or explanation not reviewed in the discussion. Ethological observations, relevant behavioral and neurobiological research, and dog behavior clinical findings are reviewed and critiqued, while various protocols, procedures and techniques are introduced and explained in detail.

Advances in neurobiology, cognitive neuroscience, and psychobiology are revolutionizing our understanding of the neural substrates mediating emotion, cognition, executive functions (attention and impulse control), and learning. In addition to studying normal function and development, brain scientists have accumulated a growing and impressive body of scientific information concerning the organic and stress-related causes of abnormal behavior. Of special interest are experimental efforts under way to tease out and trace the neural substrates mediating expressive emotional behavior and learning. According to a prominent psychobiological theory of emotion postulated by Panksepp (1998), emotional command systems interact in biologically prepared ways to modulate (inhibit or excite) and shape the expression of motivated behavior. Behavioral disturbances may result from adverse learning or traumatic events disrupting the equilibrium of emotional systems—a theory possessing significant practical value for understanding and treating a variety of dog behavior problems. Panksepp's quadrant of emotional command systems nicely dovetails with the primary drives traditionally ascribed to dog behavior. Another exciting area of basic neurobiological research that is relevant for applied dog behaviorists and trainers involves work that is tracing the neural basis of reward. For example, strong data suggest that dopaminergic reward circuits are activated or depressed in accordance with the occurrence of positive and negative predictions errors—findings that have far-reaching theoretical and practical implications. The neurobehavioral investigation of expectancy, comparator mechanisms, and prediction error is poised to revolutionize our understanding of learning and the significance of reward and punishment. Prediction and control expectancies, calibrated establishing operations, emotional command systems, and the prediction-error hypothesis figure prominently in cynopraxic training theory.

Vulnerability to emotional distress and stress appears to play a significant predisposing role in the etiology of many dog behavior problems. The ability of dogs to cope with stressful situations is influenced significantly by the type and degree of stress that they are exposed to in early development. Although some limited exposure to stress is beneficial, inappropriate stress and traumatic fear conditioning may produce a lasting adverse effect on the way dogs cope with stressful situations in adulthood. The organization and functional integrity of the brain are strongly influenced by prenatal and early postnatal stress, perhaps predisposing dogs to develop a variety of stress-related behavior problems and disorders. A very active and productive area of brain research has been dedicated to exploring the effects of adverse postnatal stress on the developing brain and behavior. Some of this research has been reviewed in the context of potential factors that predispose affected dogs to develop aggression and separation-related problems. In addition, brain scientists are closing in on the genes, receptors, circuits, and complex matrix of biochemical pathways mediating the learning and expression of emotional behaviors. This research suggests that highly effective and precisely targeted medications might be available in the not-too-distant future for controlling fear-related problems and aggression that currently remain refractory to conventional treatment. Finally, neurobiology has considerable value for identifying putative organic causes of behavioral disorder and the probable mechanisms mediating pharmacological benefits, which is information of considerable value to veterinarians requiring coherent rationales for prescribing psychotropic medications to manage behavior problems. Knowledge of neurobiology and behavioral pharmacology offers nonmedical behavior modifiers insight into the close link between brain function, emotion, and behavior, and provides an improved appreciation of the use of drug therapy in the treatment of behavior problems.

What a dog does, its propensity to learn, the range of what it learns, and the way it goes about learning it are preemptively influenced by biological constraints. These phylogenetic predispositions include both evolutionary adaptations of an ancient origin as well as more recent changes wrought by domestication and selective breeding. Although heredity exerts a powerful effect, the social and physical environment plays a decisive role in the way these biological propensities are expressed in a dog's behavioral phenotype. From conception to senescence, biobehavioral ontogeny is in a continuous process of change and adaptation, with each stage in a dog's development affecting subsequent phenotypic physical and behavioral characteristics and organization (epigenesis). Whereas normal and protective environments nurture adaptive behavior, abnormal and distressing environments facilitate the elaboration of various emotional and behavioral disturbances increasing a dog's vulnerability to serious adjustment problems. In addition to the disturbing effects of adverse early experiences (e.g., prenatal and neonatal stress, early abuse and trauma, and social deprivation), a wide range of disorganizing emotional and behavioral effects are mediated by stressful or neurotogenic environments possessing insufficient order and regularity to promote social competence and adaptive success.

Environmental pressures shape both phylogenetic and ontogenetic adaptations. Dogs are compelled by an ever-present array of internal and external environmental pressures to adjust in various ways. In addition to an assortment of relatively rigid adjustment mechanisms (e.g., reflexes and modal action patterns), dogs are biologically equipped to adjust to environmental pressures by means of behavioral changes organized by learning. Dogs possess sophisticated cognitive, instrumental, and associative learning abilities that enable them to cope with and adapt to complex and variable environmental circumstances. These abilities enable dogs to find and exploit necessary resources (comfort seeking) and to detect, escape, or avoid environmental hazards in the process of doing so (safety seeking). Competent instrumental control over significant aversive and attractive events is only possible to the extent that a dog is able to anticipate and prepare for their occurrence in advance, which requires that the environment possess a certain degree of regularity and constancy with respect to such events and that the dog possess the ability to codify the benefits of experience into a useful and accessible form. The predictive information needed is obtained by means of classical conditioning, whereby contexts and incidental stimuli that regularly anticipate significant events are associatively linked, thereby preparing the dog emotionally and behaviorally to respond effectively. Learning of this sort provides a major organizing or disorganizing influence via the formation of prediction expectancies and preparatory appetitive and emotional establishing operations. Behavior operating under excessively disordered circumstances tends to produce varying levels of conflict and stress (anxiety and frustration), attentional strain and disturbance, impulse-control deficits, insecurity, emotional reactivity and panic, and behavioral incompetence—sequelae often associated with common dog behavior problems.

Just as evolution depends on an organism's capacity to maintain stability while changing, the optimization of prediction-control efforts depends on a balance between necessity and uncertainty. Whereas evolutionary advances are the results of life and death experiments etched into a species' genome and transmitted by genetically related individuals to progeny, behavioral adaptation proceeds in accord with interactive experiments consisting of social exchanges and transactions that transmit a collective culture, whereby culturally related individuals and their progeny are able to coexist in relative harmony and security (comfort and safety). Although the attainment of enhanced prediction and control over environmental events is a significant adaptive priority of organized behavior, learning does not proceed by the confirmation of prediction and control expectancies alone, but depends on adjustments resulting from the detection of prediction errors. Logically speaking, well-predicted and well-controlled events routinely produced by the dog do not require that it learn anything else about them beyond what it already knows, at least so long as the situation remains the same. The occurrence of such anticipated outcomes may elicit strong emotions conducive to comfort and safety (e.g., gratification and relaxation) that may incidentally excite or inhibit behavioral output, but it does not produce reward or punishment unless the anticipated outcome is found to be better or less aversive than expected. Adaptive learning depends on environmental conditions that provide enough order to foster reliable predictions together with sufficient change and variety to produce prediction dissonance. Either extreme of excessive regimentation or disorder (confusion) is inimical to instrumental learning. Consequently, given the deleterious effects of either extreme order or disorder, behavior therapy and training activities should be designed to strike a balance between the dog's need for order and its need for variability.

Chapter 1 provides a foundation of procedures and techniques used for basic training and the prevention or management of a variety of behavior problems. Basic training is an important aspect of cynopraxic therapy, playing a significant role in the treatment of virtually all behavior problems by improving interactive dynamics and establishing a platform of training and conditioning that complements and facilitates the implementation of behavior-therapy procedures. Emphasis is placed on the importance of integrating training activities into the home and bringing the dog under the control of everyday rewards and play—a process referred to as *integrated compliance training* (ICT). Although food reinforcement figures prominently in many cynopraxic training and therapy procedures, strong emphasis is placed on the pivotal role of affection and play for mediating behavior change via a normalization of human-dog interaction.

Play is particularly valued for its capacity to mediate cognitive and emotional transactions conducive to fairness, mutual appreciation, and interactive harmony. In addition to providing means for integrating and elaborating complex patterns of motivated behavior, play mediates powerful therapeutic effects by balancing emotional command systems, enhancing the human-dog bond, and improving the dog's quality of life. In general, attractive motivational incentives are used to facilitate a perception of control over significant events and enhanced power (competence and confidence).

Cynopraxic training efforts are distinguished by a focus on attentional functions (attending and orienting behavior), expectancies, and emotional establishing operations. Creating a framework of mutual attention and focus between the trainer and the dog is critical for communication, emotional transactions, and the bonding process. Attention control plays an important role in most dog behavior therapy and training procedures insofar as it mediates improved impulse control, social engagement, and autonomic attunement. Focusing training efforts on attending and orienting behavior is extremely efficient for establishing control over highly motivated behavior, especially when it is combined with the activation of potent conditioned and unconditioned appetitive and emotional establishing operations. For attention control to be maximally effective, it requires timeliness, ideally linking orienting stimuli, conditioned reinforcement, and establishing operations with the earliest intentional movements in anticipation of action, the target arc. Intensive orienting and target-arc training with positive prediction error exert a number of far-reaching benefits in the context of cynopraxic behavior therapy, virtually rebooting attentional functions, invigorating the social engagement system, and modifying preattentive biases. Rather than attempting to establish direct control over highly motivated and complex behavior by head-on means, many behavioral efforts are facilitated by first training a dog to orient toward the trainer, to attend (make sustained eye contact) in response to its name, and to pursue deictic signals or commands directing the dog's attention by gesture and gaze, and then building a small repertoire of reliable basic-training modules and routines (e.g., come, sit, down, stay, and controlled walking) via reward-based efforts incorporating both attractive and aversive motivational incentives. By means of basic training, attention control is progressively integrated with behavioral adjustments incompatible with undesirable activities and gradually unlinks attentional connections with competing sources of gratification and reward (distractions).

Chapter 2 contains foundation procedures and techniques for the control of inappropriate elimination, appetitive and ingestive behavior problems, and destructive exploratory activities. These basic areas of adjustment can exert a profound and enduring adverse effect on the bond and the dog's quality of life. Dog's that habitually eliminate in the house or destroy personal belongings may foster a high degree of familial resentment, often leading to excessive confinement, abusive punishment, or relinquishment. The section on house training completes a discussion on elimination problems begun in Volume 2, where several procedures and techniques used for controlling common elimination problems are discussed. In addition to methods used for controlling destructive behavior, various techniques are explored for the management and treatment of pica and coprophagy. The eating of nondigestible items is a significant health concern because it may result in life-threatening intestinal obstructions. Coprophagy also represents a health risk, but the greatest risk of harm is the damage such behavior does to the human-dog bond. Since coprophagy is highly offensive to the average dog owner's sensibilities, the disgust for the habit is easily transferred to the dog, especially in cases where small children affectionately interact with the dog. As a result, excessive or persistent coprophagy should receive prompt medical and behavioral attention aimed at resolving it, rather than be brushed off as an innocuous canine vice.

Chapter 3 explores the functional and dysfunctional significance of fear together with a variety of techniques and procedures used to treat fear-related behavior problems. Maladaptive fear and anxiety figure prominently in the etiology of many adjustment problems as well as serious behavior problems. Once established, certain fear reactions may become virtually permanent, forming highly durable and extinction-resistant associations with conditioned eliciting stimuli. Dogs exhibiting such phobias are often treated with procedures aimed at reducing fearful arousal while exposure is organized in a way that encourages more effective coping strategies when faced with fear-eliciting situations. These procedures usually involve some form of graded interactive exposure or desensitization process carried out in combination with counterconditioning. Many fearful behavior patterns appear to operate under the influence of faulty prediction and control expectancies. Avoidance behavior occurring in association with fearful arousal may prevent a dog from discovering that its fear is unfounded, simply because the dog does not remain in the situation to recognize that it is not dangerous and that the anticipated aversive outcome does not occur. In essence, since the expected outcome never occurs, the avoidance response confirms the control expectancy. Consequently, response-prevention procedures are often used to block avoidance behavior with the goal of demonstrating to the dog that the aversive contingency no longer exists, thereby gradually extinguishing the avoidance response. Graduated exposure and response prevention are usually performed in conjunction with fear-antagonizing counterconditioning efforts and instrumental training efforts aimed at shaping behavior and expectancies incompatible with avoidance and fear. In addition to dysfunctional or faulty prediction and control expectancies, many common canine fears appear to stem from competency doubts arising in potentially dangerous or risky situations. Counterconditioning techniques are of little value in treating fears maintained under the anxiety and pessimism of competency doubts. In such cases, fear is treated by means of graded interactive exposure in combination with the progressive development of various skills needed to successfully control the feared situation (e.g.,

climbing stairs). Along with developing competent skills, the dog naturally becomes more confident and relaxed—a potent counterconditioning effect that follows from training and systematic skill development. In addition to social fears and avoidance, many aggression problems appear to stem from competency deficits, whereby the dog enters into provocative exchanges under an expectation of failure. Cynopraxic training enables dogs to cope more effectively with fear through the empowerment resulting from reward-based training. Learning to control the occurrence of attractive and aversive motivational stimuli promotes an improved sense of power that enables dogs to approach situations perceived as threats or challenges with a positive expectancy bias.

Chapter 4 addresses problems that occur in association with emotional agitation and distress at separation. The term *separation distress* has been chosen over the more commonly used term *separation anxiety* because the former term seems to capture more accurately the diversity of the emotional causes and varied presenting signs that characterize this collection of behavior problems. Although dogs distressed at separation often exhibit anxiety and worry, they also exhibit signs of frustration and panic, which are coactive states of arousal that likely arise from different causes and that may accordingly require different strategies of control and management. The term *separation distress* seems preferable to *separation anxiety* because the former is sufficiently general to encompass a varied group of coactive emotional influences, while remaining consistent with the experimental use of the term, denoting the propensity of young animals to become agitated or depressed when separated from maternal and sibling attachment objects or others with whom a state of reciprocal autonomic regulation or attunement has been established through interactive exchange. Also, separation distress appears to originate in a circuit dedicated to the generation of a special type of aversive emotional arousal associated with social loss, which is emotional activity that is sensitive to a variety of coactive excitatory and inhibitory influences, including anger, frustration, anxiety, and fear. Adopting the term separation distress also helps to distance separation reactivity in dogs from potentially misleading connotations and implications derived from the use of the term separation anxiety in child psychiatry.

Currently, the most common procedures used to control problematic separation distress are systematic desensitization and detachment training. These procedures are discussed in detail. Both procedures are hampered by compliance problems, on the one hand, due to technical and practical difficulties associated with the implementation of systematic desensitization and, on the other hand, stemming from the unwillingness of many dog owners to consistently impose restrictions on their dog's affection- and contact-seeking behavior. Various protocols emphasizing the importance of secure place and social attachments in the treatment of problematic separation distress are presented. Instead of breaking down the attachment between the owner and the dog or exclusively relying on techniques to reduce anxiety or other coactive symptoms presenting at separation, emphasis is placed on training and therapy procedures that improve the quality of the existing attachment and bond. Essentially, the goal of such training is replace dependent and insecure or nervous attachment dynamics and reactive patterns of separation behavior with a more mature and trusting bond while systematically shaping a more competent repertoire of separation behaviors. These objectives are achieved by means of various behavior therapy procedures, including the implementation of a program of variable and reward-dense separation exposures (planned departures), with the goal of organizing more secure separation expectancies and enabling the dog to endure stressful separations without becoming overly reactive or panicked. Training activities that increase social trust and secure attachments (comfort and safety) are central to the effective treatment of separation-related problems.

An increased vulnerability to separation distress (and aggression) may be causally related to stressful insults occurring at a formative stage of development. To evaluate possible causal linkages between prenatal and postnatal stress on developing behavior, relevant lines of neurobiological research are reviewed, which is a theme that is continued in the context of aggression problems in Chapter 8. Interestingly, separation-distress problems often share with serious aggression problems an element of panic (reactive incompetence) arising in association with social exchanges and transactions that threaten a loss of comfort or safety. Both sets of adjustment problems present with a similar autoprotective urgency, but, of course, operating under diametrically opposed incentives aimed at producing quite opposite effects, yet sharing equally reactive and incompetent means, namely, efforts to increase proximity (separation distress) versus efforts to decrease proximity and contact (intrafamilial threats and attacks). Separation distress and intrafamilial aggression appear to share a common hub of vulnerability and autonomic dysregulation that develops in the process of forming regulative attachments with people, making such problems and their treatment preeminently cynopraxic in nature, and underscoring the necessity of therapy and training activities to reduce social ambivalence and entrapment tensions, promote comfort, safety, and power (security), and secure place and social attachments. Although genetic and stress-related neurobiological factors probably play a predisposing role in the development of many separation-distress and aggression problems, giving owners appropriate counseling and providing at-risk puppies with supplemental training may substantially help to ameliorate or prevent some of these problems. Initiating protective and counteractive measures at an early stage in the epigenetic process is more likely to succeed than belated heroic efforts performed after the problem behavior is well established. Of particular importance in this regard is the provision of secure environmental circumstances, the development of a trusting bond, and training efforts to help the puppy or dog learn how to cope more competently with the periodic loss of comfort or safety resulting from social separation.

Chapter 5 deals with various procedures and protocols used for controlling and managing excessive behavior. Compulsive excesses are under the control of a variety of evoking and exacerbating influences, many of which remain obscure. Dogs prone to motor compulsions are often highly active and intolerant of frustration (choleric or c-type dogs), whereas dogs showing self-directed compulsions (e.g., licking) may be particularly vulnerable to the adverse effects of anxiety and depression (melancholic or m-type dogs). One theory suggests that compulsive actions may trigger reward circuits that help to maintain the activity in the absence of other sources of extrinsic reward, perhaps reflecting a failure of the dog to obtain adequate reward in more adaptive ways. Control and management programs frequently include efforts to remove or minimize adverse sources of social (interactive conflict and tension) and environmental stress, consisting of significant events perceived as uncontrollable, while introducing training activities designed to normalize executive cognitive functions (attention and impulse control). Play therapy is often employed to balance emotional command systems, provide a source of reward and gratifying interaction with the owner, and increase object interest and environmental exploratory activities. Finally, a variety of behavior-therapy and training procedures are described for the treatment of specific compulsive behaviors, including diverting or disrupting techniques, counterconditioning, shaping incompatible behaviors, bringing the compulsive behavior under stimulus control, exposure with response prevention and blocking, and, in the case of refractory or physically harmful compulsions, inhibitory techniques.

Impairments associated with compulsivity and hyperactivity appear to represent the opposite ends of a common continuum or spectrum related by functional significance. Whereas compulsive dogs tend toward introversion, repetitive self-directed activities, and intolerance for anxiety and danger, hyperactive dogs are typically extraverted, tend toward highly variable and other-directed activities, exhibit a high degree of fearless (bold) behavior, and show intolerance for frustration and a propensity toward impulsive aggression. Whereas compulsive dogs have trouble controlling autodirected activities,

hyperactive dogs exhibit difficulty controlling allodirected activities, exhibiting executive disturbances affecting their ability to regulate ongoing activity voluntarily. These correspond to passive and active modal activities launched to cope with drive-activating stimulation but disengaged from competent prediction-control expectancies, giving compulsive behavior and obsessional appearance. The compulsive-impulsive continuum may represent a significant temperament dimension that has been differentially selected and preserved during the dog's evolution. Depending on environmental conditions, the traits of compulsivity or impulsivity may be variably adaptive or maladaptive with respect to survival. Traits associated with hyperactivity and impulsive behavior may be conducive to survival under conditions of adversity and scarcity, whereas compulsive traits may be more adaptive and useful under conditions of plenty, suggesting the possibility that phylogenetic survival modes and quality-of-life factors may play a significant role in the expression of such traits (see *Phylogenetic Survival Modes* in Chapter 10).

The executive attention and impulse-control deficiencies associated with hyperactivity are improved by reward-based integrated compliance training aimed at shaping improved attending and waiting behaviors. Explicit training of attention skills appears to focus and invigorate impaired executive impulse-control functions. As a result of the hyperactive dog's preference for novelty and surprising events, attention training makes use of prediction dissonance (i.e., varying the size, type, and frequency of attractive outcomes) to build attention and impulse control. Without gaining conditioned control over attention, there is little possibility for effectively and consistently interrupting highly motivated activities, activating antagonistic appetitive or emotional establishing operations, or prompting incompatible instrumental behavior. In addition to attention therapy, time-out, response blocking, overcorrection, and posture-facilitated relaxation training are employed to help discourage behavioral excesses. Perhaps the most valuable strategy for controlling and managing hyperactivity and associated problems is to integrate attention and impulse-control training into the context of play.

Chapters 6, 7, and 8 are dedicated to exploring the etiology, safe management, and treatment of a broad spectrum of common aggression problems. Aggression problems are distinguished by a significant factor of risk and danger to the cynopraxic therapist/trainer, the client family, and the public at large. Calculating and managing these risks in an informed and professional manner is an important aspect of interventions involving aggressive dogs, particularly involving dogs with a history of delivering hard and damaging bites. Assessment, decisions on whether to accept cases, articulation of working hypotheses, selection of a course of therapy and training, evaluation of the benefits of training, and prognostic opinions require that the cynopraxic therapist possess a significant amount of technical knowledge and direct experience handling aggressive dogs. In addition to bringing competence to the situation, the cynopraxic therapist/trainer must be able to convey a realistic picture of the risks involved and the likely benefit of training. The owner needs to be made aware that the control and management of aggression problems is an art that is prone to many uncertainties and vagaries with respect to outcomes, but may nonetheless help to improve the dog's behavior and reduce the risk of aggression by instituting appropriate and effective precautions, reducing interactive conflicts and tensions, increasing the occurrence of prosocial behavior, and improving the dog's confidence and ability to relax. Nevertheless, the risk cannot be entirely eliminated, and the dog might bite at some point in the future, despite the most conscientious efforts. On principle, serious aggression problems cannot be cured but many can be successfully controlled by means of preventive and preemptive management, behavior therapy, and training. This limited prognosis is a far cry from what most owners want to hear about the fate of their aggressive dog, but it is something that needs to be driven home with no waffling or exceptions—there will always be some risk for a similar or worse bite in the future. To be successful requires of the family a lifelong commitment to preemptive management and training. In accordance with the dead-dog rule (training objectives should not be guided by assessment markers that a dead dog can satisfy), successful training and therapy are not measured merely by the absence of an aggressive episode for some period (dead dogs do not bite), but more significantly success is measured by an increase in socially competent, cooperative, and friendly behavior in situations that previously provoked reactive incompetence and aggression.

The dog's dependency on human prerogative and fickleness for obtaining its survival needs places significant pressure on it to learn how to anticipate and control human contingencies of reward and punishment. As a result, social interaction that lacks adequate predictability and controllability may produce significant conflict, stress (anxiety and frustration), and social ambivalence, potentially exerting a persistent deleterious effect on the dog's ability to organize competent social behavior and trusting expectancies regarding social change. The dog cannot simply leave a disorganized and emotionally destructive situation but is forced to cope and adjust to it (entrapment). Unable to leave the relationship and pressed to the limits of its ability to cope with its vagaries and inconsistencies, the predisposed dog may become progressively agitated, irritable, intolerant, emotionally rigid, and reactively incompetent. Consequently, the process of cynopraxic counseling and therapy is guided by a principle of fairness in which both the family's expectations and the dog's needs and limitations are acknowledged and given appropriate weight and consideration when resolving interactive conflicts and tensions that interfere with the development of a trusting bond. Finally, quality-of-life issues need to be carefully assessed and addressed, insofar as they adversely affect the dog's ability to develop a secure place and social attachments as well as predispose it to increased irritability and emotional reactivity. Dogs that are sick, in pain, improperly fed, inadequately exercised, denied play and variegated forms of environmental stimulation, excessively confined or isolated, and so forth may show signs of increasing irritability and progressive auto-protective insularity and reactive intolerance toward social interference and contact.

How dogs cope with social ambivalence and entrapment dynamics depends on a variety of predisposing factors, including heredity, prenatal and postnatal stress, and the quality of early socialization and training activities. In addition to impairing cognitive functions, excessive emotional stress, inadequate or inappropriate socialization, and abusive-traumatic handling may focalize persistent disturbances in vulnerable emotional command systems (anger/rage system). Potentially serious emotional disturbances of this kind may be produced by abusive social transactions involving the simultaneous elicitation of high levels of fear and anger. In extreme cases, a history of abusive handling may impair a dog's ability to modulate aggressive arousal in response to even mildly provocative stimulation. Under such circumstances, fear or anger may spark a spiraling and rapidly escalating state of emotional reactivity (panic), thereby setting the stage for an reactive attack arising from a dog's incompetent attempt to cope. In moderate cases, abusive transactions may predispose a dog to conflict-related stress (anxiety and frustration) associated with close social contact. Consequently, the dog may exhibit an increased sensitivity to anxiety or frustration occurring in association with minor intrusions and losses of comfort (frustration) or risks to safety (anxiety), thereby intensifying autoprotective behavior and increasing the dog's readiness to threaten or bite. In all cases, a dog's ability to form a trusting bond with humans is significantly harmed by abusive and traumatic handling. The extent of harm and the type of emotional disturbance that such handling produces depends on a dog's temperament, the severity of the emotionally destructive transaction, and the presence or absence of reconciliation efforts and ameliorating influences (e.g., supplemental socialization and training).

A failure to establish or to maintain a trusting bond appears to play a prominent role in the development or exacerbation of many domestic aggression problems. The rehabilitation of an aggressive dog is not so much about imposing a structure of dominant and subordinate roles (although the necessity of setting appropriate limits should not be neglected) as it is concerned with the restoration of interactive order and harmony by means of affectionate, appetitive, and playful interactions, with the goal of increasing interactive cooperation, familiarity, and trust between the owner and the dog. The comfort and safety associated with orderly and nurturing interaction serve to increase a dog's enjoyment of social contact as well as to improve its tolerance for intrusive interaction. In addition to facilitating fairness and friendliness, play appears to enable dogs to cope with social uncertainty in a more positive way. In general, the dog that has formed trusting expectancies toward the owner is more likely to exhibit tolerance and restraint when exposed to provocative stimulation than is the dog that is uncertain or socialized to distrust the owner. Dogs that have formed a trusting bond appear to give the owner (and others) the benefit of doubt when faced with uncertain situations rather than interpreting provocative or unexpected transactions in worst-case terms and jumping to threatening or retaliatory conclusions. In the absence of a flexible and trusting bond, human-dog interaction is prone to degenerate, resulting in varying degrees of persistent uncertainty and suspicion, anger and irritability, distrust, and reactive incompetence. These sorts of social expectancies and emotional establishing operations combine to lower reactive thresholds and increase the likelihood that the dog might threaten or attack in response to innocuous social intrusions. Identifying puppies that show reactive tendencies at an early age or exhibit other indicators of increased risk (low fear and anger thresholds) and providing puppy owners with counseling on proper training and management may protect against the development of more serious aggression problems later.

In recent years, there has been a growing professional use and interest in electronic devices for dog-training and behavior-modification purposes. Unfortunately, scant little technical information has been written on the proper use of such devices in the context of canine behavior therapy and dog training—a situation that is especially problematic with respect to radio-controlled collars. With significant trepidation and concern about the potential for abuse, Chapter 9 addresses the use of electronic devices in the context of problem solving and training. When properly used, such devices and techniques can be highly effective and humane for the control of certain otherwise intractable or difficult-to-control behavior problems. It is the author's sincere hope that cynopraxic trainers will use electronic devices, and other tools that produce aversive stimulation and startle, sparingly and with an appropriate degree of restraint and respect for the dog and not fall into the trap of reaching for an electronic collar whenever a tough problem presents itself. Aversive tools and techniques can be extremely useful as motivational incentives to promote behavioral change in the context of reward-based training efforts, but they should not become an alternative to affectionate, playful, and creative attractive incentives. Aversive procedures should be applied in conformity with the dead-dog rule (see *Dead-dog Rule* in Volume 2, Chapter 2), the least intrusive and minimally aversive (LIMA) principle, and cynopraxic goals.

As a philosophy and method for investigating natural phenomena, science is generally a powerful and productive way for acquiring, organizing, and putting knowledge to work. Scientifically informed and coherent procedures and protocols are more likely to work and survive the test of time by virtue of their explanatory value, efficacy (combining simplicity, efficiency, and effectiveness), and adaptability, that is, their ability to continuously adjust and improve in accord with scientific progress. However, despite the obvious value of the scientific method for obtaining descriptive and causal information, the scientific method suffers from a lack of serious regard and sensitivity for some of the more subjective and emotional aspects of human-dog interaction. Interactive exchanges (particularly problem behavior) are not simply factual events but emotional transactions with various levels of meaning and significance that will forever slip through the Cartesian grid. In

addition to practical criteria of success, canine behavior-therapy and training procedures must be applicable to the domestic situation, offer benefits for both the human-dog bond and the dog's quality of life, and be humane. As a result of these special requirements, scientific means are tempered and given humane direction by confining their use to the pursuit of cynopraxic goals and vision.

In writing this series, the author has directed a significant amount of attention toward developing a theory compatible with scientific and cynopraxic interests in order to establish a firm but flexible foundation for the advancement of canine behavior counseling therapy and training. Chapter 10 draws together the central elements of cynopraxic bonding, training, and biobehavioral theory. These theoretical concepts and principles have been discussed and elaborated to various degrees throughout the *Handbook of Applied Dog Behavior and Training*, and readers should refer to relevant sections in Volumes 1 and 2 for additional discussion regarding cynopraxic bonding theory, philosophy, and ethics. The goals of cynopraxic theory are to clarify cynopraxic processes, to develop an account of learning that is compatible with cynopraxic objectives, and to establish a simplified and coherent language for describing organizational learning processes associated with cynopraxic training and therapy. Cynopraxic theory incorporates a pragmatic principle of fallibility, acknowledging the possibility of error in its inferences and explanations, thereby embracing a readiness to adjust in accordance with future scientific progress; however, the dyadic goals of cynopraxic training and therapy are considered indisputable, namely, enhancing the human-dog bond while improving the dog's quality of life. The study of cynopraxic bonding, training theory, and practice arts is referred to as *cynopraxiology*.

No compendium of instructions can take the place of competent professional help for properly assessing canine behavior problems and prescribing behavior-therapy and training recommendations. The assessment procedures, instructions, guidelines, recommended devices and uses, behavior-therapy protocols, and training techniques described in Volume 3 assume that the user is appropriately experienced, knowledgeable, skilled, and qualified to apply them in a selective, competent, and safe manner. The proper selection and implementation of behavior-therapy and training procedures require that the behavior practitioner possess a thorough appreciation of their therapeutic benefits, risks, and potential adverse side effects. Aggression problems are particularly risky and problematic and should only be treated under the supervision of a competent professional qualified to give such advice and instruction. Improperly treated aggression problems may rapidly worsen, becoming more dangerous and difficult to manage or control. While Volume 3 offers educational information that may be of significant value to dog owners and others interested in dog behavior, it is not intended as an alternative to professional cynopraxic counseling and supervised treatment activities.

REFERENCES

Panksepp J (1998). *Affective Neuroscience: The Foundations of Human and Animal Emotions*. New York: Oxford University Press.

Wilson EO (1998). *Consilience: The Unity of Knowledge*. New York: Vintage.

Acknowledgments

Writing a book is the culmination of many influences and the help of many people. I have enjoyed the encouragement and support of numerous individuals who have given me valuable advice and inspiration, engaged me in useful discussion, or have simply been helpful in tracking down information or other small matters and details. Listing and individually thanking all of these wonderful people would be impossible and not without the risk of overlooking someone in the process. So, instead of thanking some of you, I hope that it suffices to thank all of you for your unselfish help. I also thank the clients who have entrusted me with the responsibility of helping them work through behavior problems with their dogs. The concept of cynopraxis and many of the procedures and protocols described in Volume 3 could not have been developed without their confidence and participation. A special thank you is due to Christina Cole for her many sacrifices on by behalf and her steadfast support of the project from its inception to completion.

HANDBOOK OF APPLIED DOG BEHAVIOR AND TRAINING

Volume Three

Procedures and Protocols

1

Cynopraxic Training: Basic Procedures and Techniques

PART 1: FOUNDATIONS AND THEORY

BENEFITS OF CYNOPRAXIC TRAINING

A coevolutionary process of mutual exchange and adjustment appears to have prepared a biological bond between people and dogs making them compatible to live together in the home (see *Coevolution, Play, Communication, and Aggression* in Chapter 6). The training process helps to perfect and intensify this evolutionary bond while enhancing our mutual appreciation of one another. In addition to enhancing the ability of people and dogs to relate, training serves the obligatory role of improving the quality of canine life under the constraints of domesticity. Learning to come reliably when called or to walk on leash without pulling, along with sundry other useful and critical behaviors, provides an effective and safe means to liberate dogs from the drudgery of excessive confinement and an overly narrow social and environmental life experience. In effect, no activity offers more potential benefit for enhancing the human-dog bond and improving the dog's quality of life than training (see *Cynopraxis:*

Training and the Human-Dog Relationship in Volume 1, Chapter 10).

The dog's close social interaction with people requires that it learn to accept certain inevitable limits and boundaries, respond reliably to a number of basic commands, and exhibit habits and manners conducive to domestic harmony. These general behavioral objectives are integrated into everyday training activities, thereby strengthening the social connection between the owner and dog as well as facilitating interactive harmony and the development of cooperative behavior. Learning to defer and comply with owner directives is essential for a dog to become a successful companion. A dog's proper adaptation to life with people demands responsible discipline and the establishment of appropriate limits and boundaries. Without boundaries and social distance, a relationship is not possible. Whereas assertions of dominance serve to establish social distance and set limits upon the expression of unacceptable behaviors, leadership promotes more acceptable and cooperative behavior by means of affectionate encouragement, play, food giving, and other nurturing activities. Deference to limit-setting actions and assertions of control promotes affectionate and voluntary cooperation, thereby providing the necessary preconditions for effective leadership. Training helps dogs to learn that deferring and following the owner's lead optimizes their ability to obtain comfort and safety. By learning to follow rules happily and obediently, social conflicts are reduced and a leader-follower bond based on affection, communication, and trust is allowed to

TABLE. 1.1. Benefits of cynopraxic training

Provides a foundation of communication based on predictable and controllable exchanges between the owner and the dog

Provides the owner with effective management and control skills

Systematically balances the triune bond consisting of dominance, leadership, and nurturance

Improves the dog's attention and impulse-control abilities

Promotes affection and mutual appreciation

Establishes habits conducive to domestic harmony

Enhances social adjustment, cooperation, and competence

Promotes relaxation and a sense of well-being

Builds confidence and trust

form—an essential foundation for the development of a healthy human-dog relationship (Table 1.1).

Training promotes behavioral change by manipulating contingencies of reinforcement and punishment. For dogs, social and environmental predictability and controllability are necessary preconditions for security, contentment, and well-being. A failure to predict and control significant attractive and aversive events adequately gives rise to varying degrees of disstress in the form of anxiety and frustration. Of course, when present in limited amounts, anxiety and frustration are conducive to enhanced adaptive success (e.g., prediction error), but in situations where excessive and persistent social conflict and interactive tensions are present, a dog's ability to function in an organized way may gradually deteriorate or break down (see *Experimental Neurosis* in Volume 1, Chapter 9). Dogs living under stressful and inescapable conditions of social disorder and adversity are vulnerable to develop a wide range of behavioral adjustment problems and disturbances (see *Dysfunctional Social and Environmental Influences* in Volume 2, Chapter 2).

Interactive conflict and tension between the owner and dog often develop in the context of antagonistic control interests. In many daily situations, the owner stands between the dog and the acquisition of a variety of highly valued rewards or prevents the dog from escaping or avoiding aversive events, often occurring as the result of engaging in rewarding activities forbidden by the owner. Dog owners often dedicate a tremendous amount of energy to regulate the appetitive interests of their dogs by employing a variety of active and passive control strategies, primarily involving interactive punishment and confinement. Active punitive strategies are particularly problematic since they are often used without much, if any, subsequent concern for showing the dog how to obtain the gratification that it is seeking while engaged in the forbidden activity. Limiting the dog's behavior by means of passive control strategies (e.g., crating and tethering) in the absence of constructive training efforts can be equally harmful to the human-dog bond and the dog's quality of life. In both instances, the dog's

ability to establish predictive control over appetitive and social rewards needed to optimize its adaptation and security (comfort and safety) are impeded or blocked. Setting limits by means of varying degrees of force (dominance) or restriction can be highly beneficial for the dog, but only if the dog is simultaneously shown alternative means to obtain the gratification that it seeks to obtain. Impeding the dog's ability to escape or avoid an aversive situation by punishing an unacceptable mode of behavior (e.g., separation distress barking or whining), but without helping it to discover an alternative way to escape, avoid, or cope (e.g., providing it with an alternative or compensatory source of reward) from the aversive state (e.g., isolation and loneliness), may only tend to generate additional distress and focalize a point of ongoing conflict and tension between the owner and dog. Thwarting the dog's ability to obtain appetitive and social rewards by punishing unacceptable behavior (e.g., jumping up, barking, digging, chewing, pulling, and mouthing), without at the same time teaching the dog more acceptable means to produce equal or better reward opportunities, only serves to focalize conflict and tension between the dog and the owner over the acquisition and control of those thwarted reward opportunities.

From the cynopraxic point of view, these interactive conflicts and tensions oppose the objectives of interactive harmony and mutual appreciation, and, as such, represent the specific target areas of therapy efforts aimed at enhancing the human-dog bond. In addition, interactive conflicts and tensions precisely define the various social and biological needs that are not being adequately met by means of the relationship, thereby offering opportunities to improve the dog's quality of life significantly. Cynopraxic training is based on the assumption that interactive conflicts and tensions are resolved by teaching the dog alternative and mutually acceptable means to obtain the sought-after activities and rewards. In the process of dog owners being counseled about the sources and causes of interactive conflict and tension, owners learn about canine needs and become progressively appreciative of them, especially as they learn how to use them constructively in the process of improving their ability to control the dog via integrated compliance training (ICT). ICT refers to a training strategy that objectifies interactive conflicts and tensions as potential sources of reward for the dog, on the one hand, and opportunities for enhancing owner control efforts, on the other—a win-win exchange in the service of cynopraxic goals. ICT promotes social competence, cooperation, and trust via the mutual success of the owner and dog to establish predictive control over each other's behavior in the process of seeking and gratifying their individual needs by means of gratifying the needs of the other. Instead of standing in the way of the dog's appetitive and emotional gratification (comfort and safety), the owner becomes a cooperative and trusted partner in the process of acquiring attractive outcomes and avoiding aversive ones. The resultant reduction in interactive conflict and tension gives rise to social competence and trust, increased confidence and relaxation (the cognitive and emotional corollaries of social competence), and a foundation for interactive harmony and mutual appreciation. These various elements and outcomes of training play a significant role in cynopraxic counseling and canine behavior therapy, providing a platform of preliminary cognitive and emotional organization for approaching a wide spectrum of canine behavior problems.

Organized training activities not only systematically influence overt social behavior, they also serve to produce a broad spectrum of emotional changes (Rolls, 2000) (Figure 1.1). Classical conditioning and instrumental learning processes interact at various levels of cognitive and emotional organization, with appetitive and emotional attractive and aversive stimuli instigating a variety of emotional and motivational changes (see Rescorla and Solomon, 1967). In addition, a dog's cumulative successes or failures to control significant attractive or aversive events are reflected in persistent emotional changes and its disposition to learn and adjust. For example, establishing reliable predictive control over attractive and aversive events appears to promote enhanced mood and optimistic expectancy biases—a "better state" of being (Wyrwicka, 1975). Finally, training activities improve

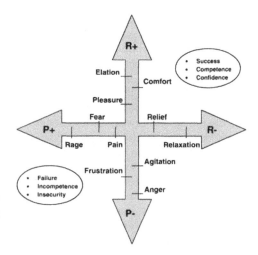

FIG. 1.1. Training events are associated with the production of a variety of emotional states that exert pronounced effects on mood and reactive behavior (see Rolls, 2000).

attentional functions and impulse-control abilities, as well as reduce adverse anxiety and frustration via increasing competence, confidence, and relaxation. Essentially, all training activities function as attention and impulse-control therapies in the context of developing useful behavior. As the result of effective training, dogs appear to adopt a more focused, relaxed, secure, and trusting attitude toward the social and physical environment, helping them to cope more effectively with conflict or emotionally stressful stimulation.

In addition to the various benefits of cynopraxic training for dogs, owners stand to gain from the experience. As the result of training their dogs, owners learn how to observe behavior, to appreciate a dog's biological and emotional needs, to communicate more effectively, and to develop a more informed estimation of a dog's cognitive capacities and limitations—all leading to a better relationship with the dog. Also, during introductory lessons, owners learn basic learning principles while practicing skills and techniques of behavior modification. In addition to reducing interactive conflict and tension, the progress and success that owners experience during these early lessons (e.g., training a dog to walk on-leash, to come when called, to sit and lie down on command, and to stay) help to generate a more constructive and optimistic attitude about the dog's responsiveness to behavior therapy efforts.

SPECIFIC BENEFITS OF VARIOUS EXERCISES

Dogs with behavior problems often benefit from systematic training before advancing to the implementation of more specialized behavioral procedures. In addition to general benefits, the practice of various trained exercises and tasks provides specific benefits relevant to the enhancement of canine behavior therapy efforts:

Orienting and Attending Response

Training the dog to reliably turn and focus its attention toward the trainer is a vital aspect of behavior control and management. In the absence of attention control, it is not possible to efficiently control impulsive behavior or responses operating under the influence of extraneous sources of reward (distractions). The direction of a dog's attention is defined by moment-to-moment motivational changes and intentional shifts preparing it to act on the environment. All purposive behavior is determined by shifts of attention, intention, and action functionally integrated and directed toward the environment in response to some motivationally significant imperative or impulse. Orienting and attending behavior promotes organized behavior. Without an ability to orient and selectively focus attention, the senses would be overwhelmed by the surrounding flux of environmental stimulation. As an adaptive interface between internal imperatives (establishing operations) and the external environment (a field of activity and choice), attention mediates action with the goal of increasing environmental predictability and control. Attention, intention, and action are intrinsically dependent on one another via a complex network of modulating interactions and feedback relations that are strongly influenced by the complementary effects of reinforcement (success) and punishment (failure). Attention therapy plays an important role in the treatment of a variety of behavior problems occurring in association with impulse-control deficits. Attention is related to impulse control as a hinge is to a door, such that the hinge defines the full range of the door's movements. Controlling a dog's attention is virtually tantamount to controlling the full-range of the dog's behavior, whereas losing a dog's attention to environmental distractions leverages control away from the trainer. In extreme cases of behavioral disorder, a dog's attention may become "unhinged" as attention and orienting responses become overstrained and disturbed, resulting in reactive and impulsive behavioral disorganization (see *Locus of Neurotogenesis* in Volume 1, Chapter 9).

Sit-Stay and Down-Stay

The sit response is an instrumental control module that every dog owner should master and practice with their dog under a wide variety of situations. Sitting on command is rapidly conditioned, produces a significant amount of control, and requires a minimal amount of instruction. Stay training strengthens inhibitory processes and impulse control, increases delay of gratification capacities, and promotes deference to owner control efforts. Training dogs to sit and stay on command for food, petting, and other rewards in everyday situations provides a simple and effective way to obtain improved cooperation and compliance. The rapid success and control produced by training dogs to sit and stay may have a highly beneficial effect on owners needing a ray of hope. In the late 1960s and early 1970s, David Tuber and Victoria Voith happened upon the value of preliminary reward-based sit-stay training in the context of treating fear-related behavior problems. As Voith recounts,

> Firstly, it gave the owners something to do between the first and second visits (which were a week apart). This gave us time to discuss the problem and develop a detailed, individual behavior modification program for that case.

Secondly, most of our programs involved a classical conditioning component designed to change the emotional/physiological response to specific stimuli, e.g., loud noises, frightening people or other animals, distress responses etc. It was advantageous to have the dog stationary as the stimuli were introduced and it was essential that learning sit-stay be fun, non-punitive, not forced in any way and pleasant. No leash correction, no stern voices. The reward for the act of sitting and then remaining so for progressively longer periods of time was a mouthwatering tidbit. Needless to say, the dogs learned to sit and stay within a few minutes. But the dogs were not only learning an operant response; they were associating pleasant experiences (delicious food, praise from owner) with the verbal cue "sit" and the act of being in a sit-stay. A week of simple sit-stays was also teaching the owner how dog's learned.

When we saw the dog a week later, the sit-stay (or down-stay) kept the dog in one spot, allowing us to gradually introduce other stimuli and to easily pair food rewards with the introduction of stimuli. In addition, the verbal cues and the act of sitting and staying also acted as conditioned stimuli, evoking pleasant emotional responses. The pleasant emotional states associated with sit-stay contributed to the classical counterconditioning paradigm and even could be a conditioned reinforcer when food was no longer presented. (Voith, personal communication, 2002)

The method was further developed and refined by Voith while she directed the Animal Behavior Clinic at the University of Pennsylvania. Voith's Sit-Stay Program involves dozens of discrete sit-stay tasks and variations of increasing difficulty (Voith, 1977b; Marder and Reid, 1996) (see Appendix A). Although not always appropriately credited to her as the originator, variations of her Sit-Stay Program and her Nothing in Life Is Free (NILIF) protocol (Voith, 1977a) are widely recommended by veterinarians, trainers, and applied dog behaviorists as a preliminary platform of control for carrying out counterconditioning procedures. Practicing sit-stay variations under varying environmental and motivational conditions promotes better attention and impulse control abilities. Together with the wait, controlled walk, coming when called, and down-stay exercise, sit-stay plays a prominent role in ICT. Finally,

the sit-stay is frequently used as an incompatible response in various instrumental countercommanding procedures.

Controlled Walking

Every dog should be trained to walk on leash and collar without pulling. Such training is imperative in the case of dogs exhibiting behavior problems associated with attention and impulse-control deficiencies. Training the dog to walk on a slack leash is a necessary step toward enhanced deference to trainer-control efforts while in the presence of highly distracting or provocative stimuli. Since the dog must actively defer to every step and change of direction that the trainer takes, without impulsively chasing after other animals or objects that may be encountered, the process yields rapid and significant attention and impulse-control enhancement, especially if it is combined with sit and sit-stay training. Controlled walking consists of training the dog to walk at the left side with its hip aligned with the trainer's left leg. Although the dog can move back from this position, it cannot move ahead of it. Training the dog to walk on leash in a controlled manner allows the trainer to move the dog about in a controlled manner. This enhanced control of movement is useful when exposing the dog to potentially provocative situations, such as during graduated exposure procedures. A dog that is responsive to leash control can be more readily moved toward or away from provocative stimulation, thereby increasing the trainer's ability to perform controlled exposures to target stimuli during counterconditioning and desensitization efforts. The ability to precisely control exposure gradients decreases the risk that a dog will react adversely during such training activities. In combination, these aspects of controlled walking significantly enhance the effectiveness of response prevention and counterconditioning procedures. Training a dog to defer to leash limits and to follow prompts and signals while on leash appears to enhance significantly the leader-follower bond and the dog's overall willingness to cooperative. Finally, a major benefit of training a dog to walk on leash without pulling is that it is likely to result in the dog getting more walks and going more places with the owner.

Quick-sit

The quick-sit is conditioned in the context of controlled walking. The dog is trained to sit rapidly and without hesitation, and remain in the sit position until the trainer releases it. Consequently, in addition to sitting rapidly, quick-sit training places a high priority on conditioning the dog to remain in the sit position regardless of environment distractions. Quick-sit is an emergency response that means "sit and stay," period. The quick-sit is practiced under a variety of increasingly distracting and adverse conditions. The training exercise promotes alertness, enhanced attention and impulse control, and readiness to respond cooperatively and obediently under adverse conditions. The exercise is useful as platform for various behavior-therapy procedures and is particularly helpful in the case of dogs exhibiting offensive aggression toward other dogs or various chasing problems.

Down, Down-Stay, and Instant-down

Down training builds on control established during sit-stay training. The down-stay is used in situations requiring that the dog defer and stay in a relaxed manner for long periods. Down training is particularly useful in the control and management of overly active and intrusive dogs. In adult dogs, resistance and oppositional tendencies may be momentarily intensified during down training. Down training provides a means to work systematically through such resistance constructively. In addition to down and down-stay, impulsive dogs should be trained to go to a spot and lie down on command without hesitation. Similar to the quick-sit, the instant-down promotes increased cooperation and compliance to command in emergency situations.

Starting Exercise

Dogs should be trained to a high degree of proficiency to move to the trainer's left side and sit there. The starting exercise requires that the dog turn away from distracting or arousing stimuli and either hook around at the trainer's left side or move to the rear of the trainer before crossing over to the left and sitting automatically. The control established by means of the starting exercise has many applications, such as establishing or enhancing control during greetings with visitors or bringing the dog back under closer control while on a controlled walk. All the basic elements of attention training are incorporated into the starting exercise.

Heeling

As an organized and coordinated activity, heeling requires that both the trainer and the dog concentrate on the actions of each other, promoting enhanced connectedness, common purpose, and leader-follower bonding. While heeling, the dog remains close at the trainer's side, keeping pace with abrupt and frequent changes of pace, following directional changes, and responding to stop and go actions by sitting or standing up. These various coordinated movements reflect the development of a signaling system of increasing subtlety and refinement. In contrast to the passive nature of static tasks such as sit-stay and down-stay, controlled walking and heeling are dynamically organized, consisting of responses sequentially entrained in accordance with the trainer's movement and body position relative to the dog. In an important sense, heeling is *moving-stay* exercise. The high level of positive reinforcement and inhibitory training associated with the conditioning of controlled walking and heeling provide a platform of control that competes with undesirable behavior, making counterconditioning efforts and the differential reinforcement of other, alternative, or incompatible behavior more efficient and likely to succeed.

Recall and Halt-Stay

A dependable willingness to walk on leash without pulling and to come when called is the mark of a successfully socialized and trained companion dog, whereas persistent pulling and refusal to come when called is the mark of an untrained or improperly trained dog. The amenable habit of staying close when off leash or coming when called despite the presence of competing distractions signifies the presence of a leader-follower bond of sufficient strength to withstand the intrusion of external diversions and temptations. Freeze training is a routine aspect of recall training. When properly introduced and conditioned, the halt-stay module serves to interrupt highly motivated behavior decisively, enhancing the trainer's control over seeking excesses and dangerous impulsive behavior. Instead of running out of control when off leash, dogs should be trained to orient, come, or halt instantly in place and wait where they stand until *reached, recalled,* or *released* by the trainer—the 3 R's of halt-wait training. Effective recall and halt-stay training provides dogs with numerous quality-of-life benefits, serving to free them to enjoy the environment while minimizing the risk of harm to them as the result of being off leash. The recall and halt modules are critical and should be trained to a high degree in advance of letting dogs off leash to play and enjoy an open or public environment. Even in the case of dogs not let off leash in such places, the recall and halt modules should be trained to a high degree of reliability to prevent accidental injury as the result of bolting from the car or house. Many common problems are obviated by solid recall and halt-stay training.

BEHAVIORAL EQUILIBRIUM

Basic training should be performed with an eye toward balancing exercises with opposites in order to prevent a dog from becoming overly expectant and reliant on some set of behaviors to the exclusion of others. A dog that is repeatedly prompted to lie down from the sit, but not the other way around, might prove more difficult to train to perform the reverse action of sitting from the down; similarly, a dog that is exclusively trained to sit, without being occasionally prompted to stand, may be more difficult to train to hold a stand or stand-stay later on. Consequently, basic exercises are balanced by patterning their sequence in various ways. For example, heeling closely at the trainer's side is balanced by opportunities to walk freely. Staying in place is balanced by opportunities for increased activity, including heeling, recall,

and release for play. Movement away from the trainer is balanced with stopping and returning exercises. Taking objects from the hand is balanced by prompting the dog to release them. Fetching objects is balance by training the dog to avoid certain objects. Waiting at doorways is balanced by release cues, move-away signals, or come-along signals. Lying down is balanced by having the dog sit or stand from the down position. The sit response is balanced by prompting the dog to stand. The automatic sit is balanced by an exception cue signaling the dog to stand or stand-stay instead of sitting. Going to heel (start and finish) is balanced by having the dog learn to go back to front from the trainer's side. A balanced repertoire of directional tasks can be extremely useful. Dogs can be easily trained with vocal signals and hand prompts to stop, back, move forward, turn left, turn right, and turn about. Not only do such activities improve a dog's attention abilities, they also enhance the trainer's ability to precisely control the dog's behavior at a distance. Many additional examples of behavioral equilibrium could be listed following the same basic pattern in which the type, direction, and function of any given item in a dog's repertoire is matched with its behavioral opposite.

Balance should also be considered when modifying common nuisance problems. When dogs are trained to limit excessive barking, they should also be trained to bark on signal. Similarly, dogs trained not to jump up should also be trained to jump up on cue under appropriate circumstances. Prompting a dog to stop some activity ("Enough") is balanced by releasing it to engage in another activity. In addition to mixing modules and routines to prevent imbalances, trainers should take care to balance emotional and sensory stimulation. For example, bouts of energetic play should be balanced with periods of inhibitory restraint (e.g., stay and wait training). Experiences causing fearful arousal should be followed by stimulation evoking relaxation or other responses incompatible with fear. Activities resulting in close attachment should be balanced by periods of separation. Assertions of control resulting in submissive behavior are balanced by affectionate reassurance and opportunities for the dog to compete in constructive ways. Competitive interaction is balanced by engaging the dog in cooperative activities, and so forth. In general, emotionally inhibitory activities are balanced by excitatory ones and vice versa. Organizing behavioral opposites to occur in close association with one another provides a significant source of reinforcement and punishment. For example, releasing the dog from a sit-stay provides a powerful reward for staying, while, conversely, having the come to sit and stay may exert a punitive effect on its willingness to come in the future when called.

SIGNALS AND COMMUNICATION

Dog-training signals use a variety of sensory modalities, with visual, auditory, and tactile signals playing a prominent role. Visual signals include all forms of bodily movement and gesture designed to influence dog behavior in some way. There are both formal and informal visual signals. Formal hand signals are used to inform or reinforce vocal signals issued at a distance. Informal signals are used to communicate an intention or expectation to a dog by directly stimulating some action; for example, running away, crouching down, or clapping the hands can prompt the dog to follow or come. Dogs are also highly responsive to directional gazing and pointing. Apparently, the dog's ability to take instruction by pointing and other gestures (bowing, nodding, and head turning) has been enhanced by selective breeding and learning (McKinley and Sambrook, 2000). Such communication represents a significant form of interspecies exchange between people and dogs (Miklósi et al., 1998). As a result, most dogs can quickly learn to follow directional cuing with minimal practice.

Ideally, training signals should be presented in an orderly way with the least informative signals preceding more informative ones and concluding, if necessary, with directive prompts and physical guidance. Besides being well organized and presented in an orderly manner, these various signals, especially vocal ones, must be well differentiated. The greatest potential for confusion arises

when signals are used inconsistently or when they are presented in a manner that makes them difficult to discriminate. To avoid this source of confusion, vocal signals are presented in distinctive tones of voice, depending on their intended purpose.

Vocal signals are used to perform a variety of functions, including conditioned reinforcement, that is, bridging a contingent response with a future reward (e.g., "Good," "Yep," "That's it," and "Yes"), conditioned punishment (e.g., "No," "Eh," "Ack," and "Nah"), and cuing or command (e.g., "Sit"). Vocal praise and directive reprimands (e.g., "Enough," "Stop it," "Leave it," and "Off") serve to produce more general activating or depressing effects on behavior via both conditioned and unconditioned effects of tone of voice on dog behavior. To minimize confusion, vocal signals are spoken in a distinctive and consistent tone. The loudness and tone of vocal signals and the way they are presented are shaped in conformity with the changes that the trainer wishes to make in a dog's behavior. The reprimand is spoken in an assertive tone of voice from the belly; the command is spoken in a clear, normal tone of voice from the chest and throat; and praise is spoken in a lively, friendly, and high-pitched tone of voice from the mouth and throat. The volume of voice is adjusted from soft to harsh for purposes of emphasis. Good communication with the voice depends on keeping these various tones and their intended functions distinct by not saying commands like praise, issuing a reprimand like a command, or delivering a command like a reprimand. Many signals function as establishing operations motivationally shifting behavioral thresholds and making the occurrence of certain classes of behavior more likely while making other classes of behavior less likely. Besides regulating a dog's behavior, tone of voice also serves to modulate the dog's mood and attitude during the training process. The lower and assertive barklike reprimand may trigger innate mechanisms mediating behavioral inhibition and deference (see *Sensory Preparedness* in Volume 1, Chapter 5).

Although dogs are surprisingly clever at deciphering the associative implications of words, they do not seem to understand words as conceptual constructs. In addition to associative meanings, words signify concepts and relations extending well beyond the reach of a dog's understanding. Concepts are mental representations of related things, and words stand in a symbolic relation to concepts. In addition, words are part of a language system articulated by grammatical rules and syntax to enable us to communicate with one another in meaningful ways. To dogs, words are auditory *images* deriving their *meaning* through associative contiguity with the regular occurrence of some thing, action, or relation in the presence or close association with the vocal signal. According to Hobbes (1651/1994), the dog shares with people an imagining faculty that facilitates such understanding and appreciation of words:

> The imagination that is raised in man (or any other creature endued with the faculty of imagining) by words, or other voluntary signs, is that we generally call understanding, and is common to man and beast. For a dog by custom will understand the call or the rating of his master; and so will many other beasts. That understanding which is peculiar to man is the understanding not only his will, but his conceptions and thoughts, by the sequel and contexture of the names of things into affirmations, negations, and other forms of speech: and of this kind of understanding I shall speak hereafter. (11)

Along with the associative meanings and implications of vocal signals, the tonal variations in which vocal signals are given help to communicate a trainer's emotional state and immediate intentions to a dog. The dog may not appreciate the symbolic or conceptual significance of a word, but it does appear to be extremely sensitive and responsive to the feeling content of vocal signals reflecting the will of the speaker.

The language barrier between people and dogs causes many dog owners to both overestimate and underestimate their dog's capabilities. Some of the difficulty can be attributed to the facility with which we transform experience into mental representations (thoughts and images) that are almost automatically arranged into logical relations and configured into concepts fitted to words. Words give us the ability to represent experience symbolically in terms of causal relations, connecting long-past events (causes) to current or future events (effects). A dog's experience is more temporally confined and limited to the immediate demands of existence surrounding the moment (Roberts, 2002). The stream of life passes by with all its disappointments and adventures, with each moment lived to the fullest or lost. A dog has little time to ruminate on past events or future possibilities, except to the extent that they directly impact on the present moment. Unlike people, dogs lack the symbolic, conceptual, and logical means to connect long-past events and actions with the present moment; that is, they appear to lack an episodic memory. Dogs exist in an ever-present and perpetually becoming *now*.

The dog is remarkable among animals by its willingness to work for affection and approval from a human handler (Kostarczyk, 1991). The dog loves to please, first of all itself, of course; but after some basic training it will work to obtain various social expressions of affection, such as petting, gentle caresses, and praise. Although a brief high-pitched vocal signal like "Good" is preferable for refined training purposes, periodic longer phrases of vocal praise and sweet talk can be extremely useful and beneficial as a means to enhance a dog's incentive to work for social rewards. The vocal bridge "Good" functions as a conditioned reinforcer and exactly refers to some specific behavior, whereas affectionate praise and sweet talk relate more generally to a dog's willingness to work and cooperate. Sweet talk both reassures and encourages dogs. Praise also keeps the training process from becoming too clinical and boring, helping to keep the atmosphere cheerful and fun for dogs and trainers. Gentle, but firm, petting and soft embracing hugs with endearing words are well received by most dogs. As a cynopraxic activity, training is always concerned with ways of maximizing bond and quality-of-life benefits; rather than pursuing the training process with excessively sterile and rigid procedures, cynopraxic training incorporates affectionate means and play whenever possible. Praising and petting is an art that should be given from the heart as a sincere expression of affection and appreciation in response to a dog's behavior and accomplishments. Nervous finger tickling, fidgeting, and hard shoulder slapping are not usually well received by dogs in training, although many do appear to enjoy a friendly shoulder pat now and then. The key to effective petting is its intention and sincerity. If the heart is not in it, it would be better not to pet the dog—the dog knows the difference. Of course, dogs exhibiting aggression problems should only be handled and touched with appropriate care and precautions.

ATTENTION AND IMPULSE CONTROL

Attention provides a selective interface between the internal and external environment, helping dogs to detect and control events and situations that have motivational significance for them (see *Attention and Learning* in Volume 1, Chapter 7). Attention, impulse (the combined activation of relevant control expectancies and establishing operations), intention, and action are closely linked by a network of classically conditioned predictive associations that inform and motivate instrumental control efforts (see *Basic Postulates, Units, Processes, and Mechanisms* in Chapter 10). When attention falls upon a motivationally significant (salient) object, a control incentive may be aroused, followed by the activation of preparatory responses and intentional movements or orientations in anticipation of overt control efforts (see *Control Incentives and Reinforcement*). Under the influence of appetitive arousal, attention functions may be recruited by control incentives to coordinate instrumental modules and routines leading to gratification (comfort seeking). As the dog commits to a course of action, its attention may be locked or *vectored* on the developing situation and dedicated to the acquisition and processing of real-time information relevant to adjustments conducive to instrumental success. Once launched, highly motivated behavior may only stop after it is consummated (confirmed), fails (disconfirmed), or is interrupted by the evocation of an antagonistic control incentive having a greater motivational significance and priority. In practice, the inhibitory control over impulsive behavior is often

accomplished by means of startle or momentary discomfort. The startling event produces a rapid diminution of appetitive arousal while at the same time establishing an incompatible control incentive aimed at escaping the unexpected and dangerous situation (safety seeking). As a result, the appetitive control expectancy is modified to include an element of danger, thereby increasing the dog's responsiveness to inhibitory signals and avoidance when engaged in similar activities in the future.

Although such control efforts are often necessary and expedient for gaining control over certain impulsive behaviors, the routine induction of fear or discomfort to establish control over impulsive behavior risks various adverse side effects, especially in cases where such training is performed incompetently or in the absence of reward-based alternatives. Once a dog is acting on a strong impulse, attempting to interrupt it by means of threats and belated punishment is analogous to grabbing an ox by the tail and whipping it in order to stop it from running away. Of course, a more sensible approach for controlling such a powerful animal is to guide it by means of a rope and nose ring while luring it forward with a clump of fresh hay. Similarly, keeping the dog on a long line or leash and conditioning a strong orienting and attending response in the context of shaping a variety of basic exercises (modules) and skills effectively facilitates enhanced attention and impulse control while reducing the amount of aversive inhibitory training needed to gain reliable off-leash control. The key for effective attention and impulse control is anticipating and capturing the dog's attention in advance of it becoming absorbed by competing environmental sources of reward. Capturing and diverting a dog's attention toward comparable or better sources of reward under the trainer's control is akin to the ox's nose ring, giving the trainer a high degree of leverage for controlling undesirable impulses. In addition to employing preemptive attention-control efforts, the intensive training of orienting and attending behaviors with techniques that produce positive prediction error can significantly improve attention and impulse control and reduce the use of aversive techniques. Attention control is established by means of both instrumental and classical conditioning mechanisms. For example, a dog's name is first and foremost learned as a discriminative stimulus for controlling the dog's attention; the dog can choose to attend or not when it hears its named called. However, attention (orienting response) is also controlled by a reflexive mechanism. Given a sufficiently salient and unexpected stimulus, such as an unusual sound, a dog—willing or not—will start and orient toward the source of stimulation. Pairing the dog's name with such unconditioned orienting stimuli (e.g., squeak, smooch sounds, clapping, and so forth) and bridging the orienting response with surprise-producing rewards can rapidly enhance the nominal signal's ability to control a dog's attention.

To attend (Latin *attendere,* to heed) and to obey (Latin *oboedire,* to listen) are functionally dependent and intrinsic aspects of the basic training process. Improving a dog's attention and impulse-control abilities by training it to actively listen to and heed human guidance and directives is among the most important core objectives of basic training. When properly understood and performed, training that establishes attention and impulse control serves to form and preserve a shared moment of mutual awareness and consideration (mutual appreciation) while reducing interactive conflict and tension via reward-based training efforts. The cynopraxic process is tantamount to leading the aforementioned ox by means of its nose ring and desire for hay, then letting go of the rope, eventually forgetting about the ox's training, and finally just enjoying the companionship and walk. The mutual exchanges and transactions between the trainer and dog that compose the training process are mediated by the establishment of an attentional nexus bringing the trainer and dog into the same time frame for the sake of mutual benefits derived from their cooperation (interactive harmony).

INTERRUPTING BEHAVIOR

Establishing control over a dog's attention often involves the use of diverters and disrupters to interrupt ongoing behavior. Divert-

ers rely on an element of surprise and attractiveness to turn a dog's attention away from some competing activity. Disrupters, on the other hand, depend on startle and alarm to gain a dog's attention. Interrupting diverters and disrupters may momentarily intensify attention and enhance learning by activating behavioral inhibition and other rapid adjustments via prediction-error signals occurring in response to the detection of a dramatic incongruence or mismatch between what the dog is accustomed to expect and what is happening. With the occurrence of surprise or startle, a brief hesitation or halt in activity may occur while the discrepant information is cognitively and emotionally processed and integrated before the dog's previous activity is resumed or another activity is begun. The effectiveness of diverters and disrupters is influenced by a variety of factors, including previous exposure to the event (see *Latent Inhibition* in Volume 1, Chapter 6), habituation and sensitization, and the presence of other stimuli (e.g., fear-potentiated startle and prepulse inhibition) (see Koch, 1999). In the case of fear-potentiated startle, a previously conditioned fear-eliciting stimulus may serve to potentiate the startle produced by the disrupter. On the other hand, the presence of a conditioned aversive stimulus may decrease the effectiveness of a diverter to attract and hold the dog's attention (see *External Inhibition and Disinhibition* in Volume 1, Chapter 6). An attenuated stimulus (distraction) occurring immediately before the disrupter is delivered may significantly decrease the startle response elicited by the event via prepulse inhibition (see *Prediction and Control Expectancies*). Despite their potential to reward or punish behavior, diverters and disrupters are not conceived of as producing reinforcement or punishment, until the dog produces behavioral efforts aimed at controlling their occurrence (see *Diverters and Disrupters* in Volume 1, Chapter 7). Diverters and disrupters function primarily as generic establishing operations serving to mobilize control incentives and to launch control modules, routines, and modal strategies in accordance with anticipated needs. Although not productive of reinforcement and punishment initially, consequent presentations of diverting and disrupting stimuli may function as reinforcers or punishers to the extent that a dog is able (reinforcer) or unable (punisher) to predict and control them. Diverters and disrupters play a major role in the control of a wide variety of dog behavior problems (see *Diverters and Disrupters*).

Particular care must be exercised when using diversionary techniques to control behavior problems, since, if improperly used, such procedures can easily result in unintentional reinforcement rather than simply diverting a dog's attention or initiating an incompatible establishing operation. If a dog is repeatedly diverted from some unwanted activity by offering it the opportunity to perform some other more desirable activity, it may gradually learn that the desirable activity can be obtained by engaging in the unwanted behavior. In this case, the diverter is no longer functioning as a diversionary stimulus but has become a positive reinforcer. This risk is always present when a diverter is repeatedly presented in the absence of other training activities, whereby other (DRO), alternative (DRA), or incompatible (DRI) behavior is reinforced following the evocation of a diversionary establishing operation (see *Differential Reinforcement* in Volume 1, Chapter 7). Diverting a dog from one activity to engage in another one usually means that the second activity is motivationally located higher up on the dog's response-priority hierarchy, making it likely that the diversionary activity could function as a positive reinforcer (see *Premack Principle: The Relativity of Reinforcement* in Volume 1, Chapter 7). For example, a dog racing through the house or grabbing personal belongings may be diverted from the activity by picking up a leash, signaling a possible walk. If a walk follows regularly at such times, the dog may learn to control the opportunity to go for a walk by engaging in rambunctious behavior. In this case, the lower-priority behavior (racing through the house) is instrumental in obtaining the higher-priority behavior (going for a walk). For owners of such dogs, it may not be clear to them that the pattern of picking up the leash is not only serving to stop the unwanted behavior but is also inadvertently helping to maintain it. In fact, an owner may be quite

gratified by the momentary success achieved by getting the leash whenever the dog appears out of control. In sum, the outcome is a *behavioral trap* in which short-term control is achieved at the expense of increased undesirable future behavior (Tortora, 1980).

Bribes and threats may be confused with diverters and disrupters, but function in very different and problematic ways. Dogs are commonly bribed after they have refused to come when called. Although the offer of a food bribe may cause a resistant dog to come, the bribe also directly reinforces the refusal behavior. As the result of repeated bribery, the refusal behavior may actually become stronger than the dog's interest in obtaining the offered food bribe, causing the owner to produce something even better to gain the dog's resistant compliance. Improving the bribe serves only to strengthen the refusal behavior further and so on, with the *bribe trap* progressively leading to a deterioration in the dog's willingness to come when called. Unenforceable threats following misbehavior or refusal to obey can be equally problematic. Under the influence of empty or inconsistently enforced threats, a dog's unwanted behavior may increase as it finds that the threatened consequence is not forthcoming, causing it to experience a significant amount of relief by evading the owner's punitive efforts successfully. Furthermore, in the case of the *threat trap*, because some percentage of threats are effective, the owner's threatening behavior is intermittently reinforced and may persist despite a progressive deterioration of overall control. Dogs exposed to such treatment quickly learn that staying away at a safe distance insulates them against any real consequences associated with threats. Consequently, rather than helping to suppress unwanted behavior, repeated and ineffectual threats may serve only to encourage a dog to misbehave at a safe distance out of the owner's reach. In an effort to counteract the dog's defensive ploy, the impatient owner may complicate matters further by enticing the dog to come within his or her reach before grabbing it and delivering a dose of belated and self-righteous punishment. Although the owner may feel privately vindicated by a belief that justice had been served or some such hokum, the only thing that a dog is likely to learn from such abusive treatment is to be more wary and difficult to catch in the future. In addition, such acts of calculated deception may rapidly train a dog to view the owner and others with distrust, thereby potentially setting the stage for more serious adjustment problems later.

TRAINING AND PLAY

In the process of describing the procedures and techniques of basic training, it is easy to lose sight of some of the subtle nuances and flavor, the sundry incidental activities and diversions (e.g., spontaneous playfulness and affectionate interaction), the rhythm and dancelike quality of the interaction between the trainer and dog, and the general presence of fun and excitement associated with training a dog. In fact, nothing is more important to successful training than play. Although food is a tremendously useful reward, excessive reliance on food should be avoided, and other sources of reinforcement should be identified and used to support training objectives, with the goal of actualizing the dog's whole emotional and behavioral potential. In addition to an appetite for food, dogs exhibit a wide range of other social and physical needs that seek gratification, but, most importantly, they need to play and they enjoy playing with people. Consequently, whenever possible, training objectives should be organized around play incentives. Playing with dogs makes them more flexible and willing to open their behavioral repertoire creative experimentation and change. In the context of play, social limits and rules are much more readily accepted and incorporated into everyday interaction. Play makes change and adaptation easier and more durable, seeming to promote a sense of joyful harmony and trust between people and dogs (The *Cynopraxic Trainer's Attitude* in Volume 2, Chapter 10). In the case of serious behavior problems, play often offers a valuable behavior-therapy modality for accessing and modulating affected emotional command systems (see *Modulatory and Unifying Effects of Play* in Chapter 6).

By means of modal play and exploratory activities, dogs interact with and adapt to the social and physical environment. In essence, dogs learn about people and their surroundings by playing and exploring (Trumler, 1973). In the context of instrumental control efforts, active modal play and exploratory strategies help to shape and entrain control modules, routines, and projects into patterns of instrumental behavior via the discovery of outcomes conducive to surprise (reward) and the avoidance of outcomes producing disappointment. Active modal strategies are activated (rewarded) or depressed (punished) by positive and negative prediction errors, respectively (see *Prediction and Control Expectancies*). Play appears to be particularly sensitive to the effects of positive prediction error, making it a potent source of reward and mood enhancement. The canine disposition to play and explore endows the dog with a high degree of curiosity and capacity for producing reward derived from the discovery of stimuli evoking positive prediction error and surprise. In addition to mediating reward, play appears to perform a special modal balancing and integrating function in relation to emotional command systems (see *Play and Drive* in Chapter 10). A lack of playfulness or an inability to sustain playful interaction is a reliable indicator of emotional imbalance, degraded mood, or disease. Given the social and quality-of-life objectives of cynopraxic training, it is natural that play should figure centrally in the process of behavioral change and adjustment (see *Fair Play and the Golden Rule* in Chapter 10). During playful interaction, both the dog and the trainer learn the value of compromise and cooperation; without mutual compromise and cooperation, playful interaction cannot be sustained. In contrast, time-out (i.e., loss of social contact and reward) has an opposite effect on modal activity and serves to mediate passive module strategies via disappointment and decreased reward incentive (de-arousal).

A spirit of affectionate playfulness should inform the training process. Training sessions frequently, but not always, start off with play, but formal sessions should always end on a playful note. Periodic bouts of play are interspersed throughout the session, bringing trained modules and routines under the motivational influence of playful incentives. Training a dog to control playful impulses by turning them on and off again in the process of rewarding compliant behavior provides a powerful means to improve impulse control. As Hediger (1955/1968) once aptly noted, "Good training is disciplined play" (139). Spontaneity does not arise out of chaos, but is born under the nurturing influence of order, discipline, and play. As trained behavior becomes reliable (i.e., well predicted and controlled), first through reward training using social and appetitive reinforcers and then directive training conducive to enhanced competence, relaxation, and safety, further refinement and integration are achieved via the unifying influence of ludic incentives and play rewards. Play rewards gradually transform the significance of trained behavior via associative processes, whereby trained responses become progressively linked with playful affects, ludic incentives, and qualities (e.g., spontaneity and joy). Under the liberating influence of play rewards, trained behavior becomes more responsive to reorganization and generalization. Play makes the training process more creative for trainers and makes work more fun for dogs. Just as training sessions are started and concluded with play, play is both the means and the end of cynopraxic therapy.

THE TRAINING SPACE

Setting appropriate social boundaries and limits is an important foundation for all training activities. All dogs must learn to respect three basic boundaries at the outset of training: limits on jumping up, limits on biting on hands and clothing, and limits on pulling against the leash. In most cases, these behaviors are not entirely suppressed but redirected or modified into more acceptable forms. Although spontaneous jumping up is not permitted, dogs may be trained and permitted to jump up on cue. Similarly, while biting on hands and clothing is discouraged, biting on tug toys is encouraged with play. Since both jumping up and tug games are highly enjoyable activities for dogs, they can be invited to

jump up or given opportunities to play tug as a reward. Similarly, from an early age, puppies should be discouraged from pulling by various means. Such boundaries are set by first causing the dog to passively defer and then to actively follow the trainer's rules of interaction, defining when it can jump up or bite. Besides learning to relinquish control and to desist from competitive challenges, the establishment of social boundaries enhances a dog's attention and impulse-control abilities. The limits and training set around jumping up, biting, and pulling form a training space within which reward-based training activities can be carried out. Without the establishment of a viable training space, training activities may be continuously frustrated by intrusive social excesses and oppositional behavior.

INSTRUMENTAL REWARD AND PUNISHMENT

Just as objects acquire the appearance of form and solidity as the result of the interplay of light and dark on their surface, behavior is shaped through the complementary influences of reward and punishment. Practically speaking, behavior is formed and structured by systematically arranging reward and punishment to occur in ways that produce controllable behavioral changes consistent with immediate (proximal) and remote (distal) training objectives. The conventional definitions of reinforcement by reward and suppression by punishment stress the complementary effects that these events have on the frequency or probability of behavior as consequences, but without much reference to the emotional or cognitive processes mediating the observed effects (see *Basic Concepts and Principles of Instrumental Learning* in Volume 1, Chapter 7). This general characterization of instrumental learning by reward and punishment, founded on Thorndike's law of effect, appears to be overly simplistic and theoretically inadequate for capturing the complex and organized nature of adaptive learning processes. The conventional view neglects critical molar and modal aspects of learning and behavioral organization, perhaps as the result of an excessively myopic emphasis on molecular relations between consequent events and isolated responses. Of particular interest from the perspective of cynopraxic behavior therapy and training are the acquired molar relations operating under the organizing influences of emotional and cognitive processes.

Control Incentives and Reinforcement

The effects of reinforcement and punishment are quantified by reference to the differential changes that the events have on response probability or frequency. However, defining reinforcement and punishment in terms of probability is rather circular and inadequate for several reasons (see *Reinforcement and the Notion of Probability* in Volume 1, Chapter 7). Alternatively, reinforcement and punishment can be viewed from the perspective of a control incentive and function. According to the control-incentive theory, behavior that enhances an animal's control over significant events produces reinforcement whereas behavior that impairs control efforts results in punishment. Changes in the frequency or probability of the reinforced or punished behavior are secondary to its success or failure to improve an animal's ability to control the environmental event prompting action. The establishment and optimization of control over attractive or aversive events appears to be an important aspect of reinforcement and punishment for dogs. Dogs work to optimize their control over attractive events by obtaining or maintaining their availability; similarly, they work to escape, reduce, or avoid aversive ones. Normally, when a dog acts, it does so with the intent of producing some specific effect on the environment; that is, instrumental behavior is purposive and shaped by the accumulated successes or failures that such efforts afford with respect to the control of significant events. To the extent that these efforts are successful, they are reinforced and integrated into a dog's behavioral repertoire, whereas efforts that fail to control attractive or aversive events adequately are punished by loss or discomfort and are gradually modified or removed from a dog's behavioral repertoire, at least in those situations where the actions have failed to enhance control efforts. In short, according to the control-incentive

theory, reinforcement occurs when purposive efforts succeed in enhancing a dog's control over some motivationally significant event, whereas punishment occurs when such purposive efforts fail to make a difference or make matters worse; that is, they result in a lack or loss of control.

Premack's interpretation of reinforcement and punishment is consistent with a control-incentive analysis (see *Premack Principle: The Relativity of Reinforcement* in Volume 1, Chapter 7). According to Premack, instrumental behavior is reinforced or punished by the occurrence of other behavior. The reward value of any particular behavior is determined by its probability of occurrence relative to other behaviors operating under similar motivational and environmental circumstances. Therefore, at any given moment, an animal's behavioral repertoire is distributed along a hierarchic continuum from behaviors that are least likely to behaviors that are most likely. Behaviors that are more likely tend to reinforce behaviors that are less likely, whereas behaviors that are less likely tend to punish behaviors that are more likely. In short, instrumental behavior is reinforced by other behavior occurring at a higher probability. Premack's response-probability hierarchy is really a control-incentive index. Obviously, responses of the highest probability are precisely those that would most likely lead to enhanced control over some immediate and motivationally significant event, whereas responses with low probability and reinforcement value are precisely those actions with the least likelihood of establishing control or those that may actually impair control efforts. Low-probability responses are potentially punitive, not because they are assigned a low probability or intrinsic hedonic value, but because they do not directly serve the animal's immediate control interests. High-probability responses are those that are most relevant or likely to succeed with respect to the control of motivationally significant events, whereas low-probability responses are those that are most irrelevant or likely to fail.

Although control incentives are functionally significant with regard to reinforcement and punishment, the gratification of a control incentive is not sufficient to explain the organizing effects of learning. In addition to control incentives, various predictive influences are at work. In an important sense, instrumental control incentives appear to emerge in the context of classical conditioning. The predictive information produced by associative learning provides a framework for instrumental control efforts. Classical conditioning provides predictive information about the occurrence of significant events and prepares a dog motivationally for them, whereas instrumental learning is concerned with optimizing a dog's ability to control the events when they occur. The orderly nature of learning suggests that it occurs within the context of prediction-control expectancies. As argued in *Prediction-Control Expectancies and Adaptation* in Volume 1, Chapter 7, reinforcement and punishment are not so much about the effects of arbitrary attractive and aversive events increasing or decreasing the future probability of some isolated response, but rather the result of the confirmation or disconfirmation of instrumental control expectancies. Control expectancies are the encoded results of past instrumental efforts to exploit or avoid attractive or aversive events. Classical and instrumental learning activities share a common organizing function, viz., to make the environment more predictable, controllable and, consequently, more comfortable and safe.

Classical Conditioning, Prediction, and Reward

Successful control over significant events depends on the accumulation of predictive information concerning their occurrence. Classical conditioning not only provides predictive information about the occurrence of attractive and aversive events, it also establishes a complex network of predictive contingency relations between antecedent and consequent events that guides instrumental control efforts (see *Relations Between the Signal, Response, and Outcome* in Volume 1, Chapter 7). In addition to providing predictive information that is incorporated into instrumental control expectancies, classical conditioning significantly influences instrumental behavior via excitatory and inhibitory

emotional influences (Rescorla and Solomon, 1967; Dickinson and Pearce, 1977). At the level of organizing functions, the conventional distinctions between classical and instrumental learning begin to dissolve. The successful control of significant events depends on the acquisition of accurate predictions regarding the details of their occurrence, size, and quality. Similarly, adequate prediction depends on feedback derived from instrumental control efforts.

Refinement of instrumental control efforts depends on information obtained from conditioned stimuli, especially those stimuli that are relevant to control efforts. In the process of training, for example, bridging stimuli (conditioned reinforcers) play an important role in the acquisition and maintenance of learned behavior. In addition to evoking various conditioned appetitive and emotional responses, bridging stimuli are informative about the size, type, and frequency of the pending attractive or aversive event. In fact, the ability of bridging stimuli to control and modify behavior appears to depend on their information value (Egger and Miller, 1962). Optimal bridging effects occur when new and surprising information is obtained about the occurrence of rewarding stimuli. The moment of reward is not when a dog ingests food or when it receives affectionate attention and petting, but, more precisely, reward occurs at the moment a dog detects some new bit of information that enhances its control over such motivationally significant events. Reward and punishment appear to depend on the detection of a discrepancy between what a dog expects to occur and what actually occurs: reward occurs when the outcome is better (more attractive) than expected (surprise), whereas punishment occurs when the outcome is worse (less attractive) than expected (disappointment). A similar relationship is obtained in the case of aversive events: reward occurs when the expected outcome is better (less aversive) than expected (relief), whereas punishment occurs when the outcome is worse (more aversive) than expected (startle). As the result of prediction discrepancies, conditioned reinforcers undergo excitatory or inhibitory changes in accordance with the Rescorla-Wagner model; that is, only when the conditioned stimulus (CS) either underpredicts (excitatory) or overpredicts (inhibitory) the unconditioned stimulus (US) does additional learning take place (see *Assumptions Derived from the Rescorla-Wagner Model* in Volume 1, Chapter 6). Three possible effects on the associative strength of the bridging stimulus occur in association with attractive and aversive outcomes:

1. If the outcome is more attractive or aversive than expected (surprise or startle), then excitatory conditioning occurs—the associative strength of the conditioned reinforcer is strengthened.

2. If the outcome is less attractive or aversive than expected (disappointment or relief), then inhibitory conditioning follows—the associative strength of the conditioned reinforcer is weakened.

3. If the outcome is exactly as expected (comfort and safety), then no additional learning occurs (the prediction is verified)—the associative strength of the conditioned reinforcer is unchanged.

Studies focusing on the response of dopamine (DA) neurons to the presentation of signals with varying temporal and predictive relations to rewarding stimuli indicate that the activation (reward) or depression (punishment) of reward-mediating DA neurons depends on the detection of discrepancies between what an animal expects and what actually occurs (Waelti et al., 2001). DA reward signals are generated in association with positive prediction errors (the attractive outcome is better than expected), whereas punitive signals are produced in association with negative prediction errors (the attractive outcome is worse than expected) (Schultz, 1998):

All responses to rewards and reward-producing stimuli depend on event predictability. Dopamine neurons are activated by rewarding events that are better than predicted, remain uninfluenced by events that are as good as predicted, and are depressed by events that are worse than predicted. (1)

In essence, the collection of DA neurons localized in the ventral tegmental area gener-

ate teaching signals in response to the detection of prediction errors, thereby facilitating improved adaptation and organized behavior via an incentive to explore, experiment, and discover. These various behavioral and neurobiological findings complement the behavioral findings of Egger and Miller (1963) and lend support to their hypothesis that "reinforcement occurs primarily at the point at which new information is delivered" (132). As such, learning appears to depend on expectancy errors that variably lead to surprise and disappointment—errorless learning is an oxymoron. Outcomes that are well predicted and expected do not support additional learning, even though the attractive outcome consistently follows the learned behavior—a fully predicted reward appears to block additional learning (plateau). Such outcomes serve to verify the control expectancy, gratify the control incentive, abolish the establishing operation, and contribute to feelings of comfort and safety, but they do not produce reward.

As instrumental behavior becomes stable under the influence of repeated bridging and reinforcement, DA release shifts to the earliest predictor of impending reinforcement, viz., the bridging stimulus (Schultz, 1998) (Figure 1.2). DA activation via bridging stimuli exhibits a preference for stimuli with a clear onset and alerting quality. Also, DA neurons are exclusively sensitive to the onset of the bridging stimulus and are unresponsive to its offset, even if the offset coincides with the delivery of the rewarding stimulus (Schultz, 1998). These findings suggest that the bridging stimulus should be brief and crisp and have an alerting quality, helping to explain the bridging efficacy of brief high-pitched vocal sounds, squeakers, whistles, and clickers. The conditioned effect of bridging stimuli may be mediated via efferent pathways originating in the amygdala (Hassani et al., 2001). The lateral nucleus of the amygdala contains neurons that are highly sensitive to acoustical stimulation, which play an important role in the detection of auditory conditioned stimuli. In addition to receiving afferent acoustical signals via the thalamus and sensory cortex, the amygdala forms strong efferent connections with DA neurons in the ventral tegmental area (Schultz, 1998), lending some credibility to the hypothesis that the amygdala may be involved in the process of conditioned reinforcement. In any case, noradrenergic pathways also probably play a role, since norepinephrine (NE)-producing neurons originating in the locus coeruleus exert a potent excitatory effect on numerous forebrain areas mediating orienting and alerting responses to conditioned appetitive and aversive stimuli, as well as novel or startling ones (see *Reticular Formation* in Volume 1, Chapter 3). As in the case of DA neurons, NE neurons

are responsive to changes associated with learning. Whereas DA neurons appear to be responsive to the appetitive and hedonic salience of significant events, NE neurons are responsive to their attention-grabbing aspects (Schultz, 1998). Conditioned reinforcement appears to involve a coordinated process involving both NE and DA circuits, with the former mediating alert and orientation to the bridging stimulus and the latter assessing its appetitive and hedonic significance. In addition to mediating orienting responses and selective attention, NE circuits appear to play an important role in

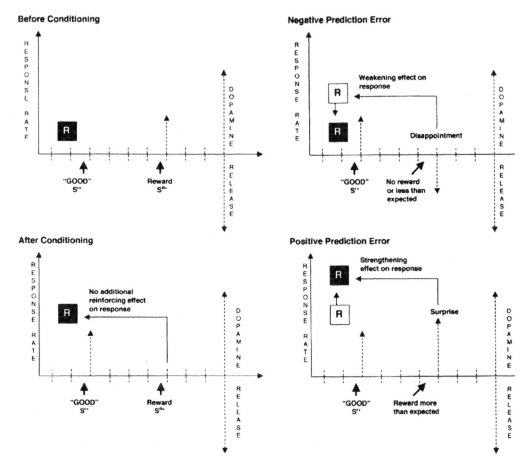

FIG. 1.2. Prior to conditioning, the vocal signal "Good" (S^{R+}) fails to provide conditioned reinforcement, as indicated by the absence of dopamine reward activity. After conditioning, however, dopamine release shifts toward the occurrence of the conditioned reinforcer and away from the predicted reward (S^{R+}). The well-predicted reward loses its capacity to activate the release of dopamine. Without a prediction error, additional learning does not appear to occur.

more flexible scanning activities (Aston-Jones et al., 1999).

Prediction and Control Expectancies

Learning appears to proceed as the result of the acquisition and refinement of prediction-control expectancies, necessitating the postulation of a hypothetical expectancy-comparator mechanism, whereby what a dog expects to occur is compared with what actually occurs (see *Neural Comparator Systems* in Chapter 10). Numerous comparator circuits sensitive to prediction error are distributed throughout the brain, mediating a variety of neural and behavioral adjustments in response to changing moment-to-moment circumstances (Schultz and Dickinson, 2000). These specialized comparator circuits appear to communicate together and orchestrate complex adaptive functions, including the detection of prediction errors conducive to reward and punishment. Prediction-error signals resulting in reward and punishment are produced when what the dog anticipates to occur as the result of an action (control module) and conditioned reinforcement turns out to be better or worse than expected. Such positive and negative prediction errors differentially produce reward or punishment by activating or depressing dopamine activity.

According to the expectancy-comparator model, predictions are processed by a complex series of feedback loops that serve to confirm or disconfirm expectancies, process error signals, calibrate appetitive and emotional establishing operations, and adjust behavioral output to control target events more effectively. In the process of confirming instrumental control expectancies, the detection of prediction discrepancies results in four possible effects:

1. Attractive outcomes that occur earlier than anticipated or are better than expected serve to produce positive prediction errors, surprise, and reward signals.

2. Attractive outcomes that are omitted or turn out to be worse than expected serve to produce negative prediction errors, disappointment, and punitive signals.

3. Aversive outcomes that are omitted or are better (less painful or frightening) than expected serve to produce positive prediction errors, relief, and reward signals.

4. Aversive outcomes that occur sooner than anticipated or are worse (more painful or frightening) than expected serve to produce negative prediction errors, startle, and punitive signals.

The practical implications of these findings are significant. Deliberately arranging reward outcomes to produce positive prediction error serves to make training efforts more efficient and effective, helping to avoid plateaus and enhancing performance reliability and quality (e.g., speed and enthusiasm), even in the presence of highly attractive distractions. However, simply varying rewards randomly is not conducive to positive prediction error and the generation of DA reward signals. Prediction discrepancies and errors can be detected only against a backdrop of an already established pattern of highly predictable outcomes. Consequently, the first step is to provide the dog with a highly predictable and controllable pattern of reinforcement, thereby establishing a standard expectancy against which deviations can be detected and compared. The destructive behavioral effects associated with unpredictable and uncontrollable social interaction may be due in part to a failure to develop a standard against which to judge outcomes and detect prediction discrepancies conducive to reward activation. Typically, variables conducive to prediction error are arranged to occur as trained responses approach or reach plateaus. Plateaus in the training process signal the need for additional reward, and the way to achieve that effect is not by providing bigger and better rewards, but by introducing prediction-error contingencies, that is, vary the size, type, frequency, and timing of the reinforcing outcome. Outcomes can be varied in a variety of ways while training the dog. During recall training, for example, as the dog turns to come in response to its name or a relevant orienting stimulus (e.g., hand clap or lip smooch), the trainer flicks the right hand out to the side with fingers wrapped in a fist around the reward. As the dog touches the closed hand with its nose, the trainer says

"Good" and the reveals the contents. Alternatively, a clicker can be closely paired with the opening of the hand (see *Introductory Lessons*). As the dog learns to come and touch the hand, the concealed reward is varied in different ways. In addition to varying the size and type of reward, the length of time the dog must wait before the hand is opened is also varied from an immediate presentation to a 3-second delay. Another method of varying rewards involves sustained reinforcement. In this case, instead of altering the amount and type of the reward and giving it to the dog all at once, it is given to the dog over a period in a piecemeal fashion. For example, after the dog comes and sits, a treat or two is broken up into a dozen small pieces and fed one piece at a time over the course of 15 to 20 seconds. Sustained-reinforcement techniques can be particularly effective in dogs with attention problems. Rewards are presented in such a way that the dog cannot predict how much food it will receive as a reward or how long it must wait. Mixed into this pattern are other types of food rewards (e.g., kibble, various meats, biscuit pieces, cheese, jerky, cereals, and soft treats). Varying the amount and type of reward appears to maximize the effect of reinforcement, causing dogs to work harder and rendering the learned behavior more resistant to extinction. Because the reward varies in size, type, frequency, and timing of presentation, the dog is alternately affected by surprise and disappointment. When reward (surprise) and punishment (disappointment) are presented in a balanced proportion, a prediction dissonance and control incentive based on hope is produced. Prediction-error contingencies that provide more reward (positive prediction error) than punishment tend to produce prediction-dissonance effects conducive to elation and increased active modal activity, whereas contingencies that limit positive prediction error tend to produce behavioral plateaus and ruts, boredom, and despair. Finally, poorly predicted contingencies that involve uncontrollable aversive stimuli or outcomes producing more punishment (negative prediction error) than reward are prone to produce maladaptive prediction-dissonance effects and neurotic passive modal activity,

with increased anxiety and frustration (behavioral stress), depression, and irritability.

A comparator mechanism associated with the septohippocampal system (SHS) appears to respond to prediction discrepancies related to novelty and startle. Prediction-error signals originating in the SHS are believed to activate a neural network mediating startle and behavioral inhibition, causing the animal to "stop, look, and listen, and get ready for action" (Gray, 1991:114) (see *Learning and the Septohippocampal System* in Volume 1, Chapter 3). The momentary pause in activity produced by novelty and startle may be the result of a sensorimotor priority given to unusual or unexpected events. Novelty and startle appear to activate increased emotional and cognitive processing, apparently with the goal of assessing the significance of unusual events and adjusting behavioral output accordingly; that is, novelty and startle are received and interpreted in terms of new information. Consistent with such a information-processing function, attenuated stimuli occurring immediately before the startling event appear to perform an automatic sensorimotor gating function (prepulse inhibition), whereby excessive or insignificant stimuli occurring at the moment of stimulation are barred from cognitive and emotional processing in order to prevent overload and help to ensure that only the most relevant stimuli present in the situation are focused upon (see Koch, 1999). The gating function associated with prepulse inhibition suggests the possibility that subtle signals immediately preceding a startling event may be preferentially associated with startle— a phenomenon confirmed by many common dog-training applications of startle conditioning. In addition to enhancing startle-conditioning effects and learning, an attenuated vocal, auditory, or olfactory signal presented immediately before a startling event appears to reduce the magnitude of the startle response significantly. Interestingly, the absence or lack of prepulse inhibition appears to be a marker associated with a variety of psychiatric disorders (Braff et al., 2001).

Gray (1991) has proposed that behavior is regulated by three focal neural systems: a behavioral approach system (BAS), a behavioral inhibition system (BIS), and a flight-fear system

(FFS). The BAS is activated by stimuli associated with appetitive arousal, reward, and the cessation of punishment, whereas the BIS is activated by unfamiliar stimuli (novelty), startle, and conditioned stimuli associated with aversive events and punishment (loss of reward). The FFS is activated by unconditioned aversive stimulation and nonreward (i.e., loss of safety and comfort) mediating escape behavior and defensive aggression. In addition to mediating rapid and disruptive startle, hesitation, or avoidance in response to startle and novelty, the BIS is activated by conditioned aversive stimuli and biologically prepared fear stimuli, loss of reward (negative prediction errors), or the disconfirmation of control expectancies. The BAS, on the other hand, is activated by conditioned and unconditioned stimuli eliciting appetitive arousal (establishing operations) and by signals of reward and the absence of punishment (positive prediction errors). Whereas the activation of the BIS by novelty/startle or loss of reward promotes increased arousal, scanning and vigilance, hesitation, and waiting, the activation of the BAS via surprise-dependent reward intensifies attention and interest, and promotes fearless seeking, searching, and exploratory activities. The BAS operates under the modulating influence of dopaminergic pathways in close association with the activation of species-typical motor programs. Under the influence of excessive BAS activation and imbalance, a dog may be made more vulnerable to compulsive-impulsive spectrum disorders. The BIS, on the other hand, appears to be under the modulating influences of noradrenergic and serotonergic pathways (anxiety-depression spectrum). Excessive activation of the BIS is associated with anxiety-depression spectrum disorders. The BAS and BIS are the rough neural correlates of active and passive modal activities and strategies.

Instrumental Control Modules and Modal Strategies

According to cynopraxic training theory, control expectancies are closely coordinated with establishing operations and adaptive modal strategies. Establishing operations are under the regulation of classical conditioning and mediate associative and motivational linkages between control expectancies and emotional command systems. Functionally speaking, establishing operations calibrate appetitive and emotional arousal in accordance with predictive information derived from instrumental control efforts. In effect, the establishing operation mediates a precise motivational state that defines in advance the sort of instrumental output needed to obtain gratification, that is, produce outcomes conducive to comfort or safety. Collectively, instrumental control incentives, appetitive and emotional establishing operations, prediction and control expectancies, and instrumental actions are referred to as control expectancy modules (control modules). Control modules, routines (linked modules and skills), and goal-directed projects operate within the context of active and passive modal strategies to form patterns of adaptive behavior. Control modules and adaptive modal strategies are postulated as the basic units of behavioral organization. Modal activities are general classes of motivated behavior consisting of active strategies (exploring, seeking, playing, searching, experimenting) and passive strategies (checking, waiting, hesitating, deferring, delaying, worrying), roughly corresponding to Gray's BAS and BIS. Control modules and routines operate in close association with modal strategies. Positive and negative prediction errors produced by the operation of control modules and routines have a differential activating or depressing influence on behavior and mood, mediating the expression of active and passive modal strategies. The various immediate and cumulative emotional and mood effects associated with positive and negative prediction error are referred to as positive and negative dissonance.

Active modal strategies develop in association with control modules and routines in the process of optimizing control efforts over aversive and attractive events. Active modal strategies organize the performance of control modules and routines into patterns of behavior that increase the likelihood of producing positive prediction errors, that is, set the occasion for surprise, discovery, and reward. Control incentives involving attractive and aversive outcomes entrain control modules and routines into patterns of modal searching, exploring, experimenting, adventure, risk taking, and daring. Active modal strategies are supported by reward (that is, better-than-expected outcomes) produced in the process of exploiting appetitive resources or controlling dangerous situations. Passive modal strategies are closely associated with the operation of well-established and orderly control modules and routines, representing the conservative, preservative, careful, and risk-avoidant patterns of organized behavior. Passive modal strategies are primarily involved in the detection and avoidance of negative prediction error (disappointment) and punishment.

Passive modal strategies develop in situations where active modal strategies fail (i.e., produce punishment and loss of reward). Under adverse circumstances, punishment may educe incompatible passive modal strategies (e.g., waiting, hesitating, deferring, delaying) aimed at avoiding negative prediction error and punishment. Although passive modal strategies are organized to preserve security (comfort and safety), they do so at a heavy potential cost that may, if performed in excess or to the exclusion of active modal success, ultimately result in progressive disorder and insecurity. Excessive passive modal activity is associated with increased worry and hypervigilance, the gradual loss of responsiveness to reward (dissatisfaction and pessimism), and increasing vulnerability to aversive arousal and emotional tone (anxiety, depression, and irritability). Active modal strategies, on the other hand, tend to pattern control modules and routines toward increasing behavioral variability and output via the search and discovery of positive prediction error (surprise and reward). In contrast to the aversive emotional tone (anxiety and depression) and inhibition of behavioral output associated with passive modal strategies, active modal strategies promote elation, excitement, enthusiasm, and diversification of behavior. However, under situations where active modal strategies operate in relative isolation from the order-enhancing influence of passive modal strategies, various imbalances involving impulsiveness, overactivity, attention deficits, loss of control, and behavioral disorganization may ensue. When functioning together harmoniously and operating under the prediction dissonance of hope, active and passive modal strategies produce a behavioral organization consisting of a balance of order and variability (see *Organizational Order and Variability*). A

clarification and elaboration of these various distinctions and their implications for dog behavior therapy and training are provided in Chapter 10.

Establishing Operations

An overarching and paramount psychological need is the optimization of predictive control over the local environment via learning and behavioral adaptation. The attainment of such goals presumes the existence of orderly and stable environmental circumstances. Dogs are motivationally affected by a variety of transient conditioned and unconditioned establishing operations conducive to enhanced prediction and control (see *Antecedent Control: Establishing Operations and Discriminative Stimuli* in Volume 1, Chapter 7). An establishing operation consists of any activity, event, or condition that renders a reward more effective. In addition to enhancing the motivational salience and effectiveness of instrumental rewards, an establishing operation sets the occasion for the occurrence of behaviors previously rewarded under its motivational influence. For example, food deprivation is an appetitive establishing operation that significantly enhances the reward value of food while at the same time encouraging dogs to offer behavior that has been rewarded previously with food. Conversely, activities, events, or conditions that reduce the effectiveness of a reward and decrease the occurrence of responses previously reinforced by it are referred to as abolishing operations (Michael, 2000). For example, satiation has an opposite effect on the value of food as a reward; that is, feeding the dog before training reduces the appetitive value of food and decreases the occurrence of behaviors that have been rewarded with food in the past. Identifying and using establishing and abolishing operations are important aspects of behavior assessment and problem solving (McGill, 1999; Iwata et al., 2000).

At the cognitive-emotional level of organization, establishing operations are postulated as performing the role of coordinating motivational arousal with instrumental behavioral adjustments via a loop of classically conditioned prediction expectancies (see *Adaptation, Prediction Error, and Distress* in Chapter

10). Establishing operations calibrate appetitive and emotional arousal to match behavioral output in terms of ongoing and anticipated situational change. The instrumental control expectancy defines in advance the sort of behavior needed to gratify the motivational state produced by the establishing operation. As such, establishing operations function as interfacing conduits between control expectancies and emotional command systems. Establishing operations are modulated by prediction-error signals coded in the process of confirming or disconfirming control expectancies. Both control expectancies and establishing operations are adjusted and refined in response to reward and punishment signals, thereby enabling dogs to better predict and exploit or avoid the detected discrepancy in the future. Active (e.g., seeking) and passive (e.g., waiting) modal strategies are highly sensitive to the activating and depressing effects of positive and negative prediction errors. Active modal strategies, including social and environmental exploring, searching, experimenting, testing, and so forth are dedicated to the search for positive prediction errors and the avoidance of negative ones. The enhanced order and security provided by instrumental control modules, routines, and patterns are the accumulated results of useful discoveries produced in cooperation with active and passive modal strategies. Modal strategies are not functionally independent of control expectancy modules, but rather depend on prediction errors arising in the process of confirming or disconfirming them. Whereas control modules and routines produce order conducive to survival and security (comfort and safety), active modal strategies promote variability, discovery, and risk taking. Passive modal strategies are likely to occur primarily under conditions of order and where active modal strategies are likely to produce loss of reward or punishment (see *Drive-related Modal Activity and Strategies* in Chapter 10).

Daily activities provide numerous opportunities to exploit establishing operations conducive to increased instrumental output and reward. Using these transient moments of heightened motivation is a central aspect to

ICT. For example, going for a walk is usually a highly valued activity for most dogs. Occasions anticipating a walk trigger significant anticipatory arousal, frenetic pacing, jumping up, and barking. The establishing operations associated with getting ready to go for a walk motivationally set the occasion for a variety of undesirable behaviors that are reinforced before a dog is let outside. If, instead of allowing the dog to engage in undesirable behavior at such times, the trainer requires that the dog perform a balanced cycle of tasks before leaving the house, the behaviors involved will undergo significant reinforcement and change over time in association with the opportunity to go for a walk. Another valuable establishing operation occurs as the result of separation. Following a long separation, a dog's interest in social attention and contact is significantly enhanced. The resulting social establishing operation can be used to promote a variety of training objectives. Social rewards can be used effectively at such times to reinforce attention and impulse control, as well as to strengthen the dog's willingness to come when called and other basic exercises. Another everyday opportunity for exploiting motivation conducive to training occurs in association with feeding times. Training that uses food reinforcement is enhanced by taking advantage of appetitive establishing operations associated with the expectation of a pending meal.

Despite the usefulness of social and appetitive establishing operations, the ultimate motivational operation for dog-training purposes is play (see *Modulatory and Unifying Effects of Play* in Chapter 6). Ludic establishing operations are resistant to satiation (abolishing operations) and conducive to the mood-enhancing effects of reward. For example, when catching a flying disk or chasing an out-of-round rubber toy, a tremendous amount of variety occurs in a dog's movements and the effects produced by them. With every chase and catch, deviations from the standard expectancy occur that are conducive to prediction error: air turbulence may cause the disk to turn up or down, float longer than usual or dive rapidly to the ground, or unexpectedly to veer off—all contributing to unusual maneuvers and catches (surprise) and misses (disappointment). The net result of such play is a high level of reward and positive dissonance (elation). Control modules and routines established in the context of play are highly durable and resistant to extinction. When properly carried out, play-rewarded behavior gradually becomes play itself, making the opportunity to perform the behavior its own reward. Play has the ability to educe and shape drive-related behaviors into unique and usable forms with a rapidity that cannot be accomplished by other means of reward. The playful eduction and entrainment of drive-related modal activities is the basis of many practical dog-training activities. Working dogs work to play and play while working.

Diverters and Disrupters

In accordance with the control-incentive theory of reinforcement, attractive and aversive events are only reinforcing to the extent that the dog is actively engaged in efforts to control them (see *Diverters and Disrupters* in Volume 1, Chapter 7). For example, tossing a dog a piece of food while it is straining on the leash in order to play with another dog would not likely strengthen the pulling response, certainly not as much as might occur by letting go of the leash (see the previous discussion regarding the Premack principle). Similarly, throwing a treat to a dog while it is aggressively barking at a passerby will not likely reinforce the barking behavior, but if the person happened to run away in response to the dog's threats, then such territorial behavior might be strongly reinforced. In both cases, the presentation of noncontingent treats may interrupt instrumental behavior by exciting motivational interests irrelevant or incompatible with the rewards being sought by the dog at the moment. If the diverter performs an establishing-operation function, the dog will subsequently exhibit instrumental efforts aimed at controlling the diversionary stimulus. Under the influence of a control incentive, the diversionary stimulus may become a reward capable of performing a reinforcement function. However, even if a

control contingency were inadvertently established between the barking behavior and the food item presented as a diverter, the barking response would be gradually stripped of its defensive significance via the classical conditioning effects of food reinforcement. Now, although a passerby might function as a discriminative stimulus for barking to get food rewards, the barking behavior would be of a very different motivational nature than aggressive barking and more readily controlled via a contingency of reinforcement now under the trainer's control. Disrupters are typically startle-producing stimuli that serve to interrupt behavior momentarily but without necessarily mediating a punitive effect. For example, in the case of a barking dog that ignores food at such times, a burst of compressed air might momentarily interrupt or briefly stop defensive barking. The brief hissing sound might immediately stop the behavior, but the effect may not last for long or significantly alter the future occurrence of the barking response. However, if the hissing startle is repeatedly presented under similar circumstances when the dog barks and is immediately preceded by some avoidance signal (e.g., "Quiet"), the dog may gradually learn to control the occurrence of the aversive event by not barking while in the predictive context or by stopping when the vocal avoidance signal is delivered. A preferable approach, though, is to follow the disrupter event with reward-based training efforts aimed at shaping responses incompatible with defensive barking (e.g., sitting or standing quietly for food and petting in the presence of the target). The combination of interruption and reward-based training can strongly enhance control efforts.

DIRECTIVE PROMPTS AND BLOCKING

Directive prompts and reprimands are the most common procedures used to enhance attention and impulse control. Although directive procedures can be highly effective and efficient, they can also produce significant fallout when used improperly or excessively (see *Coercive Compulsion and Conflict* in Volume 1, Chapter 8). Attention and directive prompts serve the purpose of limiting behavior that disrupts or interferes with reward-based training objectives, especially behavior occurring under the influence of competing distractions, that is, extraneous establishing operations and sources of reward not under a trainer's control. In addition to capturing the dog's attention and enhancing impulse control, an obvious advantage of vocal and directive prompts in training is the ease and immediacy with which a highly motivational state (establishing operation) can be produced and exploited. Directive prompts perform two functions at once: they block or inhibit undesirable behavior (compel abstention) while at the same time causing the dog to produce more acceptable alternative behavior (inducing action). Such procedures and techniques are particularly useful and beneficial for the control of harmful or potentially dangerous activities. The paradigm's simplicity and power to establish immediate motivational change and readiness to work has made the correct-and-praise method of training very popular over the years—a method that remains a standard and integral aspect of many fields of practical dog training, especially those activities requiring a high degree of control and performance reliability. The firm and unshakeable reality of dog training is that some amount of compulsion is unavoidable.

Distractions: Extraneous Sources of Reward

Since no natural environment is completely free of distractions, a significant portion of training time is dedicated to gaining control over behavior operating under the influence of extraneous rewards. In a certain sense, distractions represent a valuable source of potential rewards not yet under a trainer's control. Staging training activities so that distractions can be made available to the dog on a contingent basis represents a powerful means to reduce the disruptive effects of distractions as well as serving to advance training objectives. The combination of response-blocking and directive techniques within the context of reward-based training activities facilitates the

process of harnessing extraneous rewards to constructive goals. For example, preventing a dog from playing or chasing after another dog can be followed by an opportunity to engage safely in the activity, so long as it first waits and defers to the trainer's control prerogatives. Exploratory distractions of various kinds can be provided on a contingent basis provided that the dog periodically turns its attention to the trainer on signal, comes when called, and so forth. Since naturally occurring sources of reward are difficult to control and potentially dangerous to give on a contingent basis, motivationally equivalent activities may need to be identified and given to the dog instead. An alternative for dogs that enjoy chasing animals is the provision of tug-and-retrieve games, especially ball and flying-disk play. Dogs that engage in excessive exploratory behavior can be encouraged to play various hide-and-seek games in which toys are hidden for them to find.

Some extraneous sources of reward cannot be reliably controlled through the aforementioned procedures but may simply need to be inhibited and replaced with an alternative behavior. Directive training efforts are carried out to proof the dog's compliance under a wide variety of circumstances and distractions. Such training codes distractive stimuli into inhibitory signals, causing the dog to wait or stop when exposed to them rather than stimulating increased arousal and loss of control. Inhibitory training is recommended in the case of persistent behaviors posing significant potential harm to the dog or others. For example, dogs that chase after cars, bicyclists, joggers, and so forth may simply need to learn to avoid such activities by the application of appropriate commands, reprimands, and corrections. As the result of well-timed and appropriately impressive corrections, such dogs gradually become more responsive to commands and reprimands in the face of distracting influences. Gradually, by means of associative learning, distractions become conditioned into avoidance or inhibitory signals rather stimuli triggering arousal and chase behavior. For example, many dogs exhibiting the unacceptable habit of chasing cats quickly learn, after the delivery of a few directive leash prompts or electrical corrections, that lunging after a fleeing cat only results in discomfort and nonreward—not the attainment of the anticipated joys of the chase. As a result, the dog learns to approach cats with improved self-control, first hesitating and then gradually learning to avoid chasing them altogether, and finally learning to ignore them or to expect food rewards in their presence as the result of concurrent reward-based attention and sit-stay training efforts. The overall effect is to improve the dog's attention to the trainer's instruction whenever a cat happens to be nearby.

Least Intrusive and Minimally Aversive

Correction procedures should not be used lightly or haphazardly. The rule of thumb is to select the least aversive and intrusive procedure that is reasonably expected to succeed. According to the least intrusive and minimally aversive (LIMA) model, aversives are ranked in terms of their relative severity and intrusiveness, requiring that the trainer apply a less aversive technique before advancing to a more aversive one (see *Compliance* in Volume 2, Chapter 2). Adhering to this model and selection process ensures that the least necessary and sufficient aversive procedure is used to produce the intended behavioral objective. In addition to minimizing the potential for producing pain and discomfort, correction procedures should be governed by a principle of minimal intrusiveness. Training procedures should intrude minimally on the human-dog bond and avoid adversely affecting the dog's quality of life. Overly constrictive restraint and confinement techniques should be avoided in favor of techniques that most rapidly and humanely achieve training objectives without causing undue distress or discomfort to the dog.

PART 2: TOOLS AND TECHNIQUES

TRAINING TOOLS

The equipment used in dog and puppy training is fitted with a concern for the dog's age, size, temperament, training history, and specific needs. A wide range of products of varying quality and price are available. Training equipment should be of the best quality, remembering that cheap equipment is most likely to fail when it is needed most. All training tools have advantages and disadvantages that need to be considered carefully, and each requires a degree of expertise for proper use. Although some rather vitriolic and unproductive hyperbole bubbles up now and then against the use of various training collars, most experienced and competent trainers agree that such tools have a functional and humane place in dog training. Any standard training tool can be used abusively and cause injury, but there is nothing inherently cruel about such tools (see Delta Society, 2001). Although neck injury can result from the improper use of a slip or halter collar, I have personally never witnessed or know of a single verified case in which a dog sustained serious cervical injury as the result of a properly applied leash correction, even involving corrections that have been applied very forcefully. Some dogs (e.g., the toy poodle and Yorkshire terrier) appear to be predisposed to tracheal problems and should be trained on harnesses. If in doubt about the suitability of a specific collar for a particular dog, consult a veterinarian for advice.

Flat-strap and Martingale Collars

For many dogs, commercially available flat-strap and buckle or so-called martingale collars are sufficient for most training purposes. The flat collar is tightened just snugly enough to prevent it from slipping over the dog's head. When properly fitted, the martingale collar has the advantage of a slack fit with little risk of the dog backing out of it. Puppies under 5 months of age are typically trained with a strap collar alone or a fixed-action halter. In the case of strong puppies and dogs, a buckle-type fastener is preferred over a plastic snap-on one.

Limited-slip Collars

A highly effective limited-slip collar can be made from a single length of nylon webbing (Figure 1.3). The primary advantage of the limited-slip collar is adjustability, both in terms of the range of slip action and the pressure

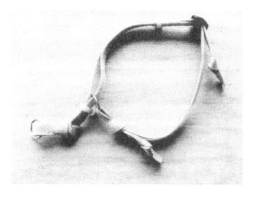

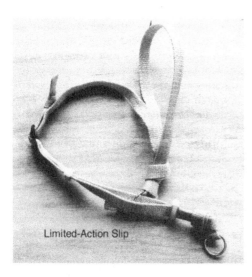

Limited-Action Slip

FIG. 1.3. Limited-slip collar (top) and limited-slip/halter combination collar (bottom) provide excellent control and adjustability.

applied to a dog's neck. The limited-slip collar features two slides that are used to make these adjustments. As in the case of full-action slip collars, the limited-action collar is placed around a dog's neck so that it forms a "p for perfect" (frontal view). Another way of making sure that the slip collar is on properly is to observe how the collar closes. When pulling the live ring (the one hooked to the leash), the collar should close dragging the dead ring clockwise around the dog's neck.

Conventional Slip Collars

Many trainers prefer using a nylon-slip or chain-slip collar—a collar that remains espe-

cially popular among working-dog trainers. The chain-slip or check collar consists of a chain with two rings, the live ring and the dead ring. The leash is attached to the live ring, causing the dead ring to travel clockwise around the dog's neck as it applies momentary pressure. The term *choke collar* is a misnomer that may have contributed to a significant misunderstanding about the use of such collars, as evident among inexperienced dog owners who purchase them to control pulling dogs. Many people use these collars under the false assumption that they work to stop pulling behavior by choking the dog. Consequently, under the belief that the choking effect will eventually discourage pulling, they allow the dog to pull continuously during walks. This belief is not only wrong with regard to the reduction of pulling behavior, but such control by choking may also produce significant physiological distress and harm (see *Walking on a Slack Leash*). The size of the chain-slip collar is estimated by measuring the widest part of the dog's head. A chain-slip collar can be made safer by placing a key ring through the chain to block the collar from closing too tightly around the dog's neck, thus limiting the amount of compression to the neck that the collar can deliver (Figure 1.4). In addition, a split ring can be attached to the chain to prevent it from sliding through the dead ring, thereby helping to keep the collar in place on the dog's neck. The training slip collar requires significant skill to be used properly and safely.

Prong Collars

The prong collar features a high degree of adjustability by way of removable prong links that are positioned to press into a dog's neck as the leash is pulled back (see Figure 1.4). A chain with two opposing rings (the center ring and swivel ring) closes the collar with an action similar to that of the martingale collar. The prong collar can be converted into a martingale collar by turning it around so that the prongs face away from the dog's skin. The leash is attached to the swivel ring. The center ring on the reciprocating chain slides from side to side. The side-to-side action of the central ring serves to direct prong pressure

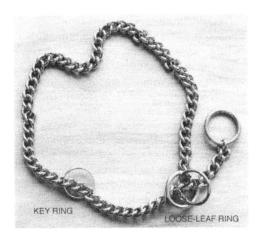

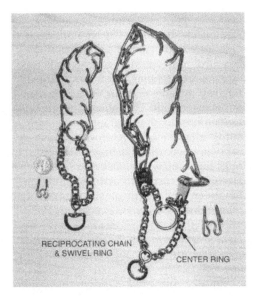

FIG. 1.4. Limited-slip chain (chain-slip) collar (top) and micro and small prong collars (bottom). The chain-slip collar can be modified to yield enhanced adjustability and safe control over the slip action.

prong collar as a shaping and polishing tool requires significant instruction, but with respect to basic control uses novice trainers can rapidly master the prong collar. It is frequently used to train high-spirited working dogs.

Halter Collars

A variety of halter collars are currently on the market. Most of these can be traced to an original concept and design fashioned by Alice DeGroot and patented in 1984 (Figure 1.5). DeGroot's K-9 Kumalong design offers significant head and muzzle control while at the same time allowing the dog to open its mouth fully. The basic logical and mechanical principle of DeGroot's collar is that "where the dog's head is led, the body is sure to follow." (DeGroot, 1985:30). In addition to improved head control, the muzzle action of the collar provides a source of negative reinforcement and jaw control. Whenever a dog

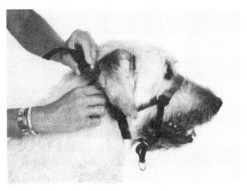

differentially to different parts of the dog's neck. When pulled straight back, the chain causes the prong collar to close evenly around the dog's neck. When the leash is pulled toward the right, the center ring shifts position and catches on prong links that direct most of the leash pressure to the left side of the dog's neck, causing it to move to the right in a highly controlled way. These actions and effects are useful for shaping and polishing precision heeling. The proper use of the

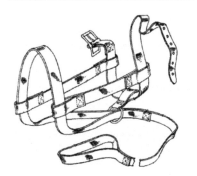

FIG. 1.5. K-9 Kumalong.

pulls back against the leash, the clamping action of the muzzle loop closes the dog's mouth, an effect that is immediately reversed when the dog stops pulling. DeGroot suggests that part of the halter's effectiveness may stem from ethological origins, in particular, from the way in which the mother disciplines or reorients her puppy by manipulating its muzzle. She argues that the Kumalong muzzle loop provides "surrogate maternal control" (31), an effect that adult and dominant dogs may resent, causing them to resist halter control fiercely when they are first exposed to it. Although some dogs may become momentarily reactive to halter restraint, others appear to become progressively relaxed and calmed as the result of it, an effect that DeGroot claims is especially prominent in hyperactive, nervous, or timid dogs. She speculates that the tranquilizing effect of halter control may be due to endorphin release, perhaps involving a mechanism similar to that attributed to the tranquilizing effect of acupuncture treatment.

With the advent of muzzling-type halters, the slip action of the traditional training collar shifted from around the dog's neck to a more vulnerable point around its muzzle. The muzzle-controlling loop effortlessly twists and turns a dog's head when it pulls, while forcefully pinning the dog's mouth shut if it attempts to struggle or back out of the collar. Of course, the capability of such collars to control the head and exert a forceful muzzling action is a desirable innovation in the case of aggressive dogs, providing trainers with increased control and safety over such situations than afforded by conventional collars. A subsequent halter design marketed under the trade names Promise and Gentle Leader was patented in 1986 by R. K. Alexander with two co-inventors, as a combination collar and muzzle training aid. Over the years, Anderson has been an enthusiastic proponent of halter training in the context of veterinary behavior management and therapy. The collar-muzzle combination provides secure control over a dog's head movements, produces a robust muzzle-clamping action, and features a fixed-muzzle capability. Releasing and moving up a plastic adjusting slide located on the muzzle loop and resetting it at a point that prevents the dog from opening its mouth produces a

partial muzzle effect. Although a muzzle set in this way prevents wide-mouthed bites, dogs can still manage to pinch with their incisors. Clamping the muzzle loop down farther to completely prevent pinching bites is not recommended, since it results in significant discomfort and distress to dogs. In such cases, or in cases involving a serious risk of attack, a mesh-sleeve or basket-type muzzle should be used instead of a muzzle-type halter.

Most dogs exposed to halter collars exhibit varying amounts of struggle and distress before finally accepting the restraint (Haug et al., 2002). After several brief sessions of introductory training with treats and patient encouragement, the vast majority of dogs calm down and learn to accept or at least tolerate the collar. The odor of orange oil (2 or 3 drops) rubbed on the hands or presented from a scented squeaker bulb can exert a potent calming effect over persistent reactivity to halter restraint when presented to the dog to sniff. The subsequent presentation of the odor of orange appears to work as both a calmative and a positive reinforcer to maintain more relaxed behavior. However, some dogs simply will not accept such restraint and react with persistent and vigorous protest and present an appearance of significant distress. Aggressive dogs (especially experienced biters) that resent the halter represent a significant risk to trainers or owners when they attempt to put the halter over the dog's muzzle.

Although one would expect to find significant differences in the biological stress exhibited by dogs wearing flat collars versus halters, a study performed at the University of Minnesota found no significant stress-related physiological differences between the Gentle Leader and a flat-strap collar (Ogburn et al., 1998). Head collars should be used with great care, since they work by twisting a dog's head and neck. Excessively hard corrections or surprise lunges by the dog could result in cervical strain or injury, especially in dogs predisposed to such injury, but to my knowledge no confirmed injuries of this kind have been reported. Halters can produce friction sores on the top of the muzzle, but careful fitting and proper use of such collars prevent most of these problems. In the case of adult aggressive dogs, halters should be used in combination with an oversized slip collar that is sufficiently long not to interfere with the clamping action of the halter. The backup collar prevents dogs from breaking free during unexpected episodes of intense struggle or when the halter might accidentally come off or fail in some unforeseen way. Alternatively, a backup collar and halter can be fastened to the same leash by hooking a small carabiner through the handle of the leash and attaching it to the collar. The leash forms a closed loop between the collar and halter and is held with both hands, the left hand controlling the collar and the right hand controlling the halter.

Another closed-loop arrangement uses a hip-hitch (see *Hip-hitch*) in combination with a flat strap or limited-slip collar and halter (Figure 1.6). A leash fitted with a small carabiner hooked to the handle of the leash is used. Alternatively, a service leash with bolt snaps at both ends can be used. The carabiner is attached to a strap or limited-slip collar, and the other end of the leash is hooked to the halter, functioning as a control lead. The arrangement provides a closed loop in which forceful pulling is blocked with the hip-hitch, while the halter is used to guide the dog rather than hold it back. This arrangement appears to be safer and more acceptable to many dogs, especially those reactive to halter control. The combination also appears to facilitate active training rather than simply controlling the dog via passive halter restraint. The undesirable clamping action produced by the conventional halter can be eliminated by the arrangement, unless the trainer wishes to produce such additional restraint with the control lead. The use of a hip-hitch and collar in combination with the halter makes the introduction of halter control less evocative and stressful. Instead of functioning as a tool to passively control pulling by forcefully twisting a dog's head, the combined hip-hitch, collar, and halter arrangement allows the halter to be used in a much more gentle way. The arrangement makes fading of halter control easier as more appropriate walking behavior is shaped under the control of the strap or limited-slip collar. Finally, a major

advantage of the hip-hitch is that it frees the trainer's hands to present various hand signals, bridges, and rewards, while minimizing the risk that the trainer might accidentally lose control of the leash.

Fixed-action Halter Collars

Although the muzzle-clamping action of most halter collars is highly effective and useful, for most basic training purposes a fixed-action halter is adequate when the added control of a halter is needed. The fixed-action halter has two significant advan-

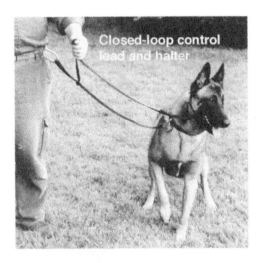

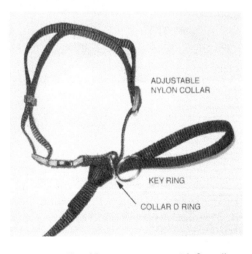

FIG. 1.6. Closed-loop arrangement with flat collar and fixed-action halter.

tages: snug fit and comfort. The nonclamping muzzle loop ensures that pressure will be appropriately delivered to the back of a dog's head when it pulls back, rather than unnecessarily clamping down on its nose. When the dog pulls ahead, the neck and muzzle loops effectively serve to turn the dog's head, but without putting any unnecessary pressure or rubbing on the dog's muzzle. Fixed-action halter collars provide an excellent transitional means to control excessive pulling in puppies and adult dogs alike. The muzzle loop is formed by tying a figure-of-eight loop or simple overhand loop into an 8-foot length of nylon webbing, leaving a short end to form a neck loop and the remaining long end to make a leash and handle (Figure 1.7). The short end forms the neck loop by slipping it through the muzzle-loop knot and then tying it off to the leash

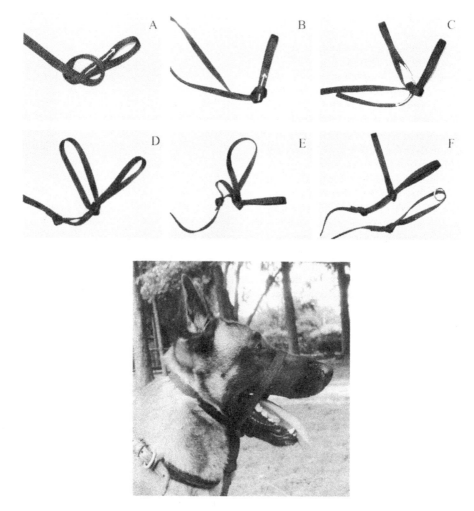

FIG. 1.7. Fixed-action halter. (A) The muzzle loop uses either a figure-of-eight or an overhand loop knot. (B) A finished muzzle-loop knot. (C) The neck loop is formed by slipping the short end through the muzzle-loop knot. (D) A finished halter with the adjusting knot binding the neck loop to the leash. (E) A fixed-action halter is opened by sliding the neck loop through the muzzle-loop knot. (F) A fixed-action halter with handle measured and ready for use as a muzzle-clamping halter.

end approximately 4 to 8 inches below the knot, depending on the size of the dog's neck and head. When fully pulled out, the neck loop should fit snugly, thus preventing the dog from backing out of it, but it should not press uncomfortably around the dog's neck. Once tied off to the leash, the neck loop can be opened by pulling it back through the muzzle-loop knot, thereby expanding it so that the neck loop can get over the dog's head. Before it is closed again, the collar loop is situated just behind the dog's head, and the muzzle loop is placed over its nose. To close the neck loop and secure the muzzle loop in place, the left hand grips the muzzle-loop knot while the right hand pulls the neck-loop knot back, thereby causing the neck loop to tighten and the muzzle loop to move back into place on the dog's nose. The fixed-action halter and leash are continuous with a handle tied into the end of the leash.

In addition to fixed-action halters, a limited-slip/halter combination collar is often used in training (see Figure 1.3). The halter/limited-slip collar combines the advantages of both the halter and slip-action collar, while minimizing some of the disadvantages of conventional slip and muzzling-type halter collars. By distributing force between the limited-slip collar and the muzzle loop, the halter/limited-slip collar provides enhanced head control without excessive clamping or twisting actions. Excessive neck twisting is prevented by the automatic transfer of force from the muzzle loop to the limited-action slip collar. The relative amount of force directed to the neck or muzzle is adjusted by moving the slip-limiting slide on the collar. The flat collar, the limited-slip collar, the fixed-action halter collar, and the halter/limited-slip collar combination are the primary collars used in cynopraxic training.

Fixed-action and Slip-action Harnesses

In cases involving dogs with a propensity for tracheal problems or a veterinary diagnosis counterindicating the use of a collar around the dog's neck, a harness can be a useful alternative. Various designs are available, and proper fitting is critical to prevent the dog from getting out of the harness. Full and half-slip harnesses can be easily made with nylon webbing.

Leash and Long Line

The best training leashes are made of harness leather with a brass bolt-swivel snap braided into the end of the leash. However, a well-stitched nylon or cotton-web leash is also acceptable, especially for puppy training. For most purposes, the leash should be about 6 feet long with a weight and width determined by the training needs, the collar, and the size of the dog. A light leash is preferred for use with a halter. The long line is a 30- to 50-foot length of cotton webbing fitted with a bolt-swivel snap or a one-quarter to five-sixteenth-inch braided white nylon rope that is tied off with a limited-slip collar and knotted handle (Figure 1.8). The white rope long line is preferred for visibility and stretch, whereas the primary advantage of cotton webbing is the absence of stretch when it is pulled taut. The long line requires careful and attentive handling if one is to avoid severe friction burns and other potential injuries resulting from the abrupt force generated by it. Long-line training should be performed in well-controlled surroundings without playing children or dogs nearby, and all observers in the situation should be

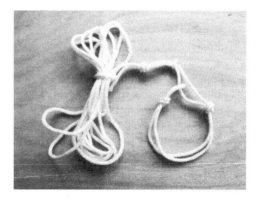

FIG. 1.8. Long-line with limited-slip collar tied with a series of overhand knots.

warned of the potential risks and dangers associated with long-line training. Observers are instructed to stay out of way and how to remain on the outside of the line. The trainer should always wear pants and appropriate shoes when working a dog on a long line. Grabbing a long line with bare hands is risky and should be generally avoided. Instead of grabbing it, the trainer should tamp or stamp on the long line to control the dog. If the long line must be handled with the hands, light leather gloves can be used to prevent friction burns. Gloves are generally a mixed blessing, however, since the safety afforded by them is achieved at the cost of losing a sensitive feel for the line. Also, the added security of gloves may cause inexperienced trainers to use the long line without proper respect, perhaps increasing the risk of other more serious injuries (e.g., fingers getting caught and broken). When holding the long line, it should be kept organized in neat folds and carefully managed to prevent it from becoming wrapped around the dog's feet, legs, or body. The long line is carefully folded at the end of training sessions. Before using the long line to control highly motivated behavior, the trainer should first become skillful with it in less demanding situations (e.g., playing ball) and acquire an appreciation for its safe use. Temporary overhand loops can be tied at various points along the line to hook into with the leash, thereby providing the trainer with a secure source of backup control if it is not possible to step on the line.

Hip-hitch

A useful tool for controlling pulling excesses is the hip-hitch and control lead. The simplest hip-hitch method consists of tying a 12- to 20-inch loop in the leash and hooking it to a carabiner held in place at the left hip by a belt. The remaining leash and handle, referred to as the control lead, is used to guide and fine tune control. The hip-hitch requires skill, coordination, and careful attention to various precautions, especially when working with large dogs (see *Controlled-leash Walking and Hip-hitch*).

Miscellaneous Items

Other items of equipment include a carpenter's apron or small treat pouch, a tennis ball with a handle, and treats (Figure 1.9). The most effective commercial dog treats are usually moist and possess a strong odor. Microwaved turkey or chicken hot dogs can make an attractive food reward. The treats are prepared by finely cutting a hot dog into pennywide slices. The pieces are spread out evenly on a paper towel or plate and cooked in a microwave for 2 to 3 minutes or until leathery to touch but not dry. Hot-dog treats are used in small pieces torn from the microwaved slices. Each slice can produce between 3 to 10 rewards, depending on the size of the dog. Chicken or turkey lunchmeat can be partially dried in the microwave and used in a similar way. Small biscuits, cheerios, cornflakes, popcorn, and so forth can be mixed in with hot-dog treats or be coated with the powder produced by microwaving hot dogs until they are dry and then crushing them. Another possibility is to mix some of the dog's kibble with a small amount of finely grated Romano or Parmesan cheese. Crated hard cheese can be sprinkled lightly on cheerios or similar treats and microwaved to give them additional value as food rewards. A tool of considerable usefulness in dog training is the shaker can, which

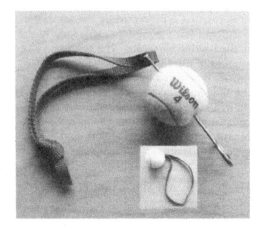

FIG. 1.9. Tennis balls used in training should be equipped with a handle.

is made from an aluminum soda can that has been rinsed and allowed to dry. Usually, two cans are made: one containing seven pennies and the other 30. Turning the finger tab around so that it covers the opening helps to block the pennies from falling out but without muffling the sound, as occurs when tape is used to close the can. Another disrupter-type device that can be very useful is the modified carbon-dioxide pump, which delivers a highly effective hissing sound for getting the dog's attention without producing pain or sensory discomfort. The modified carbon-dioxide pump can be used to deliver conditioned and unconditioned odors, giving it additional usefulness in a variety of applications.

BRIDGES, MARKERS, AND FLAGS

During the 1960s, Leon Whitney (1961 and 1963), a veterinarian, breeder, and pioneering dog trainer, first introduced clicker training to the dog-training community. The method of shaping instrumental behavior with a clicker, first described by Skinner (1951) and more recently popularized by Pryor (1985), uses the sound of a clicker that has been repeatedly paired with food to bridge successive approximations of some target behavior with a contingent, but not immediately available, food reward. Unfortunately, clicker training was largely overshadowed by other prevailing techniques that remained relatively dominant in the field until recently. Over the past decade, however, many applied dog behaviorists and trainers have rediscovered the value of the clicker and the technique of shaping. Of course, any distinctive sound (e.g., a click, squeak, or trill) can be used as a bridging signal. Although valuable and effective for purposes of conditioned reinforcement, clickers and other mechanical markers and bridging stimuli have two inherent practical drawbacks: (1) they can be unwieldy for the average dog owner to use, and (2) they are not always immediately at hand when needed. With instruction and practice, most owners can learn how to use a clicker effectively, but such devices should be not be used with the intent to replace conditioned vocal bridges

(e.g., "Good"). The squeaker and clicker are especially useful in situations requiring precisely timed conditioned reinforcement (e.g., attention training and shaping procedures) or repeated bridging (e.g., controlled-walking or heeling patterns). In addition, the clicker and squeaker can play a valuable role in the treatment of behavior problems. The clicker provides a discrete and salient stimulus that may help to obviate adverse emotional cues projected unawares in vocal signals. In the case of fearful dogs that are startled by the sharp click sound, a recording of the clicker can be made and delivered with an inexpensive digital recorder (Figure 1.10). The reduced volume of the recorded click sound is less likely to produce a startle response. A major advantage of the clicker and other mechanical bridge signals is that their effect can be conditioned and easily transferred from one person to another without losing potency.

The relative neutrality and clarity of the hiss, beep, click, or squeak can be highly effective for diverting the dog's attention or bridging orienting and attending behavior with reinforcement. Squeakers possess an added potential use obtained by putting an odor inside of them and dispensing it with or without the squeak sound. When dispensed at close quarters (e.g., as the dog sniffs the hand), the odor is released a split second before the squeak sound is generated. The

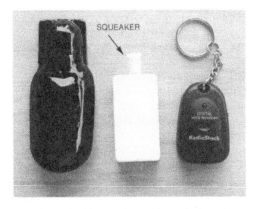

FIG. 1.10. Different clickers that produce varying levels of sound. The box clicker is equipped with a squeaker element that can be used in combination with the clicker during attention training.

odor can be deliberately arranged to precede the squeak by gently "pulsing" the squeaker bulb, so that the odor is dispensed but without the squeaker sound. Pulsing gives the odor time to reach the dog before the squeaker sound is produced, together with the delivery of a stronger odor stimulus as the squeaker bulb is more firmly squeezed. As the result of repeated pairings of the odor or the odor-squeak combination with food, taction, and other sources of reward, the odor and squeak gradually acquire unique conditioned properties that can be used in a variety of creative ways to modulate reactive thresholds and control attention. In addition to producing a distinctive sound, the squeak, unlike the click, can be varied in various ways, depending on the pattern of squeaking sounds produced or the force used to deliver them, thereby preventing habituation and enhancing its ability to grab the dog's attention. Gently pressing a small amount of air out produces a weak squeak sound, whereas forcefully pressing a full bulb of air through the squeaker valve produces a much louder and more impressive sound. In many cases, the squeaker has already undergone significant conditioning as an auditory stimulus in the context of playing with squeaker toys. Finally, the squeak sound is rapidly conditioned as a bridge or orienting signal, suggesting the possibility that it may be biologically prepared for forming associations with appetitive (seeking) or social activity. Small animals in distress often squeak in a similar way, perhaps helping to explain the apparent preferential and rapid association that can be made between the sound of the squeaker, conditioned odor, and food. Similarly, the squeaker and smooch sound (a powerful orienting stimulus) may be innately attractive and reinforcing. Ryon (1977), for example, found that a captive wolf mother called her 3-week-old pups out of the den interior to its entrance by squeaking.

Normally, dogs are first taught vocal bridging signals (e.g., "Good," "Yes," "That's it," and "Wow"), reward-delay or nonreward markers (e.g., "No," "Phooey," "Wrong," "Eh, eh," "Ack," and "Nah"), and flags (various hand and bodily movements used to momentarily direct a dog's behavior), with the goal of improving the owner's vocal control and other communication efforts. Unlike mechanical bridges or markers, voice and hand signals are charged with human emotional expressiveness—content and meaning that provide significant and valuable secondary bonding and socialization effects. Expressive affectionate talk and gestures help the trainer to transact and connect with the dog via an emotionally activated conduit of empathetic appreciation. The mélange of gross and subtle emotional expressions associated with human approval and disappointment, together with variations of touch (ranging from the gentle stroke to the abrupt shove), all contribute to a dog's fullest socialization and development as a companion. In sum, socially significant and emotionally charged consequences facilitate a profound level of mutual awareness, exchange, and bonding between people and dogs. Optimal training incorporates the broadest possible spectrum of motivational incentives and behavioral potentials of a dog.

Mechanical reinforcers and training techniques tend to promote a push-button attitude toward a dog's behavior and its modification. Although mechanistic precision and efficiency are valuable for attaining certain practical training objectives, excessively technical means may inadvertently interfere with the bond-enhancing goals of cynopraxic training. Both the clicker and other precise mechanical means (e.g., the remote electronic collar) are powerful and effective tools with which to control dog behavior. The effectiveness of these devices has caused them to become increasingly popular among trainers and the dog-owning public, with one company marketing a product that incorporates both a click feature for delivering conditioned reinforcement and an electrical stimulus for delivering negative reinforcement and punishment. With regard to the goals of cynopraxic training, the mixture of expressive voice, gesture, touch, and play are preferred to mechanical bridging stimuli or remote stimulation that target a narrow range of motivational systems. However, the clicker's simplicity and clarity provide a significant advantage for some training activities, such as walking a dog on a slack leash, shaping attention and orienting behavior, and recall—all can benefit from the immediacy and consistency of mechanical bridging stimuli.

THE TRAINING SESSION

A training session usually consists of a series of repeated trials that are performed with some goal or training objective in mind. Training trials consist of antecedent and consequent events or conditions that are arranged by the trainer to enhance predictive control over a target segment (module) or sequence (routine) of dog behavior. Trials are separated by intertrial periods, usually consisting of less controlled and more natural modal activity and interaction between the trainer and the dog. Many trials are initiated by calling for the dog's attention, whereas releasing the dog with an "OK" and clap often marks the beginning of intertrial periods. Within the context of a training session, trials and intertrial periods are organized into lessons and goal-oriented projects. The practice of modules and routines in conformity with the goals of the project is referred to as an exercise. Projects give structure and purpose to the training session and help to integrate and pattern modules and routines around active and passive modal strategies. Within the context of the training session, special modal outcomes (play and time-out) are arranged to mediate modal integration via sustained surprise and elation (active modal strategy) and disappointment and de-arousal (passive modal strategy). Training sessions organize trials, lessons and exercises (modules and routines), and projects in accordance with the objectives of the training program (e.g., solving a behavior problem). Training activities and procedures are typically introduced and broken down into a series of discrete steps, exercises, and projects (training plan) that are practiced by the owner between sessions. Finally, training activities are performed in accordance with cynopraxic goals and vision.

The steps making up the training plan are organized so that preliminary work prepares the way for the dog to learn what follows next more easily and efficiently, moving from simple modules to progressively more complex routines and skills. Ideally, the training process should proceed with minimal error

and tension, becoming a source of fun and mutual reward for both the trainer and the dog. In addition to vocal affection, petting, and food rewards, play activities of various kinds are used to activate control incentives and to reward trained behavior. A brief period of ball play is often used to initiate practice sessions. The ball is also presented periodically during the session as a surprise to enhance interest and to associatively link the trained modules and routines with play. Tug and ball play should also conclude the session to further associate trained behaviors with play, thereby gradually integrating trained behavior with modal play. The session period varies according to the dog, its age, the lesson, and other considerations (e.g., health and temperament). Puppies can benefit from very brief sessions consisting of as little 3 to 8 minutes, but can happily perform and enjoy much longer sessions, provided that the process is reward dense, affectionate, and playful. The average training session for an adult dog is around 20 minutes, including 5 to 10 minutes dedicated to play and agility activities, such as jumping over poles, hoops, and hurdles, and running through weave poles. Longer or briefer sessions are also used depending on training objectives. Training sessions can be scheduled two or three times a day. In addition to training activities performed in the context of structured sessions, a strong emphasis is placed on integrating training activities into everyday activities via ICT.

PLAY TRAINING

Basic training constrains and focuses natural learning capacities and incentives to obtain behavioral objectives that are often unnatural and occasionally unpleasant or annoying for a dog to perform. Some learning occurs rapidly, and may even be fun for the dog, because it takes advantage of innately prepared associations and drives. Behaviors occurring naturally in the process of play are most easily trained and brought under the control of ludic incentives. Teaching a dog to fetch a ball, for example, is highly prepared and easily learned by most dogs. For many dogs, the opportunity to play ball is hedonically far more valuable than getting a delicious food reward. Because such dogs love playing ball, the activity can be exchanged for the performance of other behaviors that a dog may not find as enjoyable; that is, ball play can be used as a potent incentive and source of reward. As a result, trained modules and routines can be gradually patterned into modal play activities—a procedure that is widely used in the training of working dogs, making necessary skills more enjoyable for them to learn and perform as the work becomes associatively integrated with play and its performance becomes its own incentive and source of enjoyment (see *Training and Play*).

Every dog should learn to play ball. Older dogs that have not been exposed to play at an early age may not show much interest in the activity, but many can be motivated with patient encouragement and playful stimulation. To increase interest, the trainer might tease the lackadaisical fetcher by repeatedly bouncing the ball against a wall, causing it to fly enticingly close to the reluctant player. Another useful method is to play keep away by kicking or flicking the ball just out of the dog's reach. If the dog happens to pick the toy up, it can be engaged in a gentle tug contest for possession. Interest in the ball can also be enhanced by playing "monkey in middle," keeping the ball just out of the dog's reach. At a point when the game reaches a sufficient pitch of excitement, the dog can be allowed to get the ball and keep it for a moment before being called to exchange it for a treat. Playing tug with the dog helps to improve ball drive and its willingness to chase and bring the ball back. Finally, ball drive can be enhanced by keeping the ball away from the dog at all times other than when it is used for play or training. The goal of ball play is to make the dog a fanatic about the ball! Often a few drops of a conditioned odor (e.g., lemon or orange) are put inside the ball to establish an association between the scent and the play activity. Such conditioned odors can be effectively used in the management of a variety of behavior problems.

Getting a dog to chase a ball is often more easy than getting it to bring it back. Many dogs welcome the opportunity to play keep away, especially if the owner is game and offers a chase. Keeping the dog on a long line

and giving it a treat in exchange for returning and releasing the ball helps to encourage good retrieving habits. Each time the dog returns with the ball, a food reward is offered to it, causing the dog to release the ball in order to obtain the treat. After a moment, the ball is tossed again, and the dog is encouraged to return with it by making smooch sounds, clapping, crouching down, and so forth. Training the dog to come to a closed hand for a variable food reward is a useful preliminary for dogs that habitually refuse to return with the ball. Eventually, the release of the ball is brought under the control of a release signal like "Out," spoken just before the dog releases the ball. Another way of improving the dog's willingness to return with the ball is to use a second one as a trade. The dog is required first to drop the one it has before the second one is thrown. The long line provides additional control by preventing the dog from running off with the object or refusing to come back with it.

With a foundation of ball play and retrieve in place, an improved willingness to come when called can be developed. In fact, there is no better time to introduce recall training than during ball play. After sending the dog to retrieve the ball, but just before it turns to bring the ball back, the trainer says the dog's name and waits until it turns fully around before saying "Come" in a crisp and playful tone of voice. The command is followed by encouraging praise and clapping, crouching down, or running backward in the case of hesitant dogs to encourage them to come more enthusiastically. The dog soon learns that the command "Come" is linked with a treat and the opportunity for more play. Besides learning to come on command, the dog can also be taught to wait briefly before the ball is tossed again. This is accomplished by saying "Wait" prior to each throw while having the dog focus on the ball, thereby enhancing attention and impulse control under the strong motivation of play. The act of waiting is reinforced by the whole chain of events: the opportunity to chase, fetch, and drop the ball into the trainer's hand—all eventually leading to the acquisition of food and the opportunity to play again.

PART 3: TRAINING PROJECTS AND EXERCISES

INTRODUCTORY LESSONS

The introductory lessons are largely the same for both puppies and adult dogs. The goal of these early lessons is to establish a foundation of attention and impulse control within the context of reward-based training.

Bridge Conditioning

Conditioned reinforcers serve to bridge the occurrence of some target behavior with the delayed delivery of unconditioned reinforcers (see *Shaping: Training Through Successive Approximations* in Volume 1, Chapter 7). Consequently, conditioned reinforcers are often referred to as bridges or bridging stimuli. Bridge conditioning is usually carried out under relatively distraction-free conditions in the house or yard. A variety of soft and hard treats are prepared and placed in small hip pack or belt pouch, and the web handle of the ball is passed under the belt, making it easy to access. Both food pouch and ball should be kept on the trainer's right side. The dog should be slightly hungry and rested at the start of training. Social and food deprivation is rarely necessary to heighten the appetite of a healthy and emotionally balanced dog to work for food and social rewards. The first step in the process of conditioning the bridging stimulus or bridge is to allow the dog to sample the food reward from the right hand. Food treats should be consistently given with the right hand. A tiny piece of the food reward is given to the dog first from the fingers and then from a closed hand as it approaches. A small bit of food can produce a surprisingly strong food incentive, probably as the result of the dopamine reward signal produced by the activation of an olfactory incentive system (see *Olfactory Incentive System and Prediction Error* in Chapter 10). Modal seeking activity associated with food is rapidly invigorated and is highly responsive to the activation effects of surprise. The sampling or priming process is repeated until the dog enthusiastically searches and follows the trainer, seeking the food reward. As the dog reaches the trainer, the vocal bridge "Good" is spoken in a clipped and high-pitched tone just before the food reward is delivered to the dog from the right hand. The food reward should be concealed in a closed hand, requiring that the dog touch it and briefly wait, whereupon the bridge "Good" is delivered just before the hand is opened. Gradually, the dog should be encouraged to follow the right hand actively as it is moved in various directions before the reward is delivered. The trainer should move around the training area and encourage the dog to follow; as it turns, the trainer crouches down and flicks the right hand out to the side, attracting the dog's attention and saying "Good" as soon as the dog touches it. Alternatively, a clicker can be sounded just as the dog turns toward the trainer, and followed by the vocal bridge just before the closed hand is opened. The process of pairing the bridging stimulus with food rewards is repeated until the dog shows a clear anticipatory response to the sound of the bridge.

As a standard expectancy is established, variations can be introduced to enhance bridge conditioning. For example, varying the duration between trials, so that some occur sooner than others, produces a surprise in relation to the expected timing of reward. Also, varying the length of time taken to open the hand containing the food reward can also provide a similar element of surprise. Periodically, instead of having the dog come to the hand, the food reward is tossed to it immediately after the bridge (click) is delivered. As previously discussed (see *Prediction and Control Expectancies*), significant surprise and additional bridge-conditioning benefits can be generated by varying the size, type, and frequency of the reward given to the dog. In addition to conditioning the bridge in the context of reinforcing following behavior, the association can be strengthened by using it to enhance an orienting response whereby the dog is prompted to turn its attention toward the trainer in response to a smooch or squeaker sound followed by a click or "Good." After orienting or coming to the trainer, it can be prompted to make eye contact (attending response), whereupon the bridge and food reward are delivered. Affectionate petting should be frequently given along with food rewards. Affectionate petting enhances the rewarding event as well as linking the affectionate activity with the bridge "Good."

Following and Coming

After each trial, the trainer steps back a step or two and encourages the dog to come along, guiding it to the left side with the right hand and causing it to turn about there, before stepping forward and encouraging the dog to follow along at the left side. Following behavior is bridged with the clicker, whereupon the closed hand containing a food reward is moved slowly over the dog's head, causing it to follow and sit. As the dog begins to sit, the bridge "Good" is delivered and followed by the food reward as the action is completed. Alternatively, after taking several steps forward, the trainer can call the dog's name and abruptly backpedal away from it, causing it to turn and follow along. Just as the dog turns, the trainer clicks and flicks the closed right hand off to the side. Just before the dog reaches the hand, the trainer says "Come" and then "Good" just before the hand is opened to reveal the reward. At the conclusion of this simple chain, the trainer says "OK," claps, and again guides the dog to the left side, steps away as before, and encourages the dog to follow along at the left side until the trainer once again stops and prompts the dog to sit or steps back calling the dog's name or smooching to encourage it to turn and come. As the dog turns, a click is delivered and, as the dog moves in the direction of trainer, the vocal signal "Come" is spoken in an enthusiastic command tone as the right hand is flicked to the side. As the dog reaches the hand, the bridge "Good" is spoken and the hand is opened. This pattern is repeated several times, establishing an associative link between coming and reward.

Orienting Response

Attention control is of great utility in dog training (see *Attention and Impulse Control*). Obviously, for a dog to be trained, it must pay attention to the trainer's actions. A dog's attention can be attracted by employing various unconditioned or conditioned diverters, evoking surprise and competing interest, e.g., throwing a ball or presenting a conditioned stimulus previously paired with food (e.g., a whistle). In addition, most dogs quickly orient toward unfamiliar or out-of-the-ordinary stimuli. By calling a dog's name just prior to presenting a potent diverter or disrupter, the name is gradually conditioned as a generalized orienting stimulus. As the dog learns to respond to its name by orienting its attention toward the trainer, its name can be used to interrupt distracted behavior and to serve as a preparatory cue for commands. For example, in the case of training a dog to come, its name is used to evoke an orienting response, followed by command cue "Come" and additional prompting and encouragement, as necessary. Since the distracting environment itself is rewarding, releasing the dog after it comes serves to further reinforce the habit of coming when called. Consequently, when the dog reaches the trainer, it is immediately rewarded and released with an "OK" and hand clap. As the result of repeatedly calling and releasing the dog after it comes, it gradually learns to expect that coming not only results in a food reward but also results in another opportunity to explore the environment.

A useful attention-controlling strategy is to pair a whistle or squeaker sound with treats, feeding times, and just prior to other strongly reinforcing events (e.g., access to special toys and announcing owner homecomings). Gradually, the dog learns that the squeaker announces a moment when a food reward is likely to be forthcoming. The whistle is not a recall signal, although it may be conditioned to function as one; rather, it is an establishing operation signifying an opportunity to obtain a variety of possible attractive outcomes if the dog simply orients and takes it. If the dog does not come, no matter; it has simply lost the opportunity to obtain the reward. Additional orienting control is established by bridging the orienting response with a clicker. The click is delivered just as the dog begins to orient to its name, a smooch, or a squeak. The click is followed by a flick of the hand to the right and the delivery of a variable reward conducive to surprise. For example, varying the size and type of the reward given to the dog can magnify the effect of this training.

Attending Response

Whereas orienting behavior is momentary and strongly affected by reflexive mechanisms, attending behavior occurs with some duration over time and is more directly controlled by instrumental contingencies of reinforcement. Teaching dogs to look up and hold eye contact is an important aspect of dog training and socialization. Making various nonsense sounds (e.g., clucking or lip noises of various kinds) helps to get a dog to look up into the eyes. The moment the dog makes eye contact, the response is bridged and reinforced with an affectionate smile, sweet talk, and a treat. The clicker can be used effectively to help shape attending behavior in dogs that resist making eye contact. Once eye contact is establish, the duration of the response can be gradually increased until the dog is holding it for a second or two. As the dog learns to look up and make eye contact in response to a smooch or cluck sound, its name can be paired with the orienting stimulus. Calling the dog to come and sit and look up briefly before rewarding and releasing it promotes a valuable pattern of control (Figure 1.11). In the case of highly distractible dogs, a squeaker-clicker combination can be useful for capturing and shaping the dog's attention. The squeaker device (extracted from a squeaker bulb) is inserted into a hole drilled into the clicker (see Figure 1.9). A wide range of sounds can be made with the squeaker, minimizing the effect of gradual habituation to the sound. As the dog turns, the clicker is pressed, thereby reinforcing the orienting response. This procedure is repeated under varying conditions of distraction until the dog is quickly orienting to the sound of the squeaker, at which point its name can be paired with the sound.

Targeting and Prompting

Most training activities make use of body or hand movements to prompt, lure, or target the dog's behavior. Training a dog to orient and follow the trainer's body and hand movements is an important aspect of basic training, providing a foundation for more complex and advanced control efforts. Training the dog to take food from the right hand and then requiring that it follow the hand as a contingency for getting the reward helps develop a targeting response to the hand. The dog is trained to target on the hand by holding the right hand at the dog's eye level so that it either looks at the hand (in the beginning) or actually touches it with its nose before the behavior is bridged and rewarded. As the dog learns to orient and follow the hand, the targeting behavior is shaped through successive approximations until it is a strong and reliable response. The attractiveness of the hand as a target can be enhanced by rapidly flapping the first two fingers like beating wings—a technique referred to as a birdie lure. Training the dog to target on the hand allows the trainer to guide or position it without needing to use physical prompts. Targeting provides a rapid means to facilitate the response as well as

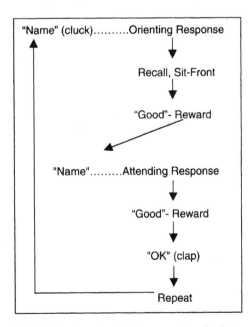

FIG. 1.11. Attention-training sequence: orienting response, recall, sit, attending response, and release.

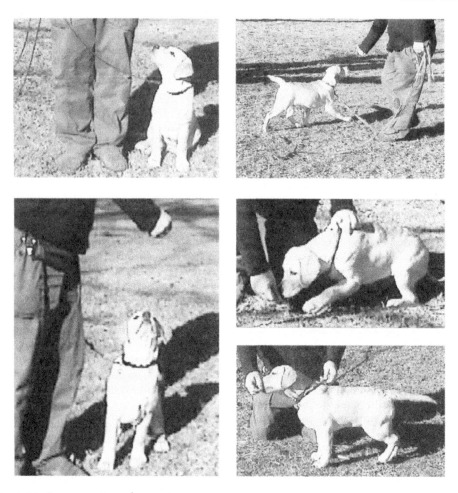

FIG. 1.12. Puppy targeting and prompting.

developing a hand signal to control it (Figure 1.12). Training the dog to reliably orient (turn toward the trainer on signal) and target on trainer's body movements and gestures is the most important objective of basic training.

As the dog's targeting behavior improves, hand and body movements can be used to guide and prompt it into various positions. For example, teaching a dog to sit is easily accomplished by moving the right hand slowly over the dog's head. As the dog follows the trajectory of the hand, there is a natural tendency for it to sit. If the dog jumps up at the hand instead of sitting, the hand can be repositioned to discourage jumping, or the trainer can simply step on the leash to prevent

the unwanted jumping behavior. The bridge "Good" is presented just as the dog begins to sit, with the food reward and affectionate petting delivered as the dog completes the action. At the conclusion of the trial, the dog is released with an "OK" and hand clap, guided to the left side, and walked out several steps before the trainer steps back and calls the dog to come again, whereupon it is prompted with the hand signal to sit and is appropriately rewarded. This pattern is repeated until it is performed fluently. Once the dog is sitting reliably in response to the prompting of the hand signal, the vocal signal "Sit" is paired with the action. After several pairings in which the word "Sit" is spoken just before the hand signal, the vocal signal alone will prompt the sit response. At this point, the hand signal can be progressively delayed or minimized, with the dog learning to respond to the vocal signal alone, gradually enabling the dog to sit in response to the vocal signal alone. If the dog fails to sit when the vocal signal is given, the signal should not be repeated; instead, the hand signal is used to prompt the action. A fairly reliable measure of a dog trainer's understanding of the process and skill can be calculated by the number of times she or he repeats vocal commands. Later on, while training the automatic sit, both vocal and hand signals are delayed or minimized, so that the dog learns to sit without aid whenever the trainer comes to a stop while the dog is heeling or at other times requiring that it sit automatically (e.g., sit-front and starting exercise). Generally, for routine training purposes, it is better to continue giving the dog a combined vocal and hand signal, since the latter helps to progressively strengthen the dog's responsiveness to the former. After rewarding the sit response, the dog is required to wait to be released with an "OK" and hand clap. If, at any point in the process, the dog appears confused or quits, the trainer should go back to the hand signal or review a previously successful step (e.g., "Come" or "Good" conditioning, attention training, and targeting on the hand) and begin again.

As the dog is guided around to left side at the conclusion of the come exercise, it can be prompted to sit at the trainer's left side and be rewarded. After a brief moment, the trainer steps off and encourages the dog to follow along with the vocal signal "Come one," sweet talk, smooches, or slaps on the leg. As the dog orients toward the left side and continues there for a few steps, the trainer stops and prompts it to sit. If the dog runs out ahead, the trainer should turn into an opposite direction while making smooches, slapping the left thigh, or crouching down to encourage it to follow along in the new direction. As soon as the dog responds, the bridge and reward follow. If the dog moves off to the left, the trainer turns to the right and encourages the dog to follow along. If the dog lags

behind, the trainer picks up the pace with gentle encouragement, perhaps bouncing a ball, making smooch sounds, or crouching down momentarily. Whenever the dog comes close to the trainer's side, the bridge and treat are delivered. After a change of pace, a turn, the dog's close walking is bridged (e.g., click) and it is prompted to sit at the trainer's left side, rewarded, and the sequence is repeated. With every successful walk-sit sequence, appropriate bridging and rewards follow. While training the dog to come along and walk close by, the trainer can mix in come and sit-front training as together with orienting and attending sequences.

Most dogs can rapidly learn to lie down from the sit. The task is usually introduced with the trainer crouching down or sitting on the floor and luring the dog down with the right hand. In some cases, the behavior may need to be shaped through successive approximations, starting with a downward bobbing movement of the dog's head, a reaching movement toward the floor and, finally, lying down. As the dog learns to follow the hand into the down, the vocal signal "Down" is paired with the hand signal. The dog should also learn to sit from the down and stand from the sit. Using a hand-targeting strategy helps the dog to learn both of these movements easily. If the dog ignores the hand, the birdie lure can be used to attract its attention. Once the dog is lying down, the trainer moves the right hand upward in front of the dog's nose, causing it to follow the movement. Similarly, the dog can be prompted in the stand position by putting the right hand in front of the dog's nose and drawing it away, thereby causing it to stand. This basic cycle of exercises (sit, down, stand, and sit) can be performed with a toy as a lure and using an opportunities to tug and fetch as a reward. As the dog masters each movement, an appropriate vocal command is paired with the hand signal. In the case of resistant dogs, a food lure (usually a small biscuit) is used to break the ice. Luring with food can be very problematic, however, and should only be used to get a response that is not likely to happen in a timely way otherwise. After two or three luring trials, the biscuit should be hidden in a closed hand and finally faded completely out.

Excessive reliance on food baiting and luring tends to produce "chow hounds," that is, dogs that will only work with the direct promise of a food reward in sight.

Stay Training

Once the dog is readily orienting, coming, sitting, and looking up on signal, the sit-stay exercise is introduced (see Appendix A). Many aspects of the stay module have already received preliminary training. For example, after coming and sitting, the dog has been required to wait a moment, steady its attention, and make eye contact as a contingency of reinforcement and release. Once these preliminaries are under control, it is an easy and natural step to train the dog to stay for longer periods and at greater distances from the trainer. The first criterion is to have the dog hold a sit-stay for a progressively longer and then variable duration before the behavior is reinforced. The variable duration of the stay response provides an interesting source of prediction error (surprise) with which to strengthen waiting and attending behavior. Releasing the dog sooner than expected relative to a standard expectancy provides a surprise and reward that can be used to steady attending behavior, especially if the dog is prompted to make eye contact in advance of being released. Similarly, vary the amount of time that the dog waits before being let outdoors, to come up on furniture, to receive a favorite toy, to be permitted to jump up, and so forth can help to strengthen waiting strategies and improve delay of gratification. The next criterion is staying as the trainer steps away a step or two. As the trainer steps back, a stay flag is presented, which is formed by extending the right arm in front of the body at chest level, with the right hand held out. The fingers should be held together and pointed up, with the palm facing the dog.

Initially, the dog is required to hold the sit-stay position for a brief period before it is rewarded. The best stay performances are built up carefully and slowly in the context of attention training. Ideally, the dog should maintain eye contact with the trainer as he or she steps back and again as the trainer

returns to the dog. The dog should also maintain steady eye contact just before being released. The release should be treated as a trained response that is brought under the control of play activities (e.g., tug and ball play). During the early phases of stay training, it is important that the trainer return to the dog instead of calling the dog to come at the conclusion of the sit-stay period. If the dog happens to break the stay position, it is lured or guided back by leash to the original spot and prompted to sit. Breaking the stay during early stages of training should be treated as a mistake of judgment on the trainer's part rather than an act of obstinacy on the part of the dog. When the dog breaks the position, it is best to simply try again at an earlier and more successful step. With every successful stay performance, the dog is rewarded (food, petting, praise) and released momentarily between trials, often engaged in play. Ideally, the process should proceed with a minimum of errors, but, in practice, learning from mistakes can also be very beneficial, so long as it does not result in excessive anxiety or frustration. The goal of sit-stay training is to enhance impulse control, not by anxious inhibition, but rather by training the dog to focus and relax. Patience in the process of training the dog to sit and stay is rewarded later on.

The most common problems encountered during the early stages of stay training involve impulsive behaviors associated with distractions. These motivations can be turned to the trainer's advantage by making access to them contingent on the dog waiting or staying first. An affirmative way to view distractions is to consider them as potential rewards not yet under the trainer's control. In the case of some highly excitable dogs, training efforts may be impeded by such distractions. Normally, distraction-dense environments are avoided until a dog's attention and impulse-control abilities are adequately prepared to meet the challenge.

Play and Controlled Walking

The controlled-walking pattern is shaped through successful approximations. The easiest way to introduce the walking behavior is through play. The first step is to encourage the dog to chase and retrieve a stick or ball. As the dog becomes excited about the toy, it is held in the right hand and used to guide the dog around to the left side. If the dog goes too far out in front, the trainer turns about while making smooch sounds and tapping a stick to the ground and encouraging the dog to follow along. When the dog returns to the trainer's side, the stick is tossed for the dog to retrieve and to come back for a tug and treat in exchange for releasing it. After a brief tug, the dog is prompted to release the stick and is lured as before to the starting position at the trainer's left side. The stick is held diagonally in front of the trainer, just out of reach of the dog, and the trainer steps off on the left leg, whereupon the stick is tapped against the front surface of the thigh, accompanied with clucking or smooching sounds to attract the dog's attention. With the dog walking close on the left side, the bridge "Good" is delivered, and the trainer comes to a stop and prompts the dog to sit by waving the stick in an upward direction over the dog's head, causing it to sit. As the dog sits, it is praised, treated, and given another opportunity to fetch the stick. Instead of using a stick, a tennis ball with handle can be used in a similar way. Gradually, the dog is required to hold the sit for longer durations before the stick is thrown. For some insecure dogs, a food lure or licking stick (e.g., a yardstick with peanut butter or crème cheese smeared on it) can be a helpful means to introduce the concept of walking close at the left side. The food lure or licking stick is held a few inches in front of the dog, allowing the dog to lick occasionally while walking or after being prompted to sit.

Clicking and Controlled Walking

Another very effective way to introduce attentive controlled walking is by using a clicker. While walking the dog on a leash, a click is delivered so long as it remains on the trainer's left and walks close by without pulling. With each click, the trainer stops

and prompts the dog to sit, whereupon the trainer says "Good" and the treat is delivered. Initially, the click-and-treat procedure is repeated every few steps, but gradually the dog should be required to walk without pulling for longer periods before delivering the bridge and reward. If the dog pulls, its name is called as the slack of the leash is let go; alternatively, a squeaker is sounded to get the dog's attention and cause it to turn around. Just as the dog turns in response to its name or squeaker, the click is delivered and the dog encouraged to return to the trainer's left side, whereupon it is prompted to sit and is given a treat. The combination clicker-squeaker is convenient for such training. Under distracting conditions, repeated and sustained reinforcers involving several small pieces of food, petting and massage, play, and vocal encouragement may be helpful to keep dogs focused and on track.

On-leash and Off-leash Practice

It is important that trainers practice the above tasks with puppies or dogs both on and off leash. Although an experienced trainer can carry out initial training efforts effectively with a dog off leash, it is usually best to work the puppy or dog on leash or long line and then gradually introduce off-leash elements as the various necessary skills are mastered. Backup leash control is particularly important in the case of dogs and puppies receiving training to curb social excesses and impulsive household behavior. Although beneficial in the early stages of training, overreliance on the leash control may cause both the trainer and dog to become dependent on it, thereby making it much more difficult to fade it out later. Reducing dependency on the leash requires that the trainer master skills needed to control a dog with vocal signals and gestural prompts alone. Also, during training periods when the leash is off, the trainer gets a more accurate picture of what the dog actually knows as the result of training. Control is meaningful only to the extent that it can be exercised both on and off leash. When the dog is worked off leash, mental notes should be kept about areas of training that may require additional work on leash.

WALKING ON LEASH

A dog's excessive pulling and lunging while on leash is perhaps the most common reason for owners to seek training help. While a confident and well-trained dog is an object of owner pride and affection, an impulsive and rambunctious one can rapidly become a source of tremendous frustration and public embarrassment for the owner (Sanders, 1999). In some cases, the owner is physically unable to walk the dog because of excessive pulling and various misbehaviors that occur while on leash, further complicating matters by giving rise to deficiencies associated with inadequate exercise and outdoor stimulation. Consequently, such dogs may become progressively difficult to handle and manage, setting the stage for the development or exacerbation of behavior problems associated with excessive activity and impulsiveness. Training dogs to walk properly on leash is vital, not only to develop and augment attention and impulse control, but to strengthen the leader-follower bond, as well. The dog that walks in close cooperation with the trainer's pace and direction takes each step and turns in acceptance and deference to that person's role as leader. Training the dog to walk properly and skillfully on leash provides a foundation for a more positive and mutually rewarding experience for both the person and the dog.

Even though pulling into a leash results in physical discomfort for a dog, forcefully holding the dog back appears to increase rather than reduce the magnitude of its pulling efforts. Pavlov (1927/1960) postulated a *freedom reflex* to help explain the dog's oppositional response to restraint. Reflexive opposition to restraint has biological significance, since, as Pavlov points out, "it is clear that if the animal were not provided with a reflex of protest against boundaries set to its freedom, the smallest obstacle in its path would interfere with the proper fulfillment of its natural functions" (12). A related phenomenon, thigmotaxis (Gk, *thigma* or touch), refers to reflexive adjustments associated with taction, but should be distinguished from Pavlov's

oppositional freedom reflex. Thigmotactic adjustments are divided into two categories, depending on whether a dog moves toward contact (positive thigmotaxis) or moves away from contact (negative thigmotaxis). Common examples of positive thigmotaxis include the rooting reflex or the tendency of fearful dogs to lean on the owner's body as a source of security. Physical opposition may also excite positive thigmotaxis, but since the dog's efforts at such times appear primarily intended to oppose the physical control, it may be more appropriate to refer to such behavior as an opposition reflex rather than thigmotaxis. Perhaps the concepts of positive and negative thigmotaxis should be reserved for describing contact behavior occurring at times when seeking comfort or safety rather than frustrated behavior associated with physical force or barriers.

When confronted with physical forces and obstacles that thwart their freedom of movement, a dog reflexively responds with commensurate oppositional behavior aimed at countering their effects. For example, the harder the owner pulls back on the leash, the more the dog will tend to pull forward (forge) against it. Similarly, if the dog is pulled forward, the dog will tend to compensate by pulling back (balk), as opposition reflexes are elicited. The motivational effect of opposition is frustration. The typical behavioral response to frustration is potentiation and persistence of oppositional behavior. The amount of oppositional effort expended by the dog depends on a number of factors, but especially upon the value of attractive incentives toward which the pulling action is directed. The primary goals of the activity appear to be the optimization of drive-activating stimulation and control of the direction and pace of the walk. Few dogs find pulling into the leash sufficiently aversive to stop doing so, even in cases where their breathing and circulation are affected by the activity or where obvious discomfort is involved.

Although holding the dog back briefly is not harmful, passively holding the dog back by a dead leash for extended periods to break its will to pull (freedom reflex) is a highly questionable practice. The theory promulgated by proponents of the method is that the dog will eventually cave in and defer to passive restraint, but actually such stimulation often evokes a persistent oppositional reflex causing the dog to continue pulling despite significant discomfort and physiological distress. Instead of discouraging pulling, such restraint often does little more than increase frustration and oppositional behavior. The procedure has become increasingly popular as a means to discourage pulling, partly because of its simple theory and application—any ambulatory person with a strong back and arms can stand like a post and hold a dog back and thwart its oppositional pulling efforts. For such methods to have a chance of success, they require a great deal of consistency and perseverance. Unfortunately, however, ordinary dog owners are often woefully deficient on both scores and will frequently ignore pulling efforts rather than consistently perform the rather tedious ritual of waiting until the dog stops pulling before taking a step forward. As a result, the pulling behavior may never get better, but instead may grow significantly worse as the result of frustration-related enhancement and intermittent negative reinforcement. Finally, given the availability of effective leash-training alternatives that work quickly and reliably to discourage pulling, letting a dog pull on leash until its will to pull is broken (i.e., the opposition reflex is fatigued) or until it becomes exhausted makes little sense. In cases where an owner is unable or unwilling to assert appropriate leash control, a halter can be introduced to passively control pulling excesses.

Not only are such leash-breaking methods questionable with respect to efficacy, they risk producing significant harm if performed on dogs that persistently pull while being exercised. Pulling continuously on a leash can impede efficient ventilation and blood circulation, thereby hampering the dog's ability to circulate and cool arterial blood before it enters the brain. While a dog is walking or running, arterial blood rapidly heats up and needs to be cooled to prevent brain damage associated with thermal stress. Blood entering the brain is cooled by passive thermal exchange between arterial and venous vessels, whereby heated arterial blood is cooled by venous blood draining from the nose and mouth of the dog (Baker and Chapman, 1977). As the result of holding a dog back by a collar around its throat, both ventilation and venous blood flow are variably obstructed, depending on the force of pulling and the sort of collar used to restrain the dog. Venous blood flow is more easily obstructed by external pressure on the neck than is arterial flow, which passes through the neck under pressure and is partially protected by the spine (vertebral artery). The net result is that heated arterial blood continues to pump into the brain while decreased ventilation and obstructed venous blood flow hamper its efficient cooling—a physiological condition capable of producing significant harm or discomfort to dogs laboring under adverse weather or exercise conditions. Intentionally allowing impulsive or oppositional dogs to pull into a dead leash is tantamount to *horizontal hanging*—a procedure that is difficult to justify as a humane means to stop or control excessive pulling by dogs.

Most dogs exhibit intense preparatory arousal whenever the owner gets the leash to take the dog for a walk. In the case of a pulling dog, the appearance of the leash functions as an establishing operation, motivationally preparing the dog to pull and to obtain reinforcement as the result of such behavior.

Dogs that engage in excessive pulling are often inordinately attracted to environmental stimuli and engage in excessive exploratory and stimulation-seeking activities. In addition, such dogs are often hyperactive and may exhibit marked impulse-control and attention-related deficits that require training efforts designed to enhance attentional focus and executive restraint. Various diverter-type and disrupter-type stimuli are employed to interrupt pulling and to refocus a dog's attention. A squeaker-clicker combination can be used to get and then reinforce attention and orientation toward the trainer. Giving such dogs an opportunity to engage in vigorous ball play before going for a walk can help to reduce pent-up energy fueling excessive pulling behavior. Moving from the play situation to a long line and then to a short leash appears to make the transition easier for many dogs because it helps to reduce oppositional reactivity and impulsive behavior when on leash.

Leash Handling

There is a certain amount of truth to the adage "Master the leash, master the dog." Before describing the basic techniques of leash training, leash-handling lore and methods need to be reviewed briefly. There are many ways to hold and handle a leash. One of the best methods for routine training purposes is first to place the thumb through the leash loop and then close the hand around it, forming a fist (Figure 1.14A). A more secure control is obtained by passing the hand through the loop and bringing the leash over the top before gripping and setting the trigger (Figure 1.13). Next, in order to take up and grip the slack of the leash, the first two fingers are extended, with the third and fourth fingers flexed firmly on the leash handle (the *grip*). The shape of the hand at this point looks like the Scout salute. A variable length of the leash

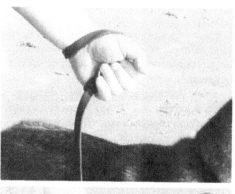

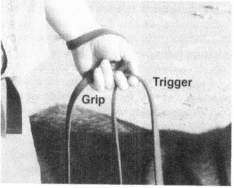

FIG. 1.13. Secure leash control.

is taken up into a single fold and held between the thumb and the index finger (the *trigger*) (Figure 1.14F and G). When walking a dog on a slack leash, the leash is held in the left hand. When practicing or performing formal exercises, however, the leash is dressed in the right hand. The leash is dressed with the dog in the starting position, and both arms are fully extended and relaxed. The *standing end* and slack of the leash is held in the right hand while the *working end* runs slackly down and across the trainer's left leg to the dog sitting at heel (Figure 1.14G).

In addition to holding and dressing a leash, trainers should be familiar with three leash manipulations: breaking, opening the leash, and changing leash hands. Breaking prevents the leash from slipping through the fingers. Many styles of leash braking are used in dog training. The most common brake is set by taking the working end of the leash with the left hand and wrapping it over the left thumb and then firmly closing the hand over the leash (Figure 1.14D). Thumb brakes are particularly useful when working with large breeds or when using nylon leashes that tend to slip through the hands. The leash is opened by taking up the working end with the left hand and setting a thumb brake before realeasing the slack held in the right hand. As the brake is applied, the left hand draws the leash open, thus freeing the right hand (leash still hung from the right thumb) to present hand signals or treats (Figure 1.14D). Besides opening the leash, trainers should know how to change leash hands properly. There are two basic ways to change leash hands. When passing the leash between hands, both its working and standing ends are gripped together just beneath the handle (Figure 1.14E). As the right hand lets go, it leaves a glovelike shape impressed into the leash fold and handle. The leash is dressed again by regripping the handle and the fold of slack as previously described. Another method for changing leash hands involves moving the thumb upward and causing the leash handle to shift up (Figure 1.14A–C). Now, the opposite thumb can hook the handle and take up the standing slack in a single fold. When the dog is located in front of the trainer or at some distance away, the leash is exchanged in a similar way between hands by the thumbs, and the standing slack is taken up as needed. The leash

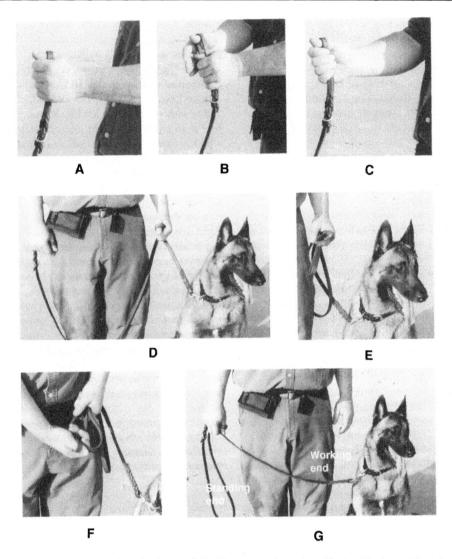

FIG. 1.14. Leash handling: basic leash control (**A–C**), opening the leash and brake (**D**), changed leash hands (**E**), setting the trigger (**F**), and dressed training (starting position) (**G**).

should never tangle to the ground—it should always have a presence of control but never be taut. Leashes should never be knotted, except as needed to form temporary looping for hip-hitching or coupling techniques in which two leashes are tied together to control a brace of dogs.

Leash-training Techniques

Choosing the appropriate method for a dog's needs is of tremendous importance. Some dogs may require very little in the way of directive or physical prompting, whereas others will require more forceful handling strategies. Four techniques are generally used, depending on a dog's needs:

1. Long-line training involves the use of reward-based attention-control techniques and avoidance cues ("Easy" and "Stay") together with stepping or tamping on a long line dragging on the ground.

2. Slack-leash training involves using an abrupt release of leash slack to simultaneously capture the dog's wavering attention and

deter future pulling with appropriate anchor and opposing thrust movements.

3. Hip-hitch training is based on a response-blocking strategy in which forward movement is interrupted by stopping, back-stepping, and otherwise preventing the dog from moving forward until it stops pulling and momentarily turns its attention to the trainer.

4. Halter training prevents pulling by using a halter-type collar and stresses positive reinforcement to shape attention and walking without pulling.

Working the dog outdoors among distractions is a major transition that often requires the addition of directive methods of control. The preliminary work done indoors and in the backyard has taught the dog what is expected of it through a reward-based training system, but knowing what to do and possessing a reliable ability to do it are two very different things. Although the dog may know how to sit or lie down and stay on signal, it may not be willing to perform the tasks as obedient acts on command, especially in situations where it would prefer to do something else. In such cases, it may be necessary at times to constrain the dog to perform the required behavior by means of directive prompting. Most importantly, however, as noted earlier, the social limit around pulling on the leash is of vital importance. The leash represents a physical extension of human will, which when properly introduced and used provides a dog with a valuable source of guidance and instruction. As such, the dog must first learn to defer to the leash and actively follow its directive movements and prompts without hesitating or resisting. A central goal of slack-leash training is to condition a dog's attention to respond to the leash so that it actively follows its guidance, thereby facilitating reward-based training efforts while minimizing exposure to leash corrections.

There are three ways that a dog is walked when outdoors, depending on the control needed at the time: slack leash, controlled walk, and heeling. Slack-leash training only entails that the dog not pull while on leash. During slack-leash walks, the dog is permitted every *reasonable* liberty, such as sniffing about,

moving from one side to the other, lagging behind, or forging ahead. The only liberty forbidden to the dog is pulling or lunging into the leash. Controlled walking adds the criterion of walking at the left side without forging beyond the point where the dog's hip aligns with the trainer's left leg. Walking at heel is an entirely different matter. Heeling is a highly structured and formal activity requiring that the dog walk in a precisely defined position at the owner's left side without sniffing or moving about. Heeling is a demanding activity requiring that the dog focus its attention on the trainer's every movement. Although restrictive and highly formal, walking at heel should not appear overly constraining or mechanical. Instead, an appearance of elegant harmony between the owner and dog should cause observers to reflect on its meditative qualities. In fact, good heeling is a meditation, bringing both dog and trainer into an attentional nexus of single-mindedness on the moment. This sort of effort requires tremendous concentration and can been done only for short periods in the beginning, with the dog heeling for longer stretches of time as its ability to focus improves with maturity and training. On an average walk, the dog should only be brought to heel periodically and released, with 90% of the walk enjoyed at ease but without pulling.

Long-line Training

Highly active dogs can be first exposed to leash control on a long line. A 30- to 50-foot length of quarter-inch braided white nylon rope is fitted with a knotted hand loop and a limited-slip collar (Figure 1.8). Alternatively, the long line (soft nylon webbing) can be fitted with a knotted fixed-action halter. The long line can be either held in hand or allowed to run freely on the ground. The long line is controlled both by tamping or stamping actions (foot braking) to limit pulling behavior and to gather and focus the dog's attention. Whenever the dog rushes beyond 10 to 15 feet away and ignores other established orienting and attention-controlling signals, the long line is tamped or stepped on and the dog prompted to return to the trainer, required to wait briefly, and released again. In addition to a free-running procedure in which the long line is let to drag on the ground, a hip-hitch and control lead are used in combination to refine control efforts. Whereas the hip-hitch provides a reliable means for blocking and countering pulling efforts, the control lead gives the trainer the ability to abruptly block and guide the dog's behavior with directive prompting. An added benefit of the hip-hitch is that it frees the trainer's hands to deliver rewards and manipulate bridging devices. During long-line training, the dog is called by name to get its attention in anticipation of tamping and stamping actions. "Easy" is paired with the tamping action, whereas a firmly spoken "Stay" command is paired with the abrupt stamping on the long line to block lunging. As the dog is brought to a halt, the trainer either goes to the waiting dog or recalls it before rewarding and releasing it to continue the walk. During long-line training, the dog is periodically called by name together with an orienting prompt (e.g., squeaker, whistle, or clap), as necessary, clicked as it alerts and begins to turn its head, and is recalled with the vocal command "Come" and hand signal. Upon reaching the trainer, the recall is bridged with "Good" and a variable reward, whereupon the dog is immediately released with "OK" and hand clap. In addition to food rewards, the dog is offered tug and ball-play activities while worked on the long line. A balking or lugging dog is encouraged with slaps on the thigh, crouching, change of pace, and enthusiastic voice and hand gestures paired with "Hurry up."

Slack-leash Walking

With the prospects of a walk, most dogs become excited and active, an enthusiasm that spills over into the walk itself. The first step, therefore, is to organize the various preliminaries to a walk in a way that is conducive to improved impulse control. Obtaining noncontingent treats at such times can help to modulate a dog's excitement by way of diversionary appetitive arousal and incompatible establishing operations. As the dog's interest turns toward the trainer in hopes of getting more treats, various behaviors that have been previously conditioned with food reinforcement are more likely to occur, making control at such times easier. The leash should not be put on the dog until the dog settles down and sits or stands quietly, thereby making the leash a contingent reward based on compliance. Further, the dog should wait at the door briefly before being released. By using a well-conditioned orienting stimulus (squeaker), the dog's attention can be turned to the trainer and bridged (click), whereupon the dog is guided from the door before the vocal bridge ("Good") and food reward are presented. The dog is gradually trained to back away from the door by calling to it "Back" before opening the door. In some cases, tossing a treat back as the door is opened will help to encourage the dog to turn or back away when the door is open. Preliminary reward training at the door should be integrated as a routine and prerequisite to going for a walk. If the dog bolts through the door, it is brought back inside, and the procedure is repeated. Directing the dog away from the door with the leash as the door is opened can be helpful. In addition to backing up as the door is opened, the dog should learn to wait in the doorway for a release signal (e.g., "OK") before exiting the house. The goal is to train the dog to back up as the door opens and then to wait at the doorway under the vocal signal "Wait," until it is released with an "OK." These compliant behaviors are gradually brought under the control of the rewarding opportunity to go for a walk.

The foregoing procedure is repeated until the dog defers and waits quietly before being allowed to go through the door. In the case of highly motivated dogs, exclusionary time-outs (TOs) can be used to reduce preparatory arousal associated with going for a walk. The reprimand "Enough" is spoken in a firm tone and the dog put outside for 30 seconds with the leash pinched in the doorjamb. The TO procedure is repeated until the dog calms down and defers to owner control efforts, whereupon reward training is reinstated. The TO procedure not only reduces preparatory arousal and undesirable behavior, it also makes it more likely that the dog will hesitate and back away as the door is opened. If, despite these training efforts, the dog charges through the door, the leash is pulled back and the door is closed on it, leaving the dog in TO on the other side. This procedure is repeated until the dog hesitates at the door and waits for the release to leave the house.

Once outdoors, pulling into the leash is handled with appropriate countermovements and directive prompts. The strength of such prompting is matched to the dog's effort to pull and its sensitivity to such stimulation. The strength of directive leash prompts is determined by the dog's forward momentum. The dog can be fitted with a limited-slip collar, strap collar, or harness, depending on the specific needs of the dog and owner. During the slack-leash walk, the leash is held in the hand closest to the dog. Approximately two-thirds of the leash is taken up in a single fold, referred to as a *bight*, and held between the thumb and first two fingers of the left hand (see the aforementioned directions for holding a leash). The properly dressed leash always has at least two points of slack (or life) in it. If both the standing and the working slack are lost, the leash is dead, and a small bight of standing slack (life) must be wrestled up before an effective leash prompt can be made. Whether on a slack-leash walk or while heeling, a small bight of the standing end of the leash is always kept in hand. In addition to standing slack, some amount of slack is kept in the working end of the leash. In some cases, a leash is held with a *bight and pinch* during controlled walking (Figure 1.15). A *pinch* is a small amount of leash slack that is taken up and held between the index finger and thumb and released as a warning in advance of dropping the standing slack. When the working slack is pulled out of the leash by the dog, the standing slack is released as both hands are brought together on the handle as one holds a bat. In the same instant, the trainer takes one step back on the left leg and firmly anchors the leash just in front of his or her belly. Alternatively, if the leash is held in the right hand, the trainer steps back on the right leg before bracing against the dog's forward momentum. Sidestepping to the left or right of the dog's line of movement can help to minimize the amount of force needed to disrupt its forward movement and turn it

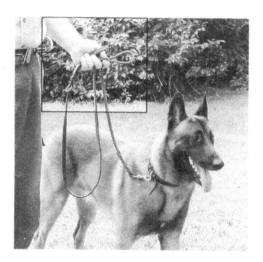

FIG. 1.15. Bight and pinch provides a third point of life in a leash.

about. Coordinating the movements of the body into one brief, unified thrust against the dog's forward momentum generates the leash prompt—not jerking, yanking, or pulling against a dead leash. If the dog charges at an awkward angle, the trainer should follow and align with the dog's direction of pulling before releasing the standing slack, anchoring the leash, and thrusting back. If the prompting action is properly applied with sufficient force, the dog will turn toward the trainer. As the dog turns, the trainer should immediately encourage it to come back and guide it to turn about at the trainer's left side, where it is prompted to sit or stand and briefly wait before being released to walk ahead again. Another variation of this method involves using a hip-hitch and stopping whenever the dog pulls for a count of 3 before the leash slack is dropped and the trainer steps back and anchors the leash, as described previously. Again, just before the standing slack is released, the owner calls the dog's name. This variation appears to be easier for some dog owners to carry out, allowing them to take one step at a time. The slow count is gradually varied so that it is delivered sooner (e.g., sometimes as soon as the dog pulls on the leash) and later than expected, thereby producing prediction error conducive to enhanced attention and avoidance of pulling.

As the result of the foregoing procedure, the dog rapidly learns to anticipate the leash prompt whenever the standing slack is loosed abruptly from the trainer's hand. The dog also learns another important lesson: the prompting action can be avoided by responding quickly and slowing down just as the trainer lets go of the leash slack. Once it is evident that the dog understands these connections, the dog's name is called just before the slack is dropped, thereby bringing the new behavior under additional stimulus control and enhancing the nominal orienting response. Now, as the dog pulls, its name is called and the leash slack is dropped, thereby causing the dog to hesitate and turn without necessitating physical prompting, whereupon it is called ("Come") and appropriately rewarded. With practice, the dog will stop pulling altogether as the result this simple procedure combining directive leash training and positive reinforcement. However, until a high degree of reliability is obtained, the trainer must remain prepared to interrupt the dog's pulling efforts every time they occur. While walking on a slack leash, the dog is permitted to move freely about, sniff, lag behind, dart ahead (unless excessive), and otherwise enjoy itself; the only requirement is that it not pull against the leash—ever. As pulling behavior is controlled, a DRO schedule can be introduced such that the dog is conditionally reinforced regardless of what it is doing at the moment so long as it has not pulled for some brief period—a duration that is progressively lengthened as the dog's behavior improves. Orienting, sit, stay, and release modules can be practiced intermittently during slack-leash walking. In this case, the dog is prompted to orient by calling its name and, if necessary, smooching or squeaking to gather its attention, bridging the orienting response with a click, and then prompting the dog to sit with a hand and vocal signal. As soon as the dog begins to sit, the vocal bridge "Good" is delivered, followed by a food reward. The dog should remain in the sit position until it is released with an "OK" and hand clap. The quick-sit and the recall routines (orienting response, click, come to closed hand, "Good," food

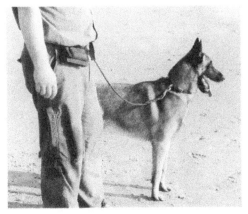

FIG. 1.16. Orientation of a dog when in the controlled-walking position.

reward, and release) are both practiced during slack-leash walking.

Controlled-leash Walking and Hip-hitch

Once a dog has learned to walk without excessive pulling, a hip-hitch and control lead can be used to help develop controlled-walking skills. In addition to not pulling, controlled walking requires that the dog stay on the left side, aligning its hip with the trainer's left leg (Figure 1.16). The hip-hitch consists of a carabiner hooked under a wide bite just behind a belt loop on the trainer's left side. A longish loop of leash is tied off 1 to 3 feet away from the bolt snap, a point determined by the size of the dog. The loop is hooked over the carabiner and attached to a halter, limited-slip collar, or prong collar, depending on need and circumstances. The hip-hitch provides a consistent source of response blocking and feedback limiting the forward movement of a dog beyond the limit set for controlled walking (Figure 1.17). Excessive pulling forward is countered by stepping abruptly back on the left leg and causing the dog to turn about. In addition, the standing end of the leash or control lead running from the knot to the handle can be manipulated in various ways to provide additional control and to transition to the heeling pattern. Only experienced trainers should use a hip-hitch on large and powerful breeds with a history of

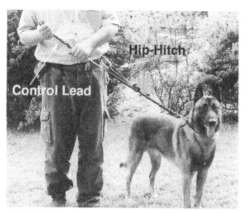

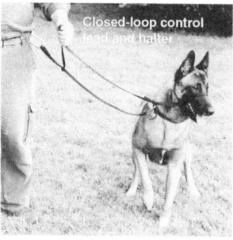

FIG. 1.17. Hip-hitch. The position of the hitch-loop knot determines the amount of action that the control lead can produce. When the loop is tied off near the carabiner, little control-lead action is possible, whereas when the knot is set closer to the to the collar, more control-lead action is available.

hard pulling. In such cases, dogs should be both hip-hitched and under the secondary control of a halter via a closed-loop arrangement (see *Halter Collars*). The hip-hitch and halter system should only be cautiously used with potentially aggressive dogs and, then, only by knowledgeable and experienced trainers familiar with the risks and techniques needed to manage and control such dogs safely. In addition to control benefits, the hip-hitch provides a means to free the hands to perform other training actions, such as squeezing a squeaker or clicker, luring and flagging, targeting, petting, and handling treats and other rewards. Controlled walking

is signaled by saying "Come on" or "Let's go," and excesses are discouraged with appropriate leash prompts paired with "Easy" or "Hurry up," as needed. The dog is released from heeling to controlled walking with the signal "OK" and released from controlled walking to slack-leash walking with "OK" and "Easy" as the dog reaches the limit set on its distance to range from the trainer. Abruptly stopping and stepping back on the left foot serves to counter the dog's pulling efforts. When hip-hitched, the action causes the dog to turn about in front of the trainer, whereupon it can be guided with the left hand to the trainer's side. Before continuing the walk, the dog is required to settle and wait for 3 to 5 seconds before continuing. The procedure is used as needed to discourage pulling and to encourage more appropriate walking behavior.

Halter Training

Halter collars can be very useful for certain dogs and owners, especially children and adults who are physically unable to control a dog otherwise. The muzzling-type halter systems are particularly useful for controlling aggressive dogs and limiting their nuisance barking when on leash. When a dog forcibly lunges into the leash while wearing one of these devices, it passively turns the dog's head around while clamping its muzzle shut if the dog attempts to back out of it. To obtain the most benefit from halter training, the trainer should make a conscientious effort to positively reinforce more appropriate slack-leash and controlled-walking behavior while the dog is restrained on the halter. DeGroot, the originator of the halter for dog training, views the halter as a tool that should be used to facilitate behavior modification with minimal discomfort to the dog. She fully acknowledges the potential abuse and misuse of such devices and stresses that the halter should not be employed as a passive means to control and restrain the dog, but used in the context of well-defined training objectives. The goal of halter control is to provide the trainer with a temporary window of opportunity for enhanced reward-based training efforts so that the dog can be gradually controlled without relying on halter restraint. The powerful head-turning and muzzle-clamping effect of the halter should not be allowed to become a way of life for the dog. The ultimate goal of halter training is to eliminate the halter (DeGroot, personal communication, 2002).

In addition to halters that exert a clamping action, fixed-action halters can be used to promote improved walking behavior. The fixed-action halter system is a versatile and effective tool for controlling excessive pulling (see Figure 1.7). The nonclamping halter has the advantage of comfort with the delivery of directive force without pinning a dog's muzzle shut. Since the fixed-action halter does not produce a muzzling effect, it is not intended or suitable for use with aggressive dogs. The design of the fixed-action halter causes pressure to be properly distributed in accordance with a dog's forward or backward movement. When a dog pulls forward, the force is directed toward the muzzle, whereas, when the dog pulls back, the force is directed to the neck loop and the back of the dog's head. In contrast, pulling back on muzzling-type halters causes the muzzle loop to clamp down on a dog's muzzle rather than primarily directing the force to the neck loop, where it is most needed for comfortable control. The muzzle-clamping action of many halter designs appears to cause some dogs a great deal of distress when they are first introduced to them. Such dogs appear to accept fixed-action halters with less resistance or struggle, making them more acceptable to concerned owners, as well. In addition to the fixed-action halter, a halter/limited-slip collar is frequently used to train adult dogs. The nonclamping, halter/limited-slip system employs both head and neck control pressure so that collar pressures are more evenly and safely distributed around a dog's neck and muzzle (see Figure 1.3). When used as a halter, it produces a very pronounced effect with a minimum of leash pressure and, since torque is distributed to both the neck and the muzzle, it can be safely used to deliver directive leash prompts. When the muzzle loop is removed, the collar becomes a limited-slip collar with a tab. In situations requiring added control, the muzzle loop can be quickly placed over a dog's nose.

Perhaps the most important consideration in halter training is proper introduction. Halters should be introduced slowly with lots of encouragement and positive reinforcement.

Efforts by a dog to struggle against or remove the collar should be immediately and firmly discouraged, however. A dog should not be allowed to flail about or scrape at the collar. Such behavior should be countered with an upward leash prompt every time it occurs, followed by positive reinforcement when it stops, until the dog accepts the collar. The scent of orange oil on the hands appears to help some dogs through the transition. A few drops rubbed on the hands and placed

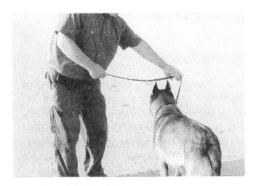

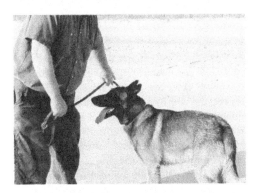

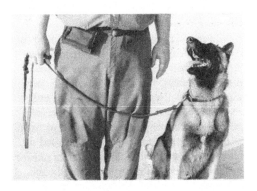

FIG. 1.18. Starting exercise.

directly in front of a dog's nose appears to produce a rapid reduction of distress. The fixed-action collar should be carefully fitted on a dog so that the muzzle loop is loose enough to allow the dog's mouth to open fully to pant and to take a ball, but not so loose that it falls off. The neck loop should be adjusted to fit closely around the back of the dog's head, with minimal slack or ability to slip over the dog's head. In the case of highly active dogs or dogs with thick necks, the fixed-action halter can be hitched to a nylon-slip or chain-slip collar for added security.

BASIC EXERCISES

Starting Exercise

In addition to coming and sitting in front of the trainer (sit-front), a dog should learn to go on signal to the trainer's left side and sit. The movement is prompted by tapping the left thigh and then taking the leash midway down with the left hand, whereupon one step is taken back on the left foot and the dog is gently guided around by the left hand (Figure 1.18). Initially, the trainer may need to take several steps backward or execute a heel-to-toe skipping movement to get the dog moving in the right direction. As the dog's head reaches a position just behind the trainer's left side, the trainer takes one or two steps forward, causing the dog to turn about and align squarely at the left side before it is prompted to sit. When the action is completed, appropriate social and appetitive rewards are delivered. After a moment, the dog is released with an "OK" and clap, and the trial is repeated. Once the exercise is mastered, the vocal signal "Heel" is paired with the hand and body signals used to prompt the behavior.

The starting exercise can be introduced by a shaping or luring procedure. Effective shaping depends on breaking the behavior down into simple steps. Initially, for example, any orientation or movement toward the trainer's left side is bridged and reinforced, especially movement occurring as the trainer steps back on the left foot. Next, the dog is required to follow the target hand a short distance toward the left before being reinforced. Finally, the dog is made to follow the hand around into

the starting position and prompted to sit. Each step should be fully mastered before moving onto the next. A birdie lure can be effectively used to draw the dog around to the starting position (see *Targeting and Prompting*). In some cases, a resistant dog can be lured into position with a ball or a biscuit. Once the dog is moving into the starting position and sitting without hesitation, the lure is faded and replaced with the appropriate voice and hand signals. Performance reliability is enhanced with directive leash prompts, as necessary to cause the dog to move in the direction of the trainer's left side and to sit. The level of force used is determined by the dog's temperament and needs to achieve reliable compliance. Compliance to the sit command can be enhanced by pulling up on the leash while squeezing, at first gently and than progressively more firmly, across the hips just in front of the hip bones. The dog's rump should not be pushed down or slapped to increase compliance.

The dog should also learn to leave the starting position and to move forward, turn, and sit squarely in front of the trainer. The dog is guided into the sit-front position by capturing its attention, saying "Front," and taking a half-step forward with the left foot. As the dog follows, it is lured with the right hand or guided around by leash to sit in front. In addition to the left-side starting exercise, the dog should learn to go to heel by moving to the right side and then continuing on behind the trainer to the starting position on the left side. This route is typically used when the dog is located somewhere toward the trainer's right side, whereas the left-side hooking movement is used when the dog is located directly in front or toward the left side. Stepping back on the right foot signals the dog to go to heel from the right side. As the dog crosses behind the trainer, the leash is transferred from the right hand to left hand, and the dog is prompted to sit with the right hand as it reaches the starting position at the trainer's left side. The starting exercise is mastered by daily practice under varying and progressively more distracting and difficult circumstances. Also, the dog should learn to hold the position for longer periods before being released. The exercise is of tremendous value for controlling dogs at times when increased close control is needed.

As the dog learns the starting exercise, an emphasis should be placed on requiring that it remain quiet and focused on the trainer for progressively longer periods. Sustained reinforcement lasting up to 15 to 20 seconds can be useful in the beginning to help keep the dog's attention in focus. Likewise, the trainer should take a moment to formally dress the leash, breathe, and concentrate on the dog and the training objectives, thereby joining the dog in the same moment of heightened attentiveness and appreciation. In the Japanese tea ceremony, the phrase *izumai o tadasu,* literally meaning to straighten one's kimono or posture, is a ritual preparation occurring in advance of preparing and serving tea, signifying an appreciation and respect for the guest and attentiveness to the moment shared with the guest in the making and taking of tea. A similar significance should be nurtured with regard to the starting exercise. As the dog comes to the trainer's side and the leash is carefully dressed, the trainer should collect the moment with an attitude of affectionate respect and appreciation for the dog's compliance and cooperation in the process of attaining interactive harmony.

Lying Down from the Sit Position

With the dog sitting in the starting position, the trainer changes leash hands and shifts in place about one-eighth turn toward the dog. The left hand (now holding the leash) is placed on the dog's shoulder and the thumb is hooked over the collar as the trainer crouches down. At the same time, the right hand is extended just in front of the dog's nose and moved downward toward the ground. As the result of the introductory lessons previously described, many dogs will naturally follow the hand's movement and lie down without hesitation. As the dog lies down, the bridge "Good" is spoken in a high-pitched tone, followed by a treat and sustained petting and massage once the dog assumes the down position. As the trainer stands upright, the left foot is placed over the leash so that the dog cannot prematurely break the down position (Figure 1.19).

The trainer should avoid pressing down on the dog's shoulder, since this may cause the dog to resist and push upward against the pressure. Lying down can be shaped through successive steps (e.g., targeting on the hand, following the hand as it moves downward, following the hand down to the floor and, finally, following the hand and lying down). Each approximation is bridged and reinforced and repeated as necessary to obtain a fluent response. In some cases, a toy or biscuit can be used as a lure to facilitate the response. The lure is kept just beyond the dog's reach as it is lowered to the ground. As previously discussed, food lures often function as a bribe; that is, luring the dog with a biscuit risks reinforcing its initial unwillingness to lie

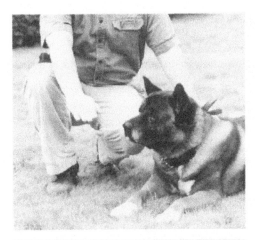

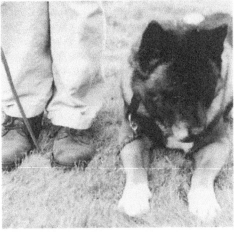

FIG. 1.19. Down exercise.

down. In a sense, the dog's refusal to lie down may be calculated to manipulate the owner into bribery. As the result of success in such efforts, the dog may quickly learn that hesitating when prompted to lie down causes the owner to offer a bribe—a pattern that the dog is only too willing to reinforce! Habitually giving the dog the biscuit after luring may lead it to hold out and refuse to perform the response unless the bribe is in hand. A useful technique for fading the lure is to close the hand as though it might contain the biscuit when giving the down signal. After the dog is rewarded, it is either released with an "OK" and clap or prompted to perform another exercise from the down position (e.g., down-stay). Once the dog is lying down rapidly and consistently in response to the hand signal, the vocal signal "Down" is paired with it. As the trainer stands up, the leash is stepped on to prevent the dog from getting up. Down is practiced in a variety of situations and contextual relations to other basic modules and routines (see Appendix B.1).

In the case of dogs that refuse to lie down despite conscientious reward-based shaping and luring efforts, the following procedure can be useful for improving compliance. The slack of the leash is dropped to the ground and stepped on with the left foot. Next, the working slack is pulled out of the leash as the left foot is angled up 3 or 4 inches, with the heel planted on the ground as a point of leverage. The down signal is given and the foot is lowered to the ground, placing pressure on the dog's neck and forcing it to lie down. If necessary, the force is increased by repeating the procedure, causing additional leash to be taken up and producing a ratcheting effect that gradually compels the dog to lie down. In some cases, squeezing across the neck muscle at the withers, gently at first and than more firmly as needed to prompt the down response, can further enhance compliance when combined with the ratcheting procedure. Forceful stamping on the leash should be avoided in favor of more controlled and measured techniques.

Sitting from the Down and Stand Positions

The dog is prompted to sit from the down position by first rocking or shuffling slightly forward on the right foot and then, as the dog begins to get up, stepping back on the left foot and, with an upward movement of the right hand, signaling the dog to sit. As the dog sits, the response is bridged and reinforced. Next, to prompt the dog to stand from the sit position, the trainer dresses the leash across the left knee and then takes one step forward into the leash with the left foot. The step forward prompts the dog into the stand position, and the response is bridged and reinforced. As the dog stands, the trainer gently restrains the dog with the left hand on the collar so that it does not move too far ahead. If the dog attempts to sit, an additional step is taken—a procedure that is repeated together with a slight downward pressure applied by the palm or fingertips of the left hand to the dog's shoulders. The slight downward pressure causes the dog to push back, thereby competing with its tendency to sit. Once steady, the dog is released with an "OK" or prompted to sit. The dog should be required to hold the stand-stay at the trainer's left side for progressively longer periods. Once the basic response is established, the vocal signal "Stand" is paired with the step forward. The reliability of stand response is gradually improved by the practice of routine variations (see Figure B.1C in Appendix B). As the dog's training progresses, sit responses occurring in association with recall and sit-front, starting and finish exercises, and heeling are often encouraged to occur automatically (see *Automatic Sit*), requiring that vocal and hand signals controlling the sit response be gradually faded. Consequently, the vocal and hand signals prompting the sit response are primarily practiced for enhanced reliability in the context of controlled and slack-leash walking, stand, and down training (see Figure B.1A–C in Appendix B).

Integrated Cycle of Basic Exercises

The basic obedience repertoire consisting of the stand, sit, down, sit from the down, and stand from sit modules is practiced as a chain of interconnected routines in order to enhance the fluency of each step and to establish a balanced and reliable pattern of performance. Not only should these routines be performed in the normal forward and reverse orders, they should also be practiced in various unexpected ways as the dog's skill and proficiency improves (see Figure B.1D in Appendix B). All the basic exercises are integrated with the stay and heeling pattern. As the dog's training progresses, the reinforcement schedule is varied so that the dog might be required to offer a series (twofers and threefers), such as sit and stand (a twofer) or down, sit, and stand (a threefer) for the same reward. Although food is given intermittently, each successful effort should receive appropriate bridging and affectionate encouragement.

STAY TRAINING

All basic exercises are performed with an implicit stay; that is, a dog should remain in the position until it is released ("OK") or prompted to perform another module or routine. It is particularly important not to allow a dog to break the position immediately after receiving affection or food rewards.

Stay from the Starting Position

The sit-stay exercise is practiced by calling the dog by name, saying "Stay," and stepping off on the right foot, whereupon the left hand is swung back to take up the leash, and the trainer turns to face the dog momentarily. As the trainer turns, the working end of the leash is dropped. The remaining standing slack is let out as the trainer steps back, with the right-hand flag (palm out and held at chest level) toward the dog. The handle of the open leash hangs from the right thumb as the trainer steps back a few steps. Once at the end of the leash, the leash handle is changed from the right thumb to the left thumb, with any excess leash slack taken up into a single fold in the left hand. Finally, the right hand is placed over the left hand at waist level. If the dog attempts to move out of position, the trainer prompts the dog back into position or returns it to the original position.

The trainer goes back to the dog by retracing previous steps or by circling behind it. If the trainer opts to go around the dog, the open leash is flipped onto the dog's right side as the trainer starts around the dog's left side. The leash is gathered and dressed as the trainer returns to the starting position at the dog's right side. At the conclusion of the exercise, the dog is either released with an "OK" and clap or reinforced and prompted to perform some another task; the dog is never permitted to break a stay without a signal (See Appendix A).

Most dogs rapidly learn to stay. However, some highly excitable ones may require vigilant handling, response blocking, and directive prompting to control. Frequent or sustained reinforcement can be a highly effective means to initially encourage excitable dogs to stay and focus on the trainer. Well-timed vocal or leash prompts can prevent dogs from breaking the position and provide an additional opportunity for reinforcement. If a dog breaks the position altogether, it is returned to the original spot and the exercise is repeated. An active-control line (ring or post) can be used to facilitate stay and recall training via response blocking and reward training. The down-stay and stand-stay are practiced in a similar way as the sit-stay. Directive procedures and blocking are minimized by gradually establishing stay routines in small well-mastered steps. Stay training consists of eight separate but interrelated criteria, each requiring explicit training:

Criterion 1 *Duration:* The dog is required to stay for progressively longer periods while the trainer stands nearby or just out in front. As the trainer's distance away from the dog increases, additional duration criteria are added in advance of every increment of distance. Reliability associated with duration is the most important foundation or anchor of stay training. The duration phase of stay is associated with training the dog to hold eye contact with the trainer for progressively longer periods. Once a standard expectancy (see *Prediction and Control Expectancies*) is established, variations with respect to the frequency of rewards and the duration of the stay period can be used to help strengthen the stay exercise. During the early stages, the dog is given frequent rewards while its stays, learning only to move out of position after it is release with an "OK" and hand clap. Since the stay exercise is mildly aversive for most dogs, providing a dog with varied and highly valued rewards can be helpful, as can the surprise generated by periodically releasing the dog sooner than normal.

Criterion 2 *Differentiation:* Differentiation refers to the systematic association of different basic exercises with stay training, until they are all equally steady and reliable, both as discrete modules (e.g., sit, stand, and down) and routines (e.g., sit from the stand, down from the sit, sit from the down, and stand) and as dynamic exercises (e.g., the walking stand-stay).

Criterion 3 *Distance:* Once the dog is holding the sit-stay, down-stay, and stand-stay for 30 seconds or so, the trainer increases the distance criterion by gradual increments. In the context of increasing distance, further differentiation and organization of basic modules and routines are continued while introducing and practicing distance exercises (e.g., sit from the stand, down from the sit, sit from the down, and stand), performed in conjunction with the walking stand-stay exercise. Initially, the trainer prompts these exercise at a distance of a step or two away from the dog, then at the end of the leash and at the end of the long line, and finally with the dog off leash (see *Walking Stand-Stay and Distance Exercises*). Practicing the recall from the sit, down, and stand-stay should be added only after a high degree of control is established over the distance exercises. Calling the dog from the stay should be calculated to produce surprise, thereby strengthening the stay and giving enthusiasm to the recall. With each step of increasing distance and differentiation, additional training and proofing of criterion 1 should be carried out, especially with respect to the proofing of the down-stay. With the trainer at a full leash distance, the dog should be reliable in a down-stay for a minimum of 1 to 3 minutes, 3 to 5 minutes at a long-line distance, and 10 minutes or more when off leash. Recall from the stay is practiced in the context of developing an interruption signal that causes the dog to stop after starting to come, to wait, or immediately to drop before being called to front and finish.

Criterion 4 *Direction:* The dog should be left to stay with the trainer walking away in various directions, for example, stepping off to the side, stepping back, stepping toward the front, and sharp turns off to the left or right. When introducing directional variations, further differentiation and reliability of basic exercises is achieved by having the dog sit, stand, or lie down from various distances, directions, orientations (e.g., facing away from the dog), and locations relative to the dog.

Criterion 5 *Difficulty:* After the dog is staying reliably at a long-line distance, various elements of difficulty are added with the dog both close by and at various distances. Additional difficulty can be introduced by leaving the dog in unusual directions and ways and doing things out of the ordinary while the dog is in the stay. For example, the trainer can crouch down or sit on the ground, walk around the dog, run by the dog, fall down, roll over, rush toward the dog, or step slowly toward the dog. Additional difficulty can be added by leaving the dog's sight (e.g., hiding behind a tree or going around the corner of building).

Criterion 6 *Diversification:* Stay is integrated into everyday activities requiring that the dog stay or wait before getting what it wants, e.g., wait before being released to fetch a toy, before getting into a car, before being permitted to jump onto furniture, and before being let outdoors. With the transition to the long line, the dog should learn to halt and stay when chasing a throw-away object (e.g., a stick or other object of no critical significance to training objectives). After giving the dog a stay command, the object is thrown and, if the dog chases after, it the command "Stay" is shouted as the trainer tamps or stamps on the long line. The dog should wait in place until the trainer recalls it or releases it to retrieve the object. The halt-and-wait response is a critical preliminary to off-leash training (see *Using the Long Line*).

Criterion 7 *Diversions:* After the dog is solid under the foregoing circumstances, increasingly distractive situations are identified to proof the dog's ability to stay in the presence of attractive diversions (e.g., children playing, wildlife, other dogs, joggers, and bicyclists) while on leash and long line. The trainer can bounce a ball with the dog in a stay exercise, finally releasing the dog to chase or catch the ball. The quick-sit and instant-down are introduced in the context of proving the stay under highly distracting conditions.

Criterion 8 *Disruptions:* In addition to attractive diversions, the dog is also gradually exposed to potentially startling or aversive events with appropriate counterconditioning and graduated exposure, as needed to reduce its reactivity (e.g., traffic and loud noises) while practicing stay variations.

Stop, Stay, and Come

Occasionally, while walking on a slack leash, the dog is signaled to "Stay." If the dog hesitates and stops, the trainer should immediately bridge the behavior and approach the dog in a reassuring way, reward it, and release it with an "OK" and clap. If the dog fails to stop, the trainer anchors the leash on the waist with both hands and abruptly stops, thereby bringing the dog to a sudden halt. Besides learning to stop and wait while walking on a slack leash or long line, the dog should also learn to come when called and to sit-front. The trainer calls the dog by name, says "Come," and delivers a hand signal consisting of a sweeping action of the right hand moving across the chest. If the dog responds, the behavior is bridged with the clicker or vocal reward "Good," and the dog is directed to sit directly in front of the trainer. Taking a few steps backward as the dog approaches the trainer can help to facilitate straight sits. Finally, the dog is prompted to finish with the command "Heel," whereupon it should sit automatically. The dog is appropriately rewarded and released to repeat the exercise.

Quick-sit and Instant-down

The quick-sit involves training the dog to sit rapidly without hesitation, regardless of the dog's disposition or environmental circumstances. The quick-sit is an emergency exercise that signifies that the dog must stop whatever else it is doing and sit immediately and remain still until it is released. The quick-sit should involve a foundation of intensive reward-based training and directive enhancement, as needed to achieve a high degree of reliability under diverse and progressively distracting and difficult environmental condi-

tions. The quick-sit is proofed in the context of intensive stay training. Like the quick-sit, the instant-down is a rapid and immediate emergency response. The dog is required simply to drop in place without hesitation. The module is introduced only after the dog is fluently lying down from a sit position. The first step involves training the dog to lie down from the stand. This task is facilitated by first training the dog to bow by targeting on a hand moving toward the ground. Once the dog is bowing on signal, instant-down while walking or heeling is much easier for it to perform. The task is prompted by turning slightly toward the dog and directing it with an excited tone of voice and downward hand signal to drop to the ground. If the dog fails to respond, the trainer lures or physically prompts the dog into the down position. As the dog complies, the behavior is bridged and reinforced, but the dog should continue to hold the down-stay until it is released. If the dog attempts to get up, the trainer stands on the leash with the left foot. At the conclusion of the exercise, the dog is either released, prompted to sit or stand, or walked out of the down position, depending on what is appropriate given the situation. This exercise is repeated several times in close succession until the dog learns to drop without hesitation. The instant-down can be facilitated with a ball lure and play following compliance.

Go-lie-down

Training dogs to go to a specific place and to lie down is a valuable exercise that all companion dogs should learn and regularly practice. The behavior consists of the dog leaving the proximity of the trainer or stopping some activity, moving to a designated spot, and lying down. This sequence of behaviors is first shaped using positive-reinforcement techniques. Training the dog to go lie down assumes a reliable and fluent down and instant-down response. Initially, the dog should be trained to go to a rug by using a shaping process. One way of accomplishing this is by using a clicker and shaping the routine via a series of approximations that train the dog to go to the rug, lie down, and stay there (Table 1.2). Once the dog is going rapidly to the rug or bed and lying down, the response is generalized to other places and contexts involving increasing distractions and difficulty (e.g., the presence of a guest or while the family is eating). Tossing a soft toy toward the spot where the dog is expected to lie down may help it to follow the pointing prompt. If necessary, the dog can be lured or ushered part of the way and then prompted to the spot by pointing and saying "Go." As the dog nears the spot, the command "Lie down" is given, and a treat is tossed to the dog as it lies down. Once the pattern is established, the whole command is given at once, "Go lie down," coupled with a pointing prompt toward the spot.

HEELING

In addition to slack-leash and controlled walking, dogs are trained to walk at heel. Formal heeling is a valuable lesson for every dog to master. When heeling, a dog remains close at the trainer's left side, without crowding or interfering with the trainer's movements. The leash is held in the right hand and dressed across the left knee. When the dog is heeling in the proper position, the working end of the leash intersects the trainer's line of movement

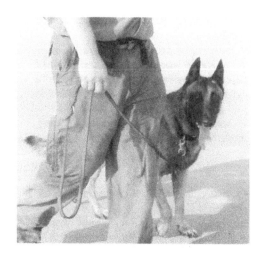

FIG. 1.20. Heeling position.

at a 90° angle; that is, the dog is squared up at the trainer's side when heeling, neither moving past nor lagging behind this reference point (Figure 1.20). Heeling is an exacting activity, with a mere inch or two of deviation out of the position representing a flaw needful of adjustment. A close approximation is not enough, the dog is either heeling or not. There is a groove that is hard to describe but known to anyone who has trained a dog to

TABLE. 1.2. Shaping contingencies for the go-lie-down response

Step 1:	Turn away from the trainer
Step 2:	Turn away and orient in the direction of the rug
Step 3:	Move in the direction of the rug
Step 4:	Move with hand signal in close proximity to the rug
Step 5:	Move in close proximity to the rug and wait for reward
Step 6:	Pair hand signal with "Go," touch the rug, and wait for reward
Step 7:	Stand halfway on the rug and wait for reward
Step 8:	Stand fully on the rug and wait for reward
Step 9:	Hand and voice signal "Go lie down," go to the rug, wait, and down on hand signal before reward is delivered
Step 10:	Go to the rug, lie down on signal, and wait for reward
Step 11:	Go to the rug, lie down (signal faded), and wait for reward
Step 12:	Go to the rug, lie down, and wait to be released before receiving the reward
Step 13:	Go to the rug, lie down, and stay for a variable length of time before being released
Step 14:	Specify different locations to lie down by vocal and directional cuing

walk squared up at heel. Although the heeling position can be defined as a geometric relationship, in reality it is more a state of mind shared by the trainer and dog. Properly understood and performed heeling is a moving meditation during which the dog and trainer *join* in an attitude of cooperative purpose and heightened awareness of each other.

Again, the importance of preliminary training using a shaping procedure and play-based luring cannot be overemphasized. The trainer should always strive toward making training efforts as affectionate and rewarding for the dog as possible. Shaping a heeling pattern is introduced in a relatively distraction-free environment. The trainer attracts the dog's attention and encourages it to orient toward the left side, whereupon the approximation is bridged and the dog given the reward after it comes to the trainer's left side and sits. Sustained reinforcement helps to strengthen an impression that the left side is a desirable place to be. Using a licking stick slathered with peanut butter is one way to deliver sustained reinforcement while the dog is walking or sitting at the trainer's left side—a method that can be useful in the context of counterconditioning fears where sustained appetitive arousal is needed. With every occurrence in which the dog orients on the left side, a bridging signal is followed by a prompt to sit, "Good," and food reward. To make handling the various paraphernalia less cumbersome, the dog can be kept on a hip-hitch, thereby freeing the hands to signal, lure, and reward its behavior. Alternatively, the dog can be worked on a loose leash dragging on the ground or, in the case of more active dogs, a long line that is controlled by stamping actions. The usual pattern is to encourage the dog to orient and walk closely at the left side of the trainer before bridging and rewarding the behavior. By crouching down, turning about, running ahead, making various lip and squeaker sounds, and otherwise attracting and keeping the dog's attention, it will be more willing to play along and follow. Attracting the dog with a ball, luring it to the left side, and encouraging it to walk closely with right turns and right about-turns and changes of pace before allowing the dog to tug or fetch the ball can be a highly effective and fun way to introduce the concept.

Although play and reward-based training is a desirable way to introduce some of the basic elements, heeling as a formal activity is rarely fully attained without some element of directive training, as required to control the influence of distractions on a dog's wavering attention and impulse control. However, by carefully preparing the dog with preliminary play and reward-based training activities and making heeling a fun thing to do, the dog is certain to require far fewer and less forceful prompts than would be otherwise necessary to control its attention

Major Faults

At the beginning of every walk, dogs should always be given the liberty to walk at ease on a slack leash or long line, giving them a moment to relax and eliminate, if necessary. In the case of highly excitable dogs, ball play can be a useful way to dissipate excess energy. Once a dog is walking without pulling, it is called to the starting position at the trainer's left side and prompted to sit. The leash is dressed and, after a brief moment of affectionate praise and petting, the trainer gathers the dog's attention with its name and the command "Heel" and steps off on the left foot, slapping the left thigh, and smooching and clucking as needed to attract the dog's attention. If the dog forges out in front, the trainer drops the leash slack and turns away from the dog. As the turn is made, the left and right hands are drawn together and anchored near the left hip. The right hand is closed firmly around the leash handle, while the left hand is held open with thumb forming a crook over the leash. If the dog lurches to the side instead, the trainer turns sharply to the right. When applying directive prompts, the leash should be adjusted up or down on the thigh to keep it level with the line of the dog's back. Careful timing is crucial; if the slack of the leash is taken up too soon or too late, the effect is diminished or lost. The collective movement of the shoulders, hips, arms, and legs are coordinated to join up just as the dog gets to the end of the leash. As the dog turns and follows, the trainer should continue walking in the opposite direction for a few steps before resuming the original direction. As the dog follows along, its behavior is appropriately bridged and reinforced, with the trainer periodically stopping and prompting the dog to sit and rewarding it with affectionate praise, petting, and food.

Minor Faults

As dogs learn to stay back, changes of direction and leash prompts are used to refine the heeling pattern further. Now, instead of dropping the standing slack, the working slack is used to generate the appropriate directive prompt. A closer approximation to the proper heeling position is obtained by making left quarter-turns and about-turns into the dog. The left turn is made by taking up the working slack of the leash with the left hand, pivoting slightly on the left foot, and turning into the dog with the right leg. Short grab-and-release leash prompts delivered with the left hand can be used to improve slight out-of-position faults. Although such corrections are useful for polishing purposes, a broader brush is needed during the early stages of training, during which the left hand should refrain from holding the leash unless a directive prompt, left turn, or stop-sit prompt is being performed. To function efficiently, the change of behavior produced by the directive prompt should be bridged and reinforced with food and social rewards (praise, petting, and play).

Lateral lurching from the heeling position is corrected by turning to the right. This maneuver simultaneously exaggerates the fault (thereby making it more explicit and evident to the dog) and corrects it. Balking and lugging are corrected by dropping the standing slack and walking into the leash, combined with enticement actions (clucking, smooching, leg slaps) and vocal encouragement. Lunging is discouraged with brisk changes of pace and efforts to enhance the dog's performance motivationally with increased positive reinforcement and play. Stepping back abruptly into the leash with the right leg and then forward again on the right leg effectively discourages the dog from crossing behind the trainer. The various left and left-about turns, right and right-about turns, and changes of pace serve to zero the

dog in on the heeling position. Throughout the training process, heeling should be continuously reinforced with vocal rewards and mechanical bridging, petting, play, and varied food treats.

Heeling Square

The quality and accuracy of the heeling pattern is gradually improved by employing various changes of pace (slow, normal, and fast) mixed with turns, directive prompts, bridging, and reinforcement. A heeling square can be used to refine and polish the heeling performance. The square can be indicated either with corner markers or by simply keeping the shape roughly in mind as one counts off steps from corner to corner. With the dog positioned on the outside of the square, the trainer says "Heel" and steps off on the left foot. After 6 to 10 steps, a sharp 90° right turn is made; this right turn is repeated three times, bringing the dog back to the starting point. As each turn is made, the trainer slaps his or her left thigh to draw the dog's attention, followed by appropriate encouragement and affectionate praise, as the turn is completed. Once back at the starting point, the trainer turns about so that the dog is now located on the inside of the square, and the dog prompted to sit and is reinforced. From this orientation, the dog is heeled around the square in the opposite direction by making a series of left 90° turns. Just before each left turn, the trainer picks up the working slack with the left hand, pivots slightly on the left foot, and steps in front of the dog with the right leg to complete the turn. As the square is completed in both directions, the trainer orients the dog toward the opposite corner of the square before prompting it to sit. The dog is walked at heel along the diagonal line between the corners and alternately prompted to make left and right about-turns. As each turn is completed, the trainer changes pace, saying "Easy" before slowing the pace or "Hurry" before speeding it up. After left and right about-turns with changes of pace, the dog is heeled around an imaginary circle traced within the square. The dog is first directed to heel around the square in a clockwise direction and then in a counterclockwise direction. Walking clockwise requires the dog to walk slightly faster to keep up at the trainer's side, whereas walking counterclockwise requires the dog to slow down to stay properly aligned. At the conclusion of the foregoing variations, the dog is walked in a spiraling direction toward the center of the square, where it is left in long down-stay. After a variable period of 1 to 3 minutes, the trainer returns to the dog, releases it with an "OK" and clap, and engages it in ball play.

Automatic Sit

When walked at heel, a dog should sit whenever the trainer comes to a stop. In addition to sitting automatically while heeling, the dog should also learn to sit automatically after starting and finishing exercises and when called to sit front. The trainer's intention to stop is communicated to the dog by taking up the leash with the left hand and making a pulsing movement two or three steps before stopping. The slight movements of the leash announce the trainer's intent to stop, thereby preparing the dog to stop in unison with the trainer and to sit neatly at the left side. As the dog sits, the response is bridged and rewarded; if the dog the fails to sit, however, the trainer prompts the response with a hand signal, shadow, or knee bend and directive prompt. Crooked or awkward sitting is most easily adjusted or prevented by prompting the dog to adjust before it completes the action. If the dog begins to sit crookedly, it can be lured into the proper position or walked a step or two forward before being prompted to sit again. Alternatively, the dog can be prompted to perform the starting exercise before being prompted to sit straight. Attentive heeling in a proper alignment with the trainer prevents or solves many problems associated with crooked or awkward sits.

Interrupting the Automatic Sit

When walked at heel, a dog is obligated to sit automatically whenever the trainer stops. However, the trainer may prefer on some occasions that the dog not sit but stand still and wait instead. With such considerations in mind, an interruption signal is introduced that serves to set aside the obligation to sit and sets the occasion for the dog to stop and stand still instead. The automatic sit is interrupted with the vocal signal "Stand" while touching or gently pushing on the dog's shoulders or the back of its neck after coming to a stop. This stand prompt has been previously used to help the dog learn to stand from the sit or down position. If the dog begins to sit, the trainer repeats the command and takes an addition step forward on the left foot. The dog rapidly learns that a light touch on the shoulder or neck signifies that it should not sit, whereas the absence of such a signal by default indicates that it must sit automatically when the trainer stops.

Releasing the Dog from the Heeling Pattern

Proper heeling requires focused attention and the exertion of tremendous impulse control by a dog. Although it is beneficial and useful for a dog to learn how to heel, it is not beneficial to force a dog to heel all the time. Most dogs have so little opportunity to go on walks that it is only fair that such opportunities be made as cheerful and pleasant as possible for them, without the owner being towed around by an out-of-control dog. Normally, dogs should be walked on a controlled or slack leash 80% to 90% of the time and be brought to heel at times when more control is needed or as a means to discourage undesirable walking behavior. In accordance with the Premack principle (see *Premack Principle: The Relativity of Reinforcement* in Volume 1, Chapter 7), releasing a dog from the heeling position to controlled-leash or slack-leash walking can be used to reinforce good heeling habits. Consequently, it is best to release the dog while it is heeling nicely without pulling, sniffing, or looking around, whereas the dog is called back to heel when it becomes difficult to control while walking on a slack leash. Moving from walking the dog on a slack leash to a heeling pattern is mildly annoying and can serve to discourage undesirable walking behavior. After a period of heeling, the dog is again released and periodically reinforced for walking without pulling with appropriate bridges, treats, and opportunities to play. The dog is released from heeling to controlled walking by saying "OK," changing leash hands, and flipping the slack leash onto the dog's back. The trainer releases the dog from controlled walking to slack-leash walking by saying "OK" and letting the slack slide out between the thumb and index fingers. When the appropriate amount of leash has been let out, the trainer says "Easy" and pinches the leash, thereby setting the distance given to the dog. The dog is brought to heel from slack-leash walking by transferring the leash from the left to the right hand, calling its name and "Heel," and delivering appropriate hand signals and leash prompts. With the left hand guiding the leash, the dog is prompted to turn about and come up sharply and squarely into the heeling position. Depending on specific needs, the dog is either allowed to sit automatically or directed to heel forward with the leash dressed neatly across the left knee.

WALKING STAND-STAY AND DISTANCE EXERCISES

The walking stand-stay is performed with the dog heeling at the trainer's left side. The exercise is initiated by saying, "Stay" and then sweeping the left hand back and taking up the leash, whereupon the trainer pivots slightly on the left foot before turning and stepping sprightly in front of the dog. As the trainer turns about, the leash slack is dropped, and the stay flag is presented to steady the dog as the trainer backs away from the dog. The exercise is practiced with the goal of training the dog to stop in midstride with the vocal and hand signals.

The walking stand-stay is introduced in the context of practicing distance exercises, including sit from stand, down from sit, stand from sit, down from stand, stand from down, and the recall routine. These various exercises are practiced at a half-leash and a full-leash distance away from the dog. As the behaviors are mastered, they are practiced with the dog on the long line and finally with it off leash. Sitting from the stand-stay is prompted by saying "Sit" and then sweeping the right hand upward to a point just below shoulder level. The down is prompted with

the dog in the sit position by saying "Down," followed by a downward sweep of the right hand. Hand signals are delivered while taking a half-step on the right foot in the direction of the dog. The stand exercise is prompted from a distance by saying "Stand," together with a hand signal presented by shifting the right hand, palm down, first toward the dog and then bringing it back toward the hip. As the right hand is pulled back toward the hip, the trainer takes a half-step back on the right leg. As the dog moves into the stand position, the stay flag is presented with a step toward the dog to prevent it from moving out of position. If necessary, a stamping action is included to discourage forward movement by the dog when it is prompted to stand. Finally, the dog is recalled by calling its name and saying "Come" as the right hand is swept across the chest. The recall signal is also performed with a half-step back on the right foot. The forward and backward half-steps

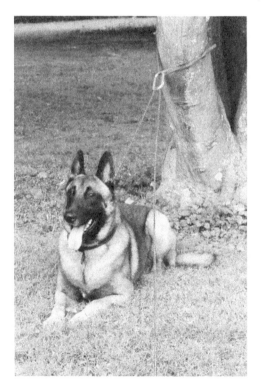

FIG. 1.21. Active-control line with carabiner and webbing.

used to introduce distance exercises are gradually faded and then used only in situations requiring additional emphasis. When hand signals are presented, the fingers of the right hand should be held together, and the signal is performed neatly and consistently. Once the dog responds reliably to the vocal and hand signal combinations, the repertoire of basic modules and routines is practiced with vocal and hand signals presented alone. These various body and hand movements are also used in association with prompting delivered at a distance via the long line. In some cases, distant exercises are introduced with the dog on an active-control line (ring or post), thereby giving the trainer added control over the dog's forward movement (Figure 1.21).

The stand, sit, and down modules are practiced in various sequences and routines to promote balance and to prevent anticipatory responding. After the completion of each trial, the trainer should return to the dog to deliver rewards and initiate another trial or to release the dog. Distance exercises can be practiced in routines consisting of two or three modules at a time before returning to the dog. These basic exercises should be practiced under a variety of conditions of increasing distraction and difficulty. The recall sequence can be performed intermittently in the context of practicing distance exercises. However, repeatedly calling a dog from the stay after completing some exercise may cause the dog eventually to start breaking in anticipation of being called. Consequently, the dog should be called infrequently while organizing distance exercises and projects. The recall is practiced with the dog in sit-, stand-, and down-stay positions. Figure B.1A–D in Appendix B contains several sets of practice variations that are gradually introduced in accordance with the dog's training level. The variations are practiced in groups defined in terms of the dog's specific training needs. It is not necessary to practice all of the variations during the same session (practice may be limited to repetitions involving three to five variations per session), nor is it necessary to follow the particular order in which the practice modules and routines as are listed. These various exercises are practiced at progressive dis-

tances from the dog on a long line and off leash, as the dog's reliability permits.

RECALL TRAINING

No training project is more important than training the dog to come reliably when called. All companion dogs, but especially dogs exhibiting problem behaviors when off leash, should be trained to come and halt-stay to a high degree of proficiency and reliability. The habit of coming when called should be established early and practiced often. Puppies not trained to come when called before week 16 are typically much more difficult to train to come reliably as adults. Early training efforts should emphasize reward and play training, thorough environmental exposure and habituation, and varied daily practice activities. An unwillingness to come is most often the result of the combination of neglectful training and interaction that inadvertently trains the dog not to come when called. One of the most common mistakes leading to adult recall problems involves chasing a puppy that refuses to come or delivering punishment after catching or trapping a puppy on the run. Such interaction invariably promotes expectancies antagonistic to the development of a reliable recall. Another source of conflict and tension involves calling the dog from highly rewarding activities to less rewarding outcomes.

For instance, a dog that is kept indoors in a crate for the majority of the day often finds opportunities to go outside very exciting and enjoyable. Calling the dog back inside before it is ready demands that it give up a highly rewarding circumstance in exchange for a much less rewarding one. In this case, it would be more constructive to have the dog stay at the door and then to call it to come outside. After the dog has gotten its fill of the outdoors, its desire to come back inside will naturally improve, especially if strong incentives to do so are presented at such times. When the dog must be called from a highly rewarding situation to a less rewarding one, two methods are usually recommended: (1) The trainer goes to the dog and secures it without calling it. (2) If the dog must be called, a 45-second period of diversionary activity and reward is provided (e.g., affection, treats, and ball play), thereby producing a buffer between the act of coming and a potential loss of reward.

Along these lines of inadvertent punishment, a common mistake is to call a dog to its crate. Crate restraint is far from pleasurable for most dogs and puppies (see *Dangers of Excessive Crate Confinement* in Chapter 2). The overall effect of calling a dog to crate confinement is to arrange a long exclusionary TO with restraint to occur when the dog comes, hardly an incentive to come when called in the future. In addition to being intrinsically aversive to the dog, the timing of crate confinement often signifies that the owner is about to leave the house, further increasing aversive associations with coming. Habitually calling a dog in order to confine it may result in its learning behaviors that are actively antagonistic to coming when called at other times, including the development of chase-and-evade contests when outdoors. Such activities are exciting, fun, and rewarding for dogs, serving to further reward the dog for not coming when called. Lastly, a poorly informed or impatient owner might fall into the foot-shooting habit of calling the dog to the site of a house-soiling or chewing incident in order to deliver a belated dose of punishment. Not only is such treatment ineffectual for producing the intended effect, it will strongly decrease the dog's future willingness to come when called, as well as adversely affect its trust in the owner.

Behavior shaped through positive reinforcement alone is reliable only to the extent that the dog is willing to work for the rewards offered by the trainer. In the case of food and petting, this readiness fluctuates widely depending on the dog's motivational state. Another important factor affecting the reliability of behavior shaped through positive reinforcement is the influence of extraneous contingencies of reinforcement (see *Distractions: Competing Sources of Reward*). For instance, a dog might find chasing a squirrel into the street much more intrinsically rewarding and immediately gratifying than anything the owner has to entice it to stay or to come. In this example, the opportunity to chase a squir-

rel may be more exciting and reinforcing than rewards controlled by the trainer (e.g., petting, food, and play). The learning theorist E. R. Guthrie (1938/1962) has nicely summarized some of the more important elements and pitfalls of recall training:

> A careful trainer follows the instructions to be found in an army manual: Never give a command that you do not expect to be obeyed. The reason for this is, of course, that a command that is followed by disobedience becomes an associative cue for the disobedient action. To train a dog to come when his name is called, the dog must first be induced to come. This can be done in various ways, and it is in his knowledge of these ways that the man who knows dogs shows his superiority. But whether he shows the dog food, or pulls the dog toward him with a check line, or starts away and trusts the dog to follow, it is the repetition of the name as the dog starts to approach that establishes the name as a cue for approach … To undo this training all that need be done is for the trainer to do as many owners do, call the dog's name while he is preoccupied with something else, or just as the dog starts off to chase a car, or in any circumstances in which the dog could not be expected to obey promptly. The name then becomes a cue for this particular form of disobedience and loses all its drawing power. (41)

Guthrie's observations are reminiscent of Thoreau's pithy journal comment: "When a dog runs at you, whistle for him." As a general rule, a trainer should never call a dog unless confident that the dog will comply or, if it fails to respond as expected, the trainer has adequate means at his or her disposal to ensure compliance. Calling the dog when one is uncertain of its compliance flirts with introducing a highly undesirable lesson, training the dog that it can sometimes escape the obligation to come when called, especially when under the influence of a highly motivational state. Ultimately, such training may teach the dog that the vocal signal "Come" signals an exciting opportunity for it to safely run away. Also, the trainer should avoid misusing the dog's name as a recall signal or reprimand. In obedience training, the dog's name should be used only to capture and control its attention—not as an alternative recall signal (Table 1.3).

TABLE. 1.3. Common activities that are counterproductive for reliable recall habits

Avoid chasing or cornering a dog that refuses to come. No advantage is derived from this effort, except perhaps in an emergency situation where no other alternative is available.

Never punish a dog that finally comes after at first hesitating or refusing to come when called.

Avoid calling a dog unless it is virtually certain that the dog will comply or that appropriate means are available to enforce the command should the dog fail to comply.

Avoid bribing or threatening. Whereas bribes reinforce the undesirable behaviors that prompt the bribes in the first place, threats are doubly inappropriate: they remove any positive incentive for the dog to come while at the same time revealing that the owner is unable to deliver on threats, so long as the dog remains at a distance.

Avoid repeating commands: repeating commands tends to associate the signal with behavior incompatible with coming when called. When running off, a dog is typically running toward something that is more rewarding at the moment than the owner. Calling a dog to come at such times may only serve to train the dog to run away on cue.

Whenever possible, avoid calling a dog from a highly rewarding activity to a less rewarding one.

One of the most challenging problems faced during off-leash training is training dogs to desist from running off after moving distractions, such as cars, bicyclists, runners, wildlife, or other dogs (see *Distractions: Extraneous Sources of Reward*). In addition to inhibitory training, proofing a dog while around such sources of stimulation is achieved through graduated exposure and counterconditioning—objectives that are facilitated by making use of a long line (see *Leash and Long Line*). The 30- to 50-foot long lines help to approximate off-leash conditions without totally relinquishing control over the dog. The dog should be given a certain fixed *search limit* that it must learn to avoid exceeding by turning back or by waiting for the trainer to approach from behind. The behavior of following, moving out, turning, and coming back (the search chain) is an innate tendency in most dogs. However, dogs not exposed to off-leash walks early in life may not show search-chain behavior, possibly because some window of opportunity or sensitive period for its expression passed in the absence of appropriate allelomimetic stimulation. In any case, as the dog reaches the limit of its range, the trainer should call its name (perhaps whistling or clapping if necessary to draw the dog's attention). Just as the dog turns, the trainer clicks and calls the dog by saying "Come" (see *Introductory Lessons*). At this point, running backward, crouching, or clapping may help to

increase the dog's willingness to come. If the dog comes, it is rewarded with a variable food reward delivered from a closed hand, affectionately praised, and released immediately with an enthusiastic "OK" and hand clap. On the occasion of some successful trials, the trainer can toss the dog a ball, play tug, prompt it to jump up, or engage it in playful roughhousing. In the case of dogs that enjoy ball play, the ball can be thrown to the dog at different points in the performance of the recall sequence (as soon as the dog steps toward the trainer, after taking five steps, and so forth). The ball can also be thrown immediately after the dog alerts to its name or as it is released from a halt-stay at a distance. If the dog fails to come, it is prompted to "Stay!" whereupon the long line is stamped on to stop the dog from advancing farther. During the walk, a ball or stick is occasionally thrown for the dog to retrieve. If the dog attempts to bolt away or refuses to return with the object, the long line is used to block the behavior and to condition a halt-stay response. Since coming is consistently followed by reward and release, dogs appear gradually to acquire an expectation that returning to the trainer not only helps to extend the time they get to walk freely, but is also associated with a significant amount of reward in the form of affection, food, and play.

Orienting is nine-tenths of the act of coming, and many dogs can be successfully trained to come by means of reward-based incentives and intensive conditioning of the orienting response. A significant population of dogs cannot be trained to a reliable off-leash criterion of control by reward-based means alone. Many of these dogs can be rapidly trained to come when in the safety of a backyard or when walked on a long line; however, this control does not evenly transfer to situations where the dog is off leash and exposed to competing sources of reward. Training can be additionally transferred by slowly and painstakingly fading the long line, but such efforts are ultimately confounded and slowly degraded by competing environmental rewards whose occurrence or nonoccurrence are not yet under the trainer's control. Although the dog can be taken to the very threshold of a reliable recall via expert and conscientious reward-based training efforts by integrating many sources of environmental reward, the process is ultimately dashed on the wall of a stubborn reality: reward-based behavioral control is only as good as the trainer's ability to control environmental rewards. The success of long-line training is based largely on its ability to block behavior seeking the gratification of competing sources of reward.

Although competing control modules and routines established by the rewards presented or withheld by the trainer can help, many

sources of environmental reward occur independently of the trainer's direction and remain a constant threat to control efforts. Since most extraneous environmental contingencies remain as they were before training was commenced, the dog's behavior relative to those contingencies remains largely intact—a fact that the trainer and dog quickly discover when the long line is finally removed. Essentially, the training process has provided the trainer with a valuable foundation of enhanced control with which to manage the dog in the context of uncontrolled sources of environmental reward. Such management is not equivalent to a recall and a halt-stay response. The recall and halt-stay responses must function reliably to control potentially dangerous or harmful behavior operating in the presence of extraneous sources of reward (e.g., bolting out of doors, charging after bicycles, cars, and passersby, or chasing other animals), not simply manage it (see *Electrical Stimulation and Chasing Behavior* in Chapter 9). Traditionally, the transition from management to recall and halt-stay control was achieved by fading the long line while at the same time introducing a variety of remote inhibitory control devices. Throw rings can be useful for this purpose: they are relatively safe and have a distinctive sound that is not easily confused with other common sounds (Figure 1.22). Unfortunately, the use of throw rings and similar tools for proofing off-leash recall is something of an art, perhaps a dying one, that requires significant skill and experience to pull off successfully. In addition to the necessity of good timing skills, the trainer must be able to throw such things with a high degree of accuracy. Few average dog owners possess the necessary skills for using throw tools properly. In any case, with the advent of sophisticated remote-activated electronic collars, proofing recall and halt-stay with throw tools is rapidly becoming an obsolete practice (see *Recall Enhancement* in Chapter 9). Electrical collars can significantly reduce many problems associated with off-leash control in a rapid and humane manner. To optimize the effectiveness of electronic training and reduce the possibility of adverse side effects, preliminary reward-based recall and halt-stay training should be thoroughly

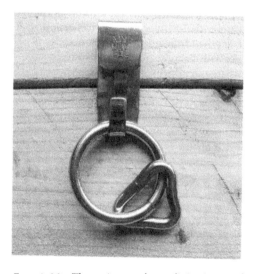

FIG. 1.22. Throw-rings produce a distinctive sound that is useful for establishing off-leash control.

carried out beforehand. Dogs that have undergone such preliminary training usually require very little electrical prompting to make the recall and halt-stay responses significantly more reliable. Finally, the goal of electronic training should be to produce an opportunity for additional reward-based training and safe exposure to the many quality-of-life-enhancing activities made possible by means of establishing off-leash control.

REFERENCES

Aston-Jones G, Rajkowski J, and Cohen J (1999). Role of locus coeruleus in attention and behavioral flexibility. *Biol Psychiatry*, 46:1309–1320.

Baker MA and Chapman LW (1977). Rapid brain cooling in exercising dogs. *Science*, 195:781–783.

Braff L, Geyer MA, and Swerdlow NR (2001). Human studies of prepulse inhibition of startles: Normal subjects, patient groups and pharmacological studies. *Psychopharmacology*, 156:234–258

DeGroot A (1985). K-9 Kumalong: A quantum leap for Irish wolfhound and owner. *Ir Wolfhound Q*, 8:28, 30–32, 34.

Delta Society (2001). *Professional Standards for Dog Trainers: Effective, Humane Principles.* http://www.deltasociety.org/standards/toc.htm.

Dickinson A and Pearce JM (1977). Inhibitory interactions between appetitive and aversive stimuli. *Psychol Bull*, 84:690–711.

Egger DM and Miller NE (1962). Secondary reinforcement in rats as a function of information value and reliability of the stimulus. *J Exp Psychol*, 64:99–104.

Egger DM and Miller NE (1963). When is a reward reinforcing? An experimental study of the information hypothesis. *J Comp Physiol Psychol*, 56:132–137.

Gray JA (1991). The neuropsychology of temperament. In J Strelau and A Angleitner (Eds), *Explorations in Temperament: International Perspectives on Theory and Measurement.* London: Plenum.

Guthrie ER (1938/1962). *The Psychology of Human Conflict: The Clash of Motives Within the Individual.* New York: Harper and Brothers (reprint).

Hassani OK, Cromwell HC, and Schultz W (2001). Influence of expectation of different rewards on behavior-related activity in the striatum. *J Neurophysiol*, 85:2477–2489.

Haug LI, Beaver BV, and Longnecker MT (2002). Comparison of dog's reaction to four different head collars. *Appl Anim Behav Sci*, 79:53–61.

Hediger H (1955/1968). *The Psychology and Behavior of Animals in Zoos and Circuses*, G Sircom (Trans). New York: Dover (reprint).

Hobbes T (1651/1994). Chapter 2: Of Imagination. In *Leviathan*. Indianapolis, IN: Hackett (reprint).

Iwata B, Smith RG, and Michael J (2000). Current research on the influence of establishing operations on behavior in applied settings. *J Appl Behav Anal*, 33:411–418.

Kaminski J, Call J, and Fischer J (2004). Word learning in a domestic dog: Evidence for "fast mapping." *Science*, 304:1682–1683.

Koch M (1999). The neurobiology of startle. *Prog Neurobiol*, 59:107–128.

Kostarczyk E (1991). The use of dog-human interaction as a reward in instrumental conditioning and its impact on dogs' cardiac regulation. In H Davis and D Balfour (Eds), *The Inevitable Bond: Examining Scientist-Animal Interactions.* Cambridge: Cambridge University Press.

Marder A and Reid PJ (1996). Treating canine behavior problems: Behavior modification, obedience, and agility training. In VL Voith and PL Borchelt (Eds), *Readings in Companion Animal Behavior.* Trenton, NJ: Veterinary Learning Systems.

McGill P (1999). Establishing operations: Implications for the assessment, treatment, and prevention of problem behavior. *J Appl Behav Anal*, 32:393–418.

McKinley J and Sambrook TD (2000). Use of human-given cues by domestic dogs (*Canis familiaris*) and horses (*Equus caballus*). *Anim Cognit*, 3:13–22.

Michael J (2000). Implications and refinements of the establishing operation concept. *J Appl Behav Anal*, 33:401–410.

Miklósi Á, Polgárdi R, Topál J, and Csányi V (1998). Use of experimenter-given cues in dogs. *Anim Cognit*, 1:113–121.

Ogburn P, Crouse S, Martin F, and Houpt K (1998). Comparison of behavioral and physiological responses of dogs wearing two different types of collars. *Appl Anim Behav Sci*, 61:133–142.

Pavlov IP (1927/1960). *Conditioned Reflexes: An Investigation of the Physiological Activity of the Cerebral Cortex*, GV Anrep (Trans). New York: Dover (reprint).

Pryor K (1985). *Don't Shoot the Dog: The New Art of Teaching and Training.* New York: Bantam.

Rescorla RA and Solomon RL (1967). Two-process learning theory: Relationship between Pavlovian conditioning and instrumental learning. *Psychol Rev*, 74:151–182.

Roberts WA (2002). Are animals stuck in time? *Psychol Bull*, 128:473–489.

Rolls ET (2000). Precis of *The Brain and Emotion*. *Behav Brain Sci*, 23:177–234.

Ryon CJ (1977). Den digging and related behavior in a captive timber wolf pack. *J Mammal*, 58:87–89.

Sanders CR (1999). *Understanding Dogs: Living and Working with Canine Companions*. Philadelphia: Temple University Press.

Schultz W (1998). Predictive reward signal of dopamine neurons. *J Neurophysiol*, 80:1–27.

Schultz W and Dickinson A (2000). Neuronal coding of prediction errors. *Annu Rev Neurosci*, 23:473–500.

Skinner BF (1951). How to teach animals. *Sci Am*, 185:26–29.

Tortora DF (1980). Applied animal psychology: The practical implications of comparative analysis. In MR Denny (Ed), *Comparative Psychology: An Evolutionary Analysis of Animal Behavior*. New York: John Wiley and Sons.

Trumler E (1973). *Your Dog and You*. New York: Seabury.

Voith VL (1977a). Aggressive behavior and dominance. *Canine Pract*, 4:11–15.

Voith VL (1977b). Sit-stay program (client handout). Animal Behavior Clinic, University of Pennsylvania, Philadelphia.

Waelti P, Dickinson A, and Schultz W (2001). Dopamine responses comply with basic assumptions of formal learning theory. *Nature*, 412:43–48.

Warden CJ and Warner LH (1928). The sensory capacity and intelligence of dogs, with a report on the ability of the noted dog "Fellow" to respond to verbal stimuli. *Q Rev Biol*, 3:1–28

Whitney LF (1961). *Dog Psychology: The Basis of Dog Training*. New York: Howell Book House.

Whitney LF (1963). *The Natural Method of Dog Training*. New York: M Evans.

Wyrwicka W (1975). The sensory nature of reward in instrumental behavior. *Pavlovian J Biol Sci*, 10:23–51.

House Training, Destructive Behavior, and Appetitive Problems

PART 1: HOUSE TRAINING

Adult elimination problems represent a significant source of distress for both owners and dogs. Not surprisingly, incomplete house training is the leading cause given by dog owners for relinquishing their dogs to the uncertain fate of the animal shelter (Salman et al., 2000), underscoring the importance of preventing and resolving house-training problems. Elimination problems are the result of a variety of causes, each requiring specific training programs to ensure effective control or management (see *Common Elimination Problems* in Volume 2, Chapter 9). The leading cause of household elimination problems, however, is improper or incomplete house training (Voith and Borchelt, 1985; Yeon et al., 1999). The majority of household elimination problems can be prevented with appropriate and effective house-training efforts begun at an early age. In general, adult dogs exhibiting improper, incomplete, or unlearned house-training habits are treated in much the same way as puppies, until they are back on track.

HOUSE-TRAINING BASICS

The two primary goals of house training are to prevent the occurrence of elimination in the house while at the same time encouraging puppies to eliminate outdoors. Prevention depends on confinement or careful supervision while the puppy is moving about in the house. The importance of confinement and close supervision cannot be overemphasized. Keeping a record of house-training activities provides a useful source of objective feedback concerning a puppy's progress. Tracking daily house-training progress is especially useful in situations where a number of family members share house-training responsibilities (Figure 2.1). The chart allows others to see at a glance whether the puppy or dog has been taken out recently. The center column is used to indicate the number of accidents that occurred during the day, showing precisely how well things are going or not.

Confinement and Supervision

Effective house training depends on a combination of constructive confinement, diligent supervision, scheduled feeding, and the provision of adequate opportunities to eliminate outdoors. Several methods of confinement are used, including a loose leash, a crate or crate-holding pen combination, and tie-out stations. Crate confinement is particularly useful for initiating preventative restraint; however, as is discussed later in this chapter, excessive crate confinement may inadvertently produce significant adverse side effects. Over reliance on crate confinement may also interfere with effective house training by preventing a puppy from learning to generalize its training to the whole house. To optimize such generalization, a puppy should be exposed to all parts of the house while under influence of varying types and degrees of restraint, depending on its abilities. An easy way to accomplish this daily exposure is to walk the puppy around the house on leash or by teth-

ering at various locations (tie-out stations) in the house. Tie-out stations consist of a length of braided nylon rope with a head loop and slide for easy fitting and removal. The puppy can be tethered in various ways, such as tying it to a piece of heavy furniture, knotting and slipping the rope under a closed door, or tying it to an eyehook screwed into molding. Initially, the length of tether should be approximately the sum of the puppy's height at the withers plus the distance from its nose to the base of its tail. Care should be taken to make sure that the puppy cannot become entangled in the tether or wrapped around something. Also, the tie-out station should not be close to valuable carpeting, furniture, or woodwork, since a puppy may chew while restrained. A blanket and toys that cannot roll away should be given to the puppy whenever it is tethered. As the puppy's reliability improves, the length of the tether can be gradually increased and finally eliminated via a fading procedure.

Although excessive crate confinement and isolation is not constructive, neither is letting a puppy run around the house unsupervised before it is ready for such freedom. In addition to inhibiting elimination, tethering offers several benefits that recommend its use. Unlike crate confinement, tethering provides more opportunities for the puppy to have close contact with family members while restrained. In addition to preventing inappropriate elimination, such restraint limits the amount of trouble the puppy can get into, thereby maximizing positive attention and socialization while helping to minimize punitive interaction. In the case of overly active or competitive puppies, tethering permits children to escape from mouthing and jumping excesses by simply scooting back out of the puppy's reach. Tethering also helps to constrain undesirable chewing activity by limiting it to appropriate chew toys left within the puppy's reach. Since tethering is frustrating for puppies, objects provided at such a time may acquire a preferential association as chew toys at times of increased frustration and emotional tension—an effect that may help to reduce destructive chewing later on when the dog is given more freedom to move about in the house.

Most accidents can be prevented if puppies are kept under careful observation and proper supervision. The owner should be instructed to watch for telltale signs both in body language and facial expression that have occurred in the past just prior to eliminating. Various signs can be used to predict and prevent future accidents (e.g., movement toward areas

		AM				**PM**			
	Location	**Time**	**U**	**D**	**Total No. Accidents**	**Location**	**Time**	**U**	**D**
M									
	FEEDING:					FEEDING:			
T									
	FEEDING:					FEEDING:			
W									
	FEEDING:					FEEDING:			
T									
	FEEDING:					FEEDING:			
F									
	FEEDING:					FEEDING:			
S									
	FEEDING:					FEEDING:			
S									
	FEEDING:					FEEDING:			
COMMENTS:									

Above table titled: **HOUSE-TRAINING CHART**

FIG. 2.1. House-training chart.

that have been soiled in the past, sniffing and circling, whining when restrained by crate or tether).

There are various times when puppies are most likely to eliminate:

> After awaking
> After bouts of play
> After any form of excitement
> After eating or drinking and again 20 to 30 minutes later
> After a significant period without eliminating

With diligent house training, most puppies can learn to eliminate outdoors with very few accidents. If a puppy is having several accidents every day, it is probably not the puppy's ability that needs to be improved, but the owner's supervisory efforts that need modification. When the occasional accident does occur, the owner should be prepared to respond appropriately and immediately to minimize adverse learning effects (see *Classical and Instrumental Learning* in Volume 2, Chapter 9). Elimination habits are under the influence of both instrumental and classical conditioning (Skinner, 1968), requiring careful attention to ensure that the behavior is brought under the control of appropriate environmental stimuli and reinforcement contingencies. Since the act of elimination is intrinsically negatively reinforcing for a puppy, allowing the puppy to eliminate in the house without a countervailing aversive consequence is tantamount to rewarding it.

Inhibitory stimulation should be sufficient to disrupt urination momentarily, but not so strong as to cause the puppy to become fearful or run away. For most puppies, an abrupt vocal shout combined with a clap or stomp on the floor is adequate to get the impression across. However, some puppies may require a stronger treatment involving the toss of some light object (e.g., a fluttering magazine) to instill a lasting impression. Whatever method is selected, it is critical that the puppy be caught in the act and then immediately rushed outdoors to finish it. Having the puppy on leash facilitates this movement outdoors. As the puppy is directed through the doorway, the owner's voice and manner should shift to a cajoling and encouraging

tone, thereby causing the puppy to relax and finish the act outside. To improve the likelihood that the puppy will finish the elimination outdoors, it is imperative to catch the puppy at the earliest sequence in the act, ideally during preparatory or intentional movements. Although disrupter-type stimulation is appropriate and useful, excessive punishment should be avoided. Punishment causing a puppy significant discomfort or fear could cause it to overly generalize the event, thereby not only inhibiting elimination indoors, but possibly reducing the puppy's willingness to eliminate outdoors in the owner's presence, as well. A surprisingly large number of dog owners still believe that rubbing a puppy's nose in its mess is a helpful house-training deterrent. In a study involving people that had relinquished their dogs to an animal shelter, nearly 32% of those responding (N = 1947) believed that it was helpful to rub a dog's nose in its mess, with an additional 11.4% indicating that they did not know whether it was beneficial or not (New et al., 2000). Finally, retroactive punishment should be eschewed as an abusive misuse of punishment.

Placement Preference and Cleanup

Although the odor of previously deposited urine may act as an elimination cue, the importance of scent is often exaggerated, overshadowing other, perhaps more important, environmental cues affecting placement preferences. Actually, odor is one of many environmental cues informing placement preferences; others include habitual context and location, substrate, and remoteness from other basic biological functions (e.g., eating and sleeping). A poorly supervised puppy may urinate dozens of times throughout the house before the problem is finally recognized and brought under control, leaving many soiled areas undiscovered and uncleaned. Despite the presence of numerous indoor scent cues, once trained to eliminate outdoors puppies are rarely attracted back to these previously used and scented areas, suggesting that factors other than smell may be of greater importance in the development of placement preferences. Scent cues appear to play a much more significant role in the control of adult elimination patterns and urine marking. Some practitioners recommend the use of black lights, moisture-detecting probes, and biological dyes to find hidden urine spots, noting that, unless such spots are discovered, house-training efforts will be frustrated. In addition, high-tech, enzyme-activated chemical odor eaters are used to attack these attractants soaked into carpeting, ostensibly perpetuating marking behavior in adult dogs (see *Household Urine-marking Problems* in Volume 2, Chapter 9).

Cleanup after accidents should be thorough to reduce unpleasant odors and potential damage to carpeting and flooring. Rather than rubbing the urine deeper into the carpet, the key to proper cleanup is to first dilute and extract the urine. The first step is to get as much urine out of carpeting as possible. Paper balls, which make excellent disposable sponges for soaking up urine spots, are made by firmly wading together several sheets of newspaper into several softball-sized balls. In addition, these newspaper balls should be covered with a few sheets of paper toweling to protect carpeting from the ink on newspaper. As soon as an accident occurs, these paper sponges are used to extract urine by stepping and rocking on them. To dilute and further remove urine, a quarter cup of warm water is poured into the spot and then similarly sponged up. Finally, a solution of warm water and baking soda is poured onto the soiled area. The solution (one-quarter teaspoon of baking soda to one-quarter cup of warm water) is left to soak into the carpet for a minute or two and then thoroughly sponged out and allowed to dry overnight. When dry, the carpet can be gently brushed and vacuumed, leaving it clean and free of odor. The common practice of using vinegar should be avoided. Vinegar is particularly hazardous in the case of fine rugs. When exposed to sunlight, the acid in vinegar may produce a photochemical reaction with sunlight, causing sensitive carpet dyes to fade or discolor.

After the spot is cleaned and dry, a tie-out station can be set up nearby and the puppy restrained there for 15 to 20 minutes during the same time of day that the accident occurred. The puppy can be fed, massaged, trained, and played with over the spot. Also,

the owner can seed the area with biscuits and allow the puppy to discover and eat them over the spot. A scent (e.g., an orange) associated with the puppy's crate can also be applied to the area. The goal of such training is to establish a number of associations with the area that are incompatible with the urge to eliminate, thereby replacing the expectations and preparatory sequences leading to elimination with those leading to the acquisition of food, toys, relaxation, and so forth.

House-training Schedule

A critical aspect of successful house training is the scheduling of meals and elimination opportunities so that they occur on a regular basis. Whenever possible, the puppy should be permitted to sleep in a bedroom. Initially, it may be necessary to confine the puppy to a crate placed next to the bed or tethered to a tie-out station. Before the puppy is confined for the night, it should be taken outside two or three times to give sufficient opportunity to evacuate fully. Giving the puppy a 10- or 15-minute walk before bedtime is a good habit for the owner to establish and maintain into adulthood. In any case, the owner should be prepared for the possibility of an early wake up, especially for the first week or two of house training. Whining in the middle of the night often signifies that a puppy is distressed by a need to eliminate. It is important for the owner to respond, but at the same time to push forward the puppy's biological clock steadily so that the puppy gradually learns to make it through the night. Instead of immediately responding, the owner should wait for a brief period before taking the puppy outside. During the first week or two, the puppy is progressively required to wait for longer periods until it can make it through the night. As the puppy's reliability improves, demonstrated by consistently making it through the night for at least 2 or 3 weeks, it can be gradually given more freedom to move about in the bedroom.

In the morning, the puppy should be taken to the same general location and vocally prompted to eliminate, using a voice signal previously paired with the act of eliminating. As the training process progresses, the puppy should be encouraged to eliminate in different locations near and away from home, thus preventing the behavior from becoming overly contextualized to particular substrates and locations. When the puppy finally performs, it is rewarded with vocal encouragement and praise. Food rewards are usually not given to reward eliminatory behavior directly, but may be presented following defecation, especially if a puppy is coprophagous. Although elimination is intrinsically reinforcing, it is useful to provide additional social-positive reinforcement to counteract the generalized effects of punishment used to discourage elimination indoors. If a puppy fails to eliminate outdoors, it should be taken back inside and tethered or crated and taken out again after 15 to 20 minutes.

The length of time spent outside should be carefully controlled, with each outing not to exceed 1 to 3 minutes. Most puppies usually eliminate within the first minute after going outside. Instead of spending long periods of unproductive time walking and waiting for a puppy to eliminate, time outdoors is more efficiently used by giving the puppy several brief opportunities rather than one or two long ones. In the morning, most young puppies require three or four closely spaced opportunities outdoors to evacuate bowel and bladder fully:

> Immediately after waking
> Immediately after eating
> 20 to 30 minutes after eating
> Again in association with outdoor play

During the day, multiple outings should be scheduled around feeding times. Between feeding times, puppies should be kept under close supervision or confinement, thereby preventing elimination from occurring inside the house. The average maximum length of time that a puppy should be expected to hold between daytime outings is calculated by dividing its age in weeks by 3. For example, an average 12-week-old puppy should be expected to hold for a maximum of 4 hours, with some puppies showing more or less control of elimination functions. Although some puppies are able to hold for longer periods, it may be stressful or unhealthful for them to do so. Initially, to minimize accidents, puppies

should be taken out on a frequent basis (e.g., every 45 to 60 minutes) to establish the desired habit, gradually lengthening the period between outings to approximate the average age-appropriate limit. In addition to scheduled brief outings, two or more daily walks should be scheduled together with play sessions and positive training activities. Although requiring a puppy to hold for excessively long periods between outings should be avoided, giving the puppy too many opportunities to go outside may prevent it from acquiring appropriate eliminatory inhibitions. The crucial goal is to train the puppy to hold in response to internal elimination signals. Puppies that are taken out too often may not acquire this aspect of house training, but instead learn to respond to such internal cues as signals to eliminate or defecate. Not only must puppies learn to defer elimination to appropriate times and place, they must also learn to cope with the mild discomfort of holding a filled bladder or bowel.

Along these lines, teaching puppies to give a signal to go outside is a common, but questionable, house-training practice. While appearing reasonable and useful at first glance, encouraging puppies to give such signals may conflict with the objective of training them to hold and eliminate in accordance with an arbitrary schedule. Again, effective bowel and bladder control require that puppies learn to endure some amount of discomfort—an aspect of house training that is not necessarily served by training puppies to perform a signal to get outdoors on demand. Furthermore, such need-to-go signals depend on the owner being present to respond—a state of affairs that can rarely be maintained on a consistent basis. An unfortunate outcome of such training is the development of common elimination problems later. Unable to get the owner's attention with the elimination-need signal, a dog may go to the door and after a moment just turn around and eliminate nearby or run off to another room before eliminating, thereby reflecting the pattern previously established in association with the need-to-go signal, viz., give signal and then eliminate. Finally, many puppies rapidly learn to extend and generalize the need-to-go signal into a need-to-whatever-whenever signal, prompting the owner to go outside for purposes other than the dog's elimination. Such puppies learn that barking or pawing at bells can get them outside for play and other activities having nothing to do with elimination.

To prevent problems, the prospective dog owner should plan to take a two-week vacation to coincide with the puppy's arrival in the home to get the house-training process on track and perform other training activities. The owner should also plan to come home at lunch to feed and exercise the puppy for several additional weeks, if possible. Alternatively, a dog walker might be hired to take the puppy outside during the day. These and many other practical issues should be carefully considered before getting a puppy.

COMMON HOUSE-TRAINING PROBLEMS

The vast majority of puppies learn to eliminate outdoors on schedule with little difficulty. Most common house-training problems are the result of the following:

> Fear
> Distraction
> Weather or surface aversions
> Inappropriate interactive punishment
> Improper house training

Fearful puppies that refuse to eliminate outdoors and prefer instead to eliminate after going back inside should receive appropriate behavior therapy consisting of graduated habituation and counterconditioning efforts. Puppies exhibiting specific fears should be exercised in locations away from fear-eliciting stimuli and only gradually exposed to such stimulation in association with counterconditioning. Fearful puppies should be provided with supplementary activities that promote feelings of safety and relaxation when outdoors (e.g., play and reward-based training). Overly active and inquisitive puppies may be excessively distracted by the novelty and excitement of being outdoors and fail to eliminate in a timely manner while on walks. Such puppies should be consistently taken to a familiar spot where exploratory interests have been habituated and only permitted to explore after eliminating (Borchelt, 1984). Puppies that refuse to eliminate as the result of weather changes or surface aversions should be provided with a surfaced area that is acceptable to them or taken to spots that are protected from the weather. Puppies should be gradually exposed to varying surfaces and weather changes to improve their willingness to eliminate. Rather than constraining its options, a puppy should be allowed to choose it spots, thereby facilitating more rapid habituation and willingness to eliminate in a timely manner. Walking the puppy to a remote part of the yard or requiring that it eliminate within a small area should be avoided, especially in puppies showing signs of inhibition about eliminating outdoors. Occasionally, as the result of inappropriate interactive punishment, the puppy may become anxious about eliminating in the presence of the owner, regardless of location, preferring to hide when back inside. In such cases, the punitive interaction should be discontinued and the puppy allowed to range away to a safe distance when taken outdoors. In addition to vocal encouragement, such puppies should be given food rewards or play after eliminating outdoors. Puppies that fail to eliminate outdoors should be taken back inside after 3 minutes and kept under close supervision on leash for 15 to 20 minutes (or longer depending on age and need) before being taken out again. This pattern is repeated until the puppy finally eliminates.

Dogs that habitually eliminate in the crate pose a significant problem (see *Elimination in the Owner's Absence* in Volume 2, Chapter 9). In cases were the behavior occurs overnight or at other times when the owner is present, increased opportunities to go outdoors may help to get the dog back on track and encourage better control. Sometimes simply making the crate smaller by inserting a divider can be helpful. However, in some cases, dogs may have simply lost their capacity to hold, perhaps as the result of repeated exposure to crate confinement exceeding their ability to hold. As a result, instead of holding in response to bladder signals, such dogs may simply learn to let go and urinate, often responding to progressively earlier signals in the sequence in advance of any significant discomfort associated with the holding effort. In other cases, the puppy may simply not exhibit sufficient inhibitory control over urinary sphincters to hold for long. Training such dogs to hold in the crate may require the use of a urine-activated alarm, giving the dog immediate feedback whenever it eliminates in the crate. The alarm consists of a moisture detector (available at most hardware stores) attached to quarter-inch cooper adhesive tape applied to a plastic crate tray (Figure 2.2). Two lines of tape are laid in parallel to each other so that a spiral form is made covering most of the tray surface. The tray is covered with a thick, open-weave blanket or a pegboard, allowing urine to run through and make contact with the copper tape. Now whenever the dog urinates a circuit is completed causing the moisture detector to activate an alarm that has been fastened to the inside of a plastic cup and appropriately muffled to match the auditory sensitivity of the dog. This arrangement is only suitable for use when the owner is at home or

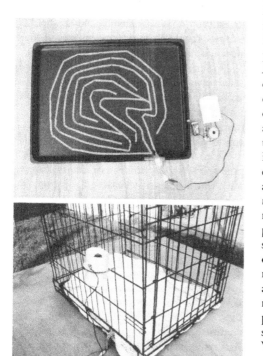

FIG. 2.2. Moisture-detector alarm.

at bedtime, providing the owner with a signal while at the same time helping to inhibit urination in midstream. Such devices do not automatically reset and need to be manually switched off and urine wiped off the copper strips, making them unsuitable for dogs that are left alone in their crates.

Another frequent source of house-training problems is preliminary paper training. Depending on the procedure used, paper training often violates both of the central imperatives of house training by allowing puppies to eliminate at will while indoors, albeit on papers or thereabouts. Owners often mistakenly choose the paper-training option to make the process easier for puppies and more convenient for themselves. A common adult elimination problem stemming from paper training is the tendency of some dogs thus trained to refuse to eliminate while on walks or when released outdoors, but instead waiting until they get back inside to eliminate—papers or no papers. Frustrated owners of such dogs are often at a loss to understand the origin of the behavior until the logic behind it is explored. Such dogs are performing in a manner consistent with the training that they received during an impressionable period of development for such learning. Although paper training is justified in the case of owners living in high-rise apartments or ones having disabilities or health problems, otherwise paper training should be discouraged. Of course, the temporary use of papers to protect flooring may be necessary if a puppy is left in a holding pen during the day. But even such stopgaps can result in problems such as the one just described, especially if such methods are used in an excessive and habitual manner. If the owner elects to paper train a puppy, the process should be performed in the same way as training the puppy to eliminate outdoors. Access to the papers should be restricted and allowed only in accordance with an appropriate house-training schedule. In most cases, efforts should be made to train the puppy to also use the outdoors, just in case such behavior becomes necessary in the future. Whenever possible, the first elimination in the morning should be performed outdoors to facilitate this dual training. Far from being easier, paper training, when properly performed, requires just as much, if not more, dedication to achieve reliable control over the placement of elimination.

PART 2: DESTRUCTIVE BEHAVIOR IN PUPPIES

A common reason for seeking canine behavioral advice is destructive behavior. All puppies and dogs engage in varying amounts of exploratory and manipulative behaviors that may become misdirected into destructive activities (Figure 2.3). The problem is not chewing or digging per se, but rather chewing and digging activity that is inappropriately directed toward valuable personal belongings or things that may be dangerous to the dog. The goal of counseling and behavioral training in such cases is sixfold: (1) increase the owner's understanding of why dogs chew and dig, (2) identify evoking situations and contributory causes (e.g., separation distress, attention seeking, and insufficient exercise), (3) stress the importance of supervision and confinement, (4) discuss appropriate outlets for chewing and digging activities (e.g., chew toys and digging area), (5) discuss and demonstrate various techniques for discouraging destructive activities, and (6) provide basic training.

Puppies possess a need for a significant amount of daily chewing. Chewing provides stimulation and exploratory outlets, psychological benefits, metabolic (e.g., it elicits

insulin secretion) and digestive effects, and a variety of homeostatic functions. Under the influence of adverse emotional arousal (e.g., barrier frustration) and inadequate exercise and social stimulation, chewing and digging activities may become exaggerated and problematic. As in the case of many other behavior problems, prevention is the key to the successful control of destructive behavior. Keeping puppies under a watchful eye and guiding their oral activities into appropriate outlets help them to develop habits incompatible with destructiveness. Strategic crate and pen confinement, tie-out stations, and leashing puppies help to reduce the likelihood that they will chew on forbidden items. Young dogs require a significant amount of social stimulation and opportunities to play, explore, and manipulate the environment with their mouths and feet. Playing various toy-oriented games (e.g., fetch, tug, and hide-and-seek) with puppies helps establish a durable preference for the toys used during such activities. Finally, puppies benefit from daily training activities consisting of following exercises, coming when called, sitting, lying down, and staying. All of these exercises can be introduced at an early age. Such training helps to improve puppies' attention and impulse control abilities, as well as enhancing their responsiveness to vocal control and direction.

ASSESSING AND CONTROLLING DESTRUCTIVE BEHAVIOR

Excessive oral activity may indicate a medical problem requiring veterinary attention. In cases involving abnormal destructive behavior and pica, a veterinary examination should be performed to exclude possible physiological causes. A general history and daily activity profile should be explored with the owner, including

Amount and type of exercise
Amount and type of play activities
Length and place of confinement

In addition, the trainer should obtain specific information about the objects chewed, the time of day when chewing is most likely to occur, and the various efforts already

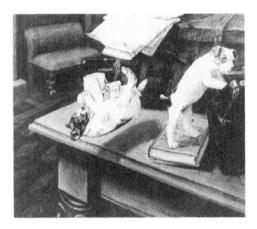

FIG. 2.3. Puppies at play (John Hayes, 19th century).

attempted to control the problem (e.g., restraint, punishment, repellents, and so forth).

SELECTING APPROPRIATE CHEW ITEMS

Once an oral attraction is established, it may persist into adulthood and become very difficult to control or suppress. Consequently, it is important to encourage puppies to adopt an acceptable chewing pattern at an early age while they are most impressionable and receptive to such learning (see *Development of Exploratory Behavior* in Volume 1, Chapter 2). In addition to directing oral activities toward acceptable items, it is important consistently to discourage chewing directed toward forbidden household items. In addition to not being easily generalized and confused with forbidden items, a chew toy should meet three basic criteria: (1) it must maintain the puppy's interest, (2) it must sustain active hard chewing without being easily destroyed or eaten, and (3) it should not evoke guarding behavior. Although a nylon bone may satisfy criteria 2 and 3, it is not likely to be among a puppy's first choices in terms of attractiveness. A nylon toy can be made more appealing by drilling several small holes into it that are filled with cheese or peanut butter. Rawhide chew toys, while much more taste appealing, may not last very long, and many puppies may become overly possessive over them. Rawhide chew toys are better if they are slightly oversized and rolled, rather than knotted at the end. Despite the dire warnings in the trade literature to the contrary, rawhide chew toys are relatively safe for most puppies, but such toys may be inappropriate for dogs and puppies that chew through them too quickly. Rawhide toys are particularly appropriate after meals as aids in keeping the puppies teeth clean and facilitating digestion. After 20 to 30 minutes, the toys can be taken up and allowed to dry out between meals. Hollow rubber toys can be made more attractive by smearing peanut butter inside of them. Such toys can be safely left with a puppy when it is left alone, perhaps helping to ease mild separation distress by occupying the puppy. In addition to hard chew toys,

most puppies, especially those prone to more severe separation distress, appear to be comforted by soft-cloth toys (Pettijohn et al., 1977), especially those scented with the owner's body odor. James (1961) studied toy preferences in puppies (2 to 3 months of age), finding that puppies exhibit definite preference toward soft or cloth-type toys:

> Those which elicited the most play were objects which could be bitten, carried in the mouth, held with the feet and pulled, and which could be held in the mouth and shaken. In general, soft objects were more attractive than hard objects. The piece of cloth with which two animals could play together definitely elicited the most play in the present study. (277)

Many puppies prize knotted ropes and fleece-type toys; however, such toys should be given only to puppies that do not destroy or eat them. For teething puppies, rope toys can be dampened and frozen.

Besides chew toys, puppies should also have access to a variety of interactive toys that can be used to play tug-and-fetch games. Training puppies to play tug games provides a constructive outlet for competitive play, with little risk of producing aggression problems (see *Play and Leadership* in Chapter 6). Consequently, tug games should be highly structured, with a beginning and end under the control of the owner. At the conclusion of a bout of tug, the puppy should release the toy (e.g., a ball with an attached loop of webbing), whereupon it is thrown a short distance away and the puppy encouraged to fetch it in exchange for another bout of tug or treat. Playing tug-and-fetch games helps to promote a positive association with toys and can be used to introduce new toys. Another useful game for introducing new chew toys is hide-and-seek. To stimulate interest, the puppy is briefly teased with a toy, which is then hidden out of sight but easy for the puppy to find. The puppy is told "Find it" and encouraged to find the toy. After repeated trials of such training, the puppy may learn to look for the item when motivated to play or chew. Another effective way to increase or maintain interest in chew toys is achieved by rotating them daily. This practice involves taking the toys up at night and giving them back at various times during the day as a reward for good behavior or during bouts of play. Giving a puppy access to only a few toys at a time, occasionally taking them up and providing others, is another way to enhance their appeal. Whatever toys are chosen are of little value unless they are available to the puppy at all times. Remember that something is always within a puppy's reach when chew toys are not—clothing, molding, corners of furniture, rugs, plaster walls, and electric wires.

Many owners inadvertently facilitate undesirable chewing habits by giving puppies poorly chosen toys. For example, an old shoe may be offered to a puppy as ersatz toy in place of other shoes lying around the house. The owner soon discovers, however, that instead of satisfying a puppy's desire for shoes, giving it a worn-out one may only further increase its interest in shoes, worn-out or otherwise. Another common mistake is to forcefully remove forbidden objects from a puppy's mouth or attempting to capture a puppy by running after it to retrieve something that it has picked up. Instead of forcing things out of a puppy's mouth, it should be prompted to release objects by offering it a food treat in exchange. If a puppy has darted off with something, it is far better to call the puppy and reward it for relinquishing the object rather than trying to chase it down.

Whereas interactive games can help to instill an enhanced interest in toys, as well as reinforce cooperative behavior, chase games in which a puppy runs off with the toy in an effort to evade capture by the owner may promote a number of undesirable side effects, including an unwillingness to come when called and increased risk of producing undesirable possessive behavior.

REDIRECTING AND DISCOURAGING DESTRUCTIVE BEHAVIOR

To integrate a puppy successfully into a home, the puppy must learn not to disturb or destroy personal belongings. Although orienting a puppy toward acceptable chew toys is helpful, such efforts may not fully train the puppy to stay away from forbidden items. Eventually, such personal items as shoes, socks, undergarments, books, and plants will attract a puppy's interest. Keeping such things out of a puppy's reach is helpful, but eventually things are forgotten and left within the puppy's reach. Practically speaking, it is important, therefore, that puppies be trained to discriminate between forbidden household items and safe chew toys. Although direct techniques may ultimately be necessary to establish a sufficiently strong and durable object-related inhibition, indirect demonstrations may be useful as a starting point. Remarkably, an action modeled by a rival for the trainer's attention can have a powerful organizing effect on an observing dog's subsequent behavior, closely resembling what one might expect to occur if the dog had been directly stimulated instead of merely observing the model/rival (M/R) responding to the trainer's instructions and actions. Given the apparent benefits of the procedure for affecting object-oriented behavior, the M/R procedure should be explored in advance of going on to direct inhibitory training methods (see *Model/Rival Method*). While the M/R procedure may not establish a lasting deterrence or redirection of chewing activity, such preliminary demonstrations may help to reorient the puppy and, perhaps, make subsequent direct training efforts more efficient and rapid.

A surprising amount of control over destructive activity can be established by employing a novel stimulus (e.g., squeaker) to avert attention from forbidden items and reorient the activity to a more acceptable chew item. Clicker training can be used to enhance the puppy's orienting response to the squeaker (see *Orienting Response* in Chapter 1). Many puppies can be discouraged by saying "Leave it" firmly or by clapping and, if necessary, applying a leash prompt sufficient to turn the puppy away from the object and to redirect it toward a more acceptable item. Playing a tug-and-fetch game with the object can further enhance the puppy's interest in it (Table 2.1). The dog's sensitivity to directional cuing (pointing and glancing) can be used to help orient it to acceptable items, as well as improve its avoidance of forbidden ones. In the case of puppies that show a persistent interest in forbidden items, more emphatic disrupter-type stimulation may be

TABLE. 2.1. Managing puppy destructive behavior

Until puppies are reliable with regard to chewing activities, they should not be permitted to move freely about the house without supervision.

Puppies should be provided with supervised exposure to the home environment and surroundings sufficient to promote habituation, familiarity, and relaxation.

Attractive chew objects should be made available to puppies at all times.

Daily play, exercise, and social attention appear to reduce tensions associated with destructive behavior.

Disrupter-type stimulation and remote deterrents may be necessary to train puppies to stay away from forbidden objects. In addition to carefully timed corrections and booby trapping, repellents are often useful for controlling destructive appetites and excesses.

Puppies should be provided with daily reward-based training activities.

necessary in combination with behavior-activated and remote deterents. Forbidden items, especially those that have been previously damaged, can be used as temptations to help discourage future chewing by means of booby trapping and other deterrent techniques using startle and olfactory avoidance conditioning.

A highly effective deterrent is the sound made by a shaker can (see *Miscellaneous Items* in Chapter 1). A seven-penny can is usually sufficient. To charge the shaker sound, the can is tossed near a puppy that is engaging in a destructive activity with an object that has been scented with a novel odor (e.g., citronella-eucalyptus mix). The can should land close enough to evoke a startle response sufficient to stop the behavior, but not so close that it overstimulates or strikes the puppy. Alternatively, the forbidden scented item can be situated under a drop can, suspended by a length of dental floss held by the trainer and arranged to drop near the item but not risk striking the puppy. The suspended can arrangement allows the trainer to more closely define the level of stimulation produced (see *Three-step Deterrence: Step 3*). The can should contain cotton balls scented with the same odor scenting the forbidden item (e.g., electrical wires). The goals are to establish a conditioned association with the odor and to sensitize the puppy further to the odor by presenting it together with the startling sound of the can. As a result, the conditioned odor can be used on other items as an olfactory deterrent, as well as potentiating the startle

effect of the shaker can, perhaps making the mere shake of the can an effective deterrent. Sniffing objects scented with a previously conditioned odor appears to cause puppies to react more keenly to the sound of the shaker as well as potentiating other sources of startle (e.g., vocal deterrents) used to control such behavior. In the case of sensitive puppies, a scented plastic vitamin bottle with holes drilled into it can be used as a shaker or a small scented beanbag can be used instead. Another way to establish a mild deterrent effect with sensitive puppies is by spraying a lightly scented stream of water toward the object at the moment the puppy approaches it.

Once a conditioned association between the olfactory stimulus and startle is established, booby traps should be set up to transfer control from situations in which the owner is present to situations in which the owner is absent or distracted. Booby traps are particularly important in the case of persistent, unhealthy, or dangerous chewing habits. A reliable method for doing this involves the use of a pull can. Tying a piece of dental floss to the ring of a shaker can and attaching it to the forbidden item rigs the pull can to fall when a puppy grabs at the object. The rigged can is placed on the edge of a shelf so that it will fall and land near the puppy but not strike it. Careful placement and testing of the arrangement can help to prevent such things from happening. A small amount of a conditioned odor is put on the forbidden item with a cotton swab. Objects can also be scented with a piece of paraffin wax that has been melted and mixed with the conditioned odor. The pull can is strongly scented so that it delivers an impressive olfactory message, echoing the subtle odor on the forbidden object and reinforcing its significance as a warning signal. The net effect is to enhance the deterrence value of the subtle odor cue placed on the object and to provide a means to generalize the effect to other items without necessitating that an aversive startle be applied in each case. Another mild remote startle device is the upside-down mousetrap. This is especially useful for discouraging chewing on paper and similar light items (e.g., socks). The scented forbidden item as attached to the back of the trap with tape, and laid on the floor. If arranged properly, there is no risk that the puppy will be hurt by the trap as it snaps shut, but the odor and sound of the trap makes a clear and lasting impression. In some persistent cases, a shaker can or mousetrap is arranged in combination with a motion-sensitive alarm, so that the alarm is activated before the pull can or mousetrap is triggered, thus magnifying the effect of the event as well as providing reliable feedback if the puppy returns to the scented object (see *Controlling Inappropriate Chewing Activities*).

Most puppies quickly learn to stay away from forbidden things when some variation of the aforementioned methods is used. Of course, puppies that engage in excessive or dangerous chewing activities should also be carefully managed with crate confinement and tethering to prevent the unwanted behavior. Severe physical punishment (slapping and spanking) for destructive chewing should be eschewed because it will do little to control the chewing problem, but may generate undesirable fear and avoidance behavior. Although commonly practiced in error, belated punishment serves no useful function in the control of destructive chewing. Deterence that does not immediately precede or contiguously overlap the unwanted chewing should be avoided. Brief gentle scolding, although technically questionable, may produce a reminder effect in dogs that have previously received inhibitory training; that is, showing the item to the puppy or dog and saying "Not yours" or "Leave it" may not be without some benefit. Even if the procedure does nothing, never-

theless, it appears to help owners by giving them a way to let off steam in a controlled and inconsequential way. Alternatively, a model/rival procedure might be suggested as a better option for responding to after-the-fact situations, offering an approach that is more likely to produce a training effect without risk of adverse side effects (see *Model/Rival Method*).

Note: Puppies vary with regard to their sensitivity to startle. Consequently, startle-producing stimulation should be carefully adjusted to levels appropriate to a puppy's temperament and age. Particular caution should be exercised with young puppies, especially those between 8 to 10 weeks of age. Such puppies may be particularly sensitive to the effects of fear conditioning (see *Learning and Trainability* in Volume 1, Chapter 2).

PART 3: DESTRUCTIVE BEHAVIOR IN ADULT DOGS

A variety of adult behavior problems are associated with excessive chewing and other destructive behaviors (e.g., digging and scratching). Storm-phobic dogs may exhibit pronounced destructive behavior directed toward walls and flooring in an apparent effort to hide or escape stimuli associated with a storm. Many juvenile and adult dogs show destructive chewing and scratching only when left alone, often as the result of separation-related arousal and distress. Other dogs may chew and engage in other destructive activities as the result of inadequate impulse control associated with hyperactivity and excessive excitability. Chewing and scratching directed toward window casements and doors may occur secondary to territorial aggression or predatory excitement evoked by animals coming into the dog's view. Destructive behavior associated with fears, separation distress, hyperactivity, compulsions, and aggression needs to be addressed in the context of treatment activities aimed at reducing the underlying causes by applying appropriate behavior therapy procedures. Dogs exhibiting unusual destructive behavior or pica may be suffering from an undiagnosed medical condition (e.g., hypothyroidism) requiring veterinary examination to detect and treat properly. The owner should be encouraged to keep a record of destructive behavior, including information on the time of day, location, presence or absence of the owner, object damaged, and possible causes (Figure 2.4).

A common source of destructive behavior in adult dogs stems from ineffective training and management of play and exploratory behavior. Highly active and inquisitive puppies rapidly learn that owner attention can be consistently obtained by bothering forbidden objects. Grabbing socks, undergarments, chil-

OWNER'S NAME:

DOG'S NAME:

RECORD OF DESTRUCTIVE BEHAVIOR
(LIST MOST RECENT FIRST)

# 1	LOCATION	TIME OF DAY	OWNER PRESENT / ABSENT	OBJEC

DESCRIBE EVENT:

POSSIBLE CAUSES:

# 2	LOCATION	TIME OF DAY	OWNER PRESENT / ABSENT	OBJECT / DAMAGE

DESCRIBE EVENT:

POSSIBLE CAUSES:

# 3	LOCATION	TIME OF DAY	OWNER PRESENT / ABSENT	OBJECT /

DESCRIBE EVENT:

POSSIBLE CAUSES:

OTHERS:

4

5

6

FIG. 2.4. Record of destructive behavior.

dren's toys, and similar things serves to evoke a reliable and often entertaining activity. Some dogs appear to seek out and then daunt the owner deliberately with forbidden object, apparently with the goal of triggering a chase escapade through the house. Despite repeated scoldings, the behavior may continue unabated. If the owner ignores the dog, it may then chew the item. Dogs that have learned to grab and run off with forbidden objects may exhibit playful oppositional behaviors that require significant training and management to modify. In extreme cases, dogs appear to respond to the owner's disciplinary efforts as a provocative challenge to compete, causing them to become progressively resistant and difficult to control.

Such dogs often behave in precisely those ways that are most likely to yield the maximum amount of owner attention, often attention concentrated in a ritual of interactive punishment. Rather than discouraging the oppositional dog's game, however, the owner's ineffective punishment only seems to have an opposite effect. Driven by distorted attention-seeking incentives, oppositional dogs seem to thrive on negative attention as something desirable and rewarding. Oppositional dogs with destructive habits are often habituated to gradually escalating forms of punishment and, ultimately, may not be reached by the owner's most severe disciplinary efforts. In the context of punishing destructive behavior, low-intensity punitive events may be linked inadvertently with high-intensity reward outcomes (e.g., escaping owner control and running about with the forbidden object). As a result, the punishing event may become a signal entraining vicious-circle behavior (Brown et al., 1964), causing oppositional behavior and destructiveness to increase over time. As punitive efforts are applied again and again, a dog may learn to tolerate progressively more aversive events while at the same time acquiring a variety of escape and avoidance strategies to stay out of the owner's reach and to maximize the reward value of the activity. Instead of deterring the dog from engaging in future destructive behavior, the forbidden object becomes a discriminative stimulus setting the stage for a cat-and-mouse game. Playful opposition is often misunderstood as dominant

behavior, but, more accurately, such dogs are most often simply incompetently and improperly trained.

Another common cause is excessive or inappropriate confinement or lack of daily stimulation. Dogs learn to become familiar with the environment by interacting with it. By sniffing, picking things up, scratching, digging, and running about, dogs gradually become comfortable with the environment via habituation. With familiarity and habituation come an increased sense of safety and a progressive ability to relax. Dogs that are excessively confined or restrained may not habituate to environmental stimulation normally, becoming highly active and inquisitive or reactive when allowed to move about freely to explore, sometimes resulting in significant damage [see *Environmental Adaptation (3 to 16 Weeks)* in Volume 1, Chapter 2]. Such dogs may get caught up in vicious cycle, such that excesses resulting from a failure to habituate cause the owner to confine and isolate the dog further, thereby making the problem worse. Dogs exhibiting excessive exploratory behavior in combination with destructiveness and pica need to be carefully supervised while gradually being given more room to move about, explore, become familiar, and habituate to the home environment. Borchelt (1984) has proposed that the space given to the puppy or dog to move about the home environment should be managed with a concern for basic behavioral and physiological priorities, adjusted in accordance with the dog's development and ability, while meeting the owner's needs to protect personal belongings, furniture, carpeting, and so forth from damage. Accordingly, space management serves three basic functions:

1. It provides for the biological and behavioral needs of a puppy.
2. It affords protection against damage to personal belongings, carpeting, and furniture.
3. It facilitates a puppy's behavioral adjustment to the human environment, appropriate to its stage of development and training.

In addition to generalizing house training to different parts of the house, space-management strategies are used to systematically discourage destructive activities and introduce alternative chew items. The process of environmental adaptation is combined with integrated compliance training (ICT) and play. The cynopraxic concern for the establishment of interactive harmony converges with quality-of-life goals in the process of mediating the dog's adjustment to the home environment. The extent to which the dog is fully integrated into familial activities and free to move about the house is an important cynopraxic indicator of adaptive success.

BASIC TRAINING, EXERCISE, AND PLAY

Dogs exhibiting destructive habits in association with oppositional behavior usually benefit from basic training, which provides a structure of communication and rules that helps to resolve interactive conflicts and tension (see *Hyperactivity and Social Excesses* in Chapter 5). Many of the problems associated with this type of dog spontaneously improve as better attention and impulse control is established. As a dog learns to work for positive attention and rewards, a more stable and satisfying bond can be formed between the owner and dog, ultimately leading to greater cooperation and harmony. The goal of basic training is to provide oppositional dogs with a set of unambiguous social boundaries and expectations; above all, though, such training serves to systematically show them how to obtain what they want by means of cooperation. Opposition is drive energy not constructively channeled and put to work by training.

The development of refractory adjustment problems associated with destructive behavior often points to environmental deficiencies and problematic social dynamics. Whereas cooperative transactions serve to promote feelings of security (comfort and safety) and trust via reward, antagonistic and domineering transactions may produce significant conflict and a variety of emotionally stressful states or interactive tensions: anxiety, frustration, anger, fear, irritability, and so forth. A common source of persistent and harmful conflict and tension occurs in the context of ineffectual efforts to control undesirable or danger-

ous impulses. Dogs respond to punitive efforts differently depending on a variety of predisposing biological and experiential factors (e.g., prenatal and neonatal stress, early trauma, and deprivation), influences that may exert a lifelong effect by altering the dog's sensitivity and reactivity to aversive stimuli and conflict. Ineffectual, excessive, or abusive punitive efforts to control undesirable behavior may adversely influence emotional and behavioral systems most sensitive and vulnerable to reactive behavioral elaborations. An important aim of cynopraxic intervention is to systematically identify these points of interactive conflict and to mediate their resolution by means of counseling, appropriate training, behavior therapy, and environmental change.

Oppositional conflict develops in situations where the owner's control interests are contested by the dog's efforts to obtain reward. Particularly problematic interactive conflict of this kind develops in situations where behavioral limits are set by aversive means that are approximately equal to the motivational arousal driving the undesirable behavior, with the net result that the dog is equally averted and attracted to the situation. Over time, conflict and frustration may gradually escalate into defiance as the dog habituates to the owner's ineffectual punitive efforts, causing the owner to gradually increase the severity of the means used to constrain undesirable behavior, while the dog's desire for the forbidden reward object or activity continues unabatedly to grow. Such oppositional conflict and frustration may become ritualized, locking both the owner and the dog in a compulsive fixation from which neither is able to escape easily without outside help. Often the key to resolving such problems is to identify what the dog is trying to achieve and then providing it, or giving the dog something equivalent in value, on a contingent basis, thereby satisfying the dog's desire for reward and the owner's desire for control. The spell is broken as the owner learns to lead and show the dog how to gratify its needs, rather than just obstinately standing in the way.

Effective training for these dogs incorporates a balance of strategic confinement and integrated compliance training. Strategic confinement consists of crating, leashing, and tie-out stations located throughout the house. Keeping such dogs on leash in the house can be a highly effective means to prevent or discourage undesirable behavior. Basic exercises, such as sit, down, stay, coming when called, and walking on leash without pulling, should be trained to a high level of reliability and worked into daily activities until it becomes a way of life for owner and dog. Desirable activities and resources (e.g., attention, walks, food, play, toys, and affection) should be made available on a contingency basis, requiring that the dog perform some trained module or routine in exchange. While undergoing remedial training, the dog should be kept under constant supervision on leash or restrained in its crate or tethered to a tie-out station, gradually obtaining more freedom to move about unsupervised as warranted by improved household behavior. Simply training the dog to turn away from forbidden objects (squeak and click) and rewarding compliance by redirecting the appetitive activity into a more appropriate outlet can help to prevent problems, as well as provide a useful starting point for approaching already established habits.

In addition to daily obedience training, destructive dogs should receive daily periods of exercise and structured play activities. The dog's need for exercise varies according to the breed and temperament, with some individuals requiring much more daily exercise than others. A typical exercise program should include at least two 20- to 30-minute walks, once in the morning and again in the evening. For active dogs, an aerobic activity (e.g., ball play) should also be provided. Playful tug-and-fetch games with chew toys can help to focus a dog's interest on them.

CONTROLLING INAPPROPRIATE CHEWING ACTIVITIES

The model/rival method can be incorporated in the context of helping. For a week, the dog should be carefully supervised and restrained to prevent access to inappropriate chew items. During this period, the dog should receive intensive attention and integrated compliance training. Emphasis is placed on training the

dog to orient to the sound of a squeaker, a response that is rapidly bridged (click) and followed by a food reward delivered from the right with "Good." The dog should be trained to sit and stay reliably and to halt-stay and wait until it is prompted to come, to sit, or is released. The dog should also learn to walk on a leash without pulling, sit-stay, down and stay, make eye contact, and generally learn to cooperate. Chewing activity is restricted to a small assortment of attractive chew toys, provided during play and used as rewards for compliant behavior. The selected chew toys should be both attractive to the dog and resistant to sustained chewing. Appropriate toys should be given to the dog whenever it is tethered or otherwise confined. After this initial training and orientation toward appropriate chew toys, previously damaged items can be gradually reintroduced as temptations. For dogs prone to pick up and run off with forbidden items, the objects can be tied off to a piece of furniture with a piece of twine or attached to active-control line that allows the trainer to snatch it away from the dog. One object should be presented at a time in the context of redirecting the appetite to a new and acceptable chew object. The forbidden object is kept in full view of the dog as the trainer encourages the dog to tug and fetch the toy.

Model/Rival Method

A rival/model method of training may be useful in the context of modifying object-oriented behavior (see *Complex Social Behavior and Model/Rival Learning* in Chapter 10). The full value and significance of the M/R procedure for dog-training purposes remains to be determined; however, preliminary experiments by the author suggest that the technique may exert a potent and under appreciated organizing effect on a dog's behavior, especially with respect to modulating object-oriented behavior. For purposes of orienting the dog toward acceptable items and away from forbidden ones, the following M/R procedure may serve to enhance subsequent inhibitory training.

A trainer (T) and model/rival (M/R) sit on the floor with a puppy or dog that is tied off on a tie-out or active-control line located a few feet away. The T and M/R stage instructive interactions around acceptable toys and forbidden objects. The T presents an acceptable toy to the M/R and says "Take it," which the M/R does, whereupon the T says "Good." The M/R puts a toy on the floor and picks it up again, and the T says "Good." Next, a scented forbidden item is held toward the M/R, saying "Leave it." In response to a vocal warning, the M/R should move slightly back, but then reach again for the object, at which point the M/R says "Leave it" in a more forceful tone of voice, causing the latter to flinch back once more. After a moment, the two objects are arranged on the floor at least 3 feet apart, and the dog is allowed to move toward them. If the dog goes to the acceptable item, it is rewarded with an excited "Good" and engaged in play. If the dog goes to the forbidden item instead, the T says "Leave it" and draws the dog back by the control line and picks up both objects. After a brief delay, the demonstration procedure is repeated, but now incorporating a seven-penny shaker can or modified carbon-dioxide pump. Again, the T offers the M/R the toy, saying "Take it" and "Good" as the M/R reaches and takes the toy. The same procedure as previously described is used when presenting the forbidden item, but now after the T says "Leave it," the can is shook once or a slight spritz of scented spray is delivered with a modified carbon-dioxide pump toward the object, and the M/R flinches back. Finally, both items are again placed on the floor and the is dog released. After choosing the toy, the T says "Good" and engages the dog in a brief period of play. If the dog goes to the forbidden item, the shaker is shook lightly or a brief spritz (not startling) from the pump is delivered, and the dog is pulled away from the object with the control line. Three trials of M/R training are performed per session.

Three-step Deterrence

In cases involving persistent appetites for forbidden objects and chewing in which other methods have failed or are inappropriate, the following method should help to ensure a lasting avoidance of forbidden items.

Step 1

With the dog on leash, the forbidden object is shown with the warning "Leave it," whereupon it is put on the floor. If the dog moves to take the forbidden item, a leash prompt is delivered with sufficient force to turn its head away from the item. In strongly motivated dogs, a fixed-action halter can be used to facilitate head control (see *Fixed-action Halter Collars* in Chapter 1). The entire procedure is repeated again until the dog shows an active avoidance toward the item. With every successful trial, the dog is praised, offered a treat, and encouraged to take an alternative item. The acceptable toy is presented to the dog, saying "Take it" in a playful tone. Prompting the dog to play tug-and-fetch with the object can be helpful at such times to enhance its interest in the item. Subsequently, the acceptable and ideally more attractive object is placed 1 or 2 feet from the forbidden object. The arrangement is intended to provide the dog with a choice between the acceptable item and the forbidden one. If the dog selects the acceptable item, the forbidden one is retrieved and removed. The dog should be petted while in possession of the acceptable chew item. This routine should be repeated in various locations throughout the house to generalize the effect.

Step 2

During step 2, leash control is gradually faded and a disrupter-type deterrent and conditioned odor are introduced to help further generalize the effect. With the leash dropped and dragging behind, the dog is taken to a room where a decoy and an acceptable chew toy had been previously left on the floor. If the dog goes for the forbidden item, the vocal signal "Leave it" is spoken in a clipped manner and a scented seven-penny shaker can is tossed next to the dog. If necessary, the leash is picked up and the dog is directed away from the object. The entire procedure is repeated, as needed, until the dog actively avoids the forbidden item and accepts the alternative one. After a toss or two of the can, a single shake may be sufficient to produce the desired inhibition. In the case of dogs that are highly sensitive to auditory startle, the pennies can be put into a large plastic pill bottle. A scented cotton ball is put inside the bottle that has had several quarter-inch holes drilled into it.

Step 3

By the end of step 2, the dog should show an active avoidance toward the forbidden item while on leash and off, but the training process is not yet complete. A significant contextual cue controlling the avoidance so far established is the presence of the owner. Joseph Call and colleagues (Ainsworth, 2000; Call et al., 2003) at the Max Planck Institute in Munich have confirmed what applied dog behaviorists and trainers have long known about the influence of an owner's presence as a contextual cue, viz., dogs behave differently when they are under the scrutiny of a watchful eye. The researchers found that dogs can be readily trained to avoid food that has been placed on the floor, so long as the experimenter stays in the room and keeps an eye on them. Dogs tended to approach forbidden food in a more stealthy and roundabout way when they were closely watched, in contrast to the more direct approach used when the observer was absent, turned away from the dog, facing the dog with closed eyes, or distracted by some engrossing activity (e.g., playing a computer game). Dogs rapidly learn to control their behavior in accordance to contextual social cues, appearing to discriminate between contexts where the risk of interference is high (owner present) and where the risk of interference is low (owner absent or distracted). Consequently, the purpose of step 3 is to counteract this expectation of safety from interference when left alone by implementing various booby-trapping procedures. The most commonly used booby trap is the pull can, consisting of a scented seven- or 30-penny shaker can that is tied to the forbidden item by a length of dental floss and rigged to fall near the dog (Figure 2.5D). The can is placed on a shelf, top of a door, or other ledge in such a way that it lands close to the dog

but without any risk of hitting it. Although the shaker should be strongly scented with a repellent odor, the item itself should only be lightly scented (e.g., stroked once or twice with a scented cotton swab). In some cases, additional stimulus dimension can be added and the startle effect magnified by placing a small paper cup on top of the pull can. The cup contains a small amount of water scented with a drop or two of the conditioned odor. In addition to protecting specific items, pull cans can also used to protect countertops and other areas, such as furniture. In this case, two or three cans are strung together along the length of the countertop with a single length of dental floss. Short lengths of dental floss can be attached to the line at various points that may then be fastened to temptations of various kinds (e.g., kitchen towels). When the dog jumps onto the counter or steals one of the booby-trapped items, the cans all come tumbling down with a convincing crash. The dog or puppy that grabs clothing hung over countertops can be strongly discouraged by hiding a shaker can inside of the item, so that when the item is disturb the shaker can tumbles down. Unrolling toilet paper is a common nuisance behavior that can be discouraged by placing a shaker can on the roll itself, often inhibiting the habit after a single startling crash of the can. Similarly, by taping the line of a pull can to the side of trash bins or directly fastening it to items inside the bin, a rapid and lasting inhibition about exploring such items can be established. In the case of persistent appetites for forbidden objects, regardless of the sort of pull-can arrangement used, the can should be rigged in combination with a motion- or movement-sensitive device that is activated in advance of the can falling down, so that the dog can avoid the startling stimulation by backing away in response to olfactory or acoustical warnings set up in close association with the protected object. The pull can is a one-time event, whereas the scent and motion-activated alarm is continuously available to deliver immediate feedback and warning to the dog.

Another important remote application of the shaker can is the drop can, which is different from the pull can in that it requires a trip line and trigger mechanism or must be directly released by the trainer. A simple arrangement involving the drop can is used to discourage dogs from entering a forbidden area. The drop can is attached to a length of dental floss that is passed through an eyehook fastened to the wall or ceiling. An alternate method involves bending an opened paper clip to form an eye and taping it securing to the ceiling or doorjamb. Another eyehook is set up at the level of the dog's legs. The dental floss is passed through both the upper and lower eyehooks, stretched across the doorway, and hooked by a knotted loop to the trigger—usually a paper clip shaped to serve the purpose and taped to

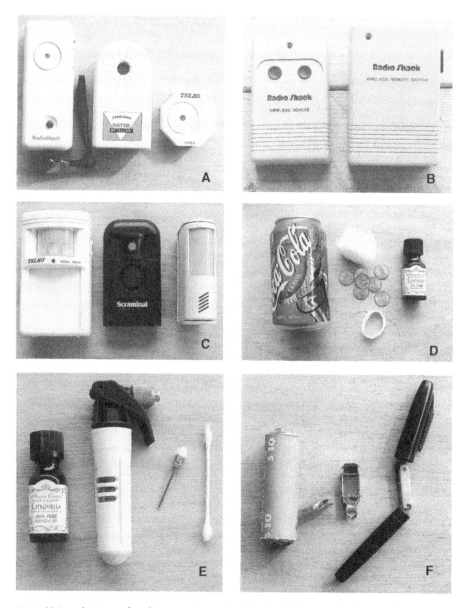

FIG. 2.5. Various devices used to discourage destructive behavior: (**A**) motion, moisture, and vibration detectors, (**B**) remote electrical switch, (**C**) infrared alarms, (**D**) shaker can with materials to make a pull can, (**E**) modified compressed-air pump, and (**F**) various spring-loaded snapping devices.

the doorjamb or wall. The arrangement allows the suspended can to fall to the floor whenever the dog trips the scented dental floss. For exceptionally difficult dogs, an identical backup arrangement can be set up on the other side of the doorway. Applying a dilute repellent scent to the floor and doorjamb and using strongly scented drop cans helps to generalized the effect and provides a means to fade the trip-line and drop-can arrangement. Drop cans are occasionally used to discourage chewing on woodwork. Here, the line is passed through an eyehook, guided across the top of the door, passed through another eyehook and then pulled down and attached to a trigger device made by slipping the looped end of the dental floss under a splinter of damaged wood. If the dog returns to the area and attempts to chew, the can is released and crashes to the floor. Drop cans should be arranged and set up so that they do not fall directly on the dog.

AVERSIVE STARTLE AND THE CONTROL OF DESTRUCTIVE BEHAVIOR

Effective aversive techniques should produce immediate and significant suppression, but not produce excessive fear or discomfort. Ideally, suppression should occur rapidly and after only a few exposures, often after a single event. Startling stimuli occurring in nature are often closely associated with potentially life-threatening events, with rapid escape and avoidance of such events serving to improve an animal's likelihood of survival. Organisms that required many exposures to a dangerous situation before learning to avoid it would be at a greater risk of injury or destruction than counterparts that rapidly learned to avoid danger as the result of one or a few exposures. Obviously, animals able to learn from a single exposure would posses a significant biological advantage over those not so prepared. Survival pressures appear to favor rapid escape and avoidance learning, especially with respect to exploratory behaviors that bring animals into contact with potentially harmful stimuli, requiring rapid appraisal and adjustments to escape or avoid them in the future. As a result, exploratory behavior appears to be highly sensitive to novelty and subtle changes that imme-

diately precede startle-evoking stimulation. An important function of exploratory behavior is to detect potentially dangerous situations in advance of an injurious exposure. Since destructive behaviors often involve exploratory and appetitive incentives, they are highly responsive to aversive stimulation, with startle and behavioral disruption playing an important role in their modification and control.

Although aversive procedures often play a prominent role in the control of destructive behavior, such efforts should be used in combination with supportive reward-based training and efforts aimed at eliminating or reducing emotional and physiological causes contributing to destructive behavior. In addition, dogs need to be provided with adequate substitute outlets to satisfy their need for oral and somatic exploratory activities. Unless aversive control is combined with constructive positive training efforts, its deterrent effects are likely to be short-lived and may require many more repetitions to maintain. Another problematic aspect of aversive control is timing. Destructive behavior is often discovered long after the fact, tempting owners to apply punishment belatedly, but interactive punishment after the fact is unlikely to produce a beneficial effect and may only cause the dog to fear or mistrust the owner rather than helping to discourage the undesirable behavior (see *Separation Distress and Retroactive Punishment* in Volume 2, Chapter 4). Dogs appear, as Roberts (2002) has noted concerning animals in general, to be stuck in time and lack the ability to form episodic memories of long-past actions connected in a causal way to present consequences. Behavior-activated devices and booby traps provide the means to deliver startling consequences at the exact moment in which the unwanted behavior occurs, making such procedures highly efficient and efficacious.

Aversive procedures should only be used to achieve cynopraxic objectives not otherwise attainable by nonaversive means alone. Further, all training procedures that produce discomfort, startle, or loss should be applied in adherence to the LIMA principle and the dead-dog rule (see *Hydran-Protean Side Effects, the Dead-dog Rule, and the LIMA Principle* in Chapter 10).

MISCELLANEOUS DEVICES AND TECHNIQUES FOR DETERRING DESTRUCTIVE BEHAVIOR

Destructive habits and various nuisance behaviors occurring in an owner's absence often require special techniques and tools to resolve them. The transition from crate confinement to free or limited access to the house is facilitated by the use of behavior-activated devices strategically placed to discourage destructiveness, jumping on furniture and countertops, and keeping dogs out of certain areas without physical barriers. Such problems are often extremely frustrating since a dog may misbehave only when the owner is out of sight or out of the house. A common method for addressing this problem is to set up booby traps or to employ various behavior-activated electronic devices that have been designed to deliver a brief spray or electrical stimulus via a dog collar (see *Behavior-activated Electronic Training* in Chapter 9). Booby traps deliver an immediate disruptive event at the instant in which the unwanted behavior occurs, regardless of the owner's presence or absence.

Modified Mousetraps

Modified mousetraps can be used to discourage dogs from jumping on furniture, from damaging potted plants, or from entering forbidden outdoor areas. While some authorities recommend the use of mousetraps without modification (Hart and Hart, 1985), good results can be obtained with upside-down mousetraps and mousetraps that are modified by wrapping 6 to 8 inches of cotton gauze around the hammer and then taping it. Such an arrangement delivers a sufficiently startling impact without risk of injury or unnecessary discomfort to the dog. A few drops of a conditioned odor can be placed on the gauze, establishing an aversive conditioned association between the odor and the startle of the trap closing shut, thereby increasing the future value of the scent alone as an environmental warning and deterrence. The usefulness of the scent as a repellent is significantly improved by using this simple conditioning arrangement. For sensitive dogs or puppies, an upside-down mousetrap may produce a sufficient deterrence to keep them off furniture and away from for-

bidden areas. Scattering a few upside-down mousetraps on forbidden furniture can be a good deterrent for the sneaky lounger. Dogs with a penchant for exploring waste bins can be discouraged with a couple of upside-down traps placed under the trash. The interior of the waste bin can be scented with a repellent odor, so that the avoidance response is maintained even after the devices are removed. The upside-down mousetrap is especially useful to deter dogs keen on paper items. The forbidden item is lightly scented and fastened to the back of a mousetrap with a ring of tape and then laid on the floor or tabletop. An empty matchbook can be placed under the mousetrap to prevent the trigger from releasing the hammer too easily.

Caps and Snappers

Many devices using cap charges can be tailored to training purposes. The pull cap is a fireworks toy that is set off when two opposing strings are sharply pulled apart. The device is a loud and effective deterrent for dogs entering forbidden rooms or closets. One end is attached to the door and the other to the doorjamb. The cap should be placed up high near the top of the doorjamb to prevent flying debris from striking the dog. Perhaps the most versatile of this group of devices is the spring-loaded snapper. These devices are available in magic supply and novelty stores as exploding pens and coin rolls (Figure 2.5F). Once set, the least movement will set off the delicate mechanism exploding the plastic cap. Since the plastic cap flies off the cap snapper with some force, precautions should be taken to cover the device or insert it in a sandwich-size zip-lock bag. Also, the powder burn of the exploding cap can damage finished surfaces. It should be emphasized that cap devices should be used only as part of an overall plan of training and in most cases as a last resort. Caps and snappers are usually set up with scented objects or placed together with a motion-sensitive alarm that is rigged to go off before the cap.

Infrared, Moisture, and Motion Detectors

Various electronic gadgets can be highly effective high-tech alternatives to the previously described booby-trap devices (Landsberg, 1994). The most useful are those that are activated by infrared detection, motion and vibration, moisture, or radio signals triggering an electrical or spray event delivered by a dog collar. Infrared detectors contain a heat-sensitive sensor that passively responds to temperature changes caused by a dog walking nearby (Figure 2.5C). When the dog enters the field covered by the infrared detector, a high-frequency alarm is triggered and continues until the dog moves out of the field, whereupon it stops and resets. Such devices can be very useful for protecting both objects and areas, such as countertops and furniture. Other devices are designed to detect photoelectric disturbances caused by a dog's movement. The photoelectric detector works by producing a beam of light that is reflected back to a light sensor. When the beam of reflected light is broken, a chime sound or loud external alarm is triggered. These devices are commonly used in stores to monitor the entrance and egress of customers. An advantage of photoelectrical detectors is that they can be used to define a highly specific area or boundary. Both passive infrared and active photoelectric detectors can be used to deter a wide variety of destructive activities. Motion- and vibration-sensitive detectors are also available with a built-in alarm and a panic-button switch (Figure 2.5A). These devices are hung on doorknobs to detect intrusion. When the door is banged or opened, the alarm is triggered, continues for 20 seconds or so, and then resets. Motion detectors can be placed on furniture or attached to forbidden items by a length of dental floss in order to deter unwanted activities. Such devices are small enough to put inside a shoe, wrap in clothing, place in trash bins, and so forth. Because such devices produce a continuous loud noise for 20 seconds, they should be used only in situations where the dog is able to move into another room away from the alarm. Moisture detectors with built-in alarms can be modified in various ways to protect areas being licked or chewed by a dog. For example, wire leads with alligator clips can be attached to the moisture-sensitive probes and fastened to two strips of

quarter-inch copper tape. The pieces of copper tape are applied to the chewed area leaving an eighth-inch gap between them. When the strips of mounted tape are shorted by lick and saliva, an alarm is triggered and continues until the dog backs away. Another simple moisture-activated device can be set up by hooking quarter-inch copper adhesive strips to a 9-volt battery. Again, an eighth-inch gap should separate the copper strips so that a short is formed between the positive and negative poles of the battery whenever the strip is contacted by the tongue and lips; the arrangement delivers a mild shock. In any case, a conditioned odor should be applied to areas and objects protected by electronic sensors and deterrents in order to help generalize the effect.

Compressed Air

The carbon-dioxide (CO_2) pump (available at bike shops or computer stores) is modified to make it a useful training tool. The modification consists of a small cotton wad that is inserted into the base of an inflation needle that is firmly screwed into the nozzle of the air pump. After screwing the inflator needle into the pump, the needle part is wiggled back and forth until it breaks off (Figure 2.5E). This simple modification serves two functions: it prevents an excessively forceful discharge of CO_2 air, and it permits the user to dispense an odor by means of highly controlled air pressure and directional flow, making it easier to direct scented or unscented air toward some nearby or distant location. The lever valve on the CO_2 pump allows the user to release a controlled amount of scented or unscented pressurized air, producing an inaudible mist, a faint spray, puff, hiss, spritz, or startling burst, depending on training needs. The CO_2 pump can be used in a variety of ways to interrupt behavior or to produce positive or negative conditioned effects. When used to limit destructive behavior, a scented spray is directed toward the forbidden item, thereby generating a significant startle while at the same blowing the object out of the dog's reach and scenting it with the conditioned odor. After two or three applications, the odor itself acquires a significant inhibitory effect and can be directly applied to forbidden objects (Otto and Giardino, 2001). In addition, olfactory startle conditioning may potentiate a dog's response to other sources of startle (e.g., the pull can), making them significantly more effective when presented in conjunction with a previously startle-conditioned odor (Paschall and Davis, 2002) (Figure 2.6). Also, once dogs are sensitized to the sound of an air pump, simply making a hissing sound can produce a mild inhibitory effect. Although the aforementioned nozzle modification helps to improve the safety of the air pump, several safety precautions should be observed when using the

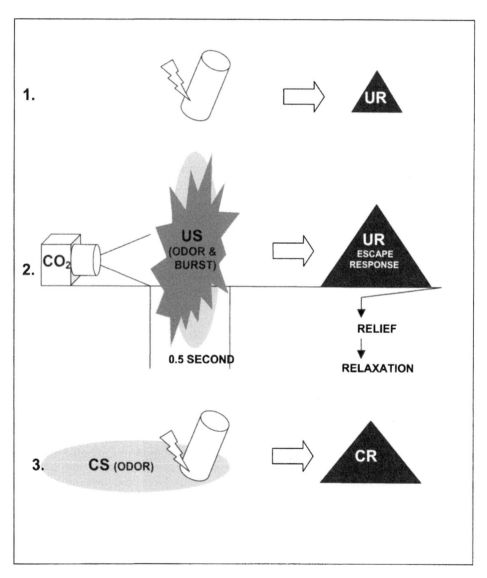

FIG. 2.6. Olfactory-mediated startle potentiation can play a valuable role in the control of destructive appetites and excesses. A previously conditioned odor applied to a forbidden item provides an avoidance cue as well as potentiating the effect of other startle events occurring in the presence of the odor. US, unconditioned stimulus; UR, unconditioned response; CS, conditioned stimulus; and CR, conditioned response.

device. The pump should never be pointed at the dog or sprayed toward the dog's face, near its ears and eyes, into its mouth, or directly against its skin. The discharge of compressed CO_2 may precipitate dry ice and cause burns if it is applied directly to the skin. Using the modified CO_2 pump safely and effectively requires some skill, and it should be kept out of the reach of children and family members not instructed on its proper use.

Repellents

Olfactory and gustatory repellents are commonly used to deter dogs from chewing and other destructive behaviors. In contrast to devices used to repel and deter dogs from engaging in destructive behaviors by stimulating auditory startle, chemical repellents serve a similar function by eliciting irritating sensations or disgust/nausea, as in the case of taste aversion (see *Taste Aversion* in Volume 1, Chapter 6). As previously discussed, conditioned odors produce a repellent event as the result of aversive conditioning in which the odor is paired with the occurrence of a startling event. A major drawback of repellents is that dogs may quickly learn to circumvent the strategy by avoiding treated objects but continue to chew objects that have not been treated with the repellent. Similarly, objects that have been scented with a conditioned odor may be avoided, but others not treated may inadvertently attract continued destructive interest. In the latter case, the absence of scent may actually help dogs to predict a degree of safety from aversive consequence. Repellents producing an acid, sour, or bitter taste do not appear to be very effective deterrents for the control of predatory behavior in wild canids (Mason et al., 2001) or scavenging garbage in dogs (Wolski et al., 1984).

Despite the aforementioned limitations, most dogs appear to respond to the deterrence produced by conditioned odors and repellents; however, when such substances are used in isolation from positive training activities, they probably do little good. Available commercial products offer varying degrees of effectiveness. With respect to repellents, odor-based substances do not appear to be very useful unless they are conditioned to evoke avoidance. The best repellents are those that directly irritate mucous membranes (Houpt et al., 1984), such as pepper derivatives (e.g., capsaicin). The most commonly used repellent substance is cayenne pepper in the form of hot sauce. Cayenne pepper can be also be applied as an alcohol extract/solution or paste. A mixture of cayenne pepper and alcohol consists of 1 tablespoon of cayenne pepper mixed into a quarter cup of alcohol. The mixture is thoroughly stirred and then let to sit for an hour or so, until the pepper granules sink to the bottom. The reddish alcohol solution that separates from the pepper is decanted and applied sparingly with a paintbrush or cotton swab to forbidden objects and areas. After application, the alcohol rapidly evaporates, leaving pepper resins behind on the treated surface. A paste of red pepper is made with water and small amounts of hair gel. The paste is typically slathered on wood objects (e.g., furniture and woodwork) that have been chewed in the past. Cayenne-pepper solution can stain or damage woodwork and fabrics, making the solution and paste inappropriate for some surfaces. Alum, an astringent, offers a mild alternative to cayenne pepper. Black pepper can be applied under the fringes of carpets or to other areas being chewed or scratched.

DIGGING

Most dogs spend large amounts of their waking time engaged in exploratory activities of various kinds, behavior that is essential for healthy development and normal environmental habituation. As the result of poor management or training, these natural exploratory interests may become exaggerated or misdirected into destructive activities, causing significant concern for dog owners. Some breeds (e.g., terriers) are more prone than others to dig. Likewise, highly active dogs (sanguine types) are more frequently presented with digging problems than more relaxed and reserved dogs (phlegmatic types). In addition to predatory incentives stimulated by insects, worms, and other creatures living in the grass and soil, some digging dogs appear to enjoy the tug stimulation of pulling out shrubbery roots. Although some dogs may bury and recover buried food items (e.g., bones), this is not as common as one might suppose from the popular literature. Interestingly, wolves dig holes to cache food and urinate over areas where food has been dug up and removed (Harrington, 1981)—a behavior pattern not reported in dogs. Most common outdoor destructive complaints revolve around chewing and digging, operating under the influence of normal canine functional and motivational systems (Odendaal, 1996). Consequently, the causes of digging are numerous and varied, requiring careful history taking and observation. The owner should be asked the pertinent questions involved in any behavioral assessment, viz., the three W's (what, when, where) and the three H's (how long, how frequent, and how severe) (see *Behavioral Fact-finding* in Volume 2, Chapter 2). Some digging activity is simply part of having a dog, requiring in some cases that owners adjust their expectations rather than attempting to suppress all digging activity. Puppies, in particular, appear to enjoy the fresh smells and tastes of tender roots and freshly turned earth. In addition to the inherent pleasures associated with digging, a dog might use the activity as a somatic outlet for the release of various tensions involving boredom, frustration, and stress. As a result, excessive digging may become a compulsive outlet for dogs living under suboptimal conditions.

The location of digging activity can offer clues about its underlying causation. Digging along fence lines and near gates may stem from efforts to escape confinement due to territorial aggressive arousal, barrier frustration, fear, or separation-related distress. Digging near resting areas, under trees and shrubs, especially during the summer, may be motivated by an urge to expose damp earth just beneath the surface to roll in and cool

down. To arrive at a successful solution, it is important that the motivational causes be identified and, if possible, removed or reduced before attempting to suppress undesirable digging. For example, bored dogs should be given additional exercise and play activities that provide adequate opportunities for stimulation, separation-reactive dogs need to learn how to cope more effectively with being left alone, and dogs digging to achieve improved thermoregulation should be provided adequate water to drink and a small plastic wading pool. Such dogs should also be provided with outdoor accommodations that provide better protection from heat when outdoors. When barrier frustration is identified as a factor, potential causes of frustration should be explored, for example, a high sex drive and desire to roam, the presence of roaming neighborhood dogs, or any other occurrences stimulating intense arousal and interest. Most digging problems appear to benefit from increased daily attention, obedience training, and exercise. Even after the aforementioned motivations and causes have been addressed, a dog may still engage in unwanted digging behavior. For many dogs, digging is inherently rewarding, providing a welcome distraction when left alone or understimulated. Because many dogs appear to possess a predisposition to dig, owners of persistent diggers should be advised to provide an area in the backyard set aside for digging activity. The digging area can be temporarily fenced off and baited with buried toys and biscuits. While digging is permitted in the designated area, excavations in other parts of the yard should be consistently discouraged. Some persistent diggers may not restrict their excavations to such areas, however, requiring the implementation of various behavior-modification efforts.

Dogs exhibiting an inordinate interest in digging should be consistently interrupted whenever they are observed engaged in the activity, and then encouraged to take up another activity such as ball play. Keeping the dog on a leash or long line can help facilitate this process. Some digging excesses can be discouraged with a vocal reprimand ("Leave it") and appropriate leash prompt sufficient to interrupt the activity. A modified CO_2 pump with conditioned odor can be highly effective as a disrupter. Tossing a 30-penny shaker can near dogs while they are digging will rapidly interrupt and potentially stop its recurrence, at least so long as the owner is present. In addition to pennies, the can should contain a cotton ball scented with citronella-eucalyptus oil or commercial repellent. The conditioned odor (e.g., citronella-eucalyptus paraffin shavings) can be placed into holes, along with a startle-producing booby-trap device. For example, a motion-sensitive alarm can be sealed in a ziplock bag and placed into holes and covered with loose dirt and grass. A repellent effect might be achieved by mixing a tablespoon of cayenne pepper into a cup of sand, which is placed into a scented plastic bag that is tightly knotted and placed into a covered hole. Another method involves placing a remote-citronella collar in the hole or forbidden area and activating it when the dog digs or approaches the area too closely. In refractory cases, electronic training can be highly effective for suppressing digging activity (see *Electronic Training and Problem Solving* in Chapter 9). A stronger booby-trap arrangement is reserved for inveterate diggers. Several spring-loaded snappers are sealed in slip-lock bags and buried at various levels together with citronella-eucalyptus wax shavings. As a result of such training, the conditioned odor may be used to help deter future digging activity by putting it other active holes.

Dogs that dig under fences can be deterred by attaching vinyl-coated wire fencing to the base of the fence and then burying it 6 to 10 inches underground. In cases where a physical modification of the fence is not practical, an electrified wire can be strung along the base of the fence to provide protection against escape efforts. Electric-fence controllers have been designed for dogs, producing a moderately strong electric shock when touched. When installing such devices, care should be taken not to allow it to come into contact with grass or other grounded objects. Another method involves stringing an electronic containment wire along the base of the fence. Either an electrical or spray boundary collar device worn by the dog should be sufficient to deter most escapists from digging or climbing over fences. Destruction of gardens and planted areas can be most effectively managed by setting up fencing that keeps dogs out of those forbidden areas.

PART 4: APPETITIVE PROBLEMS

PICA AND SCAVENGING

Scavenging forbidden food and eating nonnutritive objects (pica) are common ingestive behavior complaints, requiring both behavioral and medical assessment (see *Pica and Destructive Chewing* in Volume 2, Chapter 9). Pica may present comorbidly with compulsive or hyperkinetic disorders, perhaps requiring adjunctive pharmacological intervention to manage successfully. White (1990), for example, found that one dog in his study of acral lick dermatitis (ALD) was also a rock chewer—a behavior that ceased together with the dog's ALD following treatment with naltrexone. In some dogs with pica, the appetitive-seeking system may be overly active, resulting in hyperarousal and excessive exploratory activity, chewing, and eating of nonnutritive items—signs consistent with hyperkinesis. Dogs showing a persistent appetite for nonnutritive items need to be carefully managed and supervised to prevent alimentary blockages or poisoning. A scavenging dog should be closely controlled on walks, perhaps keeping it on a fixed-action halter collar to turn its head more easily away from found food and garbage. At such times, the vocal signal "Leave it" is combined with a leash prompt strong enough to turn the dog's head away from the object. In addition to interrupting the scavenging response directly, the owner should encourage the dog to turn its attention away from the prized item by using various vocal signals and auditory prompts (e.g., squeaker or smooch sound) and reinforcing the orienting response with a click and flick of the right hand to present a food reward. Such refocusing of attention away from the forbidden object toward the owner is consistently rewarded with treats of varying kinds and value taken along on walks. The dog also needs to be trained to release or drop anything it grabs. This phase of training is initially introduced with toys, with the dog being encouraged to take and release toys of increasing value in exchange for a proffered treat. This release-and-trade routine should be rehearsed and staged indoors and under controlled conditions before transferring it outdoors. As the dog learns to release the target item in exchange for food, the vocal signal "Out" is paired with the action as a discriminative stimulus. In addition to learning how to release toys, the dog should be trained to take them from the floor or hand on signal ("Take it").

Once the releasing and taking behaviors are under stimulus control, more compulsory safeguards are introduced to ensure that the dog avoids or rapidly releases forbidden items found on walks. The itinerary of the walk can be planted with forbidden items in advance, with their locations marked for easy recognition. An alternative method involves dropping forbidden items at various places on the outward leg of a walk and then training the dog to avoid them on the way home. Avoidance of forbidden objects is conditioned by combining directive leash prompts sufficient to turn the dog's head away together with various startle devices (e.g., the shaker can or modified CO_2 pump). As the dog approaches a forbidden object, the trainer shouts "Leave it", whereupon, if the dog fails to turn away on its own accord, a leash prompt is delivered that is strong enough to turn the dog away abruptly from the object. This procedure is repeated until the dog is reliably avoiding forbidden objects in response to the voice command "Leave it." Compliance to the limit-setting imperative is rewarded with affectionate praise and food as the dog returns to the trainer. Dogs with strong oral exploratory interests should

also be provided with frequent opportunities to chase and retrieve toys taken along on walks for such purposes. To help generalize the avoidance response to off-leash situations, a shaker can or other startle-generating objects (e.g., throw rings) can be tossed near the forbidden object with the reprimand "Leave it!" Later, as the result of sensitization, a single shake of the can may be sufficient to deter future interest in the forbidden item. Transitioning from on-leash to off-leash control often requires that forbidden items be arranged to trigger some sort of booby trap, including drop cans and various remote-activated and behavior-activated electronic devices (see *Miscellaneous Devices and Techniques for Deterring Destructive Behavior*). For example, a remote spray receiver can be concealed close to a forbidden object and activated by the trainer as the dog approaches it. In refractory cases of scavenging and pica, remote electronic collars delivering a spray or electrical deterrent can dramatically facilitate inhibitory training and aversive counterconditioning. Remote electronic collars can be highly effective, but they require significant owner instruction and preliminary training before use (see *Punishment and Aversive Counterconditioning* in Chapter 9).

Getting objects out of a dog's mouth once they have a hold can be difficult and sometimes dangerous. Many dog owners have been severely bitten in the process of prying a chicken bone out of their dog's mouth. Despite the risk presented by some dogs, the majority of dogs appear to allow owners to reach into their mouths to pull forbidden items out. Others may resist until the owner places a hand over the muzzle and gently squeezes the upper lip against the premolar teeth. Although commonly used, both of these maneuvers are risky, and it is far safer to train the dog to drop forbidden items on command and to back away (see *Aggression Associated with Guarding and Possessiveness* in Chapter 7). Dogs that persistently refuse to release dangerous objects (e.g., chicken bones) should be kept on a halter collar while on walks, as needed to prevent such behavior.

COPROPHAGY

Coprophagy is a common complaint presented by puppy and dog owners. A study using an owner questionnaire and involving 305 dogs living in Czech households found that 36% of the dogs ate feces—a habit that was more common among females (45%) than males (30%) (Baranyiová et al., 1999). Most owners are disgusted by the habit and are quick to punish such behavior. Although most dogs can be discouraged with routine prevention and training efforts, some dogs may persist in the behavior despite consistent training efforts or comply only so long as the owner is present. A wide variety of techniques have been devised to manage or suppress coprophagy. No one method is effective in all cases, but most dogs eventually respond to a combination of management and training efforts. Since coprophagia is sometimes associated with disease, the dog should be given a veterinary examination to exclude a medical cause. Persistent coprophagy is a serious problem, not just because it is potentially a health risk for the dog, but because it may threaten the human-dog bond as a result of owner displeasure and disgust with the habit. Consequently, coprophagy should be treated with sensitivity and not summarily dismissed as a normal thing that dogs do and something the owner should get over and learn to live with.

Hot Sauce, MSG, Breath Mints, and Other Concoctions

Aside from interactive punishment, the most common method used to discourage interest a dog's in feces is to contaminate the feces with hot sauce (O'Farrell, 1986). Unfortunately, the approach is rarely effective because the dog simply moves on to a fresh deposit that has not been contaminated. Recognizing the obvious shortcomings of coating feces with hot sauce, Houpt (1991) has suggested that the hot sauce be injected into the feces with a syringe and hypodermic needle. The operative assumption is that by injecting feces the dog will be unable to detect the hot sauce until it is too late, causing it to avoid untreated feces as well because it can never be sure which pile contains the repellent. However, given the extraordinary acuity of a dog's nose, it is unlikely that most dogs would be fooled by such a trick. Furthermore, even if the odor could be effectively masked inside feces, the exercise would probably still be in vain since dogs usually swallow the feces in a single gulping action, not leaving much time for the repellent to disperse into the dog's mouth before it is swallowed. Finally, many dogs will bolt down feces sloshed with hot sauce, showing little sign of aversion to the fecal condiment.

Other common remedies are given to dogs to eat in order to make feces less attractive, including meat tenderizers, monosodium glutamate (MSG)-based products, sulfur, and breath meats. There is little evidence that such methods actually work, but positive anecdotal claims have been made for meat tenderizers containing papain and products containing MSG (Carlson and Giffin, 1980). Although the usefulness of MSG for the control of coprophagy has not been demonstrated, it is frequently recommended as a way to make feces less attractive to dogs. Grinding breath mints into a dog's food has also been suggested for the control of coprophagy (Taylor and Luescher, 1996), but no data or rationale are offered to explain the treatment. Other foodstuffs that have been suggested include canned pumpkin, pineapple juice, and anise extract. Both canned pumpkin and pineapple juice are a source of papain. Sulfur-containing foods (e.g., brussels sprouts or cabbage) might be tried, based on a report suggesting that small amounts of sulfur may make the feces less attractive to a dog (Hubbard, 1989). Another alternative source of supplementation is sulfur-containing amino acids (e.g., cystine and methionine) or foods containing high levels of the same. Ferrous sulfate (iron) has also been recommended as way to adulterate feces and make it less palatable (Mugford, 1995). The addition of cooked liver (a good source of iron) to a coprophagous dog's diet might provide some benefit. Adding fiber (e.g., cellulose-containing vegetables like cooked carrots, green beans, and broccoli) to the diet may alter the texture and smell of the feces sufficiently through natural fermentation to make it less attractive to dogs. Finally, *The Merck Veterinary Manual* (Fraser et al., 1991) recommends feeding a high-protein/low-carbohydrate diet supplemented with vegetable oil twice daily, claiming that such a diet can control the problem (in many cases) within 2 months. Adding chemicals and supplements to a dog's diet can be potentially harmful and should be done only under the supervision of a veterinarian.

Nutritional and Dietary Changes

Because a dog might be attracted to partially undigested food remaining in feces, adjusting the diet in terms of its schedule, amount, and nutrient quality may be helpful. Consideration should also be given to adjusting the proportion of protein to carbohydrates and fat in the dog's diet. When possible, coprophagous dogs should be fed high-quality food provided on a multiple-opportunity feeding schedule (two or three times a day, depending on the age and needs of the dog). In addition, the diet might be supplemented with muscle or organ meat (liver or heart) on a temporary basis. Since a coprophagous dog may be seeking B vitamins in the feces, a vitamin supplement, rice bran, or brewer's yeast should be considered (Cloche, 1991). Lastly, a fish-oil supplement might also be considered and added to the dog's diet in appropriate amounts. Many practitioners recommend adding a meat tenderizer containing papain to the dog's diet. Papain can also be obtained in a pure form from most health-food stores. Dogs that prove responsive to commercial meat tenderizers should be given a trial period on papain, either from a natural fruit source (e.g., canned pumpkin) or from an extract powder mixed into their food. Alternatively, products containing a broad spectrum of digestive enzymes (e.g., Prozyme) seem to be effective in many cases.

Preliminary Training

The dog should be prevented from having access to feces for at least 2 weeks, during which time dietary changes and supplementa-tion can be introduced, if warranted, together with supplemental play, exercise, and reward-based obedience training. Ideally, a coprophagous dog should be walked on leash and distracted from feces by calling its name and smooching or squeaking to interrupt interest in the feces and divert its attention toward the owner. As the dog turns away from the feces, it is called ("Come") and rewarded with appropriate encouragement and rewards. The yard should be kept clean of feces. After eliminating, the dog should be praised and a small biscuit tossed out in front of it to pick up. Small biscuits can be covertly dropped during the walk for the dog find on the way back. Likewise, the yard can be seeded with biscuits for the dog to find when let out to play. If the dog ignores efforts to get its attention and approaches the feces, the reprimand "Leave it" is spoken in a firm tone, followed by a directive leash prompt sufficient to turn it away from the feces and toward the owner. The procedure is repeated until the dog turns away from the feces or avoids it in response to the voice signal alone. Additional training may require the use of disrupter-type stimuli, such as the toss of a 30-penny shaker can or burst of air from a modified CO_2 pump. Again, exposure is repeated until the dog shows an active avoidance of feces while on walks.

Booby Traps

Coprophagous dogs should be prevented from eating feces for at least 2 weeks before being exposed to booby-trapped feces. As already discussed, a dog's olfactory abilities mitigate the effectiveness of repellents as deterrents. Unless every feces is consistently treated, dogs will simply avoid stools treated with the repellent and look for ones that are not treated. A motion-activated alarm sealed in a zip-lock bag can be rigged so that it is triggered whenever the dog disturbs the stool. A spring-loaded snapper (see *Caps and Snappers*), which causes a small cap to explode when it is disturbed, produces a stronger startle effect and deterrence. Such "stool mines" can be hidden under the feces. The cap is glued to the underside of a 3-inch square of light cardboard. The snapper is loaded, and the cardboard is put on the ground with a stone placed on top to keep it in place, thereby preventing the loaded snapper from kicking up and going off. A fresh stool is placed on top of the arrangement, and telltale signs of cardboard are covered with bits of loose grass and dirt. For safety sake, if not placed on the underside of paper or cardboard, the snapper should be sealed in a zip-lock bag to prevent flying debris from reaching the dog.

Cat droppings are a favorite with some allocoprophagous dogs. To prevent such problems from developing in the first place, dogs should be kept away from litter pans. In some cases, a cat door or small passage cut through the base of the door can provide the cat with access to its litter but block the dog from getting inside the room. Alternatively, the door can be wedged open between two rubber doorstops, leaving an opening wide enough for the cat to get through, but blocking the dog's access. In the case of dogs exhibiting an established appetite, the first step is to prevent access to cat feces for at least 2 weeks before initiating additional training activities. Training efforts should be first performed on leash to establish an avoidance toward the litter pan, followed by the shaker-can procedure described previously. Since booby trapping risks exposing the cat to accidental stimulation, such devices are not appropriate as deterrents. In situations in which the cat's litter pan cannot be kept out of the dog's reach, electronic devices designed to activate an electrical or spray stimulus worn by the dog can be arranged in the vicinity of the litter pan. When the dog approaches too closely, the collar is activated, causing it to rapidly learn to avoid the situation.

Electronic Training

Electronic training can be used efficaciously to control coprophagy refractory to other methods of control. Both remote electrical or spray stimulation can be effective. The aversive stimulus is delivered at the moment the dog reaches for the feces, but, ideally, before it is picked up. To be effective, the training should be staged in various situations where the dog has eaten feces in the past. An electronic collar should only be used to deliver

deterrent levels of electrical stimulation after safety training is performed with low levels in the context of reinforcing attention control, recall, quick-sit, stay, and halt-stay exercises (safety training). When used to deter coprophagy, the first exposure in which the electrical stimulus (ES) is paired with feces should be of a sufficient strength to produce an immediate and durable inhibition of the activity. The level of stimulation is determined by the dog's degree of sensitivity and tolerance for the ES. Most dogs rapidly learn to avoid feces following a momentary "nick" (100 to 400 msec) of moderate to strong ES. Increasing the level of electrical stimulation gradually is problematic, since the dog may rapidly habituate to each level of ES, requiring a much more aversive event in the end to achieve the desired deterrence effect. Further, a low-level ES not only may invite or perpetuate an already established approach-avoidance conflict toward feces or risk producing vicious-circle behavior in dogs that are not deterred sufficiently by the ES, but may persist or increase the activity in the presence of the aversive event. Such dogs may learn to eat the feces rapidly, thereby foiling the owner's control efforts. Such a vicious-circle effect is often observed in the case of dogs exhibiting persistent and long-standing coprophagy. As the dog's training progresses, it should be exposed to progressively natural conditions where coprophagy might occur in the owner's absence. At such times, dogs may be tempted to find and eat forbidden feces. A well-timed electrical or spray stimulus delivered from a remote location can be very effective to deter such behavior. Until coprophagy is fully suppressed, the dog should not be let in any situation where it might find feces to eat.

Taste Aversion

Many laboratory studies have demonstrated that animals exposed to some nausea-producing event after eating consequently develop a lasting aversion toward that food item (Garcia et al., 1966). This aversion effect often occurs after a single trial and even after a long delay between eating and exposure to the nausea-producing agent. In some experiments, the nausea-producing agent was not given for several hours after the animal had eaten the food. Two aspects of taste aversion are extraordinary when compared to how associative learning usually takes place:

1. A strong and lasting aversion may occur after a single exposure.
2. The aversion develops even though the conditioning events are not closely associated with one another in time.

These characteristics are inconsistent with the usual way in which classical conditioning is believed to take place, requiring that conditioned and unconditioned stimuli be repeatedly paired together in a forward and closely contiguous fashion. The discovery of taste aversion had a profound impact on learning theory (see *Prepared Connections: Taste Aversion* in Volume 1, Chapter 5).

Taste aversion is not the same thing as the conditioned repulsion produced by aversive exposure and sensitization to olfactory and gustatory deterrents like hot sauce and commercial spray repellents. For instance, letting a dog first sniff and then squirting a repellent into its mouth is not consistent with recognized protocols for producing taste aversion (Gustavson, 1996). The procedure described by Beaver (1994) may produce significant revulsion, discomfort, and a conditioned repulsion toward the smell and taste of the substance, but despite the procedure's indisputable capacity for producing aversive arousal and sensitization, it will probably not produce a true taste-aversion effect (see *Taste Aversion* in Volume 1, Chapter 6). However, the method may rapidly cause the dog to resent having its muzzle handled or possibly make the dog refuse to let the owner open its mouth in the future, especially if the procedure is performed repeatedly. Along a similar vein, the practice of spraying concentrated or dilute repellents (e.g., lemon or vinegar) into a dog's face as a deterrent for misbehavior should be avoided, since such treatment may irritate the eyes, produce an aversive state that continues long after the unwanted behavior ceases, and perhaps overlap with more acceptable behavior and hinder efforts to reward it. Repeatedly squirting a dog in the face with dilute repellents or even plain water may rapidly cause it to become avoidant toward the owner. Rather than suppressing the unwanted behavior, dogs often learn to perform the target behavior safely outside of the owner's squirting range. In general, olfactory startle conditioning is preferred for developing chemosensory deterrent signals. Once conditioned, the odor can be used to mark forbidden objects, thereby providing the dog with a warning signal helping it to avoid booby traps set up in close association with the marked objects.

Although the efficacy of taste aversion for the treatment of refractory coprophagy remains controversial (see *Tolerance for Nausea and Taste Aversion* in Volume 2, Chapter 9), the "coprophagiac" might be beneficially treated with a series of treatments using a taste-aversion procedure, especially in cases where electronic training is not feasible or appropriate (e.g., dogs exhibiting behavioral counterindications advising against such training). Taste aversion is most effective in cases involving relatively novel food items, but this criterion is not an absolute. According to Gustavson (1996), conditioned taste aversions can be established with flavors that the animal has been repeatedly exposed to over a long period. Common emetics like ipecac and hydrogen peroxide do not perform as effectively as other taste aversion agents, since they may fail to produce nausea. The chemicals used in taste aversion must produce nausea but not necessarily vomiting. A variety of chemical substances can be used to produce nausea in dogs (see Gustavson, 1996). Taste-aversion conditioning can be established by contaminating feces in advance with the selected nauseant or inducing nausea immediately after the dog ingests feces (Table 2.2).

Caution: Taste-aversion conditioning involves administering potentially poisonous and hazardous chemicals to a dog and should be performed only under the advisement and supervision of a veterinarian familiar with the procedure and its risks, including potential adverse behavioral side effects (see Hansen et al., 1997).

PART 5: CRATE TRAINING

Crate training should always be governed by a philosophy of constructive confinement, signifying that some purposeful training objective is being accomplished by its use. In addition to the criterion of purposeful training, constructive confinement entails that a plan be devised to ensure the eventual release of the puppy or dog from confinement. Without such considerations, the crate can easily become an abusive training tool and a way of life for the dog. Even the most benign and beneficial training tool can become abusive and cruel if excessively or improperly used.

SELECTING A CRATE

Choosing the right crate involves several considerations. Two kinds of crates are typically used for house-training purposes. The most frequently used crate is constructed of heavy-

TABLE. 2.2. Program for persistently coprophagous dogs

1. Coprophagous dogs should receive a thorough veterinary exam to rule out a medical cause.

2. A broad-spectrum digestive enzyme product (e.g., Prozyme) should be considered.

3. Dietary changes may also be helpful, even in cases where the dog is eating a premium diet. Feeding more than once a day may be beneficial in some cases.

4. A determination of when and where the dog eats its stool should be established. Also, information should be recorded regarding the history of the problem. For example, when did the behavior first appear and what sort of things have been tried already to control it?

5. Possible quality-of-life contributing factors should be identified, such as excessive confinement, inadequate play or exercise, environmental stressors, and nutritional deficiencies.

6. Many dogs that exhibit coprophagy also appear to exhibit poor impulse control and attentional abilities. These deficits are addressed through integrated compliance training.

7. The owner is encouraged to walk the dog away from the yard for 2 weeks. During this period, the dog is prevented from approaching or picking up feces by keeping it on a leash and collar (halter type, if necessary). The dog's interest in feces is interrupted with diversionary efforts to capture its attention (e.g., calling its name or squeezing a squeaker) or by using directive signals ("Leave it") and leash prompts sufficient to turn the dog away from the feces. If the dog averts its attention away from the feces, the behavior is bridged ("Good" or click) and reinforced with a food reward. Gradually, the dog is trained to turn from feces and orient on the owner to obtain a food reward.

8. A small biscuit is given to the dog as soon as it leaves the house, and periodically thereafter pieces of biscuits are tossed down for the dog to find in the grass. In addition, the owner can secretly drop biscuits along the way, which the dog is encouraged to find on the way back home. The goal is to encourage the dog to focus on searching for food rather than feces while on walks. As the dog's behavior improves, the number of treats left for it to find can be gradually reduced and faded out. A similar search-and-find game can be set up in the backyard.

9. In cases where diversionary efforts fail to secure the dog's attention, more potent disrupter-type stimuli may be necessary to interrupt the coprophagous interests. A shaker can is often highly effective if thrown at the instant a dog approaches feces. The forceful hissing of the modified compressed-air pump can be highly effective, with the added benefit of blowing the feces out of the dog's reach. The modified compressed-air pump is preferred to excessively loud and startling devises, such as the compressed-air nautical horn.

10. After 2 weeks, various booby traps are introduced to discourage coprophagy when the dog is left alone in the backyard. In general, the yard should be kept clean, with the exception of one or two piles that are left with a booby trap attached to them.

11. In refractory cases, electronic training can be very helpful but should be considered only after the above preliminary efforts have been implemented. Electronic collars delivering electrical or chemical stimulation provide an exact and timely event at a distance—a critical factor affecting the effectiveness of inhibitory training.

12. A conditioned taste-aversion procedure should be considered as a last resort.

gauge metal wire. The crate should be of good quality and sturdy construction. Many dogs have seriously injured themselves attempting to escape from poorly designed and built crates. The best crates are made from panels of 1-inch grid work, but those made with 1-by 3-inch grid panels are usually sufficient for the average puppy. Another type of crate often used for house training is made of plastic and designed for air travel. The plastic travel crate can be made more comfortable by turning it upside down so that the side panels of open grid work are located toward the bottom. This arrangement improves air circulation and gives the puppy a better view of the surroundings while lying down.

An important consideration in choosing a crate is its size. The crate should be big enough to contain an adult dog with enough room for it to stand, lie down comfortably, and turn around. In many cases, this will be a medium to large crate, too big for house-training purposes. Most pet stores stock cage dividers that can be inserted inside the crate to produce the desired dimensions. In addition to a crate, an exercise pen should be obtained. The pen is composed of several interlocking panels that can be adjusted to fit various areas and size needs. It provides greater freedom of movement than provided by the crate, but prevents a puppy from wandering around too much until it is ready for such freedom. If a puppy must be left for extended periods, the crate is kept open and placed inside the holding pen or small puppy-proofed room covered with several layers of newspaper. The puppy should always be provided with a supply of fresh water to meet its needs for the day. Excessive restriction of water does not hasten good elimination habits, but could compromise the puppy's health, perhaps predisposing it to develop urinary tract problems (e.g., cystitis). In addition, puppies deprived of water may drink excessively when finally given an opportunity to drink and then rapidly excrete the excess. Once puppies are successfully crate trained, they can be gradually given more freedom of movement, first in an exercise pen, then the kitchen, and finally the entire house, as they mature and become fully reliable.

GUIDELINES FOR SUCCESSFUL CRATE TRAINING

Most puppies can learn to tolerate crate confinement with minimum distress, provided that it is introduced properly (Table 2.3). The all-too-common practice of setting up the crate and then shoving the uncooperative puppy inside of it to whine, bark, and to attempt to escape from it only risks conditioning a negative and reactive response toward confinement. Remembering that first impressions are enduring, such practices should be avoided. To produce a more positive and minimally stressful attitude toward crate confinement, several simple precautions should be taken. The crate should be set up in a well-socialized part of the house and kept open for the puppy to explore and enter on its own initiative. Putting soft bedding and toys in and around the crate can help to make it more attractive for a wary puppy. Concealing treats in bedding can further entice a puppy to explore the crate and develop a positive attitude toward it. Fetch games should be played around the crate, occasionally tossing the ball into the crate and encouraging the puppy run after it. Also, highly valued chew toys can be put in the crate at various times during the day, further increasing the attractiveness of the crate. Meals and water can also be given near or inside the crate.

Once a puppy is habituated to the presence of the crate and shows a willingness to enter on its own, further training efforts should be introduced. The following instructions are particularly useful for desensitizing and training the resistant puppy to enter and accept crate confinement.

Step 1

Small bits of an appealing food item are tossed in front or just inside of the crate. This procedure is repeated several times, gradually requiring that the puppy move closer and finally poke its head inside the crate. A familiar rug or blanket should be placed inside the crate to make it more attractive and to muffle potentially startling noises that may be produced when the puppy steps on the pan. As the puppy's confidence improves, the treats are tossed further back in the crate until the

Table 2.3. Constructive crate confinement

Do not crate a puppy wearing a collar.

Place the crate in a well-socialized part of the house.

Ensure that the crate is free of drafts and excessive heat.

Do not confine a puppy in the basement or garage.

Never use crate confinement as a form of punishment.

Never allow children to tease or play with a puppy in a crate.

Never attempt to confine a puppy for periods that exceed its ability to control elimination functions.

Provide the puppy with adequate water for its needs during the day.

Do not allow crate confinement to become a way of life.

Never use the crate as a permanent "steel straitjacket" for unresolved behavior problems.

puppy fully enters. As the puppy turns, it is tossed an additional treat, but it is not prevented from leaving the crate.

Step 2

The treat should be tossed with an exaggerated wave of the arm, with the goal of training the puppy to respond to the movement as a prompt to enter the crate. Occasionally, the gesture is made without tossing a treat, causing the puppy to move into the crate and turn about before it is given the expected reward by hand. Once the puppy reliably responds to the prompt, a vocal signal (e.g., "Crate") can be presented in combination with it. Now, as the puppy enters the crate on signal, it is rewarded and the crate door briefly closed and the puppy given several treats through the crate door. After several seconds, the puppy is released and the procedure repeated, progressively requiring that it stay in the crate for longer periods before being released. The puppy's tolerance can be improved by providing it with a beef bone or some other highly desirable chew toy (e.g., a hollow rubber toy smeared on the inside with peanut butter). It is important to vary the duration of confinement, with graduated exposures, for example: 5, 15, 25, 5, 30, 15, 45, 30, 5 seconds, thereby introducing a beneficial element of positive prediction error and reward. As the puppy learns to enter the crate

and accepts brief confinement without protest, longer periods of confinement can be introduced as well as confinement in different household locations (e.g., kitchen, bedroom, and living room), starting with a few seconds and gradually building up to 30 minutes or more, as its tolerance for confinement improves. Puppies should be crated in the bedroom at night and left in the kitchen during the day. In addition to leaving puppies with a tasty toy, the owner should provide the puppy with a scented towel or a few items of soiled clothing (e.g., T-shirt and socks) put inside of a knotted pillow case.

Step 3

Most dogs and puppies accept the aforementioned crate-training process without much anxiousness or resistance. Occasionally, a difficult dog will refuse to enter the crate no matter what efforts are employed to ease its resistance. In such cases, a leash or an active-control line is set up and passed through the opposite crate panel. The puppy or dog is hooked up and prevented from pulling away from the crate and is then slowly maneuvered closer to it through several steps of reward-based training and counterconditioning. Posture-facilitated relaxation (PFR) training may be used to help reduce resistant behavior by training the dog to relax in response to physical restraint (see Appendix C). Ideally, such dogs should be calmed before entering the crate. In some cases, mild to moderate pulling force may be needed on the control line to get the dog into the crate, but such force should be used only as a last resort. Once in the crate, the dog is repeatedly rewarded with food and reassured with affectionate praise and is immediately released. The procedure is repeated on a control line until the dog shows no resistance or hesitancy about entering the crate. In some cases, a remote feeder can be set up at the opening of the crate, delivering a soft food with a faint safety odor (e.g., orange). As the dog approaches the front of crate, the feeder is activated. Gradually, the feeder is set up farther back in the crate, requiring that the dog enter to obtain the food (see *Systematic Desensitization* in Chapter 3). The feeder enables the trainer to provide a continuous flow of repeated reward events while near the dog or while in another room and watching the dog's behavior via a remote camera.

Some puppies and dogs may protest against confinement with persistent barking and intermittent whining, despite gradual and patient desensitization efforts. In such cases, a squeaker can often be helpful as a means to interrupt barking or other vocalizations. After a brief exposure to the squeaker and clicker in the context of attention and sit-stay training, the stimuli can be used to help control excessive vocalization in the crate. As the puppy orients to the squeak sound and stops barking, the break in vocalizing is bridged with "Good" or a click, and the puppy is thrown a treat, whereupon a differential reinforcement of other behavior (DRO) schedule of reinforcement is introduced, such that a bridge and treat is delivered every so often (e.g., 2 to 5 seconds), provided that the dog does not bark during the DRO period (see *Barking* in Chapter 5). Gradually, the DRO period is increased and the vocal signal "Quiet" is paired with the initiation of every DRO period. Alternatively, the barking can be brought under stimulus control by clicking and tossing the dog a treat on each occasion it barks. As the dog's barking turns to the control of food, the vocal signal "Speak" is timed to occur just before or as the dog begins to bark, followed by the bridge and food reward;

conversely, barking off cue is followed by "Quiet" and the loss of reward (response cost). At the earliest opportunity, the trainer should prompt the dog to bark with "Speak" and then bridge and reward the behavior.

As the barking comes under stimulus control, the trainer can initiate time-outs of variable duration in response to barking off cue, thereby linking the loss of social contact with barking and its recovery with not barking. During the time-out, the dog can be ignored in the crate or the trainer can leave the room briefly (e.g. 20 to 30 seconds), requiring that the dog not bark for a brief period before bridging, returning, and rewarding the behavior. As the contingencies become clear to the dog, a drop can is set up and suspended above the crate with a line of dental floss. The drop can is arranged to fall and strike near the crate or on top of it, depending on the dog's temperament and response to such startle. The release of the can is associated with a clipped and subdued "Quiet," perhaps mediating a more rapid inhibitory association while at the same time reducing the level of startle produced by the event. (See the discussion of prepulse inhibition effects covered in *Interrupting Behavior* in Chapter 1). The strength of the event is determined by the height at which the can is dropped and the weight of the can used. In dogs with relatively high-auditory-startle thresholds, a 30-penny can suspended from the ceiling and dropped on top of the crate may be necessary, whereas dogs exhibiting low-auditory-startle thresholds may show an adequately strong response to a seven-penny can dropped 2 feet from the floor. An expedient way to discourage protest vocalizing at bedtime is to say "Quiet" and then to rattle or drop a partially suspended seven-penny shaker can, letting it fall near the crate or on top of it. The shaker should fall forcefully enough to disrupt the behavior but not evoke an excessive startle or fear reaction. If the puppy persists in the barking behavior, the can be dropped from a higher level or replaced by a 30-penny can. As a result of such training, the startle response to the rattling sound is potentiated, causing the puppy to respond to the slightest rattle of the can held by owner or produced by jiggling the suspended drop can. In the case of puppies overly sensitive to the shaker can, pennies can be put inside of a plastic vitamin bottle, thereby producing a shaker that is less noisy and startling.

Before carrying out such procedures, special care should be taken to make sure that a dog's or puppy's protests are not due to fear of confinement or separation distress. Anxious dogs and puppies need to be handled carefully, reducing their fears of crate confinement gradually by means of gradual exposure, counterconditioning, and PFR training. Crate confinement may significantly exacerbate the distress and emotional reactivity associated with separation distress (Borchelt and Voith, 1982). Separation-reactive dogs sometimes become extremely reactive when left alone in a crate, resulting in the loss of eliminatory control and panic-stricken efforts to escape. Separation-reactive and separation-phobic dogs have seriously injured themselves in their frantic efforts to escape confinement when left alone. Aggressive threats and attacks are not uncommon while an unwilling dog is being forced into a crate. If a puppy's adverse reactivity to confinement is suspected to be due to separation distress, it is imperative that appropriate training be carried out to resolve it (Voith, 2002). To prevent separation-distress-related problems, the puppy should be exposed to separation-desensitization training (see *Attachment and Separation Problems: Puppies* in Chapter 4). Such training should be carried out in parts of the house that hold positive emotional associations for the puppy, e.g., the bedroom or kitchen. Allowing a separation-distressed puppy to whimper and whine for long periods without respite should be avoided. Extended periods of separation distress, especially when occurring under unfamiliar circumstances, may predispose sensitive puppies to become overly reactive to routine separations as adults.

By gradually increasing the separation duration while confined in the crate, the puppy learns to experience the crate as a safe situation predicting the owner's eventual return. The owner should be advised of both the benefits of constructive crate confinement and the potential adverse side effects of excessive confinement. Dogs exposed to long peri-

ods of daily crate confinement should receive compensatory exercise, play, and focused attention in the form of reward-based training. A record of the amounts of time (day and night) that the puppy spends in the crate should be kept (Figure 2.7), with the goal of gradually reducing the time spent in crate confinement as training objectives are reached. In summary, constructive crate confinement can be employed as a humane and effective training tool, but it needs to be carefully introduced and never used in the absence of proper training or as an expedient way of life.

DANGERS OF EXCESSIVE CRATE CONFINEMENT

The advocacy of crate confinement as a way of life, sometimes involving 16 to 18 hours a day, for dogs is inconsistent with their biobehavioral needs and may lead to emotional and behavioral deterioration over time. Some puppies and dogs appear to develop an inordinate attachment with their crates, sometimes preferring to be in their crates rather than with the owner. The daily repeated exposure to the sterile environs of the crate may significantly undermine a developing dog's ability to habituate and adjust to the wider domestic social and physical environment. Although most puppies initially respond to crate confinement as a stressful state of affairs, with repeated exposure stress and aversion gradually give way to an odd attraction to confinement. This gradual attraction to crate confinement appears to occur in association with increased feelings of security, safety, and comfort, rather than increasing levels of vulnerability and insecurity, as one might expect from a condition of entrapment.

Bonding with the Crate

One possible explanation for this paradoxical effect is provided by opponent-process theory (see *Opponent-process Theory and Separation Distress* in Volume 2, Chapter 4). The lengthy exposure to crate confinement provides a situation in which separation distress and other reactions associated with vulnerable isolation

	DOG'S NAME:		DATE:	
	SESSION NO.:			

DAILY CRATE CONFINEMENT RECORD

D A Y	DAY	NIGHT	TOTAL	COMMENTS
1				
2				
3				
4				
5				
6				
7				

FIG. 2.7. Crate confinement chart.

eventually give way to opponent affects of comfort and safety, that is, the exact opposite to the distress and vulnerability initially evoked by crate confinement. Over the course of repeated exposures, the initial adverse reactions to confinement and isolation become weaker and gradually are overshadowed by opponent arousal involving feelings of enhanced security and contentment. In addition to providing emotional arousal incompatible with aversion and efforts to escape, these hypothesized opponent responses may provide a counterconditioning effect, further restraining and reducing aversive arousal associated with crate confinement. So far, this opponent-processing analysis does not sound like much of a problem for a dog until one considers how it may interfere with the formation of a satisfying attachment and bond between the owner and the dog. A significant aspect of the attachment object is the provision of comfort and safety, that is, security. For dogs exposed to excessive crate confinement or home environments lacking sufficient consistency and order, their search for comfort and safety may gradually turn from the family and home to the crate. Such dogs may develop a powerful bond and dependency upon the crate as a space of comfort and safety. According to the foregoing opponent-processing analysis, behavioral restraint in association with confinement may result in opponent affects associated with enhanced comfort and safety (nurturing), thereby producing a source of intrinsic reward, security, and contentment that may support passive activities occurring in association with crate confinement. As such, crate confinement minimally meets the three interactive criteria required for establishing a bond: (1) dominance (limit setting by force or threat of force), (2) leadership (prompting and rewarding alternative behavior), and (3) nurturance (comfort and safety obtained in association with deference (criterion 1) and cooperation (criterion 2). Interestingly, when dogs that have been trained to sleep in an isolated part of the house in a crate are allowed to sleep in a bedroom, they often show signs of acute distress, including increased exploratory activity, agitation, and inability to calm down and sleep. In addition, some of these dogs exhibit excessive drooling, become diarrheic, lose bladder control, and show other changes consistent with the behavioral and autonomic sequela associated with separation distress. This reactive behavior is often persistent and requires that the dog be slowly adjusted to sleeping in the bedroom at night.

So, as many owners say, it may be truer than expected that some dogs do, in fact, love their crates, perhaps in some cases more than they love the owner. According to the crate-bond hypothesis, in the absence of a secure and gratifying attachment between the owner and dog, a crate bond may preempt or interfere with the formation of a human-dog bond, possibly setting the stage for the development or exacerbation of a variety of bond-related behavior problems (e.g., separation-distress and owner-directed aggression). Interestingly, in this regard, a subgroup of social aggressors is particularly reactive when in their crates or when disturbed while engaged in activities phenomenally similar to those associated with the security afforded by crate confinement (e.g., resting). Excessive crate confinement may generally sensitize and lower reactive thresholds in predisposed dogs to signals of punishment (threat or loss of comfort) and uninvited social contact, resulting in signs of increased intolerance, irritability, and social incompetence. Excessive crate confinement may cause such dogs to become inordinately sensitive to touch contact and interference while in resting states, possibly because learning conducive to competent impulse control in response to intrusions upon such states of heightened comfort and safety requires direct interaction and tactile contact between the owner and dog, but the crate effectively blocks such interaction and learning. Although the dog may get adequate auditory and visual stimulation while in the crate to offset sensitizing effects of sensory deprivation, tactile stimulation is entirely restricted, providing the basis for a sensitization effect that may increase irritability and intolerance for frustration while lowering aggressive thresholds in response to training. Compensatory tactile stimulation in the form of PFR training is incorporated into the treatment of such dogs in order to provide the necessary direct stimulation to reduce sensitization effects and to organize expectancies incompatible with threat or loss of comfort.

Adverse Effects of Excessive Confinement

Social and environmental adaptations occurring early in life appear to moderate sensorimotor thresholds and homeostatic set points to environmental and social stimuli. Inadequate exposure to varied and complex environmental circumstances and social experiences, traumatic or abusive handling, or exposures lacking sufficient order and consistency may significantly alter reactive fear and anger thresholds, causing dogs to become progressively reactive (fearful or aggressive) or intolerant of novel or complex demands put upon them. Rearing under laboratory conditions of sensory restriction and social isolation causes a broad spectrum of devastating behavioral effects. Dogs raised to maturity under conditions of social and environment restriction tend to become increasingly excitable, reactive, and disorganized in response to environmental change. Early work carried out by Melzack (1954) identified a cluster of deleterious emotional and cognitive effects resulting from excessive sensory restriction and confinement of developing dogs. These dogs showed a persistent and excessive hyperexcitability to environmental change, reflected in durable changes in brain electrical activity (Melzack and Burns, 1965). The slightest deviation from their accustomed social and environmental conditions resulted in a dramatic increase in activity, often culminating in the expression of whirling fits. In addition to impulse-control dysregulation, restricted dogs often exhibited extreme attention deficits, preventing them from selectively attending to environmental stimuli in an organized way. Instead of exploring and interacting with objects, such dogs raced from one thing to another. Restriction-reared dogs showed a pronounced inability to learn simple avoidance tasks and reacted abnormally to painful stimuli (Melzack and Scott, 1957).

According to Melzack's analysis and model, environmental stimulation is selectively filtered at the "earliest synaptic levels of sensory pathways" in accordance with information derived from past learning—an early articulation of the sensorimotor-gating hypothesis (see *Prediction and Control Expectancies* in Chapter 1). Melzak's theory suggests that the loss of attention and impulse control exhibited by severely restricted dogs is due to a failure of the restrictive environment to provide sufficient opportunity for the dog to acquire a predictive network of associations with which to filter relevant sensory input from irrelevant static. The central nervous system of such dogs appears to crash under the overload of a sensory bombardment resulting from the restricted dog's inability to competently filter out relevant from irrelevant sensory data and to contextualize it in conformity with past memories and experiences (prediction and control expectancies). As the result of adaptive learning, the dog acquires a cognitive and emotional interface of prediction-control expectancies that rapidly appraises the significance of sensory input via a comparator function sensitive to the detection of discrepancies between what the dog expects to occur and what actually occurs (see *Prediction Error and Adaptation* in Chapter 10). Relevant information is selected from irrelevant information based upon the input's significance to operative control incentives ongoing at the moment. Sensory input that deviates from established control expectancies, resulting in surprise (reward) or disappointment (punishment), is of particular importance for the development of organized behavior. Information resulting in surprise and the avoidance of disappointment is preferentially sought in the process of learning. In addition to prediction errors related to control incentives and expectancy modules (e.g., surprise), dogs are also sensitive to discrepancies occurring in association with novelty and startle. However, instead of reacting to novelty or startle with disorganized output as in the case of Melzack's restrictively reared dogs, well-trained and socialized dogs respond to such stimuli with appropriate hesitation and curiosity before choosing a course of action. Finally, unlike restricted dogs, which respond to aversive stimuli without a clear appreciation of the event's significance as a threat, well-adjusted dogs respond to unconditioned aversive stimuli with forbearance, escape, or aggression, as appropriate and most likely to control the event successfully, perhaps in accord with a rapid cost-benefit analysis of available control modules and probable outcomes.

Even in cases where puppies have been previously well socialized, they may become progressively reactive to environmental stimuli and handling if kept under conditions of sensory and social deprivation (Fox, 1974). In such cases, sensory restriction and social isolation appear to degrade or reverse the benefits of early socialization. Dogs need a balance of sensory input to achieve behavioral homeostasis. Depending on temperament traits and early experience, environments producing too little or too much stimulation may produce an adverse effect. Environments producing too little stimulation and variety may predispose dogs to develop behavioral adjustment problems associated with intensified efforts to increase stimulation and gratification. Dogs presenting with hyperactivity are often affected by stimulation-seeking excesses, especially attention-seeking behavior that appears to continue unabated, even after the dogs get large amounts of social contact and stimulation. Environments producing too much stimulation and variety may produce changes in behavior in the direction of compulsive excesses, that is, behavior aimed at modulating excessive stimulation. Most dogs are organized with a sufficient degree of behavioral plasticity to adapt to environmental changes involving increases or decreases in stimulation, on the one hand, and increases or decreases in frustration or anxiety, on the other (adaptive types). These stable and adaptive dogs are differentiated along an extraversion-introversion continuum: the sanguine (stable extravert) and phlegmatic (stable introvert). However, some dogs, as the result genetic predisposition, adverse early experiences, or neurotogenic learning may become progressively reactive to increases or decreases in environmental stimulation and changes producing frustration and anxiety (reactive types). These unstable and reactive dogs are also differentiated along an extraversion-introversion continuum: the choleric (unstable extravert) and the melancholic (unstable introvert) (see *Experimental Neurosis* in Volume 1, Chapter 9). Whereas adaptive types are preferentially sensitive to signals of reward (sanguine) or signals of avoidance (phlegmatic), reactive types are preferentially sensitive to loss of comfort (choleric) and loss of safety (melancholic). Finally, adaptive types shown an affinity for activating the seeking and social engagement systems, whereas reactive types show an affinity for activating the anger and fear emotional command systems.

Choleric (c-type) dogs may be particularly vulnerable to the adverse effects of environmental deprivation, excessive crate confinement, and a lack of daily training and play.

Failure to provide c-type dogs (high sensitivity for frustration/low anger and attack thresholds) with appropriate daily stimulation and training conducive to organized and balanced attention and impulse control may rapidly elevate frustration levels while at the same time lowering aggression thresholds. C-type dogs may be susceptible to the sensitizing effects of restricted tactile stimulation and crate-related conflict in association with signals of loss and frustration. Such dogs may develop reactive elaborations in response to innocuous interference and loss of comfort while resting in favorite locations (see *Bonding with the Crate*). C-type dogs may also show an increased susceptibility to separation-distress reactivity as the result of sensitization occurring in association crate-related conflict and frustration. The separation-reactive c-type dog may attack as the owner leaves the house. On the other hand, melancholic-type (m-type) dogs may be more vulnerable to environmental situations or change producing too much stimulation or arousal, perhaps gradually activating behaviors aimed a reducing it (e.g., compulsive licking). Whereas c-types may become increasing reactive in response to stimulation levels falling below homeostatic set points, m-types (high sensitivity for anxiety/low threshold for fear and escape) may be affected by intolerance for stimulation that exceeds homeostatic set points. As the result of restricted tactile stimulation and conflict produced in association with excessive crate confinement and anxiety, m-type dogs may be more prone to develop reactive aggressive elaborations in response to innocuous threat signals. M-type dogs may be particularly susceptible to separation reactivity occurring in association with anxiety. Dogs presenting with an admixture of c-type and m-type propensities (high sensitivity to frustration and anxiety combined with low anger and low fear thresholds) may be prone to panic-related aggression and separation-distress reactions. Both c-type and m-type dogs tend to *react* in response to environmental changes producing frustration and anxiety, whereas sanguine (s-type) and phlegmatic (p-type) dogs tend to *adapt* to environmental changes producing frustration and anxiety. However, under conditions of excessive crate confinement, neglect (absence of training, exercise, and play), and environmental conditions lacking consistency and order, s-type and p-type dogs may become progressively unstable in the direction of c- and m-types.

The role of crate confinement in the etiology of behavior problems has not been scientifically established, but empirical impressions and logic dictate that it probably plays an important role in the development or exacerbation of many adjustment problems. In the absence of daily socialization and training, organized behavior may gradually degrade, causing a dog to lose its ability to respond competently to social signals. Even more significantly, however, under the influence of disorderly social circumstances, lacking sufficient predictability and controllability to elaborate viable prediction-control expectancies, the dog may be rendered particularly vulnerable to the stressful effects of excessive crate confinement and social isolation. Such dogs may fall victim to the disorganizing effects of inconsistent punishment and reward, causing them to become progressively incompetent and reactive to ambivalent social interaction. Given the organizing effects of learning on the development of competent attention and impulse control, it is reasonable hypothesize that a converse effect follows when dogs are exposed to excessive confinement and isolation (marginalization) in combination with disorderly or deranged social interaction—conditions that place dogs at the greatest risk of developing adjustment problems. In contrast, dogs that are integrated into a home-life situation consisting of orderly interactions are much less likely to experience an exacerbation of predisposing influences or develop an adjustment problem. Given the ubiquitous presence of crate confinement and its potential for producing stress, environmental and social deprivation, and abuse, it is odd that so little research is currently available with which to evaluate its potential role in the development of adjustment problems. Clearly, given the adverse behavioral and physiological effects associated with kenneling (Hubrecht et al., 1992; Clark et al., 1997; Coppinger and Zuccotti, 1999) and evidence of an increased risk of relinquish-

ment in situations where dogs spend most of the day in a crate (Patronek, 1996), sufficient grounds exist to justify a serious examination of the potential role of crate confinement in the etiology of behavior problems (see *Deprivation and Trauma* in Volume 2, Chapter 2). Hopefully, in the future, researchers performing relevant cynopraxic studies will routinely collect such data to help flesh out the roles of excessive confinement and social-interaction deficiencies in the development of adjustment problems.

Freedom Reflex, Loss of Control, and Restraint

Healthy dogs are endowed with a robust freedom reflex, and they accept crate confinement and other forms of restraint (e.g., halter control) begrudgingly, frequently only after a significant struggle. As such, crate confinement is not only a condition of restraint, it also represents a loss of control. The loss of control over significant events is a necessary condition for producing experimental neurosis; however, the critical factor for producing neurotic disturbances is restraint (see *Liddell: The Cornell Experiments* in Volume 1, Chapter 9). Under conditions of restraint, exposure to inescapable aversive stimulation exerts pronounced behavioral and cognitive disturbances (see *Learned Helplessness* in Volume 1, Chapter 9). The condition of crate confinement satisfies both of the requirements for inducing neurotic elaborations. The chronic inhibition of the canine freedom reflex by daily crating is probably a source of significant conflict and stress for dogs and, when occurring in combination with a social environment lacking consistency and controllability, a convergence of potent behavior-disorganizing influences may be unleashed. If exposed to crate confinement without counterconditioning, dogs and puppies often protest vigorously with distress vocalizations and persistent efforts to escape, such as scratching and biting at the cage walls. The dog's initial resistance and resentment slowly yield and, after a variable period of diminishing effort, the dog may slip into a state of depressed resignation. The dog's ability to accept such restraint may not occur without a significant risk of harm, however. In postpubertal and adult dogs, the sorts of behavior prompting owners to crate their dogs often arises from a failure to establish consistent communication and control efforts, thereby only compounding difficulties, making things much worse, and postponing the proper resolution of the problem.

ETHOLOGICAL RATIONALIZATIONS OF CRATE CONFINEMENT

A common rationalization for crate confinement is based on a questionable assumption that the dog is a denning animal, naturally prepared and well adapted for life in a crate. Despite the widespread circulation of this belief, there exists little factual evidence to support it. The belief that the dog is a denning animal is flawed in several ways, as Borchelt (1984) points out:

> The average dog book refers to dogs as "den dwelling" animals and presumes that confining imparts a feeling of security to a puppy. Dogs, in fact, are not den dwelling animals, although in a variety of canids the dam will construct a nest (often underground) for the pups. The nest is a defense against predators and protection against inclement weather. The pups use it as a "home base" from which they explore, investigate and play. There is no door on the den which encloses the pups for many hours. In many cases, "crate training" a puppy will attenuate vocalization and elimination, and prevent chewing. Unfortunately, it may also exacerbate these behaviours and sometimes leads to psychosomatic signs or hyperactivity elicited by the owner's return ... Crating or other confinement (e.g., isolating in a small room) is highly likely to exacerbate a separation problem once it has occurred for any length of time, or for a puppy with a previous attachment and separation problem. (171–172)

Although wolves do prepare dens to whelp and rear their young, they do not use such places as general sleeping or resting areas. In fact, as early as 10 to 12 weeks of age, wolf pups are generally moved from den locations to rendezvous sites ("open-air kindergartens") where they are left while adults go on hunting sorties (Young and Goodman, 1944/1964; Allen, 1979). Corbett (1995) has reported that dingoes exhibit similar den habits, moving pups from den sites at about 8 weeks of age to various rendezvous areas, usually rock ledges. Ironically, this is precisely the time when most domestic puppies are first introduced to their "four-sided" dens. Wolves normally make their beds under conifer trees or on rock outcroppings where they have an unobstructed view of the surrounding terrain (Murie, 1944/1987). After the pack has satisfied itself on a kill, they often expend a great deal of energy to find open areas to lie down and sleep (Mech, 1970):

> After feeding intensively, wolves then seek a suitable spot in which to rest and sleep. If the sun is shining and the wind is light, they prefer open areas such as ridge tops or expanses of ice, and they will travel several miles to get to such places. There they sprawl out on their sides or bellies for several hours. During windy, snowy weather, they curl up in protected areas such as beneath evergreen trees, where they remain for long periods. (190–191)

The preceding discussion is not intended to eschew crate confinement altogether or to persuade dog owners not to use crate confinement as a responsible training tool; it is intended, however, to balance the promotional propaganda of advocates recommending crate confinement as an unabashedly positive thing, a virtual utopian condition for the dog, satisfying the dog's "den instinct," and similar misunderstandings and exaggerations. Crate advocates routinely espouse crate confinement as a way of life for family dogs, without fully appreciating the harmful side effects that may occur as the result of excessive restriction and social isolation. The convenience of crate confinement and the social permission afforded by glib rationalizations has beguiled many dog owners into believing the myth wholesale. For people convinced that their dog loves its crate, keeping it confined for 16 to 18 hours a day in a laundry room is not such a bad thing: after all, the dog is a "den" animal. As a result, many dog owners have come to regard the crate as a panacea for controlling undesirable behavior. Instead of dedicating the necessary time and effort needed to socialize and train the dog properly, the crate has become a steel straightjacket for controlling untreated behavior problems.

Contrary to the popular hype, the crate is not a "home," nor is it a "den": it is a place of confinement. In essence, the crate mechanically suppresses a dog's behavior, restrains the dog's freedom of movement, and imposes a loss of control; as such, crate confinement is a condition of punishment (loss of reward) that can be highly aversive and stressful for a dog reactive to such restraint. Successful crate training requires gradual exposure and counterconditioning. Perhaps, in the future, a manufacturer will develop an inexpensive feeder and manipulandum that can be attached to the crate and interfaced with a program conducive to sustaining a dog's interest, thereby helping the dog to form a more positive association with the crate. Performing PFR training before crating a dog may help it to relax, especially if a well-conditioned olfactory-signature odor is left behind to maintain the effect. Introducing the crate slowly and making it comfortable with soft or tasty toys and objects scented with the owner's odor can help to reduce adverse side effects, but it will not eliminate them. In the case of dogs that require long-term crate confinement, appropriate compensatory stimulation and activities should be provided. The cynopraxic process is dedicated to nurturing and supporting the dog's capacity for freedom by means of training and play. As such, crate confinement is viewed as an aversive technique and used as any other aversive technique, that is, as a necessary evil toward a greater good (see *Cynopraxis and Ethics* in Chapter 10) (Table 2.4). The goal of crate training should be to get the dog out of the crate as soon as possible, and to use the crate as little as possible in the service of training and space-management objectives.

REFERENCES

Ainsworth C (2000). Dogs are a bunch of cleverclogs. *New Sci,* 168:20.

Allen DL (1979). *Wolves of Minong: Their Vital Role in a Wild Community.* Boston: Houghton Mifflin.

Baranyiová E, Holub A, Janáchová B, et al. (1999). Nutritional interactions of man and dog. In *Proceedings Mondial Vet Lyon 99* (CD-ROM), Sep 23–26.

Beaver BV (1994). *The Veterinarian's Encyclopedia of Animal Behavior.* Ames: Iowa State University Press.

Table 2.4. Summary of adverse effects of excessive crate confinement

Excessive confinement may result in deleterious sensory and behavioral deprivation.

Social and environmental deprivation provides motivational setting events for hyperactive and intrusive social excesses.

Influences of confinement-related frustration may generalize over numerous behavior systems (e.g., social, appetitive, and exploratory).

Upon release from confinement, undesirable social behavior may be strongly reinforced and integrated into the dog's postconfinement repertoire.

Excessive confinement is stressful for a highly sociable and dependent family dog.

Improper crate training may exacerbate separation distress.

Four-sided confinement (a trap) is a natural condition of vulnerability and may activate survival mechanisms associated with biological adversity.

Excessive confinement interferes with normal training, adjustment, and adaptive functioning.

Excessive confinement may socially marginalize a dog within the family system.

Since the condition of confinement is inescapable, symptoms of learned helplessness may develop especially in the case of dogs experiencing a highly level of aversive arousal while confined to a crate.

Frantic efforts to escape from the crate may result in serious injuries to the dog or its death.

Repeatedly forcing a dog into a crate may cause it to become aggressively reactive at such times.

Borchelt PL (1984). Behaviour development of the puppy in the home environment. In RS Anderson (Ed), *Nutrition and Behavior in Dogs and Cats: Proceedings of the First Nordic Symposium on Small Animal Veterinary Medicine*. New York: Pergamon.

Borchelt PL and Voith VL (1982). Diagnosis and treatment of separation-related behavior problems in dogs. *Vet Clin North Am Symp Anim Behav*, 12:625–635.

Brown JS, Martin RC, and Morrow MW (1964). Self-punitive behavior in the rat: Facilitative effects of punishment on resistance to extinction. *J Comp Physiol Psychol*, 57:127–133.

Call J, Bräuer J, Kaminski J, and Tomasello M (2003). Domestic dogs are sensitive to the attentional state of humans. *J Comp Psychol* (in press).

Carlson DG and Giffin JM (1980). *Dog Owner's Home Veterinary Handbook*. New York: Howell Book House.

Clark JD, Rager DR, Crowell-Davis S, and Davis DL (1997). Housing and exercise of dogs: Effects on behavior, immune function, and cortisol concentration. *Lab Anim Sci*, 47:500–510.

Cloche D (1991). Coprophagy. *Tijdschr Diergeneeskd*, 116:1257–1258.

Corbett LK (1995). *The Dingo in Australia and Asia*. Ithaca, NY: Comstock/Cornell.

Coppinger R and Zuccotti J (1999). Kennel enrichment: Exercise and socialization of dogs. *J Appl Anim Welfare Sci*, 2:281–296.

Fox MW (1974). *Concepts of Ethology: Animal and Human Behavior*. Minneapolis: University of Minnesota Press.

Fraser MC, Bergeron JN, Mays A, and Aiello SE (Eds) (1991). The *Merck Veterinary Manual: A Handbook of Diagnosis, Therapy, and Disease Prevention and Control for the Veterinarian*, 7th Ed. Rahway, NJ: Merck.

Garcia J, Ervin F, and Koelling RA (1966). *Learning with prolonged delay of reinforcement. Psychonom Sci*, 5:121–122.

Gustavson CR (1996). Taste aversion conditioning versus conditioning using aversive peripheral stimuli. In VL Voith and PL Borchelt (Eds), *Readings in Companion Animal Behavior*. Philadelphia: Veterinary Learning Systems.

Hansen I, Bakken M, and Braastad BO (1997). Failure of LiCl-conditioned taste aversion to prevent dogs from attacking sheep. *Appl Anim Behav Sci*, 54:251–256.

Hart BL and Hart LA (1985). *Canine and Feline Behavioral Therapy*. Philadelphia: Lea and Febiger.

Harrington FH (1981). Urine-marking and caching behavior in the wolf. *Behaviour*, 76:280–288.

Houpt KA (1991). Feeding and drinking behavior problems. *Vet Clin North Am Adv Companion Anim Behav*, 21:281–298.

Houpt K, Zgoda JC, and Stahlbaum CC (1984). Use of taste repellents and emetics to prevent accidental poisoning of dogs. *Am J Vet Res*, 45:1501–1503.

Hubbard B (1989). Flatulence and Coprophagia. *Vet Focus*, 1:51–53.

Hubrecht RC, Serpell JA, and Poole TB (1992). Correlates of pen size and housing conditions on the behaviour of kennelled dogs. *Appl Anim Behav Sci*, 34:365–383.

James WT (1961). Preliminary observations on play behavior in puppies. *J Genet Psychol*, 98:273–277.

Landsberg GM (1994). Symposium on behavior problems: Products for preventing or controlling undesirable behavior. *Vet Med*, 89:970–983.

Mason JR, Shivik JA, and Fall MW (2001). Chemical repellents and other aversive strategies in predation management. *Endangered Species Update*, 18:175–181.

Mech LD (1970). *The Wolf: The Ecology and Behavior of an Endangered Species*. Minneapolis: University of Minnesota Press.

Melzack R (1954). The genesis of emotional behavior: An experimental study of the dog. *J Comp Physiol Psychol*, 47:166–168.

Melzack R and Burns SK (1965). Neurophysiological effects of early sensory restriction. *Exp Neurol*, 13:163–175.

Melzack R and Scott TH (1957). The effects of early experience on the response to pain. *J Comp Physiol Psychol*, 50:155–160.

Mugford RA (1995). Canine behavioural therapy. In J Serpell (Ed), *The Domestic Dog: Its Evolution, Behaviour, and Interaction with People*. New York: Cambridge University Press.

Murie A (1944/1987). *The Wolves of Mt. McKinley*. Seattle: University of Washington Press (reprint).

New JC, Salman MD, King M, et al. (2000). Characteristics of shelter-relinquished animals and their owners compared with animals and their owners in U.S. pet-owning households. *J Appl Anim Welfare Sci*, 3:179–201.

Odendaal JSJ (1996). An ethological approach to the problem of dogs digging holes. *Appl Anim Behav Sci*, 52:299–305.

O'Farrell V (1986). *Manual of Canine Behavior*. Cheltenham, UK: British Small Animal Veterinary Association.

Otto T and Giardino ND (2001). Pavlovian conditioning of emotional responses to olfactory and contextual stimuli: A potential model for the development and expression of chemical intolerance. *Ann NY Acad Sci*, 933:291–309.

Paschall GY and Davis M (2002). Olfactory-mediated fear-potentiated startle. *Behav Neurosci*, 116:4–12.

Patronek GJ, Glickman LT, Beck AM, et al. (1996). Special report: Risk factors for relinquishment of dogs to an animal shelter. *JAVMA*, 209:572–581.

Pettijohn TF, Wong TW, Ebert PD, and Scott JP (1977). Alleviation of separation distress in 3 breeds of young dogs. *Dev Psychobiol*, 10:373–381.

Roberts WA (2002). Are animals stuck in time? *Psychol Bull*, 128:473–489.

Salman MD, Hutchinson J, Ruch-Gallie R, et al. (2000). Behavioral reasons for relinquishment of dogs and cats to 12 shelters. *J Appl Anim Welfare Sci*, 3:93–106.

Skinner BF (1968). *The Technology of Teaching*. New York: Appleton-Century-Crofts.

Taylor A and Leuscher UA (1996). Animal behavior case of the month (multiple problems including coprophagia). *JAVMA*, 208:1026–1028.

Voith VL (2002). Use of crates in the treatment of separation anxiety in the dog. Presented at the AVMA Annual Convention, July 13–17.

Voith VL and Borchelt PL (1985). Elimination behavior and related problems in dogs. *Compend Continuing Educ Pract Vet*, 7:537–544.

White SD (1990). Naltrexone for treatment of acral lick dermatitis in dog. *JAVMA*, 196:1073–1076.

Wolski TR, Riter R, and Houpt KA (1984). The effectiveness of animal repellents on dogs and cats in the laboratory and field. *Appl Anim Behav Sci*, 12:131–144.

Yeon SC, Erb HN, and Houpt KA (1999). A retrospective study of canine housesoiling: Diagnosis and treatment. *J Am Anim Hosp Assoc*, 35:101–106.

Young SP and Goldman EA (1944/1964). *The Wolves of North America. Part I: Their History, Life Habits, Economic Status, and Control.* New York: Dover.

3

Fears and Phobias

PART 1: ORIENTATION AND BASIC CONCEPTS

Working with fears and phobias requires considerable insight and technical skill. First and foremost, cynopraxic counseling and training activities should cultivate owner understanding and management strategies, as well as introduce and demonstrate procedures aimed at gradually reducing a dog's fear and fear-related behavior. Many common fears can be successfully treated; however, some phobias are highly resistant or intractable and may show only limited improvement despite the most conscientious training efforts. In such cases, counseling efforts should emphasize management strategies designed to help an owner cope with the challenges of living with a fearful dog.

Coping with Fear

Keeping in mind that fear is primarily under the control of Pavlovian influences (Maren, 2001; see also *Classical Conditioning and Fear* in Volume 1, Chapter 6), it is unlikely that emotional responses associated with fear (e.g., trembling and panting) are significantly influenced by reward and punishment. Nonetheless, instrumental escape and avoidance efforts associated with fearful arousal may strongly influence fear-related behavior. The way fearful behavior is managed has a direct effect on fearful arousal and its perpetuation. For example, although vocal encouragement and petting can have a calming and beneficial effect on a moderately fearful dog, such comforting efforts may also inadvertently reinforce fear-related behavior by providing the dog with a shield of safety, behind which it can escape or avoid fearful situations. Although owner attitudes and anxiety do not appear to play a particularly prominent role in the etiology and maintenance of major phobias (see *Owner Mental States and Behavior Problems* in Volume 2, Chapter 10), an owner's apprehensions about a dog's behavior when approaching fear-eliciting objects or situations may significantly influence therapeutic outcomes. In such circumstances, the dog is not likely to attribute the owner's worry to *itself* or to its behavior, but will more likely interpret the owner's worry as something bearing on the developing situation, perhaps increasing its own wariness. By adopting a confident attitude, excessive worry and apprehension about a dog's behavior can be avoided. Helping the owner to establish basic control over the dog's behavior is one of the best ways to instill confidence. As the owner's control over the dog improves, he or she will naturally feel more secure and relaxed when confronting potentially disruptive situations with the dog. Similarly, dogs under control appear to be more secure and confident, seeming to equate the owner's enhanced control over them with a safer environment.

Obviously, effective behavior therapy and training entail that both the owner and the dog learn how to cope more effectively with fear. Dogs cope with aversive situations through a variety of cognitive, behavioral, and physiological means. Appreciating the interaction between fearful behaviors and underlying physiological changes is extremely important (see *Autonomic Nervous System-mediated Concomitants of Fear* in Volume 1, Chapter 3). High levels of stress associated with fearful arousal may interfere with adaptive behavior, resulting in persistent maladaptive coping strategies that impede the extinction of fear. Emotionally stressful situations appear to contribute to the development of phobias and their expression (Jacobs and Nadel, 1985). For example, dogs exhibiting separation anxiety appear to be more prone to develop storm-related fears, perhaps as the result of an increased vulnerability to fear-eliciting stimuli stemming from emotional stress. Similarly, separation anxiety may present comorbidly with thunder phobias, requiring that both problems be addressed together. Frank and colleagues (2000) have reported that 40% of dogs with thunder and noise phobias also exhibit concomitant symptoms of separation anxiety. The threshold-lowering effects of stress can also be observed in dogs fearful of strangers and unfamiliar dogs.

When confronted with aversive situations, dogs typically cope by engaging in activities that serve to reduce the danger:

> Escape from eliciting stimulus (flee)
> Displace the source of aversive stimulation (fight)
> Increase vigilance or searching behavior (flirt)
> Wait for the situation to change (freeze)
> Tolerate or accept the situation (forbear)

Constructive coping strategies involve behavioral efforts designed to render an unfamiliar or threatening environment more predictable and controllable. Many dogs are fearful of unfamiliar things and situations because they are uncertain about their ability to predict and control them, often operating under the influence of toxic expectancies or dysfunctional learning experiences. Such dogs may *expect to fail* when faced with difficult or threatening situations (adversity). Expecting to fail when confronted with unfamiliar or adverse situations is a potent source of anxiety and frustration. Anxiety and frustration are the emotional corollaries of situations in which unfamiliarity or detrimental cognitive and learning influences undermine a dog's ability to predict and control critical events effectively (see *Anxiety* in Volume 2, Chapter 3). As an aversive or threatening situation proves unpredictable and uncontrollable, anxiety and frustration correspondingly increase and impede adaptive behavior, perhaps causing the dog to become progressively hyperreactive (choleric type) or hyporeactive (melancholic type). However, as the result of experiences in which a dog has learned that it can successfully control aversive situations and threats, it naturally acquires an enhanced sense of competency and confidence, learning to *expect to succeed* when faced with adversity (see *Efficacy Expectancies* in Volume 2, Chapter 3). Under the influence of positive efficacy expectancies, the dog is more likely to approach uncertain situations in a more confident, success-oriented, and adaptive way (sanguine and phlegmatic types). Cynopraxic behavior therapy consists of reward-based procedures aimed at reducing adverse behavioral stress (anxiety and frustration) while at the same time training the dog to cope more competently and confidently with uncertain and unfamiliar situations.

BASIC TRAINING AND FEAR

Many dogs exhibiting excessive fear or generalized anxiety appear to do so under the influence of a negative expectancy with respect to their ability to cope with aversive events effectively (see *Efficacy Expectancies* in Volume 2, Chapter 3). Threatening situations present significant prediction and control problems for fearful dogs. Following exposure to aversive events under highly controlled and predictable conditions, dogs appear to learn how to cope more competently with their presentation, showing less distress and physiological arousal than when such events occur uncontrollably or unpredictably (see *Fear and Peripheral Endocrine Arousal Systems*). As a dog's competency and confidence improves, it becomes progressively relaxed. Relaxation naturally competes with fear and anxiety, provid-

ing a significant counterconditioning influence over fearful arousal.

Competency, Confidence, and Relaxation

A chief objective in the management of fear is to promote an expectancy of success in dogs. Intensive reward-based basic training is a constructive starting point for developing such a positive attitude. The improved communication and cooperation attained by attention therapy and basic training provide numerous benefits for fearful dogs. A probable factor explaining this improvement is the high degree of consistency and order that such training affords. The enhanced control and prediction associated with basic training translate into increased competence, relaxation, and expectancies of comfort and safety. In addition to establishing instrumental control, various appetitive and ludic conditioned emotional responses are simultaneously formed between signals, responses, and outcomes that have been repeatedly linked and rewarded with affection, food, and play in the process of training. As the result of orderly and repetitious patterns of basic training, dogs learn to cope more competently and confidently with social and environmental pressures placed upon them. Basic training provides an island of order and safety that can help ground anxious and fearful dogs and provide a stable platform for graduated counterconditioning and response-prevention procedures. As standard expectancies are established, positive prediction error and dissonance effects can be used to further enhance training and therapy efforts.

The cynopraxic training process renders a dog's behavior more predictable and controllable; however, to the extent that it achieves such an effect, the dog is empowered with an enhanced ability to predict and control the trainer (see *Hitting and Missing the Mark* in Chapter 10). The combined emotional changes associated with reward and enhanced competence make the dog more receptive to approaching the surrounding environment in a correspondingly more confident and relaxed way, an extremely important transition in the management of fear. As the result of consistent and orderly reward-based training activities, insecure dogs appear to learn gradually to respond to the wider social and physical environment as though it were organized by similar rules. As training proceeds and a dog's trust grows toward the owner and the surrounding environment, playful modal activities may be educed and integrated into the training process to further extend and generalize the dog's adjustment, making it more natural and durable. Play and relaxation are the emotional antipodes of fear and anxiety. Learning to play in situations previously evoking fear is facilitated by first bringing trained behavior under the control of play rewards, gradually linking the various signals, prompts, responses, and so forth, with ludic associations. Play and reward-based training mediate a potent comfort/safety bias that is incompatible with fearful inhibition, indecision, and vigilance. By means of gradually transferring training and play activities into feared or unfamiliar situations, more competent and confident coping behavior is organized and integrated, while incompatible appetitive, social, and ludic associations antagonize or abolish situational fear and anxiety.

Sit-Stay Training and Relaxation

Reward-based attention therapy and basic training involving sit-stay and down-stay conditioning is often performed in advance of counterconditioning and desensitization efforts. During such training, appetitive and social affects elicited by the presentation of rewards may be associatively linked with contextual cues, signals, and the rewarded response itself (V. L. Voith, personal communication, 2002). Attention therapy and basic training can be particularly useful in the case of counterconditioning procedures that require dogs to remain as relaxed as possible in one place while attenuated fear-eliciting stimuli are presented and antagonized by stronger incompatible stimuli. In addition to providing an emotionally conducive platform for the reduction of fear via counterconditioning, basic training enhances a dog's ability to control significant events competently, thereby promoting expectancies conducive to enhanced confidence, relaxation, and feelings of safety (see *Benefits of Cynopraxic Training* in Chapter 1).

Victoria Voith's Sit-Stay Program was developed with this objective in mind (see Appendix A). While working with David Tuber in the late 1960s and early 1970s in Ohio, Voith found that training dogs to sit and stay afforded several therapeutic benefits for the treatment of behavior problems (Voith, personal communication, 2002). Owners presenting dogs for behavior therapy were taught how to train them to sit and stay by using a reward-only training technique. The owner-trainers were explicitly instructed not to use a stern voice or forceful means and were urged to limit training to social and appetitive rewards only. Sit-stay training not only taught dogs to sit still but also appeared to teach them how to relax. She noticed after a week of sit-stay training that many of the problems exhibited appeared to improve without any other treatment and regardless of the type of problem presented. In addition, Voith noted that the bond between the dog and the owner had changed in positive ways. Several factors may have played a contributory role in mediating these rapid behavioral and relationship changes, but Voith speculates that two general influences were probably most important:

1. Less aversive interaction between the dog and the owner may have decreased the stress, anxiety, and frustration underlying the presenting problems.
2. Enhanced mutual attentiveness occurring in association with reward-based training may have produced significant changes of affect and mood incompatible with stress, anxiety, and frustration.

Voith also observed that many owners showed attitude changes that may have also contributed to a more positive response to treatment:

> They learned how dogs learn.
> They showed increased pride in their dog.
> They became more enthusiastic and committed to the therapy process.
> They showed an enhanced appreciation of the dog's intelligence and abilities.
> They seemed less distressed and more optimistic about the resolution of their dog's problem.

Voith subsequently composed an autotutorial sit-stay program that she gave clients as a handout. The program is included in Appendix A, with some modifications. The autotutorial organizes the training process into a progression of sit-stay skills of increasing duration, distance, and difficulty. In addition, during sit-stay training, performance criteria are presented in accordance with an errorless learning format, whereby dogs are prepared for each new requirement in advance, with the goal of minimizing stressful errors and maximizing efficient acquisition.

The emphasis placed on errorless learning and positive reinforcement in the sit-stay protocol raises a number of questions with respect to the differential effects and side effects of reward and punishment on emotional behavior and stress. At least one study raises a concern about potential adverse side effects associated with inhibitory stay training (Wilhelmj et al., 1953) (see *Liddell: The Cornell Experiments* in Volume 1, Chapter 9). The researchers found that it took several weeks to months of intensive inhibitory training to quiet dogs enough to get accurate basal blood pressure readings. As a result of such training, however, many dogs showed a potent hypertensive response as well as signs of exaggerated emotional reactivity toward trivial environmental changes (e.g., strangers and noises) and changes of routine. The amount of training given to the dogs appeared to affect the severity of the dog's response adversely:

> The degree of training seems to be of considerable importance in that highly trained and conditioned animals give much greater blood pressure responses to trivial changes in the experimental environment and procedures than animals that are less highly trained. (1953:394)

In addition to the duration of training, a dog's temperament strongly influenced how it responded to inhibitory training. Dogs with stable temperaments were relatively unaffected by intensive inhibitory training, whereas dogs exhibiting unstable and emotionally reactive temperaments were most harmfully affected by it—findings consistent with Pavlov's observations concerning the vulnerability of choleric-type and melancholic-type dogs to neurotic

elaborations. On a side note, these findings underscore the importance of selecting dogs for practical training that are highly stable to begin with, since emotional reactivity and instability may not improve with training, but may in fact worsen over time under the influence of demanding inhibitory training. Highly monotonous and repetitive inhibitory training may be particularly damaging to emotionally reactive and unstable dogs as the result of overstraining inhibitory attentional and impulse-control mechanisms (see *Locus of Neurotogenesis* in Volume 1, Chapter 9). Further, these findings point to the possibility that certain forms of intensive sit-stay training and restraint may be problematic with respect to long-term behavior-therapy efforts aimed at reducing fear and enhancing a dog's tolerance for environmental stimulation. These undesirable effects may exert an especially pronounced deteriorative effect in emotionally reactive dogs, such as those with behavior problems in associated with anxiety, fear, and aggression. Unfortunately, the report does not contain a description of the procedures used to train dogs for blood-pressure testing, leaving significant questions up for debate concerning its relevance.

The sit-stay program designed by Voith has not been implicated in producing similar adverse side effects and probably does not risk doing so, but it remains to be rigorously tested and evaluated for both beneficial and adverse side effects. A major difference in the case of dogs trained in accordance with the sit-stay protocol is they are not compelled by restraint to stay; that is, they perform the response by virtue of self-imposed restraint—they want to sit and stay. The freedom of choice appears to exert a protective effect on the development of neurotic elaborations (Liddell, 1956). However, such freedom is not only a characteristic of food training but present in virtually all forms of standardized animal training:

> In the case of the seeing-eye dog or the performing seal in the circus the self-imposed restraint developed through training *enhances* their effective and skilled behavior. Although they perform at signal, they do so with zest. Spontaneity and initiative are not quelled. Such animals are not brow-beaten. Freedom of action after the work period remains unimpaired. (Liddell, 1956:35)

Without choices, a dog's adaptation to significant events may be thwarted, causing it to become rapidly inhibited or impulsively reactive. Provided that the dog can escape or avoid aversive events, a choice remains available to it, thereby minimizing adverse side effects. The most common and chronic obstruction to making choices effectively is a lack of order in the occurrence and controllability of significant training events and outcomes. Events lacking predictability and controllability are disabling to a dog essentially because they make effective choices impossible for it. The sit-stay protocol combines a freedom to choose in the context of highly predictable and controllable signals and outcomes—ideal conditions for appetitive learning.

Any behavioral procedure that is capable of producing a significant benefit should also be capable of producing adverse side effects, if used improperly. The notion that training with positive reinforcement only produces less stress and promotes beneficial emotional changes during inhibitory sit-stay training remains a hypothesis that is overdue for experimental evaluation and validation. Although the sit-stay program appears to be useful and generally beneficial, the placebo effect is a powerful and pervasive influence that can profoundly alter the perceived efficacy of behavioral procedures—an effect that can be excluded only by controlled experimentation and clinical trials. Given the widespread use of the sit-stay program in the treatment of behavior problems, it is critical that appropriate tests be carried out to confirm its efficacy in order to justify claims attributed to its use. The dramatic and in some cases almost miraculous effects anecdotally and clinically attributed to the protocol suggest that sit-stay training ought to produce a robust effect that distinguishes it from other ways of training dogs to sit and stay. The sit-stay program should also outperform procedures in which appetitive and social rewards are presented on a noncontingent basis.

A starting point for such research might be to obtain baseline behavioral and physiological indices (e.g., cortisol, blood pressure, and heart rate) and then to compare that data with measures taken at week 1, week 2, and so forth, thereby obtaining a tentative within-subject indication of stress-related behavioral changes occurring as the result of the implementation of reward-only training. In addition to short-term effects, follow-up data should be collected. Given evidence of change, additional experiments might be performed to test whether reward-only training was specifically the agent of change rather than other causes incidental to sit-stay training [e.g., increased positive attention (more petting and food rewards)], increased orderliness of interaction between the owner and the dog, or the discontinuation of aversive and provocative stimulation.

Many practitioners using the sit-stay protocol take for granted that reward-only training produces superior therapeutic effects, but does it? If it does, why does such a benefit occur? If the reward-only strategy is selected as the result of welfare or humane considerations, then that underlying intent should be made clear at the outset and not mixed with efficacy considerations, except insofar as they can be demonstrated. In other words, if the basis for using a reward-only strategy is a matter of enhanced efficacy and therapeutic outcome, then appropriate data should be provided in support of the rationale together with outcome assessments showing a superior effect. To address these issues, a series of experiments need to be performed to evaluate how sit-stay training with food and petting only, in accordance with the errorless format, performs in comparison with other methods of training that use different procedures and combine varying proportions of food, petting, manual restraint, mild leash prompting, and so forth. These comparisons should be based on established behavioral and physiological indicators of stress (e.g., cortisol and blood pressure) and emotional reactivity. For example, one experiment might involve training two groups of dogs yoked together under identical training conditions, except that one group is given intensive sit-stay conditioning in accordance with the errorless sit-stay protocol, while the other group receives an equal number of voice commands, bouts of petting, and treats, but randomly distributed over the training session on a noncontingent basis (i.e., the rewards and signals are unlinked to a sit or stay response). This sort of study could be modified and performed as a clinical single-subject reversal design, whereby the effects of sit-stay training could be systematically compared with noncontingent reward or attention therapy without a sit or stay response (i.e., conditioning of an orienting, attending, or following response). For example, dogs could be divided into two groups, with one receiving 1 week of sit-stay training followed by 1 week of attention training, whereas the second group is reversed, with dogs receiving 1 week of attention training followed by 1 week of sit-stay training. In cases where a larger number of dogs are available, a randomized, placebo-controlled, reversal design could be used, thereby obtaining the added power of a group-statistical analysis.

Another set of experiments could be performed to compare the errorless and reward-only group with two experimental groups using varying amounts of rewards, prompting, and restraint together with a control group. In one of the experimental groups (restraint), dogs might be trained with manual restraint, voice commands and hand signals to sit and stay, with leash prompting in combination with contingent appetitive and social rewards presented to reinforce sitting and staying. A second restraint group might consist of dogs trained to sit and stay in a similar way, but with appetitive and social rewards presented on a randomized noncontingent basis in accordance with a yoking procedure, whereby the same rewards given to the reward-only group are also given to the restraint group, regardless of what they are doing at the time of a reward's delivery. Finally, dogs in the control group receive no sit-stay training but are also yoked to the reward-only group, thereby receiving an identical treatment in terms of signals and reward stimulation. Additional studies could be performed to evaluate and compare the reward-only sit-stay and down-stay procedures with other techniques of sit-stay training in order to assess its relative efficacy, practical viability for use in applied settings, and relative ability to provide a conducive platform for counterconditioning. Given the rather simple and straightforward nature of such behavior studies and the widespread use of the sit-stay protocol in the professional treatment of frequently serious

and dangerous behavior problems, it is rather extraordinary that no significant studies exist to date that evaluate its rationale and claims of clinical efficacy.

NEUROBIOLOGICAL SUBSTRATES OF ANXIETY AND FEAR

A major adverse influence affecting a dog's ability to cope with fear-eliciting stimuli is early sensitization of neural circuits mediating the fight-flight response (see *Stress and Flight or Fight Reactions* in Chapter 4). Emotional stressors affecting the mother during gestation, together with excessively stressful postnatal conditions, may exert a lifelong detrimental influence on the way dogs cope with fear- and anger-provoking situations (see *Maternal Separation and Stress* in Chapter 4). Together, heredity and adverse prenatal and postnatal stressors may destine many young dogs to express reactive traits and tendencies before they open their eyes, requiring that such dogs obtain early preventive treatment to improve their ability to develop an adaptive coping style and to minimize the long-term effects of stressful sensitization to the fight-flight system. Stress-sensitized dogs may show a lowered threshold to startle and fear, rapidly learn fear-eliciting associations, and show a deficient ability to extinguish fearful associations once they are established. Knowing how fear is processed, learned, stored, and extinguished at the neural level provides useful insight into how to prevent and treat it effectively.

Startle and Fear Circuits

Startling auditory events are processed by a direct pathway between the thalamus and amygdala and an indirect pathway between the thalamus, prefrontal cortex, hippocampus, and amygdala (Figure 3.1). The direct pathway between the thalamus and amygdala serves to reflexively orient dogs toward the source of stimulation and prepare them for emergency action, whereas cortical and hippocampal inputs provide more specific information about the eliciting stimulus and its contextual significance (LeDoux, 1996) (see *Neurobiology of Fear* in Volume 1, Chapter 3). Of significance to sound-related phobias, the lateral amygdala contains neurons that are highly sensitive to acoustical stimulation. Some of these neurons are prone to rapid habituation and dishabituation, perhaps performing an important fear-related function by detecting novelty and change. Other groups of amygdala neurons are dedicated to loud noises, perhaps mediating unconditioned startle responses to threatening noises such as thunder (Bordi and LeDoux, 1992) (see *Habituating and Consistently Responsive Neurons* in Volume 1, Chapter 3). These various neurons may undergo modification as the result of learning, resulting in threshold and tuning changes that may make them selectively responsive to certain auditory stimuli and not others.

Afferent pathways from the auditory cortex and thalamus to the lateral amygdala use the excitatory neurotransmitter glutamate. Within the lateral amygdala, these glutamate tracts form synaptic connections with inhibitory GABAergic interneurons. GABA (gamma-aminobutyric acid) is known to play an important role in the modulation of fear and anxiety (see *Glutamate and GABA* in Volume 1, Chapter 3). GABA-mediated inhibition within the lateral amygdala is of tremendous interest with respect to noise-related events triggering fear. Excessive sensitivity to fear-eliciting stimuli may reflect a deficiency of GABAergic-related inhibition over glutamatergic neurons. The inhibitory modulation of glutamatergic networks generating fear and anxiety appears to be mediated by serotonin receptors expressed on GABAergic interneurons (Stutzmann and LeDoux, 1998). Serotonin (5-hydroxytryptamine or 5-HT) modu-

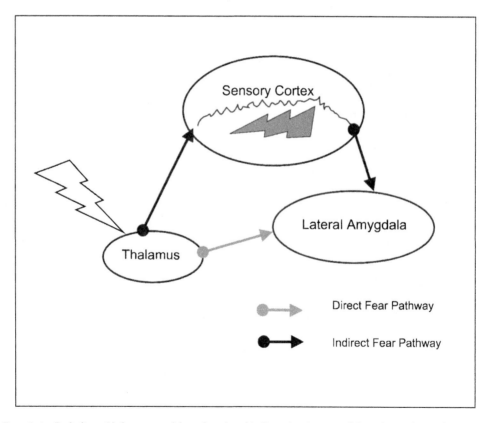

FIG. 3.1. Both direct (thalamo-amygdala pathway) and indirect (cortico-amygdala pathway) fear pathways converge on the amygdala. The direct pathway produces rapid orientation and preparation for emergency action, whereas the indirect pathway provides additional specific and contextual information about the eliciting stimulus.

lates anxiety via the 5-HT$_{1A}$ receptor, the absence of which renders affected animals vulnerable to increased anxiety-related behavior (Hendricks et al., 2002). Medications targeting GABA and 5-HT activity are frequently used separately or together to treat refractory noise and thunder phobias (see *Pharmacological Control of Anxiety and Fear*). Fear-related glutamatergic activity is also modulated in the context of fear conditioning by gastrin-releasing peptide (GRP), a glutamatergic cotransmitter that binds to GRP-receptor sites located on GABAergic interneurons (Shumyatsky et al., 2002). GRP activates a GABAergic interneuron-mediated negative (inhibitory)-feedback effect on glutamatergic neurons. In addition to dampening fearful arousal, GRP, via this signaling network, appears to exert an amygdala-specific inhibitory effect on conditioned-fear learning. Genetically modified mice, not expressing GRP receptors, show an increased responsiveness to fear conditioning, enhanced long-term potentiation, and stronger long-term fear memory (Shumyatsky et al., 2002).

Circulating glucocorticoids also appear to play a prominent role in the serotonergic inhibition of cortical and thalamic sensory inputs to the amygdala. In fact, the inhibitory effects of serotonin appear to *depend* on the presence of glucocorticoids (corticosterone) (Stutzmann et al., 1998). The production of circulating glucocorticoids is under the regulatory control of the hypothalamic-pituitary-adrenal (HPA) axis. Adrenocorticotropic hormone (ACTH) stimulates the adrenal cortex to release glucocorticoids (cortisol and corticosterone). ACTH is released into the bloodstream by the pituitary in response to corticotropin-releasing factor (CRF)—a neural hormone secreted by the paraventricular nucleus (PVN) of the hypothalamus in response to stress. In addition to releasing ACTH, the pituitary gland releases ß-endorphin under CRF stimulation. Circulating adrenal glucocorticoids exert a restraining negative feedback effect on the hypothalamus, causing it to decrease CRF release, thus completing the HPA axis (see *Hypothalamus* in Volume 1, Chapter 3). Adrenal hormones also affect hypothalamic CRF output via opponent feedback effects exerted by the amygdala

and hippocampus (LeDoux, 1996). Under the influence of glucocorticoids, the hippocampus restrains CRF, whereas the amygdala stimulates the PVN to produce more (see *Neural Stress Management System and Fear Conditioning* in Volume 1, Chapter 3).

In addition to initiating the chain of events leading to the secretion of glucocorticoids, CRF appears to coordinate a cascade of stress-related neural events that contribute to the expression of anxiety and fear. The CRF system projects to the locus coeruleus, where it exerts an excitatory influence on the production of norepinephrine (NE). Increased NE turnover is associated with increased emotional reactivity, hypervigilance, and disturbances of attention and concentration abilities (Valentino and Aston-Jones, 1995)—states consistent with clinical anxiety and fear. NE dysregulation has been clinically implicated in the development of various human anxiety disorders, posttraumatic stress disorder, and depression (Heim and Nemeroff, 1999). CRF and NE appear to interact within the central nucleus of the amygdala, with NE stimulating CRF release. Microinjections of CRF antagonists into the central amygdala significantly attenuate fear-related arousal and behavior (Koob, 1999). CRF also plays a focal regulatory role in the production and release of 5-HT. Kirby and colleagues (2000) found that CRF produces a dose-dependent, biphasic effect on 5-HT-producing neurons in dorsal raphe bodies. At high doses, perhaps, comparable to the CRF levels present during acute stress, CRF excites 5-HT-producing neurons. However, at low doses, perhaps, comparable to CRF levels associated with chronic stress, CRF exerts an inhibitory effect on 5-HT production. Price and colleagues (1998) have reported a similar biphasic effect of CRF on 5-HT activity. CRF microinjections in the striatum also affect 5-HT release in a dose-dependent manner. Again, they found that high doses of CRF increase extracellular 5-HT levels, whereas low doses decrease 5-HT levels. In both studies, the predominant effect of CRF on 5-HT activity was inhibitory. These findings suggest the possibility that acute stress associated with fear may initially increase 5-HT production and release, whereas chronic stress associated with anxiety may gradually decrease 5-HT activity. A CRF-mediated increase in NE turnover together with a reduction in 5-HT activity may impede the brain's ability to modulate stressful sensory inputs effectively and regulate behavioral responses to it. NE and 5-HT dysregulation appears to play a functional role in a wide gamut of dog behavior disorders and problems (see *Neurobiology of Behavior and Learning* in Volume 1, Chapter 3). In addition to dysregulating NE and 5-HT activity, excessive stress appears to perturb prefrontal dopaminergic functions responsible for mediating refined adaptation, selective attention, and the control of emotional behavior (Arnsten, 1998). Dopamine imbalances have been implicated in a variety of stress-related psychiatric disorders (Pani et al., 2000) and animal behavior problems (Dodman and Shuster, 1998).

The localization of long-term memories produced by fear conditioning is a complex and controversial area of research. Several brain areas appear to play contributing roles, but the actual areas dedicated to fear memories have not been completely determined. Although Pavlovian fear conditioning appears to be localized in the amygdala and depends on long-term changes localized there (Rogan et al., 1997; Maren, 2001; Shumyatsky et al., 2002), memories are also formed in other parts of the brain providing complementary fear-related functions. For example, the contextual information and motor habits associated with the expression of fear appear to be stored in the hippocampus and striatum, respectively (LeDoux, 2000). Whereas the amygdala plays a significant role in the consolidation of memories associated with inhibitory avoidance conditioning (Wilensky et al., 2000), it does not appear to modulate or inhibit (e.g., extinguish) conditioned-fear responses once they have been established. Conditioned fear originating in the amygdala is dependent on inhibitory influences originating outside of the amygdala, especially the prefrontal cortex (LeDoux, 1996). Finally, conditioned fear and anxiety appear to result from neuronal long-term potentiation (LTP) mediated by glutamate. LTP produces excitatory presynaptic changes in cortical and thalamic neurons that, in turn, exert enduring

effects on postsynaptic electrical activity in the amygdala (Tsvetkov et al., 2002). GRP appears to exert an inhibitory effect over LTP and the formation of long-term fear memories (Shumyatsky, 2002).

Once established, emotional fear memories are highly durable and may be permanent, but their expression can be restrained by extinction memories formed in the prefrontal cortex (Milad and Quirk, 2002). Training activity that successfully mediates extinction may do so by converting operative fear-related establishing operations into fear-restraining abolishing operations, whereby subcortical fear memories localized in the amygdala and thereabouts are actively inhibited and prevented from triggering fearful arousal and escape/avoidance behavior in response to the conditioned-fear stimulus. Along with revised prediction-control expectancies developed in the context of graded interactive exposure and other cynopraxic behavior-therapy efforts, emotional establishing operations are calibrated to match fear-incompatible control incentives and goals, instrumental control modules, and adaptive modal strategies (*Basic Postulates, Units, Processes, and Mechanisms* in Chapter 10). These various cognitive and emotional regulatory changes mediated by behavior therapy are theorized to take place on a preconscious level, involving a complex neural network of interacting sensory, motor, emotional, and cognitive comparator loci, and positive- and negative-feedback systems located throughout the brain, which are coordinated by executive memories (i.e., prediction-control expectancies and establishing/abolishing operations) (see *Neural Comparator Systems* in Chapter 10).

The resolution of fear-related problems depends on the integrity of executive control functions to disconfirm fear-related expectancies and to activate relevant abolishing operations as well as to consolidate new expectancies and establishing operations incompatible with fear. Fears stemming from precognitive stages of development or resulting from sensitization may dodge executive control due to the absence of prediction-control functional expectancies and establishing operations. The executive control of fear appears to depend on the formation of prefrontal linkages with sub-cortical fear circuits operating at the time in which the fear memories are formed. Fears acquired independently of executive control appear to evade executive modulation until adequate prediction-control expectancies and calibrated emotional establishing operations are integrated to regulate fearful arousal to guide functional behavioral adjustments.

The interaction between the amygdala and the cortex is bidirectional, with the amygdala exerting a significant influence on the way that fear is processed at the cortical level. In addition to modulating cortical activity, the activation of subcortical arousal systems by the amygdala indirectly affects the quality of cortical functioning (LeDoux, 2000). As a result of this close interaction, executive control systems localized in the prefrontal cortex may be adversely affected by chronic fear and persistent anxiety. Executive control systems process expectancies and contextual information associated with fear-eliciting situations, playing a major role in the way dogs respond to fear and, most importantly with respect to behavior therapy, the way in which they respond to extinction and counterconditioning efforts (see *Extinction of Conditioned Fear* in Volume 1, Chapter 3). Under the influence of chronic fear and stress, executive functions localized in the prefrontal cortex may become disturbed and hinder the dog's ability to cope effectively with conditioned fear, as well as interfere with its extinction (see *Stress-related Influences on Cortical Functions* in Volume 1, Chapter 3). In addition, the accumulated effects of acute and chronic stress may make dogs more sensitive and reactive to fear-eliciting stimulation, emphasizing the importance of early intervention. As dogs age, some may become more susceptible to noise and thunder phobias, perhaps reflecting an age-related biological degeneration of critical brain areas dedicated to the modulation of conditioned fearful arousal (see *Hippocampal and Higher Cortical Influences* in Volume 1, Chapter 3).

Fear and Peripheral Endocrine Arousal Systems

Peripheral cortisol appears to provide an objective measure of stress in dogs (Beerda et al., 1998), especially when combined with relevant behavioral changes indicative of stress. Individual differences clearly exist with respect to the way animals cope and recover from stressful experience, with some showing a rapid recovery and others recovering more slowly (García and Armario, 2001). Putatively, the ideal pattern is robust glucocorticoid release followed by rapid recovery. Stress-prone animals exhibit impaired HPA-axis recovery, with increased levels of circulating glucocorticoid hormones present long after the termination of aversive exposure. Interestingly, nervous and normal pointer dogs do not appear to exhibit significant differences with respect to HPA activity (Klein et al., 1990), a finding that appears to conflict with earlier anatomic work that found that nervous dogs had larger (hypertrophied) adrenal glands (see *Nervous Pointers* in Volume 1, Chapter 5). Nervous pointers were found to be more prone to develop severe mange, suggesting the possibility of stress-related immunosuppression. In addition, nervous pointers are typically smaller than normal counterparts, exhibiting significantly lower plasma levels of insulin-like growth factor, suggesting that chronic stress associated with fear may affect the hypothalamic-growth hormone axis (Uhde et al., 1992).

As the result of Pavlovian conditioning, adrenal glucocorticoid release can be modulated (increased or decreased) by conditioned stimuli and contextual cues paired with appetitive and aversive stimulation (Stanton and Levine, 1988). A conditioned stimulus paired with aversive stimulation tends to increase glucocorticoid output, whereas a conditioned stimulus paired with an attractive appetitive or social stimulus tends to decrease glucocorticoid output and appears to stimulate the release of oxytocin and other neuropeptides conducive to the mobilization of an antistress response (see *Origin of Reactive versus Adaptive Coping Styles* in Chapter 4). Instrumental learning also appears to have a significant effect on adrenal glucocorticoid activity and blood pressure. Dogs exposed to uncontrollable aversive events exhibit a significant increase of cortisol output in comparison to dogs that are able to escape stimulation (Dess et al., 1983). Likewise, the signaled loss of control in the context of instrumental avoidance training causes a pronounced increase in cortisol output (Houser and Paré, 1974). In addition to HPA-activity changes, the loss of instrumental control produces a significant elevation in blood pressure. Gaebelein and colleagues (1977) found that the blood pressure of dogs remained unchanged during signaled avoidance conditioning, but increased significantly when they were exposed to unsignaled avoidance conditioning. In general, dogs show a strong ability to cope and to adapt to stressful situations, as revealed by a steady decrease in cortisol output over time (Hennessy et al., 1997) and ability to adapt under suboptimal conditions (Campbell et al., 1988). Kuhn and colleagues (1991) found that both cortisol and corticosterone levels where significantly increased in dogs during transportation, but rapidly returned to baseline levels overnight once the destination was reached.

Under the activating influence of fear, various emotional, behavioral, and physiological adjustments are rapidly recruited for emergency action. Many of the coordinated responses associated with learned fear and acute fearful arousal, including startle, freezing, and fight-flight behavior, are orchestrated by the central amygdala (Van de Kar and Blair, 1999) (Figure 3.2). As previously discussed, the central amygdala also exerts a positive (excitatory) feedback effect on the release of CRF by the hypothalamus. In addition to triggering HPA-axis activity, the hypothalamus supports emergency emotional and behavioral adjustments occasioned by fear by mediating conducive physiological changes. In concert with the brainstem (medulla) and spinal preganglionic neurons, the hypothalamus activates the sympathetic division of the autonomic nervous system (ANS). Sympathetic autonomic activation produces global bodily changes in preparation for emergency action, including the secretion of epinephrine (adrenaline) by the adrenal medulla. Epinephrine complements and sustains various fear-related bodily changes set into movement by direct sympathetic arousal, including increased heart and respiratory rates and skeletal-muscle tonus and readiness for action. Epinephrine also appears to play a significant

role in the learning of fear (McGaugh, 1990; Costa-Miserachs et al., 1994) and the extinction of fear (Richardson et al., 1988). Signs of fear, such as panting and pupillary dilation, are under the control of the sympathetic division of the ANS (see *Hypothalamus* in Volume 1, Chapter 3). Sympathetic activation is followed by parasympathetic deactivation, resulting in a return to homeostatic balance. Parasympathetic opponent or rebound effects are commonly seen subsequent to fearful arousal, increased salivation, pupillary constriction, bradycardia, and loss of bladder control.

PHARMACOLOGICAL CONTROL OF ANXIETY AND FEAR

Hart and Hart (1985) have described the benzodiazepine diazepam as the drug of choice for the management of a variety of fear conditions. A significant advantage of diazepam is its rapid assimilation and attainment of therapeutically effective levels. Cohen (1981) reported that diazepam attained peak levels of effectiveness in the dog within 30 minutes. A major drawback, however, is that diazepam is very rapidly metabolized and cleared from a dog's bloodstream in a manner that far exceeds the metabolism rates observed in humans. To maintain therapeutic concentrations, dogs may require three doses per day (Löscher and Frey, 1981). Other benzodiazepines (e.g., clorazepate and alprazolam) have become more popular, in part, because they are much longer acting—a significant advantage in the treatment of fear-related problems. Benzodiazepines are not usually recommended for fearful dogs exhibiting comorbid aggression, because they tend to exert a disinhibitory effect on the fight/flight system and may lower aggression thresholds (Woolpy and Ginsburg, 1967; Marder, 1991; Dodman and Arrington, 2000). Finally, diazepam is prone to produce pronounced ataxia in dogs, including unsteady coordination and falling down, side effects that many dog owners find unacceptable. Ataxia may be particularly problematic in excitable dogs, because they may injure themselves while attempting to escape a fearful situation. With respect to diazepam's effect on escape behav-

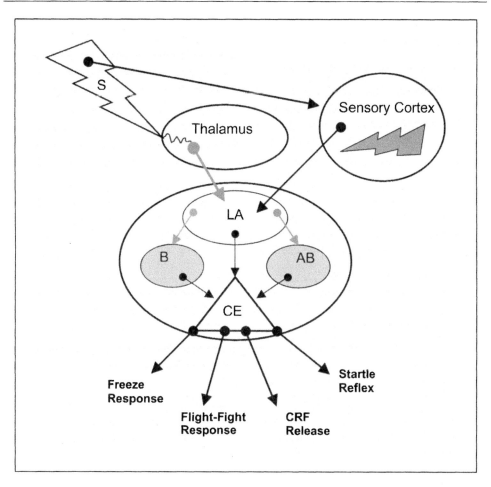

FIG. 3.2. The amygdala orchestrates the expression of a number of emotional and behavioral responses to fear via various neural connections, including the startle reflex (reticulopontis caudalis), freeze response (central gray), CRF release (paraventricular hypothalamus), and flight-fight responses. AB, accessory basal nucleus; B, basal nucleus; CE, central nucleus; CRF, corticotropin-releasing factor; and LA, lateral nucleus. After Ledoux (1996).

ior, Cohen (1981) found that it, in comparison to other drugs tested (haloperidol, chlorpromazine, thioridazine, and clozapine), exhibited a minimum effectiveness for inhibiting escape behavior at dosages not also producing pronounced ataxia.

Desensitization effects produced under the influence of benzodiazepines may be state dependent, with improvements lasting only so long as the dog is under the influence of medication. The transfer of beneficial desensitization and counterconditioning effects may be facilitated by gradually tapering off the med-

ication (Swonger and Constantine, 1983). Although tapering may help in some cases, a number of reports indicate that tapering procedures may not work in the case of highly fearful animals. For example, Woolpy and Ginsburg (1967) performed a series of experiments with various anxiolytic drugs (e.g., librium, chlorpromazine, and reserpine) in an effort to help socialize human-avoidant wolves. Although tranquilization had pronounced effects on social approach behavior, compressing into 4 days what took several months to achieve without medication, the therapeutic benefits were short lived and fully disappeared after the drugs were withdrawn:

> Thus far we have not been able to bring any animal to the fully socialized stage under drug or to maintain it at the most positive approach stage achieved under drug after the drug has been withdrawn, regardless of the variations in the tapering-off process. (362)

They also found that tranquilized wolves tended to be more aggressive and failed to offer typical threat displays, making them more dangerous to handle (disinhibition). Tranquilized wolves also did not exhibit the tail wagging, mouthing, and other social expressions shown by well-socialized counterparts. Similarly, in the case of nervous Catahoula and pointer dogs, benzodiazepines (e.g., diazepam, chlordiazepoxide, and oxazepam) facilitated the acquisition and performance of a simple instrumental bar-press task, but when the medication was discontinued the bar-press behavior was lost (Murphree, 1974). Neither gradual nor rapid discontinuation of medication had a significant effect on transferability of the bar-press task from the drugged state to the nondrugged state. Puppies receiving chlorpromazine for several weeks (weeks 8 to 15) after being socially isolated from weeks 3 to 7 showed little or no lasting social or psychological effects, even though medicated puppies appeared to extinguish trained avoidance responses more rapidly than unmedicated controls (Fuller et al., 1960). Yet, in the case of puppies exposed to longer periods of isolation (weeks 4 to 15), chlorpromazine appeared to exert a highly beneficial and lasting effect (Fuller and Clark, 1966). The researchers found that chlorpromazine in combination with handling significantly reduced the emotional arousal and behavioral disorganization (emergence stress) associated with environmental and social exposure after long-term isolation, indicating that such drug treatment, when combined with forced social contact (response prevention), might totally eliminate the postisolation syndrome in puppies expressing a "robust genotype" (Fuller and Clark, 1966:257) [see *Environmental Adaptation (3 to 16 Weeks)* in Volume 1, Chapter 2].

The experimental treatment of genetically influenced canine behavior disorders with tricyclic antidepressants has produced mixed results. Iorio and colleagues (1983) have described a strain of beagles exhibiting global behavioral disturbances. Among other things, these dogs exhibited deficits in their ability to form social attachments, appeared withdrawn and depressed (stooped posture, reduced activity, decreased alertness), and showed avoidance and failure to look at or make eye contact with human observers. Both imipramine and amitriptyline produced an improvement in 50% of the dogs after a 2-week delay, whereas benzodiazepines produced more immediate beneficial results. Dogs medicated with tricyclic antidepressants maintained improvement over the 24 hours between doses. After the medication was withdrawn, the abnormal behavior rapidly returned to pretreatment baseline levels (Iorio et al., 1983). Imipramine given daily for 4 weeks to nervous pointer dogs was ineffective against the social avoidance and fearful behavior exhibited by these dogs (Tancer et al., 1990). Chronic stress in association with fear and phobias appears to induce adverse neurobiological changes and dysregulatory influences over numerous neurotransmitter systems. Because 5-HT produces widespread neuromodulatory effects over subsystems relevant to the control of fear and the management of stress, serotonergic medications are frequently used in psychiatry to orchestrate far-reaching neurobiological changes to ameliorate depression and several anxiety-related disorders exhibited by human patients (Vaswani et al., 2003). Selective serotonin-reuptake inhibitors (SSRIs) and tricyclic antidepressants are also often prescribed by veterinary behaviorists in an effort to enhance 5-HT activity and to improve neural functions relevant to the reduction of anxiety and fear. These medications target serotonergic neurons, causing them to inhibit the reuptake of 5-HT from the synaptic cleft.

Currently, the most common medications used to treat anxiety and fear are clomipramine and fluoxetine, alone or in combination with a variety of benzodiazepines. Stein and colleagues (1994) have reported that clomipramine may be useful in the treatment of fear-related problems in dogs. All of the dogs treated were unresponsive to behavior therapy alone or in combination with anxiolytic medications (diazepam and clorazepate) or a tricyclic antidepressant lacking potent 5-HT-reuptake inhibitory effects (amitriptyline). Clomipramine proved effective in all of the dogs treated (N = 5), with three showing improvement during the first week and additional treatment benefits accruing over time. Veterinary treatment protocols combining 5-HT-enhancing medications, such as clomipramine, together with long-lasting benzodiazepines (alprazolam) appear to be effective in treating thunderstorm phobias (Crowell-Davis et al., 2001). The efficacy of this combined approach to control pathological fears (e.g., thunder phobias) may be the result of a synergistic effect produced by SSRIs and benzodiazepines on the GABAergic modulation of glutamate afferent acoustical inputs projecting to the lateral amygdala. In addition, SSRIs probably mediate a modulatory effect over central amygdala efferent tracts by way of a serotonergic mechanism. Also, experimental evidence suggests that alprazolam may exert part of its anti-anxiety effect by decreasing CRF activity in the locus coeruleus, a brain site where CRF stimulates NE production (Arborelius et al., 1999)—a neurotransmitter believed to play a prominent role in the expression of anxiety and fear. Melatonin and amitriptyline have been used in combination to treat one case involving intense and generalized fearful arousal occurring in response to various noises, including such diverse auditory stimuli as birdsong and thunder (Aronson, 1999). The combination was reported effective for delivering a rapid reduction in noise-related fear. The positive therapeutic response was subsequently maintained by treating the dog with melatonin alone, which proved effective for controlling noise-related fears, including the fear of thunder occurring over subsequent seasons of storm activity. Aronson suggests that the rapid onset of fear reduction and the ability of melatonin to maintain the effect in the absence of amitriptyline make it likely that melatonin played a prominent role in mediating the effect. Dodman (1999) has also reported some success using melatonin to

control noise-related fear (see *Pharmacological Control of Separation Distress* in Chapter 4).

Numerous physiological processes, including odor-conditioned histamine release in guinea pigs (Russell et al., 1984), odor-conditioned insulin release in rats (Woods et al., 1977), taste-conditioned immunomodulation (Ader and Cohen, 1985), and conditioned modulation of adrenal glucocorticoid release (Stanton and Levine, 1988), are influenced by classical conditioning. The sensitivity of physiological and endocrine functions to conditioning suggests the possibility that the effects of certain medications used to control fear could be harnessed or potentiated by means of Pavlovian conditioning. Many of the anxiolytic drugs prescribed to control fear exhibit rather rapid onset, producing global emotional and behavioral effects incompatible with fear. Usually such medications are given to dogs without consideration for contextual cuing and other potential conditioning effects. Perhaps by explicitly pairing a novel olfactory stimulus with medication a conditioned association between the odor and context could be established with the tranquilizing effects of the medication (Otto and Giardino, 2001). After repeated trials, the presentation of the odor alone might elicit some of the tranquilizing effects of the medication. Similarly, after repeated dosing in a certain location (e.g., a crate), a dog may learn to accept confinement there more readily.

Note: The foregoing information is provided for educational purposes only. If considering the use of medications to control or manage a behavior problem, the reader should consult with a veterinarian familiar with the use of drugs for such purposes in order to obtain diagnostic criteria, specific dosages, and medical advice concerning potential adverse side effects and interactions with other drugs.

EXERCISE AND DIET

A program of daily exercise is highly recommended for fearful dogs. Daily exercise appears to help balance neurotransmitter activity and restore efficient functioning of the brain's stress-management system (see *Exercise and the Neuroeconomy of Stress* in

Volume 1, Chapter 3). Rueter and Jacobs (1996) have reported that behavioral activity, especially rhythmic activities (e.g., walking, running, and swimming), exert a significant effect on 5-HT levels in various parts of the forebrain associated with fear conditioning, including the hippocampus, striatum, amygdala, and prefrontal cortex. The benefit of daily and long-term exercise is a heightened sense of well-being and an improved ability to cope with stressful arousal. Family dogs typically receive woefully inadequate routine exercise and may obtain significant benefits from walking, jogging, energetic play activities, and the like. Exercise activities should include taking the dog to unfamiliar places as is appropriate and safe. Another important basic consideration in the management of chronically stressed dogs is diet. Fearful dogs should be fed a high-quality, balanced diet. Hennessy (2001) found that giving shelter dogs an enhanced diet containing highly digestible protein and fat, produced a beneficial effect on HPA activity and behavioral responses to stressful situations, an effect that was augmented by brief periods of daily human contact and petting. Some evidence suggests that the manipulation of dietary protein and carbohydrate proportions (low protein/high carbohydrate) may increase the availability of tryptophan for 5-HT biosynthesis, perhaps helping to modulate certain fear-related problems associated with a 5-HT deficiency (see *Diet and the Enhancement of Serotonin Production* in Volume 1, Chapter 3). Dogs under the influence of chronic fear and stress may benefit from dietary supplementation with fish oils containing omega-3 fatty acids (Freeman, 2000). Foods enriched with the antioxidants vitamin E and alpha-lipoic acid (found in spinach) may ameliorate fear-related cognitive impairments associated with chronic stress and aging in some dogs (Packer et al. 1997; Milgram et al., 2002). Supplementation with soy protein offers another potentially useful, although currently unproven, dietary change that may exert a modulatory influence on anxiety. Soy meal contains estrogen-mimicking phytoestrogens. Phytoestrogens exert a number of behavioral and physiological effects, including the ability to bind selectively with and modulate estrogen receptors.

When evaluated in an elevated maze test, rats fed soy diets rich in phytoestrogens showed a marked reduction of anxiety in comparison to rats fed a diet low in phytoestrogens (Lund and Lephart, 2001). Diets rich in soy phytoestrogens have also been shown to enhance learning and memory significantly in both animals and people (File et al., 2001; Lephart et al., 2002). The value of soy-rich diets for the management of fear and anxiety in dogs has not yet been evaluated, but the accumulating experimental evidence warrants appropriate investigation and trials for potential clinical efficacy.

A variety of herbal supplements have been found to exert anti-anxiety effects in animals and people (see *Herbal Preparations* in Chapter 4). Passionflower (*Passiflora incarnata*) may have some value in the treatment of certain anxiety disorders. Various parts of the passionflower have been shown to exert an anxiolytic effect comparable to diazepam in mice (Dhawan et al., 2001). A randomized, double-blinded, and placebo-controlled trial found that passionflower extract performed comparably with oxazepam in the treatment of generalized anxiety in human patients (Akhondzadeh et al., 2001). Another potential herbal remedy for managing anxiety in dogs that should receive future attention with respect to efficacy and safety is kava kava (*Piper methysticum*) extract. Kava kava has been demonstrated to be efficacious as an anti-anxiety agent in several double-blinded and placebo-controlled trials to reduce anxiety in people (Pittler and Ernst, 2000). Finally, a valerian-lemon balm combination has been shown to provide a soporific effect and an improved quality of sleep in human patients (Cerny and Schmid, 1999). The combination was well tolerated and produced minimal side effects. Perhaps such a combination might offer a useful benefit for the management of certain anxiety and fear-related problems or provide a mild sedative effect to encourage sleeping in restless dogs.

Numerous anecdotes and testimonials have attributed a calming and emotion-stabilizing effect to flower-essence remedies. One veterinary author has described potent physiological effects observed as the result of administering flower essences, even the management of bleeding during surgery: "If bleeding occurs during surgery, the Trauma formula, given every 30 seconds until the situation is resolved, can be very useful" (Blake, 1998:581). The value of flower remedies for the modification of emotional or physiological states has not been scientifically demonstrated in animals. With respect to anti-anxiety effects in people, two double-blinded, randomized, and placebo-controlled studies have been performed to evaluate the effect of various combinations of flower essences to control test-taking anxiety in students (Armstrong and Ernst, 2001; Walach et al., 2001). Neither study showed any benefit, above placebo, attributable to combinations of flower remedies for the control of test-taking anxiety.

Note: Since herbal and dietary changes may produce adverse side effects if not properly dosed or balanced, such manipulations aimed at producing behavioral changes should be carried under the advisement and guidance a veterinarian.

ACTIVE AND PASSIVE CONTINGENCY MANAGEMENT STRATEGIES

The etiology and expression of fear-related behavior problems are influenced by interacting contingencies of classical and instrumental conditioning. An important aspect of the behavioral control of fear is to identify and manage these influential contingencies systematically, with the goals of reducing undesirable fearful behavior while at the same time increasing a dog's competence and confidence in the presence of fear-eliciting stimuli. Contingency management can be roughly characterized as a process in which relevant eliciting stimuli, responses, and response-produced consequences are carefully identified and then systematically manipulated to attain specific behavioral objectives. Behavioral output can be managed by both active and passive contingency management techniques. Active contingency management (ACM) refers to the collection of methods used to reliably produce overt and emotional behaviors incompatible with fear. These procedures include a wide

gamut of common behavior modification and therapy procedures. In addition to actively manipulating associative and consequent contingencies, fear-related problems are passively managed by controlling a dog's contact with and immediate response to fear-evoking situations. Passive contingency management (PCM) refers to procedures that serve two complementary functions: (1) decrease uncontrolled exposure to evocative situations and (2) prevent or block evoked behavior by various means, including direct restraint and confinement. For example, in the first case, owners are instructed to avoid activities and situations that have evoked fearful behavior in the past, at least until appropriate procedures are in place to minimize fear and to help reduce its future expression. In the second case, procedures are introduced to block fearful avoidance and escape behavior. There are significant interactions between active and passive contingency management procedures, with most behavior-therapy techniques incorporating both active and passive components.

HABITUATION, SENSITIZATION, AND PREVENTIVE-EXPOSURE TRAINING

Habituation and sensitization exert significant influences on the expression of fearful behavior (see *Habituation and Sensitization* in Volume 1, Chapter 6). Under ordinary circumstances, habituation and sensitization interact to adjust reflexive emotional behavior adaptively to environmental stimulation. Although mild fears can be attenuated by repeated exposure to a fear-eliciting stimulus or situation, pathological fears and phobias may resist habituation efforts or worsen as the result of repeated exposure. Habituation occurs when some response is repeatedly elicited—nothing more is needed than repeated stimulation. During habituation, the threshold, magnitude, and latency of the elicited response are gradually altered. For example, dogs fearful of traffic sounds may slowly learn to ignore such noises if given measured and systematic exposure to such stimulation. If, however, a dog, which has been fully habituated to traffic sounds, is frightened by a startling event, such as an accident or nearby exhaust backfire, the previously habituated fear response may reappear or be dishabituated as the result of sensitization. Following the sensitizing event, the dog may become more reactive to traffic sounds than before and respond aversively to sounds that it had previously ignored.

Although habituation results in relatively stable changes in behavior or potential, the habituated response is subject to the influence of spontaneous recovery. Spontaneous recovery occurs when the eliciting stimulus is discontinued and presented again after some test period, at which point the habituated response may rapidly recover strength. In addition, habituation is highly sensitive to contextual influences and various concurrent stimuli that may serve either to facilitate or to impede habituation (Leibrecht and Askew, 1980). Repeated presentation of weak stimuli results in more rapid habituation than strong startling ones. For example, fearful responses to loud thunder may persist despite repeated exposure to the sound of thunder and may actually increase in magnitude with repeated exposure. Instead of habituating to the thunder stimulus, dogs fearful of thunder may become progressively reactive to it. If the sound of thunder is presented in a weaker form (e.g., a low-volume recording) the dog may rapidly habituate to the sound, but if exposed to loud thunder it will immediately dishabituate and exhibit the previously habituated fear response. Desensitization by habituation involves exposing dogs to graduated fear-eliciting stimuli without the presence of a counterconditioning stimulus, a process that can be rendered more effective by introducing various training and play activities at every stage to enhance confident interaction with the feared situation.

Habituation is an important aspect of puppy training. The goal of habituation is to provide a puppy with guided experiences to familiarize it with common sources of stimulation that it will likely encounter as an adult. As the result of habituation, puppies learn to respond to such stimulation without becoming overly reactive or panicky, but perhaps more importantly such preexposure helps to prevent conditioned fears from forming as the result of subsequent aversive or fear-eliciting exposure. Early habituation and preventive-exposure training (PET) appear to help immunize dogs against fear conditioning when exposed to startling or threatening stimulation involving similar stimuli or circumstances in the future. The habituation process is basically a latent-learning process in which repeated exposure to some situation or stimulus without consequence retards or inhibits the ability of the stimulus to form conditioned associations with threatening events later on (see *Latent Inhibition* in Volume 1, Chapter 6). Latent inhibition can play a particularly useful role in the prevention of fears acquired as the result of associative learning (Lubow, 1998). Uneventful preexposure exerts a robust effect that can be easily integrated into puppy-rearing practices. For example, a fear of being inside a car can be prevented by allowing the puppy to explore it on several occasions before going on its first car ride. The first few rides should be brief and end in playful or uneventful activities. Repeated and uneventful visits to the veterinary clinic can help reduce the risk of the puppy developing conditioned fears when aversive procedures (e.g., injections) are performed. Also, repeatedly exposing the puppy to grooming tools (comb, brush, nail clipper, and so forth) before using them to perform grooming chores may produce valuable latent-inhibition effects, interfering with fearful learning occurring in association with actual grooming. PET is particularly useful in the case of noisy devices (e.g., dremel and electric shears), which may require graduated exposure and counterconditioning to prevent an unconditioned fear. Puppies exhibiting noise sensitivities, especially when belonging to a family line with a predisposition to thunder phobias, should be given PET and preventive graduated counterconditioning using storm and thunder tapes to help prepare them for their first exposure to such fear-evoking stimulation. Without the immunizing effects of PET, the first exposure to thunder and lightning may trigger an enduring sensitization and fear. Thunder phobias may be easier to prevent than cure once they are fully established. Perhaps in areas where thunderstorms are common PET should be performed as a routine procedure in conjunction with other puppy-training and socialization efforts.

Although habituation may help modulate fearful arousal and aversive conditioning, inappropriate exposure to aversive situations may result in sensitization and adverse socialization effects that dispose affected dogs to overreact to social and environmental stimulation in adulthood. In addition to habituation, socialization helps to adjust a puppy's emotional response to social encounters with people and other animals. Early experiences with varied social stimuli serve to modulate fearful arousal when a puppy makes contact with people and other dogs. Puppies deprived of adequate habituation and socialization may develop pronounced deficits in their ability to interact normally with the physical and social environment, including the development of debilitating fears as adult dogs. In addition to increased sensitivity to fear conditioning between weeks 8 to 10, later developmental periods (e.g., 4 to 5 months of age) may occasion an increased responsiveness to fear-eliciting and territorial stimuli (see Serpell and Jagoe, 1995).

SOCIAL FACILITATION AND MODELING

Dogs exhibit a wide variety of social signals and displays in an effort to influence the behavior of other dogs and people. These signals typically produce an emotional effect in the receiver, functioning as an establishing operation conducive to the desired behavioral change. In addition to affecting the emotional state of the recipient, the emotional state of the sender of signals is affected. For example, appeasement displays appear simultaneously to evoke emotions incompatible with overt attack in the receiver while stimulating emotions compatible with submission in the sender. Some signals appear to be exhibited with the intention of reducing aversive arousal without signifying appeasement (see *Cutoff Signals* in Volume 1, Chapter 10). These cutoff or "take it easy" signals promote compromise and serve to quiet fearful or aggressive arousal. Dogs also exhibit a variety of displays intended to increase social arousal and affection (e.g., greeting rituals and play solic-

itation). Not only do dogs behave in specific ways to alter the emotional arousal of others, they are also highly responsive to the emotional behavior of others. Contagious behavior and social facilitation are common among dogs. For example, in a kennel situation, if one dog begins to bark in response to a strange noise near its run, other dogs in a remote part of the kennel will also bark, even though they had not heard the noise themselves.

The ability of dogs to be affected by the emotional states of others offers a potentially useful means for modulating certain forms of fearful arousal. Unfortunately, however, contagious behavior exhibits a significant degree of biological preparedness, with some emotional states and activities being more contagious than others. For example, dogs living in the same household may respond to storm activity in distinctly different ways. One of the dogs may become extremely fearful with the approach of a storm, while another may simple curl up and ignore it. A third dog may become alarmed by the sound of thunder and bark but not show evidence of fear. These differential responses to the approaching storm reflect different coping styles—styles of behavior that appear to be highly resistant to local social influences and contagion. Similarly, two dogs living together may exhibit very pronounced differences with regard to their respective responses to separation. Whereas one of the dogs may exhibit intense separation distress, the other may simply lie down and wait for the owner's return. Interestingly, the separation-reactive dog is often oblivious to the presence of the nonreactive dog; similarly, the separation-relaxed dog is not likely to become reactive as the result of social facilitation or contagion.

The relative resistance of intense fear to modulation by incompatible social contagion makes procedures designed to aid fearful dogs with jocundity and jollity seem somewhat questionable with respect to efficacy and treatment value. The author's attempts to induce emotional playfulness in highly fearful dogs by laughing and so forth have not been successful. In the presence of intense conditioned or unconditioned fear, dogs appear confused or simply ignore laughter and other contrived efforts at jollity, and any benefit is rapidly overshadowed by growing fear. Feigned jollity may be too weak as a counterconditioning stimulus to support the effective and sustained modulation of fearful arousal. Nevertheless, in the case of mild fears associated with the introduction of new things or places or intense fears that have been reduced by other means, vocal jocundity and encouragement, together with various play activities, appear to provide useful diversions to help reduce fear (see *Play and Fear* in Volume 1, Chapter 3). For example, play can effectively promote familiarity and improved competency toward some feared activities (e.g., training dogs to swim or jump). Also, despite the aforementioned concerns regarding the efficacy of jollity as a counterconditioning stimulus, some fears may be modulated by presenting the dog with a prized toy or ball or by engaging the fearful dog in some activity that generally evokes excitement incompatible with fear, as indicated by the presence of tail wagging (Campbell, 1992). Perhaps better effects than obtained by feigned jollity may be attained by mimicking canine play signals, including play postures and sounds. Simonet and colleagues (2001) have reported that recordings of play-soliciting vocalizations (rapid huffing sounds) appear to increase the readiness of young dogs to play (see *Play and Leadership* in Chapter 6). Finally, although laughing and humoring fearful dogs may not significantly or reliably compete with fearful arousal, such vocalizing activities may help owners of such dogs to feel better by reducing their own anxiety, making such techniques useful placebos if not efficacious treatment modalities, especially in the case of owners showing high anxiety levels in response to the dog's fearful behavior. Reducing owner anxiety levels is not insignificant, since the owner's emotional state appears to affect how he or she copes with the dog's fearful behavior. Anxious owners appear to view their dogs' anxiety as more troubling or disturbing than do nonanxious owners (O'Farrell, 1997).

Some pathological fears and generalized anxiety disorders may respond beneficially to social facilitation and modeling. For example, McBryde and Murphree (1974) observed that social facilitation and modeling aided nervous pointers to become good hunting dogs. While hunting in the company of normal pointers, human-avoidant pointers became much more tolerant of human contact. Unfortunately, the beneficial effect did not endure after the dogs were returned to the laboratory. Similarly, Baum (1969) reported that the efficacy of response prevention for extinguishing fearful behavior in rats is greatly enhanced by the presence of nearby nonfearful rats. In the case of dogs living together in groups, socially fearful dogs appear to be emotionally supported by the activity of more confident dogs. Dogs that would otherwise avoid people are often much more willing to make such contact if in the presence of a people-friendly canine companion. This evidence suggests that the extinction of certain fears (especially those involving fear of people), counterconditioning, and the acquisition of prosocial behavior may be facilitated by the use of a more confident dog to model the desired behavior. In fact, dogs that are socially confident and outgoing can be very helpful as therapy assistants. The more outgoing dog provides a model of successful social behavior for the more socially inhibited one. For example, doling out treats to a confident canine cotherapist for approaching and staying near the trainer may help to lure an avoidant dog into closer proximity to obtain a share of the easy food. Seeing another dog eat may increase appetite in the fearful dog sufficient to overshadow or restrain its fear momentarily, thereby enabling it to make progressively closer and more relaxed contact with people. The model/rival procedure may possess value for momentarily altering mood or mediating rapid, but temporary, adjustments that may be subsequently strengthened and made more durable by reward training. Preliminary experiments appear to indicate that the model/rival procedure produces rapid changes in social and object-oriented behavior, perhaps having applications in the control and management of certain social and object-related fears (see *Complex Social Behavior and Model/Rival Learning* in Chapter 10).

Coping with Fear and Stress: Licking and Yawning

Voith and Borchelt (1996) have observed that licking and yawning often occur in situations involving conflict and stress. Dogs that are uneasy or fearful of approach often exhibit licking and lick-intention movements. They have also observed that yawning appears to occur in conflict situations involving a delay of gratification or frustration (e.g., waiting to be let outdoors). Licking activity may become an exaggerated or compulsive self-directed behavior, sometimes resulting in lesions to the legs (see *Licking, Sucking, and Kneading* in Volume 1, Chapter 5). They report that when a dog is restrained and exposed to an uneventful social situation in which it feels uneasy or fearful, it may involuntarily doze while sitting, standing, or lying down (sternal recumbency). Such dogs appear to fight an urge to doze that develops over time in the situation, finally losing muscle tone and slipping briefly into sleep, whereupon they start and awaken to continue the vigil. Such dogs appear conflicted between a need to maintain alertness and an opposing urge to fall asleep.

Yawning is common in similar situations of declining attention requiring an increased level of arousal and alertness. Dogs may yawn when forced to practice repetitive and monotonous training exercises, such as repeated sit-stay behaviors. In some of these dogs, yawning appears to present with penile erections, but it is not clear whether the erections are causally linked with the act of yawning or simply part of a coping response to such situations. Whether such dogs are stressed, bored, drowsy, or all three is debatable, but trainers can avoid such tedium by keeping their training sessions brief, reward dense, and playful. Yawning probably performs a cognitive-enhancement function by boosting ebbing attention under conditions in which the dog must continue to wait or defer. Similarly, yawning may help to mediate adjustments in response to unsettling social situations requiring that the dog maintain alertness while at the same time remaining inconspicuous and inactive. Yawning may also occur under certain fear-eliciting social situations. For example, Beerda and colleagues (1998) reported that yawning and stress-related oral activities (e.g., licking movements) occurred in association with fear produced by restraint or startle, but only if a person was present. These findings suggest that at least some stress-related yawning and licking may be expressed with a social intent (appeasement signal) that might not occur (or occur less frequently) in the absence of an appropriate social object. In addition, licking may perform a displacement or cut-off function, perhaps used to appease or pacify the approaching person or dog (see *Cut-off Signals* in Volume 1, Chapter 10). A pacifying function has been attributed to canine yawning, including a host of other sociosexual communication functions (Abrantes, 1997) and a controversial calming or reassuring effect that is purportedly induced when an owner yawns at a distressed dog (Rugass, 1997).

In humans, yawning is partially involuntary, socially contagious, and appears to increase alertness and arousal (Baenninger et al., 1996). Once yawning begins, it is often repeated and may facilitate yawning by others nearby, suggesting the possibility that it exerts a remote contagion effect via observation; however, merely thinking about yawning can also evoke the response. Although an increase in oxygen/carbon-dioxide exchange in the lungs has been proposed, the actual physiological function of yawning has not yet been determined. Yawning is phylogenetically ancient and is under the control of a variety of neurotransmitter systems and interactions, including stress-sensitive acetylcholine and dopamine pathways. Circulating glucocorticoids and other neuropeptides (e.g., ACTH and prolactin) exert a facilitative effect on yawning consistent with a stress-related function. Dopamine (D) appears to play a prominent role in the stress-related evocation of yawning via the release of oxytocin at the level of the paraventricular nucleus of the hypothalamus (see *Startle and Fear Circuits*), which subsequently activates an oxytocinergic pathway projecting to the hippocampus (Argiolas and Melis, 1998)—a potentially significant linkage mediating the social contagion effects of yawning.

The multifaceted role of central oxytocin in the expression of sexual behavior (perhaps explaining the occurrence of stress-related penile erections), social recognition, attachment and bonding, and the diminution of irritability and aggression (Panksepp, 1998), suggests that yawning may help to modulate aversive emotional arousal produced in association with stressful social interaction (see *Neuropeptides and Social Behavior* in Chapter 4). Among olive baboons, anxious yawning and other self-directed behaviors (e.g., touching, scratching, grooming, and shaking) increase approximately 40% if the closest group member (within 5 meters) is dominant, which suggests that such anxious behavior may sometimes possess a social significance (Castles et al., 1999). Yawning may increase attention in social transitions requiring inactivity and deference, while at the same time helping to reduce social anxiety and aggressive arousal by producing incompatible cognitive and emotional changes via the release of oxytocin (e.g., enhanced social recognition) and other neural changes conducive to peaceful social transactions. Dogs can be trained to yawn by means of instrumental techniques (Konorski, 1967), which suggests the possibility that the response might be influenced by learning and used in some instances as a deliberate signal to indicate a readiness for increased activity, waning patience, or other information. Many dogs exhibit yawns that include drawn-out high-pitched squeaking or abbreviated high-pitched howl–like sounds that conclude with chomping or clacking sounds with a sigh of apparent exasperation. Such variations in canine yawning may be produced with a signaling intent, depending on the situational and motivational context in which they occur. Audible squeaks, chomps or clacks, and sighs may be used to draw the owner's attention to the yawn and to help clarify its significance, perhaps resulting in its periodic reinforcement.

Licking and lick-intention movements serve a significant canine social communication function when performed in the context of appeasement and care-seeking situations,

but it is not clear whether licking actions performed by a person toward a fearful or stressed dog serve to produce a calming or reassuring effect or any effect at all. In the case of yawning, given its complex neurobiological nature and close association with the central release of oxytocin, one might best keep an open mind with regard to its potential value as a social signal and capacity for inducing a calming or pacifying effect. Casual experiments by the author to test the calming-signal hypothesis (i.e., the belief that yawning or licking might produce a calming effect in dogs) were without consistent effect, but some dogs do respond to human licking by licking back in return, by averting their gaze or head, by backing away, or by yawning in response to repeated licking actions, which raises the possibility that such signals might actually produce a mildly aversive effect in recipient dogs. Further, merely attracting the dog's attention repeatedly (Grahm et al., 1966) or petting it (Kostarczyk and Fonberg, 1982; Hennessy et al., 1998) may produce a calming effect of variable strength. As a result, some caution should be exercised in suggesting that such signals have special calming properties, particularly when used arbitrarily and out of context.

COUNTERCONDITIONING

Dogs experiencing fear may be functionally incapable of responding in an organized and purposive way to threatening situations. Extreme fear impedes purposive action, paralyzing the animal when it most needs to act effectively and decisively. Until the debilitating fear affecting these dogs is reduced to manageable levels, they will continue to react impulsively rather than learn how to cope in a more measured and adaptive way. The level of fear in such cases is not simply the result of some triggering event, but also reflects a dog's relative confidence and ability to exercise appropriate instrumental control over the threatening situation. To the extent that the dog is unable to control the situation, its fear may escalate into panic rendering behavioral efforts progressively disorganized and unadaptive. Under the influence of intense fear, and unable to respond in an organized way, incompetent fearful dogs may cope by relying on primitive species-specific defensive reactions. Ultimately, the goal of behavior therapy is to improve a dog's behavioral coping skills when encountering aversive situations. However, the first step toward improved behavior is the initiation of efforts designed to reduce aversive arousal to a more manageable level (see *Counterconditioning* in Chapter 7).

Most common procedures used to control excessive fear in dogs involve some element of counterconditioning (Hothersall and Tuber, 1979; Voith and Borchelt, 1985; Shull-Selcer and Stagg, 1991). Graduated counterconditioning is performed by exposing the dog to a gradual progression of increasingly feared stimuli while simultaneously evoking emotional arousal incompatible with fear (see *Counterconditioning* in Volume 1, Chapter 6). Attractive and aversive stimuli exert mutually antagonistic behavioral, emotional, and physiological effects (see Dickinson and Pearce, 1977). An aversive stimulus can be gradually cross-associated with a hedonically opposite and incompatible emotional state by means of classical conditioning. In the presence of a fear-eliciting stimulus, relaxing or appetitive activities may inhibit or overshadow fearful arousal normally produced by the stimulus, allowing it to acquire attractive significance. Another way to conceive of counterconditioning is in terms of the reduction in escape and avoidance behavior. By repeatedly presenting the fear-eliciting stimulus while emotional responses incompatible with escape and avoidance are arranged to prevail and remain unperturbed by the aversive event (e.g., appetitive arousal), the previously feared stimulus may gradually become an associative signal for emotional responses incompatible with fear. Although counterconditioning may result in the development of new associations, the permanent uncoupling of the conditioned fear stimulus does not appear to occur as the result of the procedure.

As a result of counterconditioning, the aversive stimulus is classically cross-associated with reward incentives and pleasurable hedonic emotions that are antagonistic to fear. While fear elicits escape and avoidance, reward incentives stimulate approach, making counterconditioning prone to produce

approach-avoidance conflict. Approach-avoidance conflict may be reduced by gradual exposure to a fear-evoking stimulus through small steps moving from least aversive to most aversive, until finally the dog can tolerate close contact with the feared stimulus or situation without experiencing disruptive fear. Under conditions of reduced fear, the dog can be encouraged to interact with the feared stimulus or situation more competently and confidently. The introduction of appropriate play-facilitated behavior and interactive skills is highly conducive at this point for the promotion of confident control expectancies and more natural social or exploratory modal behavior. Counterconditioning is likely to exert the most benefit in the case of fears resulting from socialization and habituation deficits or developing as the result of sensitization. Fear associated with conditioned escape and avoidance appears to be less sensitive to counterconditioning efforts.

Daily counterconditioning efforts should be recorded in a behavioral journal or chart (Figure 3.3). Methods such as interactive exposure with response prevention can be highly stressful for both dog and owner, and should be employed in combination with counterconditioning and positive-reinforcement techniques, perhaps helping to reduce adverse secondary stress and improving owner compliance. Finally, once a fear-evoking stimulus is reduced by exposure and counterconditioning, play therapy may be considered. Play is particularly useful for the acquisition of new prosocial behavior patterns or as a means to establish active interaction with a previously feared situation.

Fear Reduction and Approach-Avoidance Induction

Counterconditioning is used to alter an animal's fearfulness by associating the feared stimulus/situation with a motivationally antagonistic state. For example, dogs afraid of strangers can be encouraged to take food when people are nearby, thereby eliciting appetitive arousal incompatible with fear while in the presence of people. The attractive expectation of receiving food in the presence of nearby people motivationally competes

DOG'S NAME:			DATE:
SESSION NO.:			

COUNTERCONDITIONING RECORD

T R I A L	STIMULUS	DISTANCE	DURATION	DOG'S RESPONSE
1				
2				
3				
4				
5				
6				
7				

COMMENTS:

FIG. 3.3. Counterconditioning chart. The headings of the chart should be modified to accord with the trigger stimulus dimension being counterconditioned.

with fear otherwise triggered by their presence. After repeated trials, the approach of a stranger may gradually no longer just elicit fear, but instead cause the dog to eagerly anticipate the presentation of a tasty treat. Through gradual steps, the dog's fearful emo-tional arousal may be progressively offset with a new set of prediction expectancies, enabling the dog to interact less cautiously with strangers. Although such modifications and cross-associations may help to reduce certain aspects of the dog's response to the feared stimulus and establish new positive associations, especially in the case of fears resulting from a lack of familiarity (habituation deficit) or as the result of sensitization, counterconditioning appears to be significantly less effective in the case of conditioned fears operating under the control of expectancies that have not been disconfirmed. Although counterconditioning may establish new associations that compete with the emotional responses elicited by the feared stimulus, it may not alter the subcortical fear memory. In effect, rather than resolving the conditioned fear, counterconditioning may result in establishing an approach-avoidance conflict toward the conditioned feared stimulus (see *Partial-extinction Effects, Response Prevention, and Behavioral Blocking*)—an effect that can be particularly problematic in the treatment of dogs presenting with aggression problems associated with fear and avoidance.

In addition to the use of graduated counterconditioning and other progressive exposure techniques, instrumental avoidance behavior may need to be blocked by appropriate means (Askew, 1996). This strategy is often necessary to convince a dog that its reactive avoidance behavior is unnecessary. Consequently, response prevention is a very important aspect of fear management and modification, since allowing a fearful dog to engage in escape/avoidance behavior during graduated exposure may result in an increase of fearful behavior rather than helping to decrease it. Dogs exhibit avoidance behavior to control fear-provoking situations, and since a dog is likely to achieve some degree of success and relief from such efforts, the behavior is likely to undergo reinforcement, that is, confirm the operative control expectancy. The potential for inadvertent reinforcement under such circumstances is significant. Escape and avoidance behavior prevents dogs from learning that the feared stimulus or situation is not really a threat. By gradually bringing a dog into a closer proximity with a feared situation, sometimes against its most vigorous resistance, it is able to learn that the stimulus or situation is harmless and, further, that such contact is actually associated with pleasant things. On the other hand, letting the dog bolt out of "harms" way is contrary to con-

structive training and counterconditioning efforts. Of course, it is important that a fearful dog be gradually desensitized to the trigger stimulus with an appropriate combination of fear-reducing techniques (e.g., habituation, counterconditioning, and stimulus change).

Critical Evaluations of Counterconditioning

Despite its widespread use and apparent efficacy in the treatment of human fear and phobias (Bellack and Hersen, 1977), over the years since Wolpe's discovery of systematic desensitization (Wolpe, 1958), scientific debate has questioned its efficacy for treating phobias. In particular, the need for antagonistic arousal and carefully constructed fear hierarchies has come under question and criticism (Marks, 1987). Neither the ranking of feared samples nor the presence of a relaxing/appetitive counterconditioning stimulus have proven especially significant with respect to the overall reduction of fear and anxiety, either in laboratory animals or in human patients exhibiting fearful behavior. Marks (1978a and b), who carried out an exhaustive survey of the relevant experimental and clinical literature, came to the following conclusion:

> Arousal level during exposure does not seem crucial for improvement, which proceeds at a similar rate whether patients are relaxed, neutral, or anxious during exposure. Controlled work shows both relaxation and deliberate anxiety evocation to be redundant, time-wasting, and unnecessary for the treatment of phobias and obsessions. Systematic reward has not been found especially helpful, though it assists motivation. ... Exposure appears to be especially effective when it is interactional, with the patient actively approaching and grappling with the ES [evoking stimulus] in some way. (1978b:236)

He noted that working up the hierarchy of increasing fear arousal was just about as effective as working down in terms of final results.

Similar observations and concerns about the efficacy of graduated counterconditioning have been reported involving laboratory-animal subjects. For example, Delprato (1973) found that extinction following full exposure to a fear-eliciting conditioned stimulus (fear-CS) outperformed both graded exposure and graded counterconditioning. In the protocol used in his experiments, counterconditioning with food actually impeded the extinction of fear. These findings suggest that food may serve only to divert an animal's attention away momentarily from a feared stimulus without significantly altering its fear. Further, the resultant distraction may cause animals to miss the significance of the conditioned stimulus, thereby shielding it from extinction. The failure of counterconditioning with food to reduce fear became apparent when the fear-CS was presented in the absence of food:

> Rather than facilitating elimination of avoidance, explicit pairing of the anxiety/avoidance competing response of eating with graded exposure to the aversive stimulus was equivalent to control treatment [no exposure to the aversive CS] and, relative to graded and nongraded exposure only, actually impeded elimination of the response. (53)

Delprato suggests that the effectiveness of graduated counterconditioning may be improved by presenting the fear-CS first and allowing the animal to recognize it fully as such before presenting food and other counterconditioning stimuli.

Lastly, upon reviewing a wide array of animal (and human) studies investigating fear-reducing techniques, Thyer and colleagues (1988) concluded that, although useful, counterconditioning appeared to be the least efficacious means for reducing fearful behavior. The most effective techniques, in order of decreasing value, were response prevention, response prevention with distraction, response prevention with noncontingent reward, and response prevention with contingent positive reinforcement (shaping). Despite some of the apparent procedural and efficacy problems with counterconditioning, the authors emphasized that both counterconditioning and positive reinforcement of behavior incompatible with avoidance have a useful place in the armamentarium of a comprehensive fear-therapy program. Oddly, given the rather problematic issues surrounding counterconditioning and the refractory nature of

many fears (especially those associated with generalized anxiety and loud noises), it is rather astonishing that one author claims in a scientific journal to have a achieved a 100% success rate involving 89 fearful dogs by using a program of counterconditioning without drugs (Rogerson, 1997). Unfortunately, the study does not contain analyzable data or experimental controls with which to assess the validity of these dramatic and unexpected findings.

PLAY AND COUNTERCONDITIONING

The emotional excitement and joy produced by play are incompatible with fear, making play extremely useful for the treatment of mild to moderate social fears. If play can be produced in the presence of a fear-provoking stimulus, several potential benefits may be obtained. For one thing, play enhances a dog's confidence and willingness to take risks. Instead of the wariness, anxious vigilance, and inhibition associated with fear, play mediates a more curious, experimental, and spontaneous attitude toward the environment. Playful dogs are more free and able to behave in spontaneous ways, just because they are not overly preoccupied with the potential consequences of their behavior. Under the influence of play, fearful dogs may be more able to interact with the environment flexibly, thereby allowing them to learn and integrate new control modules, routines, and patterns under the active modal influence of play (see *Training and Play* in Chapter 1).

Trumler (1973) succinctly and correctly observed, "The dog learns by playing" (124). Playing is no less important in the case of normal skill learning than it is in the unlearning of fears. Activities associated with play and curiosity are unique in that they appear to be intrinsically reinforcing and apparently done for their own sake. The consummation of play appears to educe joy and immediate gratification. Play occurs without any apparent interest or concern for advantages in the future; the only goal of play is the perpetuation of play and the joy it produces. Play is a source of continuous reward for dogs, and behaviors used and integrated into play tend to become progressively stable and reliable. While playing, dogs can safely practice and learn numerous social skills. Both play and curiosity appear to operate on a high level of cortical organization, driving a highly flexible and experimental attitude and behavioral interface with the environment, precisely the sort of thing that is needed by fearful and aggressive dogs to overcome their biased perceptions.

Not unexpectedly, fearful dogs are usually very inhibited and reticent to play while in the presence of the feared stimulus. This play inhibition is in sharp contrast to the animation that they may ordinarily exhibit when alone with owners in the safety of familiar surroundings. Fearful dogs are unable to respond to play invitations, not so much because they are unable to play, but simply because they do not *feel free* to play; that is, they are inhibited by fear. Encouraging dogs to play in a variety of situations with both familiar and unfamiliar partners helps to promote a more generalized prosocial attitude, gradually causing the dogs to view people less suspiciously—perhaps eventually causing the dogs to view people as potential playmates. Similarly, play can help to restrain arousal associated with environmental sources of fear such as loud noises; for example, Hothersall and Tuber (1979) reported that the noise-phobic Labrador retriever "Major" could better tolerate evoking stimulation if engaged in ball play (see *Major: A Thunder-phobic Dog* in Volume 2, Chapter 3).

Several dynamics govern play behavior, making it a fitting tool for this purpose. Play is influenced by a safe-expectancy bias and can be helpful to facilitate socially risky behavior in dogs. Such features of the activity are obviously very desirable in the context of interactive exposure. The safe expectancy associated with play is the outcome of natural or species-typical boundaries and rules regulating such contact and activity, permitting interaction that might be perceived as threatening under other circumstances. As a result, play allows individuals to become more intimately familiar with one another, it promotes affectionate bonding, and it helps to establish social stratification without the risk of inciting serious combative contests. In short, play facilitates the development of a friendly and joyful relationship (see *Fair Play, Emergent Social Codes, and Cynopraxis* in Chapter 10).

INSTRUMENTAL CONTROL AND FEAR

There is some inconsistent usage of the term *counterconditioning* in the applied and veterinary behavior literature. Counterconditioning, a classical conditioning procedure, is often used to describe instrumental training efforts in which an incompatible response to fear is prompted and positively reinforced. This mixed usage is somewhat problematic and should be avoided. Instrumental control efforts typically involve obedience commands (e.g., "Sit"), prompts, and consequences that may or may not provide secondary counterconditioning benefits. Separating fearful behavior into instrumental and classical fractions is somewhat arbitrary, but the division is useful in this case since not all instrumental control efforts necessarily exert a counterconditioning effect (e.g., behavioral blocking), at least not initially. In combination with response prevention and graded counterconditioning efforts, fearful dogs are often trained to perform various obedience modules and routines incompatible with escape and avoidance. Usually, dogs undergoing counterconditioning are given intensive preliminary training to enhance attention control and to perform a variety of basic exercises (e.g., a rapid and reliable sit and down response, indoor and backyard recall, starting exercise, controlled-leash walking, and a reliable sit-and down-stay lasting for at least a full minute under distracting circumstances). When exposed to the fear-provoking situation, these various instrumental behaviors are prompted through commands and various other signals to bring the dog into closer interactive proximity with the feared situation. The social and tangible positive reinforcers used to support exposure and interaction with the evoking stimulus may perform a significant counterconditioning function. Conditioned reinforcers appear to play an important role in this regard (see *Classical Conditioning, Prediction, and Reward* in Chapter 1). When properly conditioned, bridging signals acquire potent alerting and orienting features that can be used to shape behavior incompatible with fear while at the same time eliciting antagonistic emotional arousal associated with reward. Brief and crisp vocal and mechanical sounds appear to be more effective as conditioned reinforcers than drawn-out vocal phrases. Maximal arousal of conditioned reward effects occurs with the onset of the conditioned reinforcer rather than its offset. A highly conditioned bridge can be used to introduce powerful positive prediction error and dissonance effects.

Stimulus Dimensions Influencing Fearful Arousal

The desensitization hierarchy is constructed by organizing the presentation of fear-provoking stimuli and situations along a continuum of increasing fearfulness. Several overlapping dimensions are involved, each of which should be given careful consideration when devising a hierarchy of graded exposure and desensitization. They include proximity, context, similarity, intensity (quantity), contrast (quality), duration, frequency, predictability, controllability, and stimulus continuity (Table 3.1). Desensitization can occur by counterconditioning (requiring the elicitation of incompatible emotional arousal) or habituation (repeated presentation of graduated samples of the fear-eliciting stimulus). Desensitization by habituation does not depend on the presence of a counterconditioning stimulus.

Counterconditioning Stimuli

When desensitizing fearful reactions by counterconditioning, a list of counterconditioning stimuli should be identified. A counterconditioning stimulus must be both incompatible with the feared stimulus and sufficiently strong to compete with its fear-eliciting properties (Figure 3.4). Counterconditioning stimuli usually have a calming, appetitive, or pleasurable effect on dogs. The most commonly used counterconditioning stimulus is food. A dog's relative interest in food is a sensitive measure of its emotional state, with anxious, fearful, or aggressive dogs often refusing food offered to them. Appetite and fear appear to inhibit each other reciprocally. Seeding the situation with treats that the dog

can search for and easily find appears to work better as a counterconditioning stimulus than simply feeding it by hand as it stands or sits in the presence of the fear-eliciting stimulus. Searching activity appears to help restrain fearful behavior. Also, highly motivating appetitive stimuli varied in size and type will produce a stronger effect than giving the dog a food item of low reward value and novelty (e.g., kibble). Feeding the dog a highly appetizing meal in the presence of a graduated fearful stimulus can be an effective means to reduce fear reactivity, especially if it is done over several days or weeks.

Appetitive arousal and fear typically exert a pronounced antagonistic influence over each other in dogs, perhaps stemming from a close evolutionary affinity and organization at the level of the hypothalamus controlling approach and avoidance behaviors. Counterconditioning with food probably exerts an influence at the level of the ANS, wherein food-induced parasympathetic arousal works to avert or restrain fear-related sympathetic arousal (see *Hypothalamus* in Volume 1, Chapter 3). Appetite and fear are motivationally antagonistic to each other or, as has Wolpe says, they *reciprocally inhibit* each other: the arousal of one motivational system inhibits the arousal of the other (see *Reciprocal Inhibition* in Volume 1, Chapter 6). Although food is an extremely useful counterconditioning stimulus for moderating strong fears, it is of utmost importance that the dog's appetitive response be strong enough to overshadow its fear. If food is presented to an already fearful dog, the treat may become counterconditioned in an opposite direction; that is, food may become associated with fear—a highly undesirable and common outcome. The danger of inadvertent aversive counterconditioning is minimized by gradually exposing a hungry dog to minimally evocative samples of the fear-eliciting stimulus. It is also useful to vary the kind and amount of the food given to the dog at each step: surprise is a critical factor in using food as an effective counterconditioning stimulus.

Motor activity can also produce a mild counterconditioning effect by a process that Baum (1970) has referred to as *mechanical facilitation*. The critical issue is to maintain forward locomotion without evoking a freez-

Table 3.1. Stimulus dimensions affecting counterconditioning and desensitization efforts

Proximity: Most dogs tolerate the presence of a feared object, event, or person at a distance, but become progressively more fearful and reactive as fear-eliciting stimulus comes into close proximity (Figure 3.4). For instance, a distant roll of thunder may not have any discernible affect on thunder-phobic dogs until it reaches some critical proximity.

Context: Another important factor determining the fear-eliciting stimulus's relative strength is the influence of context. Exposure to a thunderstorm while the owner is nearby may be much less aversive for a dog than exposures occurring when it is alone. In addition to social variables, the environment itself may physiologically predispose a dog to fear (see Kallet et al., 1997).

Similarity: Besides proximity and context, dogs react differentially to the relative similarity between a presented stimulus and an actual feared object or event. Dogs unable to tolerate thunder may be able to accept other loud noises sharing some similar features with thunder (e.g., loudness and surprise). Such similar surrogate items may be selected in cases where the actual feared object or event is not readily available or easily tolerated.

Intensity: Fearful stimuli of low intensity are less provocative and more easily endured or habituated than more intense samples of the same stimulus. Recorded thunder effects played back at a very low volume are obviously much less frightening to a dog than when they are presented at full volume.

Duration: The duration of the fear-eliciting stimulus has a direct and significant bearing on the desensitization process. A dog is exposed to progressively realistic exposures as its tolerance will allow, but initially brief exposure to low-intensity stimuli helps to facilitate the process.

Frequency: Many fears are associated with extremely brief stimuli occurring within a fraction of second (e.g., gunfire), requiring that they be presented repeatedly. The frequency of presentation depends on a dog's response and recovery. Repeated exposure at low intensity appears to facilitate desensitization effects.

Predictability: Aversive stimulation occurring on a predictable basis is less fear arousing than when it occurs on an unpredictable basis. Anxiety can be interpreted as a state of vigilant arousal that occurs in response to a fear-eliciting stimulus that presents unexpectedly. Anxiety serves to lower fear thresholds, thereby competing with desensitization efforts. The infrequent, brief, and unpredictable occurrence of thunderstorms may significantly contribute to the development of storm fears via anxiety occurring during times of the year when storms are more common.

Controllability: Aversive stimuli and situations presenting with a high degree of controllability are far less provocative of fear and stress than are aversive stimuli that occur on a uncontrollable basis. Many fears reflect an underlying loss of confidence stemming from a lack of appropriate experience and skill or a history of failure with respect to the control of potentially dangerous situations.

Continuity: To be maximally effective, the desensitization hierarchy should have an even flow or continuity from lower items to higher ones. Sudden discontinuous jumps between items should be avoided.

---

ing or fleeing response. Making a dog move in a beeline toward a feared situation may rapidly overshadow the relaxing effects of motor activity with fear. It is often useful to approach the fear-eliciting situation on a slight curve, moving steadily away from the situation. Repeated passes may gradually result in closer and closer passes, evidencing fear reduction and decreased avoidance. While some benefit can be obtained by merely walking a dog near a fear-provoking situation, stronger effects are attained by periodic changes of pace (excited running),

letting the dog find planted treats and engaging it in various play activities (e.g., tug games) while in the proximity of the feared situation. Mild fear can be modulated in some dogs by giving them a soft toy to carry. Toys stuffed with food can also be useful, especially if they are strategically hidden in a way that requires the dog to become progressively closer to the feared situation in order to find them. Prompting the dog to perform a series of well-conditioned obedience exercises and providing food and affection as rewards can be an extremely beneficial fear-

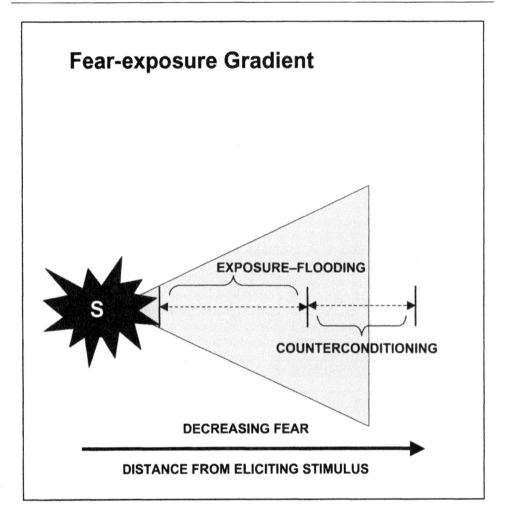

FIG. 3.4. Various stimulus dimensions, including distance, alter the capacity of a trigger stimulus to elicit fear. Effective counterconditioning is usually performed by evoking a state of arousal antagonistic to fear while exposing the dog to a minimally provocative fear-eliciting stimulus, whereas exposure with response prevention may be performed in the presence of more provocative trigger stimuli.

reducing technique, especially if a highly desirable reward is given for every correct response. Another powerful technique for modulating fear is structured postural manipulation together with relaxing massage and olfactory conditioning (see *Posture-facilitated Relaxation Training* in Appendix C), which appears to help restrain adverse emotional arousal and stress-related concomitants associated with fear. Finally, as previously noted, the presence of a confident canine cotherapist acting as a model for the desired behavior may facilitate the process through social facilitation and local enhancement (see *Social*

Learning in Volume 1, Chapter 7). Model/rival play activity in which the dog is put on a tie-out and allowed to watch the trainer and owner tossing a ball back and forth and playfully interacting may inspire some dogs to lower their guard, especially in the case of highly sociable dogs showing a keen interest in the ball.

GRADED EXPOSURE AND RESPONSE PREVENTION

Although graduated counterconditioning may not be consistently effective in all cases and may not be very efficacious as a stand-alone procedure for resolving conditioned fears, it does appear to provide benefit in many cases involving fear due to habituation deficits or adverse sensitization and remains a legitimate and useful tool for modulating fearful arousal in the context of behavior therapy, especially when used in combination with other behavioral procedures (e.g., graded interactive exposure, habituation, response prevention, attention therapy, and basic training). Perhaps the most important function of counterconditioning in the process of treating conditioned fears is to help modulate aversive arousal occurring in association with the graduated introduction of response prevention and to decrease anxiety associated with its fading and discontinuation.

Partial-extinction Effects, Response Prevention, and Behavioral Blocking

Conditioned fear is most effectively extinguished by disconfirming escape/avoidance expectancies (see *A Cognitive Theory of Avoidance Learning* in Volume 1, Chapter 8). In practice, fear is reduced under circumstances in which the escape/avoidance response is blocked, while the feared outcome is prevented and stimulation incompatible with fearful arousal is presented. Such treatment results in a condition of safety and fear reduction, but it may impede the full extinction of fear. Full extinction extends the partial-extinction effects obtained under the blocked condition to more natural unblocked conditions, thereby fully disconfirming the operative avoidance contingency. According to this interpretation, full extinction requires exposure to both blocked and unblocked conditions (see *Conditioned Fear and Extinction* in Volume 2, Chapter 3). As the result of response prevention, only the blocked condition is disconfirmed, leaving the unblocked condition untested; that is, the feared event might still occur when the blocking contingency is lifted. As such, the discontinuation of response prevention may generate significant apprehension and anxiety in response to the conditioned fear stimulus. Consequently, although response prevention may significantly reduce fear, apprehension and anxiety may occur when the safety of the blocking

contingency is removed. By slowly fading the blocking contingency in association with counterconditioning, the risk of such anxiety can be significantly reduced; in turn, graded interactive exposure with response prevention can help to reduce the approach-avoidance conflict associated with stand-alone counterconditioning. The reciprocal benefits resulting from the combined use of response prevention and counterconditioning (RP-CC) strongly recommend that they be used together as complementary therapies in a comprehensive approach to the treatment of canine fears and phobias. In addition to disconfirming fearful expectancies, intensive basic training is seamlessly integrated into RP-CC procedures, with the goal of enhancing executive control functions (attention and impulse control) and improving the dog's ability to cope more competently with feared situations.

Response prevention is essentially a punitive contingency serving to disconfirm a dysfunctional control expectancy. In addition to physical restraint, avoidance control and safety training techniques might be considered in some cases to block escape/avoidance behavior and to reinforce incompatible behavior. A major potential advantage of such training is the internal relief/relaxation effects and safety associated with successful escape and avoidance (see *Safety Signal Hypothesis* in Volume 1, Chapter 8). Persistent and refractory fears stemming from sensitization or precognitive exposure to traumatic stressors may be responsive to an approach combining RP-CC and behavioral blocking. As the result of behavioral blocking via trained avoidance responses, fears operating independently of functional prediction-control expectancies might be brought under better functional executive control, thereby helping to mediate fear extinction via the formation of cortical inhibitory restraint over subcortical emotional fear memories. In addition to potential for restraining emotional fear, such training might help to reduce fearful behavior by consolidating fear-incompatible expectancies and emotional establishing operations in the presence of the fear-eliciting stimulus, thereby helping to modulate and normalize the dog's response to it. Behavioral blocking and avoidance training may produce significant relief/relaxation, gradually causing the dog to feel safer in the presence of the previously feared stimulus or situation.

The current experimental literature indicates that graded interactive exposure and response prevention are the most efficacious means for reducing conditioned fear in animals (see *Interactive Exposure and Flooding* in Volume 1, Chapter 6). As the result of repeated safe exposures to the fear-provoking stimulus or situation (desensitization by habituation), the animal gradually learns that the feared situation is no longer predictive of aversive stimulation. Exposure works by extinguishing or habituating the fearful reaction, thereby disconfirming a dog's fearful expectancies and promoting a more adequately predictive and "reality tested" reaction to the evoking situation. When escape and avoidance efforts are blocked, many dogs eventually recognize that a threat no longer exists in the presence of the fear-evoking situation, a recognition that appears to produce relief and relaxation. Relief and relaxation following the cessation of aversive arousal provide a powerful counterconditioning influence (see *Response Prevention, Opponent Processing, and Relaxation* in Volume 2, Chapter 3). During graded interactive exposure, the dog is brought into closer and more varied contact and interaction with the evoking stimulus, thereby developing the confidence and skills needed to cope competently with the feared situation.

Graded Interactive Exposure

Graded interactive exposure is often combined with instrumental procedures in which trained behaviors incompatible with escape or avoidance are prompted and reinforced in the presence of a fear-provoking stimulus or situation. Preliminary attention and basic training consist of bridge conditioning, following and coming, orienting, sit- and down-stay, targeting, attending behavior, starting exercise, and controlled walking. The dog should be thoroughly desensitized to the fixed-action halter and kept on a hip-hitch and control lead or closed-loop system for added safety (see *Halter Collars* in Chapter 1), especially if manipulations tying up the hands are involved (e.g.,

using a squeaker, clicker, or food). In addition to prompting and reinforcing previously established control modules and routines in the presence of the feared situation, spontaneous approach behavior can be selectively reinforced via a DRO or shaping schedule of differential reinforcement while escape/avoidance behaviors are blocked. The idea is to encourage more competent behavior through successive approximations and spontaneous initiatives occurring in the absence of escape or avoidance efforts. In addition to overt dynamic and interactive behavior, shaping efforts can also be applied to static postural behaviors associated with increased confidence (e.g., tail relaxed or wagging, ears forward and alert, standing upright, leaning forward, not leaning on trainer or objects, and steady frontal orientation). Such training efforts exert both instrumental and classical conditioning effects incompatible with fearful behavior. Effective shaping depends on a well-conditioned bridging stimulus (see *Shaping Through Successive Approximations* in Volume 1, Chapter 7). The bridging stimulus is conditioned by repeatedly pairing a distinct auditory stimulus (e.g., "Good" or click) with the presentation of food and other rewards (e.g., affectionate petting and play). Both a vocal stimulus and a clicker-bridging stimulus should be conditioned to a high degree in the context of orienting training and controlled walking in advance of therapeutic applications. After several pairings, the bridging stimulus can be used to link or *bridge* desirable behavior with a spatially separated and delayed reward while at the same time evoking affects incompatible with fear. A squeaker bulb (without squeaker valve) scented with an odor (e.g., orange or lavender) is held in the right hand and squeezed just before the hand is opened to deliver treats. The conditioned odor can be subsequently used to augment appetitive counterconditioning efforts. Preliminary training should strongly focus on augmenting orienting and attending responses via the manipulation of positive prediction error and dissonance effects, using the dog's name or an orienting stimulus (e.g., a squeaker or smooching sound). Capturing the dog's attention in a decisive and timely way (i.e., at the earliest sign or link in the rapid chain of events leading to the avalanche of emotional and behavioral events associated with fear) serves to interrupt and deflect fearful behavior, while enabling the trainer to redirect it toward activities incompatible with fear (see *Target-arc Training*). Many dogs trained in such a way adopt a coping pattern in which the feared stimulus prompts them to look toward the owner for support rather than balking, fleeing, or becoming reactive (e.g., compulsive barking).

The efficacy of graded-exposure training is influenced by a number of procedural constraints. Although exposure procedures can be extremely effective, they may make things worse when improperly performed. For example, repeated, *brief* exposures to intense fear-eliciting stimuli may increase fear and make subsequent exposure efforts more difficult. Exposure to the provoking situation should continue until fear subsides or is replaced by relief and relaxation. Also, unexpected and intense occurrences of the fear-eliciting stimulus may cause increased sensitization and dishabituation. This adverse influence is especially problematic when it is coupled with repeated, brief exposures to the intense sample. Many common fears appear to persist because the dog does not remain in the presence of the provoking situation long enough to benefit from slowly emergent opponent relief and relaxations effects. When startled, the animal simply hides or runs away. Interestingly, the brevity of intense loud noises (e.g., gunshots, fireworks, or thunder) may be a major factor in the development of phobias related to loud-noise stimulation. For example, thunderstorms are seasonal, they are brief, and they may involve intense acoustical stimulation capable of eliciting pronounced fear in predisposed dogs, independently of other sources of unconditioned aversive stimulation. Thunder-phobic dogs repeatedly exposed to these brief and traumatic experiences with thunder and lightning may become progressively sensitive to them as well as other phenomena related to storm activity. The periodic and intense nature of such stimulation precludes normal habituation and strongly recommends early preventive exposure in the case of dogs and puppies exhibiting a low startle threshold to noise (see *Habituation,*

Sensitization, and Preventive-exposure Training).

Normally, following intense startle and fearful arousal, opponent relief and relaxation predictably follow the discontinuation of aversive stimulation (see *Safety, Relief, and Relaxation* in Volume 1, Chapter 3). Relief and relaxation appear to help restrain fearful arousal and to promote homeostatic adaptation following the aversive event. Relief occurs immediately after the aversive stimulus is discontinued and continues for 15 to 20 seconds. Relaxation is a more sluggish opponent process and begins to appear only after approximately 2 1/2 minutes after the aversive stimulus is withdrawn. To take full advantage of these effects, techniques involving the discrete presentation of fear-provoking stimuli should be spaced to maximize relief and relaxation effects. In addition, safety signals should overlap both relief and relaxation phases of postaversive adaptation. By pairing vocal cues (e.g., "Relax"), acoustical stimuli (continuous tones or music), various scents, and tactile signals (petting) with relief and relaxation, these combined redundant stimuli may gradually become conditioned safety signals predicting the absence of aversive stimulation (see *Fear, Cognition, and Avoidance Learning* in Volume 1, Chapter 3). Conditioned safety signals may function as conditioned inhibitors of fearful arousal (Hawk and Riccio, 1977) as well as evoke therapeutically beneficial conditioned safety-relaxation effects (Denny, 1976). As a result, conditioned safety signals provide a convenient means for reducing fearful arousal and encouraging more secure behavior when a dog is faced with a fear-provoking situation.

Rehearsal

Fearful arousal resulting in frantic escape or panic behavior is detrimental to the exposure process. If such behavior succeeds, a dog's reactive escape behavior may be strongly reinforced, leading it to respond in a similar way when exposed to the fear-eliciting situation in the future. Avoidance and escape behavior is incompatible with maintaining a progressively closer proximity with the threatening situation—a requirement for successful fear reduction. However, observing the feared stimulus or situation at a safe distance, though comfortable for the dog, may not alleviate its fearful avoidance or promote confident behavior when it is brought into closer contact with the feared situation. The fearful dog must be gradually and systematically exposed to fear-provoking situations to optimize the effects of graded interactive exposure. Since fearful arousal may be increased by repeated, brief, and uncontrolled exposures to threatening situation, it is advisable that casual exposure to the fear-eliciting stimulus or situation be minimized.

Before exposing the dog to the actual fear-provoking situation, each step in the process should be rehearsed under minimally provocative conditions. For example, if the dog is afraid of strangers when they first visit the home, the various events and activities associated with such visits can be practiced in advance. Behavioral rehearsals include such activities as ringing the doorbell, leashing the dog, calling the dog to heel, training the dog to hold a sit-stay, opening the door, and finally appropriately reinforcing the dog's behavior. Most dogs enjoy going for walks, and the opportunity for such activity is associated with keen interest and anticipatory activity. Ringing the doorbell or knocking on the door before getting the dog's leash and going for a walk can help to countercondition aversive associations evoked by the sound of the bell. Whenever possible, taking the fearful dog for a walk with unfamiliar visitors is an effective interactive exposure technique. Not only are walks enjoyable, they can last long enough to moderate fearful arousal and facilitate relatively close and sustained interactive contact between a socially avoidant dog and people. Moreover, taking the dog outdoors and away from the home to interact with the visitor obviates confounding territorial issues that may complicate the situation.

To perform these various activities, it is imperative that fearful dogs learn to walk on a controlled leash, to perform the quick-sit without hesitation, and to hold a reliable sit-stay and down-stay. Such preliminary training should be practiced in every situation where the dog might potentially encounter the fear-eliciting stimulus. Food is a convenient reward, as it can be readily used as a counter-conditioning stimulus, as well. Once all the elements have been trained and rehearsed, the next step is to stage the actual event by using a situation that is minimally provocative. Besides representing a positive in vivo exposure to a minimally evocative situation, such staging is a useful way to iron out any unforeseen difficulties that might emerge during more natural exposures later.

Staging and Response Prevention

Response prevention brings a dog into close proximity with the fear-provoking situation, thereby evoking low to moderate levels of fear that slowly undergo habituation. An important function of response prevention is to block undesirable escape and avoidance behaviors. Uncontrolled avoidance and reactive escape efforts hinder a dog's ability to unlearn the toxic emotional expectancy, thus forestalling the development of a more moderate and adjusted response to such stimulation. As the result of repeated uneventful exposures, the dog may gradually discover that its fear is unfounded and begin to experiment with more prosocial or exploratory behavior. Significant evidence suggests that the motor components of fear are localized in the basal ganglia (species-typical routines) and the cerebellum (skilled motor coordination), whereas the emotional aspects of fear are elaborated in the amygdala (Mintz and Wang-Ninio, 2001). This research suggests that fearful emotions and fear-related behavior are acquired and maintained in different parts of the brain. As the motor skills needed for successful avoidance are acquired, a significant reduction in fear arousal occurs. Motor competency appears to have a pronounced modulatory effect on emotional fear localized in the amygdala; however, reactive escape/avoidance behavior that does not provide enhanced control over the fear-eliciting stimulus may actually intensify fear. Fear-related motor output may have pronounced secondary effects on fearful arousal, especially if the animal's escape/avoidance efforts are frantic and disorganized. Consequently, such reactive responses to fear should be prevented or blocked and replaced with more competent and adaptive alternatives.

During the staging of in vivo graded exposures, a dog is presented with progressively more aversive situations, provoking arousal in amounts that won't overwhelm it with fear or panic. The reactive dog is forced to give up its escape efforts as useless by systematically blocking movement away from the feared situation. These blocking efforts are continued until the dog's escape efforts subside. Initially, keeping the dog in motion is generally superior to having it sit or lie down and stay in the presence of a feared situation; as its fear is reduced, sit-stay and down-stay exposures can be added gradually. In addition to outward curving or angling approaches from the feared situation (e.g., crossing the street), a circular or spiraling pattern can be used. As the pattern is walked off, various types of food reward are covertly dropped at varied distances from one another. As the circle is completed, the same pattern is walked off a second time and the dog is encouraged to find the planted treats. Another technique involves having a stranger walk away from the dog while dropping treats every so often, including an occasional big surprise, as the dog follows at a safe distance from behind picking them up. After repeated graded exposures with response prevention, the dog gradually discovers that there is nothing to fear, thereby becoming more receptive and responsive to counterconditioning and safety training efforts (see *Response Prevention, Opponent Processing, and Relaxation* in Volume 2, Chapter 3). Interactive exposure involves physically directing the dog to engage in behavior that it would probably not choose on its own. Restraining a fearful dog in the presence of a fear-provoking object or person is potentially risky, so appropriate precautions should be taken. Consequently, when performing response-prevention procedures, appropriate restraint and equipment should be used (leash attached to a fixed-action halter or limited-slip/halter combination). Under some circumstances involving potentially aggressive dogs, a muzzle-clamping halter or muzzle may be a necessary precaution. When highly aroused with fear or rage, dogs should not be coddled with reassurance and protective petting. Such handling is not usually productive under such circumstances,

and it may inadvertently make things worse or result in a redirected attack.

Counterconditioning and Interactive Exposure: Final Steps

Response prevention is particularly important when bringing the dog into close contact with the feared object or persons. Getting through this final barrier often requires a combination of response prevention, attention training, counterconditioning, and behavioral blocking techniques. In addition to inducing postarousal relief and relaxation effects, response-prevention procedures serve to block and extinguish instrumental escape and avoidance behavior via the disconfirmation of dysfunctional prediction-control expectancies, thereby preparing the way for additional cynopraxic behavior therapy and training efforts. Although graded exposure with response prevention may rapidly reduce overt fearful behavior, additional appetitive and emotional counterconditioning and play therapy may be needed to antagonize lingering emotional fear and prevent excessive anxiety as the blocking contingency is removed. Finally, by incorporating and reinforcing trained behavior with a composite of social, appetitive, and ludic rewards, an augmented safety bias can be developed to help generalize more confident behavior over varied situations previously eliciting fearful reactions.

Approach behavior is supported by bridging (DRO and shaping), petting, massage, food, conditioned odors, and play in order to produce new, attractive, and complex associations with the situation, to enhance attention and impulse control, to strengthen more appropriate and diversified patterns of behavior, and to establish active modal activity (exploring, investigating, experimenting, and so forth) conducive to interactive competence. Again, planting the situation with highly palatable food rewards that the dog can easily find on its own or with the aid of the trainer pointing them out can be very useful for motivating seeking and exploratory activity. A conditioned odor can be introduced to further facilitate the transitional process. For example, an odor that has been repeatedly paired with food via a scented squeaker bulb (squeaker valve removed) can be delivered quietly with a modified carbon dioxide (CO_2) pump or a scented squeaker bulb, thereby modulating aversive arousal and enhancing food-related counterconditioning efforts. The olfactory signature used to facilitate and conclude posture-facilitated relaxation (PFR) training may be incorporated to produce associations and arousal incompatible with fear and enhance counterconditioning efforts associated with tactile stimulation (e.g., long and firm strokes of petting and massage), perhaps hastening the recruitment of a relaxation response (see *Olfaction and Emotional Arousal* in Chapter 6).

Interestingly, many (but certainly not all) fearful dogs, once within close contact with the feared situation, rapidly begin to relax under the influence of response prevention and the presentation of conditioned odors. During such exposure, the dog is vocally encouraged, petted and massaged, and rewarded with different types of food presented in varied amounts and frequencies. Rewards are presented in association with a highly conditioned bridging stimulus in accord with a DRO or shaping contingency or in the context of attention training. A dog's willingness to accept food at such times is a propitious sign, because it indicates that fear is either attenuating or at least not increasing. In general, the dog's willingness to accept food is a fairly reliable, but not foolproof, way to monitor nascent emotional changes incompatible with fear, whereas the loss of appetite is a useful barometer for gauging fearful interference. Evidence of progressive relaxation in response to massage is also a promising indicator, since a dog cannot be tense and reactive while at the same time remaining relaxed and calm.

Targeting-arc Training

As the result of socialization deficits, abusive or traumatic handling, or behavioral stress (anxiety and frustration associated with disorderly social interaction), dogs may become progressively reactive, showing signs of hypervigilance, anxiousness or irritability, and an acquired inability to respond adaptively to signals of threat or loss (see *Inclusion Criteria* in Chapter 5). A chronic exposure to attractive and aversive stimulation lacking order and consistency may exhaust or degrade attentional and comparator functions, giving rise to persistent frustration, anxiety, or both (helpless-panic spectrum), and an inability to produce reward via executive mediated comparator networks and positive prediction error. As a result, such dogs may become progressively reactive to environmental stimuli, showing a preferential sensitivity toward signals of punishment (loss and threat) and an affinity for fight/flight reactivity. Such reactive-type dogs appear to be prone to develop fears as the result of aversive sensitization. Paradoxically, though, despite their enhanced sensitivity to signals of punishment, such dogs often show striking deficits with respect to avoidance learning and nociception, apparently obtaining little reward as the result of successful avoidance (see *Post-traumatic Stress Disorder* in Volume 1, Chapter 9).

Training the orienting response to a high degree of reliability is of critical importance and value in preparation for both graded interactive exposure and counterconditioning efforts (see *Attention and Autonomic Regulation* in Chapter 8). In the case of highly reactive dogs, however, a variation of attention training focusing on the targeting arc of several sensory-analyzer systems (i.e., auditory, visual, olfactory, tactile, and kinesthetic) may yield additional benefit as a starting point. Targeting-arc training (TAT) is based in part on distinctions drawn by Konorski (1967) between targeting and orientation reflexes (see *Targeting Reflex* in Volume 1, Chapter 6). The targeting arc is a rapid adjustment of a sensory analyzer to an environmental event, captured or sandwiched between an orienting stimulus (e.g., squeaker, hand movement, odor, touch, or prompt by leash) and bridge stimulus (clicker). The targeting arc is akin to a behavioral snapshot delineated by a stimulus response and a reward signal. For example, the auditory targeting arc consists of a slight sideways head movement or ocular orientation toward the source of stimulation. TAT is introduced in a relatively distraction-free environment with an ambient odor (e.g., orange or orange-lemon mix) delivered by an aquarium pump and diffuser. During TAT, the dog is first trained to take food from a closed hand flicked to the side (see *Introductory Lessons* in Chapter 1). TAT is focused on the split-second adjustment when the dog alerts to the orienting stimulus, whereupon the trainer clicks and flicks the closed right hand to the side, causing the dog to approach and take the food reward. A squeaker scented with the ambient odor is gently squeezed just before the hand is opened to deliver the reward. The targeting arc is a micro-control module consisting of reflexive and instrumental elements and organized in accordance with an appetitive control incentive. Initially, TAT is performed in the context of a varied DRO schedule, but is gradually superseded by a shaping contingency (e.g., following the trainer's body or tracking the movements of the right hand) and training the dog to come, sit, stay, and attend (i.e., make and hold eye contact in response to its name).

As a gate between the environment and executive analyzing and organizing functions, the targeting arc mediates selective attention and impulse control, providing an anchor for subsequent training and a conduit for manipulating appetitive and emotional establishing operations. If trained by ordinary means, using a repetitive orienting stimulus and a highly predicted reward, the orienting response rapidly habituates and plateaus. However, by varying the sound of the squeaker and presenting variable rewards on a DRO schedule conducive to positive prediction error and dissonance effects, a highly potentiated orienting response is produced, perhaps helping to refresh and restore attention functions and renewing the dog's interest in reward, as well. In addition, since positive prediction error is conducive to adaptive modal activity, TAT provides a viable organizing platform for reward-based training and therapy efforts (see *Instrumental Control Modules and Modal Strategies* in Chapter 1). Attention therapy with TAT may help disorganized dogs to transition gradually from a reactive cognitive and emotional orientation to a more adaptive one that shows an increasing sensitivity and

responsiveness to signals of reward and punishment.

PART 2: FEARS AND PHOBIAS: TREATMENT PROCEDURES AND PROTOCOLS

Dogs are prone to develop fears and phobias toward a wide variety of eliciting stimuli and situations (see *Phobia* in Volume 2, Chapter 3). Many of these problems are discussed in Volume 2. The purpose of the following is to examine common phobias and to explore various methods for reducing them (see *Classical Conditioning and Fear* in Volume 1, Chapter 2). Remedial training for phobic dogs follows a regular course of events regardless of the specific fear involved. The first step is to define the functional and structural limits of the problem accurately, that is, the what, when, where, and how of its occurrence (see *Assessment and Evaluation of Fear-related Problems* in Volume 1, Chapter 3). This information can then be used to select an appropriate training program. Most of the fear-reducing techniques described are based on experimental studies involving fears produced by aversive conditioning, typically involving electrical shock; that is, the studies are largely limited to understanding the acquisition and extinction of the fear of pain. Fearful behavior presented by companion dogs is typically far more complicated, and the originating causes are often unknown and may emerge quite independently of any identifiable experience of pain. Further, it is virtually impossible to duplicate the highly controlled conditions of a laboratory in a home or clinical setting (Baum, 1989). Consequently, in addition to scientific knowledge, a significant amount of common dog sense and creative problem solving is needed to treat canine fears and phobias successfully, making cookbook protocols quite beside the point.

FEAR OF PAIN AND DISCOMFORT

Common fears associated with pain include grooming, handling, nail clipping, various veterinary procedures, and improper training procedures. Many conditioned fears associated with pain can be prevented by means of latent inhibition and other habituation procedures performed early in the dog's development (see *Habituation, Sensitization, and Preventive-exposure Training*). Some dogs appear to be more sensitive to touch and prone to develop persistent fears associated with discomfort and painful handling. The usual procedures used for resolving such problems employ some combination of graded interactive exposure with RP-CC. Although conscientious efforts should be made to countercondition a fearful dog with treats and relaxing massage while it undergoes progressive exposure to the feared activity, it is imperative that avoidance and escape be blocked. Very often in such cases counterconditioning efforts will achieve only a small portion of the desired effect. Response prevention using physical restraint followed by massage as the animal begins to relax can be very useful. It is important for the dog to become relaxed before it is released from restraint. In the case of dogs that become highly reactive, they should be held in restraint (with massage) for 3 additional minutes after the last strong effort to break free. Excessive sensitivity to touch and contact aversion appear to play significant roles in the development of some aggression problems. Dogs exhibiting pain-based fears may resort to aggressive efforts to escape restraint during response-prevention procedures. Consequently, a muzzle or other adequate restraint may be necessary, at least until the dog learns to recognize that it is safe and will not be hurt during the training procedure. Persistent fears based on past painful experiences are usually responsive to graduated exposure with response prevention and counterconditioning.

STORM AND THUNDER PHOBIAS

The vast majority of noise phobias involve thunder or loud percussive sounds such gunshots or firecrackers. Shull-Selcer and Stagg (1991) reported that 93% of cases (N = 30) of dogs with noise phobias involved fear of thunder and other loud noises (e.g., gunshots, fireworks, backfiring, or cap guns). Occasionally, a critical precipitating event can be traced in a dog's history that helps to explain its fear of loud noises, such as a particularly strong

aversive event that has occurred in close association with the eliciting noise. Perhaps the most common cause is sensitization resulting from intense exposure to a loud noise (thunder, fireworks, gunfire, and so forth). Such highly aversive events may permanently alter a dog's fear and escape thresholds by sensitizing alarm-threat pathways mediating fear and startle (Koch, 1999), making it excessively reactive to noises and prone to exhibit persistent fear in response to minimal provocation. Finally, some dogs may simply exhibit a strong genetic predisposition leading to increased sensitivity to loud noises and a low-threshold acoustic startle response (Royce, 1955).

Prognostic Considerations

Unlike conditioned stimuli that acquire their fear-eliciting properties by way of startling or traumatic events, thunder phobias may develop with little or no evidence of extraordinary associative conditioning; that is, they are biologically prepared (see *Biological Predisposition and Preparedness* in Volume 2, Chapter 3). Further, in the case of noise-sensitive dogs, thunder and other loud percussive noises represent an unconditioned source of startle and fear. Stimuli that evoke fearful reactions without conditioning may do so through reflexive and hardwired neural pathways that may be shielded from the effects of graduated exposure, habituation, and counterconditioning—procedures that are notoriously prone to rebound effects, spontaneous recovery, and other savings (Kehoe and Macrae, 1997; see *Spontaneous Recovery and Other Sources of Relapse* in Volume 1, Chapter 6). Several other factors mitigate the effectiveness and efficacy provided by these procedures in the case of storm and thunder phobias. Most dogs that are afraid of thunder can learn to tolerate recordings of thunder if the sound effects are presented at sufficiently low levels while they are being massaged or eating food; they may even gradually accept more realistic recordings and loud playback of thunder sounds, but the conditioning may not transfer to other situations involving the actual sounds and ambient stimuli associated with real storms. Further, the benefits of counterconditioning are largely dependent on the presence of the owner together with unconditioned stimuli (e.g., food and massage) evoking arousal incompatible with fear.

Unlike many common fear-eliciting situations, avoidance and safe escape from storm activity are not possible, although a dog may find some degree of momentary relief by hiding or clinging to the owner. Since avoidance and escape are not practical coping strategies, it is imperative that emotional fear be modulated through a variety of means. With help, highly fearful dogs can learn to cope passively with their fear of thunder (ultimately this may be the best that one can expect), but such efforts may not result in permanent change. Controlling fear associated with thunderstorms can be extremely frustrating and subject to recovery and relapse effects. Excessive fear represents a significant welfare concern and, in cases involving extremely fearful dogs that show a refractory response to behavior therapy, veterinary medical intervention should be considered. Behavior therapy combined with appropriate anxiolytic medication can make the process less stressful for both owners and dogs. Providing thunder-phobic dogs with prophylactic desensitization and medication during times of the year when storm activity is most likely to occur may help to modulate or manage symptoms, perhaps the best that one can expect in severe cases.

The prognostic picture for moderately fearful dogs is much better. Even in the case of moderate storm phobias, though, controlling fear of thunder is complicated by a variety of difficulties. The foremost difficulty in this regard is that thunder is not easily predicted and controlled. For example, a dog may be at home alone while the owner is at work when the storm occurs, making it impossible to organize appropriate fear-reducing efforts to head off excessive fear. This consideration is particularly relevant to separation-anxious dogs, whose distress at being left alone may add to their susceptibility to thunder-elicited fear. Even under ideal conditions, with the owner present, control over the frightening event is compromised to the extent that its intensity varies widely according to the strength of the storm and where lightning

happens to strike. This lack of control also extends to various antecedent and extraneous stimuli (contextual influences) associated with the thunder itself. Ultimately, the best approach to managing thunder phobias is by means of preventive-exposure training (latent inhibition) starting at an early age (see *Habituation, Sensitization, and Preventive-exposure Training*). Since the exact causes underlying the development of storm and thunder phobias are unknown, methods for preventing them are based on reasonable speculation and training lore. Many young dogs show some degree of apprehension with the approach of a storm and may exhibit signs of growing fearful arousal during thunder and lightning. Encouraging confidence at such times by engaging them in tug games or ball play may be very useful. Going for walks in the rain, playing fetch, or having the dog perform a set of basic training exercises as the storm approaches may also help it to cope better with storms.

Behavioral Signs and Indicators

As a storm approaches, dogs may become progressively nervous and apprehensive, often seeking close contact with the owner or anxiously searching about the house. Fearful arousal intensifies as the storm nears, causing dogs to increase fearful activities and present increasing signs of restlessness and sympathetic arousal (e.g., panting and trembling). Some dogs may seek close comfort contact, leap on the owner's lap, or search frantically for a place to hide. Upon hearing a lightning strike nearby, fearful arousal may become even more pronounced and panicked. If outdoors, dogs may attempt to run off or dig back into the house (Voith and Borchelt, 1996). Other dogs kept inside the house may search for a way outside, often resulting in significant damage to window casings and door frames; some highly aroused dogs have jumped through glass windows and screens. Finding that escape is not possible, they may run to a bedroom or other areas of the house in search of safety. Many thunder-phobic dogs hide in closets, where they may cause significant damage to flooring and drywall by scratching and digging.

In an internet survey, McCobb and colleagues (2001) found that nearly 50% of those dogs that hide do so in bathrooms. Some of these dogs appear to be particularly attracted to tubs and showers as places of retreat. Theorizing about the motives compelling dogs to seek out tubs and other bathroom fixtures, Dodman (1996) has fashioned a dubious hypothesis to explain this predilection of canine thunder phobics. Based largely on reasoning from anecdotal evidence and hearsay, he speculates that static electricity may play a powerful role in the etiology of storm phobias. The theory purports that dogs may receive static electrical shocks during storms, causing them significant fear and distress. According to Dodman's hypothesis, fearful dogs may be seeking metal pipes and other grounds (water) to discharge static electricity safely from their bodies, which he believes builds up in their coats during storms. Years ago, Whitney (1964) proposed a similar theory, suggesting that some thunder phobias may be related to storm-related electrical stimulation. Whitney argued that dogs may be more sensitive to small electrical shocks than are people because dogs have greater amounts of salt in their blood. To reduce the risk of static shock, Dodman recommends various measures to prevent and reduce static buildup (Dodman, 1999), such as misting the dog with water, rubbing it down with a used sheet of fabric softener, or treating its feet with an antistatic spray. Unfortunately, very little in the way of compelling data or empirical evidence is provided to support the static electricity theory.

Social Contagion and the Fear of Thunder

Some authorities, most notably Beaver (1982, 1983), have suggested that storm and thunder phobias may be facilitated by a social contagion and reward. According to this theory, storm phobias are learned or worsened as the result of social attention given to dogs by owners during storms:

> Lightning striking nearby is a neutral stimulus and a dog continues sleeping. The frightened owner pats the dog (an unconditioned stimulus) mostly for self-assurance. The dog quickly learns that it will receive social attention during thunderstorms and that trembling will increase the amount of attention. (1982:1348)

There are a number of problems with Beaver's notion of contagion-mediated fear. First, lightning and thunder are far from neutral; actually, thunder is a potent unconditioned stimulus capable of eliciting intense fear in a sensitive dog. A fear of lightning and thunder does not need the owner's help to be learned. In fact, loud noises can be used to support fear conditioning or to rapidly suppress behavior. If anything, lightning in the aforementioned scenario is a neutral stimulus related to thunder as an unconditioned stimulus eliciting fear. The function of the owner's pat might serve as an unconditioned stimulus in so far as it evokes an antistress response (see *Origin of Reactive versus Adaptive Coping Styles* in Chapter 4), but it is extremely doubtful that such contact comfort would evoke or mediate fear. As a result of the close forward association between lightning and thunder, distant flashes of lightning in the future may evoke in the dog an anticipatory apprehension of an impending thunder event, causing it to become uneasy with conditioned fear. Second, far from evoking fear-related behavior, social attention and petting under such conditions might actually help to attenuate a dog's fear, perhaps helping to avert excessive arousal and sensitization to the sound of thunder. Third, and importantly, many signs of fear, such as trembling and panting, are bodily expressions of involuntary sympathetic arousal that are not under the control of instrumental contingencies of reward and punishment. A dog may be able to control certain aspects of its behavior when under the influence of fear, but activities such as trembling are not among them.

To the best of my knowledge, no significant evidence exists to support the belief that phobias are acquired or worsened through social rewards. Strong contrary evidence does exist, however, supporting the view that contact comfort may provide a significant source of anxiety and fear reduction for dogs and may be useful for reducing fearful arousal in the context of behavior modification (see *Effect of Person* in Volume 1, Chapter 9). The key is to provide such contact and reassurance in a constructive way that helps to modulate fearful arousal and guides the dog into more appropriate coping behavior. In some cases, it may be essential that the dog learn to seek refuge with the owner rather than pacing about aimlessly or running away to hide. The big problem with providing affectionate reassurance and petting for fearful dogs is that they may come to rely on the owner's emotional support rather than learning to cope with fear on their own. Unfortunately, this is an inherent problem with most counterconditioning efforts. While petting and vocal reassurance may inadvertently support active avoidance, the effect of social attention and contact is probably minor in comparison to the reward produced by the act of successfully moving away from or avoiding contact with the provoking stimulus or situation. For the majority of dogs, the reward maintaining avoidance behavior is the avoidance of the feared situation or stimulus. Owner-mediated reinforcement of avoidance behavior is primarily the result of allowing the avoidance response to succeed, with subsequent affection and reassurance provided by the owner paling in significance to the intrinsic relief and relaxation associated with successful avoidance (see *Fear and Instrumental Reinforcement* in Volume 2, Chapter 3).

Finally, the belief that thunder fears may be transmitted as a contagion that is transmitted from the owner to the dog is not supported by research designed to evaluate the effect of human anxiety on dog behavior problems (O'Farrell, 1997). Although anxious individuals appear to be more disturbed by their dog's phobic tendencies, O'Farrell was unable to find a significant correlation between the anxiety levels of anxious owners and the development of phobic behavior in their dogs. Social contagion may play a role in the etiology of some common behavior problems (see Speck, 1964), including some fear-related problems (Howard, 1992), but it does not appear to play a prominent role in the development of thunder or loud-noise phobias.

Evolutionary Significance of Escape Patterns

Dogs show a fairly typical profile of fear and panic behaviors associated with storm phobias, suggesting that their reactions may belong to a common phylogenetic origin. This general hypothesis suggests that phobias are not dependent on learning for acquisition (Menzies and Clarke, 1995), although learning may play a significant role in the maintenance and generalization of fear to incidental neutral stimuli present during the fear-eliciting event. The primary instinct evoked under such circumstances is self-preservation, as evidenced by the dog's extreme arousal and efforts to escape the stimulation. Perhaps, at least in some dogs, storm activity involving lightning and thunder may directly activate primitive species-typical subroutines dedicated to maximizing survival when faced with natural catastrophes associated with lightning and thunder. Trapped within a house, dogs may feel threatened and vulnerable, causing them to run about in search of cover. As their fear and vulnerability increase, they may resort to other species-typical escape activities, such as biting, digging, and scratching. The failure of these various coping and escape efforts to obtain relief may stimulate a spiraling escalation of fearful arousal. Under future circumstances, frustrated escape efforts, now conditioned predictors of failure, may become potent elicitors of escalating fear. These observations underscore the importance of response prevention in the control of fear-related behavior.

Systematic Desensitization

Playing recordings of storms and thunder at progressively louder levels while dogs are maintained under the influence of incompatible arousal of sufficient strength to antagonize fear is the most frequently recommended method for reducing thunder phobias. While thunder sounds can be recorded and played back at varying volumes and degrees of realism, many aspects of the storm situation and ambience cannot be reliably replicated: illusion of sound coming from a distance, window and wall vibrations resulting from thunder, changes in barometric pressure, dark and overcast skies, increased humidity and rain, realistic lightning flashes, sounds of wind and rain on windows, ozone level changes, and many other subtle nuances remain outside of direct manipulation or duplication. Also, given a dog's sensitive sense of smell, ambient odor changes associated with impending storm activity may play a significant role as a conditioned stimulus or contextual cue (Otto and Giardino, 2001). Furthermore, no recording can faithfully capture and duplicate the temper and violence of an actual thunderstorm. Consequently, many dogs that appear to respond positively to an artificial arrangement may do so knowing that the stimulation is not real. Most dogs rapidly learn to ignore recorded storm sounds, strobe flashes, subdued lighting, and so on, but probably do so knowing that the recorded sound and other effects originate safely within the house and while the owner is nearby. When left alone or when exposed to a real storm, previous desensitization efforts may not do much good. Since the beneficial effects of counterconditioning depend on the presence of emotional arousal that is incompatible with fear, any benefits acquired as the result of desensitization may be lost when an actual storm strikes, simply because the owner is not present to provide the accustomed appetitive stimulation, massage, and contact comfort.

The first step in the desensitization by counterconditioning is to determine whether the audio storm recording elicits a fearful response. If the recording proves effective, the next step is to find an audio level that is sufficient to evoke orientation but without eliciting fear. The thunder-phobic dog is initially exposed to the least evocative item on the list and then progressively challenged with more intense audio samples until the entire stimulus-gradient hierarchy is covered. Many variations are possible depending on a dog's temperament and the severity of its phobia. The desensitization hierarchy is treated as a guideline open to adjustment and modifications as they may prove necessary during training. The hierarchy should be as simple and short as possible, with addi-tional items added as training progresses and such alterations prove necessary. Each step of the hierarchy should be worked on until both visible and inferred (anorexia) signs of fear are extinguished.

The key to successful desensitization is gradual exposure to as many features of the evoking stimulus and situation as possible, while at the same time maintaining the dog in a motivational state that is incompatible with fearful arousal. Several stimulus and situational dimensions should be considered when constructing an artificial desensitization hierarchy: similarity to the evoking stimulus; proximity (distance from the evoking stimulus has a significant bearing on the magnitude of the response); context (the presence of the owner, for example, during desensitization has a significant effect on fear levels; this the effect of person must be faded out gradually); intensity of stimulation (a loud sound typical elicits more arousal than a soft one); contrast (relative to surrounding ambience and competing stimulation); and stimulus continuity (whenever possible, evoking samples should be presented in a smooth progression of fear-eliciting increments).

The key to effective desensitization by counterconditioning is careful progression and patience. Between regular training sessions, a previously desensitized level of recorded thunder may played for extended periods for added benefit, especially at times associated with play activities and eating. By using an electronic timer, such samples can also be presented at low and progressively louder and more natural levels while the owner is out of the house.

The controlled circumstances of crate confinement are conducive to desensitization, but the crate must be introduced gradually and patiently with counterconditioning in order to avoid negative associations (see *Guidelines for Successful Crate Training* in Chapter 2). An air-pump odor dispenser and feeder is an easy way to deliver food rewards and olfactory stimuli while a dog is in a crate (Figure 3.5). The device is constructed from an aquarium air pump and a modified water dispenser. Air pressure is directed through pliable tubing and controlled by a touch valve and a three-way valve that diverts a small amount of air pressure to a glass diffuser that is used to deliver a dilute odor. The air pressure directed to the diffuser should be adjusted to produce a minimal airflow, ensuring that most of the air pressure remains available to dispense the food. The tubing is attached to the water bottle by a plastic connector inserted into a small hole drilled into the side of the bottle. Also, to allow food to pass through the stem of the water dispenser, the steel-ball valve must be removed. As air pressure builds up in the water bottle, the soft food is forced out through the stem of the water dispenser. Since the air in the diffuser moves more freely than the air going into the water bottle, the arrangement results in the odor reaching the dog a second or two before the food is delivered, thereby providing a viable classical condition arrangement.

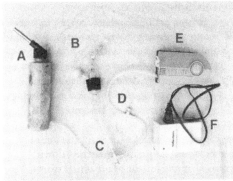

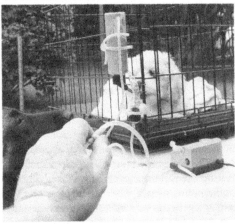

FIG. 3.5. Odor dispenser and feeder: (A) modified water dispenser, (B) glass diffuser, (C) three-way valve, (D) touch (screw) valve, (E) air pump, and (F) remote switch.

A touch valve situated in the main tubing regulates air pressure and allows the trainer to turn the odor and food presentation on or off. When the touch valve is covered with a finger, the air pressure rapidly builds and dispenses first the odor and shortly thereafter the soft food. When the finger is lifted from the touch valve, pressure is lost, and the odor and food stop dispensing. For remote operation, the touch valve can be sealed with a screw stopper, and a remote switch can be used to activate the air pump and control the delivery of food. This arrangement allows the trainer to stage desensitization conditions that more closely mimic situations when the owner is not at home—occasions when many phobic dogs are particularly vulnerable to thunder and other fears.

The persistence and resistance of storm phobias to extinction and desensitization efforts may, in part, be due to the brief duration of storm activity. Thunder storms typically roll in and roll out rapidly, perhaps not giving the dog sufficient exposure time to the stimulation to habituate naturally. As the storm subsides, the dog may experience significant emotional relief, negatively reinforcing preceding escape efforts, even though they had no effect on the storm's coming and going. Further, because the motivational arousal is extremely high, the potential effect of reinforcement at such times may be extremely strong and perhaps sufficient to establish persistent superstitious escape/avoidance behaviors. As a result, storm-associated cues may gradually become discriminative stimuli and establishing operations, setting the occasion for fear-related escape and avoidance behavior in the presence of stimuli associated with a storm. Consequently, during desensitization, dogs may be permitted to move around the room, but are not permitted to run off or hide. Efforts to hide or escape are prevented by keeping the dog on a leash or other restraint, as necessary. Some dogs may benefit from being restrained on a halter-type collar, an arrangement that enables the handler to control even very subtle escape/avoidance behaviors. Prior to performing desensitization procedures, the dog should receive intensive attention and basic training (see *Graded Interactive Exposure*).

Sample Hierarchy

Baseline information about a dog's reaction to thunder should be recorded, including various signs of fear. A chart and behavior journal should be kept to record procedures used and the dog's response to therapy. Heart rate is a sensitive measure of fear and should be measured and recorded at the beginning and end of each session. The outline of desensitization by counterconditioning described below is intended to provide a general picture; many variations and intermediate steps and subsets may be involved, depending on the specific requirements of a dog:

- The dog is exposed to low-level audio recordings of storm sounds (15 to 30 minutes or longer) while moving about, playing tug, chasing a ball, or receiving food and petting after coming when called. All efforts to leave the situation are prevented by keeping the dog on leash. Food rewards can be delivered from a hand holding a scented squeaker bulb. The bulb is squeezed just before the hand is opened to deliver the reward. Presenting the conditioned odor during simulated and real storms may augment appetitive counterconditioning effects. The conditioned odor is presented via an aquarium pump and diffuser before turning on the recording and continued for 3 to 5 minutes afterward. An easy-to-construct diffuser can be made with some rubber tubing and a small bottle with a cap (see *Taction and Olfactory Conditioning* in Chapter 4).
- The dog is exposed to low-level audio recordings of storm sounds under subdued lighting, flashes of light (camera strobe), and a fan blowing curtains while the dog moves about, plays tug, chases a ball, or receives food and petting after coming when called.
- The dog is exposed to a progression of stronger audio sounds of thunder with subdued lighting, remote flashes of light, a fan blowing curtains, and a sprinkler casting water against a window while the dog moves about, plays tug, chases a ball, or receives food and petting after coming when called. Previously desensitized levels

are presented randomly during the day while the dog is playing, eating, or sleeping.
- The dog is exposed to increasing intensities (starting at a low level) of audio-recorded sounds while receiving PFR training.
- The dog is exposed to a progression of stronger audio sounds of thunder under subdued lighting, remote flashes of light, and a fan blowing curtains while the dog is in a crate receiving treats.
- The dog is exposed to taped recordings of thunder at natural intensity along with other storm-related sounds and movements while in a crate, with the owner on the other side of the room.
- The dog is exposed to taped recordings of thunder at natural intensity along with other storm-related sounds and movements while in a crate, with the owner out of the room.
- The dog is taken outside in the presence of an advancing storm and walked and engaged in various training activities, tug games, and ball play. Attention control is maintained by calling the dog's name, squeaking or smooching, and reinforcing appropriate orienting behavior.

At the conclusion of each step, the audio storm should be gradually turned down, mimicking the retreat of an actual storm. Perhaps the most effective use of counterconditioned audio storm recordings is to present them during actual storm events, thereby providing means to continue stimulation for a sufficient time to promote habituation and extinction and to reinforce behavior incompatible with fear. Counterconditioned audio storm sounds may exert a significant restraining influence on fear occurring in the presence of actual storms. The conditioned odor is presented just before the storm appears, followed by the audio storm, and continued during the full duration of the storm. The audio storm should stay on even after the actual storm has subsided, and continue until the dog's fear attenuates. The olfactory stimulus should be continued for 3 to 5 minutes after the audio storm is gradually tapered off. The combined presentation of the counterconditioned audio storm and the conditioned odor may help to dampen fearful arousal elicited by an actual storm event (see *Safety Signal Hypothesis* in Volume 1, Chapter 8). In some cases, earplugs fashioned from pliable silicone may be helpful, at least temporarily. A short knotted string should be imbedded in the silicone wad to make its removal easier.

FEAR OF LOUD NOISES AND HOUSEHOLD SOUNDS

A dog's response to loud noises is mediated by a variety of physiological and behavioral systems. Startle to loud sounds is reflexive and depends on genetic predisposition (sensory and behavioral threshold variability) and experience. The evoked startle response triggers a cascade of biobehavioral events preparing dogs for defensive action. Dogs exhibiting a low acoustical threshold may exhibit a very pronounced startle response to loud percussive sounds (e.g., gunfire or fireworks), even when they occur at some distance away, whereas dogs with a high acoustical threshold may simply orient in the direction of stimulation or ignore it altogether unless it occurs nearby. A dog's response to startling stimulation appears to be strongly affected by genetics, but experience exerts a powerful modulatory influence over functional thresholds controlling the latency and magnitude of the canine acoustical startle response. An increased responsiveness to auditory stimulation can be produced by fear-potentiated startle and sensitization (Koch, 1999). In the presence of ambient stimuli previously paired with aversive stimulation, loud noises or unfamiliar sounds may produce a potentiated startle response even though those auditory stimuli had never been paired with aversive stimulation in the past. For example, excessive punishment may result in the owner becoming a conditioned aversive stimulus. In the presence of such an owner, a dog's response to auditory stimulation may be significantly potentiated as the result of fear. Similarly, a wide variety of aversive conditioning events can permanently alter startle thresholds to auditory stimulation. Such fear-potentiated startle can have both adverse and beneficial effects on a dog's training and adaptation.

Sensitization occurs when a dog is exposed to an intense and unexpected auditory event, which subsequently results in significantly lower acoustical thresholds in response to that sound and other loud noises, as well. Sensitization appears to have played a role in the following case described by Humphrey and Warner (1934):

> One day she stopped him for a curb at a street crossing and waited for a large truck, halted by the traffic lights, to move on. As the lights changed and the truck started it back-fired in the face of the dog. The master, who was shell shocked as well as blind, jumped backward, yanked, stepped on and fell over his dog. Thus, the ear-pain from the back-fire was followed immediately by the body-pain of the trampling. The animal was retired from blind-leading at once because it was found that she had become extremely oversensitive to sound. After a year's service as a companion in a private home she seems to have outgrown the effects of the shock and to have become again gun-sure. She has not been returned to blind guide work, however, for it is feared that in a difficult traffic situation the occurrence of another noise, even though not so loud this time, might cause her to act erratically and endanger her man. (151)

The authors attribute the dog's fear to a conditioned association between the sound of backfire and painful stimulation, but a more likely cause is sensitization and the ensuing chaos and loss of control and predictability associated with the event.

Dogs exhibit varying degrees of stress-related behavior and physiological changes in association with noisy environments. Although many dogs appear to be remarkably undisturbed by loud noises so long as they are presented in nonstartling increments, sudden and loud noises may produce a surge of adrenal hormone activity indicating HPA-axis activation (Stephens, 1980). Thalken (1971) found that laboratory beagles exposed to a total of 2 hours of loud noise (120 dB) in repeated 30-second to 5-minute doses over an 8-hour period did not exhibit a significant increase in glucocorticoid activity. Similarly, Beerda and colleagues (1997) found minimal heart-rate and cortisol changes in dogs exposed to moderate stimulation levels under 87 dB. However, one dog exposed to 95-dB auditory stimulation for several minutes showed increased cortisol activity and other signs of behavioral stress: tongue exposed, nose licking, paw lifting, and shaking. In a subsequent study involving strong, momentary auditory stimulation, the authors reported that repeated exposure to a momentary blast (1 to 2 seconds) from a foghorn (110 to 120 dB) resulted in significant physiological and behavioral evidence of stress, including a pronounced cortisol surge that returned to baseline levels after 60 minutes (Beerda et al., 1998). The researchers also found that the blast of the foghorn produced more cortisol activity than produced by moderately strong levels of repeated brief electrical stimulation delivered by a remote electronic collar (Tri-tronics 100 A set at level 8). Loud barking and other sources of noise are common in situations where dogs are housed together, with noise levels frequently exceeding 120 dB in kennel situations (Sales et al., 1997). Thalken's findings do not necessarily suggest that exposure to loud noise is not stressful; instead, the apparent absence of stress may be the result of previous exposure and habituation to loud noises in the dogs studied. Also, Thalken's failure to find evidence of stress in response to loud auditory stimulation may be attributable to breed-specific peculiarities affecting auditory arousal in beagles. As hunting dogs, beagles may have been selected to exhibit an elevated acoustical threshold for loud noises, enabling them to work in close range to the blast of a shotgun. In fact, dogs of different breeds exhibit varying levels of emotional reactivity to startle-eliciting stimulation (Mahut, 1958), making generalizations concerning fear and stress in dogs based on the study of a select breed or small group of represented breeds highly questionable. Finally, there is significant individual variability in the way dogs respond to startle- and fear-eliciting stimulation, further militating against such generalizations.

Desensitization by counterconditioning or habituation follows the same basic procedures as already described. The fear-eliciting effects of loud noises can be attenuated either by presenting them at a distance or by various muffling techniques. Hart and Hart (1985) have described a method whereby a nest of six cardboard boxes is used to muffle the sound of a starting pistol. Removing one box at a time, progressively making the sound stronger, produces a graduated effect necessary for desensitization. A more convenient method, and one that allows dogs and handlers to move about freely indoors and outdoors, is to wrap the starting pistol in a towel. Unwrapping the pistol one layer at a time gradually increases the intensity of the sound produced, thereby providing a means to present progressively louder samples of gunfire. Another way to present fear-eliciting noises on a gradient of intensity is to have a helper approach at various angles or orientations relative to the dog while periodically firing the pistol. Graded exposure can also be carried out with the dog on a 50-foot long line, allowing it to move to a safe distance before discharging the pistol or cap gun. As the dog starts in response to the stimulus, it can be called back, rewarded, and released again. In cases, where more precise control over the dog's distance is required, an active-control line can be used instead.

In addition to presenting the fear-eliciting stimuli on a gradient of increasing intensity, various conditioned and unconditioned counterconditioning stimuli are presented to offset fearful arousal. The choice of procedure depends on the magnitude of a dog's fear. Various techniques are employed, including play activities (tug and fetching) and romps, systematic desensitization by graduated counterconditioning or habituation, and response prevention. The most common method involves presenting a treat immediately after the noise is made, thereby training the dog to expect food whenever the gunshot occurs—an expectancy that is incompatible with fear. In some cases, the dog is prompted to sit, whereupon a sound stimulus just strong enough to capture the dog's attention is presented. The dog's attention is then immediately diverted from the event by calling its name, squeaking, and so forth. As the dog turns in the direction of the handler, a conditioned reinforcer "Good" or a click is presented and followed by food. Randomly altering the size and type of the reinforcer may help to magnify its effect, both in terms of conditioned reinforcement and the elicitation of appetitive and emotional arousal incompatible with fear.

Whenever possible during appetitive counter-conditioning, the dog should be kept moving forward. Forward movement and standing are preferred to having the dog sit and wait; however, sit-stay training may be a necessary transition in the case of dogs likely to show strong escape or avoidance efforts in response to the feared stimulus. Sit-stay and down-stay training is also preferred in the case of dogs exhibiting reactive aggressive behavior in association with fear. Forward-oriented movement appears to have a functional affinity with the seeking system, mediating an increased sensitivity to signals of reward and approach, whereas remaining still or turning away or walking backward are motor correlates of the behavioral inhibition system and a heightened sensitivity (hesitation or avoidance) to signals of punishment. Lightly spraying a conditioned odor from a modified CO_2 pump just prior to the presentation of the feared sound appears to facilitate appetitive counterconditioning and reduce startle reactivity (see Miltner et al., 1994). The scent of orange (Lehrner et al., 2000) and lemon (Komori et al., 1995) appears to have some intrinsic anxiety- and stress-modulating properties that might be useful in fear control and management. A dilute lavender fragrance (Motomura, 2001), chamomile (Roberts and Williams, 1992), or vanillin (Miltner et al., 1994) may also possess intrinsic properties of value for modulating fearful arousal and adjusting acoustical startle thresholds. In the case of strong and startling sounds, timing the presentation of a diminutive sound to occur immediately before the startling event may help to reduce fearful arousal via prepulse inhibition and enhanced cognitive regulation and organized processing (see *Interrupting Behavior* in Chapter 1). Further, presenting a target-arc stimulus contiguously with the onset of the feared event may produce a potent fear-incompatible orienting response (see *Target-arc Training*). Exposure with prepulse inhibition and TAT may be particularly useful for the prevention and control of noise fears involving sensitization in association with discrete eliciting events (e.g., gunshots).

In addition to loud noises, many dogs react fearfully to unfamiliar sounds. Repeated exposure with playful encouragement and response prevention can be extremely effective in such cases. Finding a constructive way to have a fearful dog interact with the object producing the unfamiliar or startling sound can also be helpful. Many dogs exhibit fear toward motor-driven household appliances; a fear of vacuum cleaners is especially common. Since these sorts of stimuli are fairly easy to control and present in a form that allows the dog to habituate gradually, they are fairly easy to resolve, perhaps explaining the relative infrequency of such fears presenting for treatment. Shull-Selcer and Stagg (1991), for example, found that, of 30 noise-fearful dogs, 7% exhibited fear toward television or stereo sounds and only 3% presented fear related to the sound of vacuum cleaners. Some dogs exhibit persistent fears associated with the switching on of furnace relays, causing them to awake at night and pace or pant nervously. A furnace-related fear should be considered in dogs exhibiting sleep disturbances that involve pacing and other signs of fear (e.g., panting and trembling).

FEAR OF SUDDEN MOVEMENT OR CHANGE

An innate expectancy bias toward sudden movement or change appears to underlie many fears expressed toward moving objects, such as cars, bicycles, joggers, and skaters. Additive effects are likely to occur when fear-evoking stimuli are both novel and encountered in unfamiliar locations (see *Expectancy Bias* in Volume 2, Chapter 3). Consequently, initial exposure and desensitization should be carried out in familiar places and gradually extended to areas progressively less familiar to the dog. A useful method is for the owner to introduce the feared object or activity as part of a play activity. For example, a ball can be thrown in the vicinity of a bike resting against a tree. Gradually, other exposure elements are added (someone standing with a bike, rolling it, running with it, and so forth) together with various counterconditioning efforts as necessary to reduce fearful arousal. Typically, the dog is prompted to sit in the presence of the fear-evoking stimulus, starting at a distance where the stimulus elicits an orienting response but does not elicit fear. With repeated exposures, the size and type of the food reward given to the dog should be varied to maximize positive-prediction-error effects. Dogs that are fearful of bicyclists or joggers can be introduced to the feared stimulus through fear-graded interactive exposures. For example, close interaction with a bicyclist helper can be accomplished by first having him or her stand next to the bike, followed by a walk in which the bike is rolled along next to the dog. If the dog tolerates this level of exposure, the next step can involve having the rider mount the bike and ride slowly nearby. Finally, the bicyclist is instructed to ride by in a progressively more natural manner. During these various exposure exercises, the dog should be kept under control by heeling, sitting, or staying at the owner's side. A variety of food treats can be given in varying amounts to facilitate counterconditioning and shaping objectives. Repeatedly capturing the dog's attention with a squeaker and click at the earliest sign of incipient arousal and redirecting its behavior into more constructive action (e.g., sitting or standing quietly in place) in the presence of the feared object can help counter established escape/avoidance behavior.

Some dogs exhibit a global panic or generalized anxiety whenever taken outdoors, behavior that parallels symptoms reported by human agoraphobics. Low behavioral thresholds for fear may persist despite patient environmental exposure efforts. Such fear may develop without the involvement of any identifiable aversive event in the dog's history. An innate dread of loud sounds (e.g., gunshots or thunder) and abrupt movement is sometimes evident in such dogs from a very early age or may appear spontaneously as such dogs mature. Fears and phobias associated with an innate predisposition may be controlled to some extent with behavioral and environmental management, but cure is not likely in these cases. Dogs exhibiting signs of global anxiety and fear should be referred for veterinary evaluation and possible treatment with appropriate medications (e.g., SSRIs) prior to the initiation of behavior therapy and training.

FEAR OF HEIGHTS

Many puppies exhibit a fear of heights when placed on a table or prompted to engage in some activity that poses a risk of falling, such as walking over a log bridge. The fear of heights, like other innate fears with phylogenetic origins, may be easily potentiated by pain associated with falling, making them prone to one-trial learning. For example, children may accidentally drop a puppy that they have picked up or frightened with awkward and insensitive handling. Another common fear associated with heights involves stair-climbing inhibitions, although such fears are probably more related to a competency deficit than a fear of heights. Such fear is particularly common in adult dogs that have not had adequate experience climbing and descending stairs. Some dogs will develop an aversion toward stair climbing or jumping in a vehicle as the result of bone- and joint-related problems, making a veterinary examination an important preliminary, especially in cases where fear or competency do not appear to be significant factors.

Intense fear is commonly associated with the acquisition of complex motor skills needed to interact safely with threatening situations. Mastering stairs is a good example of such habit learning involving a fear of heights. When first learning to climb steps, puppies are awkward and hesitant in their movements. In addition, they may show significant fearful arousal and freezing behavior. Alternately, they may race down the steps in a mad dash to escape the situation. As the result of practice, however, the motor skills needed to climb steps are gradually acquired, making their efforts progressively more natural and effortless. To some extent, a puppy's climbing behavior is reinforced by the relief and relaxation it gets as it successfully reaches the top of the steps. Gradually, the initial fear of heights is overcome by the development of skillful climbing and improved confidence. Learning to climb steps exemplifies the importance of competent control and skill to overcome certain natural fears.

Puppies are usually taught to climb stair steps by placing them on the uppermost step and luring them with treats and encouragement. As the necessary skills and confidence improve, more steps are added until the puppy can climb all of them at once. After learning how to climb up the stairs, the same general procedure is used to teach puppies to climb down. Confidence building by vocal encouragement and treats play an important role in such training and should be given to puppies following every successful trial. Successful climbing is associated with significant emotional relief and relaxation, effects that may gradually help to countercondition a puppy's initial fearful reaction to steps as well as provide a source of reinforcement for climbing behavior. During the training process, the puppy should be kept on a leash to provide physical support and prevent it from falling down the steps.

As puppies learn to maneuver themselves successfully on stairs, they become progressively relaxed and confident—fearless—when climbing steps. However, dogs not exposed to stair climbing as puppies, or dogs that have been traumatized as the result of falling down steps, may prove to be much more difficult to train by using methods based on the foregoing procedure. Inexperienced dogs may resist climbing steps even after many hours of conscientious desensitization and behavioral shaping. Misguided efforts to compel them to climb by withholding meals (sometimes for days) until they finally climb the steps to get food are usually ineffective and should be avoided. Adult dogs that are afraid of steps can benefit from playful exposure to jumping over things while on outdoor excursions, climbing inclined surfaces, walking along a curb, and repeatedly stepping up and down from a low curb. Such fearful dogs may be more willing to climb low steps (e.g., the long sort sometimes found in front of schools and office buildings) when the steps are approached at an angle and then progressively approached more directly. The process involves playful and gradual exposure to progressively more difficult step-climbing challenges.

The stairs may be altered to make them easier for the dog to climb. Borchelt (1997) has suggested laying bricks side by side in front of the stairs to make the first step easier to take. Alternatively, a length of carpeting can be attached to the first few steps and extend several feet in front of the steps to provide the dog with a secure traction and "runway" up to the steps. Finally, the steps may be made less threatening to climb by covering them with a nonslip rubber runner or carpet-

ing. Letting inhibited dogs observe a more confident dog climb steps may help facilitate a greater willingness to climb.

Given that such efforts have been attempted without success, directive exposure might be considered. In this case, the dog is physically prompting to climb by being hauled up and down the stair steps on a leash. In some cases, a wide harness can be used to support some of its weight. If a harness is used, a second leash should be attached to a strap collar for safety and enhanced control. The inhibited dog is repeatedly prompted to climb steps until relaxed compliance and enthusiastic climbing replace its resistance. Dividing the training objective into simple steps facilitates directive exposure. Initially, the dog may be prompted to climb two or three steps before being permitted to turn and climb back down again. If the dog is unwilling to climb back down, it is directed to do so with steady pressure on the leash. From the top of the steps, the dog is first prompted to climb down two or three steps before allowing it to turn and scamper back up. The opportunity to reverse directions and climb back down or up again may provide a significant source of skill and confidence building.

After a series of introductory trials, the dog is carefully hauled up and down the steps. Avoidance or resistance is consistently countered with enough leash pressure to break the dog's resistance and keep it moving. The dog's willingness to follow is reinforced with enthusiastic praise and encouragement by a helper (the owner) waiting at the top or bottom of the steps. It is imperative that the trainer does not hesitate or yield to the dog's sometimes-considerable resistance, but to drive headlong up or down the steps without taking notice of the dog's reluctance to follow. Once the dog is following the handler's lead, the directive prompt is faded and a controlling discriminative signal is added to the routine. The step-climbing behavior is repeatedly prompted over a session until the dog climbs steps with minimum prompting. With the conclusion of each successful trial, the dog is given 15 to 20 seconds of encouraging praise, petting, and treats. After a session of repeated trials, the dog is prompted into a down at the top of the steps and encouraged to relax with petting and massage for 2 to 3 minutes. The successful session is followed by vigorous ball play.

Another common fear related to falling is associated with slippery flooring. Dogs exhibiting this fear may freeze when prompted to walk across waxed linoleum or wooden floors. When compelled to walk, they may move in a very awkward and poorly coordinated way. These problems are usually approached on two fronts. First, a carpet or vinyl runner is laid down to provide a safe pathway with good footing and traction. Second, the dog is walked over a piece of the runner in other parts of the house until the fear is not exhibited. In addition, the dog is prompted to lie down, sit, stand, and stay at various points on the runner. Next, a length of runner material is laid down starting in a separate room and crossing into the room containing the feared flooring. Treats can be put on the runner for the dog to pick up and eat, though most dogs exhibiting this type of fear may not be attracted to the food. Efforts to escape the situation are blocked, and the dog is prompted to move forward by leash and encouragement. Once the inhibition begins to break down, several passes are made having the dog move both into and out of the room. Rewarding objects and activities should be made contingent on the dog crossing the feared area. For example, the dog's meals, toys, and opportunities to go outside should all be preceded by its walking across the runner. The runner is gradually pulled back little by little over several days, requiring that the dog walk on more and more of the feared surface. Trimming nails back and treating the dog's paws with products to reduce slipping may be helpful in making stair climbing and walking on smooth surfaces easier for some dogs.

FEAR OF WATER

The psychological opposite of fear is confidence and relaxation—not appetitive arousal. Relaxation is a symptom or by-product of confidence. Without confidence, a dog simply cannot feel relaxed when faced with a potentially dangerous situation. The systematic training of skills needed by dogs to control feared situations competently serves to enhance their confidence while simultaneously reducing its fear (Figure 3.6). Coping adaptively with fear entails that a dog learn how to control the fear-evoking situation (see *Efficacy Expectancies* in Volume 2, Chapter 3). Fearful dogs often appear to be tense and worried about their ability to perform a feared activity or to control a potentially dangerous situation, rather than being especially fearful of the object or situation itself. In contrast, nonfearful dogs exhibit a more relaxed and confident attitude toward such situations as the result of a history of competent interaction and success. Many persistent fear conditions are the result of dogs not knowing what to do or not possessing sufficient skills and confidence (practice) to do what they need to do to control potentially dangerous situations. For example, many dogs are fearful of water and may refuse to go into it even when in the company of other dogs who enjoy water (positive models). Other dogs may not only lack the necessary skills to control a feared situation, but may actively fear stimuli associated with it. For example, some dogs are so fright-

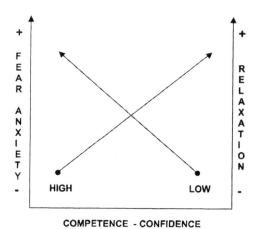

FIG. 3.6. Relaxation is a natural corollary of competence. As a dog's competence and confidence increase, fear is generally reduced as relaxation increases. Relaxation competes with the tenseness, worry, and vigilance associated with anxious and fearful states. The elation and relaxation associated with competent control over a potentially dangerous situation represent a powerful counterconditioning influence and source of positive reinforcement for dogs.

ened of water that they frantically scurry away from puddles to avoid coming into contact with it. In the case of some storm-phobic dogs, a single drop of rain can precipitate a major fearful episode.

Interactive exposure to water can be highly effective in the treatment of such phobias. Performing a variety of obedience exercises reinforced with food, play, and affection while near water is often beneficial. Gradually, the dog is progressively moved closer to the water until it is directed to walk into it or stay while standing in it. Once accepting the feel of water, stronger incentives, like an opportunity to play tug or fetch, are introduced near it. The play activity is gradually moved closer to the water until the dog is able to fetch things thrown into it. Walking at heel or fetching a ball while in water invariably teaches a dog many skills about interacting with water that can help improve its general confidence and attitude toward water. Probably the best way to prevent and overcome a fear of water is to train a dog how to swim.

FEAR OF RIDING IN CARS

The majority of dogs seem to look forward to car rides. However, some dogs, especially those that have not been exposed to car rides early in life (see *Habituation, Sensitization, and Preventive-exposure Training*), may be quite uneasy or fearful while in a car. The first step is to familiarize the dog gradually with the car. With car doors open, the dog is simply walked around the car, perhaps performing various obedience exercises or encouraged to play (e.g., tug or fetch) when near it. Any approach toward the car can be bridged ("Good" or click) and reinforced. Bonuses involving highly appetizing food items can be given in a pan that is placed progressively closer to the car. In some cases, the dog is tied to a tie-out that is attached to the car. At such times, the dog can be given a highly desirable chew item (e.g., rolled rawhide or a beef bone), and the car radio can be turned on. Graded interactive exposure and counterconditioning proceed through progressive steps until the dog willingly approaches the car. PFR training with an odorant signature can be very helpful. The conditioned scent is applied to the inside of open doors and at vari-

ous other places on the outside of the car. Since the dog is highly motivated with approach incentives during homecomings, it may be useful to arrange for someone to let the dog out of the house at such times in order for it meet the owner at or in the car. At such times, the owner should get in the rear of the car and slide across the seat, giving the dog room to jump in. The excitement elicited by the owner's homecoming may offset fearful avoidance and increase the dog's confidence. As the owner gets out of the car, both doors should be left open. Depending on the dog's response, the owner might opt to get back inside the car and encourage the dog to follow. As the dog's willingness to jump into the car improves, the owner should prompt the dog to get in first. Over several trials, a progressively more natural pattern is introduced in gradual steps and reinforced. Feeding the dog by hand or putting food on the car seats and floor may encourage the dog to move about, explore the situation, and become progressively comfortable. At the conclusion of the session, the dog is given a brief period of ball play or a walk. Another alternative is to allow the inhibited dog to play with a more confident dog close to the car with both back doors open. The confident dog can be encouraged to jump into the car to get food previously thrown there and the reluctant dog encouraged to follow. In addition, a ball or other toy can be thrown into the car, perhaps causing the reluctant dog to jump in after it. Holding the reluctant dog back for 15 seconds or so may help to build a heightened enthusiasm to follow the confident dog into the car.

An unwillingness to get into a car may be related to a lack of confidence, stemming from inadequate training. Some dogs may refuse to get into a car, as though afraid of it, but once inside not show any significant signs of anxiety or fear. In such cases, various training efforts should be carried out to teach the inhibited dog how to jump in and out of the car. As in the case of stair-climbing inhibitions, a dog that strongly resists jumping into the car may benefit from directive exposure. In this case, the dog is repeatedly prompted to jump up into the car. Any resistance is consistently countered with sufficient force to compel the dog to jump. As the dog leaps into the car, relief is associated with vocal encouragement, food, and petting. After 15 to 20 seconds, the dog is directed out of the car, and the procedure is repeated. Each trial is repeated in the same manner until the dog jumps up on its own. Once the dog is responding, a vocal cue such as "Hup" can be paired with the action of jumping into the car. At the end of the training session, the owner and the dog should remain in the car for 2 to 3 minutes, thereby obtaining benefits associated with opponent-relaxation effects. This period is associated with quiet petting, massage, listening to the car radio, and the presentation of an olfactory safety cue.

Dogs may develop fears about riding in the car as the result of traumatic events or a history of aversive consequences associated with car trips. For example, dogs that are taken in the car only for veterinary visits, especially if they have experienced painful procedures, may develop an anticipatory fear associated with car rides. When such causes are suspected, frequent rides that result in more attractive outcomes (going to the park, picking up children at school, and so forth) can help to counteract such fears. Some dogs who have been exposed to an automobile accident or abrupt stop throwing them around inside the car may develop a lasting fear that makes them uncomfortable in cars. The affected dog may pace back and forth, pant, whine, and in general appear to be unable to settle down. Such dogs may be aroused continuously during drives or become aroused only after a sharp turn or bump in the road. One advantage of this class of fears is that the duration of exposure can be controlled, making response-prevention procedures feasible. Smooth and straight rides(e.g., on expressways) can be taken during which the dog is appropriately restrained from moving about. In addition, the dog should be taught to sit and stay while in the car. As the dog shows signs of calming, the car can be pulled over and the dog taken for a walk.

FEAR OF ENCLOSED SPACES AND CONFINEMENT

Many puppies initially respond to crate confinement with intense fear and escape behav-

ior. In an important sense, crate confinement is more like a trap than a den. Under natural conditions, a situation like a crate would be a serious threat to an animal. It is little wonder, therefore, that many puppies and dogs respond with intense aversion and distress when locked inside a crate for the first time. Unfortunately, many new dog owners simply put the puppy in a crate and leave it there to work through its distress alone, with little appreciation for the potential harm done by such treatment. The puppy may subsequently eliminate in the crate as the result of ensuing distress or because the owner may neglect to take it out on a timely basis, thereby making an already problematic situation much worse. Puppies that eliminate in the crate may be further stressed by abusive after-the-fact punishment and water deprivation initiated to correct the elimination problem. Because of work and school schedules, the puppy may spend the vast majority of the day in a crate. Thus, life goes by with the puppy rapidly transitioning through extremely sensitive and influential developmental periods under the adverse and deprived conditions associated with excessive crate confinement and unsympathetic rearing practices. The net result of such treatment is sustained and inescapable stress, perhaps quietly sensitizing neuroendocrine systems in ways that may make the puppy vulnerable to develop serious adjustment problems in adulthood. As a result of such risks, crate confinement should be introduced through gradual steps involving desensitization by counterconditioning and associated with compensatory measures to offset stress associated with its use (see *Crate Training* in Chapter 2). Although gradual exposure is much better and likely to result in fewer adverse side effects, crate confinement should still be used with a proper degree of concern for potential harm. Crate confinement should be used in a limited way for specific purposes of space management and training, but not as permanent way of life (see *Adverse Effects of Excessive Confinement* in Chapter 2).

In the case of adult dogs, many show a persistent aversion toward crate confinement in association with various adjustment problems, including separation distress and fears (e.g., storm phobias). Such problems need to be addressed and ameliorated first in order to effectively modify the dog's adverse response to confinement. In the absence of contributing adjustment problems, dogs exhibiting a strong aversion to crate confinement are usually responsive to some combination of graded interactive exposure with RP-CC and shaping. For example, the dog is trained to obtain food by approaching the front of the crate. Initially, treats are dropped on the floor just in front of the crate and then gradually tossed inside of it. Some dogs appear to be afraid of the crate pan and the noise it makes as they step on it. Temporarily, removing it or laying down a blanket or rug can be very helpful in such cases. To encourage more willingness to approach the crate, a standard shaping procedure can be used to reinforce successive approximations, with the food reward being delivered closer and closer to the crate opening. In addition to such training activities, the dog should learn to find highly desirable treats and chew toys in or around the crate. Also, the dog can be fed with its bowl placed close to the crate and then in it. Once the dog is approaching the crate and entering, it is trained to wait briefly before being let out again. With progress, the gate of the crate can briefly closed and opened again to reward the dog's behavior (see *Guidelines for Successful Crate Training: Step 3* in Chapter 2).

SOCIAL FEARS AND INHIBITIONS

Social and environmental fears may be influenced by different emotional mechanisms and systems. The fear of others and the fear of unfamiliar objects are differentiated at an early age under the influence of socialization and habituation. Social and environmental fears appear to modulate or inhibit the expression of one another, suggesting that such fears are not under the control of a unitary substrate. For example, MacDonald (1983) found that a fear of unfamiliar objects and the fear of people are not summative; on the contrary, a reciprocal inverse relationship appears to influence their expression such that wolf pups afraid of unfamiliar objects tend to be less afraid of people, whereas wolf pups afraid of people tend to be less afraid of unfa-

miliar objects. These findings suggest the possibility that the fear of unfamiliar environmental events tends to promote social affiliation (excessive dependence), whereas increased social fears may tend to increase independent environmental exploration and problem-solving activities (enhanced independence).

Toward People

Dogs commonly present with varying degrees of fear toward strangers. The most common causes underlying excessive social fear and reactive behavior involve some constellation of genetic predisposition, socialization deficits, or traumatic exposure or learning. A number of techniques have proven effective in reducing social fears. Woolpy and Ginsburg (1967) have described the basic pattern of change that occurs during the treatment of excessive social fear in wolves. These stages include escape efforts, followed by avoidance, approach with aggression and, finally, friendly social interaction. It is interesting to note that, as escape and avoidance give way to approach behavior, an increased risk of aggression was observed to occur. This is consistent with the notion that fear exercises an inhibitory influence over aggression. In the case of highly aggressive animals, fear reduction may have a potential collateral effect of increasing social assertiveness.

The most beneficial techniques used for the management of social fear involve some combination of graded interactive exposure, counterconditioning, relaxation, modeling, response prevention, and play. These various procedures facilitate social contact, which serves to disconfirm aversive expectations and encourage more constructive social behavior. Deciding which procedure or combination of procedures to employ depends on the nature of the problem. Perhaps, the most common training pattern used to alter social inhibition and avoidant behavior is to train dogs to sit and accept food in the presence of people under a variety of evocative situations. As the dog's fear is reduced, closer and closer contact and interaction may be attempted. Social fears such as those directed toward visitors and other brief encounters may be facilitated by the length of exposures being insufficient to result in relaxation. Typically, persons who are not feared by the dog are those that have spent extended time interacting with the dog during visits. Going for long walks together with an unfamiliar person (a pet walker can be hired for this purpose) can be extremely helpful. The walks must be long enough to habituate fearful responding. Once the dog is showing signs of reduced fear and increased interest in obtaining social contact (food and affection), activities like ball play can be explored as a means to extend socialization efforts. Nebuhr and associates (1977) reported a case involving an "extremely shy and withdrawn" German shepherd that was exposed to interactive play activities as the primary therapy modality. After 2 weeks of patient play therapy, the owner reported dramatic improvement in the dog's behavior, indicating that the dog had become progressively relaxed and "acted like a normal dog" (11).

The use of play in such cases should be considered only after successful exposure efforts. Of course, challenging an overly fearful/aggressive dog to play with an unfamiliar person would be dangerous and not be very productive. Dogs that are unwilling to play treat social contacts as aversive events. Another possibility is that socially inhibited dogs may lack the necessary skills and confidence needed to play. As already discussed, encouraging a fearful dog to play can promote a more trusting and open attitude toward social interaction. In the case of mild social inhibitions, play (especially in puppies) can be initiated as a starting point, but only if the risk of aggression is negligible. It should be emphasized that not all dogs that show a disinterest in play are fearful; often such dogs are unresponsive because of underlying social irritability or aggressive tensions. *Prompting such dogs to play may evoke aggression.* Dogs exhibiting social aggression with fear should be appropriately restrained with a muzzle-clamping head halter or muzzle, as needed for secure control.

Graduated counterconditioning and interactive exposure can be staged in places where high levels of foot traffic can be found. City parks can be useful for this. Relaxed exposure can take place as the owner sits on a bench with the dog on a limited-slip or halter collar, depending on need. During outdoor exposure, a hip-hitch and control lead can be extremely useful for maintaining control while freeing up the hands to deliver petting and massage, squeaks and clicks, food treats, and so forth. As passersby approach, the dog can be prompted to sit, thereby obtaining various social and tangible rewards. The delivery of noncontingent rewards (priming) or rewards delivered on a DRO schedule can be very useful. During DRO training, a brief period (e.g., every 10 to 20 seconds) is set at the end of which the dog is rewarded, provided that it does not exhibit avoidance behavior during the period. Over a number of trials, a variety of prosocial behaviors will be adventitiously reinforced. In some cases, a more sustained source of appetitive stimulation may be needed. For such purposes, a large syringe can be filled with a soft delicious food reward that is slowly dispensed to the dog in a drip, blob, or continuous squeeze, depending on need. Cheese from compressed cans can be dispensed in a similar way. Finally, a licking stick, consisting of a spoon or wooden stick slathered with peanut butter, can be a convenient way to deliver a sustained reinforcer while walking a dog. Since appetitive arousal is incompatible with fear, such a procedure can be very useful for calming a dog. Attention-control exercises can also be practiced intermittently, requiring that the dog turn and focus its attention on the trainer before the reward is delivered. Training a dog to turn its attention toward the trainer at such times gives it a potential coping strategy when confronted with fear-evoking social situations. Dogs trained in this way quickly learn to look toward the trainer for support and guidance. This procedure is especially effective if the amount and type of reward are varied and attention is paired with a conditioned reinforcer. In one variation, a novel odorant is injected into a squeaker toy (e.g., a ball) that is used as a conditioned reinforcer. As a result of repeatedly pairing the scent with food and behavioral success, eventually a very potent conditioned emotional effect is produced. Together with other conditioned stimuli, the conditioned odorant can be used to help restrain aversive emotional arousal associated with fear-evoking situations. Dogs that exhibit a strong interest in play may be encouraged to play tug or fetch a ball while on leash in order to facilitate a more relaxed attitude in unfamiliar surroundings. Training efforts can also be carried out near stores, where exiting shoppers provide discrete and repeated trials for approach exposure. During such exposure training, the dog can be prompted to sit and stay as the shopper comes through the store exit.

Dogs that fear strangers are often very reactive around crowds. Exposure to groups of people should proceed very gradually, beginning with minimally provocative situations and only slowly advancing toward more challenging situations according to the dog's ability and tolerance. In the case of a moderate fear of crowds, a graded interactive exposure technique may be used. Intensive attention training as well as shaping of controlled walking and heeling skills can be performed. Every few steps with the dog in the controlled-walking position, the trainer clicks and delivers a variable reward. In addition, the dog should be prompted to quick-sit every so often after bridging controlled walking. In this case, instead of giving the dog a food reward, the vocal and hand sit signal are delivered, followed by "Good" and the delivery of a food reward. During an outdoor event, for example, where a large crowd is gathered, the dog may react with less fear if it is initially walked along the opposite sidewalk away from the gathering. After 15 or 20 minutes, provided the dog is not showing any overt signs of anxiety, it can be led across the street and walked along the adjoining sidewalk, but still kept away from direct contact with people. Finally, after another lengthy period of exposure, and provided that overt signs of fear are absent, the dog may accept more close contact and interaction with the fringes of the crowd, and so on. Incidentally, since walking is mildly anxiety reducing, it is helpful to keep the dog moving during such exposures.

Dogs exhibiting fears toward people should receive intensive basic training as a preliminary to graduated counterconditioning and response-prevention therapy. Most fearful dogs develop increased confidence, improved attention abilities, and enhanced control over

emotional behavior as the result of daily structured training activities. Sit-stay and down-stay training using a reward-based process in conjunction with attention and orienting conditioning can be very useful to promote control and fear-antagonizing internal states linked with sitting and lying down. Also, PFR training with olfactory conditioning can be useful. Once an odorant is conditioned, it can be placed on a tissue and held in the trainer's hand or dispensed with a squeaker or modified CO_2 pump. Delivering the scent during social encounters appears to help modulate a dog's emotional arousal, perhaps making social counterconditioning efforts more effective. These various preliminary attention and basic training procedures are collectively referred to as the *counterconditioning platform*.

Toward Dogs

Learning to interact confidently with other dogs begins early in a puppy's life, especially between weeks 3 and 8. Puppies that are taken too early from their littermates and mother, or otherwise inadequately socialized, may exhibit signs of increased fearfulness around dogs as they reach maturity. Undersocialized dogs may exhibit pronounced deficits in their ability to reciprocate playful overtures initiated by other dogs. They are often unable to exchange ritualized threat and appeasement displays competently and may be particularly awkward in situations involving unfamiliar dogs. The friendly approach of another dog may evoke frantic efforts to escape or cause the overly fearful dog to freeze in a trembling ball of nerves. Typically, dogs exhibiting a socialization deficit may feel equally uncomfortable in the presence of both male and female dogs, but some may show specific aversions and preferences. In addition to socialization deficits, fear of other dogs can often be traced to traumatic experiences occurring at some point in the dog's life. Young puppies are especially prone to develop persistent fears after being attacked by an adult dog. Such experiences may be especially traumatic in cases where the event occurs in an unfamiliar location or in a location already associated with distress, e.g., a veterinary clinic or kennel.

The aforementioned procedures for managing dogs fearful of unfamiliar people are modified for controlling fear of other dogs. Socialization and training efforts should be carried out that bring the socially inhibited dog into progressively more demanding encounters with other dogs. A good controlled situation for such exposure is a veterinary clinic during office hours. Dogs entering or leaving the clinic provide discrete trials of controlled exposure. As dogs exit the clinic, the trainer can prompt the dog's attention (squeak and click), signal it to sit, and reward it ("Good") with a variable treat, first at a distance and then progressively closer to the target dog. The presence of a friendly and nonthreatening canine model can also be very helpful. Using a friendly dog model to go along on walks and to participate in training sessions may provide a framework for making more positive future contacts with other dogs. The positive model may also help the dog to overcome some of its inhibition. Once some degree of control is established, the fearful dog can be taken to group training classes for additional exposure and counterconditioning.

REFERENCES

Abrantes R (1997). *Dog Language: An Encyclopedia of Canine Behavior*. Naperville, IL: Wakan Tanka.

Ader R and Cohen N (1985). CNS-immune system interactions: Conditioning phenomena. *Behav Brain Sci*, 8:379-394.

Akhondzadeh S, Naghavi HR, Vazirian M, et al. (2001). Passionflower in the treatment of generalized anxiety: A pilot double-blind randomized controlled trial with oxazepam. *J Clin Pharm Ther*, 26:363–367.

Arborelius L, Owens MJ, Plotsky PM, and Nemeroff CB (1999). The role of corticotropin-releasing factor in depression and anxiety disorders. *J Endocrinol*, 160:1–12.

Argiolas A and Melis MR (1998). The neuropharmacology of yawning. *Euro J Pharmacol*, 343:1–16.

Armstrong NC and Ernst E (2001). A randomized, double-blind, placebo-controlled trial of a Bach Flower Remedy. *Compend Ther Nurs Midwifery*, 7:215–221.

Arnsten AF (1998). The biology of being frazzled. *Science*, 280:1711–1712.

Aronson L (1999). Animal behavior case of the month: A dog was evaluated because of extreme fear. *JAVMA*, 215:22–24.

Askew HR (1996). *Treatment of Behavior Problems in Dogs and Cats: A Guide for the Small Animal Veterinarian*. Cambridge: Blackwell Science.

Baenninger R, Binkley S, and Baenninger MA (1996). Field observations of yawning and activity in humans. *Physiol Behav*, 59:421–425.

Baum M (1969). Extinction of an avoidance response motivated by intense fear: Social facilitation of the action of response prevention (flooding) in rats. *Behav Res Ther*, 7:57–62.

Baum M (1970). Extinction of avoidance responding through response prevention (flooding). *Psychol Bull*, 74:276–284.

Baum M (1989). Veterinary use of exposure techniques in the treatment of phobic domestic animals. *Behav Res Ther*, 3:307–308.

Beaver BV (1982). Learning. Part 1: Classical conditioning. *Vet Med*, Sep:1348–1349.

Beaver BV (1983). Fear of loud noises. *Vet Med Small Anim Clin*, Mar:333–334.

Beerda B, Schilder MBH, Van Hooff JARAM, and DeVries HW (1997). Manifestations of chronic and acute stress in dogs. *Appl Anim Behav Sci*, 52:307–319.

Beerda B, Schilder MBH, Van Hooff JARAM, et al. (1998). Behavioural, saliva cortisol and heart rate responses to different types of stimuli in dogs. *Appl Anim Behav Sci*, 58:365–381.

Bellack AS and Hersen M (1977). *Behavior Modification: An Introductory Textbook*. New York: Oxford University Press.

Blake SR (1998). Bach flower therapy: A practitioner's perspective. In AM Schoen and SG Wynn (Eds), *Complementary and Alternative Veterinary Medicine*. St. Louis: CV Mosby.

Borchelt PL (1997). Fear of flights: Staircase phobias in dogs. *Anim Behav Consult Newsl*, 14(3).

Bordi F and LeDoux J (1992). Sensory tuning beyond the sensory system: An initial analysis of auditory response properties of neurons in the lateral amygdaloid nucleus and overlying areas of the striatum. *J Neurosci*, 12:2493–2503.

Campbell WE (1992). *Behavior Problems in Dogs*, 2nd Ed. Goleta, CA: American Veterinary Publications.

Campbell SA, Hughes HC, Griffin HE, et al. (1988). Some effects of limited exercise on purpose-bred beagles. *Am J Vet Res*, 49:1298–1301.

Castles DL, Whiten A, and Aureli F (1999). Social anxiety, relationships and self-directed behavior among wild female olive baboons. *Anim Behav*, 58:1207–1217.

Cerny A and Schmid K (1999). Tolerability and efficacy of valerian/lemon balm in healthy volunteers (a double-blind, placebo-controlled, multicentre study). *Fitoterapia*, 70:221–228.

Cohen M (1981). Effects of orally administered psychotropic drugs on dog conditioned avoidance responses. *Arch Int Pharmacodyn Ther*, 253:11–12.

Costa-Miserachs D, Portell-Cortés I, Aldavert-Vera L, et al. (1994). Long-term memory facilitation in rats by posttraining epinephrine. *Behav Neurosci*, 108:469–474.

Crowell-Davis S, Seibert L, Sung W, et al. (2001). Treatment of storm phobia with a combination of clomipramine, alprazolam, and behavior modification: A prospective open trial. *Newsl Am Vet Soc Anim Behav*, 23(2/3):6.

Delprato DJ (1973). An animal analogue to systematic desensitization and elimination of avoidance. *Behav Res Ther*, 11:49–55.

Denny MR (1976). Post-aversive relief and relaxation and their implications for behavior therapy. *J Behav Ther Exp Psychiatry*, 7:315–321.

Dess NK, Linwick D, Patterson J, et al. (1983). Immediate and proactive effects of controllability and predictability on plasma cortisol responses to shock in dogs. *Behav Neurosci*, 97:1005–1016.

Dhawan K, Kumar S, and Sharma A (2001). Anxiolytic activity of aerial and underground parts of *Passiflora incarnata*. *Fitoterapia*, 72:922–926.

Dickinson A and Pearce JM (1977). Inhibitory interactions between appetitive and aversive stimuli. *Psychol Bull*, 84:690–711.

Dodman N (1996). *The Dog Who Loved Too Much: Tales, Treatments, and the Psychology of the Dog*. New York: Bantam.

Dodman N (1999). *Dog Behaving Badly: An A-to-Z Guide to Understanding and Curing Behavioral Problems in Dogs*. New York: Bantam.

Dodman NH and Arrington D (2000). Aggression between 2 unrelated dogs residing in the same household. *JAVMA*, 217:1468–1472.

Dodman NH and Shuster L (1998). *Psychopharmacology of Animal Behavior Disorders*. Malden, MA: Blackwell Science.

File SE, Jarrett N, Fluck E, et al. (2001). Eating soy improves human memory. *Psychopharmacology*, 157:430–436.

Frank D, Overall K, and Dunham AE (2000). Co-occurrence of noise and thunderstorm phobias and other anxieties. *AVSAB Newsl*, 22:9.

Freeman MP (2000). Omega-3 fatty acids in psychiatry: A review. *Ann Clin Psychiatry*, 12:159–65.

Fuller JL and Clark LD (1966). Genetic and treatment factors modifying postisolation syndrome in dogs. *J Comp Physiol Psychol*, 61:251-257.

Fuller JL, Clark LD, and Waller MB (1960). Effects of chlorpromazine upon psychological development in the puppy. *Psychopharmacologia*, 1:393–407.

Gaebelein CJ, Galosy RA, Botticelli L, et al. (1977). Blood pressure and cardiac changes during signaled and unsignalled avoidance in dogs. *Physiol Behav*, 19:69–74.

García A and Armario A (2001). Individual differences in the recovery of the hypothalamic-pituitary axis after termination of exposure to severe stressor in outbred male Sprague-Dawley rats. *Psychoneuroendocrinology*, 26:363–374.

Grahm FK and Clifton RK (1966). Heart-rate change as a component of the orienting response. *Psychol Bull*, 65:305–320.

Hart BL and Hart LA (1985). *Canine and Feline Behavioral Therapy*. Philadelphia: Lea and Febiger.

Hawk G and Riccio DC (1977). The effect of a conditioned fear inhibitor (CS–) during response prevention upon extinction of an avoidance response. *Behav Res Ther*, 15:97–101.

Heim C and Nemeroff CB (1999). The impact of early adverse experiences on brain systems involved in the pathophysiology of anxiety and affective disorders. *Biol Psychiatry*, 46:1509–1522.

Hendricks TJ, Fyodorov DV, Wegman LJ, et al. (2002). Pet-1 ETS gene plays a critical role in 5-HT neuron development and is required for normal anxiety-like and aggressive behavior. *Neuron*, 37:233–247.

Hennessy M (2001). Human interaction and diet affect neuroendocrine stress responses and behavior of dogs in a public animal shelter. In *AVSAB Proceedings*, Boston, July 16.

Hennessy MB, Davis HN, Williams MT, et al. (1997). Plasma cortisol levels of dogs at a county animal shelter. *Physiol Behav*, 62:485–490.

Hennessy MB, Williams MT, Miller DD, et al. (1998). Influence of male and female petters on plasma cortisol and behaviour: Can human interaction reduce the stress of dogs in a public animal shelter? *Appl Anim Behav Sci*, 61:63–77.

Hothersall D and Tuber DS (1979). Fears in companion dogs: Characteristics and treatment. In JD Keehn (Ed), *Psychopathology in Animals: Research and Clinical Implications*. New York: Academic.

Houser VP and Paré WP (1974). Long-term conditioned fear modification in the dog as measured by changes in urinary 11-hydrocorti-costeroids, heart rate, and behavior. *Pavlovian J Biol Sci*, 9:85–96.

Howard R (1992). Folie à deux involving a dog. *Am J Psychiatry*, 149:3.

Humphrey E and Warner L (1934). *Working Dogs*. Baltimore: Johns Hopkins Press.

Iorio LC, Eisenstein N, Brody PE, and Barnett A (1983). Effects of selected drugs on spontaneously occurring abnormal behavior in beagles. *Pharmacol Biochem Behav*, 18:379–382.

Jacobs WJ and Nadel L (1985). Stress-induced recovery of fears and phobias. *Psychol Rev*, 92:512–553.

Kehoe EJ and Macrae M (1997). Savings in animal learning: Implications for relapse and maintenance after therapy. *Behav Ther*, 28:141–155.

Kirby LG, Rice KC, and Valentino RJ (2000). Effects of corticotropin-releasing factor on neuronal activity in the serotonergic dorsal raphe nucleus. *Neuropsychopharmacology*, 22:148–162.

Klein EH, Thomas T, and Uhde TW (1990). Hypothalamo-pituitary-adrenal axis activity in nervous and normal pointer dogs. *Biol Psychiatry*, 27:791–794.

Koch M (1999). The neurobiology of startle. *Prog Neurobiol*, 59:107–128.

Komori T, Fujiwara R, Tanida M, and Nomura J (1995). Potential antidepressant effects of lemon odor in rats. *Eur Neuropsychopharmacol*, 5:477–480.

Koob GF (1999). Corticotropin-releasing factor, norepinephrine, and stress. *Biol Psychiatry*, 46:1167–1180.

Kostarczyk E and Fonberg E (1982). Heart rate mechanisms in instrumental conditioning reinforced by petting in dogs. *Physiol Behav*, 28:27–30.

Kuhn G, Lichtwald K, Hardegg W, and Abel HH (1991). The effect of transportation on circulating corticosteroids, enzyme activities and hematological values in laboratory dogs. *J Exp Anim Sci*, 34:99–104.

LeDoux JE (1996). *The Emotional Brain: The Mysterious Underpinning of Emotional Life*. New York: Simon and Schuster.

LeDoux JE (2000). Emotion circuits in the brain. *Annu Rev Neurosci*, 23:155–184.

Lehrner J, Eckersberger C, Walla P, et al. (2000). Ambient odor of orange in a dental office reduces anxiety and improves mood in female patients. *Physiol Behav*, 71:83–86.

Leibrecht BC and Askew HR (1980). Habituation from a comparative perspective. In MR Denny (Ed), *Comparative Psychology: An Evolutionary Analysis of Animal Behavior*. New York: John Wiley and Sons.

Lephart ED, West TW, Weber KS, et al. (2002). Neurobehavioral effects of dietary soy phytoestrogens. *Neurotoxicol Teratol*, 24:5–16.

Liddell HS (1956). *Emotional Hazards in Animals and Man*. Springfield, IL: Charles C Thomas.

Löscher W and Frey HH (1981). Pharmacokinetics of diazepam in the dog. *Arch Int Pharmacodyn Ther*, 254:180–195.

Lubow RE (1998). Latent inhibition and behavior pathology: Prophylactic and other possible effects of stimulus preexposure. In W O'Donohue (Ed), *Learning and Behavior Therapy*. Boston: Allyn and Bacon.

Lund TD and Lephart ED (2001). Dietary soy phytoestrogens produce anxiolytic effects in the elevated plus-maze. *Brain Res*, 913:180–184.

MacDonald K (1983). Stability of individual differences in behavior in a litter of wolf cubs (*Canis lupus*). *J Comp Psychol*, 97:99–106.

Mahut H (1958). Breed differences in the dog's emotional behaviour. *Can J Psychol*, 12:35–44.

Marder AR (1991). Psychotropic drugs and behavioral therapy. *Vet Clin North Am Adv Companion Anim Behav*, 21:329–342.

Maren S (2001). Neurobiology of Pavlovian fear conditioning. *Annu Rev Neurosci*, 24:897–931.

Marks I (1978a). Exposure treatments: Clinical applications. In WS Agras (Ed), *Behavior Modification: Principles and Clinical Applications*. Boston: Little, Brown.

Marks I (1978b). Exposure Treatments: Conceptual Issues. In WS Agras (Ed), *Behavior Modification: Principles and Clinical Applications*. Boston: Little, Brown.

Marks I (1987). *Fears, Phobias, and Ritual: Panic, Anxiety, and Their Disorders*. New York: Oxford University Press.

McBryde WC and Murphree OD (1974). The rehabilitation of genetically nervous dogs. *Pavlovian J Biol Sci* 9:76–84.

McCobb EC, Brown EA, Damiani K, and Dodman NH (2001). Thunderstorm phobia in dogs: An internet survey of 69 cases. *J Am Anim Hosp Assoc*, 37:319–324.

McGaugh JL (1990). Significance and remembrance: The role of neuromodulatory systems. *Psychol Sci*, 1:15–25.

Menzies RG and Clarke CJ (1995). The etiology of phobias: A nonassociative account. *Clin Psychol Rev*, 15:23–48.

Milad MR and Quirk GJ (2002). Neurons in medial prefrontal cortex signal memory for fear extinction. *Nature*, 420:70–74.

Milgram NW, Head E, and Cotman CW (2002). The effects of antioxidant-fortified food and cognitive enrichment in dogs [Abstract]. In *Symposium on Brain Aging and Related Behavioral Changes in Dogs*, Orlando, FL, January 11.

Miltner W, Marjak M, Braun H, et al. (1994). Emotional qualities of odors and their influence on the startle reflex in humans. *Psychophysiology*, 31:107–110.

Mintz M and Wang-Ninio Y (2001). Two-stage theory of conditioning: Involvement of the cerebellum and the amygdala. *Brain Res*, 897:150–156.

Motomura N, Sakurai A, and Yotsuya Y (2001). Reduction of mental stress with lavender odorant. *Percept Mot Skills*, 93:713–718.

Murphree OD, DeLuca DC, and Angel C (1974). Psychopharmacologic facilitation of operant conditioning of genetically nervous Catahoula and pointer dogs. *Pavlovian J Biol Sci*, 9:17–24.

Nebuhr BR, Levinson M, Nobbe DE, and Tiller JE (1977). Treatment of an incompletely socialized dog. *Canine Pract*, Oct:8, 10.

O'Farrell V (1997). Owner attitudes and dog behaviour problems. *Appl Anim Behav Sci*, 52:205–213.

Otto T and Giardino ND (2001). Pavlovian conditioning of emotional responses to olfactory and contextual stimuli: A potential model for the development and expression of chemical intolerance. *Ann NY Acad Sci*, 933:291–309.

Packer L, Tritschler HJ, and Wessel K (1997). Neuroprotection by the metabolic antioxidant alpha-lipoic acid. *Free Radic Biol Med*, 22:359–378.

Pani L, Porcella A, and Gessa GL (2000). The role of stress in the pathophysiology of the dopaminergic system. *Mol Psychiatry*, 5:14–21.

Panksepp J (1998). *Affective Neuroscience: The Foundations of Human and Animal Emotions*. New York: Oxford University Press.

Pittler MH and Ernst E (2000). Efficacy of kava extract for treating anxiety: Systematic review and meta-analysis. *J Clin Psychopharmacol*, 20:84–89.

Price ML, Curtis AL, Kirby LG, et al. (1998). Effects of corticotropin-releasing factor on brain serotonergic activity. *Neuropsychopharmacology*, 18:492–502.

Richardson R, Riccio DC, and Ress J (1988). Extinction of avoidance through response prevention: Enhancement by administration of epinephrine or ACTH. *Behav Res Ther*, 26:23–32.

Roberts A and Williams JMG (1992). The effect of olfactory stimulation on fluency, vividness of imagery and associated mood: A preliminary study. *Br J Med Psychol*, 65:197–199.

Rogan MT, Stuabli UV, and LeDoux JE (1997). Fear conditioning induces associative long-term potentiation in the amygdala. *Nature*, 390:604–607.

Rogerson J (1997). Canine fears and phobias: A regime for treatment without recourse to drugs. *Appl Anim Behav Sci*, 52:291–297.

Royce JR (1955). A factorial study of emotionality in the dog. *Psychol Monogr (Gen Appl)*, 69:1–27.

Rueter LE and Jacobs BL (1996). A microdialysis examination of serotonin release in the rat forebrain induced by behavioral/environmental manipulations. *Brain Res*, 739:57–69.

Rugass T (1997). *On Talking Terms with Dogs: Calming Signals*. Kula, HI: Legacy by Mail.

Russell M, Dark KA, Cummins RW, et al. (1984). Learned histamine release. Science, 225:733–734.

Sales G, Hubrecht R, Peyvandi A, et al. (1997). Noise in dog kenneling: Is barking a welfare problem for dogs? *Appl Anim Behav Sci*, 52:321–329.

Serpell J and Jagoe JA (1995). Early experience and the development of behaviour. In J Serpell (Ed), *The Domestic Dog: Its Evolution, Behaviour, and Interaction with People*. New York: Cambridge University Press.

Shull-Selcer EA and Stagg W (1991). Advances in the understanding and treatment of noise phobias. Vet Clin North *Am Adv Companion Anim Behav*, 21:299–314.

Shumyatsky GP, Tsvetkov E, Malleret G, et al. (2002). Identification of a signaling network in lateral nucleus of amygdala important for inhibiting memory specifically related to learned fear. *Cell*, 111:905–918.

Simonet O, Murphy M, and Lance A (2001). Laughing dog: Vocalizations of domestic dogs during play encounters. In *Animal Behavior Society Conference*, Corvallis, OR, July 14–18.

Speck RV (1964). Mental health problems involving the family, the pet, and the veterinarian. *JAVMA*, 145:150–154.

Stanton ME and Levine S (1988). Pavlovian conditioning of endocrine responses. In R Ader, H Weiner, and A Baum (Eds), *Experimental Foundations of Behavioral Medicine: Conditioning Approaches*. Hillsdale, NJ: Lawrence Erlbaum.

Stein DJ, Borchelt P, and Hollander E (1994). Pharmacotherapy of naturally occurring anxiety symptoms in dogs. *Res Commun Psychol Psychiatry Behav*, 19:39–48.

Stephens DB (1980). Stress and its measurement in domestic animals: A review of behavioral and physiological studies under field and laboratory situations. *Adv Vet Sci Comp Med*, 24:179–210.

Stutzmann GE and LeDoux JE (1998). GABAergic antagonists block the inhibitory effects of serotonin in the lateral amygdala: A mechanism for modulation of sensory inputs related to fear conditioning. *J Neurosci*, 19:RC8(1–4).

Stutzmann GE, McEwen BS, and LeDoux JE (1998). Serotonin modulation of sensory inputs to the lateral amygdala: Dependency on corticosterone. *J Neurosci*, 18:9529–9538.

Swonger AK and Constantine LL (1983). *Drugs and Therapy*, 2nd Ed. Boston: Little, Brown.

Tancer ME, Stein MB, Bessette BB, and Uhde TW (1990). Behavioral effects of chronic imipramine treatment in genetically nervous pointer dogs. *Physiol Behav*, 48:179–181.

Thalken CE (1971). Use of beagle dogs in high intensity noise studies. *Lab Anim Sci*, 21:700–704.

Thyer BA, Baum M, and Reid LD (1988). Exposure techniques in the reduction of fear: A comparative review of the procedure in animals and humans. *Adv Behav Res Ther*, 10:105–127.

Trumler E (1973). *Your Dog and You*. New York: Seabury.

Tsvetkov E, Carlezon WA, Benes FM, et al. (2002). Fear conditioning occludes LTP-induced presynaptic enhancement of synaptic transmission in the cortical pathway to the lateral amygdala. *Neuron*, 34:289–300.

Uhde TW, Malloy LC, and Slate SO (1992). Fearful behavior, body size, and serum IGF-I levels in nervous and normal pointer dogs. *Pharmacol Biochem Behav*, 43:263–269.

Valentino RJ and Aston-Jones GS (1995). Physiological and anatomical determinants of locus ceruleus discharge: Behavior and clinical implications. In FE Bloom and DJ Kupfer (Eds), *Psychopharmacology: The Fourth Generation of Progress*. New York: Raven.

Van de Kar LD and Blair ML (1999). Forebrain pathways mediating stress-induced hormone secretion. *Front Neuroendocrinol*, 20:1–48.

Vaswani M, Linda FK, and Ramesh S (2003). Role of selective serotonin reuptake inhibitors in psychiatric disorders: A comprehensive review. *Prog Neuropsychopharmacol Biol Psychiatry*, 27:85–102.

Voith VL and Borchelt PL (1985). Fears and phobias in companion animals. *Compend Continuing Educ Pract Vet*, 7:209–218.

Voith VL and Borchelt PL (1996). Fears and phobias in companion animals: Update. In VL Voith and PL Borchelt (Eds), *Readings in Companion Animal Behavior*. Trenton, NJ: Veterinary Learning Systems.

Walach H, Rilling C, and Engelke U (2001). Efficacy of Bach-flower remedies in test anxiety: A double-blind, placebo-controlled, randomized trial with partial crossover. *J Anxiety Disord*, 15:359–366.

Whitney LF (1964). *Dog Psychology*. New York: Howell Book House.

Wilensky AD, Schafe GE, and LeDoux JE (2000). The amygdala modulates memory consolidation of fear-motivated inhibitory avoidance learning but not classical fear conditioning. *J Neurosci*, 20:7059–7066.

Wilhelmj CM, McGuire TF, McDonough J, et al. (1953). Emotional elevations of blood pressure in trained dogs: Possible origin of hypertension in humans. *Psychosom Med*, 15:390–395.

Wolpe J (1958). *Psychotherapy by Reciprocal Inhibition*. Stanford: Stanford University Press.

Woods SC, Vasselli JR, Kaestner E, et al. (1977). Conditioned insulin secretion and meal-feeding in rats. *J Comp Physiol Psychol*, 91:128–133.

Woolpy JH and Ginsburg BE (1967). Wolf socialization: A study of temperament in a wild social species. *Am Zool*, 7:357–363.

4

Separation Distress and Panic

PART 1: NEUROBIOLOGY AND ONTOGENETIC INFLUENCES

The dog's ability to form satisfying attachments and bonds with people has secured for it a unique place in human society. Dogs are often treated as members of the family, with a level of care and affection that rivals the treatment reserved for children. For most people, the relationship formed with a dog is immensely gratifying. The majority of dogs appear to reciprocate our affection and invite close contact. Most dogs are adept at engaging people in prosocial relations by attracting attention to themselves by various means. In fact, much of what well-socialized dogs do appears calculated to maintain or enhance close contact with human companions. In addition to making bodily contact, various gestures, postures, vocalizations, and expressive rituals are used to communicate the dog's prosocial intention to interact and make contact with us. The preeminent means for promoting affiliative contact is play. Through our mutual capacities to play, people and dogs seem to transcend evolutionary barriers and open a common ground of empathy and appreciation for one another.

The powerful attraction and affiliations formed between dogs and people are a source of considerable pleasure, so long as the object of affection is present and available. When left alone, all normal dogs appear to experience some degree of discomfort by separation; however, the vast majority learn to cope with routine separation without becoming overly distressed. Many, though, respond adversely to separation, exhibiting varying degrees of despair, emotional arousal, or panic. Separation-reactive dogs may engage in a variety of undesirable behaviors, including motor excesses (pacing, running about, and jumping up on counters and window sills), excessive vocalization (persistent barking and howling), various destructive activities, and separation-related elimination problems. In extreme cases, a dog appears inconsolably worried and panicked about its inability to restore contact with the absent owner. Some dogs become separation reactive as the result of being confined to a separate room while the owner is elsewhere in the house, whereas others may exhibit signs of distress (e.g., household elimination and destructiveness) as the result of being merely denied contact and attention from the owner. Aside from the potential household damage produced by such dogs and the complaints of neighbors about excessive barking, separation-related distress represents a significant welfare concern.

Separation distress in dogs presents with a variety of behavioral signs under the influence of several coactive influences, including anxiety, fear, stress, boredom, frustration, and panic (see *Separation Distress and Coactive Influences* in Volume 1, Chapter 4).

Traditionally, borrowing from human psychiatry, the term *separation anxiety* has been adopted to name the syndrome in dogs. In the author's opinion, the notion of *anxiety* at separation has led to considerable confusion with respect to understanding the etiology of separated-related behavior and its treatment. First, separation distress appears to be mediated by a neural circuit that is functionally discrete from circuits subserving anxiety and

fear. Second, although some overlap certainly exists between separation distress and anxiety, overlap also exists with other coactive influences, such as boredom, frustration, stress, and panic. As a result of these considerations, the term *separation distress syndrome* (SDS) has been adopted to emphasize the multimodal function of behavior commonly referred to as separation anxiety.

NEUROBIOLOGICAL SUBSTRATES OF ATTACHMENT AND SEPARATION DISTRESS

Adaptive behavior is the outward appearance of an utterly astonishing and complex infrastructure of physiological processes. Understanding the evolutionary origins and biological significance of canine social behavior, attachment, and separation distress depends on some familiarity with neurobiology and the neural substrates mediating the expression of such behavior. Dogs, like other mammalian species, have evolved species-typical behavior patterns associated with maternal care (nursing), separation calls, and play. MacLean (1985) has implicated paleomammlian limbic pathways and diverse interconnections between the amygdala, hippocampus, septum, thalamus, hypothalamus, and cingulate cortex as providing the neurobiological substrates for the emergence of the mammalian capacity to give and receive care, to seek and enjoy company, and to interact playfully (see *Neurobiology of Attachment and Separation Distress* in Volume 1, Chapter 3).

Neuropeptides and Social Behavior

Humans and dogs exhibit a mutual need for social contact and comfort, providing a motivational basis for interspecies attraction and social bonding. Odendaal (2000) refers to our shared need for positive social interaction as emanating from an emotional capacity, *attentionis egens*, to give and receive affection and comfort from the company of one another—a capacity that is evident in social behavior as well as reflected in a variety of physiological changes that occur during such interaction (see *Tactile Stimulation and Adaptation* in Chapter 6). A diverse assortment of neurochemical influences mediates social attraction and affiliative behavior. For example, phenylethylamine, a centrally active amine, is believed to promote a rapid increase in alertness, activity, and positive affect (euphoria), changes that may be involved in the biology of social attraction between people and dogs. Both people and dogs show a significant increase in phenylethylamine activity, as indicated by increased levels of circulating phenylacetic acid (a metabolite of phenylethylamine) following brief periods of positive social interaction (Odendaal and Lehman, 2000).

A variety of neuropeptides that are strategically distributed throughout the paleomammalian system serve to mediate the expression of attachment, separation distress, social comfort, and a variety of other ancient social behaviors. These neuropeptides include endogenous opioids (endorphins and enkephalins), substance P, oxytocin, prolactin, and arginine vasopressin (AVP). A number of different opioid receptors are widely distributed in the canine brain, with many concentrated in areas of the brain believed to mediate the expression of separation distress and agitated-explosive behavior (panic circuit) (Panksepp, 1982). These opioid-sensitive receptors serve a number of functions, including the modulation of physical and emotional pain, the regulation of mood, the mediation of reward and pleasure, and social attachment (see *Limbic Opioid Circuitry and the Mediation of Social Comfort and Distress* in Volume 1, Chapter 3). Opioids have been shown to modulate canine social behavior (Panksepp et al., 1983; Knowles et al., 1989) and separation-distress vocalization (Panksepp et al., 1980). Opioidergic disturbances have been implicated in the elaboration of various mood and emotional deficits associated with learned helplessness and depression (Tejedor-Real et al., 1995).

The neuropeptide substance P closely interacts with opioid pathways in various parts of the brain, but in association with opposite hedonic effects. The activation of substance P pathways is closely associated with psychological stress and the experience of emotional anguish and pain. Substance P exhibits a preferential affinity for the receptor neurokinin 1

(NK-1). NK-1 receptors are concentrated in brain areas associated with aversive emotional arousal (e.g., the amygdala, hypothalamus, and periaqueductal gray). In addition to mediating anger and rage, substance P plays a role in the transmission of peripheral pain, mediates separation distress, and facilitates the addictive effects of opiates. Murtra and colleagues (2000) have reported that NK-1 knockout mice (mice lacking the gene needed for the expression of the NK-1 receptor) are unresponsive to morphine and do not show physical withdrawal symptoms when the administration of the drug is stopped. Substance P agonists generate separation-like distress vocalizations in guinea pigs—an effect that is "virtually abolished" by pretreatment with a substance P antagonist. Substance P antagonists have been shown to suppress separation-induced distress vocalization completely in guinea pigs (Kramer et al., 1998).

Another highly influential neuropeptide that closely interacts with opioid pathways is oxytocin, perhaps co-mediating emotional changes opposite to those produced by substance P. Whereas substance P is evocative of emotional anguish, social irritability, and rage, oxytocin promotes emotional comfort, pleasure, and well-being, as well as exerting potent antiaggression effects (Panksepp, 1998). In addition to mediating such biological functions as parturient contractions and the milk let-down reflex, oxytocin is involved in the expression of maternal behavior, social bonding, and the modulation of separation distress (see *Social Comfort Seeking and Distress* in Volume 2, Chapter 4). Oxytocin has been identified as playing a significant role in early olfactory learning, especially the rapid conditioning of environmental-scent stimuli associated with the mother (Nelson and Panksepp, 1996) and place attachments. Such learning may mediate the calming effects that familiar and safe places have for dogs. Place attachments associated with the mother's odor may prevent the young from wandering too far away from the nest and the mother's protection, as well as promote huddling behavior. In contrast to the formative effects of oxytocin on place attachments, substance P and substance P agonists appear to induce strong place aversions (Kramer et al., 1998).

In addition to olfactory memories associated with place attachments, oxytocin promotes the consolidation of olfactory memories needed for social recognition (Ferguson et al., 2002). In rats, the effect of oxytocin on social recognition appears to be dose dependent, with low doses facilitating social recognition learning and high doses blocking it. Knockout mice lacking the gene necessary for the production of oxytocin exhibit various social deficits, including an inability to effectively process olfactory social stimuli and to consolidate olfactory memories of conspecifics (Ferguson et al., 2000). Interestingly, these olfactory-dependent social recognition abilities are restored by the injection of oxytocin into the medial amygdala (Winslow and Insel, 2002). Knockout mice are also more aggressive as adults than oxytocin-expressing counterparts (Winslow et al., 2000). Although not yet scientifically demonstrated to my knowledge, oxytocin probably plays a central role in mediating long-term kin recognition in dogs (see *Attachment and Separation Distress* in Volume 2, Chapter 4).

Developmental Adversity and Adjustment

Affiliative behaviors and separation-distress behaviors are grounded in both phylogenetic and ontogenetic influences. Developmental influences on dog behavior take place within the context of biological constraints and timetables that roughly serve to define a dog's potentiality—a biogenetic potential that remains unactualized in the absence of appropriate experience and organizing learning. A sensitive period for socialization occurs during a time of rapid change and development early in a puppy's life. The socialization period is characterized by an inverse relationship between waning social attraction and a gradual increase in social aversion and fear (Figure 4.1). In addition to the expression of biogenetic propensities for social contact, attachment, and aversion, acquired Pavlovian expectancies and instrumental social and motor skills gradually shape the behavioral phenotype to reflect social and environmental pressures. Each step in the process necessarily influences subsequent steps (epigenesis), with disruption occurring at any point in the process potentially exerting pervasive disturbances over subsequent developmental organization and behavior.

Learning consists of various sensory and neurobiological processes whereby information and behavior are integrated and coordinated with the ultimate goal of optimizing an animal's ability to adapt and achieve a better state of being. The ability to learn and adjust enables dogs to predict and control the social and physical environment better. However, the adaptation process is not without error, adversity, and misfortune—life is relentlessly stressful and risky. Consequently, evolution has favored the perpetuation of biobehavioral stress systems that are flexible and capable of coping under the adversities of behavioral conflict, failure, and threats (e.g., fear, anxiety, frustration, anger, and irritability). Biological stress serves to mobilize a cascade of coordinated behavioral and physiological events that improve an animal's ability to survive under adverse conditions. However, as the result of disruptive early experiences or trauma, these adaptive mechanisms may become maladaptive and potentially result in lifelong disturbances in a dog's ability to cope and respond adaptively to stressful situations, especially those stressors involving emotional adversity.

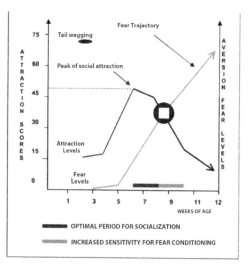

FIG. 4.1 The socialization period is associated with numerous developmental changes reflected in dramatic shifts in social attraction and fear.

During the first 16 weeks, various changes in autonomic reactivity and the propensity for social attraction and aversion follow a consistent pattern of heart-rate changes (Scott, 1958) (see *Socialization: Learning to Relate and Communicate* in Volume 1, Chapter 2). Until the onset of the socialization period, neonatal puppies exhibit a rapid heart rate before it undergoes a significant deceleration between weeks 3 and 5, possibly associated with the emergence of parasympathetic dominance—an autonomic change occurring in close association with increased social attraction and elevated thresholds for fear. After week 5, a puppy's heart rate begins to accelerate again and peaks between weeks 7 and 8, marking the emergence of sympathetic dominance. With the onset of sympathetic dominance, puppies become progressively wary about making new social contacts and begin to show increasing fear and responsiveness to aversive conditioning, especially between weeks 8 and 10. Fear thresholds continue to fall until the close of the socialization period at week 12. From weeks 7 to 16, the heart rate progressively levels out toward adult levels, representing a period of autonomic equilibrium (Figure 4.2). During periods of autonomic and developmental change, puppies may be particularly vulnerable to traumatic

conditioning and stress. Early traumatic events that increase sympathetic activity may significantly impair a puppy's ability to cope with stress and aversive stimulation as an adult, making the dog either hyperresponsive (choleric/c type) or hyporesponsive (melancholic/m type) to environmental stimulation. On the other hand, insufficient stimulation may also produce a damaging effect. The key is to provide puppies with appropriate and adequate stimulation to support their developmental needs and promote adaptive adjustments consistent with sanguine (s type) and phlegmatic (p type) typologies.

Origin of Reactive versus Adaptive Coping Styles

Traumatic stress may also exert a pronounced influence on subsequent development from a much earlier age. Deprivations and excessive stress during the first 2 weeks of life may permanently disrupt the normal pattern of neural development and result in disturbances associated with coping and impulse-control deficiencies, common features of many dog behavior problems, including separation-related problems (see *Postnatal Stimulation*). Given the potent effects of early handling and gentling on stress reactivity, emotionality, and

A N S	PRIMATIVE ORGANIZATION	PARASYMPATHETIC DOMINANCE	SYMPATHETIC DOMINANCE	INTEGRATED ANS
S O C I A L	APROACH-WITHDRAWAL	INCREASING ATTRACTION LOW FEAR	DECREASING ATTRACTION INCREASING FEAR	REGULATED SOCIAL BEHAVIOR
H R	ACCELERATED	DECELERATED	ACCELERATED	LEVELING
A G E	Birth to 3 Weeks	Weeks 3 to 5	Weeks 5 to 8	Weeks 8 to 16

FIG. 4.2. Changes in heart rate (HR) are highly correlated with behavioral changes that may reflect underlying developmental changes associated with neural development and integrated autonomic activity. ANS, autonomic nervous system.

social dominance, it is reasonable to assume that unfavorable influences during the neonatal period may adversely impact separation-distress circuits [see *Neonatal Period (Birth to 12 Days)* in Volume 1, Chapter 2]. During the first 2 weeks of life, there is a transient "overproduction" and proliferation of oxytocin and AVP receptors in limbic brain areas of infant rats that gradually moves toward adult levels as rat pups mature (Tribollet et al., 1991). The adult distribution of AVP-binding sites is established by the time of weaning. These sites include areas associated with the mobilization of fear and emotional stress in adulthood [viz., the locus coeruleus, the nucleus of the solitary tract, the central amygdala, and the septal area (an area associated with separation distress)]. On the other hand, oxytocin sites are generally located in areas of the brain associated with social attachment, reward, and the behavioral approach system (viz., the cingulate cortex, the nucleus accumbens, and the caudate putamen). Oxytocin sites undergo change in distribution and density at the time of puberty, including a proliferation into brain areas associated with social recognition (the olfactory tubercle), social fearful behavior (the posterior central amygdala), and sexual and maternal behavior [the bed nucleus of the stria terminalis (BNST)]. By day 60, there is a twofold increase of oxytocin-binding sites expressed in the central amygdala and the BNST, another site believed to play a role in the elaboration of separation distress. Finally, oxytocin-binding sites in the ventromedial hypothalamus were expressed only toward the end of the 60-day period.

The changing distribution of oxytocin-binding sites suggests the possibility that similar changes might mediate developmental changes in puppy social approach and fear patterns described previously, suggesting several interesting hypotheses concerning a potential role of oxytocin and AVP in the organization of social behavior and the integration of social-emotional stress responses. The restraint of autonomic arousal and the mediation of social approach between weeks 3 and 5 may reflect heightened oxytocin activity, whereas the increasing fear and sensitivity to avoidance learning emerging as the puppy moves into week 8 and 10 may be due to

emergent AVP dominance and the downregulation of oxytocin. In addition, although this is conjecture, early AVP activity may play a role in keeping puppies huddled together via a calming effect mediated by oxytocin produced in association with nursing and tactile stimulation with littermates, which, if discontinued by the puppy wandering too far away, might trigger distress signals via the activation of AVP and CRF painlike circuits, causing the puppy to seek contact with the mother and littermates to obtain relief via oxytocin release. In addition to mediating contact comfort, oxytocin appears to facilitate social recognition (Ferguson et al., 2002). The theme of comfort and safety seeking with familiars that is sketched out in early infancy may exert a profoundly influential effect over the epigenetic development of social behavior, attachment, and separation-related behavior. Accidental separation of a neonatal puppy over some lengthy period might result in significant sensitization of separation-distress circuits, perhaps predisposing the puppy to a heightened sensitivity to separation in adulthood. Inadvertent exposure to excessive stress or trauma in early puppyhood may play a key etiological role in the development of a variety of social and stress-related behavior problems (e.g., separation panic and owner-directed aggression).

Early epigenetic approach-withdrawal adjustments foreshadow the elaboration of increasingly sophisticated social recognition abilities, comfort- and safety-seeking behaviors, emotional complexity, and cognitive abilities that gradually unfold and enable dogs to form prediction-control expectancies and social relationships. The development of these abilities enables dogs to learn and to adapt by means of optimized control modules, modal strategies, and choice (see *Ontogeny and Reactive Behavior* in Chapter 8). As such, learning enhances a dog's ability to control social and environmental events, thereby increasing its competence and well-being, whereas a failure to learn from experience promotes incompetence, distress, and reactive behavior. The process of adaptive learning appears to be intimately linked to oxytocin and dopamine reward circuits. When eating food, dogs exhibit a rapid, steep, and extremely brief spike of oxytocin release (Uvnäs-Moberg et al., 1985). The oxytocin spike associated with eating is sensitive to conditioning, with dogs responding to conditioned stimuli that regularly occur in advance of the presentation of food. Whereas oxytocin appears to mediate reward associated with gratification, comfort, and safety, dopamine appears to mediate reward associated with surprise, heightened arousal, and increased incentive (Schultz, 1998). These differential reward effects produced by oxytocin and dopamine point to an important function of cynopraxic training and therapy, to wit: the mediation of an antistress response via physiological and neurobiological changes conducive to social attachment and bonding. However, in addition to mobilizing an antistress response, oxytocin exerts potent anti-aggression and antifear effects while promoting social approach, affectionate interaction, and calming. Consequently, in addition to shaping and modifying behavior, petting and food rewards appear to mediate numerous additive counterconditioning and socialization benefits via the conditioned and unconditioned release of oxytocin and other neuropeptides conducive to an adaptive coping style.

Although the significance of these changes in the distribution of oxytocin-binding and AVP-binding sites remains conjectural, various suggestions have been put forth, including a role in brain growth and neural elaboration, which facilitates the formation of infant-mother attachments and the modulation of separation-related behavior. In addition to developmental changes, stressful environmental influences appear to exert pronounced effects on neuropeptide-receptor density and activity. For example, the number of oxytocin-receptor sites in the hippocampus is transiently decreased in infant rats by brief repeated exposure to maternal separation (Noonan et al., 1994).

> It is interesting to speculate that even brief separations of the infant from the mother, manipulation that involves both stressing the infant and the disruption of a social bond, may have effects on oxytocinergic activity that subsequently influence the expression of social- or stress-related behaviors or endocrine function. (119)

The developmental effects of comfort- and stress-induced alterations in oxytocin-receptor proliferation has been shown to exert profound changes in adult social and maternal behavior (see *Antistress Neurobiology, Maternal Care, and Coping Style* in Chapter 8).

Stress and Flight or Fight Reactions

The close association of AVP with areas of the brain associated with the activation of emotional stress, fear, and aggression (see *Arginine Vasopressin and Aggression* in Volume 1, Chapter 3) suggests the possibility that AVP may play a significant role in the mediation of a reactive stress response, whereas oxytocin appears to mobilize an adaptive or antistress response conducive to cooperative interaction and bonding (Uvnäs-Moberg, 1997b). The finding that the central amygdala expresses both oxytocin-binding and AVP-binding sites is intriguing with respect to this general hypothesis and the notion that these neuropeptides may mediate opposite effects on the elaboration of emotional stress responses and social adjustment. Whereas oxytocin appears to activate systems conducive to what might be called an adaptive *flirt and forbear* response (see *Adaptive Coping Styles: Play, Flirt, Forbear, and Nip* in Chapter 6), AVP appears to mediate a reactive flight or fight response (social avoidance, punishment, and agitation), perhaps via epigenetic interaction with corticotropin-releasing factor (CRF), testosterone (see *Arginine Vasopressin, Testosterone, and Serotonin* in Chapter 6), and substance P.

CRF, oxytocin, and AVP are all produced by the paraventricular nucleus (PVN) of the hypothalamus. The release of CRF by the PVN activates the hypothalamic-pituitary-adrenal (HPA) system by prompting the anterior pituitary gland to release adrenocorticotropic hormone (ATCH), which, in turn, causes the adrenal cortex to secrete glucocorticoid hormones (cortisol and corticosterone) into the bloodstream (see *Startle and Fear Circuits* in Chapter 3). Circulating glucocorticoids exert a negative-feedback effect on the hypothalamic stress response. CRF-containing neurons located in the central amygdala initiate the emotional stress response via projections to the locus coeruleus and the release of norepinephrine (NE), which in turn mediates the rapid release of epinephrine by the adrenal medulla and the activation of the sympathetic nervous system. These amygdala CRF neurons show a threshold shift and potentiation in response to repeated and uncontrolled emotional stressors, possibly resulting in generalized anticipatory anxiety (Cook, 2002) (see *Stress-related Potentiation of the Flight-Fight System* in Chapter 6).

The amygdala mediates the hypothalamic stress response by means of a direct pathway via the BNST and an indirect pathway via medullary NE-producing neurons—the primary signal activating CRF production and release. The medial prefrontal cortex forms reciprocal connections with the amygdala, as well as projecting to every major system involved in the mobilization of the stress response. These various prefrontal and subcortical interactions mediate the process of organizing adaptive control expectancies and emotional establishing operations. Increased catecholamine activity associated with acute stressors enhances attention and alertness to environmental stimuli, but with a cost to cognitive functions. Increased dopamine (DA) activity under the influence of stress may reduce prefrontal efficiency, perhaps in vulnerable dogs, significantly disrupting their capacity to perform executive control functions (see *Stress-related Influences on Cortical Functions* in Volume 1, Chapter 3). In human subjects, high cortisol levels in response to moderate stressors are associated with decreased problem-solving capacity, increased arousal and focus on sensory stimuli, and negative mood (e.g., depression, anxiety, and confusion) (Al'Absi et al., 2002).

As a result of an intense threatening event or loss of control (e.g., abusive punishment), NE is rapidly released in the prefrontal cortex and the central amygdala, coordinating a shift from behavior organized in accordance with expectancies and calibrated establishing operations to one of heightened arousal and vigilance, mobilizing the flight-fight system in preparation to escape or attack, if necessary, to secure safety. Under such circumstances, behavioral output may become highly reactive and unpredictable, especially in cases involving a history of abusive treatment. Glucocor-

ticoid negative feedback helps to reverse stress-related arousal by turning off the release of ATCH and by generally quieting the flight-fight system by inhibiting CRF and NE activity while increasing mesocortical DA activity and facilitating serotonin (5-hydroxytryptamine or 5-HT) stress-management functions. Chronic stress, however, appears to gradually exert a global dysregulatory effect on prefrontal and central amygdala functions, while circulating glucocorticoids may slowly degrade the functional fitness of hippocampus (see *Hippocampal and Higher Cortical Influences* in Volume 1, Chapter 3). Chronic stress can be extremely harmful to the integrity of the brain's stress-management system and the dog's ability to adjust adaptively, producing widespread disturbances and dysregulation of DA, 5-HT, and NE systems (see *Startle and Fear Circuits* in Chapter 3). Finally, in addition to playing a central role in the mediation of behavioral stress and anticipatory anxiety, CRF produces a suppressive effect over appetite and facilitates the expression of separation-related distress (Panksepp et al., 1988).

Maternal Separation and Stress

Excessive stress early in a dog's life cycle may disrupt critical neurobiological checks and balances associated with glucocorticoid- and CRF-receptor proliferation and sensitivity, making the puppy more vulnerable to the adverse effects of uncontrollable environmental and social stressors in adulthood. Heim and Nemeroff (1999) have argued that early abuse and emotional trauma in childhood may predispose people to develop a variety of stress-related psychiatric conditions later in life, pointing to CRF sensitization and HPA-system dysregulation as decisive etiological factors. Central CRF activity in the limbic system and brainstem appears to mediate anxiety and other mood disturbances. As the result of early sensitization of the CRF system, even moderate levels of stress may produce significant perturbation of emotional and cognitive functions in adult animals. Early exposure to adverse maternal separation appears to sensitize the HPA system, causing isolation-stressed rats to produce excessive ACTH and adrenal corticosterone when exposed to psychological stress as adults.

A laboratory model for studying the effects of neonatal handling on adult stress and psychopathology has been developed in rats. Maternal separation can either improve or disturb adult coping abilities, depending on the sort of isolation used. Although brief periods of stressful handling early in life appear to have a highly beneficial effect on an adult animal's ability to cope with stress (Levine et al., 1967), more lengthy exposure to repeated stressful separation from the mother may result in increased sensitivity and vulnerability to stress as an animal matures. The perturbations appear to involve changes in the brain's responsiveness to stressful stimuli, especially central CRF-mediated activation. Plotsky and Meaney (1993), for example, reported that infant rats, when repeatedly separated from their mothers on days 2 to 14 for 180 minutes, exhibit pronounced and persistent changes in the density of CRF-receptor-binding sites and increased CRF-system activity, whereas animals exposed to briefer separation experiences (15 minutes) showed an opposite effect, exhibiting significantly less CRF-system activity than both the 180-minute separation group and the control group that had been left undisturbed during the same period. Ladd and colleagues (1996) found that infant rats deprived of maternal contact for 6 hours on days 2 to 20 exhibited a 59% increase in CRF-receptor-binding sites in the dorsal raphe nucleus, the area involved in the production of 5-HT.

CRF exerts an inhibitory effect on 5-HT production (Kirby et al., 2000)—an effect that may be significantly enhanced as the result of excessive postnatal stress. CRF proliferation in the dorsal raphe nucleus and stress-induced suppression of 5-HT production may play a significant role in the etiology of stress-related dog behavior problems. Reportedly, long-term treatment with paroxetine, a selective serotonin (5-HT) reuptake inhibitor (SSRI), attenuates or reverses the neuroendocrine and HPA-system aberrations produced by stressful maternal separation, normalizing both behavioral and endocrine aspects of the stress syndrome in rats (Ladd et al., 2000). The normalizing effects of SSRIs

on the brain's stress-management system may help to explain the therapeutic effects of such medications on stress-related behavior problems. Finally, the effectiveness of SSRIs and tricyclic antidepressants for controlling symptoms of separation distress in dogs suggests a close modulatory role of 5-HT within emotional circuits mediating social behavior and affiliation (Insel and Winslow, 1998).

The loss of familiar attachment objects and places produces significant stress in dogs. Hennessy and colleagues (1997) found that dogs entering a shelter initially exhibit increased levels of cortisol for several days, after which they progressively adapt toward control levels exhibited by dogs living in homes (Figure 4.3). Although separation from an attachment object is often associated with increased glucocorticoid output in adult animals, not all animals show signs of biological stress when they are separated from affiliative partners (Hennessy, 1997). Hennessy suggests that the sudden loss of an attachment object represents a major threat to animals, and the increase in HPA activity may provide the necessary biochemical and metabolic activation to cope with the threats associated with loss and isolation. Perhaps the most important factor determining whether an animal shows signs of stress at separation appears to be the degree of attachment or bonding between the separated animal and the affiliative partner. Dogs separated in an unfamiliar place exhibited increased glucocorticoid activity that was only slightly affected by the presence of a kennelmate (Tuber et al., 1996) (Figure 4.4). Interestingly, though, glucocorticoid levels of separated dogs in the presence of a familiar person, a caretaker who had worked with the dogs for many years, were significantly lower (see *Biological Stress and Separation Distress* in Volume 2, Chapter 4). The differential response of separated dogs to the presence of a familiar dog versus familiar person is difficult to explain. Ostensibly, the separated dog obtains more comfort from the presence of a caretaker than it does from its kennelmate. Precisely why this is so remains unknown, but one possible explanation is that humans represent a supernormal stimulus for social attraction and attachment (see *Supernormal*

Attachment Hypothesis in Volume 2, Chapter 4). Gantt (1944) found that the conditioned anxiety of a dog was markedly reduced by petting but not by the presence of a nearby dog. Perhaps, as the result of selective breeding for traits conducive to companionship with people, dogs may have acquired a genetically influenced preference for contact with people over contact with conspecifics (Feddersen-Petersen, 1994). Odendaal (1999) has reported that interaction between familiar owner-dog dyads results in significantly more oxytocin release than when the dog is exposed to an unfamiliar person, perhaps pointing to a neurobiological basis for the apparent preference of dogs for familiar humans. These physiological differences associated with contact-induced oxytocin activity probably reflect the effects of social conditioning on the mechanisms involved in the release of oxytocin. In any case, puppies exhibit a preference for human contact over canine contact from an early age. Pettijohn and colleagues (1977) found that puppies separated in a strange situation showed a significant reduction in separation distress when

in the company of a person. Whether involving active or passive contact, the proximity of a human was more comforting to the puppy than the presence of its own mother. Surprisingly, the presence of the mother was no more effective at assuaging separation distress in a strange situation than was the presence of an unfamiliar adult dog (see *Social Attachment and Separation* in Volume 1, Chapter 2). As a social stimulus, the human being may be a better activator of oxytocin activity in dogs that show a preference for humans over other dogs—a hypothesis that would be easy to test. According to Panksepp (1992), in the context of maternal care, oxytocin may centrally stimulate emotions conducive to social approach and contact:

A straightforward emotional prediction is that brain oxytocin may evoke warm positive feelings of social strength and comfort when aroused by peripheral stimuli. For instance, as mother and infant share in the nursing experience, brain oxytocin systems may be activated in both individuals through reciprocal somatosensory and gustatory stimulation. This would contribute to a sense of ease and relax-

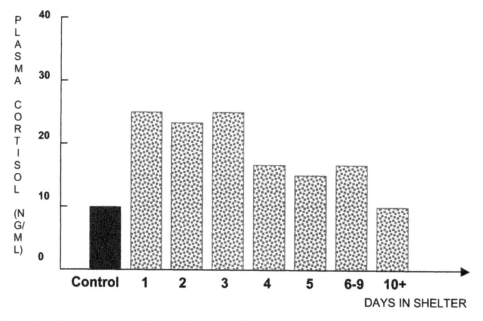

FIG. 4.3. Upon entering a shelter, dogs show a significant increase of HPA (hypothalamic-pituitary-adrenal)-axis activity. The first 3 days appear to be particularly stressful. After day 10, however, most dogs appear to be physiologically adapted to the new situation. After Hennessy et al. (1997).

ation (feelings of acceptance and nurturance) and thereby tend to promote conditional attraction (i.e., social bonding/imprinting) between caregivers and receivers. These are the types of neuroaffective changes that would also tend to counteract feelings of isolation and distress. (243–244)

In conjunction with endogenous opioids, oxytocin performs various neuroregulatory roles in the process of modulating stress responses and coordinating dynamic neurobiological changes conducive to social bonding and the development of complex social behavior (see *Oxytocin-opioidergic Hypothesis* in Chapter 6). Like endogenous opioids, oxytocin also exerts a significant inhibitory effect over separation-distress vocalizations.

PHARMACOLOGICAL CONTROL OF SEPARATION DISTRESS

Since the cascade of events leading to full-blown separation-related panic includes the activation of the brain CRF system, drugs capable of blocking CRF-receptor sites or

restraining CRF activity would probably prove beneficial in the management of separation-related problems. In addition to SSRIs, such as paroxetine, tricyclic antidepressants appear to provide such regulatory enhancement. Imipramine, for example, appears to exert a pronounced effect on CRF activity (Sternberg and Gold, 1997):

> In rats, regular, but not acute, administration of the tricyclic antidepressant imipramine significantly lowers the levels of CRH [corticotropin-releasing hormone] precursors in the hypothalamus. Imipramine given for two months to healthy persons with normal cortisol levels causes gradual and sustained decrease in CRH secretion and other HPA-axis functions, indicating that down-regulation of important components of the stress response is an intrinsic effect of imipramine. (13)

Given the complementary roles of CRF as a trigger for separation reactions and the efficacy of oxytocin to quiet them, Panksepp (1998) has suggested that medications capable of restraining central CRF activity while enhancing oxytocin activity might prove

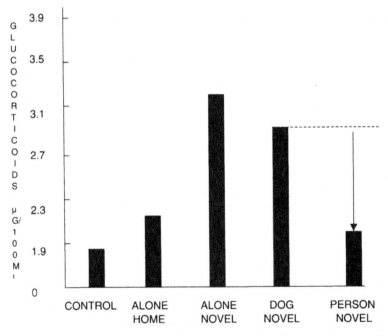

FIG. 4.4. Stress response to social contact and separation in novel and home environments. Note the increased effect of a person on a dog in a novel environment versus the effect of a familiar dog. Maximum distress occurs when the dog is left alone in an unfamiliar environment. Adapted from Tuber et al. (1996).

efficacious in the treatment of separation-related problems. Recently, promising strides have been made in the development of CRF receptor (subtype 1) antagonists (Gilligan et al., 2000; He et al., 2000). These compounds appear to have excellent oral availability, potent anxiolytic efficacy, and minimal side effects. Similarly promising advances have been made in the development of an orally available substance P antagonist (MK-869), a compound that appears to be highly effective in the management of depression and may eventually prove beneficial in the management of separation-related problems (Kramer et al., 1998). Medications with the capacity to block CRF and substance P activity offer exciting possibilities for the treatment of stress-related dog behavior problems and deserve preclinical and clinical veterinary investigation.

The preponderance of evidence supports the view that different emotional circuits mediate the expression of separation distress (panic system) and anxiety (fear system) involving the cingulate gyrus, the preoptic and ventral septal areas, the dorsomedial thalamus, the BNST, and the PAG (Panksepp et al., 1985; Panksepp, 1998). Although panic and fear systems appear to exert a reciprocal excitatory influence on one another, they are motivationally distinct systems (see *Emotional Command Systems and Drive Theory* in Chapter 6). However, certain fears, such as thunderstorm phobias, are highly correlated with separation distress (Overall et al., 2001), suggesting the possibility that the sensitization of the fear system (e.g., the occurrence of a severe thunderstorm) occurring at times when the owner—the dog's source of safety—is absent may play a role in the etiology of SDS. Many separation-reactive dogs do not show evidence of noise or thunderstorm phobias, consistent with the notion that SDS is complex in origin and affected by several causes and contributing influences. Despite the reciprocal excitatory influences exerted by fear on panic and by panic on fear, separation distress and the panic circuits mediating its expression operate with significant independence from anxiety and fear—an observation supported by both psychobiological (Panksepp, 1998) and pharmacological stud-

ies. For example, Scott and colleagues (1973) found that separation-distress vocalization in beagle puppies was not ameliorated by anxiolytic medications (e.g., chlorpromazine, reserpine, meprobamate, and diazepam), but was rapidly and consistently reduced by imipramine:

> In sufficient doses, it [imipramine] will reduce vocalization to essentially zero without producing abnormal behavior or adverse physiological side effects. Even under the largest doses, the dogs that received imipramine appeared to be no different from the controls that were given placebos, except for their vocalization rates. (17)

Imipramine produced both immediate and sustained relief from separation distress. Even though diazepam had no discernible effect on separation-distress vocalizations, treated puppies appeared to be more relaxed when handled. In the case of infant rhesus monkeys, however, diazepam has been demonstrated to produce a potent attenuating effect on separation-related stress (Kalin et al., 1987), suggesting the possibility that different aspects of the separation stress response are under the control of different regulatory neurotransmitter systems in dogs and monkeys.

Although imipramine was highly effective in controlling the separation-induced vocalizations produced by beagles and Australian terrier-beagle crosses, the drug did not control the separation-distress vocalizations exhibited by shelties and Telomians. These findings suggest that the effects of tricyclic antidepressants on SDS may be highly variable depending on the breed and temperament of dog. Observing that such drugs exert variable behavioral effects on dogs depending on breed type should not be surprising, however. Arons and Shoemaker (1992), for example, found that dogs of different breeds (e.g., Border collies, shar planinetz, and Siberian huskies) exhibit significant neurobiological variability with respect to neurotransmitter levels localized in different brain areas, as well as exhibiting differences in the expression of highly influential receptor sites (Niimi et al., 1999). These fundamental differences exert profound influences on behavioral thresholds and the dog's response to medication. Evidence of breed-related variability at the level of neural organization underscores the importance of medicating dogs according to breed-specific differences, recognizing that they are not all cut from the same neurobiological cloth.

Panksepp and colleagues (1978) found that pronounced alleviation of separation distress could be achieved in puppies with the administration of very low doses of morphine. Medicated puppies behaved normally, without signs of sedation, except that they appeared comfortable and calm while separated from mother and littermates. The benefit of morphine, however, is dose dependent, with larger doses resulting in catalepsy or, paradoxically, more separation-distress vocalization. Morphine has also been shown to control separation-distress vocalization effectively in infant rhesus monkeys, without reducing activity levels (Kalin et al., 1987). The efficacy of morphine and other opiates is dramatic, but the clinical feasibility of such medications for the treatment of SDS is limited because of the potential for abuse, rapid tolerance, and eventual withdrawal symptoms that might worsen the symptoms of SDS when the treatment is discontinued. Nonetheless, morphine in low doses (perhaps in combination with imipramine) may have a therapeutic application in the management of acute separation-related panic, especially in cases where other medications have failed.

Voith and Borchelt (1996) have suggested that a wide variety of drugs (including benzodiazepines, neuroleptics, progestins, and tricyclic antidepressants) may have some usefulness in the treatment of separation distress. Historically, the tricyclic antidepressant amitriptyline has been the most commonly prescribed medication for the control of problematic separation-related behavior. A possible added benefit of amitriptyline is a sedative effect, probably stemming from a potent blocking effect on histamines. Amitriptyline exerts a ninefold greater blocking effect on histamines than does imipramine (Julian, 1995). Benzodiazepines (e.g., clorazepate or alprazolam) are often used in combination with tricyclic antidepressants or SSRIs to enhance effectiveness, especially in cases where SDS presents comorbidly with a phobia associated with being left alone or a high level of anticipatory anxiety associated with departures. Neuroleptic medications, such as acepromazine, are occasionally used to suppress temporarily the motor expressions of acute separation distress, but they have very limited value with respect to targeting the underlying emotional arousal pathways triggering with separation distress and are generally reserved for emergencies.

More recently, the tricyclic antidepressant clomipramine, a potent 5-HT-reuptake inhibitor, has become increasingly popular for the treatment of separation-distress problems. Although clomipramine has shown promise for the management of separation-related behavior (Simpson, 1997), Podberscek and colleagues (1999) have questioned its value in the treatment of separation anxiety. In their study, the efficacy of clomipramine was evaluated as an adjunct to behavior therapy. Although clomipramine appeared to produce a significant sedative effect, it was not "any more effective than a placebo as an adjunct to behavioural therapy in the treatment of separation-related behaviour problems in dogs" (369). Hewson (2000) has criticized their study and Simpson's previous report, concluding that neither behavior therapy nor clomipramine alone or both together have been shown to control separation-related behavior problems effectively. A subsequent study, however, reported by King and colleagues (2000) indicates that clomipramine in combination with behavior therapy does significantly reduce separation-related destructiveness and elimination problems, though the combination does not significantly attenuate separation-related vocalization excesses. They suggest that the previous failure of Podberscek and colleagues to detect a reliable effect of clomipramine was due to shortcomings in the study's design (e.g., sample size).

Panksepp (personal communication, 1996) has suggested that clonidine in combination with morphine, imipramine, or a 5-HT-reuptake inhibitor (e.g., clomipramine) *might* be beneficial in the treatment of separation-related distress in dogs. Clonidine is an NE-receptor agonist that exerts mixed excitatory (postsynaptic) and inhibitory (presynaptic) effects on NE activity (Panksepp, 1998). Evidence for a beneficial role of clonidine in combination with imipramine for the control of separation distress has been reported in squirrel monkeys (Harris and Newman, 1987); in rhesus monkeys, however, clonidine alone reduced activity levels, but without influencing separation-distress vocalizations (Kalin et al., 1988). Interestingly, clonidine in combination with passionflower (*Passiflora incarnata*) has been shown to exert a significantly superior effect over clonidine alone in the management of mental symptoms associated with opiate withdrawal (Akhondzadeh et al., 2001). An SSRI that may offer significant efficacy in the control of SDS with panic is paroxetine, which appears to influence the CRF system beneficially as well as enhance serotonergic activity, with proven efficacy in the control of human panic disorder, general anxiety disorder, and obsessive-compulsive disorder (Ballenger, 1999).

Lastly, some owners have reported success using over-the-counter drugs such as melatonin, which has been shown to modulate separation distress in chicks (Nelson et al., 1994), separation anxiety exhibited by a bear that failed to hibernate (Uchida et al., 1998), and fear of noises (Aronson, 1999). Dodman (1999) has used melatonin with some apparent success in the treatment of compulsive licking and thunderstorm phobias. Melatonin appears to modulate endogenous opioid activity, perhaps providing an opioid-mediated regulatory influence on attachment processes and separation-related distress. A bidirectional feedback relationship appears to exist between melatonin and endogenous opioids, with melatonin inhibiting opioid activity and opioids stimulating melatonin activity (Barrett et al., 2000). These findings suggest that the putative effects of melatonin on separation distress may not be mediated directly by an increase in opioid activity, but via an indirect influence existing at another level of interaction between melatonin and opioids. In rats, melatonin has been shown to attenuate the adrenocortical response to stress, to increase HPA-axis responsiveness to glucocorticoid feedback effects, and may ameliorate stress-related disturbances associated with chronic stress (Konakchieva et al., 1997). Melatonin also appears to perform a protective neuroregulatory role over the immunosuppressive effects of stress by various means (Pierpaoli

and Maestroni, 1987). Finally, Pacchierotti and colleagues (2001) have conjectured that stressed animals may produce increased amounts of melatonin in an effort to stabilize internal states associated with anxiety and agitation.

Some experimental evidence indicates that melatonin may exert an inhibitory effect over thyroid activity in various animal species (Wright et al., 2000). To my knowledge, the thyroid-inhibiting effects of melatonin have not been explicitly demonstrated in dogs, but the existence of such a potential side effect warrants careful use of melatonin in the case of dogs showing borderline thyroid levels or behavioral conditions believed to be under the influence of thyroid insufficiency. Aronson (1998) has suggested that thyroid insufficiency may play a significant role in the etiology of a wide variety of behavior problems and has been associated with aggression in dogs (Fatjó et al., 2002) (see *Assessment and Identification* in Volume 2, Chapter 8). In addition, recent research shows that thyroid hormones produce an augmentative effect over cognitive functions via the enhancement of cholinergic activity, emphasizing the far-reaching influence of the hormone (Smith et al., 2002). The short-term and long-term side effects of melatonin therapy in dogs are unknown. In people, melatonin appears to be well tolerated, and the risk of toxicity is low at prescribed dosages (De Lourdes et al., 2000).

Note: The foregoing information is provided for educational purposes only. If considering the use of medications to control or manage a behavior problem, the reader should consult with a veterinarian familiar with the use of drugs for such purposes in order to obtain diagnostic criteria, specific dosages, and medical advice concerning potential adverse side effects and interactions with other drugs.

POTENTIAL ALTERNATIVE TREATMENTS

Herbal Preparations

Numerous studies (especially in Germany) have investigated the efficacy of St. John's wort, *Hypericum perforatum*, for the management of mild to moderate depression in people (Josey and Tackett, 1999). Hypericum (0.3% hypericin) has been shown to perform on a par with imipramine, amitriptyline, and fluoxetine for the treatment of depression (Bergmann et al., 1993; Vorbach et al., 1994; Harrer et al., 1999), strongly suggesting that it may have some therapeutic value for the management of SDS and other behavior problems treated successfully with SSRIs and tricyclic antidepressant medications (e.g., compulsive excesses). Pharmacological studies in rodents indicate that hypericum extracts influence dopaminergic, serotonergic, and noradrenergic reuptake mechanisms (Mueller and Rossol, 1994; Muller and Schafer, 1996; Kaehler et al., 1999). St. John's wort has been shown to increase DA and 5-HT metabolite levels, but without affecting monoamine oxidase activity, suggesting the possibility that the herb exerts its pharmacological effects by inhibiting DA or 5-HT reuptake (Serdarevic et al., 2001). Steger (1985) found that a combination of hypericum and valerium proved more effective for the control of depressive symptoms than did desipramine, a tricyclic antidepressant having pronounced noradrenergic reuptake effects. The combination of the two herbal preparations appears to produce a synergistic effect. So far, the side effects of hypericum have been repeatedly described as minimal when the herb is taken at recommended dosages, but no studies to my knowledge have been performed demonstrating efficacy or safety with dogs. The ingestion of large amounts of St. John's wort may cause gastric disturbances or phototoxicity. Although several studies have indicated that St. John's wort is an effective treatment for mild depression, Davidson and colleagues (2002) failed to detect a therapeutic benefit resulting from hypericum treatment for moderately severe-major depression in human patients. Among the patients studied, hypericum was no more effective than its matched placebo. Interestingly, however, sertraline, a potent SSRI commonly used to treat depression, failed to perform much better than hypericum in terms of primary outcome measures, leaving some questions open for future study. Finally, Fornal and colleagues (2001) have directly measured the discharge rate of 5-HT neurons in the dorsal raphe nucleus after administering St. John's wort to awake cats. They found that St. John's wort had no effect on neuronal activity, in sharp contrast to the robust effects produced by fluoxetine and sertraline. Both SSRIs produced a marked reduction of neuronal activity by increasing synaptic 5-HT levels. These findings suggest that the putative effect of St. John's wort may be mediated by a mechanism other than 5-HT-reuptake inhibition.

Two other herbal preparations that may exert some modulatory control over the distress associated with separation are ginkgo biloba and kava kava. Porsolt and colleagues (1990) reported that preventive dosing with ginkgo biloba prior to repeated inescapable shocks produced a significant protective influence against stress associated with learned helplessness. The blocking effects of ginkgo biloba against symptoms of learned helplessness were more robust than the effects produced by diazepam and did not impair passive avoidance learning—a side effect observed to occur in association with benzodiazepines. Finally, some evidence suggests that kava extract may modulate circuits controlling separation distress. Many double-blind, randomized, and placebo-controlled trials have demonstrated the efficacy of Kava extracts (30% kavalactones) for the symptomatic treatment of anxiety (Pittler and Ernst, 2000). Kava extracts have also been shown to attenuate separation-distress vocalizations and stress-induced analgesia in 8-day-old chicks (Smith et al., 2001). Whether similar effects might occur in dogs is not known. Scattered reports associating the use of kava kava with severe side effects, including liver damage, have recently called the safety of herb into question. Although serious side effects do appear to occur sporadically, they appear to be relatively rare when kava kava is taken without other drugs for short periods at recommended dosages (Stevinson et al., 2002). The potential benefits and side effects of kava kava for the management of separation-related problems in dogs is unknown; nonetheless, it is widely used, alone or in combination with St. John's wort, by dog owners seeking an over-the-counter cure for separation-related stress, often without veterinary guidance and support.

Herbal preparations that are capable of producing a clinical benefit should be considered prima facie capable of producing harmful side effects if improperly used. In addition, herbal remedies may interact synergistically with other medications in ways that could be potentially harmful to a dog, requiring that such remedies be carefully evaluated for safety before considering their use (Cooper, 2002). Consequently, like other medications used in the control and management of behavior problems, complementary herbal and dietary regimens should be introduced under the close supervision of a veterinarian familiar with the various clinical effects and side effects of such treatment programs.

Dog-appeasing Pheromone

A synthetic analogue of apaisine, a pheromone reportedly produced by lactating female dogs, may exert a beneficial modulatory effect over separation distress. The putative pheromone is believed to produce a calming effect on nursing puppies. Unfortunately, the basic scientific evidence supporting these potentially exciting and breakthrough findings remains to be published. To the best of my knowledge, the procedures used to isolate and synthesize the pheromone, its biochemical characteristics and molecular description, and evidence in support of its putative emotional and behavioral effects on puppies and adult dogs have not yet been published in a peer-reviewed scientific journal. Pheromones are captured by the vomeronasal organ and processed by the accessory olfactory bulb. Although dogs lack a true flehmen response, they do exhibit tonguing—a flehmenlike response that appears to collect pheromone molecules from the air and surfaces where they have been deposited (see *Vomeronasal Organ* in Volume 1, Chapter 4). Preliminary results of a multicenter study are promising, showing that the synthetic analogue, marketed as dog-appeasing pheromone (DAP), may produce a clinical effect comparable to clomipramine when used in combination with behavior therapy to treat separation-related behavior problems (Gaultier and Pageat, 2002). Curiously, though, given the robust release of oxytocin and prolactin during nursing (Uvnäs-Moberg et al., 1985), it seems odd that a functionally redundant pheromone would also be genetically coded to produce an appeasing effect in support of an activity that is intrinsically calming for a puppy to perform in the first place. A plug-in electric diffuser supplied with the product dispenses DAP into the air. In addition to possibly helping to calm separation-reactive dogs, DAP is believed to reduce stress and fear. Another proposed use of DAP is to facilitate a puppy's transition into the home or ease the acceptance of stressful environmental changes (e.g., moving). Perhaps the appeasing pheromone can be harvested by wiping the inter-mammary line of lactating females with gauze moistened with dilute alcohol. The collected material can then be mixed with water and dispensed from a spray bottle or other means (e.g., placed on toys). Also, sending home towels and bedding containing the odors of the mother may help to facilitate the puppy's transition into the new home. In any case, pheromone or not, maternal odors may produce beneficial emotional effects by means of conditioned associations.

Note: The foregoing information is provided for educational purposes only. If considering the use of herbal remedies, the reader should consult with a veterinarian familiar with the use of such preparations to obtain specific dosages, diagnostic criterion for their use, and medical advice regarding potential side effects.

SEPARATION DISTRESS AND DIET

In the past, dog owners were frequently advised to make various dietary changes for the purpose of altering a dog's behavior or motivation. Most of these recommendations have come and gone, leaving in the wake a high degree of skepticism about the usefulness of dietary manipulations for the management of behavior problems. Undoubtedly, the quality, quantity, and combination of foods eaten by a dog exert some influence, but the extent of these influences and the specifics involved remain to be disclosed by animal psychodietetic research (Ballarini,

1989). What little is known, however, may be useful for managing some problems associated with separation distress, anxiety, and panic. For example, the physiological arousal and aversive motivational tensions associated with hunger may increase exploratory and destructive activities when a dog is left alone. A full stomach may help dogs to relax and sleep when alone. Consequently, it may be useful to feed separation-reactive dogs in the morning rather than in the evening. In addition to morning feedings, Mugford (1987) suggests that a high-fiber diet may help to calm separation-reactive dogs and reduce destructiveness, but provides little evidence to support this claim. Growing evidence suggests that essential fatty acids (EFAs), especially omega-3 fatty acids (fish oils), may alter negative mood and alleviate depression (see *Aggression and Diet* in Chapter 7). In addition, some evidence suggests that olive oil may also exert some benefit on mood (Puri and Richardson, 2000). Olive oil is a rich source of oleic acid, the nutritional precursor of oleamide, a psychoactive lipid. Oleamide appears to play a significant role in sleep induction and the modulation of serotonergic neurotransmission (Huidobro-Toro and Harris, 1996; Thomas et al., 1998). The anxiolytic effects of diets rich in soy may be beneficial in some cases of SDS presenting comorbidly with anxiety and fear (Lephart et al., 2002). Although dietary change and supplementation may provide a nutritional benefit for the management of separation-related problems, the efficacy of such nutritional supplementation for the management of SDS remains to be clinically evaluated and should be considered on a case-by-case basis under the advisement of a veterinarian.

Various preservatives, additives, flavorings, and dyes used in the manufacture of dog food have been suspected of producing a wide variety of effects on behavior, but no solid evidence is yet available to support the widely held conviction (Halliwell, 1992). A common source of allergies among dogs is food, suggesting that certain foods might produce neurotropic allergies that could contribute to the development of behavior problems, including SDS. Excessive sugar in the diet has been frequently pointed to as a cause of hyperactivity in children, but no solid scientific evidence supports the hypothesis (see *Dietary Factors and Hyperactivity* in Volume 2, Chapter 5).

One isolated report has suggested that diet plays a dramatically significant role in the treatment of behavior problems (Anderson and Marinier, 1997). The authors claim that a significant benefit may be obtained by feeding dogs according to their preferences, that is, giving them a choice in the foods they eat. By merely adjusting the diet to reflect the dog's preferences (e.g., feeding fresh meat, well-cooked vegetables, and raw knuckle bones) and avoiding excessive exercise or excitement, they claim that behavioral complaints were drastically reduced in 98% of the 100 dogs observed in their study. Unfortunately, as a result of limited information concerning the procedures used to assess behavioral change and collect data, the absence of experimental controls, a lack of rigorous statistical analysis, and other experimental design problems, it is impossible to assess the value of these findings. For what it is worth, however, Beaver and colleagues (1992) found that most dogs prefer meat over vegetables, especially cooked fresh meat, which they prefer over raw meat. When given a choice, their top choices were fried liver with onions (see the following note) and baked chicken, followed by cooked beef and fish. Aged meats (cooked and raw) were significantly less attractive than fresh cooked meats. The least attractive food items were fruits. (*Note:* Onions are toxic to dogs and can cause hemolytic anemia, a blood disease in which red blood cells are damaged and destroyed. Dogs should not be fed onions.)

Dietary supplements that may have some merit for the management of SDS are milk products containing casein. Casein is found in milk powder and cottage cheese. The digestion of casein produces casomorphins, naturally occurring opioids that are absorbed into the bloodstream (Panksepp et al., 1985). Other exorphins (or exogenous opioids) are produced as the result of the duodenal digestion of cereal glutins (Ballarini, 1990). Since separation-distressed animals appear to be highly responsive to morphine, it would seem sensible to investigate the effect of casomorphins and other exorphins on separation distress. Perhaps the habit of sending children off to school after a meal of cereal and milk is no accident, but an unwitting nutritional remedy for the reduction of childhood separation anxiety. The notion that casein from the mother's milk might mediate social attachment by way of an opioid mechanism offers some intriguing, but as yet untested, possibilities with regard to the influence of nutrition on attachment and separation-related behavior. Whatever the specifics, attachment and separation are orchestrated by an intricate web of psychological and physiological interactions involving complex neural systems regulating emotions associated with comfort and distress.

Finally, considering the significant role of 5-HT in the regulation of impulsive behavior, the modulation of fear and anxiety, and the neural management of stress, it would seem advisable to provide separation-reactive dogs with a diet that maximizes the utilization of nutritionally derived tryptophan (see *Diet and Serotonin Activity* in Volume 1, Chapter 3). Diets combining low-protein and high-carbohydrate content appear to increase the availability of peripheral tryptophan, the amino acid precursor of 5-HT. In addition, increased exercise may stimulate increased 5-HT production and help optimize tryptophan transport across the blood-brain barrier (Meeusen and De Meirleir, 1995)(see *Exercise and Diet* in Chapter 3). In addition to providing an acceptable outlet for agitated oral activity, chewing may evoke an insulin release enhancing tryptophan access to blood-brain barrier transport molecules (see *Nutrition and Aggression* in Volume 2, Chapter 6).

EARLY STIMULATION, SEPARATION EXPOSURE, AND EMOTIONAL REACTIVITY

The successful control and management of SDS depend first and foremost on accurate diagnosis and complementary behavior therapy (Marder, 1991). Although drugs may help in some cases, the long-term benefits of drug therapy depend on the implementation of behavioral techniques designed to help improve the quality of the human-dog relationship and to enhance the dog's ability to cope with separation. Medicating dogs exhibiting separation panic and anxiety problems on a long-term basis in the absence of behavior therapy and training is a highly questionable practice and should be avoided.

As the result of prenatal and postnatal stress, social or environmental deprivation, disorderly or abusive social interaction, excessive restraint, traumatic loss of trust, or a failure to form a trust-based bond, dogs may be predisposed to show reactive rather than adaptive coping styles in response to stressful circumstances. Dogs that have lost their ability to form reliable control expectancies may fixate on reactive adjustments, that is, develop behavior problems in association with a persistent condition of behavioral stress and tension stemming from an inability to experience relief or obtain reward. From the cynopraxic perspective, the working assumption in such cases is fivefold:

1. The dog has become incompetent as the result of a failure to establish an adaptive behavioral framework of prediction-control expectancies with which to obtain its basic needs for comfort, safety, and reward.
2. The dog needs a highly predictable and controllable base of interaction with a friendly human leader to attain the behavior- and mood-modifying benefits of reward produced by positive prediction error and adaptive modal activity.
3. Effective prediction and control lead to competence, confidence, and the counterconditioning benefits of relaxation inherent to an adaptive coping style.
4. By means of affectionate and fair exchanges involving petting, food, and play performed in the context of cooperative and mutually rewarding interaction, a potent normalizing effect is produced.
5. The outcome of such interaction is a friendly and stable bond and an enhanced life experience for both the owner and the dog.

Behavioral distress is expressed in the form of anxiety and frustration, whereas tensions take the form of increased irritability, intolerance, and emotional reactivity. Anxiety and frustration are closely associated with the development and expression of dysfunctional prediction-control expectancies. Anxiety is a state in which a dog is unsure of its ability to predict a pending event, whereas frustration is the result of a failure to control the event once it occurs. Together, anxiety and frustration form a problematic axis of failure with respect to the attainment of emotional relief and reward. Competency is restored through attention and basic training, integrated compliance training, posture-facilitated relaxation (PFR) training, and other reward-based techniques and procedures, providing the dog with the means to learn and to expect relief and reward by behaving in accord with predictive signals. Training and behavior-modification strategies emphasizing intrusive and aversive loss of control in such cases may only worsen the dog's chances of recovery.

The precise causal mechanisms underlying SDS are not known, but many likely etiological factors and coactive influences have been identified (see *Separation Distress and Coactive Influences* in Volume 1, Chapter 4). Although the formation of excessive attachment and dependency appears to play contributory roles, many dogs are exposed to such influences without becoming overly reactive when left alone. Dogs unaccustomed to being left alone may not have acquired the emotional coping skills needed to accommodate the stress produced by abrupt separation. Dogs exhibiting unstable-introverted temperaments (melancholic) may be more prone to develop separation-related problems associated with anxiety (despair), whereas dogs exhibiting unstable-extraverted temperaments may tend to develop separation-related problems associated with frustration (protest). Whether SDS is associated with symptoms of anxiety or frustration, the panic emotional command system appears to mediate the expression of separation distress (Panksepp, 1998).

Numerous theories have been postulated to help explain developmental disturbances resulting in excessive distress or panic at separation (see *Attachment and Separation* in Volume 1, Chapter 4). A convincing account remains to be fleshed out, but genetics (see Lakatos et al.,

2000; and Hofer et al., 2001), early stimulation, and traumatic experiences with separation probably all play a significant role in the etiology of SDS. Neonatal traumatic handling and excessive environmental stress resulting from excessive temperature changes, nutritional deprivation, physical trauma, maternal neglect or isolation, inadequate housing, or abuse may exert a lasting adverse effect on neurobiological substrates mediating stress and stress-related coping behaviors. An absence or an excess of postnatal stress may produce long-term adverse effects on a dog's health, emotional reactivity, and its ability to cope with stressful situations, that is, situations requiring adaptive adjustments.

Prenatal Stimulation

Prenatal stress appears to affect adversely a progeny's ability to cope with environmental and psychological stress. Thompson (1957) found that exposing gestating female rats to intense fear-eliciting stimulation resulted in unstable and emotionally overreactive offspring. Human infants of depressed mothers exhibit a variety of endocrine and behavioral changes associated with increased sympathetic arousal (e.g., high cortisol and NE levels coupled with low DA and 5-HT levels). Such babies appear to exhibit depressive tendencies, including decreased orienting responsiveness, flat affect, reduced activity levels, and increased irritability. Providing the rat mother with stimulation appears to produce a beneficial effect in her offspring. Adler and Conklin (1963) found that exposing gestating rat mothers to repeated daily handling helped to reduce emotional reactivity in their offspring as adults. Prenatal stress, in the form of unpredictable noise and light stimulation occurring three times weekly, during the gestation period increases basal levels of corticosterone as well as sensitizes the sympathetic-adrenomedullary (SAM) system to stress, as evidenced by increased secretion of NE and epinephrine in response to foot shock (Weinstock et al., 1998). Animals exposed to excessive prenatal stress exhibit attentional deficits, increased anxiety, and disturbed social behavior. Prenatal stress dysregulates the HPA system. In response to aversive stimulation, prenatally stressed animals exhibit a prolonged elevation of peripheral glucocorticoid levels, together with decreased negative-feedback inhibition of CRF release by the hypothalamus. In addition, animals stressed during gestation show higher levels of CRF in the amygdala, have fewer glucocorticoid receptor sites in the hippocampus, produce fewer opioid peptides, and exhibit decreased GABA-benzodiazepine inhibitory activity (Weinstock, 1997). In combination, the effects of prenatal stress are pronounced and potentially very influential on the emotional and behavioral development of dogs. Gestating females should be shielded from excessively stressful conditions and receive regular play and other enrichment activities. Postparturient mothers showing signs of stress, anxiety, or depression may benefit from brief biweekly massage (Field et al., 1996a,b).

Postnatal Stimulation

Postnatal stimulation appears to exert pronounced effects on an animal's ability to cope with emotionally provocative situations and stress as an adult. Considerable research has demonstrated that postnatal handling of rats during the first 3 weeks of life permanently alters the way in which they cope with environmental and psychological stressors. Briefly handled rats show decreased levels of CRF, ACTH, and plasma corticosterone levels, appearing to significantly benefit from such exposure to stress. In addition, such animals show an improved ability to recover homeostatic balance (return to basal corticosterone levels) after the stressor is removed (Plotsky and Meaney, 1993). According to Denenberg (1964), an inverse relationship exists between the amount of stimulation that a neonate receives and its emotionality as an adult. High levels of neonatal stimulation are correlated with reduced adult emotionality, whereas low levels are correlated with increased adult emotionality (Figure 4.5). Dennenberg's curve holds true only with respect to stimulation occurring within an optimal range of exposure, with excessive amounts of early stress producing adverse effects on a dog's development. Puppies that receive inappropriate, insufficient, or excessive contact stimulation

and separation exposure may be more prone to exhibit problematic emotionality at separation as adults. The aforementioned studies involving stressful maternal separation show that excessive neonatal exposure to stressful isolation results in lasting disturbances in CRF and HPA activity. Maternally stressed animals exhibit an increased sensitivity to stress and show heightened emotional reactivity and anxiety when exposed to aversive situations, effects also exhibited by animals shielded from environmental stress in infancy. The effects of maternal stress appear to be dose dependent, with little or no stimulation in infancy producing similar sorts of effects as seen in the case of animals exposed to excessive stress (Plotsky and Meaney, 1993). In addition to modulating stress and emotional reactivity beneficially, early handling may improve a dog's ability to cope with adversity and thereby enhance its trainability and problem-solving abilities (see *Early Development and Reflexive Behavior* in Volume 1, Chapter 2). Unfortunately, scant data is available to

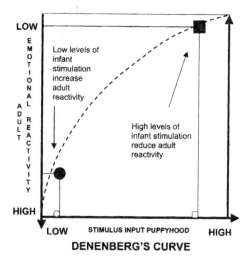

FIG. 4.5. Early infant stimulation exerts a pronounced effect on adult reactivity levels. Whereas moderate levels of tactile stimulation and environmental stress produce a beneficial effect on reactivity levels, too little or too much stimulation may produce adverse effects by increasing adult emotional reactivity levels (choleric type) or decreasing adult emotional reactivity (melancholic type), respectively. Adapted from Denenberg (1964).

confirm the benefits of early handling in dogs, but extensive research with rodents and anecdotal reports of benefits in working dogs (e.g., the Biosensor Research Team) suggest that handling may be a valuable husbandry tool in the case of military working dogs (Fox, 1978).

Handling and Gentling

Various handling procedures have been suggested for maximizing the benefits of early stimulation. The techniques vary but typically involve repeated brief periods of maternal separation from birth to 3 to 5 weeks of age, although postnatal week 1 may be the optimal period for handling effects to occur (Fox, 1971). The necessary amount of handling stress probably varies significantly from breed to breed and individual to individual, depending on genetic predisposition to stress. In addition to maternal separation, thermal stress (placing a puppy on a cold surface) and vestibular stimulation (produced by rocking a puppy side to side on a tilting board) for 1-minute periods each have been suggested by Fox (1978). Fox also recommends that thermal stress and vestibular stimulation be followed by an equal time devoted to gentle stroking. The Monks of New Skete (1991) place individual neonates into cardboard boxes and leave them there for 3 minutes, followed by a period of gentle stroking before the puppy is returned to its mother and littermates.

Perhaps, simply picking a puppy up daily and weighing it on a cold wobbly scale may provide sufficient biological stress to integrate a balanced flight-fight system. Further, given the potential long-term risks associated with maternal separation distress, perhaps adversely sensitizing stress-mediating circuits and inadvertently increasing the puppy's risk of showing stress-related problems in adulthood, the possible health and behavioral benefits of exposing puppies to such stress may not outweigh the potential harm. Consequently, without additional and unambiguous evidence concerning the benefits of such treatment for puppies, exposing neonates to maternal separation and isolation distress might best be avoided until appropriate studies are performed to show, first of all, that iso-

lation distress is beneficial, and then to precisely define the dosage needed, that is, how much isolation exposure is beneficial and at what point does it become harmful. Puppies without a mother should receive intensive neurological stimulation produced by evoking the full range of neonatal and transitional reflexes described by Fox (1965) (see Figure 2.4 in Volume 1).

Gentling refers to procedures in which a puppy is stroked while being held in various nonthreatening positions. In addition, the handler may gently blow breath around the puppy's head and face. Field and colleagues (1996b) have found that massaging infants delivered to depressed mothers exerts significant benefits on attention, emotionality, and sociability test scores. Such infants are often born with stress-related changes, including increased cortisol and catecholamine levels, both of which are significantly reduced by two 15-minute periods of massage per week. The puppy can also be exposed to brief periods of massage while restrained in various positions (stand, sit, down, and lateral roll). Brief restraint represents a mild source of stress, and massage may help a puppy learn to modulate and refine its response to it. Gentling is believed to enhance bonding and taming. Among rats, postweaning gentling has been shown to exert significant benefits, including enhanced learning and retention, increased exploratory behavior, improved competitive success (social dominance), and improved stress response (Morton, 1968). Gentling may be particularly beneficial in the case of puppies exhibiting signs of excessive fear or contact aversion.

Exposure to maternal separation distress, cold, and distressful noxious manipulations appears to integrate a potent flight-fight stress system via AVP and CRF. In contrast, the repeated nonnoxious evocation of oxytocin release appears to integrate an antistress response (see *Oxytocin-opioidergic Hypothesis* in Chapter 6), producing numerous short-term and long-term physiological benefits conducive to calming and growth (Uvnäs-Moberg, 1997a)—high priorities of early puppyhood. Rhythmic stroking, warmth, and vibratory stimuli have been shown to produce a highly beneficial release of oxytocin

(Uvnäs-Moberg, 1998). The postnatal release of oxytocin produced by repetitive massage-like stroking (strokes lasting 1.5 seconds) has been shown to have long-term beneficial effects on blood pressure and irritability thresholds (Lund et al., 2002), appearing to counter the adverse effects of prenatal stress in rats (Holst et al., 2002). Such stimulation has also been shown to exert an anti-anxiety effect (Windle et al., 1997), and repeated exposures to oxytocin-releasing stimulations help to restrain HPA-system activity (Peterrson et al., 1999). These findings strongly support the hypothesis that supplemental rhythmic massage and tactile stimulation may be of significant benefit for promoting an adaptive response to stress.

Exposure to Separation

Distress vocalization in response to separation from mother and littermates rapidly increases after 21 days and peaks at 31 days (Gurski et al., 1979). Elliot and Scott (1961) found that repeated early exposure to separation distress progressively enhanced the puppy's ability to cope with isolation in a strange place (see *Social Attachment and Separation* in Volume 2, Chapter 2). Puppies exposed to weekly 10-minute periods of separation beginning at week 3 and continuing through week 12 exhibited the least amount of distress when tested at week 12 in comparison to puppies first exposed to separation at weeks 6, 9, and 12. Twelve-week-old puppies that had not been previously exposed to separation were found to be highly reactive to isolation, showing a steady increase in separation distress over the 10-minute test period. Puppies previously exposed to separation appeared to have learned how to cope more effectively with it, exhibiting much less distress. Although puppies can habituate to isolation as the result of repeated exposure to uneventful separations, this capacity appears to develop slowly and may not be functional until a puppy is 7 or 8 weeks of age (Hetts, 1989). Interestingly, in contrast to Elliot and Scott's findings, Hetts found that 12-week-old puppies, despite a previous lack of exposure to separation, showed a distinctive pattern of inhibition involving a decrease in distress vocalization

and activity when isolated for the first time at week 12. Further, when tested at week 16, these puppies not previously exposed to isolation from weeks 4 to 12 produced significantly fewer distress vocalizations than did puppies repeatedly exposed to isolation consisting of 10 minutes/day for 6 days a week over that same period. These findings obviously conflict with those of Elliot and Scott, suggesting the need for additional research to resolve the question concerning the optimal procedure for exposing puppies to separation.

Hetts' findings seem to suggest that separation distress is relatively immune to habituation effects from week 4 to week 8, which is interesting with respect to onset of weaning. The finding that naive 12-week-old puppies showed less distress vocalization and activity during the first 30 minutes of testing at week 12 than did puppies previously exposed to isolation is consistent with an emergent inhibitory fear response associated with a strange place. Under natural conditions, distress vocalizations might attract danger, making its inhibition an appropriate response given the circumstances and the puppy's age. For example, if feral, a 12-week-old puppy might be left alone for long periods at a relatively unfamiliar rendezvous site without the mother's protection, requiring that it remain quiet and inconspicuous until her return. A genetically programmed timetable for a reduction in distress vocalization at around week 12 would make evolutionary sense. The lack of a comparable or better reduction in distress vocalization in the group of puppies repeatedly exposed to isolation might be attributable to an habituation effect reducing the puppy's fear of the isolation situation, thereby causing it to feel more relaxed to express its discontent. However, these puppies did show a significant reduction in distress vocalization as the result of habituation from week 8 to week 12, whereas a third group of puppies, isolated for 1 hour/week over the 8-week period, did not show evidence of a reduction in distress vocalization and showed no difference with respect to activity level in comparison to the frequently and repeatedly exposed group. This finding seems to indicate that while 1 hour of exposure was sufficient to habituate fear toward the isolation situation, it was not sufficient to habituate separation distress.

Finally, Hetts' results suggest that a puppy's ability to cope with separation distress may significantly improve as it matures, a finding that lends some credence to Slabbert and Rasa's suggestion that adoption delayed until week 12 is less stressful and yields health benefits (Slabbert and Rasa, 1993) (see *Adoption and Stress*). Perhaps, in the case of households in which a puppy will be exposed to a great deal of daily separation and isolation, delaying adoption to week 12 might be preferable to adoption during week 7, but only if the preadoption situation provides the puppy with adequate socialization and training in preparation for its future home life (e.g., house training).

Punishment and Separation

Increased attachment and inordinate separation distress may paradoxically result from excessive disciplinary interaction. Fisher (1955) found that puppies that were exposed to a combination of social indulgence and punishment exhibited the most pronounced dependency and proximity-seeking behavior (see *Separation Distress and Coactive Influences* in Volume 2, Chapter 4). A pattern of excessively punitive and indulgent interaction occurring early in the socialization process may predispose a dog to show social conflict and reactive behavior in adulthood. Such interaction may sensitize pathways associated with threat-avoidance behavior and produce a conflict-laden attachment with the owner. During punitive interaction, the owner, otherwise a source of comfort and safety, temporarily becomes a serious threat from which the puppy seeks protection, often by soliciting it from the owner in the form of fearful submission displays—a social conflict dynamic that may be permanently codified into a problematic stress-antistress mosaic of neuropeptide activity (see *Developmental Adversity and Adjustment*). Later, under the influence of social transactions involving emotional exchanges or loss at separation, these stress-antistress factors may express themselves in adult coping responses that may include persistently intrusive and excitable behaviors, on

the one hand, and intensely emotional, provocative, and reactive behaviors, on the other. Excessively indulgent and punitive interaction contributes to the intensification of a problematic and conflicted attachment process. Scott (1992) points out the potency of both attractive and aversive interaction to facilitate attachment by way of a general hypothesis:

> The occurrence of any strong emotion, whether pleasant or noxious, will speed up and intensify the process of attachment. (84)

Overattachment involving excessive indulgence and punitive interaction may result in a developmental fixation and a regressive dependency and intolerance for separation from the owner, or foster an adversarial and conflict-prone relationship, perhaps setting into motion social dynamics conducive to adult aggression problems, or both. Alternating between intense emotional stimulation of hedonically opposite and incompatible valences, especially when delivered indulgently and noncontingently (e.g., belated punishment) is highly destructive and without justification. Ultimately, the degree of harm resulting from such treatment depends on hereditary factors and subsequent behavioral support. Dogs genetically expressing low fear or anger thresholds may be particularly vulnerable to the lasting effects resulting from mistreatment.

ATTACHMENT AND SEPARATION PROBLEMS: PUPPIES

Adoption and Stress

Sudden changes in routine (e.g., amount of attention, exercise, or restriction) that a dog is accustomed to receive may produce significant biological stress, perhaps inducing emotional and behavioral disturbances in predisposed dogs. For example, moving a dog, accustomed to sleeping in a crate in the kitchen, to a bedroom may result in intense restlessness and inability to calm down. Some dogs pace, pant, and drool, appearing highly distressed by the change. Although puppies appear to be much more resilient and adaptable than adult dogs to change, it is reasonable to assume that separation-related distress associated with adoption may produce lasting adverse effects if not properly managed. The timing of adoption and placement of puppies may also have a strong effect on development, health, and behavior. Slabbert and Rasa (1993) found that German shepherd puppies removed from their mothers at week 6 thrived poorly and showed a significantly greater risk for disease and mortality than did puppies naturally weaned by their mother between weeks 7 and 8. They also exhibited significant behavioral deficits: "Puppies weaned before 7 weeks of age are noisy and nervous. These seem to become fixed characteristics of the dog for life" (5).

Puppies allowed to stay with their mothers through week 12 were healthier, gained more weight, and appeared better adapted. However, the significance of early adoption on the incidence of SDS has been questioned. For example, Flannigan and Dodman (2001) were unable to detect a correlation between early adoption (earlier than 7 weeks of age) and an increased risk of developing separation-related problems in comparison to other behavior problems. The authors do, however, leave open the possibility that puppies adopted at an early age may be generally more susceptible to behavior problems. Deferring adoption until week 12 conflicts with standard practice, and any potential benefit of delayed adoption would depend on the quality of socialization, habituation, and training taking place during those critical weeks while a puppy remains under the breeder's control. Ideally, a dog destined to become a family companion should be placed at around week 7, based on a number of compelling scientific considerations, practical management issues (e.g., house training), and social bonding benefits (see *Secondary Socialization (6 to 12 Weeks)* in Volume 1, Chapter 2). As previously discussed (see *Exposure to Separation*), an exception to the week 7 rule of thumb rule might involve puppies destined to households in which they will be exposed to lengthy daily separations and isolation.

From a familiar environment and social setting, a newly adopted puppy is thrust into quite a different situation of unfamiliar sights, sounds, smells, and social demands. In addition to environmental strangeness,

this new situation is probably governed by rules and expectations that sharply conflict with previous learning and social experiences. Some dogs may never fully overcome this momentous loss of filial kinship and sense of security. In combination, the abrupt loss of affiliative bonds and loss of place attachments may create a highly stressful state of disorientation and confusion, perhaps verging on helplessness when coupled with adverse rearing practices (see *Adverse Rearing Practices That May Predispose Dogs to Develop Separation-related Problems* in Volume 2, Chapter 4). Helplessness and excessive dependency are natural behavioral corollaries of excessive confinement and punishment during puppyhood.

Although many factors play a role in the development of separation-related anxiety and panic in adult dogs, the manner in which this original separation trauma is managed probably plays some role in predisposing vulnerable puppies to develop the adult disorder or helping to prevent it. Obviously, there is a natural tendency for puppies to rely on previously acquired behavior patterns in an effort to cope with the demands of family life. Some of these behaviors are conducive to a harmonious transition, while others may set the groundwork for significant interactive conflict and potential problems. Despite the potential pitfalls and difficulties, it is truly remarkable how well most puppies navigate the transition into family life, underscoring the average puppy's high degree of behavioral and emotional flexibility. Clearly, the young dog is very adaptable and, when problems do occur, more often than not they are the result of improper training or mismanagement. With these considerations in mind, it makes sense to provide newly adopted puppies with careful transitional handling and training in an effort to reduce the amount of stress associated with adoption. The first step in making a successful transition is to recognize that the puppy is probably experiencing significant stress and disorientation, despite outward signs that may seem to indicate otherwise. The energetic and rough efforts of children to play with a new puppy are probably not beneficial. What the puppy needs during the transitional period is gentle handling, nourishment, and quiet surroundings, especially for the first few days.

Coping with Stress at Separation

A significant source of emotional distress for puppies is associated with the strain and upset elicited by separation and confinement (Borchelt, 1989). The average puppy has not had very much prior experience with being left alone and may not cope well with even brief periods of separation. For many puppies, learning to cope with loneliness and isolation without excessive worry and distress is a hard lesson for them to master, and their success will depend on the patient guidance and support of understanding owners. Initially, the puppy should be allowed to sleep in the bedroom, and only gradually moved to another part of house—if such an *unnatural* arrangement is necessary. If available from the breeder, a familiar soft toy or towel possessing the odor of the mother may help to pacify the puppy at bedtime and when left alone during the daytime. One possible method for breeders to explore is to associate the mother with a distinctive dilute odor throughout the nursing period. The odor can then be bottled and given to the owner to spray on bedding and so forth, perhaps providing some relief to the puppy at times when it needs to be left alone. Alternatively, the breeder may wipe the mother from head to toe with a damp cloth and rinse it in a quart of spring water. Wiping the area of the intermammary line may be particularly useful, since it is reportedly associated with the production of appeasing pheromones in lactating dogs (see *Dog-appeasing Pheromone*). The water can be stored in a spray bottle (refrigerated) and applied to bedding and locations where the puppy is confined.

Confinement

Confinement is useful for facilitating early house-training efforts, to prevent household damage, and for the sake of the puppy's safety in the owner's absence. This will require that the puppy be introduced to some amount of crate confinement. It is important that the puppy form a positive place attachment with the crate. The crate should be equipped with soft toys (stuffed animals and knotted towels) and blanketing—all of which may help to pacify and relax the puppy. In addition, some puppies may benefit from a mirror securely attached to the outside of the crate or nearby wall. Although most puppies can be trained to accept crate confinement without too much trouble, some may rebel despite the most patient and systematic efforts to desensitize them. Such persistent and demanding puppies may find crate confinement highly frustrating and vigorously protest against it. It is important to exercise careful judgment here and not mistake frustrative protests against confinement as separation-related panic. Vocalizations associated with separation-related panic are not under the same degree of voluntary control as vocalizations exhibited by difficult and frustrated puppies. In such cases, exposure to crate confinement might be carried out via a folding pen that is gradually made smaller, while the crate is made attractive and comfortable.

Many crate-training problems can be avoided by slowly introducing such confinement through gradual steps (see *Crate Training* in Chapter 2). Finally, regardless of the reasons for confining a puppy, it should be done in a part of the house that is familiar to the puppy (e.g., the kitchen or bedroom). The highly questionable practice of isolating the puppy or family dog in the basement or garage during daily absences is associated with an increased risk of heightened separation distress and panic.

All normal puppies are stressed by separation and may vent their displeasure through intense vocalizations aimed at getting the owner's attention or engage in other activities (e.g., chewing baby gates) aimed at securing contact. Allowing a puppy to persist in such stressful isolation behavior may inadvertently potentiate separation-distress reactions. On the other hand, routinely responding to such protests with affectionate reassurance or by releasing the puppy from confinement may only serve to reinforce such unwanted behavior. Diverting the puppy with a treat or sound (e.g., a squeak) and requiring that it remain quiet for some brief period before releasing it is probably better than just rescuing it at such times. Although the puppy's sensitivity to isolation usually decreases as it matures, it is still important that the puppy learn how to cope with such situations without experiencing excessive distress. This is usually accomplished through graduated exposure and desensitization. Training a puppy to accept isolation is accomplished by scheduling opportunities for social contact, exercise, and play in exchange for short periods of confinement and separation—a process that is carried out concurrently with early crate training. Separation training instructs the puppy to anticipate regular attention and contact based on contingent waiting and quiet behavior. Although intensive affection, stroking, massage, and feeding by hand may help to counter the stress associated with adoption, social contact should gradually approximate the amounts of attention and contact that will likely be provided to the dog as an adult.

Graduated Departures

Graduated exposure to brief and nonthreatening separation experiences may help to immunize a puppy against the stressful effects of more lengthy separation (Voith, 1980; Marks, 1987). Training a puppy to accept limited exposure to separation can be accomplished by gradually exposing it to increasing periods of crate or pen confinement. The crate or pen should be placed in a room where the puppy is left when the owner is away from home. Once the puppy can tolerate being left alone in the room, the next step is for the owner to begin leaving the house for varying lengths of time, thereby gradually increasing the puppy's tolerance for owner departures and absences. The goal of such training is to help the puppy to anticipate the owner's return optimistically while systematically reducing its aversion to being left alone. These safe and relaxed planned departure activities help the puppy to learn that separation is temporary and that the owner's eventual return is certain. Gradually, the puppy develops more positive expectations about separation events, learning to tolerate departures and to wait patiently for the eventual return of the absent owner.

From the very beginning, safety stimuli or bridges should be paired with every safe departure experience. Safety stimuli can be easily established by associating short, nonanxious departures with an auditory, visual, or olfactory stimulus (e.g., a scent associated with the mother or used during massage). Safety stimuli appear to give the puppy some sense of security when it must be left alone, perhaps by forecasting the owner's eventual return or by evoking conditioned associations of comfort and safety. The goal is to establish a positive association between safe separation experiences and ambient contextual stimuli. Also, just before leaving, the puppy is given a highly prized chew item made available primarily at such times (e.g., a hollow rubber toy slathered with peanut butter). With the puppy distracted by the toy, the owner turns on a radio or television and light and exists the room. After a brief separation, the owner returns, turns off the radio or television and light, goes to the puppy, and retrieves the chew toy. At the conclusion of a safe departure, the puppy is given a brief period of tug or fetch play, especially if signs of building stress are evident.

The aforementioned pattern of departure and return is repeated again and again, increasing and randomly varying the duration of departures. Care should be taken not to proceed too quickly, and closely observe the puppy for any signs of distress. If the puppy becomes distressed, the handler should return to a previously successful step and try again. In the case of highly sensitive and reactive puppies, the process of introducing safe and relaxed departures might begin by merely scooting back a foot or 2 before returning to the puppy to reward it. Standing up and walking 2 or 3 steps back and waiting for a 5 or 10 seconds before returning might be the next step, followed by a variety of similarly gradual departure steps organized to prevent the puppy from becoming distressed. Sometimes training the puppy to sit-wait and down-wait while in the crate can be useful in the context of planned departure training, gradually training the puppy to wait for longer durations, at greater distances, and involving progressively more difficult departure exposures (e.g., going around a corner, into another room, and finally outdoors). Varying the duration of separation by interspersing short and long durations randomly is useful [e.g., 30 seconds, 15 seconds, 10 seconds, 1 minute, 20 seconds, 5 seconds, 45 seconds, 1 minute 30 seconds: variable duration (VD), 35 seconds]. The first 20 minutes of separation for a puppy are the most sensitive, with proper confinement training and desensitization focusing on the first 10 to 30 seconds providing a stable foundation and anchor for subsequent counterconditioning efforts. It is not necessary, therefore, to spend long hours desensitizing a puppy to separation, but to concentrate on the first minute or 2, gradually building up to 20 to 40 minutes. As the puppy progresses, add more varied and realistic departure experiences to the program, including picking up keys, slipping on shoes, putting on an overcoat, picking up a briefcase, and so forth (see *Graduated Departures and Separation Distress*).

Planned Separations

In addition to brief, graduated exposure to separation, other benefits may be obtained by exposing a puppy to more protracted periods of safe separation. Poulton and colleagues (2001) have reported that late-adolescent separation anxiety in children is negatively correlated with the number of overnight hospital stays away from home in early childhood, with more overnight stays away from home being associated with a reduced risk of separation anxiety. Also, as one might expect, the longitudinal study found that children exposed to planned hospital stays experienced fewer symptoms of separation anxiety in late adolescence than did counterparts exposed to unplanned hospitalization. The use of dog day care and overnight stays away from home in a safe and supportive environment may provide additional inoculation against adult SDS. Such recommendations should be seriously considered in the case of puppies showing evidence of excessive distress when left alone.

In the case of puppies that need to be left confined to a crate (e.g., needing such confinement for house-training purposes), with a high probability that heightened distress will occur while the owner is absent, a second crate might be used transitionally to avoid

associating stressful arousal with the safe crate (Voith, 2002). In preparation for such departures, the puppy should be given a high-value chew item and put in the crate for at least 5 minutes before leaving. A fragrance such as lavender or chamomile might be sprayed initially and then diffused by means of a diffuser and aquarium pump (see *Taction and Olfactory Conditioning*). Although the author has not yet evaluated the usefulness of dog-appeasing pheromone, it is reportedly helpful in the management of distress at separation in puppies and dogs (see *Dog-appeasing Pheromone*).

During stressful habituation exposures to separation, the owner should avoid returning to the puppy while it is still aversively aroused. Instead, for example, upon returning from an errand, the owner should check first and make sure that the puppy is not vocalizing before entering the house. If the puppy is vocalizing and does not stop, the owner might call the home phone with a cell phone, perhaps momentarily distracting the puppy, whereupon the owner should enter the house and initiate a brief period of attention training (i.e., orienting response to a squeak followed by a click and treat), feeding the puppy through the crate door, but refraining from immediately letting the puppy out. As the puppy shows signs of calming, it is released and tossed a ball or engaged in sit and sit-stay training with a brief attending response, whereafter it is transitioned to the scented safe crate or confinement area. The foregoing method helps to control aversive arousal, enhances attention and impulse control during greetings, and associates opponent relief and relaxation produced by the owner's return with the safe crate and the olfactory safety signal (OSS). Habitually using the cell phone to call home prior to entering the house can establish a potent conditioned safety signal by association with the owner's homecoming. Alternatively, a remote doorbell and the sound of the garage door opening can be used to serve a similar purpose. The sound of the garage opening, the doorbell, and the phone are naturally conditioned in association with increased social activity and transition and can be used in a variety of creative ways as diversionary stimuli to manage puppy and dog behavior.

Miscellaneous Recommendations

Taking measures to reduce or prevent separation distress is an important aspect of puppy rearing. In addition to the aforementioned recommendations, the following list of suggestions should be considered:

- Avoid excessively emotional interaction that might lead a puppy to become overly attached and dependent. Although a young puppy needs a great deal of attention and affection, the character of this attention need not be indulgent. Constructive interaction involving various training activities, walks, and instructive play is much better than just providing gratuitous affection and unearned treats.
- When leaving a puppy alone for extended periods, the puppy should be confined to well-socialized part of the house (e.g., the kitchen). Ideally, the puppy should be restrained in an exercise pen equipped with an open crate made comfortable with bedding. The floor of the penned area should be covered with several layers of newspapers for the inevitable accidents. *Do not restrict water.* Make an audio tape of the puppy's reaction to separation, thereby providing some baseline information about the puppy's response to it and improvement (or not) over time.
- Avoid overemotional departures and homecomings. Approximately 5 to 10 minutes before leaving the puppy, it should be placed in the pen and given a highly desirable chew item that is not provided at other times. Giving the puppy periodic treats during this time can help calm it. Puppies appear to benefit from the presence of a towel richly scented with the owner's body odor. Also, it may be useful to direct the puppy's attention to the towel as an object of play and contact when the owner returns home. Puppies prone to become overly aroused should receive 1 to 3 minutes of massage just before being confined and then again after homecomings.

- Avoid punishing a puppy for destructive behavior or elimination occurring during absences. Such punishment will not impact beneficially on the misbehavior and may make the situation worse. In general, aversive training methods should be minimized or avoided (if possible) during the transitional period immediately following adoption.

As a puppy develops, it will naturally become more confident and independent, with the puppy appearing to develop improved abilities to cope with safe separation exposure between weeks 8 and 12 (Hetts, 1989). With maturation, separation reactions usually decrease in intensity, unless—because of excessive frustration, inappropriate punishment, or inadvertent reinforcement—the puppy learns to persist in such undesirable behavior. With maturation, reactive separation behavior usually moderates as a secure and balanced social relationship is established between the owner and the dog. However, as the result of adverse interaction (e.g., social frustration, inappropriate punishment, or inadvertent reinforcement), the dog may form a problematic attachment and express persistent separation-related distress when left alone. The social competence provided by structured integrated compliance training, in combination with habituation and graduated exposure to separation events with counterconditioning, appears to exert an ameliorative and preventive effect on separation distress. However, extensive early socialization and training efforts away from the home may not be beneficial. According to Bradshaw and colleagues (2002), extensive exposure to varied social contacts at approximately month 3, involving persons not belonging to the family, strangers, or children, may predispose puppies to exhibit problematic separation-related behavior between months 6 and 9. Conversely, extensive social exposure between months 6 and 9 appears to exert a protective influence by reducing the risk of subsequent separation-related behavior. These findings suggest the possibility that socialization with varied people and situations away from the home in early puppyhood (e.g., puppy socialization classes) may not be beneficial with respect to separation-related adjustments, whereas added separation-related benefits may be obtained as the result of attending group training classes and providing diversified socialization experiences after month 5 or 6.

McBride and colleagues (1995) have reported that dogs (N = 44) rehomed from an animal shelter between 6 and 12 months may be at greater risk of developing separation-related behavior problems than dogs adopted in other age groups. Perhaps, during this important developmental transition between puppyhood and adulthood, there exists a period of increased vulnerability to the emotional effects of attachment and separation. However, another possible association may exist that should receive additional research. This time frame is commonly associated with neutering, a procedure that has been implicated as a potential risk factor in the development of separation problems. Flannigan and Dodman (2001) have found that sexually intact dogs were three times less likely to exhibit separation problems than neutered counterparts (male and female). With respect to the influence of sheltering on the incidence of separation-related problems, in addition to the traumatic loss of attachment objects suffered by the relinquished dog, the sheltered dog may subsequently form strong place and social attachments with the shelter environment and workers. In addition, the daily stimulation of cleanup, feeding, and other care activities, the presence of other dogs, periodic visits, and exercise opportunities may significantly contrast with the humdrum loneliness of the adoptive home environment. Sheltered dogs appear to form rapid attachments, requiring as few as three meetings with

a stranger consisting of 10 minutes each to show a significant increase in attachment behavior (Gácsi et al., 2001). A shelter dog may be sensitized in various ways to attachment processes that predispose it to become emotionally vulnerable when left alone.

PART 2: SEPARATION DISTRESS AND PANIC: TREATMENT PROCEDURES AND PROTOCOLS

ATTACHMENT AND SEPARATION PROBLEMS: ADULT DOGS

Most dogs appear to accept daily exposure to long periods of separation without showing excessive distress. Separation-reactive dogs, however, exhibit a distinct and persistent pattern of generalized arousal, protest, or excessive worry when left alone. SDS is identified by a cluster of diagnostic signs and symptoms involving a variety of biobehavioral modalities, including appetitive, oral, vocal, motor, eliminative, and physiological changes (Table 4.1).

Diagnostic Signs of Separation Distress

Few dogs exhibit all of the aforementioned signs listed, but many show more than one sign, and it is not uncommon for separation-distressed dogs to exhibit several of the behavioral signs of distress whenever they are left alone. Owners should be encouraged to maintain a behavioral journal, including a record of separation-related behavior in order to produce an objective assessment of the benefits of training and behavior therapy (Figure 4.6).

TABLE. 4.1. Diagnostic signs of separation-distress syndrome (SDS)

Excessive attachment (clinging behavior)

Predeparture restlessness

Separation-distress vocalization (e.g., barking and howling)

Destructive behavior only when left alone

Self-injurious behavior

Urination and defecation only when the owner leaves

Separation-related loss of appetite

Excessive greeting behavior

DOG'S NAME: DATE:

DAILY SEPARATION-DISTRESS RECORD
(ELIMINATION, DESTRUCTIVENESS, VOCALIZATION)

WEEK	ELIMINATION	DESTRUCTIVENESS	VOCALIZATION
	M T W T F S S	M T W T F S S	M T W T F S S
1			
	M T W T F S S	M T W T F S S	M T W T F S S
2			
	M T W T F S S	M T W T F S S	M T W T F S S
3			
	M T W T F S S	M T W T F S S	M T W T F S S
4			
	M T W T F S S	M T W T F S S	M T W T F S S
5			
	M T W T F S S	M T W T F S S	M T W T F S S
6			

COMMENTS:

FIG. 4.6. Daily separation-distress chart. The day of the week is checked and a brief note concerning the separation-related behavior is recorded (time of day, location, object, and duration, and so forth).

Appetitive Signs

Separation-distressed dogs are usually anorexic. Some will even ignore a fresh beef bone or other highly prized food items until the owner returns. Separation-induced anorexia can be very problematic when it involves dogs being boarded or hospitalized.

Oral Signs

Many separation-distressed dogs are destructive when they are left alone. Among 200 dogs presenting with separation-related problems at Tufts Animal Behavior Clinic, destructive behavior was the most common complaint, with 71.7% of the dogs showing some form of household destructiveness when left alone (Flannigan and Dodman, 2001). These findings roughly correspond to those reported by Voith and colleagues (1997), in which the most common complaint associated with separation anxiety was destructiveness, followed by excessive vocalization, elimination, aggression, and overactivity. McCrave (1991) has differentiated destructive behaviors occurring with separation distress from destructive behaviors associated with other common etiologies. She has noted that separation-related chewing is typically directed toward points of egress, whereas playful destructive behavior is directed toward items "that are fun to toss or shred" (252), e.g., pillows, furniture cushions, and paper. These latter items are frequently targets of separation-distressed dogs as well, requiring careful analysis of the context and the presence of other signs to determine whether the destructive appetite is due to separation or other causes (see *Assessing Separation-related Problems* in Volume 2, Chapter 4). Separation-reactive dogs often scratch doors and dig at carpets in front of doors. Miller (1966) aptly describes this behavior as *barrier frustration*: "Frustration creates tension and the dog releases this tension, causing a problem like chewing. The single greatest frustration and tension builder is found in barriers, usually the door" (104). In addition to points of egress, destructive chewing is directed toward a wide variety of socially significant objects. In some cases, the chew object chosen by the dog appears to provide a symbolic link with the absent owner. Besides clothing, shoes, books, the television remote, pillows, and the owner's bed, separation-reactive dogs may chew on woodwork, curtains, furniture—almost anything that it can sink its teeth into, except, ironically, the chew toys that have been left for such purposes. Such compulsive chewing activity appears to provide an outlet for anxious feelings. But because the dog often chooses personal belongings as objects to gnaw on, the owner is often convinced that the dog is misbehaving out of spitefulness (Lindell, 1997).

Vocal Signs

Another common complaint associated with SDS is separation-related barking. Although barking is not the most common complaint, it is extremely common among dogs becoming reactive at separation. Voith and colleagues (1997) reported that 90% of separation-anxious dogs (N = 36) barked when left alone, with 80% engaging in destructive behaviors and 55% exhibiting elimination problems. Owners of such dogs are often prompted to seek help as the result of a citation or a neighbor's complaint. Sustained barking and howling are vocalization variations that many separation-reactive dogs exhibit—some to an astonishing extent. It is amazing how long a dog can bark and howl without stopping. Many owners return home daily to find their dog soaked with slobber from hours of agitated barking and panting.

Motor Signs

Many dogs become overactive at separation, with nervous pacing and bursts of frantic motor and exploratory activity occurring periodically during the day.

Eliminative Signs

In cases where the dog exhibits normal eliminatory control while the owner is at home, but loses control only when he or she leaves the house or denies contact to the dog, separation distress should be considered as a putative causal factor underlying the problem. Flannigan and Dodman (2001) reported that 28.1% of dogs with separation anxiety showed some form of inappropriate elimination when left alone.

Physiological Signs

Separation-distressed dogs may exhibit a variety of signs indicating pervasive autonomic arousal, including trembling, panting, increased heart rate and, less frequently, profuse salivation or diarrhea.

In addition to the identification of emotional and behavioral signs of separation distress, dogs with SDS should be screened for phobias, especially noise and storm phobias. Flannigan and Dodman (2001) found that nearly half of dogs with separation-related problems also exhibit evidence of noise phobia. In cases where SDS occurs comorbidly with a phobia, the successful resolution of the separation problem requires that both problems be addressed (see *Prognostic Considerations* in Chapter 3).

Preliminary Considerations

Owners of dogs with separation-related behavior problems must first be convinced that their dog's misbehavior is not motivated by spite or vindictiveness. This is not always easy for one reason or another. Some owners may simply not want to get bogged down with behavioral explanations that portend difficult and time-consuming training efforts; they may have little patience in reserve and want immediate results. Others simply cannot rise above a heartfelt conviction that their dog is punishing them. An astonishing number of dog owners adhere to the belief that dogs often misbehave to spite the owner. In a large study, New and colleagues (2000) found that 48.3% of persons relinquishing their dogs to shelters held that dogs will misbehave to spite their owners, with nearly an equal percentage of owners (44.3%) with a dog living in the household indicating a similar belief concerning the spiteful motivation of canine misbehavior. The implications of spite and vindictiveness are distracting and misleading, but many separation-reactive dogs do appear to be more angry than anxious, appearing to protest at being left alone. Protest is a common behavioral sign of canine separation distress, resulting in persistent vocalization, increased motor activity, and destructive behavior (see *Separation Distress and Coactive Influences: Frustration* in Volume 2, Chapter 4). This situation is compounded when strong external pressures are demanding that the owner achieve results quickly or face dire consequences. Dogs are rarely brought for treatment of separation distress without some pressing behavioral complaint, including neighbor complaints, threats of eviction, or costly citations. What many of these owners want is a ready and easy means to suppress their dog's misbehavior—not a psychological explanation for it. Other owners welcome a scientific understanding of their dog's separation problems and willingly face the prospects of a daunting training process as a challenge and responsibility.

Every situation is a bit different, and it is of immense importance that problems involving separation distress be approached with an appreciation for each case's unique characteristics. Failure to take such matters into consideration will invariably impact adversely on compliance and the overall effectiveness of training efforts. Behavioral counseling is a pragmatic process based on a fluid dialogue between the trainer and the owner, often requiring compromise on minor points in order to build overall support and enthusiasm for the program. An owner's cooperation and confidence is won through a process of gradual persuasion and logical demonstration—not polarizing confrontation and criticism. Pressure tactics—no matter how accurate and brilliant—serve little purpose but to cause the owner to feel resentment toward the trainer. An experienced trainer listens to the owner's needs and assiduously avoids judgmental polemics. The cynopraxic trainer is a mediator showing the owner how to improve the situation, while avoiding narrow and one-sided prescriptions that the owner cannot accept or will not carry out. Consequently, wherever possible, the training program must be modeled to conform to the owner's needs and expectations.

Very few owners are able to implement the current planned-departure protocol for the treatment of separation distress in its entirety or apply it with the sort of diligence that the procedure requires to optimize success. The underlying premise of such training is based on systematic desensitization and graduated counterconditioning. The owner is instructed to leave the dog for progressively longer periods, starting with a few seconds and gradually building the dog's tolerance for longer and longer periods of separation. While undergoing separation desensitization, the owner is instructed never to leave the dog alone under circumstances that may evoke separation distress or panic. This most central requirement is often impossible for owners to comply with, since it may entail considerable expense (e.g., day care or pet sitting) or inconvenience. Occasionally, a neighbor or relative will volunteer to watch the separation-reactive dog while it is undergoing training, but this is usually the exceptional situation rather than the rule.

Effective behavior therapy requires a high degree of competence in the application of a highly technical and exacting methodology. Desensitization procedures, in particular, assume a psychological understanding that may be natural for an applied dog behaviorist, but are often arcane and difficult for a dog owner to master. Most owners presenting their dogs for behavior therapy do not possess the self-discipline or understanding to adhere methodically to a behavioral plan. Describing the most general aspects of the process is easy, but the actual mechanics involved require the development of special skills and knowledge that may not be realistically attained in short-term counseling. Surely, many of the required skills cannot be fully mastered after a single session of counseling, but that is precisely what is often expected of the client-owner by the busy dog behavior therapist. This shortcoming of "brief therapy" may represent a serious danger for the owners of aggressive dogs who are expected to perform advanced behavior-therapy procedures after a single session of counseling. This situation can be somewhat mollified by supplementing verbal instructions with relevant reading material. Many articles and pamphlets have been written on the subject in a language that is accessible to the average owner, but few provide the sort of detailed instruction that would help the owner to apply the procedures mean-

ingfully and consistently. Despite these shortcomings, most owners still report good results from the portion of the behavior protocol that they are able to carry out; even a few simple tips over the phone appear to help a great deal in some cases.

In addition to recording a thorough behavioral history, assessing separation distress is assisted by making an audio tape recording of the dog's reaction to separation. Besides monitoring the dog's behavior during a specific time frame and getting a picture of the sorts of things the dog does during separation, such recordings provide a baseline from which to gauge training progress or lack thereof. Although not all separation-anxious dogs bark or howl, a great many do, but even those that do not will often exhibit other signs of agitation that can be picked up by an audio recorder. A motion-activated video recorder can also be extremely useful for assessing separation behavior and tracking a dog's progress (Figure 4.7). Also, the owner should be encouraged to keep a behavioral journal for recording daily training activities and noting the dog's response to behavior-therapy efforts, such as planned-departure training. Records of planned departures should include the date and time, the length of departure, and a brief description of the dog's behavior (Figure 4.8).

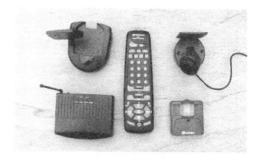

FIG. 4.7. Motion-activated remote video system. Inexpensive video devices are available to record a dog's separation activities throughout the day. A motion-sensitive infrared detector turns on a remote VCR and turns it off again after a short period. A similar device could be devised to activate an air-pump odor dispenser and feeder described in Chapter 3 (see *Systematic Desensitization*, Figure 3.5).

DOG'S NAME:			DATE:
SESSION NO.:			

PLANNED DEPARTURE CHART

T R I A L	LOCATION	DURATION	DOG'S RESPONSE	PROBLEMS
1				
2				
3				
4				
5				
6				
7				

COMMENTS:

FIG. 4.8. Planned departure chart.

Behavioral training for separation-reactive dogs involves a variant application of systematic desensitization and instrumental training (Hothersall and Tuber, 1979). Departures are planned and graduated in such a way that the dog progressively learns to anticipate the owner's eventual return without experiencing excessive worry or distress. In additon, more appropriate waiting behavior is systematically reinforced. The systematic desensitization portion of this plan may be superfluous, especially if it is determined that the dog's separation problems are motivated by frustration and protest. If fear is determined to play a role, then it may be more profitable to identify the fear-eliciting stimulus and desensitize the dog to it first, rather than attempting to desensitize the dog to separation while it continues to remain fearful of the situation. As already noted, in practice systematic desensitization by way of graduated departures is nearly impossible for the average dog owner to carry out. Very few people have the luxury to take two or three weeks away from work to administer a dog's desensitization training. Nonetheless, meaningful progress can be made by performing graduated departures while at home with the dog, counterconditioning predeparture cues, focusing efforts on shaping more appropriate predeparture behavior, and employing various techniques to improve the quality of attachment and interaction between the owner and the dog.

Summary of Behavioral Procedures Used to Modify Separation Distress

Podberscek and colleagues (1999) found that behavior modification without medication was effective for controlling behavior problems associated with separation-related distress. The eclectic program that they recommend involves four phases of therapy (Table 4.2). King and colleagues (2000) have described a similar treatment program used in conjunction with clomipramine, which they divide into these areas of focus:

At-home interaction
- Dog is ignored during greetings until it calms down.
- All forms of retroactive punishment should be discontinued.
- All interaction between owner and dog must be initiated by the owner.
- Attention-seeking efforts by the dog should be ignored.
- Touching and playing with the dog are restricted to interaction on the command and initiative of the owner.
- Dog may sleep in the bedroom at the owner's initiative.

Departure procedures
- The dog is ignored for 30 minutes prior to departure.
- The dog is confined to the location where it must stay for the day 30 minutes prior to leaving.
- The dog is provided with toys and an object impregnated with the owner's scent.
- The owner is instructed to practice false departure routines in which preparations to leave are not followed by the owner actually leaving the house.

Other common treatment recommendations include graduated departures (Voith, 1980; Voith and Borchelt, 1985), involving progressively longer and more realistic departure exposures, muzzling the dog while the owner is away from home (Polin, 1992), and lengthy daily crate confinement (Takeuchi et al., 2000). Muzzling separation-reactive dogs is of questionable value and represents a significant risk of harm to such dogs (e.g., aspiration of vomit and heat exhaustion). Separation-distressed dogs become highly excited, and panting helps to regulate building body and brain temperatures. Restricting the dog's ability to pant may result in it overheating, with devastating results. Also, highly reactive dogs may become virtually obsessed with getting the muzzle off, possibly doing significant damage to themselves in the process. The so-called *denning* method involves the following stages of crate confinement (Takeuchi et al., 2000):

- The dog is confined to its crate continuously for 2 weeks, except for elimination, exercise, and obedience training.
- The dog is confined for an additional 2 weeks except when the owner is at home and awake.
- The dog is confined for an additional 2 weeks only when the owner is away.
- The crate door is left open at all times, permitting the dog to come and go as it pleases.

The use of crate confinement for treating SDS is fraught with dangers and raises a number of welfare concerns. Voith and Borchelt (1985) have criticized the use of crate confinement for treating separation-related behavior as usually being counterproductive. In addition to persisting in the unwanted separation behavior, dogs confined in crates may severely injure themselves in an effort to escape confinement. When the crate is used, it should be introduced gradually and then faded out again as the dog's behavior improves, making every effort not to allow it to become a steel straitjacket (see *Adverse Effects of Excessive Confinement* in Chapter 2).

The methods used to treat SDS are often very restrictive and highly intrusive with respect to the human-dog relationship. Given the limited behavioral acumen of owners and questionable compliance patterns, it is hard to imagine that owners actual carry out some of the required treatment recommendations. In addition to complexity, procedures that intrude excessively upon the owner's ability to interact, play, and exchange affection with the dog spontaneously may simply be more aver-

TABLE. 4.2. Summary of separation procedures recommended by Podberscek et al. (1999)

Phase 1

Retroactive punishment is discontinued.

The dog is stopped from sitting on a lap or furniture when owner is nearby.

The dog is prevented access to the bedroom by baby gate first and then by closed door.

Gratuitous treats are discontinued.

Only the owner initiates interaction with the dog.

The dog's solicitations for attention are ignored.

Interaction between the owner and dog ceases 1 hour prior to departure.

When ready to depart, the owner waits an additional 10 to 15 minutes before leaving the house.

The dog is confined 20 to 30 minute before departure.

The dog is provided with clothing imbued with the owner's scent, given chew toys that are not otherwise available, tape recordings of owners voice are switched on, and the dog is ignored when the owner leaves the home.

Upon returning home, the owner should change clothing and wait 5 to 10 minutes before releasing the dog from confinement.

The dog's greeting behavior is ignored.

Phase 2

The dog is exposed to progressive and varying periods of separation from the owner while it is at home and awake.

The dog is separated by a door or gate (if separation by closing a door stresses the dog).

The dog is prevented from following the owner around the house.

The dog is prevented access to the upstairs (bedroom) during the day.

Phase 3

The dog is gradually removed from proximity to the bedroom at night and required to sleep in areas progressively closer to the area where the dog is confined during the day.

Phase 4

Predeparture cue desensitization and scrambling are used, e.g., picking up keys, putting on shoes or outdoor clothing, and setting burglar alarm, but not actually leaving the dog.

sive to the owner than the problem itself. In this regard, Takeuchi and colleagues (2000) found that more instructions were not necessarily associated with increased therapeutic benefit. In fact, owners given fewer than five instructions reported significantly better improvement in their dogs' behavior than owners given more than five instructions. Owner compliance was not a significant factor in the outcome of treatment. The significance of the study is hard to pin down, though, since owners who received more instruction may have presented a more severe and intractable problem in the first place. Nonetheless, a possibility exists that owners simply became progressively confused with more instructions or more inclined not to comply.

Aside from social intrusiveness, the implementation of common animal behavior-therapy procedures often involves significant changes in routine and restriction taking place over a very brief period. Stephens (1980) has suggested that abrupt changes in the direction of increased restriction or greater freedom may produce psychological stress, perhaps inclining some sensitive dogs to develop emotional and physiological disturbances. Dramatic loss of attention, contact, and freedom of movement may produce pronounced stress in already reactive separation-distressed dogs. Highly intrusive and restrictive methods of therapy may reduce undesirable behavior by generally shutting the dog down and thereby elaborating a generalized inhibitory state incompatible with separation-related excesses and distress: depression. The detachment process often recommended may not significantly alter a dog's attachment levels, as much as simply depressing the dog by the abrupt change in routine, social loss, and anxiety: previously predictable social interaction is suspended and replaced with physical and rule-based barriers designed to disrupt or prevent normal contact comfort and attention. The influence must certainly be destabilizing for highly attached and insecure dogs. To make therapeutic recommendations effective and humane, changes involving social loss and increased restriction should be implemented gradually and only after other less intrusive methods are carefully considered or tried. The

keys to successful behavior therapy are simplicity and respect for the human-dog bond.

Crate Confinement

Despite the dangers and risks involved, crate confinement may prove to be a necessary part of the management of separation-distressed dogs, especially in cases involving destructive problems. Although increased anxiety or frustration may be initially evoked by the introduction of the crate, it is often an unavoidable part of the separation training process. The key here is to introduce the crate gradually together with the provision of comfort objects and appetizing toys over several days (see *Crate Training* in Chapter 2). Treats and toys can be put inside the crate in hopes of tempting the dog to explore it. In addition, the dog can be fed in front and later inside of the crate. In some cases, food is given to the dog only when the owner is about to leave, thereby compelling it to eat while alone and in the crate. Frozen rice balls containing turkey burger and kibble may be useful for this purpose. Rubber toys can also be stuffed with moist food and frozen.

Once the dog is entering the crate on its own accord, the door can be closed for brief periods while giving it treats from the outside. As the dog learns to accept crate confinement by freely entering it, a signal can be established to control the behavior (e.g., "Crate" followed by a hand movement similar to the one used to toss a treat inside the crate). Next, the dog should learn to enter and lie down in the crate for varying lengths of time. These initial exposures to crate confinement should involve a close association with the owner. The owner may lie down next to the dog while it is crated and periodically pet or feed the dog treats. These initial nonexclusionary exposures to crate confinement help the dog to form a positive place attachment toward the crate. As training progresses, the crate will gradually become a place of security and crate confinement a safety signal predicting the owner's eventual return. The crate also offers an effective response-prevention strategy in which the undesirable destructive behavior is blocked while other counterconditioning efforts are carried out. Once the dog becomes better adapted to being left alone and the risk of destructiveness is reduced, crate confinement can be gradually faded out and the dog given more freedom to move about in the safe room.

The air-pump odor dispenser and feeder described in Chapter 3 (see *Systematic Desensitization*, Figure 3.5) can also be used to facilitate planned-departure training in separation-reactive dogs. The air pump can be used to deliver odor only or food only by clamping the tubing at appropriate points. Food-only delivery can be accomplished by completely closing the three-way valve. A remote switch can be used for remote activation. The presentation of the odor (e.g., orange or lemon-orange mixture) with safe departures and returns of the owner will gradually cause it to become an OSS. When the dog must be left alone for periods that exceeds its tolerance and is likely to result in high levels of distress, the odor should not be presented. The odor should only be used to overlap safe departures. Positive associations can also be formed between the odor and the presentation of food that may be useful for facilitating more relaxed and contented behavior. Perhaps, in the future, inexpensive timers will be available that can be used to turn on the pump periodically for brief and variable periods of time during the day to deliver the conditioned odor and food. Dilute odors such as lavender and chamomile may exert unconditioned mood-enhancing effects when delivered by diffuser.

Graduated Departures and Separation Distress

Many separation problems can be worked out without crate confinement, but usually some room or safe area (e.g., pen) is selected where the dog can be kept when left alone. In some cases, however, the crate may provide a secure place attachment from which to organize separation-related treatment activities. Before staging actual departures, the dog is first exposed to a series of planned-departure rehearsals while confined or crated in a separate room and the owner waiting in another part of the house. The room chosen for this purpose should be the same one used for con-

finement purposes when the dog is left alone during the day. Usually, a bedroom or kitchen is selected for such purposes, mainly because the dog has probably already formed significant place attachments or other positive associations with those areas. Both places appear to evoke strong and beneficial contextual effects. The bedroom, for example, may elicit relaxation and other effects associated with sleep, while the kitchen may be associated with a number of social and appetitive interests for the dog. The room is provided with a rug or blanket, a towel scented with the owner's odor, and other accoutrements to create a safe, comfortable, and relaxing ambience. Isolating a separation-reactive dog in a remote part of the house (e.g., the basement or garage) or outside on a chain is not only counterproductive, but may be dangerous and should be avoided. During rehearsal departures, the dog is left in the safe room for progressively longer periods, as determined by its tolerance and ability to cope with separation. It is important to keep these programmed separations brief enough to prevent the dog from becoming overly distressed or frustrated. Responding to the dog at such times by releasing it or attempting to calm it should also be carefully avoided. Frustrative persistence can be maintained on a surprisingly lean schedule of reinforcement. On the other hand, allowing the dog to persist in demanding barking or frenetic efforts to escape confinement is also inappropriate.

Barking behavior can often be interrupted with a squeaker followed by a click and treat when the dog defers its attention. Subsequent rewards are delivered in accordance with a DRO schedule such that the reward is produced only if barking does not occur during some brief period (2, 3, 10, 5, 7, 3, 5, 8, 15 seconds, and so forth on a variable basis). The only requirement put on the dog is that it not bark during the no-bark period. Alternatively, the barking behavior can be brought under stimulus control before off-cue barking is extinguished in accordance with instructions discussed in Chapter 5 (see *Barking*). If barking occurs, "Quiet," the vocal signal discriminating the no-bark contingency, is introduced or a firm "Enough" is spoken in a sharp and clipped manner, if a stronger impression is needed. Again, at brief intervals, the dog is prompted to "Speak" and rewarded. The procedure is repeated many times in order to establish the necessary associative linkages. However, if despite such efforts the dog continues to bark, it may be necessary to employ a disrupter-type event or startle technique to stop the behavior from escalating (see *Guidelines for Successful Crate Training: Step 3* in Chapter 2).

Although many more or less sophisticated procedures can be employed for this purpose (e.g., a remote-activated citronella collar), the most simple and effective tool is a shaker can. The following recommendations assume that the dog has been habituated to the crate or safe room and that the undesirable behavior is likely driven by frustration. The shaker can (see *Miscellaneous Items* in Chapter 1) is introduced by tossing it near the dog while it is barking or attempting to escape confinement. The startling experience will sensitize the dog to the sound of the can, making its rattle an effective disruptive stimulus. Punishment of this sort briefly disrupts and inhibits the barking pattern so that the owner can return and positively reinforce more appropriate behavior. If allowed to bark, many dogs appear to become progressively distressed as the barking continues, but may immediately show signs of relaxation and contentment soon after an effective startle deterrent is applied. The disruptive startle elicited by the shaker can interrupts the cycle of increased arousal and demanding behavior, thereby allowing the owner to reward more cooperative behavior. Some separation-related barking that occurs when the owner is out of sight or outside of the house can be controlled by connecting an inexpensive remote-activated switch to an alarm, radio, or cassette player with a recorded message left on it. The remote switch provides an effective means to disrupt the undesirable behavior without requiring that the owner return to the dog while it is still barking—a potentially highly reinforcing event for a separation-frustrated dog. When the dog stops barking, the owner can return to the dog and reinforce quiet waiting behavior. Ideally, however, programmed separations should progress so gradually that the dog is not unnecessarily challenged or distressed, but

if it does become reactive, the shaker can provides an expedient source of inhibitory control. In balance, allowing a dog to bark at such times may be much more stressful than the inhibitory effects produced by the sound of a shaker can or other moderate deterrents, as necessary to establish control (see *Separation-related Problems and Punishment*).

Once the dog is accepting brief periods of separation without signs of distress, safety stimuli such as a radio, light, or odorant can be introduced. For many dogs, the sound of a radio appears to offer some comfort prior to explicit conditioning efforts, perhaps stemming from an association of such stimulation with the presence of the owner. For some dogs, the television is particularly effective, especially in cases where the owner spends more time watching TV than listening to the radio. However, to obtain maximum benefit of safety signals, they should be systematically associated with minimally stressful separations and returns. The radio and light should be turned on just before the owner leaves the room and turned off just before the dog is released from confinement. A tape recording composed of everyday sounds and activities, such as the owner speaking on the telephone, washing dishes, watching television, vacuuming, or whatever else the owner might do while at home, might be made and turned on during departures. The safety tape is played on a continuous loop behind the door or otherwise out of the dog's sight, both during planned departures and when the dog is left alone for longer periods. During planned departures, the dog is given an especially desirable chew toy, such as a hard-rubber toy smeared on the inside with peanut butter or baby food (creamed meats) and stuffed with a biscuit. A nylon bone with several holes drilled into it can be stuffed with hard cheese or other canine delicacies. Such items offer an appetizing diversion for some dogs; however, other dogs seem to prefer the contact comfort of a soft item like a stuffed animal or towel saturated with the owner's smell. In addition to showing a preference for soft toys and cloth items, some evidence suggests that a mirror can provide relief against separation distress (Pettijohn et al., 1977). The mirror is securely fastened to a wall adjacent to the crate.

A session of planned-departure training involves several trials consisting of graduated and variable durations of separation. A sample session might include the following variable duration (VD) exposures to separation: 5, 45, 10, 60, 20, 30, 45, 5, 120, and 50 seconds (VD, 39 seconds). Care should be taken not to progress too quickly or abruptly from one step to the next, since excessive separation exposure might intensify a dog's distress rather than help to reduce it. Notice that the progression is not a linear one, but varied so that the dog is unable to make any definite predictions about when the owner is likely to return; it only knows that the owner will eventually return after some variable period of separation. From a cognitive-emotional perspective, the aforementioned pattern of exposure results in varying degrees of surprise (the owner returns sooner than expected) and disappointment (the owner returns later than expected), but, ultimately, the owner does return. The combined effect of planned departures is to replace despair and loss at separation with hope, with the dog learning that patient waiting results in the eventual return of the owner. The expectant anticipation of the owner's eventual return appears to compete with adverse separation distress and frustration. For example, it has often been noted that many separation-reactive dogs are not apparently distressed when left in a car. Such dogs appear to have learned that calmly waiting for the owner's return eventually pays off. Apparently, the intermittent schedule of the owner's departures and returns to the car are sufficiently brief, frequent, and variable to facilitate a state conducive to separation security. Such dogs have learned to expect that their owners will eventually return and are comforted during periods of separation by a sense of hopefulness or positive anticipation about their owners' eventual return.

The time between exposure trials (intertrial interval) also appears to be an important variable. During the early stages of training, when very brief and unstressful separation exposures occur under the counterconditioning influence of an attractive or appetitive stimulus, the influence of the intertrial interval may not be significant. However, separation exposures involving durations of a minute or longer may require a more lengthy recovery period between separation-exposure trials. The recommended interval between trials of separation exposure ranges between 1 and 3 minutes, depending on the dog's response.

The success of planned departures is not based solely on the absence of separation distress, but also depends on before-and-after separation behavior. Ideally, the dog should gradually accept separation exposures without showing evidence of worry or other efforts aimed at forestalling separation. During actual departures, the dog should be given 5 to 10 minutes of basic obedience training and confined at least 15 or 20 minutes before the owner leaves, with the owner periodically returning to the confinement area to give the dog a treat. In some cases, massage and the presentation of a conditioned olfactory stimulus can be very beneficial as transitional aids to help reduce excessive arousal before departures and after homecomings (see *Taction and Olfactory Conditioning*). To forestall excessive greeting activity, a dog can be trained for a minute or 2 while remaining in the crate, requiring that it orient and attend briefly before bridging and rewarding the behavior. As the dog becomes more focused and calm, it is released and the training activity is continued outside of the crate for additional 5 to 10 minutes. Appetitive arousal produced by conditioned reinforcers and food appears to help restrain social arousal, perhaps by means of an oxytocin-mediated calming effect occurring in response to food reinforcement and social rewards (see *Origin of Reactive versus Adaptive Coping Styles*).

Counterconditioning Predeparture Cues

As already noted, separation-reactive dogs may show pronounced signs of rising apprehension whenever the owner prepares to leave the house. Such anticipatory arousal is the result of the dog recognizing a predictive relationship between certain of the owner's habits and separation. These predeparture activities (putting on shoes, picking up keys, and similar things) motivationally prime a dog to exhibit various comfort-seeking or separation-delaying behaviors. In addition to setting the occasion for such behavior, if the behavior happens to be even marginally effective at forestalling the separation event, the underlying motivational arousal present at the time makes it certain that the behavior will undergo marked reinforcement. At such times, any efforts by the owner to calm or to compensate the dog otherwise for the impending separation will likely result in an increase in undesirable preseparation behavior. In addition, this anticipatory arousal to impending separation sets into motion the preliminary conditions for the expression of more intense separation distress or panic when the owner actually leaves the house.

Essentially, predeparture cues are conditioned stimuli that elicit preparatory emotional arousal in anticipation of heightened distress and panic that usually ensue whenever the dog is exposed to separation. Preseparation arousal and activities involve complex operant-respondent interactions. Consequently, the process of changing the associative, behavioral, and motivational implications of predeparture stimuli involves the use of both instrumental shaping and classical counterconditioning techniques. Predeparture cues are counterconditioned in various ways:

- *Engage the dog in some highly attractive activity while simultaneously exposing it to predeparture rituals.* One way to do this to give the dog an appetizing chew item that will occupy it while pretending to get ready to leave.
- *Explicitly pair predeparture cues with antagonistic attractive or appetitive stimuli.* In this case, items such as keys or a briefcase are picked up and immediately followed by giving the dog a food treat. Another situation might be staged where the owner picks up car keys and umbrella only to sit down again, tossing the incredulous dog a treat. Another possibility involves the owner putting on work clothes before feeding the dog. Other possibilities include picking up a briefcase or performing some other predeparture sequence and surprising the dog by taking it for a walk, initiating a brief play session with a favorite toy or ball, or massage.

- *Condition predeparture cues as discriminative stimuli for cooperative behavior.* The owner puts shoes and coat on and then has the dog lie down and stay for several minutes while periodically receiving treats. At other times, a session of basic training could be carried out.
- *Extinguish aversive associations by repeatedly performing predeparture sequences without actually leaving home.* For example, the owner periodically picks up keys only to put them back down again. A variety of predeparture sequences are initiated and concluded without the owner leaving the house. The overall effect is to scramble associations so thoroughly with regard to predeparture activities that the dog is unable to predict when separation is likely to occur. *Note:* Scrambling predeparture cues may help to dissociate them from the actual departure event, but some separation-anxious dogs may become significantly worse as the result of the scrambling procedure. In such dogs, scrambling may raise anxiety levels by decreasing the dog's ability to predict when the owner will leave the house, appearing to cause them to become more vigilant for the event. Many dogs showing separation distress with anxiety or panic appear to do better if predeparture cues are left unscrambled.
- *Shape more appropriate behavior occurring in the presence of evocative predeparture cues.* After putting on work clothes, the owner systematically reinforces behavior such as turning away or laying down.

In general, the goal of these procedures is to alter the dog's expectations about the significance of preseparation events or to reinforce more appropriate preseparation behavior.

Practical Limitations and Compliance Issues

Performing graduated departures and counterconditioning or scrambling predeparture cues appears to be effective, but the precise value of these procedures for the control of SDS is not known. Although most dog behavior therapists seem to agree that graduated departure training is beneficial, some have criticized the complexity and difficulty of the method for the average dog owner to implement. The success of graduated departure training depends on highly controlled circumstances of exposure and diligent owners willing to commit the necessary time to make the process work. The biggest obstacle is ensuring that the dog is not left alone for too long during the treatment program—a commitment that can last several weeks. Although some dedicated dog owners can find time to carry out planned departures while at home in the evening or on weekends, they must inevitably leave the dog alone. In principle, lengthy exposures to separation should adversely impact the positive gains achieved by desensitization efforts.

Several methods might be considered to address this difficulty. The owner might be fortunate enough to find a neighbor or friend with whom the dog can stay for the first few days or weeks of training. Another method involves hiring a dog walker to carry out graduated departures after the owner leaves for the day. Finally, the owner might borrow a friend's dog (perhaps also left alone during the day), which the resident dog knows and likes, to stay with the distressed dog on a trial basis. Although such an arrangement may sometimes work (Houpt, 1979), it often does not (Voith and Borchelt, 1985) and may be highly stressful for the visiting dog. The arrangement should be discontinued if the distressed dog continues to exhibit a high degree of separation distress. In some cases, the owner might be able to take the dog to work temporarily, but this option does little to improve the dog's behavior when it must be left alone at home. Other options include kenneling or dog day care. Lastly, various medications may be considered as a temporary means to control excessive distress, especially if the dog must be left alone while undergoing desensitization (Voith and Borchelt, 1985).

QUALITY OF SOCIAL ATTACHMENT AND DETACHMENT TRAINING

Attachment and Detachment

The difficulties associated with the graduated departure procedure have prompted the development of techniques designed to alter attachment levels via the implementation of interactive stressors (e.g., ignoring care-seeking behavior, refusing the dog physical contact, removing the dog from the bedroom, and continuous crate confinement). Detachment procedures are premised on the belief that SDS is the result of a dog's poorly regulated attachment behavior. Presumably, as the result of excessive and unregulated social contact, the dog becomes exceedingly and problematically attached to the owner, making separations evocative of disruptive distress and a gradual breakdown of the dog's ability to cope at separation. According to this view, the amount of distress shown by the dog at separation is proportional to the degree of attachment between the dog and the owner.

The significance of attachment levels and proximity seeking in the etiology of adult separation distress has been questioned by various authors [Voith et al., 1997; Goodloe and Borchelt, 1998 (see *Attachment, Proximity Seeking, and Family Size* in Volume 2, Chapter 4)]. In addition, Bradshaw and colleagues (2002) failed to detect any relationship between the amount of owner-dog interaction and the probability of separation-related behavior from month 3 to month 18, further questioning the attachment hypothesis. These reports suggest that it is not a dog's overt attachment or the amount of interaction between the owner and dog that underlies separation-related problems, but rather the way in which the dog copes with being left alone. Most dogs develop strong attachments toward their owners, but only a small percentage of them go on to exhibit clinical separation distress. Many separation-reactive dogs are quite content at separation so long as some human is nearby, even someone with whom the dog has not formed a particularly strong attachment.

The attachment hypothesis appears to confuse effects with causes. Attachment excesses may follow more directly as the result of agitation and distress at separation and a compromised capacity for coping with stress adaptively (see *Origin of Reactive versus Adaptive Coping Styles*), rather than as the result of unregulated affiliative interaction between the dog and owner. The daily agitation and distress at separation followed by relief by the owner's return probably results in the evident contact-seeking behavior exhibited by separation-reactive dogs. In other words, separation-reactive dogs may follow their owners around and seek contact, not because of unregulated affiliation, but rather because of a history of unregulated separation distress and agitation. According to this view, excessive attachment is not the cause of separation distress; on the contrary, excessive attachment is more likely the result of heightened agitation and distress at separation. Consequently, the arbitrary reduction of proximity seeking and attachment behavior between the owner and dog may not serve to alter significantly the causes of separation reactivity and dysregulation, but may instead inadvertently increase social contact needs and problematic attachment behavior. Consequently, detachment procedures and interactive stressors aimed at reducing contact and attachment behavior may inadvertently increase attachment levels via the emotional agitation, frustration, and insecurity produced by the detachment procedure itself, many components of which are highly punitive and restrictive with regard to a dog's social initiatives. The use of interactive stressors to modify attachment behavior is contrary to the enhancement of social competency, confidence building (intrinsic counterconditioning by relaxation), and reward-based stress modulation via enhanced comfort and safety-security. Ultimately, the best way to reduce excessive and insecure attachment behavior is not by arbitrarily implementing interactive stressors designed to unilaterally limit contact between the dog and the owner, but rather by reducing the amount of agitation and distress the dog experiences at separation, while at the same time training it to respond more adaptively to stressful situations, and, most importantly, improving the quality of the social bond between the owner and dog—not weakening or dismantling it.

Despite some disagreement on the matter of how attachment levels influence the development of SDS, evidence suggests that close and exclusive attachments probably do play a significant role in the etiology of some sepa-ration-related problems (see *Attachment, Proximity Seeking, and Family Size* in Volume 2, Chapter 4). Dogs exhibiting a strong attachment toward a particular family member appear to be at an increased risk of developing separation problems (McBride et al., 1995). Topál and colleagues (1998) found that dogs living in large family groups exhibit less separation distress when tested than dogs coming from families with fewer members. Data from a clinical population indicated that most separation-reactive dogs live in small family groups containing two adults and no children (Podberscek et al., 1999). Flannigan and Dodman (2001) have confirmed that family size is a significant risk factor associated with separation-related behavior problems, finding that dogs kept by a single owner are 2.5 times more likely to exhibit separation problems—a risk factor previously missed (McBride et al., 1995). Surprisingly, the presence of another dog in the household does not appear to reduce the risk of separation problems (Flannigan and Dodman, 2001). This finding seems odd since dogs generally appear to cope better with separation when living with another dog or cat. As already discussed, the presence of another dog does not ensure that canine company will comfort an already separation-distressed dog, but one would expect some preventive benefit as the result of the formation of bonds with other animals in the household. Nonetheless, consistent with the findings of Flannigan and Dodman, McBride and colleagues (1995) also found that the incidence of separation-related problems among dogs adopted from an animal shelter was not significantly related to the presence of another dog in the new home. Dogs placed in homes with at least one cat, though, were less likely to exhibit separation-related problems—a curious finding needing additional study.

In a sense, many treatment protocols seem to have misidentified the social symptoms of SDS as the causes of the problem. Although modifying and managing symptoms may exert some beneficial influence, whenever possible treatment efforts should focus on primary causes—not effects and symptoms. Unless agitation and distress at separation are reduced, heightened levels of attachment and contact needs will probably continue unabated, perhaps worsening as the result of implementing intrusive detachment procedures (Table 4.3).

Detachment training may be transitionally useful in some cases involving extreme attachment disorganization, but the necessity of interactive stressors to reduce separation-related problems has not been scientifically established. Further, there is no significant evidence supporting the belief that spoiling activities or permissiveness with respect to attachment behaviors (e.g., sleeping on the bed) are causally related to separation-related problems (see Flannigan and Dodman, 2001; and Voith et al., 1992). Also, the common belief that excessive fussing during departures and greetings is causally related to separation problems is not supported by the current data (McBride et al., 1995). For highly attached dogs, the introduction of detachment training may introduce additional conflict and confusion, resulting in further disruption and distress at separation, perhaps making matters worse and the problem more difficult to resolve in some cases. In general, the key is not to detach the dog from the owner arbitrarily and unilaterally, and possibly further undermine its social confidence and make the relationship more unstable and the dog more reactive, but to enhance the bond between the owner and dog through training. The dog's need for contact and proximity can be directed into constructive training activities that support interactive harmony, enhanced confidence, and social indepen-dence. Rather than emphasizing detachment training as a way of life, behavioral efforts are much better dedicated to independence training, whereby the dog learns to cope more competently and confidently with separation and aloneness (see *Cynopraxis and the Human-Dog Bond* in Volume 1, Chapter 10). Finally, detachment procedures are often highly intrusive, perhaps being more aversive to some owners to carry out than coping with a dog's separation problems. Consequently, even in the event that detachment procedures work, it is unlikely that the owner will want to indefinitely maintain the interaction needed to support the detachment effect.

Dynamics of Bonding: Nurturance, Dominance, and Leadership

Since the quality of attachment and bonding (mutual ties) between the owner and dog appears to play a prominent role in the development of SDS, it makes sense to build on the dog's affection and attachment, taking what one finds and guiding it into a more healthy and mutually satisfying form. In other words, treatment should focus on repairing disorganized aspects of attachment behavior, rather than suppress and impede attachment behavior in general. The relationship between humans and dogs is formed under the influence of three fundamental and complementary bonds that dynamically interact with one another: (1) nurturer-dependent bond, (2) dominant-subordinate bond, and (3) leader-follower bond. Note that each bond consists of two modes of

TABLE. 4.3. Summary of common detachment procedures

The owner must ignore all of the dog's social solicitations for contact.

Proximity-seeking behavior is discouraged by command or confinement.

The dog is separated for progressively longer periods while the owner is at home.

The dog is forbidden from sitting on the owner's lap or to share furniture.

The dog is not permitted to sleep or be in the bedroom at night.

The dog must earn all appetitive and social rewards.

The dog's greeting behavior is ignored or discouraged.

mutual reciprocation by which the owner and the dog relate to each other. A healthy human-dog relationship is based on a balance of nurturance and dependency, dominance and submission, and leadership and cooperation. Inadequacies or excesses in any of these three basic binary dimensions of social interaction may cause disharmony and disturbance in the social relations between people and dogs.

A common source of confusion is distinguishing between dominance and leadership. Many authors seem to treat dominance and leadership as synonyms meaning approximately the same thing. Dominance-related interaction involving covert, subtle, or overt threats of force or the use of actual force of varying degrees (e.g., holding the dog back from some activity or shoving it off as it jumps up) and submissive acknowledgment by the dog serve to set social limits and define what a dog cannot do. The effect of submission is primarily inhibitory, causing a dog to avoid certain behaviors, at least while in the owner's presence, but without specifying what the dog ought to do instead. Dominant-subordinate interaction involves overt contests or threat-appeasement displays, activities that appear to enhance affectionate tolerance (dominant role) and affectionate attraction (subordinate role). Affection arising from dominant-subordinate interaction causes the subordinate paradoxically to seek closer proximity with the dominator (see *Social Distance and Polarity* in Volume 2, Chapter 8). Attention seeking and proximity seeking reflect a highly submissive and inhibited orientation in which the dependent subordinate is looking for leadership and guidance—it literally needs to be shown what to do. The direction of social interaction between the dominator and the subordinate is highly directional or polarized. Social polarity is manifested in care-seeking activities, such as attention-seeking, affection-seeking, and proximity-seeking behavior. The establishment of dominant-subordinate relations prepares the subordinate to become a dependent and cooperative follower if adequate leadership is provided.

However, a highly submissive dog, in the absence of leadership, may be vulnerable to develop insecure attachment, especially if the dominator is primarily a source of nurturance and fails to *own* the responsibility of leadership. Social dominance without leadership is a formula for behavioral and emotional imbalance and insecurity, potentially giving rise to extremes of abusive domination, on the one hand, and careless indulgence, on the other.

Whereas transactions involving the exchange of threat and appeasement displays establish that certain behaviors are forbidden, leadership helps to guide the dependent subordinate into activities that are acceptable and lead to various sources of appetitive and social gratification. Leadership is associated with the initiation and coordination of cooperative activities that result in benefit for both the leader and the follower. Whereas submission exerts an inhibitory influence, following provides an excitatory influence on behavior. The result of dominance is submission, affection, and dependency, whereas leadership provides the basis for social cooperation and interactive harmony. With respect to the human-dog bond, it would seem that excessive proximity seeking and affection seeking are not symptoms of attachment excess, but reflect a submissive and dependent search for leadership. The relation between dominance, leadership, and nurturance is reflected in the moment-to-moment ebb and flow of social interaction, defining what is not done, what is done, and the sorts of appetitive and affectionate gratifications that accrue as the result of cooperative and harmonious interaction. The process of obedience training incorporates all three dimensions of the bonding triune in a balanced relationship. Basic training defines what a dog may not do (e.g., jump up, bite on hands and clothes, and pull on the leash), shows the dog what it may do (jump up on signal, play tug and retrieve, controlled-leash walking, sit, stay, come, and so forth), and provides contingent nurturance (e.g., affectionate petting and food) based on cooperative behavior.

Owners of separation-distressed dogs need some specific things to do, but more importantly they need principles (more than rules and recipes) to guide their daily interactions with the dog. Having a separation-distressed dog perform repetitive sit-stay exercises and other unilateral and arbitrary detachment initiatives (rejection of attention and contact, blocking of proximity seeking, and cessation of noncontingent affection and rewards) may fully miss the point unless the owner is led to a better appreciation of the dynamic interplay between dominance, leadership, and nurturance in the process of balanced and healthy bonding. An important step in this direction is to teach owners to appreciate their dog's behavior as form of communication needing thoughtful interpretation and understanding.

BASIC TRAINING AND SEPARATION DISTRESS

One of the best ways to restore appropriate limits and balance to the human-dog relationship is basic training. Not surprisingly, obedience training has been correlated with a reduced incidence of separation-related complaints (Goodloe and Borchelt, 1998; Jagoe and Serpell, 1996; Flannigan and Dodman, 2001), possibly as the result of organized attachment behavior and the enhanced confidence promoted by obedience training. Clark and Boyer (1993), also noting that obedience training appears to have a pronounced effect on separation-related behavior problems, speculate that obedience-trained dogs appear to be more secure in their attachments—a security that may be the result of enhanced owner-dog communication and interaction. Dogs without a viable channel of communication may be unable to relate to the owner as an independent affiliative partner, a failing that may predispose it to develop a persistent and regressive reliance on direct contact and vulnerability at separation:

> Ainsworth (1972) found that separation distress becomes less significant as children become better able to sustain attachment in abstentia and that close proximity and contact may, to some extent, be supplanted by communication and interaction across a distance. Thus obedience training may be the communication tool for

the owner to provide security in the relationship and improve the human-canine relationship. Obedience training may facilitate feelings of security for dogs, because training communicates proper behavior by reinforcing appropriate behavior and punishing inappropriate behaviour. (157)

In addition to preventing or reversing problematic dependency and enhancing an owner's leadership, basic training improves a dog's attentional and impulse-control abilities—two vital cortical executive functions necessary for effective adaptation under stress. Most importantly, though, for purposes of separation-distress problems, no other activity improves a dog's confidence and sense of security better than basic training. Training activity should be integrated into the everyday interaction between the owner and dog. A "no pay, no play" philosophy may be instituted in which the dog learns that attention and affection are earned most effectively by cooperative behavior. The heightened social contact needs associated with homecomings should be harnessed to the furtherance of training objectives (see *Establishing Operations* in Chapter 1). At such times, dogs are acutely sensitive to petting and praise as rewards. Instead of ignoring or simply giving a dog the attention and contact stimulation that it craves, a cycle of basic training exercises can be performed in exchange for social and appetitive rewards. Because all dogs, like people, are different and require training designed to meet their specific needs, basic training is best carried out under the supervision of an applied dog behaviorist or a skilled trainer familiar with the needs of the separation-reactive dog.

Although basic training may not directly modify separation distress or frustration, it offers a useful and proven means for clarifying social boundaries and establishing general control that may be extremely beneficial. Takeuchi and colleagues (2001) found that owners with separation-anxious dogs tended to indulge them and used verbal discipline rather than physical means to control undesirable behavior. Separation-reactive dogs are often very skilled at getting their way by emotionally or physically manipulating their owner. These tactics and schemes may entrap a naive owner in a subtle web of obligatory expectations and emotional pressures to concede to the dog's demands. Having maneuvered into a position of emotional leverage over the owner, the dog may find it extremely difficult to cope with situations where its control is compromised or forfeited, as occurs at separation. A dog that is accustomed to getting and controlling the owner's attention and proximity on demand may be more prone to become frustrated when the behavior fails to work, as occurs when the owner must leave the dog alone. Under the influence of frustration and secondary distress at separation, separation-reactive dogs may exhibit and intensify protest behaviors that have succeeded in past to get the owner's attention (e.g., barking, scratching on doors, or grabbing personal belongings).

From an early age onward, dogs may learn that certain undesirable behaviors are a sure way to get attention, albeit not always the most desirable attention. For some dogs, the preponderance of the daily interaction and attention received during puppyhood may have been primarily obtained by way of disciplinary interaction directed at suppressing such problematic attention-seeking behavior. Many of these behaviors are similar to the array of protest behaviors occurring at separation. As previously discussed, punitive interaction may potentiate dependency and attachment behavior in dogs (see *Early Trauma and the Development of Behavior Problems* in Volume 2, Chapter 2). Faced with separation frustration and distress, dogs may resort to those same behaviors that have worked in the past to protest and get the owner's attention. Retroactive punishment (punishment directed against past deeds), which is common in the case of separation-reactive dogs (see *Separation Distress and Retroactive Punishment* in Volume 2, Chapter 4), is highly undesirable and problematic, appearing to increase the dog's dependency and vulnerability to emotional distress at separation, potentially setting into action a vicious cycle of punishment and increased separation-related reactivity. Since retroactive punishment is relatively unpredictable and uncontrollable, it may impair the dog's ability to trust the owner as a source of safety and consistency, leading in extreme

cases to significant cognitive and emotional disorganization.

SEPARATION-RELATED PROBLEMS AND PUNISHMENT

Separation distress is potentiated by a number of coactive motivational and emotional influences, especially frustration, boredom, fear, and panic. The role of these various contributing motivational influences in the expression of separation-related behavior should be carefully assessed before considering the use of punishment. Obviously, punishment would be an entirely inappropriate option in the case of highly unstable and reactive dogs. Also, it must be emphasized that punishment may worsen some separation-related problems, especially those presenting under the influence of panic, making the use of punishment risky and requiring careful monitoring. As mentioned previously, inappropriate or excessive punitive treatment may paradoxically enhance attachment behavior and risk increasing separation-related problems. Further, without appropriate support conditioning aimed at reducing the dog's aversive emotional response to separation, a possibility exists that the dog, unable to find relief in its preferred modality, may redirect its distress-reducing impulses into other, perhaps even more undesirable and difficult-to-control, activities. Despite significant concerns and reservations, some forms of separation-related behavior, especially barking problems and destructiveness resulting from protest at separation, appear to be highly responsive to certain punitive procedures. Although the method is not popular with some and despite some authoritative opinions to the contrary, separation-related barking is often highly responsive to aversive treatment procedures involving the use of bark-activated collar devices. Barking problems may require timely intervention and modification, with the owner facing imminent eviction or costly nuisance citations. Many owners who have independently resorted to the use of bark-activated collars to treat such behaviors have reported a high degree of success. The use of bark-activated collars to suppress barking is risky and can result in disaster in the case of panic-related separation problems, which appear to escalate dramatically under the excitatory influence of fear (see *ES and Excessive Barking* in Chapter 9). Although crating or penning a dog can control destructive habits temporarily, eventually the dog is released from confinement and exposed to at least part of the house. Giving such a dog increased freedom and comfort may result in undesirable exploration and destructive behavior. Various techniques involving repellents, booby traps, and electronic devices are used selectively to prevent or suppress such behavior in the owner's absence. The details of these various procedures are described in Chapter 2 (see *Miscellaneous Devices and Techniques for Deterring Destructive Behavior*).

MASSAGE, PLAY, AND EXERCISE

Taction and Olfactory Conditioning

Massage and relaxation training have many applications in the management of dog behavior, especially in situations involving aversive emotional arousal such as separation distress (Tuber, 1986). The first systematic effort to quantify the calming effect of human taction on dogs was performed by Gantt and colleagues (1966), who observed that many dogs in distress are calmed by social contact, exhibiting a significant decrease in both heart and respiratory rates while being petted. The authors referred to this phenomenon as the *effect of person* (see *The Effect of Person* in Volume 1, Chapter 10).

In conjunction with tactile stimulation, olfactory stimulation appears to play a significant role in the formation of social attachments and bonds (see *Biological and Social Functions of Smell* in Volume 1, Chapter 4). Among rat pups, odors appear to facilitate huddling behavior, with olfactory incentives developmentally supplanting thermal and tactile ones in the regulation of such behavior (Rosenblatt, 1983). Unfortunately, the full emotional significance and value of the sense of smell for dogs remain elusive and conjectural. There is little doubt that olfaction plays an important role in emotional learning and attachment (see *Social Comfort Seeking and Distress* in Volume 2, Chapter 4). The social

significance of olfactory information is highly durable in dogs. They exhibit evidence of recognizing the scent of the mother and the breeder after years of separation, social memories that may persist throughout a dog's life cycle (Hepper, 1994; Appel et al., 1999). By way of limbic system projections, olfactory information may exert significant conditioned and unconditioned effects involving various neuropeptide systems (e.g., opioid, oxytocin, and AVP) believed to play a role in the expression of social emotions and memories. As the result of direct connections with the amygdala, strong links between olfaction and social aversion may be established. The amygdala plays a central role in fear learning and exercises a powerful modulatory influence over the expression of fear via connections with hypothalamic nuclei dedicated to elaboration of fear, startle, and stress responses (see *Limbic System* in Volume 1, Chapter 3). Olfactory stimulation is easily and rapidly conditioned to produce emotional alarm. Through interconnections with the amygdala (emotional memory) and hippocampus (contextual memory), olfactory learning may exert a significant conditioned influence over the release of CRF and the cascade of events associated with biological stress. In addition to these subcortical influences, olfaction reaches cortical representation through interconnections among the amygdala, the hippocampus, the thalamus, and the prefrontal cortex, where the information is further processed, accessed by the working memory, and coordinated with goal-directed activities. The role of olfaction at the level of cognition has received very little attention in dogs, but in rodents there is growing evidence to suggest that they may "think" with their noses (Slotnick, 1994; Slotnick et al., 2000).

The canine olfactory system provides a powerful means to influence separation distress through conditioned associations with safety (relief), physical and emotional relaxation, appetitive stimuli, and play activities. Olfactory stimuli associated with predeparture activities appears to exert significant preparatory influences on a dog's emotional response to separation. Odors (e.g., the smell of coffee or the owner's cologne or deodorant) repeatedly present at departure may become potent conditioned olfactory stressors, perhaps contributing significantly to a dog's reaction at separation. Like other conditioned predeparture stimuli, olfactory stressors need to be identified and counterconditioned whenever possible. On the other hand, olfactory stimuli associated with the owner homecomings may acquire potent conditioned relief and safety associations that can be used to counter agitation and distress associated with separations. The apparent efficacy of the owner's scent on towels and so forth to quell separation distress may be derived largely from olfactory conditioning that occurs during greetings. Putting on a scent used during safety conditioning and PFR training (e.g., orange or lemon-orange mix) just before entering the house to greet the dog or puppy after a long separation may help to intensify the effect of the odor as a conditioned source of security for the dog.

Massage is a useful way to calm a separation-reactive dog while performing graduated departures. Dogs that become overly aroused at departures and homecomings are often highly responsive to 3 to 5 minutes of PFR training just before the owner leaves and again after the owner returns home. The method used follows the guidelines and procedures described in Appendix C. Although not all dogs are equally responsive to massage, most appear to benefit from the experience. For many dogs, massage produces a pronounced and easily replicated relaxation response. In addition to the direct benefits of massage-induced relaxation, the focused and unambiguous contact comfort produced by massage may exert ancillary therapeutic benefit by modulating the production and release of neuropeptides (e.g., oxytocin, endogenous opioids, and CRF) involved in the mediation of contact comfort and separation distress. To capture the benefits of massage and optimize the ability to generalize the benefits across contexts, an olfactory stimulus is paired with massage-induced relaxation. Once conditioned, the odor can be used during graduated departures and predepartures as an OSS. Performing massage in the presence of other safety signals (e.g., music, radio, and light) can help to

support and augment the effect of such signals. To help transfer and generalize the olfactory association, the owner can place a drop or two of the fragrant oil on the hands while carrying out planned departures.

Various odor diffusers are available that can be used to present the OSS over time. A diffuser is made by drilling two small holes into the cap of a small bottle and inserting rubber tubing into the holes, with one of the tubes (the outlet) extending to the vicinity of the crate and the other (the inlet) attached to the aquarium pump. The tubes should form an airtight seal with the lid. A dilute fragrant odor can be put on several cotton balls that are placed on top of the inlet tube or the odor can be diluted in water and released by a bubbling action. The outlet tube should be situated an inch or so below the lid so that it does not touch the water. A ceramic ring that is heated by a light bulb can also be used to diffuse fragrant oils. The dilute essential oil is simply dripped onto the ceramic ring before leaving the house. When graduated departure activities are performed, the light is switched on, thereby combining the effects of two safety signals in one action. Alternatively, a plug-in room freshener can be modified so that the conditioned OSS is released instead of the packaged odorant coming with the unit.

Play and Exercise

Play and exercise appear to exert a positive influence on the treatment of separation-related problems. Play offers a ready means to normalize the social interaction between the owner and dog, reduce stress, and enhance affiliation, confidence, cooperation, and emotional flexibility, thereby helping to harmonize human-dog interaction. Engaging the dog in object-oriented play (e.g., tug and fetch) also provides a source of highly enjoyable aerobic exercise. The provision of supplemental exercise may be particularly important in the case of active, working, or sporting-type dogs with separation-related problems. Exercise appears to exert a variety of neurobiological effects, including a robust influence on serotonergic activity (see *Exercise and the Neuroeconomy of Stress* in Volume 1, Chapter 3).

Separation-reactive dogs should be exercised daily. An excellent exercise plan incorporates a combination of long walks and playing fetch with a ball or soft disk. Walks as brief as 20 minutes or so can be very beneficial, but some dogs may require much more exercise to produce a benefit (Radosevich et al., 1989). The crucial consideration with regard to exercise is that it be provided on a consistent and daily basis. Exercise scheduled erratically or on impulse may result in additional problems. For example, taking the dog for a 5-mile walk 1 day, skipping 2 or 3 days, and then jogging the dog for a week, followed by a week without any exercise—this sort of pattern may be more stressful and tension producing than relaxing for the dog. The best rule of thumb is to provide the dog with adequate exercise, play, and training on a consistent basis every day.

REFERENCES

Adler R and Conklin PM (1963). Handling of pregnant rats: Effects on emotionality of offspring. *Science*, 142:411–412.

Ainsworth MC (1972). Attachment and dependency: A comparison. In JL Gewirtz (Ed), *Attachment and Dependency*. Washington, DC: VH Winston.

Akhondzadeh S, Kashani L, Mobaseri M, et al. (2001). Passionflower in the treatment of opiates withdrawal: A double-blind randomized controlled trial. *J Clin Pharm Ther*, 26:369–376.

Al'Absi M, Hugdahl K, and Lovallo WR (2002). Adrenocortical stress responses and altered working memory performance. *Psychophysiology*, 39:95–99.

Anderson G and Marinier S (1997). The effect of food and restricted exercise on behaviour problems in dogs. In DS Mills, SE Heath, and LJ Harrington (Eds), *Proceedings of the First International Conference on Veterinary Behavioural Medicine*. Potters Bar, Herts, Great Britain: Universities Federation for Animal Welfare.

Appel J, Arms N, Horner R, and Carr WJ (1999). Long-term olfactory memory in companion dogs. Presentation at the Annual Meeting of the Animal Behavior Society, Bucknell University, Lewisburg, PA, June 27–30.

Arons CD and Shoemaker WJ (1992). The distribution of catecholamines and ß-endorphin in the brains of three behavioral distinct breeds of dogs and their F1 hybrids. *Brain Res*, 594:31–39.

Aronson LP (1998). Systemic causes of aggression and their treatment. In N Dodman and L Shuster (Eds), *Psychopharmacology of Animal Behavior Disorders*. Malden, MA: Blackwell Science.

Aronson L (1999). Animal behavior case of the month: A dog was evaluated because of extreme fear. *JAVMA*, 215:22–24.

Ballarini G (1990). Animal psychodietetics. *J Small Anim Pract*, 31:523–553.

Ballenger JC (1999). Current treatments of the anxiety disorders in adults. *Biol Psychiatry*, 46:1579–1594.

Barrett T, Kent S, and Voudouris N (2000). Does melatonin modulate beta-endorphin, corticosterone, and pain threshold? *Life Sci*, 66:467–476.

Beaver BV, Fischer M, and Atkinson CE (1992). Determination of favorite components of garbage by dogs. *Appl Anim Behav Sci*, 34:129–136.

Bergmann R, Nuessner J, and Demling J (1993). Treatment of mild to moderate depressions: A comparison between *Hypericum perforatum* and amitriptyline. *Neurologie/Psychiatrie*, 7:235–240.

Borchelt PL (1989). Behaviour development of the puppy in the home environment. In RS Anderson (Ed), *Nutrition and Behavior in Dogs and Cats*. New York: Pergamon.

Bradshaw JWS, McPherson JA, Casey RA, and Larter IS (2002). Aetiology of separation-related behaviour in domestic dogs. *Vet Rec*, 151:43–46.

Clark GI and Boyer WN (1993). The effects of dog obedience training and behavioural counselling upon the human-canine relationship. *Appl Anim Behav Sci* 37:147–159.

Cook CJ (2002). Glucocorticoid feedback increases the sensitivity of the limbic system to stress. *Physiol Behav*, 75:455–464.

Cooper LL (2002). Alternative medicine and behavior. *Clin Tech Small Anim Pract*, 17:50–57.

Davidson JRT, and the Hypericum Depression Trial Study Group (2002). Effect of *Hypericum perforatum* (St. John's Wort) in major depressive disorder: A randomized controlled trial. *JAMA*, 287:1807–1814.

De Lourdes M, Seabra V, Bignotto M, et al. (2000). Randomized, double-blind clinical trial, controlled with placebo, of the toxicology of chronic melatonin treatment. *J Pineal Res*, 29:193–200.

Denenberg VH (1964). Critical periods, stimulus input, and emotional reactivity: A theory of infantile stimulation. *Psychol Rev*, 71:335–351.

Dodman N (1999). *Dog Behaving Badly: An A-to-Z Guide to Understanding and Curing Behavioral Problems in Dogs*. New York: Bantam.

Elliot O and Scott JP (1961). The development of emotional distress reactions to separation, in puppies. *J Genet Psychol*, 99:3–22.

Fatjó J, Stub C, and Manteca X (2002). Four cases of aggression and hypothyroidism in dogs. *Vet Rec*, 151:547–548.

Feddersen-Petersen D (1994). Social behavior of wolves and dogs. *Vet Q*, 16:51S–52S.

Ferguson JN, Young LJ, Hearn EF, et al. (2000). Social amnesia in mice lacking oxytocin gene. *Nature Genet*, 25:284–288.

Ferguson JN, Young LJ, and Insel TR (2002). The neuroendocrine basis of social recognition. *Front Neuroendocrinol*, 23:200–224.

Field T, Grizzle N, Scafidi F, and Schanberg S (1996a). Massage and relaxation therapies' effects on depressed adolescent mothers. *Adolescence*, 31:903–911.

Field T, Grizzle N, Scafidi F, et al. (1996b). Massage therapy for infants of depressed mothers. *Infant Behav Dev*, 19:107–112.

Fisher AE (1955). The effects of early differential treatment on the social and exploratory behavior of puppies [Unpublished PhD dissertation]. University Park: Pennsylvania State University.

Flannigan G and Dodman NH (2001). Risk factors and behaviors associated with separation anxiety in dogs. *JAVMA*, 219:460–466.

Fornal CA, Metzler CW, Mirescu C, et al. (2001). Effects of standardized extracts of St. John's wort on the single-unit activity of serotonergic dorsal raphe neurons in awake cats: Comparisons with fluoxetine and sertraline. *Neuropsychopharmacology*, 25:858–870.

Fox MW (1965). *Canine Behavior*. Springfield, IL: Charles C Thomas.

Fox MW (1971). *Integrative Development of Brain and Behavior in the Dog*. Chicago: University of Chicago Press.

Fox MW (1978). *The Dog: Its Domestication and Behavior*. Malabar, FL: Krieger.

Gácsi M, Topál J, Miklósi A, et al. (2001). Attachment behavior of adult dogs (*Canis familiaris*) living at rescue centers: Forming new bonds. *J Comp Psychol*, 115:423–431.

Gantt WH (1944). *Experimental Basis for Neurotic Behavior: Origin and Development of Artificially Produced Disturbances of Behavior in Dogs*. New York: Paul B Hoeber.

Gantt WH, Newton JE, Royer FL, and Stephens JH (1966). Effect of person. *Cond Reflex*, 1:146–160.

Gaultier E and Pageat P (2002). Treatment of separation-related anxiety in dogs with a synthetic dog appeasing pheromone: Preliminary results. In *Annual Symposium of Animal Behavior Research, AVSAB Proceedings*, Nashville, TN, July 14, pp 7–10.

Gilligan PJ, Baldauf C, Cocuzza A, et al. (2000). The discovery of 4-(3-pentylamino)-2,7-dimethyl-8-(2-methyl-4-methoxyphenyl)-pyrazolo-[1,5-*a*]-pyrimidine: A corticotropin-releasing factor (hCRF1) antagonist. *Bioorg Med Chem*, 8:181–189.

Goodloe LP and Borchelt PL (1998). Companion dog temperament traits. *J Appl Anim Welfare Sci*, 1:303–338.

Gurski JC, Davis K, and Scott JP (1979). Interaction of separation discomfort with contact comfort and discomfort in the dog. *Dev Psychobiol*, 13:463–467.

Halliwell REW (1992). Comparative aspects of food intolerance. *Vet Med*, Sep:893–899.

Harrer G, Schmidt U, Kuhn U, and Biller A (1999). Comparison of equivalence between the St. John's wort extract LoHyp-57 and fluoxetine. *Arzneimittelforschung*, 49:289–296.

Harris JC and Newman JD (1987). Mediation of separation distress by alpha 2-adrenergic mechanisms in a non-human primate. *Brain Res*, 410:353–356.

He L, Gilligan PJ, and Zaczek R (2000). 4-(1,3-Dimethoxyprop-2-ylamino)-2,7-dimethyl-8-(2,4-dichlorophenyl)pyrazolo[1,5-a]-1,3,5-triazine: A potent, orally bioavailable CRF(1) receptor antagonist. *J Med Chem*, 43:449–456.

Heim C and Nemeroff CB (1999). The impact of early adverse experiences on brain systems involved in the pathophysiology of anxiety and affective disorders. *Biol Psychiatry*, 46:1509–1522.

Hennessy MB (1997). Hypothalamic-pituitary-adrenal responses to brief social separation. *Neurosci Biobehav Rev*, 21:11–29.

Hennessy MB, Davis HN, Williams MT, et al. (1997). Plasma cortisol levels of dogs at a county animal shelter. *Physiol Behav*, 62:485–490.

Hepper PG (1994). Long-term retention of kinship recognition established during infancy in the domestic dog. *Behav Processes*, 33:3–15.

Hetts S (1989). The effect of differential separation periods on separation distress in domestic dog puppies (abstract) [PhD dissertation]. Fort Collins: Colorado State University.

Hewson CJ (2000). Clomipramine and behavioural therapy in the treatment of separation-related problems in dogs [Letter]. *Vet Rec,* 146:111–112.

Hofer MA, Shair HN, Masmela JR, and Brunelli SA (2001). Developmental effects of selective breeding for an infantile trait: The rat pup ultrasonic isolation call. *Dev Psychobiol,* 39:231–246.

Holst S, Uvnäs-Moberg K, and Petersson M (2002). Postnatal oxytocin treatment and postnatal stroking of rats reduce blood pressure in adulthood. *Auton Neurosci,* 99:85–90.

Hothersall D and Tuber DS (1979). Fears in companion dogs: Characteristics and treatment. In JD Keehn (Ed), *Psychopathology in Animals: Research and Clinical Implications.* New York: Academic.

Houpt KA (1979). Destructive behavior in dogs. *Compend Continuing Educ Small Anim Pract,* 1:191–197.

Huidobro-Toro JP and Harris RA (1996). Brain lipids that induce sleep are novel modulators of 5-hydroxytryptamine receptors. *Proc Natl Acad Sci USA,* 93:8078–8082.

Insel TR and Winslow JT (1998). Serotonin and neuropeptides in affiliative behaviors. *Biol Psychiatry,* 44:207–219.

Jagoe JA and Serpel JA (1996). Owner characteristics and interactions and the prevalence of canine behaviour problems. *Appl Anim Behav Sci,* 47:31–42.

Josey ES and Tackett RL (1999). St. John's wort: A new alternative for depression? *Int J Clin Pharmacol Ther,* 37:111–119.

Julien RM (1995). *A Primer of Drug Action,* 7th Ed. New York: WH Freeman.

Kaehler ST, Sinner C, Chatterjee SS, and Philippu A (1999). Hyperforin enhances the extracellular concentrations of catecholamines, serotonin and glutamate in the rat locus coeruleus. *Neurosci Lett,* 262:199–202.

Kalin NH, Shelton SE, and Barksdale CM (1987). Separation distress in infant rhesus monkeys: Effects of diazepam and Ro 15-1788. *Brain Res,* 408:192–198.

King JN, Simpson BS, Overall KL, et al. (2000). Treatment of separation anxiety in dogs with clomipramine: Results from a prospective, randomized, double-blind, placebo-controlled, parallel-group, multicenter clinical trial. *Appl Anim Behav Sci,* 67:255–275.

Kirby LG, Rice KC, and Valentino RJ (2000). Effects of corticotropin-releasing factor on neuronal activity in the serotonergic dorsal raphe nucleus. *Neuropsychopharmacology,* 22:148–162.

Knowles PA, Conner RL, and Panksepp J (1989). Opiate effects on social behavior of juvenile dogs as a function of social deprivation. *Pharmacol Biochem Behav,* 33:533–537.

Konakchieva R, Mitev Y, Almeid OFX, and Patchev VK (1997). Chronic melatonin treatment and the hypothalamo-pituitary-adrenal axis in the rat: Attenuation of the secondary response to stress and effects on hypothalamic neuropeptide content and release. *Biol Cell,* 89:587–596.

Kramer MS, Cutler N, Feighner J, et al. (1998). Distinct mechanism for antidepressant activity by blockade of central substance P receptors. *Science,* 281:1640–1645.

Lephart ED, West TW, Weber KS, et al. (2002). Neurobehavioral effects of dietary soy phytoestrogens. *Neurotoxicol Teratol,* 24:5–16.

Ladd CO, Owens MJ, and Nemeroff CB (1996). Persistent changes in corticotropin-releasing factor neuronal systems induced by maternal deprivation. *Endocrinology,* 137:1212–1218.

Ladd CO, Huot RL, Thrivikraman KV, et al. (2000). Long-term behavioral and neuroendocrine adaptations to adverse early experience. In EA Mayer and CB Saper (Eds), *Progress in Brain Research.* New York: Elsevier Science.

Lakatos K, Toth L, Nemoda Z, et al. (2000). Dopamine D4 receptor (DRD4) gene polymorphism is associated with attachment disorganization in infants. *Mol Psychiatry,* 5:633–637.

Levine S, Haltmeyer GC, Karas GC, and Denenberg VH (1967). Physiological and behavioral effects of infantile stimulation. *Physiol Behav,* 2:55–59.

Lindell EM (1997). Diagnosis and treatment of destructive behavior in dogs. *Vet Clin North Am Prog Companion Anim Behav,* 27:533—547.

Lund I, Yu LC, Uvnäs-Moberg K, et al. (2002). Repeated massage-like stimulation induces long-term effects on nociception: Contribution of oxytocinergic mechanisms. *Eur J Neurosci,* 16:330–338.

MacLean PD (1985). Brain evolution relating to family, play, and the separation call. *Arch Gen Psychiatry,* 42:405–417.

Marder AR (1991). Psychotropic drugs and behavioral therapy. *Vet Clin North Am Adv Companion Anim Behav,* 21:329–342.

Marks I (1987). *Fears, Phobias, and Ritual: Panic, Anxiety, and Their Disorders.* New York: Oxford University Press.

McBride EA, Bradshaw JWS, and Christians A (1995). Factors predisposing dogs to separation problems. In SM Rutter, J Rushen, HD Randle, and JC Eddison (Eds), *Proceedings of the 29th International Congress of the International*

Society for Applied Ethology. Potters Bar, Herts, Great Britain: Universities Federation for Animal Welfare.

McCrave EA (1991). Diagnostic criteria for separation anxiety in the dog. *Vet Clin North Am Adv Companion Anim Behav,* 21:247–255.

Meeusen R and De Meirleir L (1995). Exercise and brain neurotransmission. *Sports Med,* 20:160–188.

Miller D (1966). *The Secret of Canine Communication: HI-FIDO.* Brentwood, CA: Canine Behavior Center.

Monks of New Skete (1991). *The Art of Raising a Puppy.* Boston: Little, Brown.

Morton JRC (1968). Effects of early experience "handling and gentling" in laboratory animals. In MW Fox (Ed), *Abnormal Behavior in Animals.* Philadelphia: WB Saunders.

Mueller WE and Rossol R (1994). Effects of hypericum extract on the expression of serotonin receptors. *J Geriatr Psychiatr Neurol,* 7(Suppl 1):S63–S64.

Mugford RA (1987). The influence of nutrition on canine behavior. J Small Anim Pract 28:1046–1085.

Muller WE and Schafer CS (1996). St. John's wort: In-vitro study about hypericum extract, hypericin, and kampherol as antidepressants. *Dtsch Apoth Ztg,* 136:1015–1022.

Murtra P, Sheasby AM, Hunt SP, and De Felipe C (2000). Rewarding effects of opiates are absent in mice lacking the receptor for substance P. *Nature,* 405:180–183.

Nelson E and Panksepp JB (1996). Oxytocin mediates acquisition of maternally associated odor preferences in preweanling rat pups. *Behav Neurosci,* 110:583–592.

Nelson E, Panksepp, and Ikemoto S (1994). The effects of melatonin on isolation distress in chickens. *Pharmacol Biochem Behav,* 49:327–333.

New JC, Salman MD, King M, et al. (2000). Characteristics of shelter-relinquished animals and their owners compared with animals and their owners in U.S. pet-owning households. *J Appl Anim Welfare Sci,* 3:179–201.

Niimi Y, Inoue-Murayam M, Murayama Y, et al. (1999). Allelic variation of the D4 dopamine receptor polymorphic region in two dog breeds, golden retriever and shiba. *J Vet Med Sci,* 61:1281–1286.

Noonan LR, Caldwell JD, Li L, et al. (1994). Neonatal stress transiently alters the development of hippocampal oxytocin receptors. *Dev Brain Res,* 80:115–120.

Odendaal JSJ (1999). A physiological basis for animal-facilitated psychotherapy [PhD thesis]. Pretoria: University of Pretoria.

Odendaal JSJ (2000). Animal-assisted therapy: Magic or medicine? *J Psychosom Res,* 49:275–280.

Odendaal JSJ and Lehman SMC (2000). The role of phenylethylamine during positive human-dog interaction. *Acta Vet Brno* 69:183–188.

Overall KL, Dunham AE, and Frank D (2001). Frequency of nonspecific clinical signs in dogs with separation anxiety, thunderstorm phobia, and noise phobia, alone or in combination. *JAVMA,* 219:467–473.

Pacchierotti C, Iapichino S, Bossini L, et al. (2001). Melatonin in psychiatric disorders: A review on the melatonin involvement in psychiatry. *Front Neuroendocrinol,* 22:18–32.

Panksepp J (1982). Towards a general psychobiological theory of emotions. *Behav Brain Sci,* 5:407–467.

Panksepp J (1992). Oxytocin effects on emotional processes: Separation distress, social bonding, and relationships to psychiatric disorders. *Ann NY Acad Sci,* 652:243–252.

Panksepp J (1998). *Affective Neuroscience: The Foundations of Human and Animal Emotions.* New York: Oxford University Press.

Panksepp J, Herman BH, Connor R, et al. (1978). The biology of attachment: Opiates alleviate separation distress. *Biol Psychiatry,* 13:607–618.

Panksepp J, Herman BH, Vilberg T, et al. (1980). Endogenous opioids and social behavior. *Neurosci Biobehav Rev,* 4:473–487.

Panksepp J, Conner R, Forster PK, et al. (1983). Opioid effects on social behavior of kennel dogs. *Appl Anim Ethol,* 10:63–74.

Panksepp J, Siviy SM, and Normansell LA (1985). Brain opioids and social emotions. In M Reite and T Field (Eds), *The Psychobiology of Attachment and Separation.* New York: Academic.

Panksepp J, Normansell L, Herman B, et al. (1988). Neural and neurochemical control of the separation distress call. In D Newman (Ed), *The Physiological Control of Mammalian Vocalization.* New York: Plenum.

Panksepp J, Nelson E, and Bekkedal M (1997). Brain systems for the mediation of social separation-distress and social-reward: Evolutionary antecedents and neuropeptide intermediaries. In CS Carter, II Lederhendler, and B Kirkpatrick (Eds), *The Integrative Neurobiology of Affiliation. Ann NY Acad Sci,* 807:78–100.

Petersson M, Hulting AL, and Uvnäs-Moberg K (1999). Oxytocin causes a sustained decrease in plasma levels of corticosterone in rats. *Neurosci Lett,* 264:41–44.

Pettijohn TF, Wong TW, Ebert PD, and Scott JP (1977). Alleviation of separation distress in 3 breeds of young dogs. *Dev Psychobiol*, 10:373–381.

Pierpaoli W and Maestroni GJM (1987). Melatonin: A principal neuroimmunoregulatory and anti-stress hormone—Its anti-aging effects. *Immunol Lett*, 16:355–362.

Pittler MH and Ernst E (2000). Efficacy of kava extract for treating anxiety: Systematic review and meta-analysis. *J Clin Psychopharmacol*, 20:84–89.

Plotsky PM and Meaney MJ (1993). Early, postnatal experience alters hypothalamic corticotropin-releasing factor (CRF) mRNA, median eminence CRF content and stress-induced release in adult rats. *Mol Brain Res*, 18:195–200.

Podberscek AL, Hsu Y, and Serpell JA (1999). Evaluation of clomipramine as an adjunct to behavioural therapy in the treatment of separation-related problems in dogs. *Vet Rec*, 145:365–369.

Polin DM (1992). Canine separation anxiety. *Vet Tech*, 13:403–405.

Porsolt RD, Martin P, Lenegre A, et al. (1990). Effects of an extract of ginkgo biloba (EGB 761) on "learned helplessness" and other models of stress in rodents. *Pharmacol Biochem Behav*, 36:963–971.

Poulton R, Milne BJ, Craske MG, and Menzies RG (2001). A longitudinal study of the etiology of separation anxiety. *Behav Res Ther*, 39:1395–1410.

Puri BK and Richardson AD (2000). The effects of olive oil on omega-3 fatty acids and mood disorders. *Arch Gen Psychiatry*, 57:715.

Radosevich PM, Nash JA, Lacy B, et al. (1989). Effects of low- and high-intensity exercise on plasma and cerebrospinal fluid levels of ir-beta-endorphin, ACTH, cortisol, NE, and glucose in the conscious dog. *Brain Res*, 498:89–98.

Rosenblatt J (1983). Olfaction mediates developmental transition in the altricial newborn of selected species of mammals. *Dev Psychobiol*, 16:347–375.

Schultz W (1998). Predictive reward signal of dopamine neurons. *J Neurophysiol*, 80:1–27.

Scott JP (1958). Critical periods in the development of social behavior in puppies. *Psychosom Med*, 20:42–54.

Scott JP (1991). The phenomenon of attachment in human-nonhuman relationships. In H Davis and D Balfour (Eds), *The Inevitable Bond: Examining Scientist-Animal Interactions*. Cambridge: Cambridge University Press.

Scott JP, Stewart JM, and De Ghett VJ (1973). Separation in infant dogs. In JP Scott and EC Senay (Eds), *Separation and Anxiety: Clinical and Research Aspects*. AAAS Symposium, Washington, DC.

Serdarevic N, Eckert GP, and Müller WE (2001). The effects of extracts from St. John's wort and kava kava on brain neurotransmitter levels in the mouse. *Pharmacopsychiatria (Stuttgart)*, 34(Suppl 1):S134–S136.

Simpson B (1997). Treatment of separation-related anxiety in dogs with clomipramine: Results from a multicentre, blinded, placebo controlled clinical trial. In DS Mills, SE Heath, and LJ Harrington (Eds), *Proceedings of the First International Conference on Veterinary Behavioural Medicine*. Potters Bar, Herts, Great Britain: Universities Federation for Animal Welfare.

Slabbert JM and Rasa OA (1993). The effect of early separation from the mother on pups in bonding to humans and pup health. *J S Afr Vet Assoc*, 64:4–8.

Slotnick BM (1994). The enigma of olfactory learning revisited. *Neuroscience*, 58:1–12.

Slotnick BM, Hanford L, and Hodos W (2000). Can rats acquire an olfactory learning set? *J Exp Psychol Anim Behav Processes*, 26:399–415.

Smith KK, Dharmaratne HR, Feltenstein MW, et al. (2001). Anxiolytic effects of kava extract and kavalactones in the chick social separation-stress paradigm. *Psychopharmacology*, 155:86–90.

Smith JK, Evans AT, Costall B, and Smythe JW (2002). Thyroid hormones, brain function and cognition: A brief review. *Neurosci Biobehav Rev*, 26:45–60.

Steger W (1985). Depressive moods. *Z Allg Med*, 61:914–918.

Stephens DB (1980). Stress and its measurement in domestic animals: A review of behavioral and physiological studies under field and laboratory situations. *Adv Vet Sci Comp Med*, 24:179–210.

Sternberg EM and Gold PW (1997). The mind-body interaction in disease. *Sci Am* (Special Issue: Mysteries of the Mind), 7:8–15.

Stevinson C, Huntley A, and Ernst E (2002). A systematic review of the safety of kava extract in the treatment of anxiety. *Drug Saf*, 25:251–261.

Takeuchi Y, Houpt KA, and Scarlet JM (2000). Evaluation of treatments for separation anxiety in dogs. *JAVMA*, 217:342–345.

Takeuchi Y, Ogata N, Houpt KA, and Scarlett JM (2001). Differences in background and outcome of three behavior problems of dogs. *Appl Anim Behav Sci*, 70:297–308.

Tejedor-Real P, Mico JA, Maldonado R, et al. (1995). Implication of endogenous opioid system in the learned helplessness model of depression. *Pharmacol Biochem Behav*, 52:145–152.

Thomas EA, Carson MJ, and Sutcliffe JG (1998). Oleamide-induced modulation of 5-hydroxytryptamine receptor-mediated signaling. *Ann NY Acad Sci*, 861:183–189.

Thompson WR (1957). Influence of prenatal maternal anxiety on emotional reactivity in young rats. *Science*, 125:698–699.

Topál J, Miklósi A, Csányi V, et al. (1998). Attachment behavior in dogs (*Canis familiaris*): A new application of Ainsworth's (1969) strange situation test. *J Comp Psychol*, 112:219–229.

Tribollet E, Goumaz M, Raggenbass M, and Dreifuss JJ (1991). Appearance and transient expression of vasopressin and oxytocin receptors in the rat brain. *J Recept Res*, 11:333–346.

Tuber DS (1986). Teaching Rover to relax: The soft exercise. *Anim Behav Consult Newsl*, 3(1).

Tuber DS, Hennessy MB, Sanders S, and Miller JA (1996). Behavioral and glucocorticoid responses of adult dogs (*Canis familiaris*) companionship and social separation. *J Comp Psychol*, 110:103–108.

Uchida Y, Dodman NH, and De Ghetto D (1998). Animal behavior case of the month: A captive bear was observed to exhibit signs of separation anxiety, decreased fear of human beings, and stereotypical activity. *JAVMA*, 212:354–355.

Uvnäs-Moberg K (1997a). Oxytocin linked antistress effects: The relaxation and growth response. *Acta Physiol Scand Suppl*, 640:38–42.

Uvnäs-Moberg K (1997b). Physiological and endocrine effects of social contact. In CS Carter, II Lederhendler, and B Kirkpatrick (Eds), *The Integrative Neurobiology of Affiliation. Ann NY Acad Sci*, 807:78–100.

Uvnäs-Moberg K (1998). Antistress pattern induced by oxytocin. *News Physiol Sci*, 13:22–26.

Uvnäs-Moberg K, Stock S, Eriksson M, et al. (1985). Plasma levels of oxytocin increase in response to suckling and feeding in dogs and sows. *Acta Physiol Scand*, 124:391–398.

Voith VL (1980). Destructive behavior in the owner's absence. In BL Hart (Ed), *Canine Behavior*. Santa Barbara, CA: Veterinary Practice.

Voith VL (2002). Use of crates in the treatment of separation anxiety in the dog. In *AVMA Convention Notes*, July 13–17, Nashville, TN.

Voith VL and Borchelt PL (1985). Separation anxiety in dogs. *Compend Continuing Educ Pract Vet*, 7:42–53.

Voith VL and Borchelt PL (1996). Separation anxiety in dogs: Update. In VL Voith and PL Borchelt (Eds), *Readings in Companion Animal Behavior*. Trenton, NJ: Veterinary Learning Systems.

Voith VL, Wright JC, Danneman PJ, et al. (1992). Is there a relationship between canine behavior problems and spoiling activities, anthropomorphism, and obedience training? *Appl Anim Behav Sci*, 34:263–272.

Voith VL, McCrave E, Marder AR, and Lung N (1997). Environmental and behavioural profiles of dogs with separation anxiety. In DS Mills, SE Heath, and LJ Harrington (Eds), *Proceedings of the First International Conference on Veterinary Behavioural Medicine*. Potters Bar, Herts, Great Britain: Universities Federation for Animal Welfare.

Vorbach EU, Huber WD, and Anoldt KH (1994). Effectiveness and tolerance of the hypericum extract LI 160 in comparison with imipramine: Randomized double-blind study with 135 outpatients. *J Geriatr Psychiatr Neurol*, 7(Suppl 1):S19–S23.

Weinstock M (1997). Does prenatal stress impair coping and regulation of hypothalamic-pituitary-adrenal axis? *Neurosci Biobehav Rev*, 21:1–10.

Weinstock M, Poltyrev T, Schorer-Apelbaum D, et al. (1998). Effect of prenatal stress on plasma corticosterone and catecholamines in response to footshock in rats. *Physiol Behav*, 64:439–444.

Windle RJ, Shanks N, Lightman SL, et al. (1997). Central oxytocin administration reduces stress-induced corticosterone release and anxiety behavior in rats. *Endocrinology*, 138:2829–2834.

Winslow JT and Insel TR (2002). The social deficits of the oxytocin knockout mouse. *Neuropeptides*, 36:221–229.

Winslow JT, Hearn EF, Ferguson J, et al. (2000). Infant vocalization, adult aggression, and fear behavior of an oxytocin null mutant mouse. *Horm Behav*, 37:145–155.

Wright ML, Cuthbert KL, Donohue SD, et al. (2000). Direct influence of melatonin on the thyroid and comparison with prolactin. *J Exp Zool*, 286:625–631.

5

Compulsive and Hyperactive Excesses

PART 1: COMPULSIVE BEHAVIOR DISORDERS

Dogs exhibit a variety of compulsive behavior problems. Compulsions typically involve species-typical behavior patterns that are performed repetitively, excessively, and out of normal context. Many common compulsive habits appear to involve disturbances of the seeking system and the exaggeration of normal canine behavior, occurring under the influence of frustration, anxiety, and conflict, especially social conflict. Frustration of the seeking system caused by environmental constraints that thwart the animal's ability to explore, hunt, and obtain normal daily gratification of species-typical appetitive interests may prompt a variety of compensatory compulsive or adjunctive behavior excesses [e.g., schedule-induced licking (see *Displacement Activities and Compulsion* in Volume 2, Chapter 5)]. Self-directed stimulation and injurious behaviors (e.g., self-licking, chewing, scratching and sucking), self-directed motor stereotypies (e.g., tail chasing, whirling, and air snapping), appetitive compulsions (e.g., pica, excessive eating and drinking, destructive chewing, and floor licking), social excesses (attention seeking, barking, licking, and pawing), and loco-motor excesses (pacing, jumping in place, and ground or carpet digging) can all be traced to origins in the seeking system. Behaviors belonging to the sexual system can be liberated to become compulsive excesses (e.g., mounting and thrusting on people or inanimate objects). Like tail chasing, mounting and thrusting behavior resists interruption and may in some cases evoke an aggressive response when dogs are restrained or interrupted while engaging in the behavior. Such behavior may be directed against family members or guests despite intensive inhibitory training and castration. While not customarily described as a compulsion, such behavior presents with many characteristics consistent with a compulsive etiology. The displacement behavior is prevalent during social transitions, especially during greetings and departures, or at other times of increased excitement.

Dogs most prone to develop compulsive behavior problems are frequently high strung and impulsive, temperament dimensions that are exacerbated by adverse environmental conditions. Highly motivated and high-strung dogs that are intolerant of conflict and frustration seem to be particularly at risk for developing compulsive habits. Many dogs appear to exhibit compulsive behaviors at moments of high excitement, suggesting that in some cases compulsions may serve an energy-releasing function. Diagnostically, there is significant overlap between compulsive and impulsive behavior. Differentiating between the two is particularly difficult in the case of repetitive excessive behaviors exhibited by high-strung and excitable dogs. A similar diagnostic difficulty exists in the case of hyperactive versus hyperkinetic dogs (see *Hyperactivity versus Hyperkinesis* in Volume 2, Chapter 5). In general, compulsive behaviors are more exaggerated and resistant to behavior-control efforts than impulsive ones, but even here significant variation exists.

A number of phylogenetically significant behavior systems have been implicated in the development of compulsive stereotypies and rituals, including agonistic, territorial, predatory, grooming, locomotor, and social communication systems. Additionally, separation-related excesses often possess a compulsive character (e.g., repetitive and stereotypic vocal, oral, and motor activities), suggesting that the separation-distress syndrome may involve a similar etiology and functional disturbance (see *Compulsion* in Volume 2, Chapter 4). O'Farrell (1995) has reported evidence suggesting that some compulsive excesses may be linked to owner emotional attachment levels and anthropomorphic attitudes. Licking excesses frequently present in close association with separation-related distress and excessive

confinement (Goldberger and Rapoport, 1991). Instrumental modules and modal activities performing agonistic or territorial functions may be compulsively activated under the influence of adverse social or environmental conditions. Tail-chasing behaviors may involve some degree of self-directed aggression (see *Vacuum Behavior* in Volume 2, Chapter 5), with such dogs frequently barking, growling, and snapping at their tails. Interrupting tail-chasing episodes or even standing nearby while one is ongoing may evoke redirected aggressive threats or attacks by the dog, further supporting the notion that an aggressive motivation may underlie the tail-chasing behavior. Among monkeys exposed to prolonged isolation, self-directed biting and head slapping are frequently observed. Jones and Barraclough (1978) have suggested that these compulsive and self-injurious behaviors may involve an aggressive motivation turned against the animal's body. Rapoport (1989) has observed that the checking rituals common to human patients with obsessive-compulsive disorder (OCD) may involve territorial subroutines dedicated to the maintenance of territorial boundaries and order. Recent studies appear to support the notion that territoriality may underlie human checking compulsions. Joiner and Sachs-Ericsson (2001) have detected a significant correlation between high territoriality scores and the severity of obsessive-compulsive symptoms. The excessive scent marking exhibited by some male dogs may reflect a compulsive exaggeration of a territorial module dedicated to checking and marking over urine deposits left behind by other male and female dogs. In some cases, sniffing and marking rituals may become so engrossing that other behaviors are largely displaced by its performance. Under adverse conditions, highly territorial dogs may develop a variety of compulsive excesses associated with the expression of exaggerated or maladaptive territorial subroutines (e.g., excessive barking and environmental vigilance).

Unable to engage in preferred activities, frustrated dogs may cope with the situation by compulsively engaging in alternative behaviors. In addition to conflict and frustration, stress and boredom appear to play a role in the etiology of compulsive behavior (see *Conflict and Coactive Factors* in Volume 2, Chapter 5). Boredom as the result of insufficient stimulation may be less problematic than boredom resulting from the frustration of exploratory behavior and the reward derived from such activity (see *Separation Distress and Coactive Influences* in Volume 2, Chapter 4). In the case of highly active and unstable extraverts (choleric type), thwarting their ability to explore the environment freely may be intensely aversive. Among such dogs, repetitive compulsive actions may represent a diversion and a significant source of comfort and relief. Boredom in the case of more retiring and introverted types may be less problematic, although unstable introverts (melancholic types) that show anxiety and depressive symptoms at separation may be particularly prone to develop compulsive behaviors aimed at obtaining comfort via lingual stimulation. Dogs expressing relatively balanced and stable temperaments (sanguine and phlegmatic types) appear to be much less at risk for developing compulsive habits under ordinary conditions. These observations are consistent with the supposition that temperament plays a significant predisposing role in the etiology of compulsive behavior disorders (CBDs) in animals (Dallaire, 1993). Temperament also appears to play a prominent role in the development of OCD in humans. Human subjects diagnosed with OCD frequently exhibit comorbid anxiety, depression, and biogenetic temperament dimensions conducive to compulsive disorder, including strong harm-avoidance tendencies, reduced novelty seeking, and impairments in goal-directed activity. The variable presence or absence of these contributory influences significantly affects the severity of symptoms and the patient's response to pharmacological therapy (Lyoo et al., 2001).

Many canine compulsive behaviors appear to develop in close association with increased aversive arousal (e.g., anxiety and frustration) and concomitant physiological changes associated conflict-dense situations and stress. Disruptive behavioral changes are commonly associated with a lack or loss of prediction and control over the social or physical environment. The emotional corollaries of environmental unpredictability and uncontrollability are increased anxiety and frustration. In cases where the environment is disordered, adaptive efforts are stymied by varying levels of conflict-related stress, generalized anxiety, and global behavioral disturbances. The average dog is exposed to a number of intrinsic and inescapable sources of stress stemming from a loss of control over vital interests, including reproductive prerogatives, expression of species-typical activities, free movement, private-space needs, conspecific interaction and company, and other stressors naturally accruing as the result of interspecific interaction and associated prohibitions. Compulsions are often expressed in the form of drive-related behavior (see *Emotional Command Systems and Drive Theory* in Chapter 6). Both compulsive behavior and drive-related behavior are resistant to extinction. Drive activity occurs when a critical arousal threshold is reached in the presence of an appropriate object or target. Similarly, under adverse motivational conditions involving frustration or conflict, disruptive compulsive modules and routines may be launched as critical arousal and frustration levels are exceeded. In addition to drive-related intrinsic reinforcement and gratification, compulsive behavior may be maintained by negative reinforcement insofar as the resulting behavior serves to reduce aversive arousal.

NEUROBIOLOGY AND COMPULSIVE BEHAVIOR DISORDERS

Efforts to localize the brain areas responsible for the expression of compulsive behavior have generally focused on the basal ganglia (Wise and Rapoport, 1989) (see *Neurobiology of Compulsive Behavior and Stereotypies* in Volume 1, Chapter 3). The basal ganglia, also referred to as the striatal complex, consists of several integrated structures, including the caudate nucleus, globus pallidus, nucleus accumbens, ventral tegmental area, and the substantia nigra (Panksepp, 1998). According to the basal ganglia hypothesis, species-typical behaviors stored within the striatal complex as innate motor programs are inappropriately activated under the influence of stressful conflict or frustration. CBDs may ensue when the gating function controlling sensory inputs impinging on the basal ganglia is disrupted. Among humans exhibiting OCDs, positron-emission tomography indicates that the caudate nucleus of patients exhibiting OCDs is more active than in controls not diagnosed with the disorder (Baxter et al., 1987). Under the influence of biological stress, a cascade of neurobiological changes occurs, including the release of adrenocorticotropic hormone (ACTH) and ß-endorphins by the pituitary. ACTH is a potent elicitor of self-grooming activity in rats when it is injected intracranially. ACTH-elicited grooming behavior can be decreased by opioid antagonists (e.g., naloxone or naltrexone) or increased by administering low doses of morphine (Swedo, 1989). Increased opioid release in response to stress has been demonstrated to sensitize dopamine (DA) receptors to apomorphine-induced stereotypies in mice (Cabib et al., 1984)—an agonist effect that is reversed by the administration of naloxone. Opioid receptors are distributed in close association with dopaminergic and serotonergic circuits believed to mediate the expression of compulsive stereotypies. The interaction between these neurochemical systems remains to be fully elucidated, but it is likely that opioids exert a facilitatory influence over DA activity, at least in some substructures of the striatal complex (e.g., the ventral tegmental area), whereas serotonin (5-hydroxytryptamine or 5-HT) appears to perform an inhibitory function. According to this hypothesis, in combination, opioids and 5-HT serve to functionally modulate striatal DA activity; however, things are far more complicated than the foregoing simple relation would suggest. For example, the interaction between opioid and DA systems in the basal ganglia is complementary, with endorphins producing both excitatory and inhibitory effects, depending on the substructure involved (Panksepp, 1998). Nonetheless, chronic exposure to opiates and ß-endorphins has been shown to sensitize the dopaminergic system, as evidenced by increased stereotypic activity in response to DA agonists following treatment with opiates (Cabib et al., 1984). Interestingly, the efficacy of selective serotonin (5-HT)-reuptake inhibitors (SSRIs) to control compulsive stereotypies may be, in part, due to secondary modulatory effects that they have over opioid activity. Rats exposed to chronic treatment with clomipramine exhibit significant changes in opioid function. Clomipramine has been shown to reduce central opioid levels (met-enkephalin), downregulate opioid receptor sites (mu and kappa), and reduce morphine-induced analgesia (see McDougle et al., 1999).

Opioids via their interaction with DA reward circuits in the ventral tegmental area (VTA) may mediate reward signals that serve to support repetitive stereotypies in the absence of external sources of reinforcement. Many compulsive behaviors belong to the seeking system and presumably operate under the stimulatory influence of DA, especially involving the D2 receptor subtype. DA mediates a variety of neuromodulatory functions, including a central role in making reward pleasurable. Although the relationship between increased DA activity and compulsive behavior is not without ambiguity (Goodman et al., 1992), significant evidence does suggest that DA dysregulation may play a functional role in etiology of some CBDs. Psychostimulants (amphetamines) and a variety of DA agonists injected into the ventrolateral striatum have been shown to induce oral stereotypies (biting, gnawing, and paw nibbling) in rats, an effect that is attenuated by inactivating areas of the substantia nigra (Canales et al., 2000). Amphetamines have also been shown to induce self-directed biting, head tossing, and increased vocalization in horses (Shuster and Dodman, 1998). Similar induction effects have been known to occur in domestic animals (sheep, cattle, and horses) in response to injections of the DA agonist apomorphine for many years (see Fraser, 1985). In bank voles, dose-dependent licking can be induced by apomorphine, but not jumping stereotypies (Vandebroek and Ödberg, 1997), suggesting that stress-related jumping may occur independently of the DA system or depend on a DA receptor subtype not affected apomorphine. The D_2 agonist quinpirole can induce repetitive checking behavior in rats—a behavioral compulsion that has been recently proposed as an analogue of human OCD (Szechtman et al., 2001). Just as some repetitive stereotypies can be pharmacologically induced by increasing DA activity in the striatum, agents blocking or inhibiting DA activity can reduce the expression of such behavior. The differential effects of DA agonists and antagonists depend on the DA receptor subtypes that they specifically target. For example, whereas the D_2 antagonist haloperidol exerts an inhibitory effect over repetitive jumping stereotypies in bank voles (Kennes et al., 1988), clozapine, a D_4 antagonist, does not reduce captivity-induced vole stereotypies (Schoenecker and Heller, 2001). Treatment with haloperidol may result in DA receptor hypersensitivity when the DA antagonist is removed, an enhanced sensitivity that is expressed by increased stereotypic activity in response to DA agonists (e.g., apomorphine)—a modulatory effect that may be mediated by DA presynaptic autoreceptors (Martres et al., 1977).

Stress-induced dysregulation of the 5-HT system is regarded by many authorities as playing a prominent role in the etiology of CBDs. The stress-related activation of the HPA system is initiated by corticotropin-releasing factor (CRF). In addition to precipitating a cascade of peripheral hormonal changes, CRF exerts a pronounced influence on a variety of brain areas, including the inhibition of 5-HT-producing cells localized in the dorsal raphe bodies (Kirby et al., 2000). Price and colleagues (1998) found that intracranial injections of CRF produced a biphasic (inhibitory-excitatory) effect on 5-HT release. Although relatively high doses of CRF appear to increase 5-HT release, the predominant effect of CRF on the dorsal raphe bodies appears to be inhibitory, resulting in decreased 5-HT release in the striatum. In addition, Price and coworkers found that high doses of CRF produced compulsion-like behavioral changes, including intense grooming, burying, and head-shaking activities, behavioral effects that may be mediated via CRF fibers innervating the substantia nigra—the source of DA entering the striatal complex. Acute and chronic stress-related release of CRF appears to exert a significant dysregu-

latory effect over serotonergic and dopaminergic systems, changes that may render dogs vulnerable to compulsive disorders and other problems associated with impulse-control deficits.

Chronic overproduction of adrenal glucocorticoids may also have a pronounced effect on serotonergic activity. Smythe and colleagues (1994) have reported that brief maternal separation of infant rats (15 minutes per day) during the first 2 weeks of life has a pronounced effect on 5-HT turnover in the frontal cortex and hippocampus, an effect that appears to shadow the proliferation and distribution of stress-related postnatal glucocorticoid-receptor sites localized in these brain areas. Interestingly, however, 5-HT levels in the frontal cortex of separation-stressed animals are significantly lower in adulthood than nonstressed counterparts. The authors speculate that postnatal handling, and the temporary increase in 5-HT activity produced by it, may trigger the proliferation of glucocorticoid receptors while at the same time reducing the number of 5-HT terminals in the frontal cortex and hippocampus of adult animals, perhaps by means of a 5-HT autoinhibitory signal that impedes the ontogenetic elaboration of the serotonergic system. These findings emphasize the close involvement of the serotonergic system in the modulation of stress, as well as provide a possible explanation for the efficacy of SSRIs in the treatment of stress-related disorders. SSRIs, such as fluoxetine and paroxetine, may assist affected areas of the brain to compensate for the decreased proliferation of cortical and limbic 5-HT terminals by conserving synaptic 5-HT, thereby increasing 5-HT activity and improving the overall capacity of the serotonergic system to cope with heightened stress activity resulting from increased glucocorticoid-receptor expression. Developmental and adult exposure to stress may further exacerbate the situation. In rats, chronic corticosterone administration results in the proliferation of neocortical 5-HT_{2A} receptors and an increase of a behavior anomaly specifically associated with increased 5-HT_{2A} activity known as "wet-dog shakes" (Gorzalka et al., 1998). Interestingly, melatonin has been shown to attenuate the wet-dog shakes associated with chronic corticosterone treatment, suggesting that mela-tonin may have some potency as a 5-HT$_{2A}$ antagonist and potential use in some compul-sive disorders associated with chronic stress.

Attention, Dopamine, and Reward

The dog's ability to orient, select, and contin-uously attend to changes in the environment is a critical aspect of behavioral adaptation (see *Attention and Learning* in Volume 1, Chapter 7). The orienting response is dimin-ished or augmented by the influences of habituation and sensitization, respectively, underscoring its reflexive nature, whereas attending behavior involving the discrimina-tion or continuous sensory tracking of events appears to be strongly influenced by instru-mental contingencies of reinforcement (Cata-nia, 1998). Both classical and instrumental attention-related activities interface along a respondent-operant axis transforming the environment into a predictable and control-lable field of activity—or not (see *Defining Insolvable Conflict* in Volume 1, Chapter 9). Environmentally produced disturbances of attention have been hypothesized as playing a central role in neurotogenesis (see *Locus of Neurotogenesis* in Volume 1, Chapter 9). As a result of exposure to environments lacking predictability and controllability, attention abilities may be strained, with behavioral out-put becoming progressively disorganized and ineffective. As the result of chronic exposure to adverse environments, dogs may, on the one hand, become progressively vulnerable to the elaboration of compulsive rituals or, on the other, fall victim to cognitive and output deficiencies associated with learned helpless-ness. Under the conditioning influence of unpredictable and uncontrollable events (insolvable conflict), affected dogs may gradu-ally acquire a negative cognitive set, whereby they come to act as though significant conse-quences occur independently of what they do or believe. Such dogs may simply give up and stop trying altogether. According to this gen-eral hypothesis, some compulsive rituals and impulsive behaviors may stem from an impairment of central mechanisms control-ling behavior via consequences (e.g., reward and punishment) produced by it, with the net result that repetitive stereotypies and rituals displace organized and goal-oriented behavior. This is consistent with the relative resistance of compulsive behaviors to modification by the arrangement of consequences. These observations underscore the importance of providing affected dogs with training based on highly predictable and controllable out-comes, aimed at restoring a positive cognitive set and convincing such dogs that what they do makes a difference in what happens to them. In general, a history of orderly training and reinforcement results in optimism, com-petence, confidence, and elated mood, whereas a history of excessive and unpre-dictable punishment results in pessimism, increased incompetence and insecurity, depressed mood, helplessness, and increased vulnerability to behavioral disturbance.

Dopaminergic activity appears to enhance attention, positive motivation, and learning. Mills and Ledger (2001) found that dogs treated with selegiline, a DA agonist, focus significantly better on tasks and are less dis-tracted than controls not treated with the drug. They attribute the beneficial effect of the drug to the enhancement of positive incentive. Sensory inputs that attain selective prominence and attention do so through a variety of interacting pathways. Attractive ori-enting stimuli (conditioned and uncondi-tioned appetitive stimuli) appear to converge on midbrain DA neurons located in VTA (see *Catecholamines: Dopamine and Norepinephrine* in Volume 1, Chapter 3). When animals are presented with appetitive stimuli (food), DA neurons normally respond with brief, phasic activations (Schultz et al., 1997). These DA neurons are also activated by the presentation of novel stimuli eliciting an orienting response, but this pattern of activation quickly habituates unless the stimulus is fol-lowed by the presentation of food. After repeated pairings of an auditory or visual stimulus (i.e., a conditioned stimulus or CS) with food (i.e., an unconditioned stimulus or US), the onset of increased DA neuron activ-ity occurs immediately after the presentation of the CS, with no additional DA activity being evident when the food is actually pre-sented (see *Classical Conditioning, Prediction, and Reward* in Chapter 1). These findings suggest that the primary locus of positive reinforcement occurs with the presentation of the conditioned reinforcer—not the ingestion of food, which appears to be of secondary importance, at least with respect to the activation of DA reward circuits. These findings help to explain the power of conditioned reinforcement to shape behavior and the potent incentive value of bridging signals (e.g., "Good", squeak, or click). The study also provides some clues regarding the neurobiology of extinction. After a predictive association is established between the CS and US, the omission of the customary US results in a significant depression of baseline DA activity, appearing precisely at the time (relative to the CS) when rewards were presented in the past (Schultz et al., 1997).

Compulsive excesses often consist of repetitive preparatory behaviors, liberated and functioning in relative independence from consummatory goals. In such cases, the preparatory action may possess more intrinsic reward value for the dog than the actual consummatory action or object itself (see *Instinctive Drift and Appetitive Learning* in Volume 1, Chapter 5; and *Contrafreeloading*, Volume 1, Chapter 5). Dogs may be disposed to develop compulsive excesses in situations where preparatory sequences are repetitively expressed without resulting in the procurement of the attractive object, underscoring the significance of conflict and frustration in the etiology of compulsive disorders. In the case of conflict, preparatory behaviors are repeatedly expressed but unable to achieve the consummatory objective as the result of building anxiety or fear. Under the influence of frustration, preparatory behaviors are repeatedly practiced but not gratified by access to the attractive object or activity. Finally, some repetitive rituals and stereotypies may be acquired as negatively reinforced behaviors, mediating the escape and subsequent avoidance of an *internal* aversive state by responding to antecedent signals originating in the body or environment. In other words, some compulsive behaviors— apotropaic rituals—may serve to ward off, delay, or attenuate an aversive psychophysiological state originating in the body—an action that may also produce significant sec-

ondary gratification associated with increased DA and endogenous opioid activity. Such rituals may evoke parasympathetic effects aimed at modifying aversive physiological states associated with stress. Tongue playing, for example, causes a significant decrease in heart rate in Japanese black calves (Seo et al., 1998). Similarly, rhythmic leg swinging produces a reduction in heart rate among children (Soussignan and Koch, 1985). Canine apotropaic rituals correspond roughly to human obsessive-compulsive rituals, but without reference to the cognitive attributes (e.g., intrusive thoughts and irrational worries).

Dopamine imbalances have been implicated in the etiology of impulse-control deficiencies in people, in association with what Blum and colleagues (1997) have called the reward-deficiency syndrome (RDS), a condition in which an organism is unable to obtain satisfying reward gratification from everyday activities. RDS presents with increased excitability and stimulus-seeking activities, hyperactivity, and compulsivity—all behavioral changes calculated to obtain increased reward gratification. Genetic studies in people and dogs show that alterations in the expression of DA receptors have a pronounced effect on temperament and behavioral thresholds. The seeking-rage axis appears to be strongly influenced by the D_4 receptor, with the short allele being associated with reduced novelty seeking, slowness to anger, and calmness (characteristic of the phlegmatic type), whereas the long allele is associated with increased stimulus-seeking behavior (novelty), compulsiveness, excitability, and lowered thresholds for anger and aggression (characteristic of the choleric type). Niimi and coworkers (1999) have found that golden retrievers and shibas predictably differ in terms of their expression of short versus long D_4 alleles, with golden retrievers being more likely to exhibit the short allele and shibas expressing the long D_4 allele more often (see *Neural and Physiological Substrates* in Volume 2, Chapter 5).

In line with the foregoing observations, training activities incorporating highly predictable and controllable events may help to enhance a dog's general behavioral effectiveness. The use of diverting stimuli and distinct conditioned reinforcers signaling the conclusion of a simple sequence of discrete behaviors leading to positive reinforcement appears to be useful in the management of compulsive behaviors. The activation of DA activity through conditioned reinforcement of behavior incompatible with conflict and stressful arousal may exert a significant neuromodulatory effect. Once the dog is well conditioned with food, the sound of a brief tone or click produces a pronounced orienting effect while serving to activate incompatible appetitive-incentive and appetitive-seeking activities that serve to maintain continuous tracking and attending behavior. Longer-lasting olfactory stimuli, tones, or audio recordings (music) may be paired with the presentation of meals and periods of massage. Presenting novel stimuli alone also exerts a significant disruptive or diverting effect over compulsive activity, but the use of conditioned appetitive stimuli may offer significantly more powerful effects with the added advantage of providing a means for shaping behavior incompatible with the compulsive ritual. Although conditioned appetitive stimuli ("Good", smooch, click, and so forth) may produce a stronger activating effect on DA neurons than merely giving the dog food, if such conditioned stimuli are repeatedly presented without a tangible reward, the enhanced effect is rapidly extinguished. Further, as the bridge signal becomes progressively predictive of the attractive outcome, its ability to activate dopamine neurons is reduced. Dopamine reward activation depends on prediction error, such that the attractive outcome turns out to be better than expected, whereas punishment (depression of dopamine activity) results when the outcome is worse than expected. The detection of prediction error depends on a reference or standard for comparison. To optimize the benefits of reward training, the first step is to establish a control-expectancy standard based on the arrangement of highly predictable and controllable antecedent and consequent training events. In the context of such a backdrop, outcome variations can be used to produce significant changes in the activation and depression of dopamine reward-producing circuits, changes that are of considerable usefulness in the context of canine behavior therapy

(see *Prediction and Control Expectancies* in Chapter 1)

Dopamine: Behavioral and Emotional Regulatory Functions

Growing evidence suggests that stress-related modifications and imbalances of dopaminergic activity profoundly influence cognitive and emotional competence in such diverse areas as selective attention and gating functions, information processing (comparator functions, expectancies, and establishing operations), impulse control, and regulation of emotional behavior (Pani et al., 2000), and compulsive behavior. These various functions are vital aspects of adaptive learning and adjustment. Under adaptive conditions, a network of coordinated interactions between phylogenetically ancient neural substrates and more recent elaborations are integrated to achieve a harmonic organization conducive to adaptive success. Under adverse conditions of escalating stress and disorganization, this harmonic organization may become unstable or break down, thereby liberating primitive defense reactions and abnormal behaviors, ranging from compulsive excesses to impulsive aggression. DA imbalances at the level of prefrontal cortex may significantly impair a dog's ability to cope with stressful situations and to exercise effective executive control over subcortical impulses. Instead of responding in a functional and adaptive way, stress-perturbed prefrontal influences may result in a persistent failure of the dog to respond normally to frustration- and anxiety-producing stimuli, leading to over- (compulsive) or under- (hyperactive) impulse-control impairments (compulsive-impulsive spectrum). DA dysregulation of prefrontal glutamatergic circuits projecting to the striatal complex has been proposed as playing a differentiating role in the etiology of hyperactivity and obsessive-compulsive disorders (Carlsson, 2001) (see *Hyperactivity and Neurobiology*).

PHARMACOLOGICAL CONTROL OF COMPULSIVE BEHAVIOR

A prominent theory suggests that CBDs are primarily the result of disturbances affecting the 5-HT system—a position supported by the clinical efficacy of medications that enhance 5-HT function in the treatment of canine compulsive disorders. SSRIs appear to be most effective in cases where the compulsive behavior is associated with evidence of stress and adverse emotional concomitants (e.g., anxiety). For example, among bank voles exhibiting captivity-induced stereotypies (backward somersaults), citalopram, a potent and highly selective SSRI, showed no effect until acute stress was induced, whereupon a sharp increase in compulsive activity was observed. With the onset of acute stress, citalopram produced a significant modulatory effect over the frequency of motor stereotypies (Schoenecker and Heller, 2001). Animals trained to work under stressful reinforcement schedules may also exhibit a variety of behavioral excesses. Rodents working for food presented on a fixed–interval schedule (1 to 3 minutes), show a variety of behavioral excesses [e.g., polydipsia (Falk, 1971), wood gnawing (Roper and Crossland, 1982), and paw licking (Lawler and Cohen, 1992)]. Woods and colleagues (1993) have shown that schedule-induced polydipsia is significantly reduced by SSRIs (fluoxetine, clomipramine, and fluvoxamine). Adjunctive behavior has been proposed as an experimental model of compulsive behavior (see *Adjunctive Behavior and Compulsions* in Volume 2, Chapter 5).

Significant evidence suggests that SSRIs can be effectively used to manage excessive licking, especially licking that results in local lesions of the skin known as lick granuloma or acral lick dermatitis (ALD). In hopes of obtaining an animal model for investigating human OCDs, several research psychiatrists have investigated the efficacy of SSRIs in the treatment of canine excessive licking. Judith Rapoport and colleagues (1992) at the National Institute of Mental Health (Bethesda, MD) were the first to conduct sound experimental trials to evaluate the efficacy of clomipramine and fluoxetine to control the excessive licking associated with ALD. The researchers found that clomipramine, fluoxetine and, to a lesser extent, sertraline significantly reduced the frequency of compulsive licking exhibited by dogs diagnosed with ALD (N = 37), thereby confirming previous

results of an exploratory study indicating that clomipramine exerted a beneficial effect in the treatment ALD (Goldberger and Rapoport, 1991). More recently, Wynchank and Berk (1998), working with a larger sample of dogs (N = 58), have reported similar benefits resulting from the use of fluoxetine therapy. A pilot study performed by Stein and colleagues (1998) has indicated that citalopram may also be effective in the control of excessive licking, with 66.7% of the dogs treated (N = 9) showing significant improvement. In addition to demonstrated efficacy for the management of ALD, clomipramine appears to reduce tail chasing in dogs (Hewson et al., 1998; Moon-Fanelli et al., 1998; Seksel and Lindeman, 2001). The beneficial effects of SSRIs for controlling canine compulsive disorders appear to be confined to amelioration rather than cure, emphasizing the importance of concurrent behavior therapy.

Although SSRIs frequently help to ameliorate the magnitude and frequency of compulsive behaviors, they are not likely to produce a complete suppression of the target compulsive activity. For example, Rapoport and colleagues (1992) found that the SSRIs studied reduced compulsive licking by less than half in comparison to baseline measures: clomipramine (43%), fluoxetine (39%), and sertraline (24%). Only two dogs (N = 37) showed a complete remission of symptoms, and both dogs were treated with fluoxetine. This pattern of partial efficacy is comparable to the therapeutic effects of SSRIs in the treatment of human OCD. In the case of refractory OCD in human patients, fluvoxamine in combination with haloperidol, a D_2 antagonist, has been proven effective for the treatment of resistant OCD symptoms presenting with comorbid tics (McDougle et al., 1994). The interaction between 5-HT reuptake inhibitors and haloperidol appears to synergistic. For example, 5-HT-enhancing drugs have been shown to potentiate the ability of haloperidol to block DA receptor activity in the rat striatum (Sugrue, 1983). McDougle and colleagues (2000) have also found that risperidone (a potent antagonist of 5-HT_{2A} and DA_2 receptors) in combination with fluvoxamine is effective in the treatment of refractory OCD, with or without tics. In addition to efficacy, a major advantage of risperidone as a treatment adjunct is that it appears to produce fewer adverse side effects than observed in the case of haloperidol.

Other veterinary clinical protocols have targeted the opioid system. The suppressive effects of opioid antagonists (e.g., naloxone, naltrexone, and nalmefene) on compulsive habits have been clinically demonstrated in dogs (Brown, 1987; Dodman et al., 1988; White, 1990; Shuster and Dodman, 1998). Opioid antagonists have been found effective for reducing excessive self-directed licking (Dodman et al., 1988; White, 1990). In a clinical study involving 11 dogs with ALD, over 70% exhibited significant improvement when treated with naltrexone (White, 1990). Adverse side effects were minimal, with only one dog showing drowsiness and social withdrawal symptoms. One report, however, has noted the occurrence of significant dermatologic side effects (acute, intense, and generalized pruritus) in a dog treated with naltrexone (Schwartz, 1993). Brown (1987) found that naloxone proved efficacious in the control of tail chasing in a bull terrier, whereas phenobarbital was ineffective. Control over tail chasing was maintained by combining pentazocine (a mixed opioid agonist-antagonist) and naloxone. After 18 months of treatment, the owners reported that tail chasing rarely occurred, so long as the medication was maintained. Blackshaw and colleagues (1994) have evaluated a variety of regimens (e.g., synthetic progestins, diazepam, and naloxone) for the treatment of refractory tail chasing. An emaciated bull terrier treated with naloxone showed significant improvement while on the medication. The dog was also given a narcotic drug (meperidine), whereupon it became more agitated and lunged at its shadow. All of the dogs (N = 32) were ultimately euthanized. Dodman and colleagues (1996) have reported that several bull terriers with tail-chasing stereotypies (N = 6) and other behavior problems [e.g., unprovoked aggression (N = 1) and intense fear (N = 1)] were affected by seizures (epileptiform spiking) and varying degrees of hydrocephalus. The electroencephalograms of all of the dogs tested were abnormal. Phenobarbital showed some efficacy in four of the tail-chasing dogs and the one dog exhibiting extreme symptoms of fear. Phenobarbital

treatment of tail chasing may produce an increased risk of aggression associated with episodes (Dodman et al., 1993 and 1996). At the moment, the drug treatment of choice for the control of compulsive licking or tail chasing is clomipramine or fluoxetine (Landsberg, 2001).

Note: The foregoing information is provided for educational purposes only. If considering the use of medications to control or manage a behavior problem, readers should consult with a veterinarian familiar with the use of drugs for such purposes in order to obtain diagnostic criteria, specific dosages, and medical advice concerning potential adverse side effects and interactions with other drugs.

POTENTIAL DIETARY TREATMENTS

Serotonin production and activity may be modified via dietary means and supplementation. Diets low in protein content (e.g., 16% to 18%) and high in carbohydrate levels appear to facilitate improved transport of the 5-HT precursor tryptophan through the blood-brain barrier (see *Diet and Enhancement of Serotonin Production* in Volume 1, Chapter 3). Tryptophan supplementation has been suggested as a possible treatment alternative for the management of compulsive behavior in horses (Luescher, 1998). Another potentially valuable way to improve 5-HT metabolism involves treatment with 5-hydroxytryptophan (5-HTP). Unlike tryptophan, 5-HTP freely passes through the blood-brain barrier and bypasses a critical rate-limiting step in the metabolism of 5-HT; also, it is readily available for purchase over the counter, unlike tryptophan (see *Nutrition and Aggression* in Volume 2, Chapter 6). Finally, some evidence suggests that inositol may provide a significant therapeutic effect in the treatment of human depression, panic disorder, and OCD. In a double-blind crossover trial, OCD patients (N = 13) not effectively treated with SSRIs were given inositol or placebo for a 6-week period (Mendel et al., 1996). The results indicate that inositol exerted a significant benefit, comparable to that produced by fluvoxamine and fluoxetine. Chronic treatment with inositol has also been shown to reduce behavior associated with anxiety and depression in rats, with some evidence indicating that inositol may exert a strong attenuating effect over anxiety following acute stress (Einat and Belmaker, 2001).

DIAGNOSTIC CONSIDERATIONS

Inclusion Criteria

A variety of criteria have been suggested to assist in the formal diagnosis of compulsive disorder in dogs. A study by Hewson and Luescher (1999) was performed to validate some of these diagnostic criteria. They compared the diagnoses made by an animal behavior expert with diagnoses based on a set of formal criteria. The owners of dogs (N = 84) with possible compulsive disorders were interviewed on two separate occasions. The first interview involved the completion of a behavior-history questionnaire, with the diagnosis of compulsive disorder requiring that the dog satisfy seven formal criteria (Table 5.1). A veterinary behavior expert whose diagnosis was based on clinical experience performed the second interview. The resulting statistical analysis showed a surprising lack of diagnostic agreement between the two methods. Of 60 dogs providing sufficient information to apply the seven formal criteria, there was agreement between the formal diagnosis and the expert's opinion in only 20% of the cases. Among these 12 cases of agreement, eight agreed on the absence of compulsive disorder and four agreed on the presence of compulsive disorder. Among the 48 cases in which disagreement occurred, 12 dogs diagnosed with compulsive disorder by the expert were excluded as not having CBD by the absence of all three formal inclusion criteria believed to be highly significant (see criteria 3, 4, and 5 in Table 5.1). Other dogs diagnosed with CBD by the expert but excluded as not having CBD by formal diagnostic criteria, included 13 dogs that met criterion 3, three dogs that met criteria 3 and 4, six dogs that met criteria 3 and 5, on dog that met criterion 4, eight dogs that met criterion 5, and five dogs that met criteria 4 and 5. Among those dogs (N=4) presenting with signs matching all three formal diagnostic criteria, there was complete agreement between the inclusion criteria and the expert's opinion regarding the diagnosis of CBD. Taken together, the lack of correspondence between the expert's diagnosis and formal diagnostic inclusion criteria suggests that the process of diagnosing such behavior problems involves a great deal of contingent fuzziness and subjective judgment.

The finding of a significant independence between the two methods of diagnosis with respect to the presence of conflict and contextual generalization is surprising, given the prominence attributed to conflict and frustration in the etiology and situational generalization of compulsive disorder (Hewson and Luescher, 1996). Even so, as a diagnostic inclusion criterion, a history of precipitating conflict and frustration is problematic, not because it lacks etiological significance, but simply because the owner may not be aware of such an influence (Wynchank and Berk, 1998). Undoubtedly, behavioral conflict and stress play an important role in the etiology and maintenance of many compulsive behavior problems, but some influence other than conflict and stress is obviously at work and

TABLE 5.1. Formal criteria for diagnosing compulsive behavior disorder (Hewson et al., 1999)

1. The dog has normal findings on physical examination.

2. The dog shows compulsive behavior (e.g., tail chasing, air snapping, and excessive licking).

3. Conflict or frustration is associated with the etiology of the behavior or present in a current situation (e.g., conflict, separation anxiety, inadequate stimulation, physical restraint, or social change).

4. The number of contexts in which the compulsive behavior has increased since it was first observed.

5. The frequency of the behavior has increased since it was first noticed.

6. The behavior is not dependent on conditioning and occurs both in the owner's presence and absence.

7. The behavior is not due to seizure activity.

needs to be clarified to complete the picture. A major problem with the conflict hypothesis is that conflict and frustration are ubiquitous and commonplace but compulsive stereotypies are comparatively rare. Why do some dogs develop compulsive stereotypies while the vast majority do not?

First and foremost, there is probably a genetic predisposition involved, and perhaps a specific genetic marker may be eventually identified to help predict, diagnose, and prevent compulsive stereotypies and related adjustment problems. Of course, this is all speculative at the moment, but such a genetic marker may not be too far off in the future. One potential candidate involves genetic variants associated with the expression of dopamine receptors (see *Attention, Dopamine, and Reward*). Among humans, individuals expressing the A_1 allele for the D_2 receptor (particularly those homozygous for it) are significantly more likely to show adjustment problems in association with impulsive and compulsive behavior (Blum et al., 1997). The A_1 allele reduces the expression of the D_2 receptor up to 30% in comparison to individuals expressing the A_2 allele, perhaps significantly impeding the carrier's ability to normally experience reward and respond to reward signals. Another potential marker of interest involves the long and short alleles expressing the D_4 receptor. Among humans, the long allele is associated with novelty seeking, compulsive-impulsive behavior, excitability, and aggressiveness, whereas the short allele is associated with hesitation, reserve, and tolerance (slow to anger) (see Ebstein et al., 1996).

According to this hypothetical model, dogs prone to compulsive behavior involving a strong locomotor and aggressive component (e.g., tail chasing) would be most likely to express a dopamine-receptor profile consistent with the choleric temperament (e.g., A_1 and long alleles). On the other hand, dogs showing self-directed compulsive behavior (e.g., licking) would be most likely to express a dopamine-receptor profile consistent with the melancholic temperament (e.g., A_1 and short alleles). Finally, dogs expressing the A_2 allele in combination with the long or short alleles for the D_4 receptor would tend to differentially exhibit propensities consistent with the sanguine (e.g., A_2 and long alleles) and

the phlegmatic (e.g., A_2 and short alleles) types. These four types, corresponding to Pavlov's typology (see *Experimental Neurosis* in Volume 1, Chapter 9), are hypothetically differentiated by their relative sensitivity to signals of reward and punishment (risk and loss):

Adaptive types
Sanguine (stable extravert) or s-type: Preferentially sensitive to signals of reward, much less so toward signals of successful avoidance; prone to adaptive approach.
Phlegmatic (stable introvert) or p-type: Preferentially sensitive to signals of successful avoidance, less so toward signals of reward; prone to adaptive hesitation.

Reactive types
Choleric (unstable extravert) or c-type: Preferentially sensitive to signals of loss, much less so toward signals of threat; prone to reactive frustration.
Melancholic (unstable introvert) or m-type: Preferentially sensitive to signals of threat, less so toward signals of loss; prone to reactive fear (see Figure D.1 in Appendix D).

Dogs showing a heightened sensitivity to signals of punishment, falling along the choleric-melancholic spectrum, are generally predisposed to respond to stressful conflict and frustration by reacting (e.g., attacking, repeating, persisting, or withdrawing). Conversely, dogs showing a heightened sensitivity to signals of reward, falling along the sanguine-phlegmatic spectrum, are generally predisposed to respond to stressful conflict and frustration by adapting (e.g., approaching, searching, experimenting, and waiting). According to this hypothesis, dogs fitting the choleric-melancholic profile are more prone to develop compulsive stereotypies as the result of stressful conflict educing frustration (c-type) and anxiety (m-type). The relatively fearless c-type may respond paradoxically to punishment. In such cases, rather than suppressing ongoing compulsive activity (e.g., tail chasing), punishment may increase it. C-type dogs appear to be vulnerable to vicious circle behavior, responding to signals of punishment by increasing behavioral output rather than inhibiting it (Melvin, 1971).

Excessive or inappropriate punishment or early trauma and stress may sensitize s- and p-type dogs to signals of punishment, causing them to become progressively vulnerable to develop reactive elaborations consistent with c- and m-types. Such reactive s-type dogs are often highly sensitive to both reward and punishment signals and may show extremes of intrusive playfulness and excitability, on the one hand, and inhibition and withdrawal, on the other, with little else in between. Under the influence of excessive punishment, s- and p-type dogs may become progressively unstable and reactive to signals of punishment (threat and loss), making them more vulnerable to develop compulsive stereotypies and other adjustment problems. The disruptive sensitization and polarization of behavioral approach and inhibition systems are hypothesized to result in the dysregulation of adaptive functions (see Gray, 1994), causing the dog to become inappropriately reactive to signals of reward and punishment. The alternating bipolar impulsive excitability and depressive inhibition exhibited by reactive s-type dogs is resolved by therapy efforts aimed at reintegrating behavioral approach and inhibition systems via orderly and consistent reward-based training and play. A significant function of cynopraxic training and therapy is to promote social exchanges that reliably succeed in producing reward signals in the context of reducing interactive conflict and tension. As a result of such training, maladaptive reactivity and adjustment problems are often ameliorated or resolved while at the same time improving the human-dog relationship.

Exclusion Criteria

Differential diagnosis should distinguish compulsive behavior from transient responses to conflict, learned behaviors, and behavioral sequela associated with disease. Although stereotypical activity resulting from medical conditions (e.g., partial onset seizures) is excluded, some physical injuries and traumas may set the stage for the subsequent development of compulsive behavior. Wynchank and Berk (1998) reported that although most owners could not give a reason underlying their dogs' excessive licking, 22.4% of the dogs (N = 58) began licking after a trauma or injury to the affected area. The comfort and anxiety reduction derived from repetitive licking on an injury may establish a network of conditioned associations linking the action of licking with the elicitation of feelings of comfort and safety. As a result of the intrinsic gratification produced by licking, it may be emancipated from the original function of soothing an injury to become a generalized strategy for coping with aversive emotional arousal. Emotional distress (frustration and anxiety) is essentially an aversive state involving the loss of comfort and safety. Signals of loss and suspense may function as establishing operations activating episodes of licking behavior. Licking itself may be maintained by enhanced feelings of comfort and safety, on the one hand, and an incentive to avoid signals (internal cues) portending loss and uncertainty, on the other. In short, excessive licking is an escape or brief vacation from stressful arousal. In addition to physical injuries and trauma, excessive licking may develop in association with allergies, foreign objects, arthritis, and infections (Veith, 1986) and possibly with hypothyroidism (Aronson, 1998). As the medical cause of excessive licking is discovered and treated, the licking activity may simply stop; however, in some cases, the licking may continue and become a compulsive activity.

Air-snapping behavior, an activity giving the appearance of biting at flies, has been attributed to sensory hallucinations (Voith, 1979) and vitreous floaters, that is, particulate matter suspended in a gel-like substance behind the lens of the eye (Cash and Blauch, 1979), but no clinical evidence has been reported to date establishing such a causal relationship. Another hypothesis suggests that some cases of air snapping may stem from food sensitivities or allergic reactions affecting central nervous system activity (Voith, 1979). For example, Brown (1987) reported a case (a 1-year-old, male, cavalier) in which air snapping was rapidly resolved by feeding the dog a low-protein diet consisting of fish and milk proteins. When again fed red meat, poultry, or rabbit, the air-snapping activity recurred. This report gives some support, albeit anecdotal, to the notion that food sensitivities or allergies may contribute to the development of certain stereotypies. Behavioral stereotypies involving episodic air snapping (Voith, 1979), tail chasing (Dodman et al., 1996), and air snapping with excessive licking (Crowell-Davis et al., 1989) have been linked to focal seizure activity. Although partial onset seizure activity may be an occasional factor in the development compulsive behavior, it appears to be relatively rare. Nonetheless, such possible causes should be excluded, along with other medical problems that might adversely affect the dog's behavior and hamper therapy efforts. The exclusion of medical causes requires a veterinary examination and appropriate diagnostic testing.

EVALUATION, PROCEDURES, AND PROTOCOLS

The treatment of compulsive behavior combines a variety of behavior-modifying strategies. The selection of specific techniques depends on a number of factors, including the severity of the compulsive behavior and the owner's ability to comply with the recommendations. In all cases, it is valuable to obtain a thorough history and medical background. Since environmental deficiencies and stressors appear to play a role in the etiology of compulsive excesses, it is necessary to evaluate such influences and make recommendations based on a subjective assessment of each situation. If environmental sources of significant conflict, stress, or frustration are identified (e.g., separation-related distress, excessive crate confinement, disorderly training, or mistreatment), efforts to reduce or eliminate such influences should be considered (see *Compulsive Behavior Problems* in Volume 2, Chapter 5). In many cases, an environmental cause is not readily identifiable, suggesting the involvement of a biological mechanism or an internal cue controlling compulsive behavior in response to generalized or conditioned frustration or anxious arousal (see *Assessment and Evaluation* in Volume 2, Chapter 5).

Many compulsive dogs are highly active and usually benefit from additional vigorous exercise, especially activities involving physical exertion but requiring a high degree of attentional focus and impulse control. Ball and flying-disk play, agility exercises (weave poles and jumps), and play-oriented obedience training may also be beneficial. Situations

evocative of stress-induced compulsive behavior should be avoided as much as possible, unless ongoing behavior-therapy efforts are in place. Although many compulsive behaviors respond to behavior therapy, some pathological compulsions may persist despite the most conscientious training efforts, suggesting the presence of neurobiological disorder and the need for adjunctive pharmacological intervention. Finally, some compulsive behaviors may be a nuisance or aesthetically displeasing but not harmful to the dog. For example, sucking, kneading, and licking compulsions directed toward inanimate objects (e.g., blankets or flooring) are often best left alone unless the compulsive behavior results in damage or harm to the dog.

In addition to general contextual and motivational factors, information concerning specific triggers, the frequency of the behavior, and its duration, and time and place should be noted. Information about persons present and their proximity to the dog as well as ongoing activities should be explored. Of particular importance is the ease with which the dog can be distracted from the activity and the interval between recurring bouts. Compulsive behaviors and rituals that can be easily interrupted are typically more responsive to behavior-therapy efforts. Stereotypic repetitive behaviors that cannot be safely interrupted or that require physical restraint to stop may benefit from pharmacological intervention in conjunction with intensive behavior therapy and training efforts. By combining behavior and drug therapy approaches, there is a better likelihood of achieving more durable changes when the medication is discontinued.

Together with the objective of resolving specific complaints, counseling and therapy activities should be performed with cynopraxic goals in mind (see *Cynopraxis: Training and the Human-Dog Relationship* in Volume 1, Chapter 10). From the cynopraxic perspective, the behavioral complaint is an opportunity for owners to enhance their relationship with the dog and to improve the dog's quality of life. Ostensibly, the behavior problem brings the trainer and dog owner together for the purpose of modifying the dog's behavior, but the true intent and measure of success for cynopraxic counseling and therapy efforts is the furtherance of cynopraxic bonding and quality of life objectives. As the result of such emphasis, even in cases where training efforts are not entirely successful in the short-term, a significant benefit is nonetheless achieved by fostering a better understanding of the problem and helping the owner to better cope with it. In addition to increasing the owner's appreciation of the dog's needs, the training and management skills acquired by the owner lay the groundwork for the long-term improvement or successful resolution of the problem as well as facilitating a more fulfilling and rewarding experience of the dog as a companion and family member.

Diversion and Disruption

Some compulsive behaviors can be effectively managed with the use of diverters and disrupters aimed at interrupting the compulsive sequence (see *Diverters and Disrupters* in Volume 1, Chapter 7). For example, tossing a ball just as the dog begins to chase its tail can be a useful diversion. Subsequent access to the toy can be made contingent upon the absence of the tail-chasing behavior. In addition to the presentation of play objects, target-arc training can be used to generate an effective diverter stimulus (squeaker, smooch, or whistle) having considerable value in the context of treating CBDs (see *Attention and Play Therapy* in Chapter 8). Savory treats can also be used to divert the dog from the compulsive ritual and to subsequently reward attending behavior or to reinforce actions incompatible with the compulsive habit. Since the dog is not performing the ritual with the purpose of controlling access to food, the provision of food as a diversionary stimulus is not likely to strengthen the undesirable compulsive behavior. Instead the diversionary presentation of food functions as an establishing operation that is more likely to set the occasion for the dog to show behavior incompatible with the compulsive action, that is, actions that enabled the dog to successfully control food-sharing exchanges with the owner in the past (e.g., attentive (begging and simple obedience modules). Disrupter-type stimuli can also be useful, especially in cases where diverters are not effective alone or in cases where the dog resumes the compulsive excess after being

diverted from it. A rolled sock or one containing a small amount of popcorn and knotted is very effective in the case of mild compulsive behaviors. The sound of throw rings thrown near the dog can rapidly acquire a conditioned inhibitory effect, subsequently making them effective when tossed up and down in the hand. Similarly, a shaker can, push-button alarm, or compressed-air device can be effectively used for such purposes.

Response Prevention, Interruption, and Shaping Incompatible Responses

When excessive repetitive behavior is associated with a specific environmental event or situation, the first step, whenever possible, is to modify the environment in order to eliminate such adverse influences. In cases where environmental modification is not possible, the dog's response to the stimulation must be modified. Compulsive rituals unresponsive to interruption efforts may benefit from response-prevention techniques. During response prevention, the compulsive behavior is blocked by various means, including physical restraint. Exposure with response prevention has been proven to be effective in the treatment of a variety of human OCDs. Chasing shadows and flecks of light are common behavioral excesses among highly excitable and reactive dogs. The origin of such compulsions can often be traced to teasing games involving flashlights or laser pointers. Such behavior can be highly disruptive and disturbing, especially if it is associated with barking or destructive behavior. Since specific classes of stimuli consistently evoke such behavior, they are typically highly responsive to exposure with response prevention, counterconditioning, differential reinforcement of incompatible behavior (DRI), inhibitory training using disrupter stimuli (e.g., a modified carbon-dioxide pump or shaker can), and time-out (TO) procedures. In extreme cases, however, such behavior can be highly persistent and resistant to behavior-control strategies. For example, in one case, an English bulldog developed a highly stereotypic and compulsive aggression ritual in response to lights being turned on. The dog jumped, barked, and snapped at ceiling lights until they were turned off or until becoming physically exhausted. The ritual was extremely energetic, persistent, and aggressive. Any efforts to restrain the dog during such episodes resulted in redirected aggression, making treatment efforts dangerous and unproductive. The dog had undergone veterinary testing and treatment, including various antiseizure medications, to no avail.

Leash prompts and directives leading to the reinforcement of alternative behaviors can be helpful as a means to interrupt and diminish compulsive excesses that habitually occur in the owner's presence. For example, a dog that engages in excessive licking can be kept on a leash and collar or halter at times when it is likely to lick. When licking occurs, the action is interrupted by saying "Stop" and directing the dog's mouth away from the licked area by pulling on the leash. The licking dog can also be trained to perform an incompatible response via DRI training, such as turning its head away from the licked area on signal, perhaps redirecting the dog's interest toward a toy. A clicker can be used to bridge the occurrence of the incompatible response with a food reward or toy. In cases where the compulsive behavior occurs at a high rate, differential reinforcement of other behavior (DRO) can be introduced (see *Differential Reinforcement of Other Behavior* in Volume 1, Chapter 7). The DRO procedure provides contingent reinforcement based on the absence of behavior during some fixed or variable length of time. The primary criterion for reinforcement to occur is that the dog refrain from the compulsive activity during the preset DRO time period. An advantage of the DRO technique is that it provides a high frequency of reward and support for a variety of alternative behaviors occurring in the absence of the compulsion, more specifically those behaviors whose occurrence happens to coincide with the offset of the DRO period. Eventually, as the rate of compulsive activity is reduced, a response incompatible with licking can be brought under the control of a DRI schedule.

Bringing the Compulsive Habit Under Stimulus Control

A common complaint involving compulsive attention seeking is excessive pawing directed at family members or guests—a social excess that is prevalent among golden retrievers. Social pawing, which can be a persistent habit that resists corrective efforts, is most commonly exhibited in situations in which a dog is conflicted by opposing motivations between attention-seeking needs and unstable boundaries established to control excesses associated with it. Pawing has a controlling and obnoxious quality about it that becomes especially evident and transparent if the owner or guest attempts to stop or restrain the dog while it is performing the attention-seeking excess. Direct punishment is not recommended because of the social nature of the behavior, and many owners are justly reluctant to punish such behavior. Extinction (ignoring the behavior) is of little value for controlling such excesses.

An effective approach for resolving this problem involves bringing the pawing behavior under stimulus control. The first step is to reinforce every pawing action with the presentation of food. As the dog learns that its pawing action turns on the presentation of a treat, a vocal signal like "Paw" or "Shake" can be overlapped with the action or just slightly in anticipation of it. Once the behavior is actively under the control of the vocal signal, pawing actions that occur off cue are ignored, blocked, or suppressed by TO (the owner gets up and walks away). Pawing action occurring off cue is followed by "Stop." If necessary, progress can be facilitated by employing a response-prevention procedure, whereby a leash is used to shift the dog's weight toward the side left unsupported during pawing actions. Another method is to grasp the dog's paw and hold it firmly but without producing discomfort. At the moment when the struggle to break the control reaches a peak, the paw is released as the owner shouts "Stop." This procedure is repeated every time the dog extends his paw. Grasping the dog's paw is mildly aversive, while the act of successfully withdrawing it is negatively reinforced. By shouting the word signal "Stop" at the moment of release, the signal is associated with the subsequent paw-withdrawal behavior. As the signal becomes conditioned, it can be used to interrupt future pawing efforts. Despite conscientious training efforts, it is sometimes necessary to interrupt the behavior with an appropriate disrupter stimulus (e.g., low-pressure compressed air) or the presentation of a scent previously paired with a compressed-air startle.

Once a dog hesitates and inhibits pawing, the owner should challenge-dare the dog by slapping a knee and delivering the words "Do you want!" in a forbidding tone of voice. The challenge-dare provokes a conflictive choice point, whereby the dog is tempted to paw but hesitates and chooses not to paw in deference to the owner's forbidding tone. If the dog resists the challenge-dare temptation, the appropriate hesitation and choice is rewarded with affection and an opportunity to give its paw on command, "Paw." The pawing response is subsequently stopped with the command "Stop" and the dog's compliance rewarded with food and petting. If the dog fails to stop or attempts to paw off-cue it is diverted, reprimanded, restrained, or timed out, as appropriate.

EXCESSIVE LICKING AND TAIL CHASING

Excessive Licking

A dog's excessive licking directed toward its body or inanimate objects (e.g., floor, carpeting, or furniture) is a relatively common compulsive habit. Since licking is often secondary to a variety of medical causes, it is crucial that a veterinary differential diagnosis be performed to exclude such factors and provide necessary treatment. Licking excesses that result in hair loss and sores (e.g., ALD) to the extremities are best approached by the application of a combination of behavioral techniques, selected on the basis of a dog's needs and response to therapy. Modifying social and environmental sources of stress and conflict can be helpful but rarely completely resolve the problem. If licking activity is found to occur in association with an identifiable stimulus, a process of graduated exposure in conjunction with counterconditioning or exposure with response prevention might be helpful. Distracting the dog or prompting and reinforcing alternative activities incompatible with the compulsive activity may also be beneficial (e.g., fetching a toy). Excessive licking toward the body or inanimate objects often occurs when the dog appears relaxed and when little else is going on in the household

(Hewson et al., 1998)—a finding that seems to suggest that such dogs lick to obtain stimulation or to comfort themselves. In such cases, supplemental massage, play, and exercise may be particularly beneficial.

A scented squeaker can sometimes be effectively used to control excessive licking. The compound squeak-and-odor stimulus is delivered at the earliest moment in the licking sequence, causing the dog to turn away from the licked area and direct its attention toward the trainer. In mild cases, the squeaker-odor combination alone may be sufficient to interrupt licking, especially in cases where the odor has been previously associated with play and posture-facilitated relaxation training. In cases requiring more control, a previously conditioned click is used to strengthen behavior that turns the dog's attention away from the licking site. Initially, the dog's orienting response to the squeaker is immediately bridged with a click and food reward. As the training process proceeds, a variable DRO schedule of reinforcement is introduced requiring that the dog not orient back toward the site of licking for some varied period followed by the click and food reward. The size and type of the food reward should be varied to maximize its reinforcement effect. Although any response other than licking is reinforced at the conclusion of the DRO period, gradually the licking behavior can be channeled into some other activity (e.g., licking peanut butter from a hollow rubber toy). Also, DRO scheduling can be followed by a series of attention and basic training exercises reinforced with food, petting, and play. The DRO schedule generates a reward-dense training situation that is highly compatible with a variety of TO procedures. For example, if a dog licks before the end of the DRO period, the schedule can be reset following a brief TO, during which licking is prevented or blocked and rewards are withdrawn for 30 seconds or so.

Many compulsive licking habits do not occur reliably under the elicitation of specific social or environmental stimuli that can be controlled or changed. For example, excessive licking activity sometimes develops in association with separation distress or boredom (i.e., frustration of the seeking system). Also, some compulsive licking may be performed as an apotropaic ritual and maintained by the anxiety-reducing effects produced by the activity. So long as the dog is able to perform the repetitive action, it will not likely adopt other ways to cope with stress. Consequently, it is often necessary to block or prevent the licking behavior by physical restraint. In mild cases, covering the area with an elastic bandage can be a useful way to prevent licking when the owner is absent. Alternatively, in more severe cases, the dog may need to be fitted with an Elizabethan collar to prevent licking activity. When the owner is present, a leash and collar, halter, bandaging, or muzzle can be used to prevent the dog from licking or performing similar compulsive behaviors. The dog should never be left alone while wearing a leash, halter, or muzzle. Muzzle restraint can be applied contingently in response to licking episodes. If the dog licks and fails to respond to the interruption signal "Stop," the muzzle is placed on the dog. After a brief period of response prevention, the muzzle is removed, and the dog is given an appetizing chew toy (e.g., a rubber toy slathered inside with peanut butter) used to redirect licking activity. In this case, licking turns on muzzling while not licking turns it off—a contingency that may gradually help to reduce compulsive licking. At such times, massage and the presentation of an olfactory stimulus (e.g., orange, chamomile, or lavender) previously associated with safety and relaxation can be used to support arousal incompatible with anxiety. Diffusing an olfactory safety signal (OSS) into the room may also yield some benefit (see *Olfactory Conditioning* in Chapter 6).

In the case of refractory or self-mutilative compulsions, the trainer might consider various aversive counterconditioning and aversion-relief procedures. In general, aversive procedures should be applied only after less intrusive and nonaversive methods have failed. In some cases, a repellent may be applied to the licked area or to bandages, but such approaches do not appear to be very effective. Another approach that may be more effective involves the use of a taste-aversion procedure (Gustavson, 1996). Many studies have demonstrated the efficacy of taste aversion for inducing a lasting repulsion toward tastes and foods associated with nausea (see

Taste Aversion in Volume 1, Chapter 6). In this case, a novel tasting substance is applied to the licked area. After licking the treated area, the dog is exposed to a nausea-producing agent. It is reasonable to suppose that taste-aversion therapy might produce a lasting repulsion toward the substance, perhaps sufficient to deter the dog from licking on areas treated with it. To my knowledge, this procedure has not been tested for efficacy, but it would seem to represent a possible means for controlling severe and refractory self-mutilative behavior. It should be noted, however, that the viability of taste aversion for controlling canine appetitive behavior has not proven to be very effective or durable, and the procedure is not free of potential undesirable side effects (see *Tolerance for Nausea and Taste Aversion* in Volume 2, Chapter 9).

Although various remote startle devices (e.g., shaker can, compressed air, and alarm devices) can momentarily interrupt licking episodes, the behavior tends to recover rapidly. Compressed air delivered through a modified carbon-dioxide (CO_2)-charged air pump (see *Modified Carbon-dioxide Pump* in Chapter 2) can be scented with an odor (e.g., citronella-eucalyptus mix). After the dog is sensitized to the odor, it can be applied to the licked area to produce a more lasting effect. A brief burst of scented air is directed toward the area being lick, both startling the dog and leaving a scented reminder on the spot. The diluted scent can be subsequently applied to the area with a cotton squab. Odors previously associated with startle may directly inhibit licking or potentiate the effect of other (weaker) startling events, thereby making them more effective. A remote-activated citronella collar can be used to produce a similar result. Again, a dilute citronella scent can be applied directly to the area, taking care not get the material into open sores. Finally, a scented seven-penny shaker can is sometimes used in a similar way to disrupt excessive licking. When the can is first used, it should be tossed near the dog to produce a sensitized response to the sound and odor. After a few such exposures, a shake or rattle of the can will evoke a strong inhibitory response. Such techniques should only be used in the context of reward-based training efforts in which alternative behavior is prompted and reinforced after licking is inhibited (e.g., giving the dog a hollow rubber toy smeared with peanut butter).

An aversive technique that has shown efficacy for inhibiting excessive licking is remote-electrical training. Eckstein and Hart (1996) were able to suppress compulsive licking in four dogs (N = 5) after delivering an average of 12 brief shocks per dog. The suppressive effects of electrical stimulation were rapid and highly durable (see *ES and Refractory Compulsive Behavior* in Chapter 9).

Tail Chasing and Whirling

Since tail chasing often occurs in situations involving increased excitement and frustration, it may be useful to anticipate such behavior by using a response-prevention procedure or by increasing obedience control at such times. Also, some dogs may benefit from compensatory stimulation (e.g., ball play) or the presentation of various anticipatory diverters or disrupters. An orienting response to a squeaker-odor stimulus is used to interrupt whirling momentarily in anticipation of initiating a DRO procedure. A well-conditioned click and food reward can be used to support the orienting response, with subsequent clicks and food rewards following after varying brief periods of abstinence from whirling activity in accordance with DRO schedule requirements. The DRO schedule provides reinforcement after a fixed or variable interval, provided that the dog does not chase its tail. If the dog does whirl, the vocal cue "Stop" is presented and the compulsive action is interrupted, whereupon the dog is restrained to a tie-out or TO area. When interrupting tail-chasing behavior, great care and caution should be taken, since some dogs may respond aggressively when interfered with at such times. In cases where a risk of attack exists, added precautions should be taken, e.g., muzzling or keeping the dog on a leash and muzzle-type halter that produces a clamping action on the dog's jaws. During TO, the dog's leash is pinched in the doorjamb, leaving it with enough room to stand and sit but not chase its tail (response prevention). The TO should not exceed 1 minute, with 30 seconds often being sufficient. At the

conclusion of TO, the dog is returned to the evoking situation and the DRO schedule reinstated. In the early stages of DRO training, the compulsion-free period should be adjusted to maximize the flow of rewards and reinforcement of behavior incompatible with tail chasing. In addition to the suppressive effects produced by the loss of food and social rewards, the contingent application of a brief TO appears to help de-arouse such dogs.

Another method of some value for the control of compulsive whirling involves bringing the behavior under stimulus control. Waving a hand in a wide circular direction above a dog's head can often evoke tail chasing. In cases were this does not initially evoke the whirling response, a vocal or visual signal can be paired with spontaneous tail-chasing events. After several repetitions, the signal itself will gradually evoke the whirling response. As the dog starts turning, a conditioned reinforcer (e.g., click) is delivered and a treat is tossed to the floor in front of the dog. If the dog stops, the training procedure is repeated; if not, the behavior is interrupted with the vocal cue "Stop" followed by appropriate disruptive stimulation (e.g., toss of a shaker can or compressed air with deterrent odor) or restraint. This pattern is repeated until the dog starts and stops whirling on signal. Tail chasing is interrupted at the earliest sign or intentional movement, whereupon the whirling response is countermanded by a response incompatible with tail chasing (e.g., stay or sit). All tail chasing or whirling off cue is either blocked or suppressed. This procedure is carried out until the dog's impulse to chase its tail is replaced by an incompatible response or reduced sufficiently to employ a DRO and TO procedure, as already described.

In cases where a dog fails to stop on signal or is unresponsive to disruptive stimuli, electronic training may be useful. Whenever remote electronic devices are used, the dog should first receive appropriate safety training. Initially, the least aversive electrical (e)-stimulus sufficient to stop tail chasing is used. During the escape phase, a continuous stimulus is applied until the dog stops whirling, at which point a conditioned negative reinforcer is delivered just before the e-stimulus is turned off. The avoidance phase is initiated by presenting the vocal signal "Stop" just before the e-stimulus is delivered. Once the dog demonstrates an ability to control the tail-chasing behavior in response to low-level e-stimulation, a stronger e-stimulus can be introduced with the goal of suppressing it. The vocal signal "Stop" is coupled with the immediate delivery of a momentary e-stimulus set at a moderately high level. To produce an effective reminder to deter future tail chasing, a novel odor (citronella) is applied beforehand to the dog's tail or rear end. Later, the deterrent odor can be administered contingently by using a CO_2 pump sprayed in the direction of the dog's tail (see above) or via a remote citronella collar.

Automated Training

Given the common incidence of canine licking and tail-chasing compulsions, future research efforts should explore the viability of automated devices designed to detect compulsive activity and to deliver appropriate consequent events. Such devices are especially needed in the case of compulsions that occur when the owner is absent. Behavior-activated devices are in widespread use for the control of boundaries and barking excesses, providing a foundation of technology for more sophisticated behavior tools for measuring and treating behavior problems. For example, in the case of excessive licking, a pressure- or moisture-sensitive device could be programmed to detect both the absence and presence of licking, thereby keeping track of the behavior objectively. Such a device could be designed to interface with a treat dispenser for the purpose of DRO training or for shaping an incompatible response (e.g., lever pressing). The device could also be programmed to deliver lick-activated aversive stimulation as well as safety odors, thereby making the process of inhibitory training more efficacious and lasting. In the case of excessive tail-chasing and whirling compulsions, a movement-sensitive device could detect whirling movements, record their duration and frequency, and provide appropriate consequent events to promote DRO training, shape incompatible

behavior, deliver whirling-contingent aversive stimulation, and the release of safety odors.

PART 2: HYPERACTIVITY AND HYPERKINESIS

Behavioral complaints involving overactivity and impulsivity are common with dogs, with certain breeds (e.g., hunting and working dogs) tending to exhibit such adjustment problems more often, suggesting that a strong genetic factor may be involved. As the result of conscious and unconscious selection pressures, hunting and working breeds have undergone various biogenetic changes conducive to working functions, including increased activity levels, low-threshold attention and orienting responses, and rapid behavioral adjustments to environmental stimulation (impulsivity). From the perspective of utility, such traits may significantly enhance the performance of hunting and working dogs. Such dogs are often required to search large areas as rapidly as possible, making traits conducive to high activity and energy of tremendous value. A high degree of excitability and rapid attentional shifting and sifting through environmental stimuli would also enhance the ability of hunting dogs to search for game. The best detector dogs are highly energetic, impulsive, and driven to locate hidden objects. Guarding dogs benefit from increased attentional shifting and hyper-vigilance in the detection and anticipation of potential threats. Impulsive and fearless action may serve hunting dogs in the pursuit of game and provide a significant advantage to working dogs when faced with risky or threatening situations requiring immediate and uncalculated action. Impulsive behavior is particularly advantageous in situations requiring split-second decisions. However, when comorbid oppositionality (fairly common among hyperactive dogs) and impulse-control deficiencies present together with a tendency toward rapid behavioral adjustments and fearlessness, the risk of aggression may be increased. A more common characteristic of hyperactive dogs is playfulness, with such dogs appearing to obtain pleasure from drive-related modal activity that involves environmental and social exploration, novelty seeking, and the search for positive prediction error, that is, a preoccupation with reward seeking.

Although high activity and excitability levels may be desirable in the case of hunting and working dogs, such traits often result in significant disruptive behavior and training problems when expressed in the home (Voith, 1980). Hyperactive dogs often exhibit intense greeting rituals involving sustained jumping up, running about, and other behavior indicating a high level of arousal (e.g., barking and mouthing on hands and clothing). Such dogs may persist in such behavior despite repeated efforts to correct or restrain them. In addition to social intrusiveness and oppositional behavior, overactive and impulsive dogs frequently exhibit numerous control-related behavior problems (e.g., jumping on counters, destructive behavior, and reckless behavior around children). Hyperactive dogs often appear to be possessed by an insatiable desire to play and explore, grabbing virtually anything that they can get into their mouths, occasionally swallowing objects that cause gastrointestinal distress or blockage that requires veterinary treatment. When walked, such dogs often become extremely active, excited, and distracted, forcefully pulling into the leash, barking, and exhibiting various other impulsive behaviors that greatly distress their frustrated owners. These impulsive excesses on leash frequently lead to exercise and stimulation deficits simply because owners give up trying to walk and exercise them. When transported by car, overactive dogs may frantically pace back and forth, pant continuously, and bark at passersby and other dogs. These various excesses and adjustment problems almost invariably result in the use of inappropriate punishment and confinement further depriving hyperactive dogs of needed stimulation and exercise. Hyperactive dogs are exposed to excessive crate confinement or banishment to the backyard, where they dig, destroy plants and shrubbery, and engage in nuisance barking.

Although the crate can be an effective management tool, when used excessively or inappropriately it can become the hub of a vicious cycle of restraint and escalating compensatory activity and other adverse side effects. The use of a plaster cast for mending a broken arm offers an apropos metaphor for appreciating the benefits and risks of crate confinement. When used properly, the cast provides a highly beneficial effect by keeping the arm in a fixed position. However, if the cast is left on the arm for too long, significant adverse side effects will gradually overshadow its benefits, with the muscles of the arm gradually atrophying and losing strength. Similarly, the constructive use of crate confinement can be highly effective and beneficial, but if it is used as a substitute for training or employed excessively or inappropriately (e.g., as a place for time-out), crating may produce a variety of undesirable side effects (see *Dangers of Excessive Crate Confinement* in Chapter 2).

COMPULSIVITY AND HYPERACTIVITY: EVOLUTIONARY CONSIDERATIONS

Compulsive disorders and hyperactivity appear to be phenomenological opposites sharing a common axis of impulse-control impairment and behavioral excess but in opposite directions. Whereas compulsive dogs appear to take pleasure in repeating certain sequences of behavior to the point of excess, hyperactive dogs appear to be intolerant of repetitive routines, showing a preference for behavioral change and novelty. Dogs tending toward compulsivity appear to be more routine oriented, whereas the behavior of hyperactive dogs tends toward a high level of variability (see *Cognitive Interpretations and Speculation* in Volume 2, Chapter 5). Compulsive dogs tend toward introversion (self-directed), avoidance of danger, and the performance of repetitive routines (phlegmatic-melancholic axis), whereas hyperactive dogs are more extraverted (other-directed), outgoing, reward seeking, fearless, and variable in their behavior output (sanguine-choleric axis). The evolutionary differentiation of traits tending in the complementary directions of compulsivity and impulsivity would provide an adaptive hedge against changing environmental circumstances. Under stable circumstances of plenty, compulsive traits associated with repetitive tasks, routines, and security seeking would be adaptive whereas, at times of crisis and starvation, increased behavioral impulsiveness, variability, fearlessness, and tolerance for disgust would provide a significant advantage. Interestingly, hyperactive dogs often engage in pica and coprophagy, suggesting the possibility that such vices and hyperactivity may be linked by a common evolutionary function—survival under adverse conditions (see *Encoded Survival Habits* in Volume 2, Chapter 9). Hyperactive traits may serve to increase survivability during times of adversity, starvation, and upheaval, whereas compulsive traits would be more conducive to settled and relatively stable circumstances. Under highly organized and stable conditions, disruptive hyperactive behavior becomes a source of social concern and the focus of behavioral control efforts in both humans and dogs.

HYPERACTIVITY AND NEUROBIOLOGY

A dog's nervous activity can be conceptualized as resulting from the dynamic interplay of excitatory and inhibitory neurotransmitters, especially gamma-aminobutyric acid (GABA) and glutamate, respectively, operating under the modulatory influence of monoamine neurotransmitters (e.g., DA, 5-HT, and NE), a host of neuropeptides (e.g., CRF, opioids, oxytocin, and arginine vasopressin), and other psychoactive substances (e.g., lipids and fatty acids). Normally, cortical inhibitory processes actively modulate excitatory subcortical neuroactivity. The result is organized and highly regulated activity. In hyperactive dogs, cortical inhibitory processes appear to be insufficient to regulate excitatory impulses. Hyperactivity, inattentiveness, and impulsivity may persist despite repeated punishment involving both aversive stimulation and the loss of reward, suggesting that the disorder may involve an impairment of executive control functions. Current research emphasizes the involvement of frontostriatal circuits—

including prefrontal and orbitofrontal areas, the striatal complex, and the anterior cingulate—in the etiology of hyperkinetic impulsivity. When functioning properly, each of these areas contribute to the expression of integrated and organized behavior, providing the when-what-where mechanisms by which dogs establish control over the environment and optimizes their ability to exploit it.

Executive impulse-control abilities only gradually acquire full functional activation and capacity (Rubia et al., 2000). Young dogs frequently exhibit hyperactivity and impulse-control problems that improve with age, implicating an ontogenetic normalization of attention and impulse-control abilities. In the case of hyperkinetic dogs, impaired or reduced cortical activity may persist, stemming from an organic impairment affecting the frontostriatal system. Carlsson (2001) has suggested that obsessive-compulsive disorder (OCD) and attention-deficit hyperactivity disorder (ADHD) are conditions that stem from the dysregulation of prefrontal glutamatergic activity. According to this hypothesis, OCD and ADHD are cognitive and behavioral antipodes, with obsessions and compulsive behavior resulting from prefrontal overactivity, whereas hyperkinetic inattentiveness and impulsivity are the result of prefrontal underactivity. Treatment with psychostimulants appears to increase prefrontal activity via dopaminergic activation of glutamate circuits, thereby normalizing function. Interestingly, normoactive dogs given D-amphetamine exhibit increased stereotypic activity (Bareggi et al., 1979), a finding consistent with Carlsson's hypothesis that cortical overactivity may underlie the elaboration of compulsive rituals. Various lines of research are currently under way to isolate the neurobiological causes of ADHD, with most theories focusing on disturbances of 5-HT and DA neurotransmission. Both serotonin and dopamine serve to modulate excitatory (glutamate) and inhibitory (GABA) systems governing emotional and motor activity (see *Neural and Physiological Substrates* in Volume 2, Chapter 5). In addition to stimulating dopaminergic activity, psychostimulants increase alertness and cortical arousal via noradrenergic circuits.

PHARMACOLOGICAL CONTROL OF HYPERKINESIS

Generally, hyperactivity is differentiated from hyperkinesis by identifying behavioral indicators and the performance of a stimulant-response test (see *CNS-stimulant Response Test* in Volume 2, Chapter 5) (Luescher, 1993). Unlike hyperactive dogs, hyperkinetic dogs show a paradoxical response to psychostimulant therapy; that is, instead of becoming more active under the influence of stimulants, hyperkinetic dogs become less active and impulsive and more responsive to inhibitory control (see *Hyperactivity versus Hyperkinesis* in Volume 2, Chapter 5). Psychostimulant therapy appears to reduce symptoms of human ADHD in approximately 80% of diagnosed cases (Paule et al., 2000). Although hyperactivity is common in dogs, stimulant-responsive hyperkinesis appears to be much less common in dogs than in people, but good epidemiological studies are lacking in this area. Whether the disorder is actually rare or underdiagnosed remains to be determined. Criteria for identifying impulsive and overactive dogs that may be hyperkinetic (and warrant stimulant-response testing) remain to be developed and validated. Luescher (1993) has suggested that hyperkinesis often presents with multiple and serious behavior problems.

In the past, D-amphetamine was the most common drug used to control hyperkinesis, but other medications have also been effectively used to control the problem in both children and dogs. Arnold and colleagues (1973) have compared the efficacy of D-amphetamine with L-amphetamine for the control of hyperkinesis and aggression in dogs. They found that the D-isomer was approximately three to four times more effective in the control of hyperkinesis than was the L-isomer. However, both drugs proved equally effective in the control of aggression associated with hyperkinesis. The only significant difference between the two drugs was that the effect of L-amphetamine lasted only half as long that of D-amphetamine. The

most common alternative drug for the control of human ADHD is methylphenidate. Although effective and perhaps producing fewer side effects (less agitation and fewer stereotypical behaviors), the drug wears off more rapidly and does so precipitously—a potentially dangerous pharmacokinetic feature in the case of aggressive dogs (Drastura, 1992). Voith (1980) reports success using the tricyclic antidepressant amitriptyline for the control of hyperactive symptoms not responsive to central nervous system (CNS) stimulants.

Another medication that may offer some additional benefits in the treatment of hyperkinetic symptoms is clonidine, which has shown promising efficacy with children diagnosed with ADHD not responsive to CNS-stimulant therapy. The drug appears to enhance impulse control and improve frustration tolerance in overactive and uninhibited children (Riddle, 1991). When clonidine is given with methyphenidate, the combination may produce beneficial synergistic effects and be particularly useful in the treatment of impulsive aggression presenting comorbidly with hyperkinesis (Connor et al., 2000)—a potential treatment regimen that remains to be evaluated for safety and efficacy in dogs. Also, when given together, a smaller dose of methylphenidate may be required to produce a therapeutic effect.

Schnackenberg (1973) has reported that caffeine works about as well as methylphenidate in children diagnosed with ADHD. Subsequent studies were not been able to confirm these observations (Garfinkel, 1975). Krushinskii (1960), who performed several experiments exploring the effects of caffeine on excitability in dogs, arrived at two general conclusions concerning the effect of caffeine on general excitability:

> It was shown, first, that excessively large doses of caffeine, causing a sharp increase in the process of excitation, produce limiting inhibition. Consequently, the conditioned reflexes are not increased; on the contrary, they are depressed ... Second, it was shown that the effect of caffeine on the process of excitation is largely dependent on the typological properties of the nervous system. In animals with a weak type of nervous

system, administration of only small doses of the drug leads to an increase of the conditioned reflexes; larger doses depress conditioned reflex activity. Just as during weakening of the nervous system by excessive nervous strain, castration, or old age only the slight increase in excitability obtained by the use of small or average doses of caffeine leads to an increase in the conditioned reflexes. The administration of large doses depressed them. (57)

Despite these intriguing observations, as things currently stand, caffeine has no "real place in pharmacotherapy" (Werry, 1994:327). Caffeine probably offers little or no benefit in the treatment of canine hyperkinesis; however, to my knowledge, the potential value of caffeine for controlling hyperkinesis in dogs has not been clinically evaluated.

Essential fatty acids (EFAs) are necessary for healthy brain development and function. Children with EFA deficiencies, especially omega-3 fatty acids, may be more prone to exhibit learning difficulties and behavior problems associated with ADHD (Stevens et al., 1996). Supplementation with EFAs has been shown to alleviate ADHD-related behaviors and improve cognitive function in children. The value of EFA supplementation in dogs exhibiting hyperactivity, inattentiveness, and impulsivity has not been clinically evaluated, but given the apparent benefits of such supplementation in human psychiatry (see *Aggression and Diet* in Chapter 7), such investigation appears to be warranted.

Note: The foregoing information is provided for educational purposes only. If considering the use of medications to control or manage a behavior problem, readers should consult with a veterinarian familiar with the use of drugs for such purposes in order to obtain diagnostic criteria, specific dosages, and medical advice concerning potential adverse side effects and interactions with other drugs.

BEHAVIOR THERAPY

Hyperactive dogs exhibit several cognitive and behavioral characteristics that may impair their ability to organize behavioral output and effectively adjust. In addition to increased activity levels, hyperactive dogs are easily dis-

tracted, impulsive, and lack the ability to rapidly stop or inhibit motivated behavior. The sheer volume of searching and impulsive activity exhibited by such dogs can be daunting and extremely frustrating for dog owners. Since hyperactive dogs show a characteristic inability to respond to conditioned inhibitory signals, an excessive reliance on interactive punishment is common, often making matters worse. A hyperactive dog's inability to stay still for long appears to be a function of emotional impulsivity (seeking-system imbalance), driving the dog to seek drive-activating stimulation or intensify gratification. As a result, performing tasks requiring a delay of gratification or response inhibition places an onerous demand on such dogs. Instead of hesitating, appraising the situation, and selecting an optimal course of action (control module), hyperactive dogs appear to respond swept up by transient impulses in search of immediate gratification. In addition to emotional impulsivity, the behavior of such dogs appears to be dominated by insatiable modal searching routines operating under exploitative incentives. Many of these dogs exhibit a low-threshold orienting response, causing them to scan the environment rapidly and without lingering for long on any one source of stimulation.

Reinforcement and Extinction Peculiarities Associated with Hyperactivity

Sagvolden and colleagues (1998) have proposed that normoactive and hyperactive animals (spontaneously hypertensive rats) and ADHD children respond differently to reinforcement and extinction procedures. ADHD children appear to be averse to reinforcement delays, preferring the accumulation of small rewards delivered immediately to the receipt of larger rewards requiring them to wait. In contrast with hyperactive counterparts, normoactive children appear to prefer schedules of reinforcement in which rewards are gradually maximized and presented as large accumulated earnings. Also, the behavior-strengthening effects of delayed and immediate reinforcement significantly differ between normoactive and hyperactive animals and children. In normoactive animals, not only are behaviors that directly result in reinforcement strengthened, but so are other responses leading up to the reward. More formally stated, a delay of reinforcement gradient is formed as a function of the time elapsing between the emission of a response and the delivery of reinforcement, such that behaviors occurring early in the sequence are strengthened but to a lesser extent than those occurring immediately before the reinforcing event (Figure 5.1). In the case of hyperactive animals, only those behaviors occurring in close proximity with the delivery of reinforcement are affected, gradually resulting in their exaggeration and predominance over behaviors occurring earlier in the sequence. After repeated trials, reinforcement causes hyperactive animals to differentiate from normoactive counterparts in interesting ways. For example, the behavior of normoactive animals tends to be more goal oriented and organized in comparison to the hyperactive animal's impulsive and massed response bursts primarily occurring just before reinforcement is anticipated to occur. These findings suggest that the

impulsivity associated with hyperactivity may be acquired as the result of the distinctive way hyperactive animals respond to reinforcement. In addition, hyperactive rats appear to respond differently to extinction procedures than do normoactive ones. Although hyperactive rats initially exhibit a reduction of behavior during signaled extinction trials, they rapidly resume responding and persist in doing so at high levels despite the absence of reinforcement. Hyperactive rats appear to recognize when reinforcement is no longer forthcoming, but are unable to maintain response inhibition during signaled extinction periods. Similarly hyperactive dogs exhibit intolerance for waiting and respond best to immediate reinforcement. During the training of such dogs, it is important that rewards be presented on a frequent basis rather than requiring them to wait too long or perform several responses for a deferred reward. Consistent with findings from experiments with hyperactive animals and children diagnosed with ADHD, extinction procedures (ignoring intrusive and impulsive behavior) are not usually very effective in the behavioral treatment of hyperactive dogs.

These various impairments of reinforcement and extinction processes impede a hyperactive dog's ability to adjust to changing circumstances, with the consequent breakdown of integrated behavior. Impulse control develops as the result of goal-directed behavior and inhibitory conditioning processes occurring naturally as organisms interact with the environment. Normally, dogs learn from an early age that certain behaviors are either dangerous or do not pay off, and consequently learn to stop exhibiting those actions—a process that is gradually internalized as impulse control. Dogs also learn that some behaviors alter the environment in ways that produce pleasurable or rewarding outcomes. Consequently, two general alterations occur during the process of behavioral adaptation: (1) response inhibition (impulse control) and (2) response excitation (goal-directed and integrated behavior). Adaptive behavior is motivated to avoid aversive events, on the one hand, and to optimize control over attractive ones, on the other. Practically speaking, socially acceptable behavior is acquired and

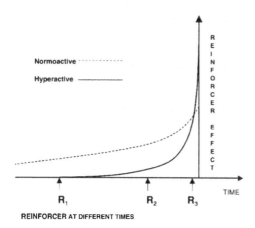

FIG. 5.1. Theoretical delay of reward gradient comparing hyperactive and normoactive animals. Hyperactive dogs appear to be affected by a number of learning impairments, including a delay of reinforcement deficiency that impedes their ability to produce goal-directed and organized output. Unlike normoactive counterparts, hyperactive dogs tend to concentrate impulsive behavioral efforts to occur immediately before the anticipated reward is delivered. After Sagvolden et al. (1998).

maintained by structuring the dog's activities in accordance with various contingencies of reward and punishment. Training procedures consist of attractive and aversive events presented in accordance with controlling signals (e.g., discriminative stimuli and conditioned reinforcers) in order to systematically shape behavior toward some behavioral objective. In the case of disruptive hyperactive behavior, the goal of behavior modification and training is to promote the development of a regulated and organized repertoire of cooperative behavior. Training activities serve to establish instrumental control modules and routines that are incompatible with disruptive impulsivity to enhance attention and impulse control, and to generally increase the dog's ability to effectively organize its behavioral output. A dog's ability to control impulsiveness involves at least four aspects: the ability to restrain a preferred response at the level of intention, to stop an action that has been initiated but not fully consummated, to continue an action despite environment interference, and the ability to delay a response (see Rubia et al., 1998). All of these aspects are addressed in the training of hyperactive dogs.

Reward-based Training and Play

The training of hyperactive dogs involves shaping instrumental control modules (e.g., sit, down, and stay) and improving attending and waiting behaviors. The strengthening of enhanced attention and impulse control is most practically and beneficially attained through highly structured and reward-based training efforts in combination with TO and response-blocking procedures. Such training should focus on developing a repertoire of compliant behaviors integrated into everyday activities. First establishing a set of highly consistent predictive control expectancies and then varying the type, size, frequency, and timing of attractive outcomes against this control expectancy standard helps to optimize reward-based training efforts by introducing positive prediction error (surprise) and a variety of beneficial dissonance effects. Not only does basic training induce a significant calming effect in most hyperactive dogs, it also provides owners with more constructive

means for controlling impulsive and oppositional behavior. In addition to basic training and attention therapy, providing hyperactive dogs with contingent access to vigorous play activities can further enhance control efforts while providing overactive dogs with beneficial ways for obtaining high levels of quality stimulation and reward. Ball play can be structured so that the opportunity to chase the ball is made contingent on the dog waiting by standing, sitting, or lying down, thereby improving impulse control and reinforcing more cooperative behavior. Playful activities that involve jumping up, biting and tugging on toys, running about, and wrestling (in the case of friendly dogs) can be provided contingently as a reward following the performance of basic exercises. Also, repeatedly turning play on ("Okay") and off ("Enough" or "Out") appears to help overactive dogs to learn better self-control over playful social excesses and impulsive behavior.

Time-out, Response Prevention, and Overcorrection

The most common means used by dog owners to control hyperactive excesses are extinction and punishment. Efforts to extinguish hyperactive behavior by ignoring it are rarely successful, and the punitive measures often used by owners are inconsistent and ineffective, usually only serving to exacerbate the situation. Disruptive hyperactive behavior may be so pervasive and persistent that reward strategies may be thwarted, requiring complementary inhibitory training efforts aimed at restraining oppositional or intrusive excesses. The most successful programs of behavior therapy and training combine reward-based training, punitive procedures (e.g., exclusionary and nonexclusionary TO), and various response-blocking techniques. Keeping the dog on leash while in the house enhances the owner's ability to interrupt and redirect unwanted behavior, effectively apply TO procedures, and prevent many common excesses associated with hyperactivity.

In combination with TO and response blocking, overcorrection can be highly effective. The overcorrection procedure requires that the dog repeatedly perform a behavior that is incompatible with hyperactivity [see *Negative Practice, Negative Training, and Overcorrection (Positive Practice) Techniques* in Volume 1, Chapter 8]. One overcorrection procedure requires that the dog perform a long-down stay (1 to 10 minutes) whenever it exhibits a loss of impulse control or target-intrusive excess. Initially, the dog is frequently rewarded with affection and food while staying in place, with the reward frequency gradually tapering off until it is delivered only at the end of the stay period. Massage can help encourage a dog to relax, especially if the dog needs to be manually restrained in the down position. Another overcorrection technique requires that the dog repeatedly perform a series of obedience exercises (e.g., sit, down, sit from the down, and stand). Each behavior is positively reinforced, and the full overcorrection cycle of exercises is slowly repeated 5 to 10 times in a row, as needed to restore attention and impulse control. Similarly, hyperactive dogs can be exposed to integrated compliance training, which requires dogs to sit, stay or wait, and make eye contact before engaging in various preferred everyday activities. For example, hyperactive dogs should be routinely required to sit, wait, and make eye contact before being let outdoors, before being let indoors, before receiving treats and meals, before going up or down stairs, before getting into the car, before being released to play, before being permitted on furniture, and before receiving affection and petting. The idea is to use everyday rewards as opportunities to enhance attention and impulse-control abilities.

By defining (and adjusting as necessary) a continuum of progressive compliance, owners are better able to direct behavioral change in an efficient and goal-directed way, minimizing negative interaction and reactive resistance—undesirable outcomes that are more likely to occur in cases where more difficult demands are made too hastily. The next important step in the process is to generalize learning to a broader range of situations that provide greater environmental and social stimulation of the dog. For example, once training is mastered in the home, it can be gradually transferred to other more uncontrolled situations. Enrolling the dog in an obedience class can be extremely useful at this point. To be most effective, all family members need to play an active and consistent role in the training process.

Posture-facilitated Relaxation Training

Few activities are more beneficial than posture-facilitated relaxation (PFR) training and massage for promoting calmness and composure in hyperactive dogs. The musculature of such dogs is often stiff with anticipation and readiness to act, especially in the case of dogs operating under the influence of heightened sympathetic arousal. Hyperactive dogs often reach a deep state of relaxation more rapidly than normoactive counterparts. The procedure incorporates nonthreatening prompting movements together with sustained massage toward the induction of a pronounced relaxation response. The postural prompting and restraint associated with PFR training appears to play an instrumental role in the relaxation process (see *Posture-facilitated Relaxation* in Chapter 6 and Appendix C). As the result of such handling, opponent tensing and releasing of muscles produces a progressive calming and enhanced receptivity to massage. The induction of relaxation by systematically tensing and releasing of muscle groups plays a prominent role in the treatment of human fear and anxiety disorders by systematic desensitization. Grandin (1992) has reported some relaxation benefits associated with sustained squeezing in the treatment of human autism and hyperactivity. In addition to postural restraint and manipulation, taction helps to support and promote relaxation. Gantt and colleagues (1966) and others following him have emphasized the pronounced effect that touch contact has on dogs via the parasympathetic branch of the autonomic nervous system (see *Taction and PFR* in Chapter 7). Touch lowers blood pressure, decreases heart and respiration rate, reduces stress-activated hypothalamic-pituitary-adrenocortical (HPA) axis activity, and generally appears to promote homeostatic equilibrium. The combination of 10 minutes of reward-based training and 20 minutes of vigorous play, followed by a 5-minute session of PFR training, is a positive prescription for change in the case of many hyperactive dogs.

HYPERACTIVITY AND SOCIAL EXCESSES

Hyperactivity and intrusive behavior appear to develop in the context of unresolved competitive conflicts and tensions. These interactive sources of conflict usually revolve around situations in which the mutual control interests of dogs and owners converge upon and conflict over the access to everyday rewards. Under the influence of owner interference and ineffectual control efforts, a puppy's behavior may become progressively organized around competitive modal strategies fueled by the intermittent reinforcement of intrusive and oppositional behavior. Problematically, the relationship between the owner and dog gradually takes form around these points of conflict and tension. Instead of producing harmonious and cooperative interaction, competitive exchanges and transactions between the owner and dog generate a variety of undesirable emotional and behavioral outcomes. In the dog's case, its behavior may become progressively hyperactive, intrusive, and disruptive. The owner may interpret the dog's emergent competitive behavior as dominating and threatening social order, but, in fact, these dogs are more aptly described as dependent and incompetent subordinates in search of a leader. Furthermore, the greatest actual threat to social order in such cases is the owner's failure to assume an appropriate leadership role and help the dog learn more acceptable ways to gratify its needs. Operating under the delusion of a dominance challenge, the frustrated owner may reactively turn to ineffectual and inconsistent punitive efforts to control disruptive behavior. Punishment in such cases may only serve to further complicate interactive conflicts and tensions, amplify competitive arousal, and further differentiate the dog's incompetent efforts to gain control over everyday sources of comfort and safety (reward). Instead of finding a leader, the dog finds a punitive adversary impeding its ability to adjust and succeed. In addition to exaggerating undesirable active-submission behaviors

(e.g., jumping up, barking, and begging), the chronic reliance on punishment may cause the hyperactive and intrusive dog to gradually lose its ability to truly submit and defer, but nonetheless refrain from openly competing with the owner. Instead, the dog may engage in a variety of socially flirtatious and ambiguous behaviors involving obnoxious submission and defiance, especially when interacting with the owner around contested boundaries and limits. The dog may become progressively demanding, clever, and evasive in the process of learning how to get around the owner's control efforts. Instead of learning how to defer and wait, under such circumstances, the intelligent dog learns to sneak and steal what it needs.

Dogs need a balance of dominance, leadership, and nurturance in order to form healthy social bonds with people and to develop well-adjusted behavior. In cases where social conflict is implicated as a potential factor underlying hyperactivity and intrusive excesses, efforts should be taken to promote a voluntary subordination strategy (see *Social Competition, Cooperation, Conflict, and Resentment* in Chapter 7) by means of reward-based training, play, and PFR training. Leadership is established by showing the dog how to succeed in its efforts to obtain reward and avoid punishment. The various points of disruptive social conflict and tension should be interpreted and explained to the owner in terms of potential sources of reward and opportunities for leadership and interactive growth. Rather than interfering with the dog's control efforts and needs, the goal of training is to show the dog how to get what it wants by following rules and cooperating with the owner's directives. Through cynopraxic training, the dog learns that the owner can help it to achieve control over its interests rather than represent an impediment standing in the way of them. Integrated compliance training (ICT) is used to attain these objectives. The ICT protocol integrates training activities with everyday sources of reward (e.g., food, play, affection, going outside, coming up on furniture, jumping up, and barking) in order to defuse and resolve interactive conflicts and tensions that have developed between the owner and the dog around these activities. Reward-based ICT efforts improve owner control efforts, reduce social ambivilence (adverse anxiety and frustration), enhance affectionate bonding processes, promote interactive harmony and mutual appreciation, and restore trust and respect between the owner and the dog. As the interaction between the owner and the dog becomes more competent and cooperative, a spontaneous reduction in oppositional and intrusive behavior, adjunctive attention seeking, and hyperactivity naturally follows.

Conventional wisdom asserts that behavior maintained by intermittent reinforcement is more resistant to extinction than behavior maintained by continuous reinforcement. Intermittent reinforcement is a potent source of prediction error and dissonance. The process of reducing or omitting reinforcement (negative prediction error) for a variable number of times serves to set the stage for the occurrence of positive prediction error and reward when the reinforcer is again delivered. Many adjustment problems appear to be maintained by intermittent and inadvertent (bootleg) reinforcement, generally reducing the value of extinction as a behavior-control procedure (see *Extinction of Instrumental Learning* in Volume 1, Chapter 7). One way to address this problem is to first bring the target behavior under the control of continuous reinforcement before initiating the extinction procedure (Ducharme and Van Houten, 1994). Switching from intermittent to continuous reinforcement prior to extinction appears to reduce the baseline level of the inappropriate behavior while at the same time facilitating subsequent extinction efforts (Lerman et al., 1996). For example, in the case of jumping up, dogs can be rewarded each time they jump up until a noticeable flattening or decline in response frequency is observed (plateau), whereupon the behavior can be brought under stimulus control by rewarding only those jumping responses that occur in the presence of the jump-up signal ("Hup"). Jumping-up responses that occur off signal are ignored (extinguished) or blocked. The type, size, and frequency of attractive outcomes are varied to maximize surprise in association with jumping up on signal, thereby encouraging the dog to defer and wait for the signal giving it permission to jump up.

Jumping Up

Jumping up is among the most common behavioral complaints presented in association with hyperactivity. Often initially invited and permitted as an expression of affection, owners rapidly learn to regard this common greeting excess as a nuisance, particularly when large dogs persistently jump on unappreciative guests. Dogs that jump up represent a significant risk of injury to young children and elderly adults, who may be knocked down when bumped into or jumped on. Owners of such dogs are often forced to isolate their rowdy dogs when guests arrive—a procedure that may eventually generate more problems and do nothing to improve the dog's intrusive greeting behavior.

Early training consisting of sit-stay and other exercises promoting impulse control when the puppy seeks attention or other rewards helps to encourage more acceptable and organized social behavior. From an early age, jumping up and other intrusive social excesses should be limited, redirected, and brought under stimulus control. During greetings, the owner should crouch down or sit on the floor and allow the puppy to nuzzle and press in closely, but not permit it to climb up on the lap without an invitation. While sitting on the floor with the puppy, the owner can practice various basic obedience exercises (sit, down, and stand) using petting and treats to reward cooperative behavior prompted by voice and hand signals. Providing the puppy with an occasional opportunity to play tug and fetch with a ball or soft toy can help to redirect excessive energy into play activities and further encourage cooperative behavior. When the puppy is greeted from a standing position, stepping on the leash and diverting its attention toward the floor by dropping treats or tossing it a soft toy can help to prevent jumping up while simultaneously encouraging more desirable behavior (see below). Training the puppy to jump up and off again on cue can be a useful way to establish better control over the behavior. If the puppy becomes overly aroused and excited, repeated brief TOs (30 seconds) can exert a pronounced de-arousing effect. Consistent discouragement of off-cue jumping up by turning away or by applying brief TOs serves to gradually weaken the puppy's enthusiasm for the habit. In general, the best results are obtained by shaping alternative behavior with reward and play rather than focusing excessively on suppressing undesirable behavior. Keeping in mind the dead-dog rule (see *Dead-dog Rule* in Volume 2, Chapter 2), training objectives involving jumping up should be organized in affirmative terms, that is, shaping alternative behaviors incompatible with jumping up rather than training the puppy not to jump up—dead dogs do not jump up.

Overly excitable and active puppies often benefit from PFR training. The postural control and taction techniques of PFR training are described in Appendix C. An abbreviated cycle of PFR training is initiated by taking the puppy by the collar and briefly massaging the jaw muscles, followed by the stand control, whereupon a focused and rhythmic massage is delivered on the neck and shoulder muscles. The massage should continue for 20 to 30 seconds before prompting the puppy to sit by gently squeezing just in front of the hip bones or by pressing forward behind the knees and guiding the puppy into the sit position. With the puppy sitting, the massage continues along its neck, spine, and lumbar areas. Next, the puppy's right leg is lifted up and forward from the elbow while it is gently and steadily lowered to the floor. The massage is continued in a calming and soothing manner. Lastly, the puppy is rolled over onto its side. Rubbing the jaw and temporal muscles can help to strengthen the relaxation response. Next, massage is directed toward the earflap, various muscled parts of the body, and the feet. As the puppy relaxes, the owner can present an odor (e.g., orange or lemon-orange mix) paired with the growing relaxation response. The puppy is released with an "Okay" and soft clap.

Controlling jumping up through extinction alone—that is, ignoring the dog or turning away from it—is not usually very effective. As a component of the greeting ritual,

jumping up appears to be intrinsically reinforcing for dogs to perform. Also, given the adverse effects of periodic bootleg reinforcement and the impaired ability of hyperactive dogs to respond to extinction procedures makes procedures relying on extinction relatively ineffective for the control of hyperactive greeting excesses. The control difficulties arising in association with the intrinsic reward value of jumping up and intermittent reinforcement can remedied in four preferred ways:

1. Put the behavior on a continuous schedule of reinforcement and then bring it under stimulus control.
2. Block or correct jumping up whenever it occurs.
3. Teach the dog an alternative greeting behavior that pays off more than jumping up does.
4. Allow the dog to jump up as a reward for not jumping.

Training procedures often include all four methods of control applied in varying proportions as required by the situation and the needs of the dog.

Building improved attention and impulse control during greetings is facilitated by focusing training efforts on orienting and attending behaviors. The first step is to train the dog to reliably orient toward the trainer in response to hearing its name or the sound of a squeaker. If the dog fails to orient when its name is called, the squeaker or other sources of attention-grabbing stimulation (e.g., repeated smooch sounds) are used to evoke the orienting response. As soon as the dog turns its head, a click or "Good" bridge is delivered, followed by a food reward as the dog approaches the trainer. Next, the dog is trained to sit-front, look up, and hold eye contact with the trainer for variable periods (0.5 to 2 seconds) before the bridging signal and reward are delivered. After the food reward is delivered, the dog should remain in the sit position and wait to be released with an "Okay," whereupon the orienting, sit-front, and attending response are repeated. While the dog is waiting to be released, food rewards are delivered periodically contingent on the dog looking up and making brief eye contact with the trainer. As the dog becomes steady in its ability to wait, a stay component can be added with the trainer maintaining eye contact as he or she steps back away from the dog. Numerous variations and elements of distraction and difficulty can be introduced to temper attention and impulse-control abilities (see Appendix A and Figure B.1A in Appendix B). Providing such training around the doorway establishes a useful platform for other reward-based training procedures used to control greeting excesses and other problems associated with greeting behavior.

Establishing control over excessive jumping behavior is facilitated by training dogs to jump up ("Hup"), to get off ("Off"), and to stay off ("Do you want this!") on cue. Dogs readily learn to jump up on signal after the behavior is brought under the influence of continuous reinforcement. Stimulus control is established by differentially reinforcing jumping responses that occur in the presence of the "Hup" signal and ignoring, blocking, or punishing (TO) jumping responses that occur in the absence of the signal. Off-cue jumping is associated with the vocal signal "Off," together with appropriate inhibitory prompts and rewards once the dog gets down. Impulse control associated with jumping up is significantly improved by using a challenge, especially at times when a dog is most likely to jump up off cue. The challenge serves to *dare* the dog to jump up, but without actually causing it to do so, whereupon the dog is rewarded for inhibiting the jumping-up response. The challenge consists of a prompt (e.g., slapping the legs or waist) that tempts the dog to jump up, together with a vocal signal delivered in an assertive tone of voice ("Do you want this!") belying the apparent invitation and causing the dog to hesitate. The dog's momentary hesitation is bridged and rewarded. This preemptive control procedure can be used to anticipate jumping up and promote a more reward-based approach to the problem. For example, when jumping up is highly probable, the owner can take the initiative by challenging the dog with the thigh or waist slap while saying "Do you want this!" Most dogs rapidly learn to hesitate in the presence of the challenge-dare, whereupon

they are appropriately rewarded with affection, a treat, or an opportunity to jump up on signal. The challenge-dare is combined with other integrated compliance-training activities (waiting to go through doorways or to climb up and down stairs, sitting and staying for treats, waiting for permission to jump on furniture, and so forth). Such training is essential in cases where a habit of jumping up has been strongly established in a dog's greeting repertoire.

Staging actual greeting encounters with guests is a necessary part of retraining a problem jumper, but the first step is to train the jumper not to jump up on the owner during greetings. Most control efforts should be carried out with the dog on a leash. However, if the dog is off leash and jumps up, the owner should simply shout "Off!" and turn sharply away, thereby sloughing the dog off. Another method involves taking one or two steps backward and then stepping aside to throw the jumping dog off balance with a body block or sideways shove. Grasping the front paws momentarily and releasing them only after the dog struggles to break free can be effective (Mathews, 1983), but grasping the paws or legs should be done only in the case of dogs that are unlikely to mouth or bite as the result of such restraint. Alternatively, the legs can be grasped and the dog walked backward before shoving it off to the side with a reprimand "Off" delivered just as the paws are released. In any case, the dog should be immediately put on leash, whereupon directive control, challenges, response blocking, and TO procedures can be carried out in conjunction with the reward-based training of alternative behavior.

When greeting visitors, the dog should be kept on leash, giving the owner better control and the ability to apply response prevention and blocking (e.g., stepping on the leash) and TO procedures. Before opening the door, a treat (e.g., a small biscuit) is tossed, making a sharp tapping sound as it strikes the base of the door. As the dog takes the treat, the owner steps on the leash. Additional treats are dropped to the floor as the guest enters the house. Presenting noncontingent rewards during greetings generally has a calming effect on socially excitable dogs, perhaps by evoking incompatible appetitive incentives that compete with social motivations driving greeting excesses. Treats may also perform an establishing operation function, thereby causing the dog to offer behavior that has been rewarded with food in the past. After receiving the noncontingent treats, the food can be withheld to reinforce sitting and waiting or presented according to a differential reinforcement of other behavior (DRO) schedule (see *Differential Reinforcement of Other Behavior* in Volume 1, Chapter 7). When using the DRO schedule, a bridged reward is delivered after a brief period (2 to 10 seconds initially), provided that the dog does not jump up. After establishing a control expectancy standard, the length of the DRO interval and the rewards given to the dog can be varied to produce better-than-expected and worse-than-expected outcomes (e.g., shorter DRO intervals or alterations of reward type and size), thereby mobilizing potent prediction-dissonance effects. Over time, the DRO schedule results in the strengthening of a varied spectrum of social behaviors that happen to occur coincidentally with the delivery of the bridge and reward. In general, presenting rewards in accordance with a DRO schedule is highly effective for managing and controlling the intrusive social excesses of highly excitable and active dogs at greetings, thereby reducing the need for punitive measures. Once intrusive greeting excesses are reduced via DRO and TO, a behavior incompatible with jumping up can be shaped (e.g., sitting or standing quietly) and reinforced according to a DRI schedule of reinforcement (see *Differential Reinforcement of Incompatible Behavior* in Volume 1, Chapter 7). Finally, because the doorbell often elicits intense conditioned preparatory arousal in association with greetings, it may be necessary to countercondition a new set of anticipatory emotions in response to the ringing of the doorbell. An electronic doorbell can be installed that allows the owner to ring the bell from inside the house. In addition to providing constructive countyerconditioning effects, such an arrangement helps to shape and practice the various modules and routines needed to control the dog effectively during actual greetings.

For dogs that actively resist such training efforts and continue to jump up, an additional assertion of control may be necessary. With the dog on leash, it is caught midair and reprimanded "Off" and shoved to the side. The procedure is immediately followed by a "Do you want this" challenge and dare, and the dog is rewarded if it refrains from jumping up again. If, instead, the dog jumps up again, the reprimand "Enough!" and a directive leash prompt are delivered just as the dog jumps up, whereupon it is briskly removed to TO. During greetings, the dog is most effectively timed-out on the other side of the same door that the guest used to enter the house, with the leash pinched in the doorjamb. During the TO, the dog should be given enough slack to stand and sit comfortably but not be able to move around or lie down. After a brief TO (approximately 30 seconds), the dog is brought back inside and permitted to have close contact with the guest. If it jumps or becomes overly excited, the TO procedure is repeated, as necessary. With each TO, a significant decrease in arousal and jumping should be observed, thereby complementing DRO training efforts. If the dog jumps during DRO training, the response can be blocked by stepping on the leash or punished by additional TOs. Once the dog stops jumping, it is challenged (as described previously) and rewarded when it hesitates and inhibits the jumping response. After a few repetitions of TO, most dogs not only learn to inhibit the jumping response, they also learn to move away from the doorway as guests enter the house, perhaps in an effort to reduce the risk of being put outside. This method can be surprisingly effective with even the most recalcitrant jumpers. To further improve greeting behavior, the dog should learn to withdraw from the door by backing up as it is opened. This behavior can be mastered by practicing it before walks or whenever else the door is opened. If a treat is consistently tossed back from the door as it is opened, gradually the hand movement will become a signal controlling the backing or turning-away response. If necessary, the dog is directed away from the door with directive prompts. Before exiting the house, the dog should wait for a release signal to move through the doorway. Training overactive and impulsive dogs to approach and to go through doors without pulling is an indispensable aspect of establishing control over greeting excesses. Dogs that charge through the door can be discouraged from the habit by bringing them to a dead halt and then closing the door on the leash and leaving them outside for 30 seconds, before bringing them back inside and repeating the procedure again.

Especially difficult dogs can be conditioned to stay within the area of a rug located near the entryway. Training the dog to go to the rug and stay on it should be accomplished to a high degree of reliability before it is used to control a dog around guests. The safe rug should be large enough for the dog to turn around without stepping off. During greetings, the dog should be kept under close supervision and restrained by leash and collar or halter in order to block or correct jumping attempts, whereupon the guest initiates a brief nonexclusionary TO by backing away from the dog. At the conclusion of the TO period, the guest approaches the dog again and continues to reward it with food and affectionate attention, so long as it does not become overly intrusive or jump up. Once the dog calms down, it can be released from the confinement area and permitted to move about more freely with the guest. If the dog jumps up, appropriate leash and physical prompts and exclusionary TOs are applied as needed to discourage the behavior. Throughout the process, frequent rewards are delivered on a DRO or DRI schedule in order to encourage and support more acceptable greeting behavior. In addition to performing sit-stay and down-stay training on the rug, PFR training can be performed on it as well, thereby developing a number of convergent associations conducive to impulse control and relaxation.

Once a dog has mastered the basic pattern of greeting without jumping, a variety of startle tools may be used to further strengthen the inhibition against jumping up. Most dogs can learn not to jump up without resorting to startle, but some may need such treatment to become fully compliant and reliable. For some dogs, tossing keys on the floor can be convenient and sufficient for such purposes,

but other dogs may require a more impressive startle event. For example, the startling rattle produced by a seven- or 30-penny shaker can tossed to the floor can be highly effective. Ideally, the shaker can is tossed without the dog observing the action. As a result, merely tapping on the shaker can will often produce a potent inhibitory effect over the impulse to jump up. In the case of dogs possessing a high startle threshold, a brief burst of compressed air dispensed by a modified carbon-dioxide pump (with or without odorant) can produce a potent startle response, but the device needs to be used carefully to avoid overstimulating the dog (see *Modified Compressed-air Pump* in Chapter 2 for precautions). The delivery of compressed air should be concealed from the dog by applying it from behind or sprayed lightly under the jaw toward the ground: it should never be pointed and sprayed at the dog. A dilute odor sprayed from the nozzle of the pump will linger in the air and provide an olfactory reminder to the dog not to jump up again. As the result of olfactory conditioning, a squeaker bulb (without squeaking element) containing the odor can be subsequently used to deter jumping up. Presenting the conditioned odor appears to make other startle devices more effective via a startle-potentiating effect. Once sensitized to the hissing sound of the pump, a similar sound produced by blowing air between the tongue and front teeth may function as an effective warning. The use of devices producing extreme auditory startle or that risk damaging the ears of the dog or people standing nearby (e.g., a compressed nautical horn) should be avoided. Squirting the dog in the face with a spray bottle or squirt gun is not recommended, since it appears to promote undesirable avoidance behavior in many dogs. In some cases, the delivery of a dilute odor (e.g., orange or lemon-orange mix) from a working squeaker bulb can have a potent diversionary effect that is frequently sufficient to reduce jumping without needing to resort to more startling procedures. The presentation of the odor together with the squeaker sound appears to produce a strong momentary disrupting effect, but without generating significant startle, making the technique useful in the case of emotionally sensitive dogs.

In rare and extreme cases of persistent jumping that is not otherwise controllable, in cases where jumping-up behavior represents a significant threat of injury (e.g., to elderly dog owners), or in cases involving persons unable to perform the necessary leash controls and prompts, TO procedures, and so forth, the use of a remote electronic procedure may be warranted. Both chemical (citronella) and electrical devices are highly effective deterrents, but each requires proper introduction. Electrical collars require preliminary training that allows the dog to learn how to control the electrical stimulus (e-stimulus) by way of various exercises and response-enhancement procedures (see *Remote Electronic Training* in Chapter 10). Electronic training procedures should be used only after a dog has had sufficient instruction with reward-based procedures to understand what is expected. Electrical stimulation (ES) is primarily used to train a dog to back away from the door and remain away at some distance as a guest enters the house. Remote electrical training can be used to support training efforts to keep the dog on the safe rug during greetings. Throughout the process, the dog should receive frequent rewards in response to more desirable and cooperative greeting behavior. Although low-level and medium-level electrical stimulation (LLES and MLES) are unlikely to elicit aggression in a normal and friendly dog, nonetheless ES should not be delivered while a dog is in the act of jumping up or while it is in direct contact with a visitor. The close control of social excesses should be performed with a leash and collar or halter. An experienced and skilled trainer familiar with the risks and benefits of ES should supervise such training activity. Highly aversive ES in such circumstances is unwarranted and could result in undesirable fear, conflict, or the elicitation of pain-elicited aggression in predisposed dogs. Electronic and startle-producing devices should be used with the goal of providing a window of opportunity for additional reward-based training.

Barking

The causes underlying barking problems are varied, requiring that provoking situations, controlling antecedent variables (establishing operations), and contingencies of reinforcement be carefully identified and assessed. Many barking problems appear to be motivated by attention-seeking incentives, inappropriate or frustrated communication efforts, and a history of inadvertent reinforcement. Barking and other canine vocalizations are strongly influenced by heredity and perform a variety of species-typical communication functions (see *Barking, Motor Displays, and Autonomic Arousal* in Chapter 8). Barking activity is clearly increased by a history of positive reinforcement (Salzinger and Waller, 1962) and reduced by punishment. Many barking dogs have learned to place the gratification of their needs on demand: they may bark to go outside and to come back in, to demand food and its timely delivery, to badger the owner into playing with them, to wake the owner up in the morning or in the middle of the night (should they become lonely or bored), or to divert the owner's attention away from guests during greetings. An important aspect of training dogs not to bark is to remove the incentives to bark, that is, discontinuing the reinforcing consequences maintaining the barking behavior. Owners should discourage inappropriate barking and train their dogs to show more acceptable behaviors as a means to get what they want. Many barking problems can be managed or prevented by taking care to provide the dog with adequate daily exercise, training, and play. Defusing or redirecting heightened arousal into other activities (e.g., tossing the dog a soft toy or ball) or leaving it with a special toy or chew item when it is confined can significantly curb excessive barking. Many hyperactive dogs are insatiable enthusiasts for ball play. As the result of structured tug-and-fetch games, the ball can be made into a potent source of reward and diversion. Many hyperactive dogs prefer to have a ball in their mouth rather than bark, unless they happen to learn how to hold a ball and bark at the same time (not an uncommon canine skill). Aside from humor, the consolation in such cases is that at least the barking is muffled.

In active and excitable dogs, excessive barking may be evoked by environmental triggers having innate or species-typical significance, such as territorial intrusion, sudden movements, auditory startle, or the presence of animals beyond their reach (e.g., seeing a squirrel run across the lawn from a window). Such barking may occur independently of the owner's presence or absence. In many cases, barking appears to obtain reward from the effects it has on the object setting the occasion for the barking response. For example, barking at passersby or dogs roaming the neighborhood may be coincidentally reinforced when the target stimulus moves away—a change that reliably occurs when the dog barks, even though the action does not actually depend on the dog's barking response. Situations evocative of approach-avoidance conflict or frustration (e.g., fence lines shared with another dog) may generate high levels of barking. Finally, in situations involving more than one resident dog, barking excesses may develop as the result of social facilitation (see *Social Facilitation* in Volume 1, Chapter 7).

As in the case of jumping up, it is often useful to begin the training process by introducing attention and impulse-control training, thereby developing in advance strong orienting and attending responses, viable bridges (click and "Good" conditioning), a sit-stay module, and waiting behavior. Controlling excessive barking often involves bringing the nuisance barking behavior under stimulus control, that is, training the dog to bark on command (e.g., "Speak"). At first glance, such a training recommendation may seem odd to the average dog owner; nevertheless, it is a very effective means to help reduce unwanted barking. As a preliminary to stimulus-control training, barking is briefly put on a continuous schedule of reinforcement by clicking and rewarding barking behavior whenever it occurs. The instrumental barking module is then brought under the control of a vocal signal by saying "Speak" just as or before the dog barks, followed by the bridging signal and a food reward. Initially, the dog will bark both on cue and off cue, but as it learns that rewards are presented only when barking occurs in the presence of the vocal signal, barking off cue will gradually weaken as the result of extinction. In some cases, DRO

training can be combined with stimulus-control efforts to help reduce excessive barking off cue. At the end of the DRO period, the bridge "Good" or a click is delivered with a food reward, provided that the dog has not barked. Alternatively, the dog can be prompted to bark on cue at the end of the DRO period. If the dog barks during the DRO period, the vocal signal "Enough" is delivered and the DRO period is reset or the dog is briefly timed-out. By combining DRO and stimulus-control training, the dog gradually learns that both waiting without barking and barking on cue results in positive reinforcement.

Exclusionary and nonexclusionary time-outs (TOs) can be useful when applied in the context of DRO and stimulus-control procedures. TO exerts the dual effects of reducing arousal and causing a dog to learn that barking leads to the loss of rewards and attention, whereas refraining from barking results in release from TO and their reinstatement. Barking that continues in TO can be gradually extinguished by ignoring it or by opening the door slightly and snatching upward on the leash with the reprimand "Enough." The TO should typically last 30 seconds, although longer TOs may be necessary for some dogs, but rarely more than 1 minute. After the 30-second TO, provided that the dog has not barked for at least 10 seconds, it is released with the vocal signal "Quiet" and returned to the evoking situation. For TO to be optimally effective, the training situation should be reward dense, making restraint and isolation unfavorable in comparison. If the training environment is excessively punitive, TO may not work as well or perhaps not work at all. In effect, under aversive circumstances, involving a high level of punishment and too little reward, TO from the situation may be experienced in terms of relief rather than punishment (see *How to Use Time-out* in Volume 1, Chapter 8).

While a dog is tethered, kept behind a gate, or crated, leaving the dog with a highly valued chew item or tossing it noncontingent rewards in accordance with a DRO procedure can often help to reduce excessive barking. In some cases, barking can be interrupted by evoking an orienting response with the sound of a squeaker or whistle that has been strongly conditioned as orienting stimulus in the context of basic training activities. The cessation of barking is followed by a bridge ("Good" or click) and food reward, thereby linking the expectation of reward with orienting and the discontinuation of barking. Gradually, the vocal signal "Quiet" is paired with the orienting and bridging sequence. Although such techniques can help to frame, process, and modulate barking activity, the control attained by such means may not be reliable or durable. In most cases involving excessive and persistent barking, effective control requires an element of deterrence. The startle produced by a seven- or 30-penny shaker can is often sufficient to generate the necessary inhibitory effect. The shaker can is tossed in the direction of the barking dog so that it lands close enough to evoke a startle response, but not so close that it risks hitting the dog. Ideally, the dog should not see the trainer throw the can. After two or three tosses, the dog may show an inhibitory response to a brief rattle of the can alone. An alternative method involves arranging a drop can to fall nearby on the floor from the vantage of a remote location. The drop can is set up by tying a length of dental floss to the ring of a soda can and then passing the line through a small eyehook fastened to the ceiling. The line should be long enough to allow the owner to move away, even to a remote part of the house, as needed. Initially, the can is dropped onto the floor by releasing the line, whereupon it is hoisted up to the ceiling again by pulling the dental floss. After two or three sensitizing trials in which the can is dropped, a brief shake or slight movement of the suspended can is frequently enough stimulation to interrupt barking. The owner should periodically return to the confined dog to reward it with affection, food, and release, so long as it remains quiet during the period of confinement.

Barking problems that are under the influence of specific eliciting stimuli can be managed by altering the environment (stimulus-change procedure) or counterconditioning. By arranging the environment so that provocative stimulation is prevented from reaching the dog (e.g., keeping windows closed and blinds shut that face on the street), the amount of daily barking can be substantially reduced. If the barking problem primarily occurs outdoors, bringing the dog indoors when the provoking stimulus is present also helps to reduce frequency and duration of barking episodes. Bringing the dog inside at such times may function as a TO event, thereby potentially helping to reduce future barking activity. In situations where environmental conditions cannot be changed, bark-provoking stimulation may be responsive to counterconditioning efforts. Counterconditioning is performed by pairing bark-eliciting stimuli with food or other sources of incompatible stimulation, thereby producing new associations and raising the bark threshold. For example, ringing the doorbell and immediately throwing a piece of food toward the door can gradually help to reduce excessive barking associated with greetings. The counterconditioning effect is augmented by repeated trials in which the size and type of the food treat are varied from trial to trial. Counterconditioning can be combined with a variety of instrumental training techniques, including DRO, stimulus control, and shaping procedures, whereby more appropriate behavior is strengthened and brought under control with positive reinforcement.

Barking excesses that occur outdoors or when the owner is not present pose significant challenges. Dogs that bark when outdoors should be trained to orient to a whistle and come when called (see *Recall Training* in Chapter 1), whereupon they are released and diverted into some other activity (e.g., ball play). Barking that takes place while the dog is alone is most frequently treated with bark-activated deterrents (see below). However, an automated application of the orienting and DRO procedures previously described might be useful in some cases of barking nuisances occurring in the owner's absence. A signaling and feeding device could be programmed to deliver an alerting stimulus whenever the dog barks, followed by a bridge and a small predictable reward when the dog stops barking in the presence of the signal. The device could also be programmed to deliver a better and varied reward in accordance with a variable DRO schedule, with the bridge and food reward automatically occurring after some period of time, provided that the dog does not bark. After a number of successful DRO trials, indicating that the barking episode is over, the program could automatically reset. In addition to reward-based procedures, remote and bark-activated punishment and avoidance training can be useful (see *Electrical Stimulation and Excessive Barking* in Chapter 9). Although both bark-activated citronella and electronic collars can be effectively used to suppress barking excesses (Juarbe-Diaz and Houpt, 1996), citronella-type collars appear to be more prone to habituation effects, a factor that may limit their usefulness in situations involving repeated bark-provoking stimulation (Wells, 2001). Barking excesses associated with fear, aggression, and separation distress need to be appropriately assessed and addressed with suitable behavior therapy procedures, with remote or behavior-activated devices being used cautiously in such cases, if at all.

Excessive Attention-seeking, Begging, and Demanding Behavior

The causes of excessive attention-seeking behavior are varied, and each case requires individual assessment and evaluation before deciding on a course of treatment. Attention-seeking excesses may stem from exercise deficits, excessive confinement, social deprivation, interactive conflict and adjunctive influences, inappropriate social stimulation, or inadvertent reinforcement. A close phenomenological relationship appears to exist between attention-seeking and active-submission behavior (see *Attention Seeking* and *Adjunctive Generation of Hyperactivity* in Volume 2, Chapter 5). Many dogs that exhibit attention-seeking and intrusive excesses are often prevented from sleeping in the company of family members—a potentially significant etiological factor. Simply allowing the dog to sleep in a bedroom, providing it with more exercise, and developing a daily play and training routine often results in a rapid reduction of inappropriate attention-seeking behavior. Many overactive and excitable dogs exhibit impaired abilities to exert inhibitory control over stimulation-seeking impulses. Seeking behavior in such dogs may be dysfunctional, operating independently of normal inhibitory regulation, consummatory objectives, and reward gratification. Instead of being satisfied with the acquisition of the reward object and stopping, such dogs repeatedly entrain the seeking sequence without appearing to obtain gratification. Although punishment may momentarily blunt the seeking excesses exhibited by such dogs, the punished behavior often rapidly recovers or actually increases over time. Attempting to directly punish or extinguish modal activity without providing adequate alternative outlets is highly problematic (see *Autonomic Arousal, Drive, and Action Modes* in Chapter 10). Although control modules and routines associated with modal seeking (i.e., searching for drive-activating stimulation) can be extinguished, the modal-seeking propensity itself is highly resilient and relatively immune to the consequent effects of risk and loss. The mismanagement of normal attention-seeking and proximity-seeking behavior with positive and negative punishment may produce significant social conflict (affection-fear) and exaggerated active-submission behavior in the dog. A natural outlet for attention-seeking excesses is provided by play, especially play activities consisting of a balance of competitive and cooperative components (e.g., tug and fetch). Play integrates the active-submission aspect of attention seeking and gives it purposeful direction and function, helps to reduce social conflict, and provides an active modality for supporting basic training activities.

Attention seeking and begging behavior appear to be governed by a shared set of stimulation-seeking incentives. Like distractions, which really amount to environmental reinforcers not yet under the trainer's control, begging and demanding behavior reflect motivational states not adequately directed toward the enhancement of cynopraxic goals. Just as one may introduce and use attractive environmental stimuli (distractions) as contingent reinforcers to support training objectives, begging and demanding behavior point to appetitive and social rewards not yet in the service of more cooperative behavior. From this perspective, attention seeking and begging (active-submission behaviors) are nuisances only to the extent that they have not yet been constructively redirected into more acceptable outlets. Just as environmental distractions represent a source of untapped reward for future training efforts, socially intrusive behaviors represent untapped opportunities for reward-based training activities. Training gives active submission (that is, attention seeking and begging) leadership and direction via nurturance. Many hyperactive dogs are simply *seeking and begging* for human leadership. Dogs of this nature are typically highly responsive to play-based and reward-based training efforts. When combined with appropriate limit setting and directive training efforts, play and reward training can be highly successful and should be earnestly encouraged in such cases.

Dogs appear to possess an innate tendency for begging, species-typical behavior that may have aided their survival as they became dependent on humans for food. As a result, begging is highly prepared and rapidly conditioned. By occasionally giving a dog food from the table, it may gradually learn to beg and subsequently develop various other pestering behaviors in other situations. As a nuisance, begging is a modal strategy that develops under the influence of a variable duration (VD) schedule of intermittent reinforcement and an element of punishment. A VD schedule provides reinforcement after the target behavior has occurred continuously for a variable length of time. VD schedules promote hopeful persistence via positive and negative prediction errors. Begging commonly produces two sources of significant positive prediction error: sooner than expected and better than expected outcomes. Demanding behavior operates under the influence of a similar prediction dissonance, but usually without a significant history of punishment. Hope, as a concomitant emotion associated with VD schedules, appears to be an outcome or function of a dynamic history of surprise (success) and disappointment (failure) occurring as the result of begging (see *Hope, Disappointment, and Other Emotions Associated with Learning* in Volume 1, Chapter 7). Hope facilitates the continuation of behavior in the face of suboptimal reinforcement conditions and punitive contingencies, with the expectation that the conditions of reinforcement will eventually change, as they have in the past. Under the influence of hope, frustration and fear are restrained, perhaps explaining the resistance of begging behavior to extinction and punishment efforts. Introducing an alternative modal strategy is the best way to control excessive begging. Such training usually involves a strong component of integrated compliance training, whereby the dog learns to earn attention and food and other everyday rewards by means of deferring, waiting, and cooperating. Instead of allowing the dog to get attention and food as the result of begging, the dog is trained to leave the situation, lie down, and stay (see *Go-lie-down* in Chapter 1). After a variable period of time, the dog is rewarded with food, affection, or release from the down-stay. During the early stages of training the go-lie-down routine, the dog is often put on an active-control line to facilitate the moving-away response and staying at a distance. The active-control line allows the owner to direct the dog away from the table without needing to get up—a feature that is particularly useful at dinnertime. To help prevent begging problems, dogs should not be fed from the table or other locations associated with food preparation.

NUISANCE OR GEM IN THE ROUGH

Dogs that exhibit an intense and persistent interest in social contact, appetitive and social rewards, and play activities, such as retrieving games and finding hidden objects, are often gems in the rough waiting to be developed. These highly active, sociable, and curious sanguine extroverts are in an almost constant state of readiness to work and play, which really amount to the same thing for them. Although tending toward excessive and impulsive behavior, such dogs are able to learn self-control and to behave in cooperative ways, provided that such training exploits their drive to play and their exaggerated predilection for social and appetitive stimulation. The athletic drive and energy, playfulness, and *obsessive* single-mindedness of such dogs are often misinterpreted and mismanaged. As a result, many of these dogs remain gems in the rough or become gems lost to neglect or abuse because of mishandling or inappropriate training or punishment efforts. To succeed with such dogs, their behavioral potential needs to be actualized rather then suppressed, while at the same time shaping social behavior and skills compatible with domestic expectations.

Dogs of this sort are essentially normal, and there are no drugs or behavioral protocols that can transmute this sort of living gold into a baser substance without simultaneously destroying it. For dogs born to leap at life with passion, being trapped in a home with little appreciation or understanding of such a dog's capabilities and needs is simply a tragic state of affairs having significant welfare implications. From the perspective of many dog owners, however, the behavior of such dogs is an unbearable nuisance that is frequently treated in the worst possible ways. As a result, such dogs may develop a variety of secondary behavior problems that further complicate things, making their lives even more untenable and miserable. Owners living with these spirited sanguine-type dogs must truly accept the challenges associated with their training and exhibit a sincere appreciation of the extraordinary potential that such dogs represent; otherwise, hard decisions might need to be made. In situations in which an owner is unwilling to provide the sort of conscientious training and nurturance required to socialize and train such a dog properly, serious consideration should be given to counseling the owner to rehome the dog.

REFERENCES

Arnold LE, Kirilcuk V, Corson SA, and Corson E O'L (1973). Levoamphetamine and dextroamphetamine: Differential effect on aggression and hyperkinesis in children and dogs. *Am J Psychiatry*, 130:165–170.

Aronson LP (1998). Systemic causes of aggression and their treatment. In N Dodman and L Shuster (Eds), *Psychopharmacology of Animal Behavior Disorders*. Malden, MA: Blackwell Science.

Bareggi SR, Becker RE, Ginsburg BE, et al. (1979). Neurochemical investigation of an endogenous model of the "hyperkinetic syndrome" in a hybrid dog. *Life Sci*, 24:481–488.

Baxter LR, Phelps ME, Mazziotta JC, et al. (1987). Local cerebral glucose metabolic rates in obsessive-compulsive disorder: A comparison with rates in unipolar depression and normal controls. *Arch Gen Psychiatry*, 44:211–218.

Blackshaw J, Sutton RH, and Boyhan MA (1994). Tail chasing or circling behavior in dogs. *Canine Pract*, 19:7–11.

Blum K, Cull JG, Braverman ER, et al. (1997). Reward deficiency syndrome: Neurobiological and genetic aspects. In K Blum and EP Noble (Eds), *Handbook of Psychiatric Genetics*. New York: CRC.

Brown PR (1987). Fly catching in the cavalier King Charles spaniel. *Vet Rec*, 120:95.

Cabib S, Puglishi-Allegra S, and Oliverio A (1984). Chronic stress enhances apomorphine-induced stereotyped behavior in mice: Involvement of endogenous opioids. *Brain Res*, 298:138–140.

Canales JJ, Gilmour G, and Iversen SD (2000). The role of nigral and thalamic output pathways in the expression of oral stereotypies induced by amphetamine injection into the striatum. *Brain Res*, 856:176–183.

Carlsson ML (2001). On the role of prefrontal cortex glutamate for the antithetical phenomenology of obsessive compulsive disorder and attention deficit hyperactivity disorder. *Prog Neuropsychopharmacol Biol Psychiatry*, 25:5–26.

Cash WC and Blauch BS (1979). Jaw snapping syndrome in eight dogs. *JAVMA*, 175:709–710.

Catania AC (1998). *Learning*, 4th Ed. Englewood Cliffs, NJ: Prentice-Hall.

Connor DF, Barkley RA, and Davis HT (2000). A pilot study of methylphenidate, clonidine, or the combination in ADHD comorbid with aggressive oppositional defiant or conduct disorder. *Clin Pediatr (Phila)*, 39:15–25.

Dallaire A (1993). Stress and behavior in domestic animals: Temperament as a predisposing factor to stereotypies. *Ann NY Acad Sci*, 697:269–274.

Dodman NH, Shuster L, White SD, et al. (1988). Use of narcotic antagonists to modify stereotypic self-licking, self-chewing, and scratching behavior in dogs. *JAVMA*, 193:815–819.

Dodman NH, Bronson R, and Gliatto J (1993). Tail chasing in a bull terrier. *JAVMA*, 202:758–760.

Dodman NH, Knowles KM, Shuster L, et al. (1996). Behavioral changes associated with suspected complex partial seizures in bull terriers. *JAVMA*, 208:688–691.

Drastura J (1992). Taming aggression with amphetamines: Drug therapy and obedience training help a Lhasa apso with temperament problems become more amenable. *Dog World*, Nov:18–25.

Ducharme JM and Van Houten R (1994). Operant extinction in the treatment of severe maladaptive behavior. *Behav Modif*, 18:139–170.

Ebstein RP, Novick R, Umansky B, et al. (1996). Dopamine D$_4$ receptor (D4DR) exon III polymorphism associated with the human personality trait of novelty seeking. *Nat Genet*, 12:78–80.

Eckstein RA and Hart BL (1996). Treatment of acral lick dermatitis by behavior modification using electronic stimulation. *J Am Anim Hosp Assoc*, 32:225–229.

Einat H and Belmaker RH (2001). The effects of inositol treatment in animal models of psychiatric disorders. *J Affective Disord*, 62:113–121.

Falk JL (1971). The nature and determinants of adjunctive behavior. *Physiol Behav*, 6:577–588.

Fraser AF (1985). Background to anomalous behaviour. *Appl Anim Behav*, 13:199–203.

Gantt WH, Newton JE, Royer FL, and Stephens JH (1966). Effect of person. *Cond Reflex*, 1:146–160.

Garfinkel BD, Webster CD, and Sloman L (1975). Methylphenidate and caffeine in the treatment of children with minimal brain dysfunction. *Am J Psychiatry*, 132:723–728.

Goldberger E and Rapoport JL (1991). Canine acral lick dermatitis: Response to the anti-obsessional drug clomipramine. *J Am Anim Hosp Assoc*, 27:179–182.

Goodman WK, McDouglas CJ, and Price LH (1992). The role of dopamine in the pathophysiology of obsessive compulsive disorder. *Intern Clin Psychopharmacol*, 7(Suppl 1):35–38.

Gorzalka BB, Hanson LA, and Brotto LA (1998). Chronic stress effects on sexual behavior in male and female rats: Mediation by 5-HT$_{2A}$ receptors. *Pharmacol Biochem Behav*, 61:405–412.

Grandin T (1992). Calming effects of deep touch pressure in patients with autistic disorder, college students, and animals. *J Child Adolesc Psychopharmacol*, 2:63–72.

Gray JA (1994). Framework for a taxonomy of psychiatric disorder. In SHM van Goozen, NE van de Poll, and JA Sergeant (Eds), *Emotions: Essays on Emotion Theory*. Hillsdale, NJ: Lawrence Erlbaum.

Gustavson CR (1996). Taste aversion conditioning versus conditioning using aversive peripheral stimuli. In VL Voith and PL Borchelt (Eds), *Readings in Companion Animal Behavior*. Philadelphia: Veterinary Learning Systems.

Hewson CJ and Luescher UA (1996). Compulsive disorder in dogs. In VL Voith and PL Borchelt (Eds), *Readings in Companion Animal Behavior*. Philadelphia: Veterinary Learning Systems.

Hewson CJ, Luescher UA, and Ball RO (1998). Measuring change in the behavioural severity of canine compulsive disorder: The construct validity of categories of change derived from two rating scales. *Appl Anim Behav Sci*, 60:55–68.

Hewson CJ, Luescher UA, and Ball RO (1999). The use of chance-corrected agreement to diagnose canine compulsive disorder: An approach to behavioral diagnosis in the absence of a "gold standard". *Can J Vet Res*, 63:201–206.

Joiner TE and Sachs-Ericsson N (2001). Territoriality and obsessive-compulsive symptoms. *Anxiety Disord*, 15:471–499.

Jones IH and Barraclough BM (1978). Automutilation in animals and relevance to self-injury in man. *Acta Psychiatr Scand*, 58:40–47.

Juarbe-Diaz SV and Houpt KA (1996). Comparison of two antibarking collars for treatment of nuisance barking. *J Am Anim Hosp Assoc*, 32:231–235.

Kennes D, Ödberg FO, Bourquet Y, and De Rycke PH (1988). Changes in naloxone and haloperidol effects during the development of captivity-induced jumping stereotypies in bank voles. *Eur J Pharmacol*, 153:19–24.

Kirby LG, Rice KC, and Valentino RJ (2000). Effects of corticotropin-releasing factor on neuronal activity in the serotonergic dorsal raphe nucleus. *Neuropsychopharmacology*, 22:148–162.

Krushinskii LV (1960). *Animal Behavior: Its Normal and Abnormal Development*. New York: Consultants Bureau.

Landsberg GM (2001). Clomipramine: Beyond separation anxiety. *J Am Anim Hosp Assoc*, 37:313–318.

Lawler C and Cohen PS (1992). Temporal patterns of schedule-induced drinking and pawgrooming in rats exposed to periodic food. *Anim Learn Behav*, 20:266–280.

Lerman DC, Iwata BA, Shore BA, and Kahng SW (1996). Responding maintained by intermittent reinforcement: Implications for the use of extinction with problem behavior in clinical settings. *J Appl Behav Anal*, 29:153–171.

Luescher UA (1993). Hyperkinesis in dogs: Six case reports. *Can Vet J*, 34:368–370.

Luescher UA (1998). Pharmacologic treatment of compulsive disorder. In NH Dodman and L Shuster (Eds), *Psychopharmacology of Animal Behavior Disorders*. Malden, MA: Blackwell Science.

Lyoo IK, Lee DW, Kim SY, et al. (2001). Patterns of temperament and character in subjects with obsessive-compulsive disorder. *J Clin Psychiatry*, 62:637–640.

Martres MP, Costentin J, Baudry M, et al. (1977). Long-term changes in the sensitivity of pre- and postsynaptic dopamine receptors in mouse striatum evidenced by behavioural and biochemical studies. *Brain Res*, 136:319–337.

Mathews S (1983). Paw grasping. *Canine Pract*, 10:13–22.

McDougle CJ, Goodman WK, Leckman JF, et al. (1994). Haloperidol addition in fluvoxamine-refractory obsessive-compulsive disorder: A double-blind, placebo-controlled study in patients with and without tics. *Arch Gen Psychiatry*, 51:302–308.

McDougle CJ, Barr LC, and Goodman WK (1999). Possible role of neuropeptides in obsessive compulsive disorder. *Psychoneuroendocrinology*, 24:1–24.

McDougle CJ, Epperson CN, Pelton GH, et al. (2000). A double-blind, placebo-controlled study of risperidone addition in serotonin reuptake inhibitor-refractory obsessive-compulsive disorder. *Arch Gen Psychiatry*, 57:794–801.

Melvin K (1971). Vicious circle behavior. In HD Kimmel (Ed), *Experimental Psychopathology: Recent Research and Theory*. New York: Academic.

Mendel F, Levine J, Aviv A, and Belmaker RH (1996). Inositol treatment of obsessive-compulsive disorder. *Am J Psychiatry*, 153:1219–1221.

Mills D and Ledger R (2001). The effects of oral selegiline hydrochloride on learning and training in the dog: A psychobiological interpretation. *Prog Neuropsychopharmacol Biol Psychiatry*, 25:1597–1613.

Moon-Fanelli AA and Dodman NH (1998). Description and development of compulsive tail chasing in terriers and response to clomipramine. *JAVMA*, 212:1252–1257.

Niimi Y, Inoue-Murayam M, Murayama Y, et al. (1999). Allelic variation of the D4 dopamine receptor polymorphic region in two dog breeds, golden retriever and shiba. *J Vet Med Sci*, 61:1281–1286.

O'Farrell V (1995). The effect of owner attitudes on behaviour. In J Serpell (Ed), *The Domestic Dog*. New York: Cambridge University Press.

Panksepp J (1998). *Affective Neuroscience: The Foundations of Human and Animal Emotions*. New York: Oxford University Press.

Pani L, Porcella A, and Gessa GL (2000). The role of stress in the pathophysiology of the dopaminergic system. *Mol Psychiatry*, 5:14–21.

Paule MG, Rowland AS, and Ferguson SA (2000). Attention deficit/hyperactivity disorder: Characteristics, interventions, and models. *Neurotoxicol Teratol*, 22:631–651.

Price ML, Curtis AL, Kirby LG, et al. (1998). Effects of corticotropin-releasing factor on brain serotonergic activity. *Neuropsychopharmacology*, 18:492–502.

Rapoport JL (1989). The biology of obsessions and compulsions. *Sci Am*, 260:83–89.

Rapoport JL, Ryland DH, and Kriete M (1992). Drug treatment of canine acral lick: An animal model of obsessive-compulsive disorder. *Arch Gen Psychiatry*, 49:517.

Riddle MA (1991). Pharmacokinetics in children and adolescents. In M Lewis (Ed), *Child and Adolescent Psychiatry: A Comprehensive Textbook*. Baltimore: Williams and Wilkins.

Roper TJ and Crossland G (1982). Schedule-induced wood-chewing in rats and its dependence on body weight. *Anim Learn Behav*, 10:65–71.

Rubia K, Oosterlaan J, Sergeant JA, et al. (1998). Inhibitory dysfunction in hyperactive boys. *Behav Brain Res*, 94:25–32.

Sagvolden T, Aase H, Zeiner P, and Berger D (1998). Altered reinforcement mechanisms in attention-deficit/hyperactivity disorder. *Behav Brain Res*, 94:61–71.

Salzinger K and Waller MB (1962). The operant control of vocalization in the dog. *J Exp Anal Behav*, 5:383–389.

Schnackenberg RC (1973). Caffeine as a substitute for schedule II stimulants in hyperkinetic children. *Am J Psychiatry*, 13:796–798.

Schoenecker B and Heller KE (2001). The involvement of dopamine (DA) and serotonin (5-HT) in stress-induced stereotypies in bank voles (*Clethrionomys glareolus*). *Appl Anim Behav Sci*, 73:311–319.

Schultz W, Dayan P, and Montague PR (1997). A neural substrate of prediction and reward. *Science*, 275:1593–1599.

Schwartz S (1993). Naltrexone-induced pruritus in a dog with tail-chasing behavior. *JAVMA*, 202:278–280.

Seksel K and Lindeman MJ (2001). Use of clomipramine in treatment of obsessive-compulsive disorder, separation anxiety and noise phobia in dogs: A preliminary, clinical study. *Aust Vet J*, 79:252–256.

Seo T, Sato S, Kosaka K, et al. (1998). Tongue-playing and heart rate in calves. *Appl Anim Behav Sci*, 58:179–182.

Shuster L and Dodman NH (1998). Basic mechanisms of compulsive behavior and self-injurious behavior. In NH Dodman and L Shuster (Eds), *Psychopharmacology of Animal Behavior Disorders*. Malden, MA: Blackwell Science.

Smythe JW, Rowe WB, and Meaney MJ (1994). Neonatal handling alters serotonin (5-HT) turnover and 5-HT$_2$ receptor binding in selected brain regions: Relationship to the handling effect on glucocorticoid receptor expression. *Dev Brain Res*, 80:183–189.

Soussignan R and Koch P (1985). Rhythmical stereotypies (leg swinging) associated with reduction in heart-rate in normal school children. *Biol Psychol*, 21:161–167.

Stein DJ, Mendelsohn I, Potocnik F, et al. (1998). Use of the selective serotonin reuptake inhibitor citalopram in a possible animal analogue of obsessive-compulsive disorder. *Depress Anxiety*, 8:39–42.

Stevens LJ, Zentall SS, Abate ML, et al. (1996). Omega-3 fatty acids in boys with behavior, learning, and health problems. *Physiol Behav*, 59:915–920.

Sugrue MF (1983). Do antidepressants possess a common mechanism of action? *Biochem Pharmacol*, 32:1811–1817.

Swedo SE (1989). Rituals and releasers: An ethological model of obsessive-compulsive disorder. In J Rapoport (Ed), *Obsessive-Compulsive Disorder in Childhood and Adolescence*. Washington, DC: American Psychiatric Press.

Szechtman H, Eckert MJ, Tse WS, et al. (2001). Compulsive checking behavior of quinpirole-sensitized rats as an animal model of obsessive-compulsive disorder (OCD): Form and control.

BMC Neurosci, 2:4. http://www.biomedcentral.com/1471-2202/2/4.

Vandebroek L and Ödberg FO (1997). Effect of apomorphine on the conflict-induced jumping stereotypy in bank voles. *Pharmacol Biochem Behav*, 57:863–868.

Veith L (1986). Acral lick dermatitis in the dog. *Canine Pract*, 13:1522.

Voith VL (1979). Behavioral problems. In EA Chandler, JB Sutton, and DJ Thompson (Eds), *Canine Medicine and Therapeutics*. Oxford: Blackwell Scientific.

Voith VL (1980). Hyperactivity and hyperkinesis. *Mod Vet Pract*, 61:787—789.

Wells DL (2001). The effectiveness of a citronella spray collar in reducing certain forms of barking in dogs. *Appl Anim Behav Sci*, 73:299–309.

Werry JS (1994). Pharmacotherapy of disruptive behavior disorders. In LL Greenhill (Ed), *Child and Adolescent Psychiatric Clinics of North America: Disruptive Disorders*. Philadelphia: WB Saunders.

White SD (1990). Naltrexone for treatment of acral lick dermatitis in dog. *JAVMA*, 196:1073–1076.

Wise SP and Rapoport JL (1989). Obsessive-compulsive disorder: Is it basal ganglia dysfunction? In JL Rapoport (Ed), *Obsessive-Compulsive Disorder in Children and Adolescents*. Washington, DC: American Psychiatric Press.

Woods A, Smith CP, Szewczak MR, et al. (1993). Selective serotonin reuptake inhibitors decrease schedule-induced polydipsia in rats: A potential model for obsessive-compulsive disorder. *Psychopharmacology*, 112:195–198.

Wynchank D and Berk M (1998). Fluoxetine treatment of acral lick dermatitis in dogs: A placebo-controlled randomized double blind trial. *Depress Anxiety*, 8:21–23.

6

Neurobiology and Development of Aggression

PART 1: EVOLUTION AND NEUROBIOLOGY

Competition and aggression are virtually universal among highly evolved social animals.

The wide phylogenetic distribution and prominence of competition and aggression among social animals attests to their adaptive value. Although competition and aggression are of tremendous value for enhancing reproductive fitness and survival, excessive competition and aggression are risky and waste energy. Consequently, animals have evolved various means for regulating agonistic interaction in order to maximize benefits and minimize costs.

DOMINANCE AND THE REGULATION OF AGGRESSION

Of particular importance is the evolution of communication systems. Dogs have evolved a wide variety of social signals, displays, and rituals involving every sensory modality in order to exchange information and communicate (see *Communication and the Regulation of Social Behavior*, Volume 1, Chapter 10). An important function of social communication is to limit competition and prevent overt aggression. Various strategies have evolved to regulate aggressive tensions arising between individuals belonging to the same group as well as reducing competition between groups living in the same general area. Competition between individuals belonging to the same social group is regulated by the formation of hierarchically organized dominant and subordinate relations based on outcomes resulting from past competitive exchanges and contests. As a result of accumulated competitive successes or failures, group members take on various dominant or subordinate roles, consisting of attitudes and social behaviors consistent with their social rank. Social rank is advertised by the exchange and observance of social rituals consisting of threat and appeasement displays, the formation and exercise of stabilizing social alliances, and numerous other complex social customs (e.g., greeting and play behaviors) (Figure 6.1). An important function of threat and appeasement displays is to make competitive interaction more predictable and less socially disruptive and violent, thereby setting the framework for more cooperative interaction based on mutual tolerance and affiliative partnering. In well-organized and friendly groups competition is redirected into cooperative ventures serving the mutual interests of both dominant and subordinate group members. However, failure to observe the rules of dominance and priority (e.g., reproductive rights) may prompt pun-

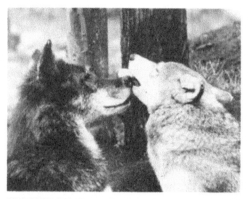

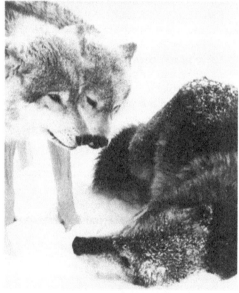

FIG. 6.1. Wolves exchange a variety of threat and appeasement displays in the process of establishing and maintaining a dominance hierarchy. Alliances between pack members are formed to stabilize the status structure and to promote peaceful and cooperative member relations. The display of direct eye contact and other gross and subtle expressions of rank causes a subordinate to avert eye contact, lower ears, and display an appeasement lick—behaviors that are also exhibited by dogs in response to assertions of social dominance. (Photos courtesy of Monty Sloan and Wolf Park, www.wolfpark.org.)

ishment in the form of strong aggressive threats or overt attacks.

COEVOLUTION, PLAY, COMMUNICATION, AND AGGRESSION

The concepts of social dominance and territorial defense are often suggested to help explain aggressive behavior in dogs, especially aggression directed against humans. This is a subject of considerable complexity and controversy that has been discussed at some length in Volume 2 (see *Dominance and Social Harmony* in Chapter 7). Of course, competition between humans and dogs occurs, occasionally escalating into overt aggression, but the causes of aggression are not limited to dominance-related ones (see *Antipredatory Strategy and Autoprotection versus Dominance* in Chapter 8). The relationship between humans and dogs is unique and of a different order than the relationship between dogs. Just as humans view and treat dogs differently than they treat other humans, dogs appear to have evolved specialized behaviors facilitating enhanced affiliative partnerships with human companions, often appearing to prefer contact with humans over dogs (see (see *Supernormal Attachment Hypothesis* in Volume 2, Chapter 4). Dogs have been lifted out of nature and placed into the human family by a transformative process of artificial selection, socialization, and training. Over the course of the dog's domestication, powerful evolutionary influences appear to have mutually altered both human and canine behavior and our propensity for close affiliation with each other. As dogs and humans engaged in convergent hunting activities aimed at exploiting similar food resources, their ability to cooperate and communicate with each other probably underwent significant change. In addition to evolutionary convergence, humans and dogs may have been brought into closer affinity as the result of coevolutionary pressures selecting for social propensities and roles that enhanced their cooperation and biological fitness. Coevolution presupposes the existence of reciprocal selection pressures such that the evolution of one species is partially dependent on the evolution of another species. The close historical interaction between dogs and people seems to fulfill this requirement. Cooperative hunting and many other uses made of dogs may have exerted pronounced coevolutionary pressures gradually making dogs more like humans and humans more like dogs (Schleidt, 1999; Taçon and Pardoe, 2002). Schleidt (1998) has argued that the wolf's highly developed packing behavior, involving cooperation, risk sharing among pack members, pair bonding, and affiliative partnerships among like-gendered individuals, enabled wolves to move to the top of the food chain. By adopting wolflike social habits, Schleidt argues, early humans may have obtained a variety of advantages that enabled them to diversify survival strategies, thus becoming better equipped to exploit nature and coevolving together with the dog rise to a heightened position of power and social complexity.

Play and Affiliation

Under the influence of coevolution, humans and dogs appear to have brought play to a high level of expression. The augmented ability of humans and dogs to initiate and sustain play activities appears to be an essential trait mediating cooperative activity as well as enhancing our desire to stay in close proximity with each other. Perhaps, in the absence of the rigors and travail attendant to surviving under natural conditions, play takes on an ascendant trajectory relative to other more serious activities aimed at self-preservation. The home provides a high degree of safety and security and is highly conducive to play. Play is the living meaning and essence of the human-dog relationship; without play, there is nothing much of value left over to maintain a connected, harmonious, and friendly relationship. Play is forgiving and mediates affectionate tolerance by various means. Play contextualizes actions and exchanges in a way that *in-earnest* implications are overshadowed by an *in-fun* interpretation and abiding trust that all is just play and not what it might otherwise denote under more serious circumstances. Playful contextualization helps smooth over our mutual failings to communicate unambiguously in the language of the other species, thereby installing an affiliative bias of trust that competes with other possible interpretations that might lead otherwise to socially disruptive behavior, including aggression. Play allows humans and dogs to interact and enjoy each other without worrying too much about the implications of interactive vagaries or ambiguous communication. Play nurtures social trust and tolerance within the context of the home. The dog's normal environment—the home—selects for playfulness, just as humans tend to select mates based on such things as a good sense of humor.

Paedomorphosis, Dependency, and Affection

In addition to playfulness, a number of other evolutionary changes occurring over the course of the dog's domestication have combined to enhance the dog's ability to bond, cooperate, and coexist peacefully with humans. These various changes are often collected under the heading of *paedomorphosis*, an evolutionary process in which youthful morphological and behavioral characteristics are retained into adulthood (see *Paedomorphosis* in Volume 1, Chapter 1). In addition to increased playfulness and dependent behavior, behavioral thresholds controlling fear and aggression have undergone significant alteration (Gariépy et al., 2001), making close interaction and affiliative partnering between humans and dogs possible. As a result of these various biobehavioral changes, dogs have generally become more tame and docile, submissive, and dependent on humans, making dogs more adaptable and responsive to human behavioral control efforts. Dogs appear to crave human contact and attention, exhibiting a comparable response to petting and praise as they do to the presentation of food as a reward for cooperative behavior (Fonberg et al., 1981). Tactile gratification and willing submission to human authority are highly prepared propensities in the vast majority of dogs. Dogs appear to be equipped with specialized adaptations that enable them to cope effectively with social stressors. Many dogs are so docile and compliant that they will endure intense physical pain and threatening restraint without resorting to aggression, and those

that do attack often do so in an inhibited sort of way. In general, dogs appear to be biologically prepared to exhibit dependent, cooperative, and submissive behavior and inhibit disruptive competition and aggression toward humans. Perhaps, most significantly, with respect to the dog's tolerance for aversive stimulation and readiness to submit, is an innate and socially actualized propensity to recognize humans as a source of safety and comfort.

Enhanced Communication Abilities

In addition to docility, dependency, and playfulness, dogs are highly responsive to human communication—a propensity that enables them to form close cooperative bonds and work under the direction of people in a wide variety of occupations. Most dogs appear to assign meaning to human actions; that is, they view much of what we do in relation to them as having significance and value as information (Soproni et al., 2001). Dogs have been shown to exhibit a pronounced ability to follow directional cues provided by gaze, pointing, and attend to extremely subtle movements (see *Nora, Roger, and Fellow: Extraordinary Dogs* in Volume 1, Chapter 4) (Candland, 1993). Further, although dogs possessing a propensity for playful environmental exploration are capable of independent problem solving of a high order (Sarris, 1938–1939), they are apt to defer to human guidance rather than rely on their own initiative to solve problems when a human is present (Topál et al., 1997). As a result of their enhanced dependency and reliance on human guidance, dogs appear to have acquired a highly sensitive faculty for responding to and giving directional cues. Dogs use a variety of human signals (e.g., pointing, bowing, head nodding, head turning, and gaze) to locate hidden food (Miklósi et al., 1998; Hare and Tomasello, 1999). Well-socialized dogs are also capable of getting us to help them solve problems by employing various *showing* strategies, whereby they simultaneously attract our attention and direct it to some object or place of interest (Miklósi et al., 2000). Showing is accomplished by bodily orientation and gaze alternation in which dogs look back and forth between the owner and the place or object of interest. Dogs often combine gaze alternation with vocalization, apparently in an effort to capture and direct the owner's attention to the object or activity of interest. For example, dogs commonly engage in showing behavior, when they want to go outside to play or relieve themselves, by barking or alternately looking at the owner and glancing toward the door or leash hanging on a hook.

A dog's ability to exploit human attention as something to use to achieve private ends, together with its ability to follow human directional cues accurately, suggest the existence of a high degree of social attunement and appreciation of humans as a source of information and environmental control. Dogs appear to be cognizant of the functional significance of attention as a means to enhance their control over the environment, perhaps reflecting an underlying evolutionary change associated with domestication, whereby assessment of information (attention) and intelligent hesitation (impulse control) are brought to the forefront, while spontaneous instinctive action, depending on the activation of innate releasing mechanisms, is pushed into the background. By becoming reliant on attention and impulse control, dogs are exposed to a double-edged sword offering great potential for benefit or harm (see *Locus of Neurotogenesis* in Volume 1, Chapter 9). Behavior regulated by attention and impulse control may be highly adaptable and effective in environments that are relatively predictable and controllable; however, if the environment is deranged, then dogs risk experiencing high levels of anxiety and frustration, potentially leading to increased irritability, intolerance, emotional and behavioral reactivity, and disorganization.

EMOTIONAL COMMAND SYSTEMS AND DRIVE THEORY

Panksepp (1982 and 1998) has described four major emotional command systems mediating behavior: seeking, fear, panic, and rage (Figure 6.2). These various emotional command systems share modulatory interconnections that interact to mediate adaptive behavior.

Emotional balance and organized activity are achieved by the complementary excitatory and inhibitory influences produced by these various systems working together in relative harmony. For example, the seeking system is influenced by positive incentives and appetitive behavior, activities that becomes less active as the result of satiation (feedback) or as the result of inhibitory influences produced by other emotional systems. Activation of the fear and rage system exerts a strong inhibitory effect on the seeking system; for example, fearful or enraged dogs typically refuse food. Also, fearful dogs are less likely to explore the environment for reward, but may become highly vigilant for signals of punishment. Under the influence of conflict-related stress, the seeking-rage axis may become progressively disorganized [unstable extravert (choleric or c type)] and susceptible to frustration-related compulsions (e.g., tail chasing) and aggression problems. On the other hand, the stressful activation of the fear-panic axis [unstable introvert (melancholic or m type)] may result in increased phobic reactivity, separation distress, and anxiety-related compulsions (e.g., excessive licking) (see *Inclusion Criteria* in Chapter 5).

Drive as a Higher-order Class of Behavior

Panksepp's emotional command systems closely correspond to the basic components of drive theory. According to drive theory, dog behavior can be divided into four interconnected primary drives: prey drive (social bonding/seeking system), social drive (panic system), defense drive (fear system), and fight drive (rage system). Drive pertains to a higher-order class of behavior containing a set of sequences or routines sharing a common motivational substrate and function (see *Higher-order Classes of Behavior* in Volume 1, Chapter 7). The nature of drive as a higher-order class of behavior denotes broad scope and biogenetic significance. In contrast to simple reflexive behaviors that are elicited by conditioned and unconditioned stimuli, drive-related behavior consists of complex species-typical sequences and routines that are educed (from Middle English *educen*, to direct the flow of; also, Latin *educere*, to lead) and guided into expressions and form. Behaviors belonging to the same class are normally educed by a common set of learned or innate triggers subserving the drive function. For example, behaviors belonging to the higher-order class subsumed under the prey drive share with one another (among other things) the motivation to chase and grab moving things. The performance of drive-related behavior is frequently intrinsically reinforcing for dogs; for example, finding and taking food or detecting and escaping/avoiding a threat are strong sources of reward. Drive activities possessing less tangible sources of gratification are also often highly reinforcing for dogs to perform (e.g., chasing a ball or playing tug games).

Social play is a special modal activity wherein integrative projects are rapidly exchanged between play partners to produce

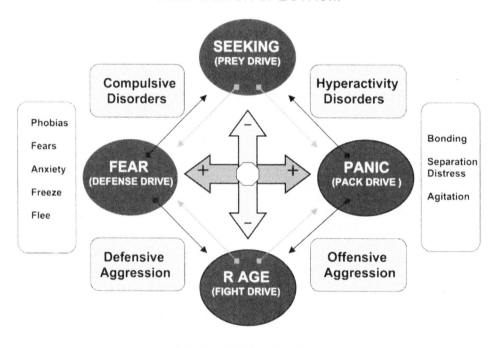

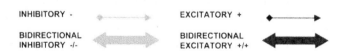

FIG. 6.2. Drive and emotional command system. According to Panksepp, behavior is under the influence of four interactive emotional command systems involving fear, seeking, panic, and rage. Panksepp's emotional command systems closely correspond to the traditional drive or instinct systems ascribed to dog behavior by trainers (see Most, 1910/1955). The activation of these various systems exerts an excitatory or inhibitory effect on other systems. The seeking and rage systems exert a reciprocal inhibitory effect, whereas fear and panic produce a reciprocal excitatory effect. Panksepp's system provides a framework of scientifically validated neurobiological influences for understanding the dynamic interrelations between emotional systems and the expression of adaptive and aberrant behavior.

mutual surprise and excitement conducive to elation and joy. Play-guided training exerts pronounced influences on the expression and form of drive-related behavior. Under the influence of ludic-establishing operations (see *Establishing Operations* in Chapter 1), sequences of behavior belonging to one drive class can be linked with behavior belonging to other drive systems, resulting in unique combinations and forms. Through the agency of play and conditioning, predatory sequences may be educed in combination with a variety of other behaviors belonging to other drive systems (e.g., social, defense, and fight). This process is most plainly apparent in the training of working dogs, whereby innate drive systems and behaviors from diverse origins are combined and harmonized into functionally useful routines via the combined influences of play, drive eduction, and conditioning. *Drive conditioning* refers to a process whereby drive-related activities are progressively focused, refined, redirected, or suppressed via the educement of other drives. The training process serves to shape and playfully entrain drive-related behaviors under the influence of ludic-establishing operations, giving their performance a high degree of intrinsic reward value for dogs. Behavioral thresholds controlling the eduction of drive-related behaviors are affected by both biogenetic and ontogenetic influences. As a whole, an individual dog's propensity to behave in drive and the behavioral thresholds controlling the eduction of drive activity are the elemental dimensions of a dog's temperament. In addition, a dog's trainability is determined by its capacity for playful drive eduction and the entrainment of the drive-related behavior needed to serve the training objective. From the cynopraxic point of view, training incorporates play and drive eduction as a source of intrinsic motivation with the purpose of actualizing a dog's potential and enhancing the human-dog relationship. Play is the substance and means to attain cynopraxic joy.

Drive Systems, Aggression, and Behavior Problems

The seeking system or prey drive consists of appetitive activities involved in searching for food (hunting and tracking), capturing and killing prey, and feeding. The searching system is also involved in the mediation of various grooming (self-stimulatory) activities (e.g., licking, scratching, and biting). The seeking system recruits various forms of locomotor activities (walking, running, stalking chasing, pouncing, and shaking) and sensory modalities (visual, olfactory, and auditory). Seeking behavior is controlled by a variety of reflexive and positive incentive systems influencing environmental exploration, excitement, and learning. When the seeking system is suppressed, its ability to restrain fear, panic, and rage may be impeded. Bilateral ablation of the olfactory bulbs results in increased emotional reactivity and aggressive behavior, suggesting that olfactory tracts projecting to the amygdala and hypothalamus may perform an inhibitory function over excessive emotional and aggressive arousal (Cheal and Sprott, 1971). This finding is consistent with the general inhibitory effect that the seeking system is believed to exert over the rage system.

Preparatory behaviors (e.g., sniffing, scanning, searching, and stalking) belonging to the prey drive system are under the influence of a positive feedback mechanism that makes their performance intrinsically reinforcing for dogs. Working dogs that track persons or search for hidden substances may be motivated to continue despite adverse reinforcement conditions because the olfactory incentive system keeps them going in the absence of immediate extrinsic rewards (see *Autonomic Arousal, Drive, and Action Modes* in Chapter 10). Under the influence of stress associated with excessive conflict or frustration, the seeking system may become pathologically overactive, leading to various disorders associated with behavioral excess and impulsivity (e.g., hyperactivity and compulsions). The seeking system is under the opposing or inhibitory influence of the rage system or fight drive. The axis between seeking and rage normally mediates reciprocal inhibition, keeping both systems in relative balance and stability. Under adverse conditions, the seeking-rage system may become unstable and disordered, perhaps by forming disruptive excitatory interconnections with fear and panic systems.

The fear system (defense drive) mediates escape/avoidance behavior (freezing and fleeing). The panic system (social drive) is activated by loss of social contact (separation distress) and is associated with agitation and intense care- and proximity-seeking behavior.

In addition to mediating reactive separation distress following the loss of social contact, the panic system is activated by the loss of social safety and trust. The axis between the panic and rage systems appears to mediate offensive aggression via the evocation of anger (see *Loss of Safety, Depression, Panic, and Aggression* in Chapter 7). Frustration and irritation preferentially arouse the rage system, triggering affective attack, biting, and fighting. A prominent factor associated with owner-directed aggression appears to be conflict associated with the loss of safety. Owners, as both attachment figures and disciplinarians, are prone to represent some degree of conflict to dogs. Normally, dogs are reared with a significant amount of training and exposure to varying degrees of aversive handling and stimulation that prepares them to cope with adversity at the hands of owners without losing their trust or sense of safety. However, in some cases, involving a history of aversive stimulation resulting in the evocation of significant physical discomfort (irritability) or repeated resource loss (frustration), heightened levels of conflict and loss of social safety and trust may ensue. Alternatively, and perhaps more frequently, dogs that have been raised permissively and indulgently, having not been properly socialized and habituated to the adversities and vicissitudes of social life, may overreact to minor intrusions, as if their social safety and trust toward the owner had been violated. And, of course, it has been violated, at least with respect to the dog's expectations of safe and trusting interaction. As the result of excessive dependency, such dogs may be especially vulnerable to panic-anger conflict in response to the owner's relatively innocuous intrusions. Many of these dogs have never been physically punished in their lives. Aversive stimulation, which obviously is relative, at the hands of a familiar and affectionate attachment figure may generate significant panic-anger conflict and autonomic arousal that, in some cases, may result in

panic-evoked aggression. Although familiarity and affection are natural and powerful inhibitors of aggression, insofar as they promote social safety and security (trust), they also appear to represent the necessary conditions for panic-evoked aggression. The sufficient condition for panic-evoked aggression is a violation of trust and a loss of social safety. Dominance-related aggression frequently is exhibited in ways that are consistent with a panic-evoked scenario in which the bond between the owner and the dog is threatened by a loss of safety and trust. Fear-related aggression, on the other hand, does not depend on social familiarity, but results in situations in which preferred escape or avoidance actions are blocked or unavailable. If successful, fear-related aggression may become a preferred means to control similar threats in the future. Approach-avoidance conflict associated with strangers and territorial transitions is prone to evoke defensive aggression (e.g., bark threats, lunging, and snapping).

In combination, these various emotional command systems and the neural circuits supporting their activity have evolved under environmental and social pressures held relatively constant over the course of the dog's phylogenetic history. Appropriate species-typical behavior patterns (instinctive activities) are intimately related to these emotional systems and their activation. The natural triggers activating command or drive systems are strongly influenced by genetically encoded thresholds and self-regulating feedback mechanisms. In addition to activation resulting from unconditioned stimulation, emotional command systems may be brought under the selective control of novel triggers or conditioned stimuli as the result of classical conditioning. Although behavioral thresholds are strongly influenced by biogenetic factors, the excitatory and inhibitory thresholds controlling drive-related behavior are variable and responsive to modification and modulation through learning. Hunger, pain, thermal extremes, fatigue, and other sources of biological need produce significant modulatory influences over emotional drive systems. Chronic and acute stress can exert a particularly pervasive effect on the conditioned and unconditioned excitation or inhibition of emotional command systems.

Under the influence of acute and chronic emotional stress, the various thresholds controlling the seeking, panic, rage, and fear command systems may undergo significant change, making behavior dependent on those systems more unstable and disorganized. Stress, however, also exerts highly beneficial and adaptive effects on behavioral thresholds and learning. Upon recognizing that a disjunction exists between what the dog expects to occur and what occurs in fact, surprise or startle is evoked, enhancing its attention to the event and increasing its readiness for behavioral change. Surprise and startle mediate significant modulatory influences over trigger thresholds controlling emotional activity. In the case of surprise, fear and rage thresholds may be significantly elevated, whereas seeking thresholds may be lowered and activated in order to exploit the unexpected resource maximally. On the other hand, startle may elevate seeking thresholds while lowering fear, panic, and rage thresholds, depending on the sort of trigger stimulus involved. Beneficial stress associated with startle may help the animal escape or avoid dangerous situations by rapidly lowering thresholds of emotional command circuits controlling species-typical defensive reactions (see *Species-specific Defensive Reactions and Avoidance Training* in Volume 1, Chapter 8). In both cases, the alteration of emotional thresholds serves to compel the animal into specific courses of action, defining in advance the sort of behaviors most likely to occur and to undergo reinforcement if they do occur (see *Antecedent Control: Establishing Operations and Discriminative Stimuli* in Volume 1, Chapter 7). However, under stressful circumstances in which the dog's normal coping efforts fail because of environmental or social constraints, emotionally reactive and unorganized behavior may emerge.

Cognition and Emotional Command Systems

Emotional command systems are modulated by cortical control systems that process experience and prepare dogs to act in ways consistent with past experience on ongoing events. Under optimal conditions, prediction-control expectancies are formed that promote adaptive behavior, but, under the influence of disorderly environments, faulty expectancies and dysfunctional behavior may develop. Particularly malignant influences may originate in traumatic events or result from habitual exposure to social and environmental events that lack adequate predictability (resulting in anxiety) or controllability (resulting in frustration). A lack of predictability over significant appetitive and aversive events may disrupt emotional activity associated with the fear-panic axis, possibly contributing to the development of phobias, compulsive disorders, and separation problems. On the other hand, a routine lack of controllability over significant events may adversely affect activities mediated by emotional circuits associated with the seeking-rage axis, perhaps playing a role in the etiology of various forms of affective aggression and behavioral excesses. When behavioral events are relatively predictable and controllable, emotional command systems function optimally to promote adaptive behavior and a better state of being. However, when behavioral events occur independently of a dog's ability to predict or control them, then various pervasive cognitive and behavioral perturbations may follow (see *Learned Helplessness* in Volume 1, Chapter 9). Another source of disturbance is the conflict resulting from the simultaneous activation of incompatible emotional command systems by the same stimulus—a common occurrence in the case of severe and unpredictable punishment, whereby the owner becomes an object of both affection and fear. Lastly, early socialization and habituation efforts may exert profound and lasting influences on the activity of emotional command systems. Whether such ontogenetic influences result in the development of abnormal coping behavior appears to depend on biogenetic influences (e.g., temperament traits) affecting the way the dog processes and responds to environmental adversity. Many dogs are exposed to suboptimal and stressful environments, but only some of them ultimately develop behavior problems. Furthermore, some dogs may exhibit severe problems in the absence of a known history of significant stress and may continue to do so despite improved social interaction and environmental enhancements, underscoring the important role played by heredity in the etiology of certain behavior problems.

Modulatory and Unifying Effects of Play

The activation of care (contact comfort and affection) circuits and play drive (joy system) produces significant modulatory effects on primitive emotional command systems. Tactile stimulation has been shown to restrain aversive arousal associated with stressful situations (see *Effects of Touch* in Volume 1, Chapter 4). Contact comfort associated with touch exerts an inhibitory influence over both fear and panic (separation distress), apparently by mobilizing a potent oxytocin-mediated anti-stress response (Uvnäs-Moberg, 1998a; Holst et al., 2002; Lund et al., 2002). In addition, somatosensory stimulation may enhance social familiarity and exert a significant inhibitory effect over aggression (Panksepp, 1998). The usefulness of petting and affectionate praise has been well established in dog training. Play offers many therapeutic benefits for the management of arousal and behavioral output deficiencies and excesses associated with emotional command systems. The eduction of modal play enables trainers to access species-typical motor subroutines that are normally under the exclusive control of specific emotional command systems. Playing fetch appears to access behavior associated with the seeking system (prey drive), whereas tug and roughhousing games may access behaviors associated with the rage system (fight drive) while remaining in the play mode. Under the influence of play, virtually the entire repertoire of motor and expressive actions associated with threat (snarling, growling, and barking) and attack (lunging, biting, and shaking) can be evoked in many well-trained dogs with little risk of a scratch to bare skin. The activation of modal play can help a dog overcome a variety of the fears associated with new places and things, whereas activation of social modal activities (care seeking, following, and begging) can be used to reduce social inhibitions, aversions, and aggression. Play therapy specifically aims to access these various behavioral and emotional systems in order to modify activity

associated with them. Combining play therapy and training provides an extremely powerful means for modifying dog behavior and enhancing social trust. Virtually all training and behavior-modification efforts take place with the dog *in drive*, that is, in a phylogenetic mode of activity, whether it be food reward (seeking system), escape/avoidance (fear system), praise and petting (social bonding/panic system), or aggressive play (rage system). Modal play is unique in that it is able to recruit activity from a variety of emotional systems and produce unique variations and modifications through learning (i.e., projects), helping to bring these diverse elements and novel connections into harmony. In doing so, play appears to liberate species-typical behavior patterns from primitive emotional systems, allowing dogs to safely practice skills and engage in novel projects that might not otherwise occur. Play promotes the activation of affects associated with enhanced harmony, balance, and joy (see *Fair Play and the Golden Rule* in Chapter 10).

Play appears to be inhibited by increasing levels of aggression or heightened exploratory or seeking activity, as well as fear and social loss. As play approaches the extremes of evoking actual aggression, fear, or separation distress, it is rapidly inhibited:

> Play may help animals project their behavioral potentials joyously to the very perimeter of their knowledge and social realities, to a point where true emotional states begin to intervene. Thus, in the midst of play, an animal may gradually reach a point where true anger, fear, separation distress, or sexuality is aroused. When the animal encounters one of these emotional states, the playful mood may subside, as the organism begins to process its predicaments and oppositions in more realistic and unidimensional emotional terms. (Panksepp, 1998:283)

Play is most likely to occur in familiar places and between familiar persons and dogs (Mitchell and Thompson, 1990). The balancing effects of play make it useful in the treatment of a variety of behavior disturbances. Play therapy is particularly useful in the management and treatment of behavior problems involving social stress and impulsive behavior. Like play, behaviors associated with drive appear to be maintained by motivational states immediately produced by behaving in drive. The mere opportunity and *choice* to behave in drive appears sufficient to support the future occurrence of the behavior, and, consequently, drive-related behavior does not depend on reinforcement derived from other activities (e.g., obtaining food or affection), that is, extrinsic or adventitious sources of drive gratification. Behaving in drive is intrinsically reinforcing and self-perpetuating.

ADAPTIVE COPING STYLES: PLAY, FLIRT, FORBEAR, AND NIP

During the process of domestication, selection pressures appear to have favored a genotype expressing a configuration of neuropeptides, neurotransmitter, and receptors conducive to a highly adaptable and sociable canine phenotype. These evolutionary changes at the neurobiological level are assumed to exert a profound organizing effect at the social level, shifting behavioral thresholds toward increased tolerance (e.g., elevating fight and flight thresholds) and affiliation (e.g., lowering care-seeking and care-giving thresholds), altering the dog's responsiveness to social signals, perhaps making the human a supernormal stimulus for bonding and forming friendly relations (see *Supernormal Attachment Hypothesis* in Volume 2, Chapter 4). This general hypothesis is supported by neurobiological and behavioral changes exhibited by silver foxes selected for tameness (see *The Silver Fox: A Possible Model of Domestication* in Volume 1, Chapter 1). Tame foxes express a significantly altered hypothalamic-pituitary-adrenal (HPA) system, exhibiting reduced reactivity to social stressors; they also show evidence of increased serotoninergic and catecholaminergic activity conducive to enhanced impulse control and a reduction of defensive behavior.

Under natural circumstances, animals expressing elevated fear and aggression thresholds would be at considerable risk and disadvantage with respect to mobilizing defensive measures against threats; under the protective influence of domesticity, however, such a pattern of reduced fear and aggressive reactivity would be an advantage to a dog, whereas an opposite pattern of heightened flight-fight system (FFS) activity would be highly problematic and incompatible with domestic relations and activities. In response to the unique social stressors experienced by dogs living in close association with people, dogs appear to have evolved novel adaptations enabling them to live in harmony with human companions. The dog's capacity to form social bonds with humans is of such magnitude that it overshadows social attraction toward other dogs, even its mother (see *Maternal Separation and Stress* in Chapter 4). Under contemporary circumstances, this ancient adaptation is a mixed blessing for the average dog left alone all day. Such dogs are at a risk of developing insecure or excessively strong and exclusive social attachments, making them vulnerable to suffer distress at separation. During the dog's early domestication, staying close to its keepers would have been a source of security, with the human keeper taking on the role of benefactor and protector (tend-and-befriend adaptions), allowing human and dog to form close bonds, and allowing the protodog to progressively shed its FFS reactivity and evolve flirt-play and forbear-nip adaptive strategies. In an important sense, when a dog is left alone, it loses its guardian shield of protection and security.

Phylogenesis, Polymorphism, and Coping Styles

Dogs appear to have evolved two relatively independent but overlapping and complementary defensive systems and styles for coping with disappointing, threatening, stressful, or aversive social situations. These hypothetical systems are present in varying degrees in all dogs, depending on heredity and activating experience. The adaptive coping styles (flirt-play and forbear-nip) are largely composed of the self-preservative and self-protective strategies of the young, reflecting a paedomorphic social adaptation. When presented with a threatening social situation, such dogs tend to exhibit an admixture of two general patterns: (1) stable introversion, a variety of attention-seeking, care-seeking, and submissive behaviors (not necessarily authentic), a genuine appetite for and enjoyment of close social contact and interaction, and a passive "grin and bear it" strategy to aversive stimulation or escape when pushed too far; or (2) stable extraversion, showing a genuine love of rough-and-tumble play and object play, a variety of playful escape and evade tactics, and a "bite the bullet" strategy to aversive stimulation or inhibited nip when pushed too far. The vast majority of dogs appear to combine these various adaptive strategies in varying proportions to form adaptive coping styles with which to manage stressful interaction with human companions. For the sake of simplicity, the term *flirt-and-forbear* system is used to designate this antistress, antifear, and antiaggression system of domestic adaptations.

In addition to fostering a heightened capacity for social affiliation, cooperation, and play, novel physiological mechanisms have evolved to support the flirt-and-forbear and tend-and-befriend styles of human-canine adaptive coping and bonding. Although the exact neurobiological substrates integrating these adaptive coping styles are not known, phylogenetic changes to the oxytocin-opioidergic system, the serotonergic stress-management system, and the dopaminergic reward system appear to be likely focal points of coevolutionary change. In any case, biobehavioral changes conducive to enhanced playfulness, social reward, social cognition, and emotional adjustment appear to have taken place in a process of phylogenetic enculturation, to borrow and extend Hare's term (Hare et al., 2002), whereby humans and dogs have mutually accommodated the other via a unique coevolutionary process (see *Coevolution, Play, Communication, and Aggression*). Over the course of 135,000 years of coevolution (Vilà et al., 1997), humans and dogs appear to have exerted a profound social and emotional transformation upon one another, mutually evolving changes conducive to close affiliation. Many of these changes appear to have taken place in the direction of social, cognitive, and behavioral neoteny; that is, humans and dogs have coevolved in a way that has caused each species to retain more juvenile characteristics into adulthood (see *Paedomorphosis* in Volume 1, Chapter 1), giving rise to our mutual appreciation and capacity for

affection and our love of play, among other things. As incredible as the notion may seem, the human-dog capacity for affiliative bonding and play appears to be organized and integrated at the level of mutual modifications of the human and canine genome, a phylogenetic testament to an ancient and perennial bond etched forever into our respective genotypes, as friends might scrawl their initials side by side on an old tree.

Accordingly, humans and dogs appear to have evolved complex and genetically polymorphic adaptations as the result of this evolutionary convergence and phylogenetic enculturation process—changes that should be evident in the matrix of physiological and neurobiological processes from which social cognition, emotion, and adaptive coping styles emerge. This general theory suggests that among dogs there is not a single species-typical nature, but rather an assortment of multiple canine natures that emerge under the influence of polymorphic variations, ontogenetic stressors, and epigenetic organizing influences (see Bittner and Friedman, 2000). Biological adaptations conducive to harmonious human-dog interaction are expressed at the level of an infinitely complex array of biogenetic and neurobiological processes from which functional and structural systems of biobehavioral organization gradually emerge, giving rise to the capacity for cognition, emotional, and the capacity to adapt by means of learning and goal-oriented initiative. Of particular interest from the practical vantage of cynopraxic training and therapy are the neurobiological changes that resulted in the development of the previously discussed canine adaptive coping styles.

Oxytocin-opioidergic Hypothesis

Brown and colleagues (2001) may have discovered a potentially significant link pertaining to the dog's adaptive abilities and capacities for social attachment and bonding in a unique modification of the canine oxytocin-opioidergic system. As discussed in Chapter 4 (under *Maternal Separation and Stress*), oxytocin and endogenous opioids appear to interact in the process of forming social attachments. Opioids also play a major role in modulating distress and pain. In adult animals, opioids appear to exert an inhibitory effect on central and peripheral oxytocin release. In dogs, however, opioids appear to inhibit central oxytocin release while at the same time stimulating peripheral release—a phenomenon that appears to be unique to dogs. The physiological implications of this finding are not clear, but given the strong correlation between increased peripheral oxytocin activity and social approach, attachment, and antistress effects, this apparently novel adaptation may contribute to the dog's ability to cope physiologically with social stressors unique to living in close association with humans. Oxytocin appears to exert an agonist effect on endogenous opioid activity (Lund et al., 2002), and facilitates exogenous opiate activity by reducing tolerance effects and by attenuating withdrawal symptoms (Sarnyai and Kovacs, 1994). Oxytocin has also been shown to enhance active avoidance learning, perhaps by reducing emotional arousal (Uvnäs-Moberg et al., 2000). Together with arginine vasopressin (AVP) and corticotropin-releasing factor (CRF), oxytocin appears to play a role in the acute integration the stress response, but after repeated release of oxytocin, perhaps in association with endogenous opioids, mediates an antistress and calming effect (e.g., reduces anxiety, decreases blood pressure, and decreases glucocorticoid release) (Uvnäs-Moberg, 1997), whereas AVP and CRF continue to mobilize stress-related physiological changes conducive to increased anxiety, glucocorticoid release, and blood pressure.

Uvnäs-Moberg and colleagues (1997 and 1998a and b) at the Karolinska Institute, Stockholm, have intensively investigated the antistress effects of oxytocin, reporting several lines of compelling evidence in support of the antistress hypothesis. Peripheral oxytocin promotes parasympathetic normalization via enhanced vagus-nerve tone, modulates irritability, decreases sympathetico-adrenal tone, promotes anabolic metabolism, and exerts a calming effect and a host of other effects consistent with an antistress function. For example, oxytocin plays a central role in the regulation of heart rate and coronary flow, cardiovascular effects that are mediated by oxytocin terminals acting on the vagus nerve

at the level of nucleus of the solitary tract (Higa et al., 2002) and by means of a direct bradycardial action on the heart itself, among other routes (Petersson, 2002). The central and peripheral effects of oxytocin on canine blood pressure and heart rate are complicated, with oxytocin and AVP appearing to have complementary roles in the regulation of cardiovascular activity (Montastruc et al., 1985). Although the blood-brain barrier shows a low permeability to oxytocin, some passive transport may occur in the case of high peripheral concentrations in association with injections (Ermisch et al., 1985; Uvnäs-Moberg et al., 2000).

Together with cardiovascular benefits, peripheral oxytocin appears to enter the brain to exert a negative-feedback effect on FFS arousal, thereby mediating a calming influence and elevating thresholds associated with irritability and pain (Lund et al., 2002). In addition to antinociceptive effects occurring at the level of the periaqueductal gray, systemic administration of oxytocin has been shown to increase central α_2-adrenoceptor responsiveness at the level of the locus coeruleus (Petersson et al., 1998), the amygdala, and the hypothalamus (Diaz-Cabiale et al., 2000). Although generally excitatory, norepinephrine (NE) acting at α_2-adrenoceptor sites produces a potent inhibitory effect, appearing to play a crucial role in helping dogs to cope adaptively to social stressors by preventing or ameliorating stress-related dysregulation at the level of the prefrontal cortex (Birnbaum et al., 2000).

Oxytocin is hypothesized to play a major role in the expression of somatic feelings of enhanced comfort and safety (well-being) resulting from the occurrence of conditioned and unconditioned rewards (e.g., vocal encouragement, petting, and food) obtained in the process of adaptive control efforts (see *Origin of Reactive versus Adaptive Coping Styles* in Chapter 4). The social benefits of oxytocin appear to be cumulative, developing as the result of repetitive stimulation of oxytocin release. The oxytocinergic benefits of petting and food rewards appear to exert a potent therapeutic effect over stress, fear, and aggression. On the other hand, complementary dopamine reward circuits appear to encode cerebral teaching signals that optimize adaptive control efforts by means of detecting and coding positive prediction discrepancies (Schultz, 1998), thereby mediating surprise and cortical reward, play, active modal strategies (e.g., exploring, experimenting, and discovering), and feelings of joy and freedom.

Not all dogs respond to petting with a decreased heart rate, but those that do are also responsive to petting as a reward (Fonberg, 1981). Dogs that exhibit an increased heart rate when petted are typically unresponsive to petting as a reward. Manual restraint also appears to exert a significant heart-rate deceleration effect in dogs, perhaps as the result of parasympathetic rebound effects, a cardiac effect that may be amplified by petting. In the case of nervous pointer dogs, restraint-induced deceleration is not appreciably enhanced by petting (Thomas et al., 1972). These findings suggest that petting may offer a valuable diagnostic tool for differentiating dogs exhibiting adaptive versus reactive coping styles. Dogs responding to petting with an increased heart rate may be vulnerable to stress associated with the activation of the FFS and show an increased propensity for emotional reactivity, social avoidance, and defensive behavior, traits consistent with reactive vulnerability, whereas dogs showing a reduced heart rate when petted may exhibit an antistress response consistent with an adaptive coping style, correlating with traits such as friendly approach and attachment, social dependency, playfulness, and calm. Kostarczyk (1991) found that the administration of atropine to dogs results in significant heart-rate acceleration and abolishes petting-related cardiac deceleration, with dogs becoming avoidant of petting and showing increased excitability, tenseness, and aggressiveness—results consistent with the loss of oxytocinergic regulatory influence over parasympathetic functions. Atropine is a potent oxytocin antagonist shown to block oxytocinergic-mediated bradycardia (Mukaddam-Daher et al., 2001). The reactive emotional responses exhibited by dogs medicated with atropine appear to reflect a loss of control over sympathetic arousal, at least in part due to blocking the antistress effects of oxytocin. As previously mentioned, massagelike tactile stimulation appears to mediate an antinociceptive effect

via increased levels of oxytocin at the level of the periaqueductal gray (PAG) (Lund et al., 2002) (see *Neural Circuits Mediating Anger and Rage*). This finding underscores the value of posture-facilitated relaxation (PFR) training for helping to attenuate irritability and contact intolerance.

Cyonopraxis, Antistress, and a Tend-and-Befriend System

Cynopraxic training is performed with the goal of reducing interactive conflict and tension arising from antagonistic control interests. Instead of reacting in accordance with the FFS when exposed to social stressors associated with owner limit-setting actions and periodic separations, the dog learns to adjust to stressors under the calming influence of the flirt/play-forbear antistress system. Cynopraxic therapy organizes interactive transactions and emotional exchanges between the owner and the dog with the goal of bringing a flirt-and-forbear antistress system on-line. The compromise and mutual appreciation associated with cynopraxic training promote interactive harmony and friendly interaction akin to what Taylor and colleagues (2000) have referred to as *tend and befriend* adjustments; unfortunately, the authors seem to assume that such a capacity is the special providence of the female nervous system. On the contrary, the potential for adaptive organization in accordance with the tend-and-befriend system is probably the result of an asexual neural plasticity shared by both male and female humans alike, perhaps arising in the course of human-canine coevolution, giving human beings the capacity for affectionate bonding, supportive and comforting interaction, and intensified feelings of well-being as the result of bonding and sharing a home with a dog. According to this hypothesis, both humans and dogs have jointly evolved specialized antistress capacities conducive to close social interaction and affectionate bonding.

Cynopraxis is essentially an expression of the human capacity to tend (provide the dog with an improved quality of life) and befriend (establish and enhance the human-dog bond), a capacity that dogs learn to reciprocate as the result of socialization and training. The natural orientation of the human being toward the dog is one of tending and befriending, whereas the dog has evolved a heightened capacity for dependent behavior and friendly reciprocity, operating under the influence of an antistress, antifear, and antiaggression system evolved to cope with stressful interaction and conflict associated with close association with humans, viz., a flirt/play-forbear-nip or, more simply, a *flirt-and-forbear* system. Although male dogs appear to exhibit a greater propensity (as a group) for reactive adjustments in association with the activation of the FFS than do females, under the influence of play, reward-based training, and social interaction conducive to the activation of the flirt-for-bear system (e.g., human tending and befriending), both male and female dogs show an extraordinary capacity for adaptive coping and adjustment, allowing the natural canine aptitude for reciprocating human tending and befriending behavior to emerge in the form of interactive harmony, mutual appreciation, and a loving and trusting bond.

OLFACTION AND EMOTIONAL AROUSAL

Olfaction appears to play a major role in the process of emotional learning and memory. The importance of olfactory learning on emotional behavior is suggested by neuroanatomic evidence showing that olfactory projections reach the amygdala more directly than do other sensory inputs. In addition, olfactory stimuli appear to form rapid and lasting conditioned associations with both attractive and aversive emotional states—associative learning that is mediated from an early age by the amygdala (Sullivan and Wilson, 1993). Oddly, though, neonatal rats exposed to odor-shock conditioning prior to postnatal day 10 show a paradoxical approach response toward the odor instead of avoiding it as one might expect. After day 10, rat pups learn to avoid the odor as the result of aversive conditioning, provided that they had not received prior odor-shock conditioning. Most interestingly, however, if the infant rats have been previously exposed to odor-shock conditioning, they continue to show an approach response toward it, even

though they are now neurologically able to learn an avoidance response. Paradoxical conditioning resulting in persistent approach behavior toward a conditioned aversive stimulus may help to facilitate infant bonding and attachment under adverse or socially abusive conditions (Sullivan et al., 2000). These findings may help to explain the tendency of dogs to respond to aversive stimulation by emitting avoidance/escape responses and then engaging in attention-seeking and comfort-seeking behavior toward the person delivering the stimulation (Fisher, 1955) (see *Early Trauma and the Development of Behavior Problems* in Volume 2, Chapter 4). The search for safety in human contact and comfort giving appears to be a significant aspect of the bonding and socialization process.

Recalling that oxytocin exerts an antinociceptive effect (see *Oxytocin-opioidergic Hypothesis*), Ågren (1997) found that rats injected with the peptide appeared to secondarily influence the pain thresholds of untreated cagemates. Further study of the phenomena, revealed that when the untreated cagements were rendered anosmic they no longer showed the change in pain sensitivity, suggesting that olfaction may mediate the effect. This finding offers an interesting olfactory hypothesis to test with respect to the increased playfulness exhibited by puppies at weeks 5 and 7 toward female handlers (Scott, 1992a). Finally, olfactory cues might also play a role in the evident gender bias shown by dogs toward human males and females, with dogs seeming to be more friendly (Lore and Eisenberg, 1986) and less defensive and aggressive toward females than males (Wells and Hepper, 1999). These findings may also have practical value, indicating the possibility that an oxytocin-related substance with antistress properties might be secreted on the skin (sebaceous) or in the sweat of animals treated with oxytocin. Conceivably such material, if it exists, could be isolated, concentrated, and tested for antistress effects. Finally, it is interesting to speculate that some potential benefit may be derived from repeated exposure to an aerosol oxytocin mist, perhaps periodically delivered by a spray dispenser controlled by a timer and attached to a crate or kennel to assist dogs under stress at home or while under hospitalization.

Olfaction, Fear, and Anger

Many dog owners and trainers have reported anecdotally that dogs appear to smell fear, perhaps helping to explain why some dogs react aggressively toward the diffident approach of nervous people (Sommerville and Broom, 1998). A fearful person would undoubtedly present a significantly different scent picture than a relaxed person. The belief that dogs can discriminate emotional states as the result of scent messages emanating from the pores and breath of humans has not been tested; however, it is highly likely that dogs can detect odors associated with highly emotional and stressful states. Detecting odors associated with human anger and fear would be highly advantageous to dogs. The scent aura at times of intense anger or frustration would likely produce a strong and lasting impression, especially if such odors were followed by severe physical punishment. Exposure to the odors associated with anger or fear may sensitize olfactory attentional processes localized in the amygdala—an area that that is strongly activated by the presentation of olfactory stimuli (Hudry et al., 2001) and prominently involved in emotional learning. Seizure-alert dogs may rely on scent-related changes occurring in advance of epileptic seizures, thereby enabling them to anticipate such activity (see *Ability to Detect and Discriminate Human Odors* in Volume 1, Chapter 4). Many dogs appear to react in a highly emotional manner to seizure activity, becoming fearful or aggressive as the result of such events (Strong and Brown, 2000). Edney (1993) found that dogs anticipating seizure activity typically exhibited signs of increased anxiety and restlessness. At such times, these dogs appeared to act strangely and were more difficult to control than usual.

Donovan (1967) has tested the hypothesis that dogs may express their anal glands in order to facilitate escape from threatening restraint. After manually expressing anal sac fluids, he presented the material to various puppies and dogs to sniff. He found that puppies showed no response to the anal flu-

ids, whereas adult dogs "recoiled and appeared apprehensive" (1048) when presented the fluids smeared on plastic gloves:

> Dogs that previously dashed enthusiastically to the opened gate of the exercise pen, turned back as if halted by an electric shock when the gloves were held in the opened doorway. (1048)

The fact that puppies showed little reaction to the odor suggests that the fearful response might have been acquired as the result of learning. As the result of expressing anal fluids consequent to intensely threatening events, dogs may associate such odors with the fear and escape behavior that occurred at such times. When another dog, perhaps under the distress of an attack, subsequently releases the odor, it may evoke a conditioned escape response in the attacker, thereby possibly turning the attacker away and protecting the loser from injury. Similarly, the deposition of anal secretions in feces may exercise a conditioned repellent effect helping to ward off intruders. In summary, according to this hypothesis, anal fluids are not inherently repellent, but may rapidly become so as the result of aversive conditioning. The scent of anal secretions may be highly prepared for association with fear and escape behavior, making biological extracts or synthetic analogues of anal fluids potentially useful for the management of certain aggression problems (see *Threat and Appeasement Displays* in Volume 2, Chapter 8).

Chemosignals, Social Behavior, and the Modulation of Emotional Thresholds

In addition to conditioned social odors, it is reasonable to assume that various chemosignals and pheromones are exchanged between dogs to modulate emotional thresholds (motivational readiness). Social chemosignals may serve to amplify the significance of other social signals present at the time of their expression, as well as promote positive mood states conducive to friendly social interaction. These modulatory effects of olfactory signals on social behavior and mood may help to explain the significance of the canine custom of mutual anogenital presentation and exploration exhibited by most dogs during close encounters with other dogs, especially unfamiliar ones. Chemosignals and pheromones may offer a valuable means for promoting affiliative interaction by increasing positive affect and mood while elevating aggression thresholds. Reportedly, a dominance pheromone may be contained in the cerumen of dominant dogs—a substance that appears to facilitate submission behavior in subordinates (Pageat, personal communication, 2001; Pageat, 1999). Interestingly, the steroids estratetraenol and antrostadienone have been shown to produce modulatory effects on human affect and mood consistent with a social function (Jacob and McClintock, 2000).

Olfactory Conditioning

Odors are rapidly conditioned and appear to exert pronounced effects over emotional behavior. Although experimental evidence is lacking in dogs, research with human subjects has shown that ambient odors presented during stressful or frustration-inducing experiences exert lasting effects. For example, Kirk-Smith and colleagues (1983) found that odors present while adults worked at a stressful task acquired the capacity to elicit increased anxiety when they were encountered again. Similarly, children exposed to an ambient fragrant scent while working on an insolvable maze task generating emotions of failure and frustration showed increased problem-solving deficits when exposed to the same odor while working on a solvable cognitive problem (Epple and Herz, 1999). The children exposed to the conditioned odor performed less efficiently on the problem than children exposed to another fragrant scent or no scent at all.

Olfactory conditioning for the purpose of reducing aversive emotional arousal in dogs has proven to be useful in a variety of training and behavior-therapy contexts. By pairing a dilute odor with relaxing massage and petting, or other sources of reward, relaxation, and safety, the odor stimulus gradually becomes conditioned to produce similar emotional effects independently of the unconditioned stimulus used. The close ontogenetic relationship between olfaction and tactile sensory development may prepare odors for rapid association with taction-elicited emotional states (see *Social Comfort Seeking and Distress* in Volume 2, Chapter 4). The pairing of an olfactory stimulus with taction-induced relaxation establishes a conditioned association between the odorant and relaxation so that the odor alone can either facilitate or independently evoke the relaxation response (see *Posture-facilitated Relaxation Training* in Chapter 7).

Practitioners of aromatherapy attribute special psychological and medical benefits to fragrant oils (Tisserand, 1977), but few of these claims are supported by scientific studies, especially in the case of animals (Wynn and Kirk-Smith, 1998). However, several studies in humans do indicate that aromatherapy may augment a modest and transient reduction in anxiety when combined with massage (Cooke and Ernst, 2000). Traditionally, many fragrant oils have been reputed to have relaxing and calming attributes; however, the beneficial effects of odors on mood and emotions probably depend more on conditioning than an inherent property of the scent. Some odors, though, do appear to exert benefits on mood, aversive states, and stress-related changes independently of conditioning (Shibata et al., 1990 and 1991). For example, the odor of lemon has been shown to produce an antidepressant effect in rats (Komori et al., 1995), and the odor of orange has been shown to reduce anxiety while promoting a more calm and positive mood in people receiving dental treatment (Lehrner et al., 2000). Lavender, chamomile, and vanillin have also been shown to exert central effects consistent with improved mood and anxiety reduction (see *Fear of Loud Noises and Household Sounds* in Chapter 3).

Although a particular fragrant oil may be pleasing to a human nose, it may not be equally attractive to a dog. Whatever odor is selected should not be aversive to the dog or presented at a concentration too strong for the dog's sensitive nose. The odorant should be delicate and faint to the human nose and, ideally, evoke interested sniffing by the dog. Odors that cause the dog to turn its nose away should not be used. Many dogs appear to be actively attracted to sandalwood, which has a soft mellow quality that provides an adequate odorant for most dogs when diluted 1:30–50 in a carrier vegetable oil. Citrus odors (e.g., lemon or orange) and lavender may have some additional advantages in the treatment of separation distress, phobias, and various anxiety-related problems.

In addition to pairing an odor with taction-induced relaxation, other scents can be paired with the presentation of food rewards and other sources of attractive stimulation. A highly effective method involves putting 1 or 2 drops of a fragrant oil or extract inside a squeaker used as conditioned reinforcer. With each squeak, the odor is dispensed into the air, thus pairing the odorant stimulus with success and reward. This same odor can be presented just before feeding the dog, as well. A play odor can be developed by putting a scent on play objects or presented in advance of getting the dog's leash to go for a walk. An olfactory safety signal can be paired with the opponent relief and relaxation associated with the discontinuation of an aversive state [e.g., an odor can be delivered under the door just before concluding a time-out (TO) period]. The idea is to pair odors with activities that access specific behavioral and emotional systems having value for specific behavior-modification objectives. Conditioned olfactory relaxation, reward, and safety stimuli provide useful means to modulate emotional states associated with undesirable behavior operating under the influence of aversive arousal (e.g., frustration, fear, anger, or irritability). Finally, using scents creatively, such as training the dog to find scented play objects, provides valuable environmental enrichment and stimulation to the dog.

NEUROBIOLOGICAL REGULATION OF AGGRESSION

Stress-related Potentiation of the Flight-Fight System

Conditioned threats and stressors are processed by a complex network of reciprocal cortical and subcortical pathways, projecting to and from the amygdala, the hippocampus, the hypothalamus, the PAG, and several other areas (Panksepp, 1998). The medial prefrontal cortex appears to perform a goal-oriented appraisal function based on prediction-control expectancies and calibrated establishing operations, whereby autonomic arousal is continually matched to expected adjustment needs. In the case of aversive events, behavioral adjustments that produce better-than-expected outcomes result in de-arousal and a reduction of autonomic activation (relief and reward), whereas worse-than-expected outcomes result in increased arousal, alertness, readiness, and agitation. In the case of unpredicted or uncontrollable aversive events, subcortical pathways may rapidly mobilize neurobiological changes conducive to emergency adjustments, including the instigation of the FFS, with the release of CRF and the activation of the HPA system (see *Stress and Flight or Fight Reactions* in Chapter 4). The amygdala appears to play a central role in the orchestration of the FFS, operating in coordination with the prefrontal cortex, where executive organizing functions and activities are momentarily overshadowed by a priority to attend to immediate sensory information and to adjust rapidly to the threat. As a result, behavior output shifts from an adaptive interface, based on prediction-control expectancies and establishing operations, to a reactive interface based on species typical modal escape-attack behaviors.

Instrumental control over aversive events is reflected at the level of autonomic arousal, with blood pressure increasing in response to uncontrolled aversive events while remaining steady during signaled avoidance (Gaebelein et al., 1977). In addition, dogs that are unable to escape aversive stimulation show a significantly stronger adrenocortical stress response than dogs that are able to escape (Dess et al., 1983) or when instrumental control over an aversive event is lost (Houser and Paré, 1974) (see *Fear and Peripheral Endocrine Arousal Systems* in Chapter 3). Cook (2002) has studied the stress response of sheep when exposed to the threat of a barking dog while under an escapable condition and under a nonescapable condition. Sheep show a two-phase change in CRF concentrations in the amygdala. The first phase involves a sharp CRF spike attributed to central arousal effects, which is followed by a slower and smaller-magnitude spike of CRF activity that closely shadows blood cortisol concentrations. Whereas the injection of a glucocorticoid antagonist just prior to stimulation had no effect on the first sharp spike of CRF, it abolished the second smaller spike, a finding that supports the hypothesis that cortisol may exert an acute activating effect on the central amygdala. The researcher found that repeated and inescapable exposure to a barking dog produced a pronounced sensitizing effect on amygdala-CRF activity when the sheep were subsequently exposed to a novel aversive event (1 second of shock).

In the case of sheep belonging to the nonescape group, a very pronounced and sustained activation of second-phase CRF activity occurred, indicating a potentiated responsiveness of the CRF neurons in the amygdala. As a result of repeated exposure to the threatening dog, the nonescape group showed signs of adapting with decreasing amounts of first-spike CRF activity, but showed a steady increase of blood cortisol levels over the course of the experiment. This evidence of habituation with regard to the first spike may indicate a modulatory prefrontal influence, whereas the increasing cortisol levels and evident sensitization of amygdala-CRF circuits may indicate a maladaptive elaboration akin to what Gannt has call schizokinesis (see *Gantt: Schizokinesis, Autokinesis, and Effect of Person* in Volume 1, Chapter 9). The sheep belonging to the escape group also showed signs of adapting in response to the acute phase of stress, and, unlike the nonescape group, the escape group showed a steady decrease of blood cortisol activity after repeated exposures to the barking dog. These findings support the hypothesis that behavioral stress associated with the loss of control over aversive events exerts a lasting potentiating effect on subsequent exposures to stressors (anticipatory anxiety), perhaps via sensitized amygdala-CRF circuits and schizokinetic elaborations. As a result, uncontrollable stressors may gradually cause dogs to become sensitized (irritable and intolerant) to aversive stimuli, perhaps causing them to respond to innocuous social threats with exaggerated emotional and reactive output that persist-

ently mismatches executive prediction-control expectancies.

Neural Circuits Mediating Anger and Rage

The amygdala plays a prominent role in the rapid processing of ambiguous and potentially dangerous stimuli (Adolphs, 2001). Modulatory signals leaving the amygdala converge on both cortical and subcortical destinations, with amygdaloid pathways both facilitating and suppressing defensive rage behavior (Siegel et al., 1997). The pathways producing anger and rage appear to originate in the medial amygdala, whereas suppressive influences originating in the central amygdala project directly to the midbrain PAG, where inhibitory connections are formed with opioidergic receptors. The PAG mediates a variety of changes conducive to affective attack, including autonomic changes (increased respiration and heart rate), increased alertness and excitability, and facial expressions associated with threat and biting actions (Panksepp, 1998). Anger-rage pathways originating in the medial amygdala reach the medial hypothalamus via the bed nucleus of the stria terminalis (BNST). From the medial hypothalamus, the anger-rage signal is relayed to the PAG. The neuropeptide substance P appears to play a prominent role in the expression of anger and rage. Psychological stress is believed to stimulate the release of substance P in the amygdala (Kramer et al., 1998). In cats, a substance P pathway between the medial amygdala and the medial hypothalamus promotes defensive rage via interaction with excitatory glutamate neurons projecting to the PAG (Siegel et al., 1997; Gregg and Siegel, 2000)—behavior that is blocked by neurokinin 1 (NK-1) antagonists. The NK-1 receptor mediates central substance P activity and is found throughout the brain, with concentrations located within the limbic system and hypothalamus. Knockout mice lacking the NK-1 receptor show a significant reduction of territorial aggression and other measures associated with acute stress and injury (De Felipe et al., 1998). Currently, a promising orally assimilable NK-1-receptor antagonist is under development for the treatment of depression

(Kramer et al., 1998). The substance, MK-869, produces potent antidepressant effects comparable to paroxetine but with fewer side effects. Given the involvement of substance P in the mediation of aversive arousal and aggression, MK-869 may eventually prove of value in the treatment of canine aggression problems, but at the moment its clinical efficacy and safety as an antiaggression agent in dogs is unknown. Interestingly, antidepressants have been shown to downregulate the biosynthesis of substance P in rats, suggesting the possibility that the apparent beneficial effect of such medications may be due, in part, to alterations of the neurokinin system (Kramer et al., 1998).

Threatening stimuli activate the sympathetic branch of the autonomic nervous system (ANS) via various direct and indirect pathways between the amygdala, lateral hypothalamus, locus coeruleus, and sympathetic preganglionic neurons terminating in various parts of the body, with the prefrontal cortex playing a prominent modulatory role at virtually every level of central organization (see *Stress and Flight or Fight Reactions* in Chapter 4). The resulting widespread sympathetic arousal prepares the organism for emergency flight or fight action. As the result of sympathetic arousal, epinephrine (adrenaline) and NE are rapidly released into the bloodstream by the adrenal medulla (see *Hypothalamus* in Volume 1, Chapter 3). Epinephrine and NE have widespread energizing effects on the body, including pronounced effects on cardiovascular activity. Although epinephrine cannot cross the blood-brain barrier, some researchers have reported that epinephrine appears to play a significant role in the consolidation of aversive memories (see *Neural Stress Management System and Fear Learning* in Volume 1, Chapter 3). The memory-enhancing properties of epinephrine may be mediated indirectly by way of afferent vagal nerve transmissions. Le Doux (1996) has suggested that vagal afferent signals triggered by peripheral epinephrine might help to explain how epinephrine facilitates the formation of memories about aversive events. The vagus nerve at the nucleus of the solitary tract forms reciprocal connections with the hypothalamus and the locus coeruleus. The nucleus of the solitary tract performs a host of integrative

functions in the process of modulating autonomic arousal via direct reflexive feedback effects on various organ systems, as well as a diffuse network of reciprocal feedback links with the lateral hypothalamus, the central amygdala, and the BNST, among other sites. The locus coeruleus is composed of NE-producing neurons that form widespread interconnections throughout the brain, including the amygdala and the hippocampus. These areas are believed to be closely involved in the consolidation of aversive memories, leading to Le Doux's hypothesis that epinephrine via vagal enervation might play a significant role in their formation. In addition to mediating the formation of aversive memories, NE has been shown to influence the expression and regulation of affective aggression (see *Monoamines and the Control of Aggression* in Volume 1, Chapter 3) (Eichelman, 1987). Defensive behavior in cats is associated with the activation of NE-producing neurons, an effect that appears to help prepare the animal to respond to threatening situations (Levine et al., 1990). Anger-induced changes in heart rate and blood pressure may activate aggression-mediating circuits (NE and otherwise) via a similar afferent vagal feedback mechanism postulated to facilitate aversive memories.

Biogenetic influences strongly affect sympathetic and parasympathetic nervous activity. These antagonistic arousing and de-arousing autonomic influences differentially affect a wide variety of behavioral thresholds, with sympathetic-dominant dogs tending to be more reactive to provocative stimulation than parasympathetic-dominant counterparts (see *Genetic Predisposition and Temperament* in Volume 1, Chapter 5). Sympathetic-dominant dogs can often be differentiated from parasympathetic-dominant ones by the degree of skeletal muscle tonus that they exhibit. The medulla mediates normal resting muscular tonus and produces tonus changes in response to sympathetic arousal. Increased muscle tonus may reflect an increased standing readiness for emergency action resulting from neurobiological predisposition and learning associated with aversive arousal (e.g., fear and anger). Dogs that exhibit the rigid muscular tonus consistent with sympathetic-dominance are often the most responsive to the muscle-relaxing effects of PFR. Alterations in blood pressure are a sensitive indicator of autonomic tone in response to environmental and social stressors (Wilhelmj et al., 1953; Kallet et al., 1997). The expression of sympathetic and parasympathetic typologies appears to be strongly influenced by gender. Significant gender-related differences in blood pressure have been reported in dogs (N = male, 67; female, 80) and in female dogs (N = 80) (Van Liere et al., 1949), perhaps reflecting underlying gender-related autonomic differences modulating emotional responsiveness to environmental stimulation. According to the gender hypothesis, males and females may be biologically different on the level of autonomic responsiveness, with males tending toward sympathetic dominance and females being more inclined toward parasympathetic dominance. The gender hypothesis is consistent with the findings of Hart and Hart (1985), indicating that male dogs are rated to be more prone to exhibit reactive behaviors (sympathetic dominance), whereas females tend to be more affectionate and trainable (parasympathetic dominance).

Amygdala-mediated emotional interpretation of social and environmental stimulation appears to be coordinated with the impulse-control functions of the prefrontal cortex and contextualizing influences emanating from the hippocampus. Sudden change or situations requiring rapid assessment of threat may result in inappropriate aggressive responses in animals possessing a strong agonistic tone. Compromised attention resulting in startle may also precede a rapid transition from a state of vulnerability to defensive aggression. A common situation involving aggressive arousal in dogs occurs when they are disturbed while asleep or in a hypnagogic state just preceding the induction of sleep. Such dogs may misinterpret the owner's actions, and without the benefit of fully alert and functional executive attention and impulse control, they may become enraged and bite.

Autonomic Arousal, Heart Rate, and Aggression

Aggressive dogs frequently exhibit a collection of exaggerated autonomic responses to social threats, including increased behavioral excitability, panic, and fear. Canine domestic aggression (CDA) is usually expressed under the influence of significant autonomic arousal—catastrophic arousal that often appears to be out of proportion to the eliciting situation (see *Loss of Safety, Depression, Panic, and Aggression* in Chapter 7). These autonomic changes, similar to symptoms of panic, appear to take control of the dog. In significant ways, dogs that attack their owners despite the presence of strong affectionate and familiar ties resemble human perpetrators of domestic violence. In fact, panic-evoked aggression may represent a viable animal model of domestic violence. Studies investigating perpetrators of domestic violence indicate that such individuals experience intense autonomic arousal and various symptoms of panic (e.g., palpitations, fear, increased respiration, feelings of losing control, and tremors) at the time of attacks. Among dogs, enhanced control over aversive events has a potent moderating event over blood pressure, heart rate, and glucocorticoid release, whereas the loss of control exerts a pronounced disinhibitory effect on physiological markers of sympathetic autonomic arousal (Houser and Paré, 1974). Perpetrators of domestic violence appear to cope differently with autonomic arousal than do nonviolent counterparts, exhibiting neural differences in the way heart rate is regulated (Umhau et al., 2002). In addition to exhibiting differences in the way their heart rate is regulated, perpetrators exhibit a pronounced autonomic response to sodium lactate infusions (George et al., 2000). The potentiating effects of sodium lactate on the autonomic arousal and panic-rage behavior exhibited by perpetrators of domestic violence suggest the possibility that canine aggressors might show a similar pattern of autonomic and behavioral responsiveness to a panicogenic agent. Monitoring and comparing the vagal tone of nonaggressors and aggressors in response to neutral, stressful, and relaxing stimulation might yield potentially valuable clues concerning the etiology of panic-evoked aggression.

People exhibiting antisocial and aggressive behavior often exhibit significantly reduced autonomic responsiveness to social stressors, as measured by heart rate and skin conductance. Adult criminals and antisocial adolescents tend to exhibit lower resting heart rates, perhaps reflecting a reduced responsiveness to fear-provoking stimulation or a lack of normal sensitivity to hedonic or nociceptive stimuli (anhedonia), a common sign of post-traumatic stress disorder (PTSD) (see *Post-traumatic Stress Disorder* in Volume 1, Chapter 9). The significance of fearlessness is based on an assumption that many aggressive actions depend on a reduced level of fear and anxiety. Fear and anxiety may directly inhibit aggressive behavior or facilitate its inhibition via punishment and other conditioning efforts. The presence of autonomic hyporesponsive suggests that antisocial and aggressive behaviors are driven by an aversive physiological state associated with low arousal. According to the stimulation-seeking theory, antisocial behavior is emitted to bring autonomic arousal up to normal levels; that is, the behavior serves a homeostatic function. Fearlessness and stimulation seeking appear to interact in the case of antisocial and violent individuals (Raine, 2002) and dogs: fearlessness and stimulation seeking are the defining characteristics of c-type dogs. Another indicator linking autonomic hyporesponsiveness with aggressive behavior is the presence of low cortisol levels (see *Stress, Low Cortisol, and Aggression*). This combined evidence strongly suggests the need for basic research dedicated to evaluating and comparing the autonomic activity and reactivity of canine aggressors and nonaggressors.

Aggressive arousal is associated with sympathetic activation and release of epinephrine by the adrenal medulla. One effect of epinephrine is to accelerate heart rate, a change that may be interpreted by the brain as signifying danger and setting into action a variety of neurobiological changes that prepare dogs to take offensive (anger) or defensive (fear) action. Social and contextual stimuli associated with aggressive arousal may result in conditioned cardiovascular changes that prepare dogs for offensive or defensive action via the FFS. In addition, certain conditioned *signature* cardiac changes occurring in association with aggressive episodes in the past may trigger aggressive preparatory responses, motivationally increasing a dog's readiness to threaten or attack. These conditioned changes in heart rate, blood pressure, and coronary

flow may mediate the activation of metered norepinergic activity, resulting in varying degrees of aggressive arousal. Heart-rate patterns appear to differ according to an animal's social rank. Among squirrel monkeys (Candland et al., 1970) and chickens (Candland et al., 1969), the highest-ranking and lowest-ranking individuals exhibit the highest heart rates, whereas middle-ranking animals show the lowest heart rates. The influence of social status on heart rate may reflect divergent motivational effects of competition on sympathetic tone, increasing the propensity of dominant dogs to fight (anger-induced acceleration) and subordinates to flee (fear-induced acceleration). Differences in heart rate have been shown to provide valuable markers with respect to the identification of emotional traits and temperament dimensions exhibited by dogs (Cattell and Korth, 1973), suggesting that a strong biogenetic component may affect arousal threshold and heart-rate changes. Cardiovascular differences associated with anger and fear may provide useful diagnostic indicators for differentiating offensive and defensive aggression, as well as help to identify evocative conditioned social and contextual stimuli associated with its expression.

The heart rates of dogs exposed to anger-inducing arousal undergo significant change indicating pronounced autonomic arousal. Verrier and colleagues (1987) found that anger evoked in association with food protection produces pronounced effects on heart rate, blood pressure, and coronary flow in dogs. On average, during aggressive episodes, heart rate increased from 112 ± 6 to 210 ± 15 beats/minute, arterial blood pressure rose from 95 ± 4 to 142 ± 5 mm Hg, and coronary blood flow increased from 31 ± 5 to 72 ± 9 ml/minute). These values returned to baseline levels after 2 to 4 minutes, suggesting that dogs do not immediately de-arouse following aggressive episodes involving anger. The time course is consistent with Denny's (1976) relaxation phase following the determination of aversive stimulation (see *Safety Signal Hypothesis* in Volume 1, Chapter 8). The extent to which canine aggressors differ autonomically from nonaggressors in the way that they respond to anger-inducing stimulation is not known; however, it is known that stressful avoidance conditioning exerts an unexpected divergence between heart rate and blood pressure. Anderson and Brady (1971) found that dogs exhibit a significant and stable reduction in heart rate while at the same time showing an increase in blood pressure during a 1-hour waiting period immediately preceding a 2-hour period of stressful shock-avoidance training. The divergence between heart rate and blood pressure steadily increased over the course of the 1-hour waiting period, with heart rates becoming lowest and blood pressure becoming highest just before the onset of shock-avoidance training.

Other studies evaluating the effects of auditory orientation and startle on heart rate have generally found that novel stimuli appear to have a decelerating effect on heart rate, whereas startle generates a rapid acceleration followed by vagal braking and deceleration (Graham and Clifton, 1966). Some human evidence suggests that many antisocial and aggressive individuals are affected by an attentional deficit that impedes their ability to orient toward neutral stimuli and to respond appropriately to startling stimuli in anticipation of aversive events (Raine, 2002). Whether auditory orientation and responsiveness to startle significantly differ in the case of canine aggressors and nonaggressors is not known, but given the findings from studies involving human antisocial and violent behavior, the possibility of such differences related to autonomic arousal and attentional behavior should be seriously investigated.

These sorts of attentional and learning deficits are consistent with a dysregulation of prepulse inhibition (PPI), a sensorimotor gating function that enables dogs to cope effectively with startling events and to sort out their significance (see *Prediction and Control Expectancies* in Chapter 1). Many studies have linked impairment of PPI function with several major psychiatric disorders (Braff et al., 2001). PPI tests are easy to perform, and the results appear to correlate with adaptive cognitive processing. Together with comparisons between standing heart rate and heart rates during petting or massage and heart rates occurring immediately after such stimulation (see *Adaptive Social Coping Styles: Play, Flirt, Forbear, and Nip*), PPI may provide a complementary measure for assessing a dog's relative fitness with regard to cognitive and emotional

tone, degree of autonomic reactivity, and vulnerability to stress. For example, a flat or increasing heart rate in response to petting and massage, together with a reduced PPI response, may indicate the presence of a stressful coping style, whereas a decreased heart rate, together with a robust PPI result, may be indicative of a more adaptive coping style and a functional antistress response. Interestingly, oxytocin has been shown to normalize drug-induced dysregulation of PPI (Feifel and Reza, 1999).

Vincent and Leahy (1997) have demonstrated a close relationship between reduced heart-rate variability in response to environmental and social stimulation and a calm/nonstress-prone temperament type in dogs. They found that dogs showing an excitable/stress-prone temperament exhibited a more sharply reactive and variable cardiac response when exposed to environmental and social stimuli. However, the determination of heart rate may not be particularly meaningful and useful as a marker with respect to aggressive behavior. As previously discussed, low heart rates may occur concurrently with divergent high blood-pressure measures resulting from stressful aversive learning (Anderson and Brady, 1971). Perhaps, at least in some cases, the acceleratory change in heart rate occurring in response to petting may reflect a touch-mediated reduction of blood pressure and an autonomic shift resulting in disinhibition. The propensity of some dominance aggressors to attack while being petted or when they are approached in situations that are routinely associated with affectionate contact or comfort may be related to a stress-related dysregulation of central oxytocin or AVP activity (Engelmann et al., 1999). Peripheral and central oxytocin and AVP perform complex regulatory cardiovascular functions influencing heart rate and blood pressure (Montastruc et al., 1985). A divergent low heart rate and high blood pressure may be context sensitive, emerging during specific social interactions and situations associated with aggressive reactivity. A stress-related divergence between heart rate and blood pressure may offer a viable diagnostic marker, a possibility that warrants future investigation. Given the potential importance of cardiovascular function as a diagnostic indicator, such data should be routinely collected and analyzed, especially in the case of impulsive CDA directed against family members.

Stress, Low Cortisol, and Aggression

Various other physiological and behavioral influences associated with stress may strongly affect aggression thresholds. For example, hungry dogs may be more aggressively reactive to interference when they are eating. A large array of potential stressors—including loud noises associated with household construction activities, thermal changes, lack of exercise and social contact, inadequate play, and excessive punishment occurring on a relatively unpredictable and uncontrollable basis—may lower aggression threshold. Such environmental and interactive influences may further destabilize predisposed dogs to aggressive behavior, whereas more stable environments and interaction conducive to harmonious interaction may produce a compensating or protective effect against the development of aggression problems. The reliance on excessive punishment, especially physical punishment, may produce particularly damaging effects via stress-related changes. Significant biobehavioral stress appears to accrue in animals in association with repeated exposure to social defeat and inability to fully avoid contact with the dominant victor (Blanchard et al., 2001)—a state of allostatic load that may play an important role in the etiology of some cases of CDA involving a history of excessive punishment. Chronic social stress appears to produce global neurobiological changes in major neurotransmitter and neuropeptide systems, as well as mediating stress-related bodily changes via sympathetic arousal and disturbances of the HPA system.

Stress is frequently cited as playing a major role in the etiology of intrafamilial aggression and other behavior problems, but little in the way of significant data has been reported in support of a causal relationship between stress and aggression in dogs. A potentially useful focus for future research involves collecting and profiling the adrenal output of aggressive dogs. One might assume that aggressive dogs with HPA-system disturbances associated with stress would be inclined to exhibit elevated plasma glucocorticoid levels. However, animal studies involving a variety of species, including wolves (McLeod et al., 1995), olive baboons (Sapolsky and Ray, 1989), guinea pigs (Haemisch, 1990), and squirrel monkeys (Manoque et al., 1975), have shown that cortisol levels are typically lower in more aggressive and dominant animals and higher in more submissive and subordinate ones. Rats that have been isolated for long periods (13 weeks) show significant changes in monoamine activity as well as lowered plasma cortisol levels, despite an increase in adrenocorticotropic hormone (ACTH) secretion (Miachon et al., 1993). Social isolation is associated with increased aggressiveness. Recently, Hennessy and colleagues (2001) found that low cortisol levels were a better predictor of problem behavior in puppies adopted from an animal shelter than were high cortisol levels.

A similar association between low cortisol levels and aggression has been reported in children (McBurnett et al., 2000; Pajer et al., 2001). Kagan and colleagues (1987) found a striking difference in cortisol levels correlating with behavioral inhibition in young children (5 1/2 years). Children described as inhibited showed consistently higher levels of cortisol than did uninhibited children. In human adults, high cortisol levels are closely associated with depression (Krishnan et al., 1988), perhaps reflecting a trajectory of HPA-axis dysregulation originating in childhood behavioral inhibition. At the other extreme, low cortisol output has also been reported in association with violent criminal offenders (Virkkunnen, 1985) and with people diagnosed with post-traumatic stress disorder (Yehuda et al., 1990). Other research has found that children exhibiting conduct and oppositional disorders show elevated levels of dehydroepiandrosterone sulfate (DHEA-S) and ACTH without a corresponding increase in cortisol (Dmitrieva et al., 2001). Increased DHEA-S and low cortisol levels have been reported in the case study of a 13-year-old boy exhibiting refractory problems associated with high levels of anxiety, anger, and aggression (Herzog et al., 2001). Treatment aimed at reducing DHEA-S levels (ketoconazole) resulted in marked improvement in both anxiety and aggression symptoms.

Stress, Serotonin, and Aggression

Although the mechanism responsible for the increase in oppositional behavior and aggression in association with low cortisol levels is unknown, the dysregulation of negative-feedback control over CRF and ACTH production may be involved. Chronically low cortisol levels may dysregulate hypothalamic CRF output, possibly causing central stress-related changes, including the inhibition of serotonin (5-hydroxytryptamine or 5-HT) production by the dorsal raphe bodies (Kirby et al., 2000) (see *Startle and Fear Circuits* in Chapter 3). Another influence localized at the level of the dorsal raphe bodies is the facilitatory effect of peripheral glucocorticoids on the efficiency of tryptophan-hydroxylase activity, the rate-limiting factor involved in the production of 5-HT (Azmitia and McEwen, 1974). Under the influence of low glucocorticoid levels, both 5-HT synthesis and its modulatory effects are impeded. Research involving wild house mice provides some intriguing potential clues suggesting a genetic influence mediating the association between low glucocorticoid levels and aggression. Korte and colleagues (1996) studied two groups of mice selected for high-offensive (short-attack latency) and low-offensive (long-attack latency) aggression. High-offensive aggressors exhibited significantly lower levels of corticosterone than did low-offensive aggressors. In addition, they found that high-offensive aggressors exhibited increased postsynaptic 5-HT$_{1A}$-receptor expression in the frontal cortex and hippocampus—an effect that the authors believe is secondary to lower-circulating corticosterone in the more aggressive mice.

There appears to be significant positive correlations between enhanced 5-HT activity and increased glucocorticoid activity. Supplemental 5-hydroxytryptophan (5-HTP), the immediate biochemical precursor of serotonin, appears to elevate glucocorticoid levels in rats (corticosterone) (Fuller, 1981). In addition, the selective serotonin-reuptake inhibitor (SSRI) fluoxetine produces a significant increase in plasma corticosterone via hypothalamic serotonergic pathways, an effect that is synergistically enhanced when rats are treated with both 5-HTP and fluoxetine (Fuller et al., 1996). The apparent close rela-

tionship between low glucocorticoid levels and reduced 5-HT activity suggests that cortisol levels might be diagnostically useful for teasing out subtypes of CDA and perhaps helping to determine appropriate treatment protocols. The role of low cortisol in the etiology and treatment of canine aggression problems is an exciting area that warrants future research.

Serotonin and Aggression

A great deal of animal research implicates the serotonergic system in the control of anxiety and aggression (Olivier et al., 1991). Evidence supporting the modulatory role of 5-HT over anxiety and aggression has been obtained in animals selected for reduced aggression and tameness. Wild Norway rats that had been selected for reduced aggressiveness toward humans exhibit significant alterations involving 5-HT activity. The tame rats exhibit significantly higher levels of 5-HT and 5-hydroxyindoleacetic acid (5-HIAA) in the hypothalamus, as well as a 25% increase in tryptophan-hydroxylase activity in comparison to fearfully reactive and aggressive rats (Popova et al., 1990). The behavioral reactivity of genetically tame and aggressive rats was shown to differ significantly in response to stressful handling and aversive stimulation (Nikulina et al., 1992). When pushed with a gloved hand, aggressive rats frequently attacked the glove, whereas tame rats showed no defensive reaction. When exposed to shock, tame rats launched fewer attacks toward one another than did aggressive counterparts. Predatory attacks directed toward mice were not differentiated between tame and aggressive rats: both groups killed mice within 1 to 3 minutes. Selection for tameness in silver foxes has resulted in similar modifications of the serotonergic system (Popova et al., 1991). Tame foxes show increased 5-HT levels in the midbrain and hypothalamus and higher levels of 5-HIAA in the midbrain, hypothalamus, and hippocampus. Tame foxes also exhibit a significant increase in tryptophan-hydroxylase activity in comparison to captive and aggressive foxes. Tame foxes produce 34% more tryptophan hydroxylase than do aggressive counterparts.

Dogs exhibiting impulsive CDA have been found to exhibit evidence of reduced 5-HT activity (Reisner et al., 1996). The cerebrospinal fluid (CSF) of aggressive dogs contains lower levels of 5-HIAA than that of nonaggressive controls (aggressive dogs, 202.0 pmol/ml, versus nonaggressive controls, 298.0 pmol/ml). 5-HIAA is a product produced by the breakdown of serotonin, with decreased CSF levels indicating reduced serotonin activity. A further reduction in CSF 5-HIAA levels was found in dogs that did not give a warning before biting (aggressive dogs not giving a warning, 196.0 pmol/ml, versus dogs that gave a warning, 244.0 pmol/ml). Low levels of CSF 5-HIAA have also been repeatedly found in people prone to exhibit impulsive aggression and violence. Mehlman and colleagues (1994) found that the severity of aggression exhibited by rhesus macaques was inversely correlated with CSF 5-HIAA levels, with monkeys having low levels of CSF 5-HIAA being more likely to exhibit severe aggression and other signs of decreased impulse control. Similar findings have been reported in the case of vervet monkeys in which decreased 5-HT levels are associated with increased irritability and aggression, irrespective of the monkey's status (McGuire and Raleigh, 1987).

Low levels of CSF 5-HIAA suggest the presence of some degree of dysfunction in the serotonergic system, perhaps involving the stress-related depletion of 5-HT, a chronic failure of affected dogs to produce adequate amounts of it, or other influences reducing its use and metabolism in the brain. In addition to serving a negative-feedback function restraining CRF output, circulating glucocorticoids appear to prime the impulse-controlling effects of 5-HT over cortical and thalamic sensory inputs via GABAergic (gamma-aminobutyric acid) interneurons (Stutzmann et al., 1998) (see *Startle and Fear Circuits* in Chapter 3). Hypothetically, in dogs where low cortisol levels present together with reduced 5-HT activity, one would expect to find an increased propensity to show impulsive aggression and other signs of emotional disturbance. Much of the current research seems to support the idea that 5-HT plays a significant role in the modulation of aversive arousal via GABAergic interneurons at the level of the amygdala—the emotional interpretive center of the anger-rage circuit:

> Decreased serotonergic functioning might result in deficient GABAergic modulation of excitatory sensory efferents, perhaps allowing innocuous sensory signals to be processed through the LA [lateral amygdala] as emotionally stimulating events. Overall, the net effect of 5-HT acting through GABAergic mechanisms in the LA appears to be inhibitory and may therefore serve as a modulator of affective sensory processing. (Stutzmann et al., 1998:3-4)

A variety of 5-HT-receptor subtypes have been identified, with at least 15 different ones currently known (Roth et al., 2000). The HT_{1B} receptor appears to mediate an inhibitory effect over aggression, whereas the $5-HT_{1A}$ receptor appears to mediate an antianxiety effect, at least in the case of mice and rats. The expression of these serotonergic receptors is dependent on a transcriptional factor, Pet-1 ETS, which is expressed in the embryo just before the first 5-HT neurons appear in the hindbrain. Mice lacking the ability to express Pet-1 do not develop normal 5-HT neurons. Interestingly, though, despite the absence of an effective serotonergic system, Pet-1 null mice show a surprising lack of abnormal structural or behavioral effects, other than becoming more aggressive and anxious as adults. Pet-1 nulls not only attacked more often than controls, they delivered significantly more bite wounds, suggesting a loss of bite inhibition. Consistent with these findings, Reisner and colleagues (1996) reported that, among dogs diagnosed with dominance aggression, those dogs delivering hard and injurious bites tended to have lower levels of CSF 5-HIAA and CSF homovanillic acid (HVA), a dopamine metabolite. Although 5-HT neurons generally exert an inhibitory influence, $5-HT_2$ neurons appear to be an exception to this rule. For example, $5-HT_2$-receptor agonists appear to facilitate the expression of defensive rage in cats (see Gregg and Siegel, 2001). Interestingly, in this regard, Sugrue (1983) has noted that one of the effects of antidepressants is gradually to downregulate the $5-HT_2$ receptor. Recent neuroimaging studies of nonaggressive and aggressive dogs performed by Peremans and colleagues appear to support the hypothesis that impulsive CDA may be linked to an aberrant upregulation of the 5-HT_{2A} receptor in the frontal cortex (see *Stress, 5-HT*$_{2A}$ *Receptor Upregulation, and Aggression* in Chapter 10).

Serotonin and Dominance

Raleigh and colleagues at UCLA (1991) performed a valuable study that appears to significantly question the role of aggression in the acquisition of social dominance, at least in the case of vervet monkeys. Vervet monkeys were observed interacting in 12 socially organized troops consisting of three adult males, three or more females, and a variable number of young. In each troop, one male had assumed a dominant rank. The alpha male was removed from the troop, and the remaining monkeys were differentially treated, one receiving a 5-HT agonist or antagonist and the other given a placebo. Two treatment programs were implemented: one to increase 5-HT activity with fluoxetine or tryptophan, and the other to decrease it with 5-HT antagonists. During the various treatment phases, the pair was observed for changes in social behavior and rank. The experiment consisted of several phases and a treatment reversal in which monkeys receiving the agonist were given the antagonist and vice versa. The results showed that monkeys treated with fluoxetine or tryptophan consistently became dominant over cagemates given a placebo. Conversely, monkeys treated with a serotonin depleter (fenfluramine) or antagonist (cyproheptadine) consistently became subordinate to placebo-treated controls. The monkeys treated with fluoxetine or tryptophan consistently achieved a dominant status, even though they became less overtly aggressive, more friendly, and less active as the result of the treatment protocol. On the other hand, the monkeys treated with the antagonists were markedly more aggressive, less sociable, more active, and consistently became subordinate to placebo-treated cagemates. The monkeys treated with fluoxetine or tryptophan appeared to become socially dominant because of an improved ability to interact with other monkeys; that is, they became more socially competent. In an earlier study, Raleigh and coworkers (1985) found that the

affiliation-enhancing effects of fluoxetine and tryptophan were facilitated by the social status of the monkeys treated. Dominant males were much more responsive to treatment with fluoxetine and tryptophan than were subordinate males. The researchers conclude that a high degree of independence exists between dominance and aggressiveness, with competent social interactions appearing to mediate social dominance.

Similar findings have been reported by Fonberg (1988). She found that previously submissive cats became dominant under the influence of chronic treatment with imipramine. The medication did not appear to have an effect on social dominance by raising aggression levels, but by some other mechanism, perhaps associated with an increase in predatory motivation and enhancement of the hedonic reward:

> Direct correlations between the gaining of dominance status and aggressive display were not found. Cats that became submissive as the result of DMA damage [dorsomedial amygdala lesions] regained their dominance under imipramine. It was suggested that imipramine enhanced dominance rather by increasing predatory motivation, and hedonic aspect of reward, than by raising the level of aggression. Some kind of "confidence" in the efficacy of action may also play an important role. The beneficial effect of imipramine in the treatment of depressive patients may reflect a similar mechanism. The increase of predatory behavior in normal or LH [lateral hypothalamus lesions] nonkillers under imipramine may also support the assumption that imipramine enhances predatory motivation. (208)

Not only is aggression not always necessary to establish and maintain dominance status, dominance maintained without aggression may result in more stable social relations. Fonberg concludes,

> The only conclusion which I can suggest is that aggression is not an indispensable factor for gaining and sustaining dominance, and that some unknown "dominance factor" is also a very important both for human subjects and other animals. (211)

Dominant dogs appear to be possessed by a dominant attitude and social competence, whereas aggressive dogs frequently lack confidence, appear to be socially incompetent, and bite reactively under the disorganizing influence of confusion, irritability, frustration, or anger (see *Dominance: Status or Control* in Volume 2, Chapter 8). Fuller (1973) has reported that puppies exposed to early isolation suffer disturbances of attention, increased reactivity, and reduced abilities to habituate to environmental stimulation. He observed that isolated puppies were consistently dominated by better-socialized counterparts. Dominance is far more a matter of attitude than physical attributes, as stressed by Trumler (1973):

> Mental rather than physical superiority, whether in another of his kind or in man, is far more impressive to a dog. Between dogs which know each other well physical strength is always being measured, whereas authority remains unquestioned. (198)

Arginine Vasopressin, Testosterone, and Serotonin

In dogs, arousal and de-arousal patterns may be significantly different in the cases of predatory behavior, dominance aggression, and affective attacks motivated by anger and rage. In addition to relatively discrete circuits dedicated to quiet and affective attack, conspecific aggression exhibited during dominance contests between males appears to be mediated by a dedicated circuit, perhaps involving the combined influences of AVP and testosterone under the modulatory influence of 5-HT (Ferris et al., 1997). Whereas affective attack is strongly associated with anger and rage, dominance aggression between males competing for status and breeding rights does not appear to rely on anger and rage for its expression (Panksepp, 1998).

Various lines of research suggest a prominent role of AVP in the development of conspecific intermale agonistic behavior (see *Arginine Vasopressin and Aggression* in Volume 1, Chapter 3). The aggression-facilitating effect of AVP appears to depend on the presence of testosterone and testosterone metabolites (e.g., estradiol and dihydrotestosterone). Both vasopressin and testosterone are perinatally active, suggesting that they interact early in an animal's development and set the stage for dimorphic sexual and behavioral differentiation. The basic organismic plan of mammals is based on female characteristics, with the appearance of maleness depending on the influence of testosterone at various points in the development of an animal's ontogeny. In dogs, just before and after birth, the testes produce a surge of testosterone that exerts a pronounced differentiating influence on neural tissue via the aromatization of testosterone into estradiol by brain aromatase (Kelly, 1991). Estrogen-sensitive neurons are widely distributed in the brain, including limbic and cortical areas, exerting pervasive nonreproductive dimorphic influences on behavior. The perinatal influence of testosterone on neural organization becomes most evident at puberty, when another surge of testosterone occurs in the dogs at 6 to 8 months (Hart, 1985) and the emergence of dimorphic behavior associated with maleness, notably increased scent-marking behavior and intermale aggression, and secondary male characteristics begin to emerge. Under the influence of maternal stress, fetal changes associated with androgenization may be significantly disturbed (Panksepp, 1998), perhaps explaining somewhat the variable expression of male-characteristic behavior in adult dogs.

Testosterone and its metabolites interact with various neuropeptides. Most important, though, in terms of the expression of male-characteristic behaviors is its interaction with AVP. Along with CRF and the closely related peptide oxytocin, AVP is produced in the paraventricular nucleus of the hypothalamus. Oxytocin and AVP are also released into the bloodstream via the pituitary gland. AVP is also synthesized by neurons in the medial amygdala and the BNST. AVP production is sexually dimorphic, with males producing more AVP than females and expressing a greater number of androgen receptors in the medial amygdala (Cooke et al., 1998). Recall that the medial amygdala and BNST are closely involved in mediation of affective aggression, with the medial amygdala playing a central role in the rapid emotional interpretation of potentially dangerous situations. Males appear to be more risk prone, perhaps reflecting changes in the medial amygdala and other related neural areas influenced by the interaction of testosterone and AVP. The distribution of AVP receptors in the brain varies significantly from species to species, which suggests that the neuropeptide plays a significant role in the differentiation of species-typical social behavior (Young, 1999).

In golden hamsters, AVP facilitates scent marking and offensive aggression, an effect that is dependent on the presence of testosterone in the ventrolateral hypothalamus (Delville et al., 1996). Earlier studies found that AVP mediates scent-marking behavior (flank marking) in hamsters when it is injected into the anterior hypothalamus. This behavior appears to be influenced significantly by social dominance, with dominant animals marking more frequently than subordinates. However, when subordinate hamsters are stimulated to exhibit more scent-marking behavior, the increased marking in the presence of a more dominant conspecific does not evoke offensive attacks or an increase in marking by the dominant animal (Ferris and Delville, 1994). Aggression can also be evoked by AVP in the anterior hypothalamus, an area enervated with a high concentration of 5-HT terminals and 5-HT$_{1B}$-binding sites interacting with AVP-responsive neurons. 5-HT is believed to perform an inhibitory role over offensive aggression and scent marking. Ferris and colleagues (1997) found that enhancement of serotonin activity with fluoxetine exerted a significant inhibitory effect on offensive aggression in experienced fighters. In addition, fluoxetine exerted a strong inhibitory influence over AVP-induced aggression directed against conspecific intruders. In the hamsters treated with fluoxetine, scent-marking behavior was completely suppressed.

Early stress may dramatically affect the activity of AVP and CRF. As previously noted, both AVP and CRF are produced in the same area of the hypothalamus and appear to interact at various levels of neural organization. As the result of postnatal stress, excessive AVP/CRF activity via the proliferation of AVP and CRF receptors in areas of the brain involved in the expression of affective aggression (e.g., medial amygdala, BNST, and PAG) may dispose some dogs show lower aggression thresholds. Stress associated with maternal separation has been shown to exert profound and lasting effects on the proliferation and density of CRF-binding sites, HPA dysregulation, and various functional disturbances of interacting neurotransmitter systems (see *Maternal Separation and Stress* in Chapter 4). In dogs, decreased glucocorticoid levels result in an increased release of peripheral AVP, with cortisol infusions producing a significant reduction of plasma AVP (Papanek and Raff, 1994). Cortisol may also restrain central AVP activity via negative feedback, a function that could be significant in dogs exhibiting aggression in association with low cortisol levels. Further, a cortisol-mediated reduction of AVP, the anti-diuretic hormone, may help to explain the loss of bladder control among many separation-reactive dogs and dogs experiencing stressful social and environmental transitions.

Immune Stress and Cytokines

Adverse emotional and mental states have been implicated in a variety of somatic disorders (McMillan, 1999), including gastric dilatation-volvulus in dogs—a condition that large, depressed, and fearful dogs appear to be at increased risk of developing (Glickman et al., 2000). Health and disease may also exert adverse effects on behavior. Serpell and Jagoe (1995) have reported the existence of a significant correlation between sickness in puppyhood and the subsequent development of behavior problems, including owner-directed and stranger-directed aggression, increased social fearfulness and reactivity, separation-related barking, and excessive mounting behavior by male dogs. A similar association between sickness in puppyhood and adult aggressiveness was detected among English cocker spaniels (Podberscek and Serpell, 1997). In both studies, the authors attribute the increased incidence of behavior problems associated with early sickness to various socialization deficits or excesses accruing as the result of the way sick puppies are treated by their owners (e.g., increased attention, care, and indulgence). However, another interpretation is also possible. Perhaps the positive correlation between early disease and an increased risk of behavior problems stems from the same root causes; that is, pediatric disease and adult behavior problems may be the short-term and long-term effects of early ontogenetic stressors. Murphree (1973) reported that nervous pointer dogs were prone to develop mange between months 3 and 9, suggesting the possible involvement of stress-related immunosuppression (see *Nervous Pointers* in Volume 1, Chapter 5). Recently, Guy and colleagues (2001) have reported that dogs treated for pruritic skin disorders are at twice the risk of biting someone than are counterparts not exhibiting such problems.

Ongoing psychoneuroimmunological research indicates that a system of bidirectional communication exists between the brain and the immune system. Numerous classical conditioning experiments have demonstrated that the central nervous system exerts a conditioned modulatory influence over immune activity (Ader and Cohen, 1985). The immune system appears to interact closely with the FFS, perhaps as the result of an evolutionary process in which the stress system has co-opted by immune mechanisms that are conducive to supporting rapid preparation for emergency action (e.g., HPA activation) and promoting recuperation or reducing risk of infection from injuries incurred from fighting or other dangerous activities (Maier and Watkins, 1998). As the result of injury or invasion by a foreign substance, immune cells are activated. Immune cells perform a variety of complementary functions, requiring communication between cells and the rest of the body. This communication function is performed by a variety of substances called *cytokines*. Cytokines mediate immune responses to bacteria, viruses, and foreign proteins. Animals exhibit both specific and nonspecific immune responses. Specific immune responses take time to develop, but eventually provide the organism with lasting protection against the target antigen by producing antibodies. In contrast, nonspecific immune responses occur much more rapidly (within 1 to 2 hours). One type of nonspecific immune response involves the activation of a class of phagocytes known as *macrophages*. Activated macrophages perform many functions, including the synthesis and release of proinflammatory cytokines (e.g., interleukin 1, interleukin 6, and tumor-necrosis factor). In addition to facilitating a local inflammatory reaction, cytokines produce far-reaching changes throughout the body and brain. Within the brain, cytokines appear to increase

NE and 5-HT turnover significantly—effects comparable to those produced by environmental stress (Dunn et al. 1999). These neural changes result in numerous affective, behavioral, and cognitive symptoms associated with sickness (e.g., fever, chills, reduced activity, increased sensitivity to pain, depression, and increased HPA-axis activity).

Since cytokines cannot freely pass through the blood-brain barrier, cytokine-mediated neural changes probably occur via another pathway, perhaps an active transport mechanism dedicated to specific cytokines. The exact route or routes of communication between cytokines and the brain is controversial (Blatteis and Li, 2000), but at least some communication between peripheral cytokines and the brain is mediated via afferent vagus-nerve transmissions (Romanovsky et al., 1997)—a pathway that may have been co-opted by epinephrine (adrenaline) to mediate the central changes associated with flight-fight activation. Whereas afferent vagal signals may activate central responses to immune stress, efferent vagal signals appear to modulate the effects of immune stress on the body (Borovikova et al., 2000), mirroring the opponent parasympathetic effects (decreased heart rate and so forth) that the vagus nerve exerts over sympathetic arousal and the FFS. According to this hypothesis, cytokines trigger afferent vagal signals that are carried to the brainstem (medulla) and relayed to various parts of the brain (e.g., hypothalamus and hippocampus), where they stimulate the synthesis and release of central cytokines. These substances, in turn, trigger a cascade of cytokine-dependent neural events that collectively produce the symptoms of sickness and distress. Studies examining the sensitization effects of cytokines on central monoamine neurotransmitter systems have shown that 5-HT activity in the central amygdala undergoes significant sensitization following exposure to immune stress, as does dopamine activity in the prefrontal cortex. Animals exposed to cytokine activation also show a marked increase in HPA-axis responsiveness to subsequent immune stress (Hayley et al., 2001). The sensitization mediated by immune stress, affecting neurotransmitter activity in brain areas associated with executive control, fear, and aggression, suggests that sickness and disease might produce a lasting dysregulatory effect in some predisposed dogs, even after the sickness has completely passed. Further, perhaps chronic subclinical infections (e.g., Lyme disease) resulting in persistent immune stress and cytokine activation may alter behavioral thresholds controlling flight-fight reactions and adversely affect a dog's ability to cope with environmental stressors. Although nothing very persuasive has been published on the subject, adverse psychiatric symptoms of Lyme disease have been anecdotally reported in human patients (Fallon et al., 1993).

The possibility that immune stress in association with disease may produce lasting epigenetic changes in the dog's behavior offers an alternative explanation for Jagoe and Serpell's findings (Dreschel, 2002). Human psychiatric research indicates that some forms of rapid-onset obsessive-compulsive disorder in children may be related to a history of streptococcal infection (Swedo et al., 1998). In addition to obsessive-compulsive disorder and tic disorder, affected children often exhibit a variety of comorbid symptoms, including emotional and cognitive deficits, separation anxiety, hyperactivity, and increased oppositional behavior. Granger and associates (2001) have reported that stressing the immune system of neonatal mice causes them to become more socially reactive and fearful as adults. Conceivably, and this is a speculative leap, some predisposed dogs may be adversely affected by the immune stress associated with vaccinations—a hypothesis that deserves clinical and experimental attention (Dreschel, 2002). In the case of human patients, immune stress resulting from vaccination with live attenuated rubella virus has been shown to induce depressive symptoms in socially vulnerable teenage girls for up to 10 weeks following vaccination (Yirmiya et al., 2000). Since the neural response to immune stress is markedly sensitized by repeat exposure at a 1-day interval and not after a 28-day interval (Hayley et al., 2001), vaccinations given on a frequent schedule may be more prone to produce adverse cumulative effects than are vaccinations spread out over time. Even when dogs are vaccinated once a year, however, they show increased levels of fecal cortisol metabolites (417% above baseline levels) 1 to 2 days

following injections (Palme et al., 2001), indicating an association of the procedure with stress-related activation of the HPA system. Finally, extrapolating from these investigations, one might reasonably assume that dogs and puppies may be more reactive to environmental and behavioral stressors for 24 to 48 hours following vaccination. Adverse behavioral effects following vaccination may be more likely in the case of dogs and puppies exhibiting unstable and reactive temperaments, especially when under the influence of heightened behavioral stress prior to vaccinations. The relationship between early stress, disease, immune-system activation, vaccinations, and behavior problems is an important area for future basic and epidemiological research.

PHARMACOLOGICAL CONTROL OF AGGRESSION

Serotonergic medications are frequently prescribed to treat aggression problems in dogs, but the efficacy of such drugs to moderate or inhibit canine aggression remains controversial, with most studies to date indicating that tricyclic antidepressants (TCAs) perform on par with placebo. In addition, no compelling evidence currently exists showing that SSRIs perform any better. The TCAs most commonly prescribed to ameliorate behavior problems are amitriptyline and clomipramine. Amitriptyline appears to block the presynaptic reuptake of 5-HT and to an even greater extent the reuptake of NE, but its therapeutic effect appears to follow primarily from the sensitization of postsynaptic neurons. Clomipramine, on the other hand, is much more specific with regards to the inhibitory effect it exerts on serotonin reuptake. Whereas amitriptyline produces a twofold greater effect on NE reuptake than it does on 5-HT reuptake, clomipramine produces a fivefold greater effect on 5-HT reuptake than on NE reuptake, exceeding the potency of fluoxetine as a serotonergic agent by over twofold (Julien, 1995). Clomipramine appears to inhibit the reuptake of serotonin by means similar to that of SSRIs. As a result of elevated 5-HT activity associated with treatment, 5-HT$_{1A}$ autoreceptors located on the 5-HT neuron are gradually desensitized, thereby causing it to release more 5-HT at the presynaptic terminal. Clomipramine, like other TCA drugs, may produce some typical side effects (e.g., mild sedation) and anticholinergic effects (e.g., dry mouth, urinary retention, and constipation), but to a lesser extent than amitriptyline, which can produce a potent histamine-related sedation effect (Julien, 1995). Despite an evident effect on 5-HT activity, neither clomipramine (White et al., 1999) nor amitriptyline (Virga et al., 2001) have been proven to be of clinical value for the treatment of owner-directed aggression. This is the conclusion of two double-blind and placebo-controlled trials performed to evaluate the efficacy of these commonly prescribed drugs. Neither study showed any significant benefit attributable to either medication; that is, dogs exhibited nearly the same behavioral course of change whether they were given the placebo or the TCA.

Perhaps the most commonly prescribed SSRI for the control of aggression in dogs is fluoxetine. The potential benefits of fluoxetine probably stem from a two-prong effect it appears to exert on 5-HT activity: decreased anxiety and lowered aggression thresholds (Olivier et al., 1991). Although probably effective in the case of aggression associated with impaired 5-HT function, no controlled study to date has shown that fluoxetine works any better than clomipramine for the control of owner-directed aggression or intermale aggression in dogs. Only one clinical trial to date has been performed to evaluate the effectiveness of fluoxetine for the control of dominance aggression (Dodman et al., 1996), but the quality of the study has been seriously questioned (White et al., 1999). The study involved nine dogs that were selected based on a history of owner-directed aggression. All of the dogs were given a placebo 1 week before commencing a 4-week course of treatment with fluoxetine. A significant reduction in aggression was found in all of the dogs after the treatment program was completed. Despite these promising results, the researchers failed to achieve their stated objective: "to determine the efficacy of fluoxetine in the treatment of owner-directed canine dominance aggression by means of a placebo-controlled blind study" (Dodman et al.,

1996:1585). In fact, the study was neither blind nor placebo controlled, but rather an "incomplete-crossover design" (Simpson and Simpson, 1996:106), throwing into doubt the value of the results reported (White et al., 1999). Given the lack of efficacy shown by TCAs and the absence of more compelling evidence regarding the value of SSRIs, as things currently stand, the use of serotonergic drugs have not been definitively shown to be an effective treatment for household aggression problems.

TCAs and SSRIs may be more effective in cases where a significant disturbance of 5-HT or NE activity is indicated by the presence of high levels of anxiety and excitability, panic, and impulsiveness (Landsberg, 2001). When TCAs are given to normal humans, their mood is not enhanced by the medication; it is only in the presence of neural disturbances affecting 5-HT and NE functions that a benefit is obtained by their use. Although a previous study showed a strong relationship between decreased levels of CSF serotonin and dopamine metabolites and dominance aggression (Reisner et al., 1996), this potential endophenotype (i.e., a quantifiable physiological marker predicting risk or presence of disorder) predicting dominance aggression has turned out to be of limited clinical usefulness. Mertens and colleagues (2000) failed to find any significant differences in the plasma or CSF 5-HIAA or 5-HT concentrations of dogs presenting with dominance aggression (N = 9) and a control group of nonaggressors (N = 20), concluding that such markers are of little value for confirming the diagnosis of dominance aggression. Nevertheless, given the earlier work of Reisner and colleagues, such laboratory tests may still be of value for helping to detect the subgroup of dogs that might exhibit a deficiency of 5-HT activity and are most likely to respond beneficially to serotonergic agents. In their study, springer spaniels were disproportionately represented in the experimental group, suggesting the possibility that aggression problems exhibited by this breed may show an increased responsiveness to serotonergic medications.

SSRIs often take weeks to become fully effective, even though the presynaptic reuptake inhibition produced by such medications (e.g., fluoxetine) appears to occur within minutes (Blier and De Montigny, 1994). The rapid increase of 5-HT occurring as the result of treatment with fluoxetine causes 5-HT$_{1A}$ autoreceptors at the level of the midbrain raphe nuclei to slow down the release of serotonin at the terminal, where 5-HT$_{1B}$ autoreceptors also exert an inhibitory effect on the release of serotonin. This braking effect is gradually reduced as 5-HT$_{1A}$ autoreceptors are slowly desensitized, thereby attenuating their negative-feedback control over 5-HT release. To induce a more rapid onset of therapeutic effect, pindolol, a mixed ß-adrenoceptor/5-HT$_{1A}$ antagonist has been used in combination with SSRIs to treat human depression. Reportedly, the combination both accelerates and enhances the effects of SSRIs. Pindolol may facilitate SSRI actions by partially inhibiting 5-HT$_{1A}$ autoreceptors and other modes of action (Artigas et al., 2001), for example, central ß-adrenoceptor blockade (Cremers et al., 2001). Since pindolol exerts an inhibitory effect over 5-HT$_{1A}$ receptors, it *may* elevate anxiety levels while exerting a more rapid onset of modulatory control over aggressive impulse.

Given the effectiveness of fluoxetine to modulate offensive aggression, scent marking, social dominance, and affiliative behavior in several animal species, perhaps 5-HT-enhancing drugs would be useful to control dog-dog aggression, especially aggression between dogs sharing the same home (Houpt, 2000). Also, fluoxetine or 5-HTP might offer significant benefit for the control of refractory canine urine marking, as Pryor and colleagues (2001) have convincingly shown in the case of fluoxetine for the control of feline urine-marking behavior. Both fluoxetine and 5-HTP have been shown to stimulate an increased production of glucocorticoids, an effect that may be beneficial in cases of aggression associated with low cortisol levels. Finally, a potent selective 5-HT-reuptake inhibitor that may have potential value for the treatment of stress-related behavior problems occurring in association with dysregulated 5-HT activity is paroxetine. Paroxetine may be particularly beneficial in the case of dogs exhibiting signs of chronic stress or abnormalities involving the HPA system (e.g., low cortisol). Report-

edly, paroxetine exerts a pronounced effect on central CRF, helping to normalize the HPA axis and promoting a more adaptive response to stress (Ladd et al., 2000).

In accordance with the dead-dog rule (see *Dead-dog Rule* in Volume 2, Chapter 2), most treatable aggression problems are best approached by training owners and dogs how to get on together more competently and affectionately, rather than targeting aggression with physical punishment, mechanical restraint, or pharmacological suppression. Given that the mere absence of aggression is not a particularly reliable predictor of risk, emphasis is placed on mediating changes conducive to more competent, playful, relaxed, and friendly interaction between the owner and family members. Establishing a pattern of behavior, with or without the support of drugs, that is incompatible with aggression appears to provide a far better predictor of relative aggression risk, but nothing is fail-safe in such matters. Many drug-study protocols appear to be overly preoccupied with the suppressive effect of medication rather than focusing on the subtle nuances and changes occurring in the dog's emotional tone and emergent organizing processes that may, in fact, be facilitated by the medication but remain undetected by the assessment instrument used to monitor change. Medications such as SSRIs may steadily enhance a dog's ability to cope more adaptively with stressful situations and to interact more competently and affectionately with the owner. Many of the neurobiological effects of SSRIs, in particular, appear to be mostly subtle, working slowly and thereby integrating a complex attunement process involving a dauntingly complicated network of serotonergic processes and neural interactions. For the full benefits of such therapy to develop and mature, perhaps the medication needs to be maintained for much longer periods than typically found in current protocols. Drug trials lasting only a few weeks—that is, ending just at a point when the drug is becoming most potent and active—may not be provide enough time to reveal the full merit of SSRI therapy on dog aggression problems. Further, more sensitive and standardized assessment instruments may need to be developed for detecting and tracking gradual behavioral changes. Finally, it seems crucial that efforts be taken to develop sharper diagnostic inclusion criteria and endophenotypic markers for sorting out aggressive phenotypes in order to determine which ones might benefit most from SSRI therapy:

> It is possible that in dogs, aggression that is a typical, albeit problem, behavior will not be affected by serotonergic drugs, but abnormal aggressiveness, which develops less frequently in dogs, may be affected. (White et al., 1999:1290–1291)

Note: The foregoing information is provided for educational purposes only. If considering the use of medications to control or manage a behavior problem, the reader should consult with a veterinarian familiar with the use of drugs for such purposes to obtain diagnostic criteria, specific dosages, and medical advice concerning potential adverse side effects and interactions with other drugs.

PLACEBO EFFECTS, ENDOPHENOTYPES, AND THE DEAD-DOG RULE

White and colleagues' (1999) data revealed a robust placebo effect occurring precisely in the treatment time course when one might *expect* to observe maximum benefits resulting from treatment with clomipramine or SSRIs, a pattern consistent with the positive findings reported by Dodman and colleagues (1996). Interpersonal expectancy effects in the treatment of aggression problems can be extremely powerful and sometimes even welcome and beneficial, appearing to exert a constructive influence that a skillful behavior therapist can use to promote positive change. However, in the case of research, placebo effects make it impossible to interpret the significance of the data collected, essentially making the work useless or, at best, stimulating additional research with appropriate controls to limit placebo and experimenter-bias effects.

Most veterinary behavior data are collected secondhand via questionnaire instruments, filtered through the owners' perception of their dog's behavior and its response to treatment. In addition, the owner is typically asked to perform some set of procedures, not to interact with the dog in some specified ways, or not to change their behavior toward the dog in any way. In a sense the owner becomes a coexperimenter, often fully aware of what the experimenter is trying to achieve by way of the study. Naturally, the owner's involvement jeopardizes the objectivity of the study at various points. Many owners desperately want their dogs to improve and may do things unconsciously to facilitate that improvement or begin to see changes where none have actually occurred, thereby potentially skewing what they observe with an overly optimistic bias. As a result, three basic concerns are raised by such studies: (1) owner reports may lack objectivity, (2) owners may not follow instructions competently or compliantly, and (3) study results will tend to confirm the experimental hypothesis. Without the safeguards afforded by a randomized, double-blind, and placebo-controlled experimental design, findings derived from such investigations are extremely difficult to analyze and interpret, perhaps ending up being a waste of time and money. Even with the proper controls in place, problems might still stem from items 1 and 2. These almost insurmountable difficulties point to the need for objective physiological or neurobiological markers or endophenotypes correlated with serious behavior problems and their resolution. Studies evaluating PPI testing, heart-rate changes in response to petting and massage, stress-related heart-rate and blood-pressure divergence (*see Autonomic Arousal, Heart Rate, and Aggression*), oxytocin levels in response to social contact/petting, cortisol response to mild stressors, blood-pressure and vagus-nerve monitoring, and so forth may prove useful in this regard. For example, SSRIs appear to mobilize an oxytocinergic-antistress response (Uvnäs-Moberg et al., 1999), an effect that may alter a dog's PPI and cardiac response to touch, thereby potentially establishing an objective marker (endophenotype) for gauging the efficacy of such medications. A chronic effect of clomipramine is to downregulate kappa- and mu-opioid receptors, suggesting the possibility that one therapeutic effect of the medication is to reduce opioid-mediated inhibition of central oxytocin

(McDougle et al., 1999), an effect that should be reflected in changes of peripheral oxytocin levels (see Brown et al., 2001).

The stated goal of cynopraxic therapy and training is to promote interactive harmony and to enhance the human-dog bond, but how can one quantify such an objective? For practical purposes, success is quantified by informal and formal assessments and comparisons of pretraining and post-training expectancy divergence and convergence indicators (see *Puppy Profile Sheet* in Volume 1, Chapter 2). For example, during pretraining interviews, the owner may be instructed to list on one side of a sheet of paper all of the dog's minor and major adjustment problems and on the other side a collection of corresponding positive statements about what the owner would consider the best possible outcome of training efforts. The owner is then instructed to draw lines between the two sets of items, connecting related items and thereby establishing a series of expectancy continuums between the owner's ideal and the dog's actual behavior. These items can then become the topic of counseling to form realistic objectives and means to attain the owner's goals. A major advantage of this approach is that it establishes a personalized profile of the dog's specific adjustment difficulties from the owner's perspective and in terms relevant to the owner's goals. Not only do dogs exhibit significant variability, relationships between people and dogs are also affected by tremendous variation. What may be a problem for one person may be a source of joy for another. The profile helps to contextualize the dog's behavior within a relationship and a home, thereby enabling the cynopraxic therapist to provide counseling and rational training relevant to improving the human-dog bond while simultaneously working to enhance the dog's quality of life.

This procedure not only provides vital information about the adjustment problem, but allows the owner to think through carefully what he or she wants to achieve as the result of training and behavior therapy. The set of expectancy continuums given by the owner can be formalized and used to construct a worst-case and best-case grouping of related items with a 10-point scale between

them, as used in the puppy profile questionnaire. With regard to experimental applications and data collection, the owner's items might be included in a standardized and validated owner-expectancy assessment developed for research purposes—something that remains to be done. At a glance, the owner can quickly note where the dog currently stands on the scaled continuum with an X and indicate what he or she would like to accomplish through training by placing an O over the appropriate point. The divergence between these two points on the scale is the expectancy-divergence score. Upon completion of the training and therapy program, a second owner-expectancy assessment is performed, and a training outcome score is assigned by comparing and recording differences between the pretraining scores and the post-training scores. By adding these scores together and then dividing the sum by the total number of items in the assessment, a social-conflict score is yielded. Success is measured in terms of a progressive trend toward a convergence between the owner's expectations and what the dog does, indicating a reduction of interactive conflict. In addition, quality-of-life improvements (e.g., time in crate, time on walks, time playing, and time training) are tracked by having the owner keep relevant records. This method of assessment is consistent with the dead-dog rule and seems to provide a valid measure of change relevant to the improvement of the human-dog bond.

PART 2: DEVELOPMENT AND CONTROL OF PUPPY COMPETITIVE BEHAVIOR

TEMPERAMENT AND AGGRESSION

Organized activity depends on the presence of an emotional balance produced by the complementary influences of inhibition and excitation. In addition to adverse developmental experiences, some dogs appear to be influenced by a genetic predisposition toward emotional instability and reactivity, corresponding to what Pavlov described as the choleric temperament (c type) (see *Experimental Neurosis* in Volume 1, Chapter 9).

Such dogs may be significantly more prone to exhibit behavioral disturbances associated with social environmental stressors (see *Temperament Testing* in Appendix D). These differences appear to express themselves at an early age in wolves (MacDonald, 1983) and dogs (Senay, 1966). Senay found that puppies prone to high levels of emotional arousal and reactivity were more avoidant and aggressive when approached than were puppies showing a more relaxed and organized response to human contact. These temperament differences were apparent at an early age and persisted throughout the first year, suggesting that they may due to inherited deviations affecting arousal levels and stimulus-reactivity thresholds. A proneness to excessive excitability and reactivity may cause dogs to engage in more disorganized and reactive behavior (withdrawal, avoidance, and aggression) when stimulated by social contact, whereas dogs functioning under the influence of moderate arousal and relaxation may be more prone to engage in organized behavior (approach, affiliation, and cooperation) under the influence of similar social stimulation. In addition to social avoidance and aggression, puppies exhibiting emotionally reactive behavior showed physiological signs of autonomic arousal (e.g., tachycardia and submissive urination). Puppies genetically prone to disturbances associated with excitability and reactivity excesses may also be more susceptible to the harmful influences of adverse rearing practices and biological stress.

TACTILE STIMULATION AND ADAPTATION

Tactile experiences and emotions share a number of common characteristics that suggest an ontogenetic link between taction and the development of emotional responsiveness and tone. Both touch and emotion are hedonically valenced and associated with varying degrees of subjective pleasure or pain; they both produce motivationally short-lived arousal prompting immediate behavioral adjustment (attraction or aversion) or more lasting and inescapable discomfort (e.g., throbbing pain or hurt feelings); they both function to direct dogs to attend to and respond to environmental stimulation selectively in order to perpetuate or terminate it; and they both can function as means to reinforce or suppress behavior.

Early tactile stimulation in the form of handling and gentling exerts profound and long-lasting influences on health (resistance to disease), activity levels, learning and problem-solving abilities, confidence, and emotional reactivity. Tactile stimulation is a significant source of potential reward for puppies and dogs (Fonberg et al., 1981), cats (Wenzel, 1959), and rats (Burgdorf and Panksepp, 2001). Rats seem to enjoy tactile stimulation as a prelude to play, with tickling of certain skin areas inducing ultrasonic chirping (Panksepp and Burgdorf, 2000). Among puppies, tactile stimulation associated with play enhances affection, social expressiveness, empathy, and restraint (bite inhibition). Just as tactile stimulation can produce disorganized and reactive behavior as the result of neurotogenic or traumatic experiences, therapeutic procedures using tactile stimulation appear to be highly effective in treating emotional disturbances originating in adverse somatosensory experiences (see *Posture-facilitated Relaxation Training* in Chapter 7).

Somatosensory systems promote attachment and social bonding via proximity seeking contact comfort and affect attunement. Puppies exhibit a strong preference for contact with soft objects, spending more time with cloth surrogate mothers versus time spent with wire surrogates providing milk (Igel and Calvin, 1960). Other studies have shown that contact with soft objects produces a significant reduction in separation distress in isolated puppies (Pettijohn et al., 1977). Petting has been shown to modulate adverse emotional reactions (Gantt, 1944; Fuller, 1967), restrain HPA-system activity (Hennessy et al., 1998), and decrease physiological arousal associated with aversive stimulation (Lynch and McCarthy, 1967 and 1969). Tactile stimulation mediates a potent effect on emotional learning and reactive thresholds via the autonomic nervous system and endocrine activity. The emotions associated with touch selectively activate and organize a puppy's behavioral output in the opposing directions of approach or withdraw in response to social and environmental sources of tactile stimulation. Tactile-related emotions exert a pervasive influence on social behavior and development. Close social contact and tactile stimulation produce conditioned and unconditioned effects on attractive (e.g., affection) and aversive (anxiety, fear, irritability, and anger) arousal thresholds, mediating the expression of both organized and reactive behavior. Gantt (1971) observed that close contact and tactile stimulation produce three general patterns of arousal in dogs, depending on temperament and past experience: calming, agitation, and autistic (little or no response as observed in many genetically nervous pointer dogs). These differences in responsiveness are reflected in overt behavior, canine cardiovascular activity (e.g., heart rate and blood pressure), respiration rate, and endocrine activity.

As a result of the close and active social interaction with the mother and littermates, puppies may acquire somatosensory set points for a certain type and quantity of tactile stimulation not provided in the new home. Failure to obtain sufficient tactile or locomotor stimulation may represent a significant source of stress for newly adopted puppies, perhaps inducing a variety of compensatory behavioral changes, including hyperactivity, excessive contact-seeking and proximity-seeking behavior, overexcitability, and increased aggressiveness associated with frustration and irritability. Slabbert and Rasa (1993) have reported that German shepherd puppies removed from their mothers at week 6 failed to thrive and showed a significantly greater risk for disease and mortality than did puppies naturally weaned by their mothers between weeks 7 and 8. They also exhibited significant behavioral deficits: "Puppies weaned before 7 weeks of age are noisy and nervous. These seem to become fixed characteristics of the dog for life" (5). Puppies allowed to stay with their mothers through week 12 were healthier, gained more weight, and appeared better adapted. The cause of these disturbances in early-weaned puppies may be related to the premature loss of tactile stimulation and comfort contact.

Early adverse stress may exert immunological effects (e.g., immunosuppression) that could compromise a puppy's ability to fight infection. Although it is difficult to estimate the effect of postnatal stress on puppy development and the etiology of behavior problems, perhaps some important clues may be obtained by the confluence of early disease conditions, immune stress, and the incidence of adult behavior problems (see *Immune Stress and Cytokines*).

PLAY, DISCIPLINE, AND DOMINANCE

Dog owners typically establish dominance by asserting authority and setting behavioral limits on their puppies' activities. When confronted assertively, most puppies acknowledge the owner's authority and submit to owner directives. Although puppies are capable of learning at an early age, mature impulse-control abilities probably do not fully develop until dogs are 8 to 10 months of age. The most prominent ways in which owners respond to inappropriate behavior is by physical assertion (dominance) or by encouraging cooperation (leadership). Whether an assertion of physical force or encouragement is used largely depends on the owner's perception of the problem and the sort of motivations attributed to it. Ben-Michael and colleagues (2000b) found that assertions of force were most likely to occur in situations where the dog was perceived as being disobedient or out of control, both of which frequently evoked anger and irritability in owners. Encouragement and comforting strategies were most common in the case of fearful and submissive dogs and were motivated by feelings of compassion and anxiety. Some owners, however, may perceive fear-related behavior as personally aversive or offensive (e.g., a submissive dog urinates), thereby intensifying feelings of anger and irritability and reducing the likelihood of comforting activities toward the dog. The most common techniques used by dog owners to handle problematic behavior were mostly punitive (e.g., demand obedience, yell at the dog, or distract it). Comforting and encouraging the dog or ignoring the problematic behavior was less common. The least commonly used strategy was reward—findings that appear sharply at odds with the data and assumptions elaborated by Hiby and colleagues (see *Owner Control Styles and Welfare Agendas* in Chapter 10). Physical punishment was mostly used in the case of aversive behavior (e.g., chewing on personal belongings or jumping on a bed) or disobedience. Punishment was avoided in situations where the dog was overexcited or fearful, in which cases owners were more likely to use distraction techniques (Ben-Michael et al., 2000a).

A significantly different picture of training and disciplinary activities has been presented by Koda (2001b) with regard to the ways in which guide-dog puppy raisers cope with inappropriate behavior. A series of direct observations of puppy raisers indicated that they rarely hit puppies and relied primarily on diversionary activities (e.g., play) or rejecting behavior (e.g., brief withdrawal of contact from the puppies) to control social excesses (e.g., mouthing). During observation periods, rejecting and, to a lesser extent, ignoring were considered to be effective in controlling biting, whereas distraction, talking to the puppy, initiating play, restraint, and showing objects to the puppy were all ineffective. These findings are difficult to interpret because of the way in which the observations were made. The presence of the observer, together with specific instructions from the guide-dog association not to use physical punishment, may have caused the puppy raisers to behave differently during observation periods than at other times when alone with the puppy. Koda has noted, however, that Japanese mothers typically avoid making their children behave by asserting authority, as "compared with American mothers" (86) (and apparently Dutch ones, too), suggesting the possibility that, in fact, the puppy raisers did avoid the use of physical punishment. Of particular interest was the finding that puppies may have exhibited an ontogenetic decline in biting and destructive activity as they matured, showing increased gentleness and willingness to cooperate. These maturational aspects of social interaction are particularly evident in the development of play behavior. Koda (2001a) found that, as puppies grew older, they tended to engage in play activities that evidenced improved impulse-control abilities. Unfortunately, it is impossible to determine whether these enhanced abilities for cooperative play are the result of ontogenetic changes or the result of puppy-raiser training activities occurring between observation periods.

Establishing dominance by setting limits on a puppy's behavior is typically accomplished by the application of varying amounts of punishment, a method of social control that is widely practiced by animals (Clutton-Brock and Parker, 1995) and the most common strategy used by people to control dog behavior (Ben-Michael et al., 2000a). Although assertive disciplinary interaction may be necessary and helpful to prevent problems (Hart and Hart, 1997), excessively harsh or frequent punishment is inappropriate and should be avoided. In response to such treatment, puppies typically show varying degrees of fear and submission, but some may be stimulated by frustration or anger and fight back. Defining and enforcing social rules for a puppy is critical for the development of appropriate adult social behavior, but excessive punitive interaction may cause the puppy to become progressively insecure and dependent on the owner or more reactive and aggressive. The risk of forming insecure attachments and excessive reactive coping styles is especially likely in situations where punishment is also associated with high levels of indulgent pampering, something that often follows severe punishment as the owner is moved by pangs of compunction and sympathy for the emotionally injured puppy.

Given the puppy's immature abilities with respect to exercising impulse control, punishment is unlikely to control social excesses effectively. As a result of limited success and growing frustration and irritability, owners and trainers may be tempted to escalate punitive efforts beyond what is appropriate and beneficial. Assertions of control using restraint, response prevention, abrupt stimulus change, assertive blocking, and loss of social contact may be effective, but physical punishment (e.g., hitting) should be avoided. Most importantly, in addition to defining what a puppy must not do, it is imperative to guide the puppy toward the expression of behaviors that it can do. Ideally, inhibitory training should be minimized. The puppy trainer should follow a philosophy of maximum overt differentiation (MOD) and systematic canalization of behavior into more socially acceptable variations through structured play activities. Gradually, behavior-selection pressures involving contingent reinforcement and punitive actions can be used to shape a more precise and predictable behavioral repertoire. Young puppies are particularly receptive to incentive-based training, especially activities that involve play, small treats, and affectionate encouragement. Play provides an ideal means for controlling social excesses and inappropriate behavior by guiding puppies into alternative activities (canalization) to obtain gratification for otherwise socially unacceptable behavior (e.g., biting and jumping up). Play training promotes cooperative interaction based on a leader-follower bond, mutual appreciation, and heightened interactive joy. Disruptive, aggressive, or impulsive behavior is best controlled through the differential reinforcement of incompatible behaviors, response prevention, restraint, and brief TO. In addition to play, affectionate petting, vocal encouragement, and food rewards given in exchange for the performance of basic exercises (e.g., sit, down, stand, come, and stay) help puppies to learn how to communicate and cooperate with people. Integrated compliance training (ICT), whereby training is integrated into everyday household activities, helps to structure a puppy's behavior in accordance with general rules and expectations.

PRECOCIOUS AGGRESSION PROBLEMS

Although severe aggression problems are seldom seen in puppies, occasionally puppies do exhibit serious problems requiring behavioral intervention (see *Social Competition, Development, and Aggression* in Volume 2, Chapter 8). A common form of pediatric aggression involves possessive guarding of objects or food—a significant concern for families with children. Overly possessive puppies may guard food or other prized objects and threaten to bite if they are approached at such times. Training puppies to drop ("Drop it"), back away ("Leave it"), and resume possession ("Take it") of highly attractive toys and chew items is among the most important early lessons for such puppies to learn. Possessive-aggressive behavior in puppies may be indica-

tive of a temporary developmental impulse-control deficit and may not necessarily predict adult possessive-aggression problems. Many puppies exhibiting possessive aggression appear to grow out of it (Marder, personal communication, 2000), but many also continue to exhibit the behavior as adults. Dunbar (1978) reported that adult male beagles rarely attempt to take bones away from young puppies, but always take them away from 7-month-old ones. This observation may be related to the ontogenetic emergence of improved impulse-control abilities in adolescent dogs. Adult dogs may recognize that puppies simply cannot control the impulse to protect such possessions.

As the result of biogenetic and experiential causes, some puppies may show more ominous signs at an early age (e.g., low fear and aggression thresholds). Evidence of excessive fear, irritability, and aggressiveness may reflect inchoate epigenetic processes, possibly prefiguring adult aggression problems (see *Behavioral Thresholds and Aggression* in Volume 2, Chapter 8). Puppies exhibiting such behavioral signs should be identified as early as possible and provided with appropriate supportive training and behavior therapy. Adult aggression problems depend on both genetic and experiential factors to incubate. Although genetic influences may put a dog at risk of developing a serious aggression problem, the risk can be significantly reduced by the presence of ameliorating or protective influences (Figure 6.3). In contrast, adverse social and environmental influences may significantly increase a dog's risk of developing aggression problems.

COMPETITIVE SOCIAL EXCESSES

Arguably the most common reason for seeking behavioral advice and training is aggressive play, including mouthing, biting, and chase-grabbing activities (see *Play and Aggression* in Volume 2, Chapter 8). Competitive playful excesses do not appear to be significantly correlated with adult aggression problems (Goodloe and Borchelt, 1998); however, such behavior may forecast oppositional tendencies, hyperactivity, and various discipline problems, stressing the importance of early behavioral training to head off secondary

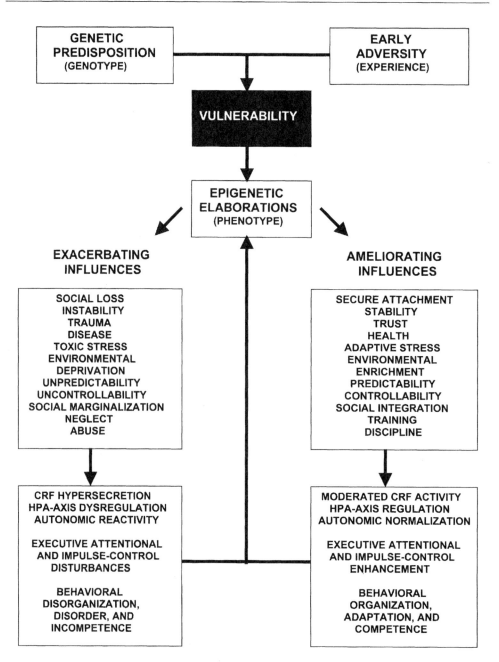

FIG. 6.3. Biogenetic and developmental predisposing influences may make a dog vulnerable to exhibiting aggression or other serious behavior problems in adulthood. Such problems are not inevitable, however, since subsequent experience (epigenesis) exerts a pronounced influence on how the predisposition manifests itself, determining whether a stable or unstable behavioral phenotype emerges. Serious behavioral problems are expressed through several layers of causation (biogenetic, ontogenetic, and epigenetic), resulting in physiological, neurobiological, and behavioral changes. Ameliorating influences may exert a protective effect against the development of aggression problems, whereas exacerbating influences place a dog at greater risk. CRF, corticotropin-releasing factor; and HPA, hypothalamic-pituitary-adrenocortical.

problems associated with excessive or disruptive competitive behavior. The key to successful puppy training is to occupy the puppy with structured play and positive learning activities. Even in cases where signs of aggression are not evident, training puppies to actively defer to human leadership should still be a prominent aspect of everyday handling and socialization. Many puppy problems involving overactivity and excessive playfulness can be rapidly improved by a combination of play therapy and increased opportunities for exercise.

The causes underlying disruptive competitive behavior are numerous and varied. Social learning is undoubtedly a factor, but difficult puppies may also be affected by a genetic predisposition and temperament traits that compete with the acquisition of behavior needed to adapt successfully to the home environment. In addition to reduced thresholds for fear, frustration, irritability, and aggression, some puppies appear to exhibit an inability to achieve sufficient reward stimulation from everyday activities (see *Neural and Physiological Substrates* in Volume 2, Chapter 5). These puppies cannot seem to get enough attention and contact and may be driven by an exaggerated and insatiable appetite for reward gratification. Stimulation-seeking puppies exhibit excessive attention needs, impulsive competitive tendencies, signs of inappropriate appetitive interests (pica), and an overall inability to achieve a normal degree of gratification and contentment from reward-producing activities, suggesting a developmental reward-processing deficiency. In such cases, it is especially important to use methods emphasizing positive reinforcement and ICT. Unfortunately, disruptive puppies are often treated with abusive physical punishment. Although limit-setting actions and TO may be useful, physical punishment involving the slapping or hitting of difficult puppies should be avoided. Most puppy owners are searching for answers that will give them enhanced control without resorting to abusive or excessively aversive techniques.

Mouthing, biting, and pawing on hands and clothing are common puppy nuisances. These playful competitive habits are normally acquired as the result of play fighting between littermates. Playful sparring and other contests involving the use of the mouth and feet constitute the most frequently observed active interactions between puppies. This playful interaction serves many vital functions, ranging from physical and sensory development to the elaboration of various social and competitive skills. Much of what puppies do during play facilitates learning how to use ritualized threat and appeasement displays competently. An important function of competitive play is to ritualize aggressive contests, thereby bringing about a more or less stable social organization among littermates. Puppies learn how to restrain their aggressive impulses and bite in order to perpetuate the joys of play. Under the influence of competitive play and social feedback, a puppy learns to be affectionate and restrain its aggressive impulses toward its playmates. In several respects, the interactive dynamics embodied in the litter are prototypical social behavior patterns exhibited by adult dogs and wolves. Playful fighting allows canine competitors to practice skills that might otherwise result in injury, increase social conflict, or disrupt the unity of the group. Puppies are conditioned to play fight affectionately, and significant benefits for the human-dog relationship may be obtained by engaging them in structured play activities.

However, some puppies may develop a rather compulsive interest in competitive behavior, engaging in persistent rough mouthing and biting whenever handled by the owner. Even though the presence of heightened excitability and competitiveness does not necessarily prefigure adult aggression problems, it appears to represent a significant risk factor (Guy et al., 2001) that warrants training and preventive efforts introduced at an early age. Competitive excesses may make puppies less enjoyable and adversely impact on the bonding process. A competitive puppy may intimidate children, frustrate adults, and create significant household tensions, gradually becoming the object of escalating punishment. Owners seeking help with disruptive puppies are often distressed and worried about the behavior. Some owners may express regrets about having obtained a dog, further emphasizing the potential injury that such behavior can have on the developing bond between the family and puppy. Instead of moving toward the center of family life, a highly excitable and disruptive puppy may be swept outward on a trajectory of progressive rejection and isolation. Instead of spending constructive time with the family as a source of affection, comfort, and entertainment, a difficult-to-control puppy may spend the majority of time in a crate, behind gates, or kept outdoors. Under such circumstances of excessive confinement and isolation, a puppy's undesirable behavior may worsen and threaten to result in its removal from the home unless something can be done rapidly to ameliorate the situation.

Restrain and Train

Obviously, it is critical to offer such families immediate and effective means for establishing control. Suggesting that they keep the puppy on a leash while indoors can be extremely beneficial. Surprisingly, many inexperienced dog owners may not have thought of this simple solution. For disruptive and hyperactive puppies, the leash facilitates control by means of passive restraint, response blocking, and limit-setting directives. Overly active puppies appear to learn much more effectively and rapidly when the range of possible actions that they are free to perform is limited. Leash control limits the amount of behavior that fails while increasing the amount that succeeds. Rather than the owner engaging in pointless yelling and other reactive and ineffectual expressions of frustration, the leash offers a more direct and communicative means to establish control and guide a puppy's behavior. In an important sense, the leash represents a reification of the human will, helping to constrain and conform the puppy's behavior toward a more acceptable social ideal. Actions prompted by the leash can be reinforced and brought under the control of vocal signals. For example, stepping on the leash can easily block common jumping-up excesses. Pairing the word "Off" just as a puppy attempts to leap up becomes associatively linked with the thwarted action. Combining such mild avoidance training and response-blocking techniques with positive reinforcement of alternative behavior, such as

standing or sitting, encourages puppies not to jump up when excited or seeking attention. Instead, puppies learn that obtaining attention or contact is best achieved by waiting or sitting or by exhibiting some other behavior that has worked in the past to produce positive reinforcement.

In addition to leashing puppies, tie-out stations can be set up throughout the house, especially in places where family members frequently gather to spend time together. Tie-out stations can be particularly useful for children, who might otherwise be overwhelmed by an overactive and uppity puppy. Such restraint provides sufficient control for them to get close to the puppy to feed it small treats by hand, pet it, and play with a toy. Initially, the puppy is trained to lick a closed hand to produce a concealed treat. As the puppy licks, the child can say "Kiss" and "Good puppy," thereupon giving the puppy the treat. In addition, with very little instruction, the puppy can be taught to sit and lie down by closely following the child's closed hand and getting a treat after completing the action. If the puppy becomes overly active or intrusive, the child can simply scoot back out of the puppy's reach, thereby initiating a brief nonexclusionary TO. As the puppy subsequently calms down, the child can return and continue the gentling process. Under the influence of such contingent pressures, the puppy soon learns that excessive or intrusive behavior results in the withdrawal of contact and the opportunity to obtain more food and affection, whereas self-control and cooperation result in the resumption of contact and the chance to get more food and attention. For puppies that engage in persistent mouthing or precocious aggression problems, more assertive procedures may be necessary. An active-control line can be set up enabling the trainer to turn the puppy away and restrain it at a distance for a brief TO period before allowing it to approach again and initiating reward-based training activities incompatible with biting. If the puppy engages in the undesirable behavior, it can again be turned away briefly (e.g., 20 to 30 seconds). Play activities, orienting and attending training, sit-stay, and down-stay training can be highly effective in helping to organize the behavior of such puppies.

Learning to Succeed

All normal dogs strive to optimize their control over the social and physical environment in order to attain adaptive success and security. Fundamentally speaking, behavior is purposive and organized to achieve some useful goal, usually involving the enhanced prediction and control over significant attractive or aversive environment events. Consequently, behavior is selected (punished or reinforced) in accordance with its relative success or failure to predict and control significant events: behavior that fails is modified, extinguished, or suppressed, whereas behavior that succeeds is perpetuated. Obviously, success is preferred over failure, but failure is not without benefit. Without Pavlovian prediction errors and instrumental failures, learning to predict and control the environment would not proceed efficiently. Prediction errors and failures provide information that can be used to improve future efforts, which ultimately serve the purpose of enhancing an animal's adaptive success. Nonetheless, dogs do not set out to fail when they purposively interact with the environment, and when they do fail to predict or control some significant event causing them loss or discomfort, they may experience a variety of hedonically aversive emotional states (e.g., disappointment, irritability, frustration, anxiety, or fear). Normally, behavioral efforts that fail are usually followed by additional attempts and variations emitted under the potentiating influences of frustration or fear. Depending on a puppy's temperament and motivational predisposition, the quickening influences of frustration and fear may result in either adaptive or reactive efforts to control the environment. Although some failure is instructive and beneficial for learning, excessive and persistent failure together with adverse concomitant emotional arousal may lead to attentional and behavioral disturbances. In the case of overly active and disruptive puppies, excessive frustration and anxiety may adversely affect their ability to adjust effectively. Structured play and ICT provide the puppy with events and activities that are highly predictable and controllable, giving it beneficial opportunities to succeed and to obtain the emotional benefits associated with success (e.g., elation). Nothing more consistently promotes enhanced well-being and contentment than repeated success with periodic surprises (positive prediction error).

Bond Considerations

The concept of dominance has received some criticism and revision in recent years, especially as it regards the human-dog relationship (see *Concept of Dominance* in Volume 2, Chapter 8). Despite some significant limitations, the notion of social dominance remains a useful and viable construct. The positive implication of social dominance is that the owner must establish sufficient authority to limit a puppy's behavior and guide it into more appropriate directions. Most disruptive and socially competitive puppies are in search of a leader and a relationship based on cooperation and safety. In contrast, many dog owners are in search of an affectionate care-bond object. The end result of these divergent interests is often confusion, conflict, and discontentment. To succeed, the owner must defer care-bonding needs to the establishment of appropriate social limits and rule-based interaction with the puppy, whereupon care bonding naturally follows as the result of the nurturance during the training process. For its part, the puppy must learn to willingly submit to owner directives and to take pleasure from following the owner's instructions, a process that is facilitated by the presentation of affection, play, food, and other desirable things to the dog in exchange for its cooperative behavior. Social dominance does not imply, nor necessitate, rigid and hostile actions, nor does submission entail fear. Healthy dominant-subordinate relations, in fact, are characterized by a relative absence of overt aggression and fear. Although the assertion of dominance may include assertive gestures and ritualized aggressive actions, the intent of such behavior is not to evoke excessive fear. Similarly, the fawning body postures and submissive displays of the subordinate may overlap topographically with behaviors expressive of fear, but fear does not properly characterize the motivational significance of such behavior. Both the dominant and subordinate partners appear to be influenced by affection for each other, with anger and fear being effectively constrained, thereby limiting overt aggression and other escape reactions associated with aversive emotional arousal (see *Affiliation and Social Dominance* in Volume 2, Chapter 8). Living in close social contact with each other, frequent and intense exchanges of aggression and reciprocal defensive behavior would be highly stressful and energy consuming for both the dominant dog and the subordinate. In an important sense, both the dominant dog and the subordinate are benefited by an affectionate impulse leading them to cooperate and tolerate close interaction with each other. The dominant dog's threats are tempered by increasing affection and familiarity, stimulating protective tolerance and responsibility for the group. Any fear that the subordinate may feel in response to the dominant dog's assertive displays is offset by a growing affectionate need to maintain contact in a search of social comfort and safety, a tendency facilitating a following and cooperative social role. In essence, establishing dominant-subordinate relations is a matter of enhancing mutual tolerance and affection for the sake of the greater good and benefit of the group. The subordinate's submissive displays may function as an escape/avoidance strategy aimed at evading the dominant dog's wrath, while at the same time stimulating its nurturance and protection.

Play and Leadership

Cynopraxic training promotes a balance of dominance, leadership, and nurturance in order to promote a healthy and successful human-dog bond (Figure 6.4) (see *Dynamics of Bonding: Nurturance, Dominance, and Leadership* in Chapter 4). A natural way to facilitate this process is through structured play activities. Leaders are not threatening or provocative; they are playful and fun. Just as assertive and submissive displays are modulated by affection, play activities similarly involve the exchange of behavioral sequences under the influence of affiliative motivations. Play activities early in life prepare dogs to

advertise and acknowledge assertive and submissive displays in a socially constructive way, facilitating an affectionate and harmonious social existence. Protoplay activities emerge almost as soon as puppies can walk (Cairns, 1972). The ascendant emotion controlling play is joy, making playful interaction highly rewarding and conducive to the enhancement of social affection, competence, and trust.

Play is unique in that it has no apparent goal other than the perpetuation of itself, perhaps as the result of play-activated reward circuits producing elation and exuberance, even in the absence of a play companion or object. Young dogs commonly exhibit various forms of solitary play. In addition, some dogs exhibit a form of frenetic solitary activity, perhaps functioning as a compensatory release in situations providing insufficient opportunities for play. The spectacle may cause first-time dog owners to suspect that their dog has momentarily lost its mind. Dogs exhibiting such behavior appear to be possessed by a torrent of spontaneous locomotor impulses. They rush about as though careening around obstacles or fleeing from a nonexistent pursuer closing in from behind. Occasionally, a dog may appear to scramble forward faster than its body can follow, creating a hunched-up appearance as it steers wildly along its fre-

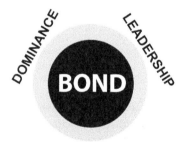

FIG. 6.4. Effective training promotes a balance of dominance, leadership, and nurturance. Dominance involves the imposition of appropriate limits on a dog's behavior in order to reduce socially intrusive excess and oppositional behavior. Leadership, on the other hand, shapes effective social behavior by means of structured play and integrated compliance training. The appetitive and social rewards used to support leadership contributes a nurturing aspect to the cynopraxic and training process.

netic path. As the playful release reaches a climax, the dog may display a wide open-mouthed smile, wedging its ears back. Meanwhile, like the baton of a drunken conductor, the tail wags excitedly one moment or, depending on the dog's passing mood and fancy, may be pressed up between its legs as though protecting it from the jaws of an imaginary pursuer. To my knowledge, a formal term has not yet been given to this kind of play behavior, but, given its solitary, spontaneous, and undirected character, perhaps the term *soliludic* would be a good choice. Soliludic activity nicely combines the Latin elements *solus* (alone) and *ludic* (spontaneous and undirected play).

Competent social play between people and dogs is expressed in two general forms: competitive and cooperative. Competitive play usually involves some element of contest (e.g., tug games and wrestling), whereas cooperative play involves sharing in the pursuit of some common activity (e.g., retrieving games). These functional aspects of play reflect the complementary dynamics facilitating harmonious group social organization and activity. Although excessive or agitational play may enhance undesirable behavior in dogs (see *Inappropriate Play and Bootleg Reinforcement* in Volume 2, Chapter 2), structured play in moderation may be highly beneficial. Tug-of-war games have been considered problematic with respect to the facilitation of dominance tensions, but little evidence supports the assumption that such games result in an increased risk of aggression in dogs not already exhibiting aggressive tendencies (Figure 6.5). Rooney and Bradshaw (2002) have attempted to test the effects of competitive play on dominance and other social behaviors. They exposed 14 golden retrievers to brief (3 minute) tug-of-war bouts involving 40 contests over 2 weeks. During the tests, the dogs were allowed to win at least two-thirds of 20 bouts and caused to lose at least two-thirds of the remaining 20 bouts. The authors found that such play had little effect on confidence levels (a measure they equated with dominance), even though the dogs reportedly became more playfully attentive, socially intrusive, and demanding as the result of repeated competitive play bouts. Observing

that the win-lose outcome of tug contests had little effect on confidence levels, the authors concluded that, at least among the group of dogs tested, human-dog play is not a "major determinant of dominance relationships" (175). A number of problems with this study deserve mention. First, the assumption that brief tug-of-war contests are enough to alter canine social behavior significantly or, more specifically, that the differential effect of winning or losing such tug contests is capable of producing significant modifications of relative social dominance is highly questionable. Consequently, just because the study failed to detect a measurable effect does not necessarily mean that more lengthy or frequent bouts of tug-of-war, perhaps performed in a more agitating fashion, would not produce significant change in such behavior. In any case, the puppy is not really winning, but is being permitted to win and compelled to lose; the

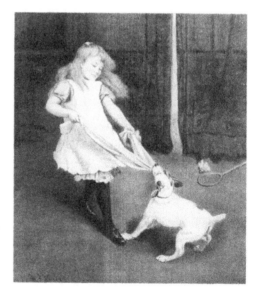

FIG. 6.5. *A Tug of War* by W. J. Hardy (1891). Tug-of-war has long been a popular play activity between people and dogs. Although shunned by some trainers as being instigative of aggression, no compelling evidence links the activity with aggression problems in dogs. Competitive games can be a potent way to facilitate controlled aggression in the case of working dogs, but special agitational techniques are used in combination with ludic incentives to achieve such ends.

handler remains the locus of control through-out, that is, the play partner maintains their control status or social dominance whether the puppy wins or loses. Second, since the experimenter performing the tug contest was relatively unfamiliar to the dogs and not a member of their primary social system, such playful interaction probably did not denote the same social significance for them as it might if performed by a family member. In fact, under the parameters of the study, com-petitive play may be irrelevant to the dogs' social dominance interests (if such interests, as defined by the authors, exist) and, as the authors point out, may only lead the dogs to view the experimenter as a "favourable play partner" (175). Third, the experiment appears to be inadequately controlled to show that the independent variable (tug-of-war) is exclu-sively responsible for the behavioral effects observed. To show a causal relationship, the concurrent effects of increasing familiarity would need to be experimentally separated from the effects of tug-of-war, an experimen-tal objective that would require the inclusion of additional control groups, a larger number of dogs, a functional and quantifiable (i.e., operational) definition of social dominance and a set of unambiguous interactive markers identifying it. Fourth, in any case, social dom-inance is probably a nonstarter with respect to puppy behavior and interaction with people. Puppy behavior appears more accurately described in terms of changes involving rela-tive social subordination or dependency/attachment levels. Most puppies are happy to be obligate subordinates, exhibiting a high degree of dependency toward the owner and others, whom they seem to view as parental surrogates—not social adversaries.

In addition to learning about one another, play appears to help individuals learn to restrain immediate competitive self-interests for the sake of advantages resulting from social cooperation. To maximize the therapeu-tic benefits of play, it is necessary to structure play activities carefully. Dogs are responsive to a variety of play signals, including facial (play face), postural (play bow), and vocal expres-sions dedicated to the solicitation of play (see *Play and Aggression* in Volume 2, Chapter 8) (Rooney et al., 2001). In combination with the play face and bow, dogs may use a huffing or rapid panting sound to indicate playful intentions (Fox, 1971). Pere Bougeant (1739) long ago recognized the capacity of dogs for laughter and joy in association with play:

> Is it not evident that beasts laugh very heartily? See a couple of young puppies romping together in a field, catching, toying, and fighting one another in jest. Can all this be done without laughing? Is it essential to laughing, that it be done, as in man, by a motion of the lips and mouth, with a convulsive sound of voice? Laughing is no more than an expression of joy, and that expression is necessarily different in the different species of animals. Man laughs after his own manner, and the dog after his. No matter whether it is by a sudden bursting of the voice, or by a simple motion of the ears or tail, or by some other like expression. (196)

Recently, Simonet and colleagues (2001) made recordings of these play sounds and found that playing them back to young dogs evokes a heightened readiness to engage in play behavior. Fox reported that, the play sound (e.g., hhuh, hhuh, hhuh) was imitated, dogs became highly aroused, causing them to withdraw, bark, or solicit play. The panting sound may serve to elicit generalized arousal and, when combined with play signals, help to educe play behaviors. Repetitive sounds appear to evoke increased activity in dogs (see *Sensory Preparedness* in Volume 1, Chapter 5), a finding that is consistent with the notion that such sounds may play a role in the process of evoking play behavior.

All episodes of play should have a clearly defined beginning and end. Normally, it is best that some object be the focus of play. A tennis ball with a handle is ideal for this pur-pose (see *Training and Play*, Chapter 1). A small amount of an odorant (e.g., orange or orange-lemon) can be put inside the ball, per-haps helping to generalize playful associations to other contexts and thereby helping to lower play thresholds. Although structured competitive play is beneficial, highly arousing or provocative tug-of-war games, associated with growling and hard sustained biting and snapping at the toy, may result in accidental scratches and bites. Competing over a tug object produces frustration, causing the puppy to pull harder and more aggressively. Systematically raising frustration levels or introducing an agitational element (e.g., tweaking) during bouts of competitive play can lead to an excitement overload in some dogs, perhaps precipitating an aggressive episode. This sort of behavior occurs and warrants appropriate precaution, but it is not the norm, and its occurrence may indicate the presence of significant emotional conflict, reactive dysregulation, or socialization deficits. When a trainer escalates the intensity of such behavior in conjunction with a puppy's increasing frustration and irritation, the puppy may learn to increase competitive output, becoming progressively tenacious and fearless. Under the influence of skilled training, such playful behavior can be gradually shaped into more serious and controlled aggression (e.g., police-dog training). Not fully recognizing the potential risks involved in playful competitive excesses, inexperienced dog owners may inadvertently promote excessive competitiveness in predisposed puppies. Despite the risks when improperly performed, tug games appear to provide a constructive outlet for competitive play, as stressed by Borchelt (1984):

> Although most puppies do growl during these games, it is a "play-growl" of quite different tone, intensity and significance than growls exhibited in an aggressive context. Conducted properly, the tug of war game will exhaust play behaviour and teach the puppy that mouthing and biting occur only with the toy in its mouth. Moreover, the interaction with the puppy (holding and pulling on the toy) eventually can be presented in brief bursts such that play is used to reward short durations of quiet, non-play behaviour. (172)

Enhancing the Leader-Follower Bond

Among young puppies, social relations and interactive boundaries are only loosely defined, exhibiting significant fluctuation and instability. As a result, hierarchical social distance between littermates may be weakly developed or vague, perhaps explaining the high levels of playful competitive interaction that typically occurs between them. The quality of early social competition appears to exercise a pronounced influence on how a puppy will later interact with people and other dogs after it is homed. As a consequence of early socialization experiences, most puppies come into the home with a set of established biases about what to expect from contact with others as well as possessing a well-practiced repertoire of playful competitive skills. The young dog does not naturally know or respect human social boundaries, but must learn directly from its interaction with people what is, and what is not, appropriate. The mother has given her puppies a solid foundation for inculcating such social learning, but everything depends on the owner taking over this canine educational process.

Upon coming into the home, the puppy may show a definite inclination to continue behavior that it has already learned and to refine its competitive skills further, often at the expense of the hands and clothing of family members. Since playful competitive activities appear to be highly reinforcing for puppies, it is of utmost importance that such behavior be blocked and redirected into more appropriate outlets. This is sometimes a hard-won step in a puppy's social education, but one that most certainly must be taken in order to ensure that the puppy becomes a welcome member of the family. To achieve this goal, the owner must provide the puppy with structured guidance, limit-setting directives, and positive instruction. Unfortunately, this process of social learning and adaptation is one that is commonly neglected, either as the result of misunderstanding or poor advice. Instead of becoming the object of affection and deference, the owner, failing to achieve the necessary social distance to become a leader, becomes a target of inappropriate social excesses. Owner contact needs, permissiveness, and tolerance provide an environment in which competitive behavior becomes exaggerated and progressively more difficult to control. In relatively gentle breeds (and individuals), the detrimental effects of such interaction may be limited to disrupting the leader-follower bond and impeding the acquisition of basic lessons needed to adapt harmoniously to life with people. However, in the case of more aggressive breeds and individuals, failure to exercise appropriate discipline, impose social distance, and assert leadership prerogatives may produce long-lasting and potentially serious consequences.

Establishing leadership does not entail or imply the use of hostile or provocative actions to dominate a puppy. Stimulation of excessive fear is counterproductive and destructive of social cooperation and trust. Scott (1992b) has argued that physical punishment is inappropriate for discouraging excessive competitive behavior in puppies. Instead of applying painful methods of physical punishment, he suggests that better inhibitory effects can be attained by the surprisingly simple means of restraint:

> In some of our experiments with dogs, we reared hundreds of puppies without using punishment, and were never attacked by them. What we did was to pick up the puppies almost daily, for various reasons. This began long before they were able to resist or fight, and they formed strong habits of relaxing peacefully in our arms. We could even break up a dogfight by picking up one or both of the contestants. (15)

Although submission and fear share some motivational overlap, they possess very different functional characteristics. In general, fear represents an adverse side effect of inappropriate techniques used to inculcate a subordinate attitude.

Good Things Must Be Earned

Among the most important lessons for oppositional puppies to learn are that *good things are better when earned* and, secondly, that *waiting is a canine virtue*. These central themes of puppy training entail that the desirable outcomes be made contingent on compromise and cooperation, in accordance with what Voith calls the Nothing In Life Is Free (NILIF) program (Voith, personal communication, 2002). The strategy includes controlling access to food, affection, exercise, opportunities for outings, play, and chew toys—in short, everything that a puppy may want can be used to shape more cooperative behavior. This training activity is integrated into everyday situations by exchanging rewards for compliance—thus the term *integrated compliance training* (ICT). Puppies should be trained from an early age to follow instructions and to develop a habit of compliant

waiting, training that helps to form a solid foundation of impulse control for all future training and socialization efforts. In addition, young puppies can easily master basic obedience skills, such as walking on leash, sit, down, come, and stay. Training puppies to obey with positive incentives involving affection, play, and encouragement is much more effective and enjoyable for both the puppy and the owner than using force to compel cooperation and compliance.

Establishing a strong orienting response is an important first step. A squeaker is used to capture the puppy's attention and, just as it orients toward the trainer, a click is delivered and immediately followed by a flick of the right hand to the side. As the puppy approaches the bridge, "Good" is delivered and the hand is opened for the puppy to take the treat. This pattern is repeated again and again until the orienting response is strongly conditioned. The next phase involves pairing the squeak, orienting response, click, and "Good" with positive prediction error, whereby the size, type, and timing of the reward are varied to produce surprise. In addition, the squeaker sound is varied by squeezing it sometimes once or twice, sometimes firmly, sometimes softly, sometimes very briefly, and so forth. Sometimes, instead of having the puppy come back to the hand, the trainer tosses the treat to the puppy just as it turns its head. At other times, the treat is concealed under the last two fingers so that when the first two fingers open the hand appears empty, but then, just at the moment the puppy appears to recognize the discrepancy, the trainer says "Good" and opens the last two fingers to reveal the treat. Orienting and bridge training provide an anchor from which an almost limitless set of modules, routines, and patterns of tremendous variety and complexity can be trained.

DIFFICULT PUPPIES: ESTABLISHING THE TRAINING SPACE

Establishing a training space is achieved by setting limits on three common disruptive excesses: jumping, biting, and pulling (see *The Training Space* in Chapter 1). In addition to limiting disruptive aspects of a puppy's behavior, this process results in the development of a beneficial degree of social distance between the owner and the puppy. Social distance emerges in the context of dyadic interaction and the formalization of social *roles* and *relations*. These social roles and relations are organized in accordance with various *rules* that govern the budgeted delivery of rewards and punishment. Intrusive excesses, such as biting and jumping up, behaviorally reflect a lack of organized social distance between the owner and the puppy—a necessary precondition for organizing rule-based roles and relations. Without the formation of appropriate social distance, a dog is prone to exhibit reactive social adjustments and develop an overly dependent attachment—not a harmonious relationship. On the other hand, extrusive excesses, such as pulling on the leash, strain the training space outwardly in the direction of attractive environmental stimuli competing for the puppy's attention and causing it to become distracted and pull. Fixing regulatory limits around intrusive and extrusive excesses is an essential step toward effective reward-based training efforts.

Pulling

A functional training space involving difficult puppies begins by training them to walk on a long line and a leash (see *Walking on Leash* in Chapter 1). Countless problems can be avoided or resolved by training puppies to actively follow the prompting of a leash. Pulling on the leash is inconsistent with the development of a healthy leader-follower bond and is productive of significant frustration and oppositional behavior. Pulling on walks has been associated with aggression problems in dogs (Podberscek and Serpell, 1997). Essentially, the leash is a physical representation or reification of the trainer's will. Instead of walking in a controlled and deferential manner, a pulling puppy is in continuous competition and conflict (opposition) with the owner for control. In contrast, a puppy that learns to walk with, rather than against, the owner appears to derive social bonding benefits from the exercise of

increased impulse control. The reward-based techniques used to encourage slack-leash walking or controlled walking serve to enhance the leader-follower bond, improve attention, and increase impulse-control abilities. The puppy first learns to walk on a long line in the context of attention and recall training. A well-conditioned squeaker or similar attention-controlling stimuli can be used to override most distractions. Using a squeaker and clicker can rapidly help to shape the habit of walking on leash without pulling. For most puppies, a flat collar and leash is adequate, whereas, in the case of more assertive puppies that pull hard, a fixed-action halter can be very helpful. The clamping action of muzzling halters seems to produce unnecessary distress in puppies, and since there is no real need for such clamping action, a nonclamping halter is better suited for puppy-training purposes. Gradually, by limiting pulling and by selectively reinforcing appropriate walking behaviors, the halter control is eliminated. As with crate training, the goal of halter training is to get rid of the head halter as soon as possible.

Body Boundary

In practice, the training space is defined by the establishment of limits around biting and mouthing, jumping up, and pulling on the leash. Social limits are first set around the trainer's body. Both puppies and dogs should learn not to jump onto the trainer's lap, back, or arms, or leap at the face. As the body boundary is respected, puppies can then be trained to jump up on signal, as a reward for waiting and respecting the limit being set on the behavior. During social boundary training, puppies should be kept on leash. With the handler sitting cross-legged on the floor, any effort by the puppy to come up on the trainer's lap is countered with "off!" and a forearm block, as needed to prevent access to the lap. The force of the action is determined by need, with some puppies requiring very little direction and others requiring a more assertive impression. Gradually, the prompting action is delayed and faded to a slight movement of the forearm as a warning, but the action may need to be reinstated if the puppy fails to respond to the faded prompt.

At the earliest sign of deference, the puppy is comforted and reassured with petting, gentle words, and food rewards (Figure 6.6). In the case of puppies showing a strong proclivity for biting on hands and clothing, a treat is held in a closed hand. As the puppy presses its nose against or licks the hand, the owner says "Good" in an affectionate tone and gives the treat to the puppy. This procedure is repeated with both right and left hands. Next, the puppy is encouraged to play tug with a tennis ball attached to a hand loop or other soft toys appropriate to the puppy's size and interest. After a brief tug game, a treat is offered to the puppy in exchange for the ball. When the ball is released, it is immediately thrown a few feet away and the puppy encouraged to retrieve it. As the puppy turns with the ball in its mouth, the owner should

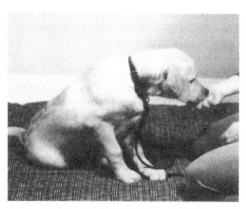

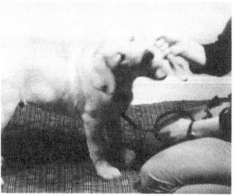

FIG. 6.6 Feeding by hand and ball play.

flick the closed right hand (containing a food reward) to the side to attract the puppy's attention. The puppy is encouraged to hurry back and to release the ball ("Out") in exchange for a treat. Again, the puppy is encouraged to play tug, release the ball, retrieve it, and is rewarded with a treat concealed in a closed hand. Once the pattern is well established, vocal signals can be presented at appropriate points in the process to help bring the pattern under stimulus control. For example, just before the puppy turns, the handler should say its name and smooch; as the puppy moves toward the trainer, "Come" is spoken in a friendly tone and, finally, the trainer says "Good" just before giving the treat to the eager retriever.

At some point, the ball is left on the trainer's lap. If the puppy attempts to jump up to take it without invitation, the trainer asserts "Off," followed by a delayed slight forearm movement or thrust prompt, as needed to defend the boundary. If the puppy defers, it is given a treat by hand and the ball play is resumed; if not, appropriate blocking actions are repeated until the puppy actively defers to the body boundary again. Once the puppy shows a stable deference to the limit set around the lap, it can be given permission to come up by the trainer snapping thumbs and gesturing upwardly toward his or her body and saying "Hup" as the puppy is lifted onto the lap. Permission to get up on the lap is periodically given as a special reward. While on the lap, the puppy is petted, massaged, and vocally reassured. If the puppy begins to mouth, it is immediately pushed off and is let up again only after deferring to the biting rule. Such puppies can often be calmed by petting under the neck and on the chest between the front legs.

Jumping Up

In addition to controlling the body boundary while sitting on the floor, puppies should also learn to refrain from jumping up while the trainer is standing upright. Since jumping up is normal and friendly behavior that is acceptable under certain circumstances, the goal of training is not to suppress jumping up, but rather to bring the jumping response under stimulus control, that is, establish a rule for its occurrence in the context of cooperative relations with the trainer. Puppies should be trained to jump up on signal (e.g., "Hup," with a thumb snap and upward movement of the hands) and to get off on signal (e.g., "Off," followed by downward movement of the hands). Puppies that jump up excessively can be trained with a differential reinforcement of other behavior (DRO) procedure, combined with a response-blocking procedure (e.g., stepping on the leash) and TO (see *Jumping Up* in Chapter 5). An alternative DRO training procedure involves delivering a click and treat after some variable but brief period (e.g., 2, 5, 3, 7, 2, and 3 seconds) and then occasionally dropping several small treats on the floor as a surprise. The treats should be very tiny and blend in with the flooring, thereby making it difficult for the puppy to find them. After dropping the treats, the trainer then helps the puppy locate them by pointing over the spots and making smooch sounds. Occasionally, as the puppy reaches the spot, the trainer might drop a choice treat, as though by accident, from the pointing hand to the floor. Dogs appear to have evolved an uncanny capacity to exploit our oversights, foibles, and clumsy moments, appearing to derive great pleasure when they do so successfully. The puppy is next trained to orient and make eye contact in response to its name, smooch, and click.

Once the foregoing introductory phase of training is carried out, the trainer should set the situation up in a way that the puppy might be tempted to jump up, but just as it prepares to do so, the trainer says "Off" in a firm buy quiet tone of voice. The trainer then abruptly glances to the side and tosses a treat to the floor in an exaggerated manner and then points until the puppy finds it. Next, the puppy is challenged to jump up with the challenge-dare "Do you want!" followed by a tap on the thigh or chest. But before the puppy has a chance to decide, the trainer says "Good" and tosses a treat to the side in the manner just described. Keeping the puppy on leash and stepping on the leash, as needed, in anticipation of the puppy jumping up can help to make this lesson easier to learn. For overly active and intrusive puppies, this pro-cedure trains a habit of moving away from guests in response to the pointing signal and is good preliminary training for the go-lie-down exercise.

Mouthing and Biting

Like jumping up, puppy biting and mouthing on hands and clothing are usually playful social behaviors that have become excessive, often as a result of inappropriate control efforts or inadvertent reinforcement. Whenever possible, the best strategy is to shape gradually an acceptable playful outlet while simultaneously discouraging biting with means appropriate to the puppy's temperament and responsiveness to training. Although most puppies can rapidly learn to limit their tugging and biting to play objects, some may exhibit a persistent preference for biting on hands and clothing. Setting the lap and body boundary as previously described is a constructive first step toward controlling this common nuisance behavior. By establishing a body boundary, the owner can simply withdraw the hands to the safety of his or her lap, thereby setting up a response cost contingency to further discourage mouthing or biting. Also, various reward-based training procedures can be used to cause puppies to emit behavior incompatible with mouthing and biting. Puppies showing a strong oral avidity should be transitionally trained to interact with the owner via a toy (e.g., a ball or soft toy). The toy provides a triangulated object relation by which some of the puppy's playful social competitiveness and energy can be deflected or reorganized. In a sense, dog toys serve a similar function as transitional objects, as teddy bears do for young children. Dogs appear to treat toys as though they are partially animated, becoming joy-producing prey or objects of competition, especially as the result of interactive play with the trainer. Interactive object play appears to stimulate canine fantasy, mediating an object relation with the dog that the trainer can connect up with and guide to gradually transition the puppy toward a more realistic and rule-based relationship.

For some puppies, a startling tone of voice or expression of discomfort followed by the introduction of some other activity (e.g., prompting the puppy to play a tug-and-fetch game) may be sufficient to control mouthing and biting excesses, whereas, in the case of more aggressive and competitive puppies, more assertive means may be necessary to discourage the activity. An active-control line can be used to turn the puppy away (TO) when it becomes overly intrusive and bites at the hands. As the puppy calms down, it can be called by name and tossed a ball to retrieve before being called back to engage in a bout of tug. Again, the amount of force used during such training is determined by a puppy's response and need. Often a reprimand ("Enough") or gentle prompt on the control line is sufficient to interrupt the activity and to turn the puppy's attention toward a more appropriate outlet (e.g., ball play). The prompting action should be sufficient to turn the puppy away, but need not be overly threatening or fear eliciting. Following such events, the trainer should challenge the puppy with the back of the right hand, held just in front of its nose, and in a daring and clipped tone state firmly "Do you want!" At such times, the puppy should yield an appeasement lick or avert its head, at which point the handler should reassure it with affectionate petting, gentle talk, and a food reward. Allowing the puppy to gnaw on a biscuit held so that only a small portion of it can be taken at a time provides a source of sustained reward, during which time the trainer can pet the puppy under its neck and chest. Subsequently, the challenge-dare can be used preemptively whenever there is an increased likelihood that the puppy is about to mouth or bite. The challenge can also be used to interrupt low-grade mouthing efforts. Whenever practical, mouthing on hands is best handled by reducing it gradually, granting the puppy some playful and affectionate mouthing allowance, so long as it shows a reliable willingness to defer when required to do so and it properly respects limits with regard to bite inhibition.

In the case of persistent or highly competitive puppies that escalate their efforts when thwarted, repeated 15- to 30-second TOs are used to reduce arousal and to discourage the behavior (see *Using Time-out to Modify Behavior* in Volume 1, Chapter 8). At the conclusion of each TO, the puppy is returned to the situation, prompted to sit, challenged, and reinforced with affectionate petting and other rewards, such as a tug-and-fetch game, when it defers. However, if the puppy attempts to bite instead, the trainer says "Enough, Time-out," and the TO procedure is repeated again and again (e.g., three to four times), until a de-arousal effect is observed. Rhythmic stroking on the neck and underside of the chest can also be helpful to induce a calming effect in many puppies. In some cases, a DRO procedure can be extremely useful as a means to moderate arousal levels. As control is established, a tug-and-fetch game can be offered as an alternative outlet for competitive play. In other puppies, an orienting response to a squeaker is formed in the manner previously discussed (see *Good Things Must Be Earned*). Once the squeaker is conditioned as a strong orienting stimulus, the squeaker can be used to interrupt mouthing. Just as the puppy stops, a click is delivered and a treat is given from a closed hand. To accomplish this training, the squeaker is held in the left hand under the last two fingers while the clicker is held between the first two fingers and the thumb. The back of the right hand is presented to the puppy and, as it orients, a click and treat is delivered. This pattern is repeated, and the puppy gradually learns to orient on the hand as a targeting stimulus. After taking food rewards, the trainer should pet and rub the puppy under its neck and chest. Repeated rewards involving food and petting appear to recruit a calming effect, perhaps via the conditioned and unconditioned release of oxytocin (see *Origin of Reactive versus Adaptive Coping Styles* in Chapter 4). As the puppy learns to follow the hand, it can be held over the puppy's head to prompt it to sit, moved downward to cause it to lie down, and so forth. The puppy is trained to sit, lie down, sit from the down, and stand from the sit, with vocal signals, bridge, and treat delivered at each step. If at any point the puppy attempts to mouth, the squeaker is used (sometimes softly and sometimes with a sharp squeeze) to interrupt the behavior, whereupon the trainer clicks, rewards the puppy, and initiates another series of basic training exercises or a tug-and-fetch game.

A collar control-and-thrust procedure can also be used in some persistent cases where less coercive methods have failed. The collar control is established by taking the leash at about 10 inches from the collar. The leash is wrapped once over the thumb and then gripped by closing the last two fingers of the left hand over it. Next, as the puppy continues to bite, the collar is abruptly taken with the right hand at approximately 4 o'clock and held with all four fingers closed around it. The left hand is then opened (except for the last two fingers holding the leash) and placed securely behind the puppy's head. Care should be taken not to grab the puppy's skin or fur while setting the collar control. With the collar control in place, the trainer makes direct eye contact and delivers a barklike reprimand "Enough," followed by a forward thrusting action. The thrusting action is delivered by tightening and immediately relaxing the muscles of the hands, arms, shoulders in an abrupt and concerted movement. If the puppy defers, it is then challenged to produce a submission response (e.g., appeasement lick or head-averting action)—behavior that is immediately followed by affectionate reassurance and petting. If the puppy escalates in response to the collar-control thrust, the control is released and the puppy is abruptly hauled off to TO. As the puppy defers and accepts petting without biting, the collar control is taken up periodically; however, instead of following it with a direct stare and assertive forward thrust, it is paired with affectionate eye contact, a smile, and rhythmic massage around the jaw muscles with the thumbs. In addition to reinforcing submissive behavior, affectionate petting and gentle talk can help to reassure the puppy that the handler remains a source of comfort and safety. At this juncture, a cycle of PFR training should be initiated. PFR training promotes relaxation and subordination to manual control (Figure 6.7) (see Appendix C).

Although hard mouthing and biting should be discouraged, the puppy should be gradually taught to mouth and bite on the hands in more gentle ways, by using the vocal signal "Gentle" to modulate the pressure of biting actions. Also, the puppy should be frequently encouraged to lick the trainer's cheek, or ear, with appropriate care

taken and common sense exercised at all times to avoid taking unnecessary risks in this regard with puppies exhibiting unusually strong or aggressive mouthing and biting

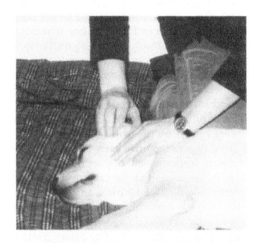

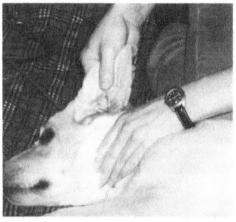

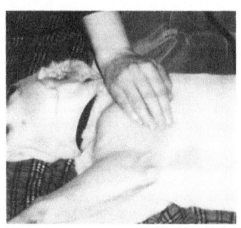

FIG. 6.7 Puppy massage.

proclivities. Any nipping at the face should be promptly and firmly discouraged, while at the same times rewarding licking with sweet talk and an affectionate caress. Most puppies, even the most persistent and excitable ones, show a clear differentiation of behavior toward the hands and face. At one moment, they can be vigorously mouthing on hands, but immediately stop as the cheek is offered to them to kiss, whereupon they often lick or nibble at the ear, as well. Puppies that lack this apparent species-typical differentiation of biting and licking behavior—that is, biting equally on the hands and face—should receive intensive early training. Another developmental marker that should trigger concern and initiate appropriate training and socialization efforts is an active unwillingness to establish and to briefly hold eye contact (see *Social Engagement and Attunement* in Chapter 8). The presence of such behavior may represent a significant adjustment marker and should be the topic of future study.

OLFACTORY CONDITIONING AND EXCESSIVE BITING

The introduction of an exciting food odor by a squeeze bulb can be useful in the control of some mouthing excesses that occur in association heightened emotional arousal. The activation of the olfactory system with the smell of an exciting food appears to exert a modulatory effect over the amygdala and hypothalamus, while strongly stimulating the ventral tegmental area, a brain area believed to play a prominent role in mediating reward. A strong-smelling cheese such as Romano or Parmesan can be cut into fine slivers and put inside a baby aspirator bulb. Sniffing the odor may interrupt the unwanted behavior briefly as well as perform an establishing-operation function, making the puppy more likely to show behavior previously conditioned with food reinforcement. For a hungry animal, the opportunity to smell food represents a significant incentive and potential source of reinforcement. With regard to the potency of appetitive olfactory stimuli, Long and Tapp (1967) found that hungry rats exhibit a pronounced increase in responding when reinforced with the smell of a familiar food:

The response rates elicited by the deprived animals for the odor of powdered food were quite high in comparison with most other rewards. To the authors' knowledge, no other rewarding events, except electrical stimulation of the brain and escape from foot shock, have been shown to be such effective reinforcers when delivered on a similar schedule. (18)

In other cases, a novel odor can be delivered from a squeaker bulb or modified carbon dioxide (CO_2) pump. Orange and lavender appear to exert mild focusing and calmative influences on many puppies; chamomile, ylang-ylang, and sandalwood also appear to be useful, but adequate research is lacking. The fragrant odor appears to produce an abrupt, if only temporary, modulation of competitive tone, sometimes producing a rather dramatic effect when presented together with the squeaker or modified CO_2 pump (see *Olfactory Conditioning*). Olfactory control appears to work better when it is delivered in the form of repeated discrete odor puffs rather than as a continuous background odor. In addition to odors that appear to exert transient focusing and calming effects, odors can be used to mediate a conditioned inhibitory effect. A conditioned inhibitory odor is established by pairing a dilute odor (e.g. citronella-eucalyptus or eucalyptus-cedarwood) with the hissing sound of a modified CO_2 pump. The selected odor is diluted 1:30-50, and a small amount of it is dabbed on a cotton wad packed gently inside the base of a inflator needle that has had the needle removed (see *Compressed Air* in Chapter 2). The scented oil is blown out of the cotton into a tissue, leaving the cotton scented but dry.

The conditioning procedure is carried out by carefully squeezing the pump lever to release an inaudible or barely audible airflow, concealed from the puppy's view and directed toward the floor—not toward the puppy. The scented airflow is continued for approximately 2 to 3 seconds before a half-second puff/hiss of compressed air is delivered to interrupt mouthing (Figure 6.8). The startle used for such training can be very effective when delivered at relatively low levels of stimulation. The puppy is immediately challenged with the back of the hand, "Do you want!" If the puppy averts its head, the response is bridged and rewarded; whereas, if the puppy fails to defer, the conditioned odor is presented again via a squeaker bulb (squeaker valve removed). If the puppy continues to mouth, a second conditioning event is delivered using a hiss/spritz level of compressed-air startle, followed by the same challenge-dare procedure. Once the puppy defers, the behavior is rewarded, and the puppy is brought up on the trainer's lap. If the puppy begins to bite or mouth while on the trainer's lap, the conditioned odor is delivered from a squeaker bulb, and it is pushed away. The challenge-dare procedure is performed and, if the puppy defers, it is rewarded; if not, the odor is delivered from the squeaker bulb, and the puppy is rushed off to TO, followed by training activities, as described previously. A crumpled tissue scented with the conditioned odor can be placed in the TO room in advance to further integrate the significance of the odor as an inhibitory signal. Once the conditioned odor is established, it can be used to produce a

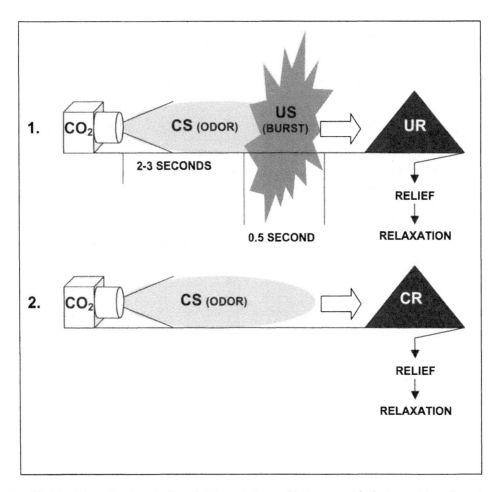

FIG. 6.8. Classical conditioning of odor and air burst. Odors are highly prepared for both appetitive and aversive classical conditioning in dogs. In cases involving persistent biting excesses not responsive to other training efforts, an olfactory conditioning procedure can be highly effective as a means to interrupt such behavior. After one or two conditioning bursts, the odor delivered at a low pressure or from a squeaker bulb (without the squeak mechanism) may cause a puppy to become more responsive to other control efforts. US, unconditioned stimulus; UR, unconditioned response; CS, conditioned stimulus; and CR, conditioned response.

direct inhibitory effect (Otto et al., 1997) or to potentiate other startle techniques (Paschall and Davis, 2002).

Posture-facilitated Relaxation

Before coming into the home, the average puppy is exposed to a tremendous amount of competitive interaction with littermates, somatically attuning and sensitizing it to respond to tactile stimulation and manual control with increased arousal, excitement, and playful competitive behavior. In addition, the puppy may be accustomed to a high level of social stimulation no longer available to it, thereby triggering unwelcome attention-seeking excesses and intrusive competitive behavior. The owner may be confused and frustrated by the puppy's incessant search for stimulation and its prodigious appetite for competitive play, possibly leading to improper disciplinary practices, excessive crate confinement, and other practices inimical to healthy socialization and habituation. There is no justification for slapping or spanking an overly competitive or aggressive puppy, especially since such actions may only cause the puppy to retaliate with even more vigorous aggressive behavior or become progressively insular and avoidant. Threatening dominance procedures wherein a puppy is flipped on its back and pinned there against its fearful or angry protests should also be avoided unless necessitated by extraordinary circumstances requiring such restraint. Although occasional mild to moderate assertions of manual control may be expedient to avert an escalation of aggressive tensions, excessively forceful or threatening handling does little to inhibit aggressive behavior constructively. Such puppies should be provided with appropriate play and exercise, daily reward-based training, and routine limits set on inappropriate behavior via TO and response-blocking procedures. In addition, competitive and stimulation-seeking puppies should be exposed to graduated relaxation exercises aimed at reducing agitation and modulating competitive tensions. Instead of relying on excessively forceful or threatening tactics, submissive behavior can be gently and efficiently facilitated through graduated

posture control and relaxation training, a process known as PFR training. When properly and routinely performed, PFR training produces several benefits (see *Basic Guidelines and PFR Techniques* in Appendix C):

1. Facilitates bonding process
2. Enhances trainability
3. Exerts beneficial counterconditioning effects
4. Promotes affection, cooperation, and trust

Taction and Posture-facilitated Relaxation

Tuber (1986) has emphasized the value of massage for promoting calmness and relaxation in dogs, advising that massage and training dogs to relax should be just as important as other training activities. Petting and massage have long been recognized as exerting significant effects on canine cardiovascular activity indicative of reduced sympathetic arousal (see *Effect of Person* in Volume 1, Chapter 9). Petting provides a potent source of reward for many dogs. Kostarczyk and Fonberg (1982) found that dogs that respond to petting as a reward exhibit cardiac deceleration while being petted, followed by rapid acceleration when petting is discontinued. The experimenters report that dogs failing to respond to petting as a reward exhibited cardiac acceleration when petted (Figure 6.9). These observations suggest the possibility that heart-rate changes in response to petting may provide useful diagnostic markers pertaining to contact aversion and proneness to irritability as the result of tactile stimulation. In the case of dogs that are responsive to petting as a reward, petting may induce sympathetic de-arousal and cardiac deceleration via the recruitment of an antistress response (see *Oxytocin-opioidergic Hypothesis*).

Odendaal (1999 and 2000) has reported that close social interaction between people and dogs results in a cascade of neurobiological events that facilitate enhanced attachment and comfort. Close social contact and petting produce an elevation of circulating neuropeptides (ß-endorphin, oxytocin, and prolactin) and other neurochemicals believed to mediate pleasure (e.g. phenylethylamine), affiliative emotions, and social attachment. Oxytocin is

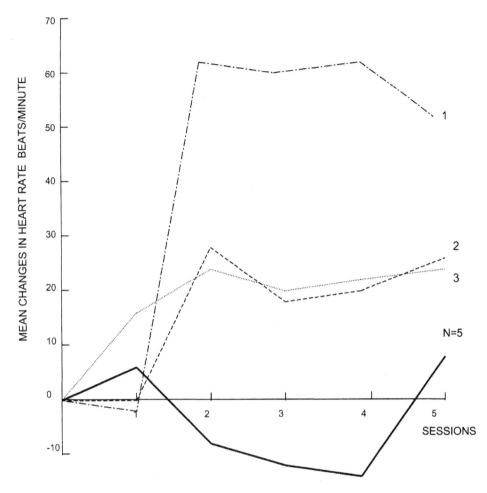

FIG. 6.9. When petting is effective as an instrumental reward, it produces a deceleration effect on heart rate. Dogs that do not respond to petting as a reward exhibit an opposite response. When petted, such dogs may exhibit pronounced heart-rate acceleration. The solid line shows the mean heart-rate changes calculated for five dogs that were responsive to petting. Broken lines 1, 2, and 3 indicate the acceleration effects of petting exhibited by three dogs not responsive to petting.

believed to actively mediate social bonding and to exert pronounced cardiovascular changes and antistress effects (Uvnäs-Moberg, 1998b), while exerting a potent diminutional effect over irritability (Lund et al., 2002) and aggression (Panksepp, 1998), "reducing all forms of aggression that have been studied" (257).

Hennessy and colleagues (1998) have reported that it is not just petting, but the way in which petting is done, that yields the best stress-reducing effects. They found that petting consisting of long, firm strokes pro-

duces the strongest effect on HPA-axis activity (Figure 6.10). Whereas light touch tends to increase arousal (e.g., tickling effect) or irritation, firm and continuous touch appears to produce a calming effect. Grandin (1992) has noted that deep-touch pressure (massage and firm petting) appears to alleviate the touch aversion exhibited by many autistic persons. Grandin, an autistic person, developed a "squeeze machine" to deliver continuous pressure over large areas of the body. She claims that the machine produces benefits, partly because one cannot pull away from it

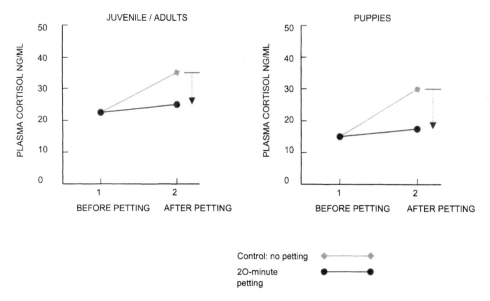

FIG. 6.10. Effect of petting on stress response to venipuncture. Petting involving firm, long, and slow strokes helps to restrain physiological stress when taking blood. Both control and petted groups had blood taken at point 1. Controls were returned to their kennels, while the other received 20 minutes of petting. Adapted from Hennessy et al. (1998).

(response prevention), making a previously aversive experience a more enjoyable one. In addition to becoming less aggressive and tense, she reported becoming more receptive of human touch and gentler in her own touching contacts with others, including a pet cat:

> Using the machine enabled me to learn to tolerate being touched by another person.... It made me feel less aggressive and less tense. Soon I noticed a change in our cat's reaction to me. The cat, who used to run away from me now would stay with me, because I had learned to caress him with a gentler touch. I had to be comforted before I could give comfort to the cat. (66)

Field (1995) found that premature babies given tactile stimulation consisting of light stroking failed to gain weight, whereas babies given massage consisting of firm stroking gained weight. In addition, Field and colleagues (1996) also demonstrated that massage therapy helps to alleviate stress-related physiological and behavioral symptoms exhibited by babies born to depressed mothers. Brief massage performed twice a week for 6 weeks significantly reduced cortisol, norepinephrine, and epinephrine levels while increasing serotonin activity. These physiological changes were associated with increased contact responsiveness and sociability in the infants. Massage has been shown to reduce anxiety and symptoms of depression in child and adolescent psychiatric patients, further reinforcing the value of massage as a therapeutic modality (Field et al., 1991). Gantt (1944) observed that petting exerted a potent inhibitory effect over conditioned anxiety in severely disturbed dogs (see *Tactile Stimulation and Adaptation*).

Posture, Response Prevention, and Posture-facilitated Relaxation

Together with supplemental environmental enrichment, exercise, play, daily training activities, and guided tactile stimulation, gentle manual control and restraint efforts help modulate a puppy's social competitive and stimulation needs. The aim of manual control is to shape behavior conducive to progressive submission and relaxation. Posture communicates behavioral intention and reflects underlying emotional and motivation states. Body posture and emotion exert a reciprocal influence on each other via somatic feedback. Consequently, the expression and experience of emotional states necessarily involve postural and gestural changes—*there are no disembodied emotions*. The manipulation of posture through guided controls, prompts, and position shifts is associated with the controlled evocation of a variety of emotional states. Response prevention assists in this process by blocking bodily responses incompatible with submissive relaxation. In addition, manual restraint exerts a pronounced calming effect and deceleration of heart rate—an effect that is magnified by petting and massage.

Gradually, instead of evoking competitive reactivity and resistance, the puppy learns to submit to handling as a source of increased comfort and safety. Response prevention and restraint assist in this process by blocking responses incompatible with submissive affection and relaxation. During the imposition of gentle manual restraint, the puppy is exposed to mild limit-setting actions (dominance) in the presence of the counterconditioning influence of massage and vocal reassurance. Postural restraint in combination with relaxing massage helps to reduce agitation by promoting more organized and compliant responsiveness to human control and manipulation.

Most puppies actively enjoy massage and accept PFR training without incident. However, in the case of difficult puppies, depending on individual differences, one of three typical responses to gentle manual restraint and massage may occur: submissive forbearance, competitive struggle, or efforts to escape. The manual restraint at such times should be consistent and clear but not overtly intimidating or threatening. Further, the level of force used to restrain the puppy should be immediately responsive to the puppy's willingness to defer. In cases involving extreme reactivity, preliminary desensitization and instrumental shaping procedures should be used first to encourage compliance and trust. The presentation of a fragrant odor (e.g., orange, chamomile, or sandalwood) may exert a useful calming or diversionary effect. Throughout the PFR process, the puppy is reassured and comforted

with relaxing massage. The operative idea is to use response prevention and the accumulative effects of relaxing massage to help the puppy accept the next level of control with minimum reactivity, thereby improving its willingness to submit and, ultimately, achieving enhanced feelings of affection, comfort, safety, and relaxation. Over the course of several cycles of PFR training, the puppy learns to accept and enjoy the systematic, highly structured, and predictable manual control efforts composing the PFR ritual, becoming progressively relaxed and compliant. PFR training can be effectively incorporated into routine care and grooming activities. All puppies should learn to accept being brushed and combed, having their eyes and ears examined and cleaned, and having their feet handled and cleaned, and submit to nail clipping and filing. Massage-induced relaxation makes these grooming chores easier to perform and less stressful for puppies and dogs.

REFERENCES

Ader R and Cohen N (1985). CNS-immune system interactions: Conditioning phenomena. *Behav Brain Sci*, 8:379–394.

Adolphs R (2001). The neurobiology of social cognition. *Curr Opinion Neurobiol*, 11:231–239.

Ågren G (1997). Olfactory cues from an oxytocin-injected male rat can induce anti-nociception in its cagemate. *NeuroReport*, 8:3073–3076.

Anderson DE and Brady JV (1971). Preavoidance blood pressure elevations accompanied by heart rate decreases in the dog. *Science*, 172:595–597.

Artigas F, Celada P, Laruelle M, and Adell A (2001). How does pindolol improve antidepressant action? *Trends Pharmacol Sci*, 22:224–228.

Azmitia EC and McEwen BS (1974). Adrenal cortical influence on rat brain tryptophan hydroxylase activity. *Brain Res*, 78:291–302.

Ben-Michael J, Korzilius HPLM, Felling AJA, and Vossen JMH (2000a). Disciplining behavior of dog owners in problematic situations: The factor structure. *Anthrozoös*, 13:104–112.

Ben-Michael J, Korzilius HPLM, Felling AJA, and Vossen JMH (2000b). An exploratory model of dog disciplining. *Anthrozoös*, 13:150–163.

Birnbaum SG, Podell DM, and Arnsten AF (2000). Noradrenergic alpha-2 receptor agonists reverse working memory deficits induced by the anxiogenic drug, FG7142, in rats. *Pharmacol Biochem Behav*, 67:397–403.

Blanchard RJ, McKittrick CR, and Blanchard DC (2001). Animal models of social stress: Effects on behavior and brain neurochemical systems. *Physiol Behav*, 73:261–271.

Blatteis CM and Li S (2000). Pyrogenic signaling via vagal afferents: What stimulates their receptors? *Auton Neurosci*, 85:66–71.

Blier P and De Montigny C (1994). Current advances and trends in the treatment of depression. *Trends Pharmacol Sci*, 15:220–226.

Borchelt PL (1984). Behaviour development of the puppy in the home environment. In RS Anderson (Ed), *Nutrition and Behavior in Dogs and Cats: Proceedings of the First Nordic Symposium on Small Animal Veterinary Medicine.* New York: Pergamon.

Borovikova LV, Ivanova S, Zhang M, et al. (2000). Vagus nerve stimulation attenuates the systemic inflammatory response to endotoxin. *Nature*, 405:458–462.

Bougeant P (1739). On the language of beasts. *Gentleman's Mag*, 9:194–196.

Braff L, Geyer MA, and Swerdlow NR (2001). Human studies of prepulse inhibition of startle: Normal subjects, patient groups, and pharmacological studies. *Psychopharmacology*, 156:234–258.

Brown DC, Perkowski SZ, Shofer F, and Amico JA (2001). Effect of centrally administered opioid receptor agonists on CSF and plasma oxytocin concentrations in dogs. *Am J Vet Res*, 62:496–499.

Burgdorf J and Panksepp J (2001). Tickling induces reward in adolescent rats. *Physiol Behav*, 72:167–173.

Cairns RB (1972). Fighting and punishment from a developmental perspective. In *Nebraska Symposium on Motivation.* New York: University of Nebraska Press.

Candland DK (1993). *Feral Children and Clever Animals: Reflections on Human Nature.* New York: Oxford University Press.

Candland DK, Taylor DB, Dresdale L, et al. (1969). Heart rate, aggression, and dominance in the domestic chicken. *J Comp Physiol Psychol*, 67:70–76.

Candland DK, Bryan DC, Nazar BL, et al. (1970). Squirrel monkey heart rate during formation of status orders. *J Comp Physiol Psychol*, 70:417–423.

Cattell RB and Korth B (1973). The isolation of temperament dimensions in dogs. *Behav Biol*, 9:15–30.

Cheal ML and Sprott RL (1971). Social olfaction: A review of the role of olfaction in a variety of animal behaviors. *Psychol Rep*, 29:195–243.

Clutton-Brock TH and Parker GA (1995). Punishment in animal societies. *Nature*, 373:209–216.

Cook CJ (2002). Glucocorticoid feedback increases the sensitivity of the limbic system to stress. *Physiol Behav*, 75:455–464.

Cooke B and Ernst E (2000). Aromatherapy: A scientific review. *Br J Gen Pract*, 50:493–496.

Cooke B, Hegstrom CD, Villeneuve LS, and Breedlove SM (1998). Sexual differentiation of the vertebrate brain: Principles and mechanisms. *Front Neuroendocrinol*, 19:323–362.

Cremers TIFH, Wiersma LJ, Fokko J, et al. (2001). Is the beneficial antidepressant effect of coadministration of pindolol really due to somatodendritic autoreceptor antagonism? *Biol Psychiatry*, 50:13–21.

De Felipe C, Herrero JF, O'Brien JA, et al. (1998). Altered nociception, analgesia, and aggression in mice lacking the receptor for substance P. *Nature*, 392:394–397.

Delville Y, Mansour KM, and Ferris CF (1996). Testosterone facilitates aggression by modulating receptors in the hypothalamus. *Physiol Behav*, 60:25–29.

Denny MR (1976). Post-aversive relief and relaxation and their implications for behavior therapy. *J Behav Ther Exp Psychiatry*, 7:315–321.

Dess NK, Linwick D, Patterson J, et al. (1983). Immediate and proactive effects of controllability and predictability on plasma cortisol responses to shock in dogs. *Behav Neurosci*, 97:1005–1016.

Diaz-Cabiale Z, Petersson M, Narvaez JA, et al. (2000). Systemic oxytocin treatment modulates alpha 2-adrenoceptors in telencephalic and diencephalic regions of the rat. *Brain Res*, 887:421–425.

Dmitrieva TN, Oades RD, Hauffa BP, and Eggers C (2001). Dehydroepiandrosterone sulphate and corticotropin levels are high in young male patients with conduct disorder: Comparison for growth factors, thyroid, and gonadal hormones. *Neuropsychobiology*, 43:134–140.

Dodman NH, Donnelly R, Shuster L, et al. (1996). Use of fluoxetine to treat dominance aggression in dogs. *JAVMA*, 209:1585–1587.

Donovan CA (1967). Some clinical observations on sexual attraction and deterrence in dogs and cattle. *Vet Med Small Anim Clin*, Nov:1047–1051.

Dreschel NA (2002). The effects of the immune system on behavior. In *Annual Symposium of Animal Behavior Research, AVSAB Proceedings*, July 14, Nashville, TN.

Dunbar I (1978). The development of social hierarchies in domestic dogs [Abstract]. *Appl Anim Ethol*, 4:290–291.

Dunn AJ, Wang J, and Ando T (1999). Effects of cytokines on cerebral neurotransmission: Comparison with the effects of stress. *Adv Exp Med Biol*, 461:1117–1127.

Edney ATB (1993). Dogs and human epilepsy. *Vet Rec*, 132:337–338.

Eichelman B (1987). Neurochemical bases of aggressive behavior. *Psychiatr Ann*, 17:371–374.

Engelmann M, Ebner K, Landgraf R, et al. (1999). Emotional stress triggers intrahypothalamic but not peripheral release of oxytocin in male rats. *Neuroendocrinology*, 11:867–872.

Epple G and Herz RS (1999). Ambient odors associated to failure influence cognitive performance in children. *Dev Psychobiol*, 35:103–107.

Ermisch A, Barth T, Ruhie HJ, et al. (1985). On the blood-brain barrier to peptides: Accumulation of labeled vasopressin, des-glyNH$_2$-vasopressin, and oxytocin by brain regions. *Endocrinol Exp*, 19:29–37.

Fallon BA, Nields JA, Parsons B, et al. (1993). Psychiatric manifestations of Lyme borreliosis. *J Clin Psychiatry*, 54:263–268.

Feifel D and Reza T (1999). Oxytocin modulates psychotomimetic-induced deficits in sensorimotor gating. *Psychopharmacology*, 141:93–98.

Ferris CF and Delville Y (1994). Vasopressin and serotonin interactions in the control of agonistic behavior. *Psychoneuroendocrinology*, 19:593–601.

Ferris CF, Melloni RH Jr, Koppel G, et al. (1997). Vasopressin/serotonin interactions in the anterior hypothalamus control of aggressive behavior in golden hamsters. *J Neurosci*, 17:4331–4340.

Field T (1995). Massage therapy for infants and children. *Dev Behav Pediatr*, 16:105–111.

Field T, Morrow C, Valdeon C, et al. (1991). Massage reduces anxiety in child and adolescent psychiatric patients. *J Am Acad Child Adolesc Psychiatry*, 31:125–131.

Field T, Grizzle N, Scafidi F, et al. (1996). Massage therapy for infants of depressed mothers. *Infant Behav Dev*, 19:107–112.

Fisher AE (1955). The effects of early differential treatment on the social and exploratory behavior of puppies [Unpublished doctoral dissertation]. State College: Pennsylvania State University.

Fonberg E (1988). Dominance and aggression. *Int J Neurosci*, 41:201–213.

Fonberg E, Kostarczyk E, and Prechtl J (1981). Training of instrumental responses in dogs socially reinforced by humans. *Pavlovian J Biol Sci*, 16:183–193.

Fox MW (1971). *Behaviour of Wolves, Dogs and Related Canids*. New York: Harper and Row.

Fuller JL (1967). Experiential deprivation and later behavior. *Science*, 158:1645–1652.

Fuller JL (1973). Genetics and vulnerability to experiential deprivation. In JP Scott and EC Senay (Eds), *Separation and Depression: Clinical and Research Aspects* [Symposium Proceedings]. Washington, DC: American Association of Advanced Sciences.

Fuller RW (1981). Serotonergic stimulation of pituitary-adrenocortical function in rats. *Neuroendocrinology*, 32:118–127.

Fuller RW, Perry KW, Hemrick-Luecke SK, and Engleman E (1996). Serum corticosterone increases reflect enhanced uptake inhibitor-induced elevation of extracellular 5-hydroxytryptamine in rat hypothalamus. *J Pharm Pharmacol*, 48:68–70.

Gaebelein CJ, Galosy RA, Botticelli L, et al. (1977). Blood pressure and cardiac changes during signaled and unsignalled avoidance in dogs. *Physiol Behav*, 19:69–74.

Gantt WH (1944). *Experimental Basis for Neurotic Behavior: Origin and Development of Artificially Produced Disturbances of Behavior in Dogs*. New York: Paul B Hoeber.

Gantt WH (1971). Experimental basis for neurotic behavior. In HD Kimmel (Ed), *Experimental Psychopathology: Recent Research and Theory*. New York: Academic.

Gariépy JL, Bauer DJ, and Cairns RB (2001). Selective breeding for differential aggression in mice provides evidence for heterochrony in social behaviors. *Anim Behav*, 61:933–947.

George DT, Hibbeln JR, Ragan PW, et al. (2000). Lactate-induced rage and panic in a select group of subjects who perpetrate acts of domestic violence. *Biol Psychiatry*, 47:804–812.

Glickman LT, Glickman NW, Schellengerg DB, et al. (2000). Incidence of and breed-related risk factors for gastric dilatation-volvulus in dogs. *JAVMA*, 216:40–45.

Goodloe LP and Borchelt PL (1998). Companion dog temperament traits. *J Appl Anim Welfare Sci*, 1:303–338.

Graham FK and Clifton RK (1966). Heart-rate change as a component of the orienting response. *Psychol Bull*, 65:305–320.

Grandin T (1992). Calming effects of deep touch pressure in patients with autistic disorder, college students, and animals. *J Child Adolesc Psychopharmacol*, 2:1992.

Granger DA, Hood KE, Dreschel NA, et al. (2001). Developmental effects of early immune stress on aggressive, socially reactive, and inhibited behaviors. *Dev Psychopathol*, 13:599–610.

Gregg TR and Siegel A (2001). Brain structures and neurotransmitters regulating aggression in cats: Implications for human aggression. *Prog Neuropsychopharmacol Biol Psychiatry*, 25:91–140.

Guy NC, Luescher UA, Dohoo SE, et al. (2001). Risk factors for dog bites to owners in a general veterinary caseload. *Appl Anim Behav Sci*, 74:29–42.

Haemisch A (1990). Coping with social conflict, and short-term changes of plasma cortisol titers in familiar and unfamiliar environments. *Physiol Behav*, 47:1265–1270.

Hare B and Tomasello M (1999). Domestic dogs (*Canis familiaris*) use human and conspecific social cues to locate food. *J Comp Psychol*, 113:173–177.

Hare B, Brown M, Williamson C, and Tomasello M (2002). The domestication of social cognition. *Science*, 298:1634–1636.

Hart BL (1985). *The Behavior of Domestic Animals*. New York: Freeman.

Hart BL and Hart LA (1985). Selecting pet dogs on the basis of cluster analysis of breed behavior profiles and gender. *JAVMA*, 186:1181–1185.

Hart BL and Hart LA (1997). Selecting, raising, and caring for dogs to avoid problem aggression. *JAVMA*, 210:1129–1134.

Hayley S, Lacosta S, Merali Z, et al. (2001). Central monoamine and plasma corticosterone changes induced by a bacterial endotoxin: Sensitization and cross-sensitization effects. *Eur J Neurosci*, 13:1155–1165.

Hendricks TJ, Fyodorov DV, Wegman LJ, et al. (2002). Pet-1 ETS gene plays a critical role in 5-HT neuron development and is required for normal anxiety-like and aggressive behavior. *Neuron*, 37:233–247.

Hennessy MB, Williams MT, Miller DD, et al. (1998). Influence of male and female petters on plasma cortisol and behaviour: Can human interaction reduce the stress of dogs in a public animal shelter? *Appl Anim Behav Sci*, 61:63–77.

Hennessy MB, Voith VL, Mazzei SJ, et al. (2001). Behavior and cortisol levels of dogs in a public animal shelter, and an exploration of the ability of these measures to predict problem behavior after adoption. *Appl Anim Behav Sci*, 73:217–233.

Herzog AG, Edelheit PB, and Jacobs AR (2001). Low salivary cortisol levels and aggressive behavior. *Arch Gen Psychiatry*, 58:513–515.

Higa KT, Mori E, Viana FF, et al. (2002). Baroreflex control of heart rate by oxytocin in the solitary-vagal complex. *Am J Physiol Regul Integr Comp Physiol*, 282:R537–545.

Holst S, Uvnäs-Moberg K, and Petersson M (2002). Postnatal oxytocin treatment and postnatal stroking of rats reduce blood pressure in adulthood. *Auton Neurosci*, 99:85–90.

Houpt KA (2000). Animal behavior case of the month: Two dogs were evaluated for sibling or "roommate" rivalry. *JAVMA*, 217:1468–1472.

Hudry J, Ryvlin P, Royet JP, and Mauguiere F (2001). Odorants elicit evoked potentials in the human amygdala. *Cerebral Cortex*, 11:619–627.

Igel GJ and Calvin AD (1960). The development of affectional responses in infant dogs. *J Comp Physiol Psychol*, 53:302–305.

Jacob S and McClintock MK (2000). Psychological state and mood effects of steroidal chemosignals in women and men. *Horm Behav*, 37:57–78.

Julien RM (1995). *A Primer of Drug Action*, 7th Ed. New York: WH Freeman.

Kagan J, Reznick JS, and Snidman N (1987). The physiology and psychology of behavioral inhibition. *Child Dev*, 58:1459–1473.

Kallet AJ, Cowgill LD, and Kass PH (1997). Comparing of blood pressure measurements obtained in dogs by use of indirect osillometry in a veterinary clinic versus at home. *JAVMA*, 210:651–654.

Kelly DD (1991). Sexual differential of the nervous system. In JC Kandel, JH Schwartz, and TM Jessell (Eds), *Principles of Neural Science*. Norwalk, CT: Appleton and Lange.

Kirby LG, Rice KC, and Valentino RJ (2000). Effects of corticotropin-releasing factor on neuronal activity in the serotonergic dorsal raphe nucleus. *Neuropsychopharmacology*, 22:148–162.

Kirk-Smith MD, Van Toller C, and Dodd GH (1983). Unconscious odour conditioning in human subjects. *Biol Psychol*, 17:221–231.

Koda N (2001a). Development of play behavior between potential guide dogs for the blind and human raisers. *Behav Processes*, 53:41–46.

Koda N (2001b). Inappropriate behavior of potential guide dogs for the blind and coping behavior of human raisers. *Appl Anim Behav Sci*, 72:79–87.

Komori T, Fujiwara R, Tanida M, and Nomura J (1995). Potential antidepressant effects of lemon odor in rats. *Eur Neuropsychopharmacol*, 5:477–480.

Korte MS, Meijer OC, De Klost ER, et al. (1996). Enhanced 5-HT$_{1A}$ receptor expression in forebrain regions of aggressive house mice. *Brain Res*, 736:338–343.

Kostarczyk E (1991). The use of dog-human interaction as a reward in instrumental conditioning and its impact on dogs' cardiac regulation. In H Davis and D Balfour (Eds), *The Inevitable Bond: Examining Scientist-Animal Interactions*. Cambridge: Cambridge University Press.

Kostarczyk E and Fonberg E (1982). Heart rate mechanisms in instrumental conditioning reinforced by petting in dogs. *Physiol Behav*, 28:27–30.

Kramer MS, Cutler N, Feighner J, et al. (1998). Distinct mechanism for antidepressant activity by blockade of central substance P receptors. *Science* 281:1640–1645.

Krishnan KRM, Ritchie JC, Manepalli AN, et al. (1988). What is the relationship between plasma ACTH and plasma cortisol in normal humans and depressed patients? In AF Schatzberg and CB Nemeroff (Eds), *The Hypothalamic-Pituitary-Adrenal Axis: Physiology, Pathophysiology, and Psychiatric Implications*. New York: Raven.

Ladd CO, Huot RL, Thrivikraman KV, et al. (2000). Long-term behavioral and neuroendocrine adaptations to adverse early experience. In EA Mayer and CB Saper (Eds), *Progress in Brain Research*. New York: Elsevier Science.

Landsberg GM (2001). Clomipramine: Beyond separation anxiety. *J Am Anim Hosp Assoc*, 37:313–318.

Le Doux JE (1996). *The Emotional Brain: The Mysterious Underpinning of Emotional Life*. New York: Simon and Schuster.

Lehrner J, Eckersberger C, Walla P, et al. (2000). Ambient odor of orange in a dental office reduces anxiety and improves mood in female patients. *Physiol Behav*, 71:83–86.

Levine ES, Litto WJ, and Jacobs BL (1990). Activity of cat locus coeruleus noradrenergic neurons during the defense reaction. *Brain Res*, 531:189–195.

Long CJ and Tapp JT (1967). Reinforcing properties of odors for the albino rat. *Psychon Sci*, 7:17–18.

Lore RK and Eisenberg FB (1986): Avoidance reactions of domestic dogs to unfamiliar male and female humans in a kennel setting. *Appl Anim Behav Sci*, 15:261–266.

Lund I, Yu LC, and Uvnäs-Moberg K, et al. (2002). Repeated massage-like stimulation induces long-term effects on nociception: Contribution of oxytocinergic mechanisms. *Eur J Neurosci*, 16:330-338.

Lynch JL and McCarthy JF (1967). The effect of petting on a classically conditioned emotional response. *Behav Res Ther*, 5:55–62.

Lynch JJ and McCarthy JF (1969). Social responding in dogs: Heart rate changes to a person. *Psychophysiology*, 5:389–393.

MacDonald K (1983). Stability of individual differences in behavior in a litter of wolf cubs (*Canis lupus*). *J Comp Psychol*, 97:99–106.

Maier SF and Watkins LR (1998). Cytokines for psychologists: Implications of bi-directional immune-to-brain communication for understanding behavior, mood, and cognition. *Psychol Rev*, 105:83–107.

Manoque KR, Lesher AI, and Candland DK (1975). Dominance status and adrenocortical reactivity to stress in squirrel monkeys (*Saimiri sciureus*). *Primates*, 16:457–463.

McBurnett K, Lahey BB, Rathouz PJ, and Loeber R (2000). Low salivary cortisol and persistent aggression in boys referred for disruptive behavior. *Arch Gen Psychiatry*, 57:38–43.

McDougle CJ, Barr LC, and Goodman WK (1999). Possible role of neuropeptides in obsessive compulsive disorder. *Psychoneuroendocrinology*, 24:1–24.

McGuire MT and Raleigh MJ (1987). Serotonin, social behavior, and aggression in vervet monkeys. In B Olivier, J Mos, and PF Brain (Eds), *Ethopharmacology of Agonistic Behavior in Animals and Humans*. Dordrecht, The Netherlands: Martinus Nijhoff.

McLeod PJ, Moger WH, Ryon J, et al. (1995). The relation between urinary cortisol levels and social behavior in captive timber wolves. *Can J Zool*, 74:209–216.

McMillan FD (1999). Influence of mental states on somatic health in animals. *JAVMA*, 214:1221–1225.

Mehlman PT, Higley JD, Faucher I, et al. (1994). Low CSF 5-HIAA concentrations and severe aggression and impaired impulse control in nonhuman primates. *Am J Psychiatry*, 151:1485–1491.

Mertens PA, Lentz S, Fischer A, et al. (2000). Serotonin and 5-hydroxyindolacetic acid in cerebrospinal fluid, serum, and plasma in dominant-aggressive dogs and non-aggressive dogs. *Newsl AVSAB*, 22:11–12.

Miachon S, Rochet T, Mathian B, et al. (1993). Long-term isolation of Wistar rats alters brain monoamine turnover, blood corticosterone, and ACTH. *Brain Res Bull*, 32:611–614.

Miklósi Á, Polgárdi R, Topál J, and Csányi V (1998). Use of experimenter-given cues in dogs. *Anim Cogn*, 1:113–121.

Miklósi Á, Polgárdi R, Topál J, and Csányi V (2000). Intentional behaviour in dog-human communication: An experimental analysis of "showing" behaviour in the dog. *Anim Cogn*, 3:159–166.

Mitchell RW and Thompson NS (1990). The effects of familiarity on dog-human play. *Anthrozoös*, 4:24–43.

Montastruc P, Dang Tran L, and Montastruc JL (1985). Reduction of vagal pressor reflexes by neurohypophyseal peptides and related compounds. *Eur J Pharmacol*, 117:355–361.

Most K (1910/1955). *Training Dogs*. New York: Coward-McCann (reprint).

Mukaddam-Daher S, Yin YL, Roy J, et al. (2001). Negative inotropic and chronotropic effects of oxytocin. *Hypertension*, 292–296.

Murphree OD (1973). Inheritance of human aversion and inactivity in two strains of pointer dogs. *Biol Psychiatry*, 7:23–29.

Nikulina EM, Avgustinovich DF, and Popova NK (1992). Role of 5HT$_{1A}$ receptors in a variety of kinds of aggressive behavior in wild rats and counterparts selected for low defensiveness towards man. *Aggressive Behav*, 18:357–364.

Odendaal JSJ (1999). A physiological basis for animal-facilitated psychotherapy. PhD thesis, University of Pretoria.

Odendaal JSJ (2000). Animal-assisted therapy: Magic or medicine? *J Psychosom Res*, 49:275–280.

Olivier B, Tulp MTM, and Mos J (1991). Serotonergic receptors in anxiety and aggression: Evidence from animal pharmacology. *Hum Psychopharmacol*, 6:S73–S78.

Otto T, Cousens G, and Rajewski K (1997). Odor-guided fear conditioning in rats: 1. Acquisition, retention, and latent inhibition. *Behav Neurosci*, 111:1257–1264.

Pageat P (1999). Biological treatments of aggressiveness in the dog [Abstract]. In *Proceedings Mondial Vet Lyon 99* (cd), Sep 23–26.

Pajer K, Gardner W, Rubin RT, et al. (2001). Decreased cortisol levels in adolescent girls with conduct disorder. *Arch Gen Psychiatry*, 58:297–302.

Palme R, Schatz S, and Mostl E (2001). Effect of vaccination on fecal cortisol metabolites in cats and dogs [Abstract]. *Dtsch Tierarztl Wochenschr*, 108:23–25.

Panksepp J (1982). Towards a general psychobiological theory of emotions. *Behav Brain Sci*, 5:407–467.

Panksepp J (1998). *Affective Neuroscience: The Foundations of Human and Animal Emotions*. New York: Oxford University Press.

Panksepp J and Burgdorf J (2000). 50-kHz chirping (laughter?) in response to conditioned and unconditioned tickle-induced reward in rats: Effects of social housing and genetic variables. *Behav Brain Res*, 115:25–38.

Papanek PE and Raff H (1994). Physiological increases in cortisol inhibit basal vasopressin release in conscious dogs. *Am J Physiol*, 266:R1744–R1751.

Paschall GY and Davis M (2002). Olfactory-mediated fear-potentiated startle. *Behav Neurosci*, 116:4–12.

Petersson M (2002). Cardiovascular effects of oxytocin. *Prog Brain Res*, 139:281–288.

Petersson M, Uvnäs-Moberg K, Erhardt S, et al. (1998). Oxytocin increases locus coeruleus alpha 2-adrenoreceptor responsiveness in rats. *Neurosci Lett*, 255:115–118.

Pitner GD and Friedman BX (2000). Evolution of brain structures and adaptive behaviors in humans and other animals. *The Neuroscientist*, 6:241–251.

Pettijohn TF, Wong TW, Ebert PD, and Scott JP (1977). Alleviation of separation distress in 3 breeds of young dogs. *Dev Psychobiol*, 10:373–381.

Podberscek AL and Serpell JA (1997). Environmental influences on the expression of aggressive behaviour in English cocker spaniels. *Appl Anim Behav Sci*, 52:215–227.

Popova NK, Kulikov AV, Nikulina EM, et al. (1991). Serotonin metabolism and serotonergic receptors in Norway rats selected for low aggressiveness towards man. *Aggressive Behav*, 17:207–213.

Pryor PA, Hart BL, Cliff KD, and Bain MJ (2001). Effects of a selective serotonin reuptake inhibitor on urine spraying behavior in cats. *JAVMA*, 219:1557–1561.

Raine AD (2002). Biosocial studies of antisocial and violent behavior in children and adults: A review. *J Abnorm Child Psychiatry*, 30:311–326.

Raleigh MJ, Brammer GL, McGuire MT, and Yuwiler A (1985). Dominant social status facilitates the behavioral effects of serotonergic agonists. *Brain Res*, 348:274–282.

Raleigh MJ, McGuire MT, Brammer GL, et al. (1991). Serotonergic mechanisms promote dominance acquisition in adult male vervet monkeys. *Brain Res*, 559:181–190.

Reisner IR, Mann JJ, Stanley M, et al. (1996). Comparison of cerebrospinal fluid monoamine metabolite levels in dominant-aggressive and non-aggressive dogs. *Brain Res*, 714:57–64.

Romanovsky AA, Simons CT, Szekely M, and Kulchitsky VA (1997). The vagus nerve in the thermoregulatory response to systemic inflammation. *Am J Physiol*, 273:407–413.

Rooney NJ and Bradshaw JWS (2002). An experimental study of the effects of play upon the dog-human relationship. *Appl Anim Behav Sci*, 75:161–176.

Rooney NJ, Bradshaw JWS, and Robinson IH (2001). Do dogs respond to play signals given by humans? *Anim Behav*, 61:715–722.

Roth BL, Lopez E, Patel S, and Kroeze WK (2000). The multiplicity of serotonin receptors: Uselessly diverse molecules or an embarrassment of riches? *Neuroscientist*, 6:252–262.

Salazar MR (2000). Alpha lipoic acid: A novel treatment for depression. *Med Hypotheses*, 55:510–512.

Sapolsky R and Ray JC (1989). Styles of dominance and their endocrine correlates among wild olive baboons. *Am J Primatol*, 18:1–13.

Sarnyai Z and Kovacs GL (1994). Role of oxytocin in the neuroadaptation to drugs of abuse. *Psychoneuroendocrinology*, 19:85–117.

Sarris EG (1938–1939). Individual difference in dogs [four parts]. *Am Kennel Gaz*, Nov 1938, Dec 1938, Jan 1939, Feb 1939.

Schleidt WM (1998). Is humaneness canine? *Hum Ethol Bull*, 13:1–4.

Schleidt WM (1999). Apes, wolves, and the trek to humanity: Did wolves show us the way? *Discovering Archaeol*, 1:8–10.

Schultz W (1998). Predictive reward signal of dopamine neurons. *J Neurophysiol*, 80:1–27.

Scott JP (1992a). The phenomenon of attachment in human-nonhuman relationships. In H Davis and D Balfour (Eds), *The Inevitable Bond: Examining Scientist-Animal Interactions.* Cambridge: Cambridge University Press.

Scott JP (1992b). Aggression: Functions and control in social systems. *Aggressive Behav*, 18:1–20.

Senay EC (1966). Toward an animal model of depression: A study of separation behavior in dogs. *J Psychiatr Res*, 4:65–71.

Serpell J and Jagoe JA (1995). Early experience and the development of behaviour. In J Serpell (Ed), *The Domestic Dog: Its Evolution, Behaviour, and Interaction with People.* New York: Cambridge University Press.

Shibata H, Fujiwara R, Iwamoto M, et al. (1990). Recovery of PFC in mice exposed to high pressure stress by olfactory stimulation with fragrance. *Int J Neurosci*, 51:245–247.

Shibata H, Fujiwara R, Iwamoto M, et al. (1991). Immunological and behavioral effects of fragrance in mice. *Int J Neurosci*, 57:151–159.

Siegel A, Schubert KL, and Shaikh MB (1997). Neurotransmitters regulating defensive rage behavior in the cat. *Neurosci Biobehav Rev*, 21:733–742.

Simonet O, Murphy M, and Lance A (2001). Laughing dog: Vocalizations of domestic dogs during play encounters. Presented at the Animal Behavior Society Conference, Corvallis, OR, July 14–18.

Simpson BS and Simpson DM (1996). Behavioral pharmacology. In VL Voith and PL Borchelt (Eds) *Readings in Companion Animal Behavior.* Trenton, NJ: Veterinary Learning Systems.

Slabbert JM and Rasa OA (1993). The effect of early separation from the mother on pups in bonding to humans and pup health. *J S Afr Vet Assoc*, 64:4–8.

Sommerville BA and Broom DM (1998). Olfactory awareness. *Appl Anim Behav Sci*, 57:269–286.

Soproni K, Miklósi Á, Topál J, and Csányi V (2001). Comprehension of human communicative signs in pet dogs (*Canis familiaris*). *J Comp Psychol*, 115:122–126.

Strong V and Brown SW (2000). Should people with epilepsy have untrained dogs as pets? *Seizure*, 9:427–430.

Stutzmann GE, McEwen BS, and Le Doux JE (1998). Serotonin modulation of sensory inputs to the lateral amygdala: Dependency on corticosterone. *J Neurosci*, 18:9529–9538.

Sugrue MF (1983). Do antidepressants possess a common mechanism of action? *Biochem Pharmacol*, 32:1811–1817.

Sullivan RM and Wilson DA (1993). Role of the amygdala complex in early olfactory associative learning. *Behav Neurosci*, 107:254–263.

Sullivan RM, Landers M, Yeaman B, and Wilson DA (2000). Neurophysiology: Good memories of bad events in infancy. *Nature*, 407:38–39.

Swedo SE, Leonard HL, Garvey M, et al. (1998). Pediatric autoimmune neuropsychiatric disorders associated with streptococcal infections: Clinical description of the first 50 cases. *Am J Psychiatry*, 155:264–270.

Taçon PSC and Pardoe C (2002). Dogs make us human. *Nature Aust*, 27:53–61.

Taylor SE, Klein LC, Lewis B, et al. (2000). Biobehavioral responses to stress in females: Tend-and-befriend, not fight-or-fight. *Psychol Bull*, 107:411–429.

Thomas KJ, Murphree OD, and Newton JEO (1972). Effect of person and environment on heart rates in two strains of pointer dogs. *Cond Reflex*, 7:75–81.

Tisserand RB (1977). *The Art of Aromatherapy: The Healing and Beautifying Properties of the Essential Oils of Flowers and Herbs*. Rochester, VT: Healing Arts.

Topál J, Miklósi Á, and Csányi V (1997). Dog-human relationship affects problem solving behavior in the dog. *Anthrozoös*, 10:214–224.

Trumler E (1973). *Your Dog and You*. New York: Seabury.

Tuber DS (1986). Teaching Rover to relax: The soft exercise. *Anim Behav Consult Newsl*, 3(1).

Umhau JC, George DT, Reed S, et al. (2002). Atypical autonomic regulation in perpetrators of violent domestic abuse. *Psychophysiology*, 39:117–123.

Uvnäs-Moberg K (1997). Physiological and endocrine effects of social contact. In CS Carter, II Lederhendler, and B Kirkpatrick, *The Integrative Neurobiology of Affiliation*. Ann NY Acad Sci, 807:78–100.

Uvnäs-Moberg K (1998a). Oxytocin may mediate the benefits of positive social interaction and emotions. *Psychoneuroendocrinology*, 23:819–835.

Uvnäs-Moberg K (1998b). Antistress pattern induced by oxytocin. *News Physiol Sci*, 13:22–26.

Uvnäs-Moberg K, Bjokstrand E, Hillegaart V, and Ahlenius S (1999). Oxytocin as a possible mediator of SSRI-induced antidepressant effects. *Psychopharmacology*, 142:95–101.

Uvnäs-Moberg K, Eklund M, Hillegaart V, and Ahlenius S (2000). Improved conditioned avoidance learning by oxytocin administration in high-emotional male Sprague-Dawley rats. *Regul Pept*, 88:27–32.

Van Liere EF, Stickney JC, and Marsh DF (1949). Sex differences in blood pressure of dogs. *Science*, 109:489.

Verrier RL, Hagestad EL, and Lown B (1987). Delayed myocardial ischemia induced by anger. *Circulation*, 75:249–254.

Vila C, Savolainen P, Maldonado JE, et al. (1997). Multiple and ancient origins of the domestic dog. *Science*, 276:1687–1689.

Vincent IC and Leahy RA (1997). Real-time non-invasive measurement of heart rate in working dogs: A technique with potential applications in the objective assessment of welfare problems. *Vet J*, 153:179–184.

Virga V, Houpt KA, and Scarlett JM (2001). Efficacy of amitriptyline as a pharmacological adjunct to behavioral modification in the management of aggressive behavior in dogs. *J Am Anim Hosp Assoc*, 37:325–330.

Virkkunnen M (1985). Urinary free cortisol secretion in habitually violent offenders. *Acta Psychiatr Scand*, 72:40–44.

Walsh MT and Dinan TG (2001). Selective serotonin reuptake inhibitors and violence: A review of the available evidence. *Acta Psychiatr Scand*, 104:84–91.

Wells DL and Hepper PG (1998). Male and female dogs respond differently to men and women. *Appl Anim Behav Sci*, 61:341–349.

Wenzel BM (1959). Tactile stimulation as reinforcement for cats and its relation to early feeding experiences. *Psychol Rep*, 5:297–300.

White MM, Neilson JC, Hart BL, and Cliff KD (1999). Effects of clomipramine hydrochloride on dominance-related aggression in dogs. *JAVMA*, 215:1288–1290.

Wilhelmj CM, McGuire TF, McDonough J, et al. (1953). Emotional elevations of blood pressure in trained dogs: Possible origin of hypertension in humans. *Psychosom Med*, 15:390–395.

Wynchank D and Berk M (1998). Behavioural changes in dogs with acral lick dermatitis during a 2 month extension phase of fluoxetine treatment. *Hum Psychopharmacol Clin Exp*, 13:435–437.

Wynn SG and Kirk-Smith MD (1998). Aromatherapy. In AM Schoen and SG Wynn (Eds), *Complementary and Alternative Veterinary Medicine*. St. Louis: CV Mosby.

Yehuda R, Southwick S, Nussbaum G, et al. (1990). Low urinary cortisol excretion in patients with posttraumatic stress disorder. *J Nerv Ment Dis*, 178:366–369.

Yirmiya R, Pollak Y, and Morag M (2000). Illness, cytokines, and depression. *Ann NY Acad Sci*, 917:478–487.

Young LJ (1999). Oxytocin and vasopressin receptors and species-typical social behaviors. *Horm Behav*, 36:212–221.

7

Canine Domestic Aggression

PART 1: SOCIAL COMPETITION AND AGGRESSION

INTERACTIVE CONFLICT, STRESS, AND SOCIAL DOMINANCE

Social dominance is frequently posited as a formative principle organizing social behavior. Animals living in close groups are hypothesized to regulate their social interaction and aggressive impulses in accordance with social rank and status. According to this model, the cumulative victories and defeats resulting from competition over valued resources gradually result in a hierarchy of dominant-subordinate relations. Rowell (1974), a primatolo-gist, has criticized the social dominance hypothesis on several grounds and rejects it as a social organizing principle. Although often bordering on diatribe, her analysis offers a number of valuable insights pertaining to social relations and organization developing under the influence of stressful conditions. She argues that rigid linear dominance hierarchies primarily develop under the influence of unnatural and conflictive conditions. Rowell, arguing that subordinate animals most often initiate conflictive interaction, turns the social dominance concept on its head by positing instead a subordinance [*sic*] hierarchy. She suggests that conditions of captivity produce unnatural levels of interactive conflict and tension, increased aggression, and the dysregulation of the hypothalamic-pituitary-adrenal (HPA) system. The submission behavior of subordinates toward dominant animals is not reciprocated by affectionate tolerance (as might occur under natural conditions), but instead is met by aggressive threats and challenges. Instead of submitting and integrating friendly relations, animals living under such conditions appear to succumb gradually to stress and develop involuntary subordination strategies, thereby losing their capacity or desire to compete effectively. The long-term adverse effects of involuntary subordination have been implicated in the etiology of depression (see Gardner, 1982). As such, Rowell's subordinance hierarchy is an index of stressful reactivity and involuntary subordination, referencing an animal's ability to cope with stressful social conflict and environmental adversity with relative social rank. Under adverse conditions, animals showing a blunted response to stressful conflict (i.e., fearlessness/low cortisol) may obtain a competitive advantage over other animals exhibiting heightened emotional reactivity (i.e., fearful/high cortisol) and vulnerability to social and environmental stressors (see *Autonomic Arousal, Heart Rate, Aggression*, and *Stress, Low Cortisol, and Aggression*, in Chapter 6):

> Submissive behavior, on the other hand, can be related to hyperfunctioning of the adrenal gland in response to environmental stress, and occurs in its most extreme form in captivity. It seems that whereas adrenal responsiveness may

be advantageous under normal conditions, the unusually high levels of stress encountered in captivity may lead to a higher-than-useful response level. Thus a rigid hierarchy may with some justification be regarded as a pathological condition of a society brought on by too high stress levels ... Whereas the concept of dominance has apparently little to offer beyond its use as a shorthand description suggested above [predicting competitive outcomes], the concept of subordinance, as seen in submission hierarchies, may still provide helpful insights, especially in relating endocrine function to behavior. (Rowell, 1974:151)

According to the subordinance hypothesis, conflictive interaction initiated by subordinate group members results in varying degrees of HPA dysregulation and adrenal exhaustion, depending on each animal's ability to cope with the stress accruing as the result of repeated activation of the flight-fight system (FFS) (see *Social Competition, Cooperation, Conflict, and Resentment*). Rowell's hypothesis predicts that higher-ranking animals should show the lowest glucocorticoid levels, whereas the lower-ranking animals should show the highest glucocorticoid levels. A social organization based on individual differences with respect to their ability to cope with social stress is reminiscent of Calhoun's experiments (1962 and 1963); however, Calhoun's findings flatly contradict Rowell's assumptions concerning the functional significance of social dominance. Calhoun's research supports the necessity of a social dominance structure in order to promote social and territorial order, to facilitate physical health, and to increase reproductive fitness (see *Calhoun's Rat Universe* in Volume 2, Chapter 7). Under conditions in which social organization was based on social dominance, Calhoun found that stressful interaction and conflict were prevented or reduced (insiders), whereas under *outsider* conditions in which social behavior differentiates in accordance with each animal's ability to cope with stress, a state of social disorder and disintegration followed.

Rowell's hypothesis is probably better described in terms of involuntary subordination and mutual intolerance resulting from unfriendly exchanges between individuals operating under the socially disintegrative

influences of conflictive arousal and reactive coping styles. Dominance by threat and attack and subordination by fear generates escape/avoidance behavior, aggressive reprisals, and resentment in association with the activation of the FFS and an involuntary subordination strategy (ISS). These reactive behaviors are neither dominant nor submissive but reactive coping styles operating under the influence of the FFS. Social interaction operating under the influence of the FFS tends to promote social intolerance, irritability, disintegrative discord, and hostility.

Fear-related behavior and obtrusiveness are explicitly excluded from the classical concept of subordination and submission as described by Schenkel (1967). Antagonism and fear are incompatible with the affectionate and affiliative intent of active and passive submission. Submission behavior is basically an expression of filial love and desire to achieve an integrated and harmonious relationship within the family/pack unit. Typically, aggression problems are not the result of a dog acquiring a dominant attitude toward the owner, but rather such problems most often stem from a failure of the owner to respond to the dog's submissive solicitation for dominant tolerance and care. Instead, the owner may respond to active-submission behavior with punishment by ignoring, confining, or hitting the dog, thereby prompting adjustments based on an ISS. In contrast, when the owner responds in a friendly and constructive way to active-submission behaviors, an affiliative process based on a voluntary subordination strategy (VSS) and the integration of a trust-based bond between the owner and dog is initiated. Dominance is solicited, if not elicited, by the care-seeking and begging (active submission) behavior of the subordinate. Schenkel nicely describes the nature of submission in dogs and wolves in a manner that resonates with cynopraxic objectives:

We may conclude that submission is a contribution by the inferior to harmonic social integration on the basis of social hierarchical differentiation. It does not elicit a stereotyped automatic response. Integration asks for a contribution by the superior also, that is, tolerance. The superior's contribution may even exceed submission in its competence to shape the social contact or relation. (325)

Wolf Model of Dominance and Submission

Many problematic training strategies used to force submission by physical punishment are derived from the popular depictions of dominance and submission portrayed by Lorenz (1955). According to this view, submission results when an opponent is defeated; however, this notion appears to be relatively alien to the social organization of dogs and wolves. Mech (1999 and 2000) has strongly criticized this popular misconception of wolf social behavior and dominance. Drawing upon observations of wolves living under natural conditions, he argues that force-based concepts of social dominance are derived from the social behavior of wolves living under captive conditions. According to Mech, social dominance and submission is an integral aspect of wolf social behavior and family life. He rejects the notion of the "alpha" wolf, arguing that such an attribution is comparable to calling a human parent an alpha. Further, since wolf offspring are generally subordinate to the breeding pair, referring to the parents as alphas or the alpha pair is redundant and adds nothing informative to the picture. The term may still have descriptive value in the case of wolf relations formed within groups containing multiple families or the hierarchical relations formed by wolves living under captive conditions (Van Hooff and Wensing, 1987). The origin and meaning of social dominance in wolves is closely associated with reproduction, a division of labor, and the formation of cooperative and harmonious family relations (Mech, 1999). These cooperative relations serve to hold the family/pack unit together and are dedicated to the service of various basic survival and reproductive priorities, including the support and protection of progeny via group-coordinated hunting and defensive activities, occurring under the leadership of the alpha pair (Mech, 2000). In the wolf family/pack, reproduction and territorial defense are the prerogative of the breeding pair (Mech, 1970), further supporting the hypothesis that dominant-subordinate relations are closely tied to incentives associated with reproduc-

tion (Derix et al., 1993). The pack is usually little more than a family group, consisting of a breeding pair and progeny. As the result of parental socialization and food begging, the progeny are trained from an early age to exhibit active-submissive behavior toward the breeding pair and other adults, perhaps helping to account for the infantile characteristics of many submission displays. Although Mech rejects a rigid and "force-based dominance hierarchy" (Mech, 1999), he acknowledges that the breeding pair dominate and lead the behavior of their young (Mech, 2000).

The progeny are typically obligate subordinates with respect to the parents, upon whom they are socially and physiologically dependent. The social competition between progeny is organized from an early age onward around the control of valued resources. These sibling rights and privileges are maintained by the exchange of ritualized threat and appeasement displays and the formation of a social hierarchy that prefigures adult status relations (MacDonald, 1983 and 1987). Competition and dominance tensions (squabbles) appear mostly to involve transient situational disputes, especially involving contests over food. The reproductive and familial origin of social dominance is reflected in the reduced tendency of male and female wolves to fight with each other (Schenkel, 1967), with the male typically dominant over the female and the rest of the pack, while the female is dominant over all pack members except the male (Mech, 1999). As wolves reach sexual maturity, they eventually leave the natal group and join up with other dispersed wolves to reproduce and form new packs, thereby reducing the risk of disruptive competition within the group. Most wolves leave the family/pack before they reach 2 years of age, with virtually all of them dispersing before they turn 3 years of age (Mech, 1999).

Dispersal Tensions and Household Aggression

Some forms of canine domestic aggression (CDA) may be related to the activation of dispersal-related tensions in adulthood. As previously discussed, wolves disperse between 1 and 3 years of age, a time frame that is frequently cited as significant with regard to the expression CDA (Borchelt and Voith, 1996). Although the lupine dispersal instinct appears to be reduced in dogs by virtue of paedomorphosis, some dogs may express polymorphic variations that support dispersal tensions in association with the formation of overly exclusive and dependent bonds with one particular person in the household, perhaps setting the stage for persistent interactive tensions, intolerance, and a failure of affected dogs to integrate submissive and friendly relations with other family members. Hypothetically, under conditions in which dispersal and breeding activities are thwarted, social dominance, bonding, and symbolic reproductive imperatives may coalesce in novel ways, facilitating social dynamics conducive to asexual-pair bonding, thereby forming an *insider* satellite group within the family system. As a result, the dog may become increasing intolerant toward other family members and may threaten or attack them as intruding *outsiders*, thus symbolically dispersing and establishing a territorial boundary within the context of the home (e.g., a bed or the favored owner's lap). Such dogs may gradually threaten a husband or wife when he or she enters the bedroom or while getting into the bed. More rarely, the aggressor may threaten a parent who approaches or shows affection toward a child. These dogs often show exaggerated territorial behavior, becoming highly reactive and threatening toward visitors and strangers coming into the house or approaching them while in a car. Owners may be flattered by the dog's close attention, affection, and protectiveness, and may inadvertently reinforce it. These sorts of aggression problems are often surprisingly well tolerated by the household and held as something akin to an innocent idiosyncrasy, at least until someone gets seriously bitten. Frequently, it is the "protected" person who gives first blood while daring to restrain the dog during one of its aggressive episodes.

DYNAMIC MODAL RELATIONS AND SOCIAL DOMINANCE

Basic Concepts of Cynopraxic Training Theory

According to cynopraxic training theory, well-organized and functional prediction-control expectancies and coordinated emotional establishing operations are subject to refinement via the coding of positive and negative prediction errors (see *Basic Postulates, Units, Processes, and Mechanisms*, in Chapter 10). A prediction error occurs when a control expectancy is confirmed but in association with an unexpected result, such that the anticipated outcome turns out to be better or worse than expected. Such discrepancies between predicted outcomes and actual outcomes produce exciting or depressing cortical reward/punishment effects via an activating or suppressing effect on dopaminergic reward circuits (see *Classical Conditioning, Prediction, and Reward* in Chapter 1). Better-than-expected outcomes resulting in positive prediction error produce surprise (reward), whereas worse-than-expected outcomes resulting in negative prediction error produce disappointment (punishment). Outcomes that match prediction-control expectancies and calibrated establishing operations are verified (reinforced) and result in enhanced comfort or safety. Verified actions are referred to as *control modules*. Control modules are under the motivational influence of appetitive and emotional establishing operations calibrated to meet the anticipated needs of a dog as it acts in accordance with functional expectancies and control incentives. Control modules form routines and patterns of goal-oriented behavior within the context of adaptive modal activities. The collection of control modules, routines, and patterns of behavior formed in association with adaptive modal activity is referred to as *culture*. Control modules and routines are maintained by the gratifying and relaxing effects (somatic reward) produced by verifying prediction-control expectancies and calibrated establishing operations. These integrative learning experiences and adjustments occurring in accordance with positive and negative prediction error and verification are mediated by a complex network of comparator loci, set points, positive- and negative-feedback systems and regulatory neural networks hypothesized to operate at a preconscious level of cognitive organization. Control modules and routines that fail to produce expected outcomes result in the disconfirmation of the instrumental prediction-control expectancy and calibrated establishing operation. Disconfirmed control modules are extinguished by means of a revised set of incompatible prediction-control expectancies and abolishing operations (see *Startle and Fear Circuits* in Chapter 3).

Adaptive Modal Strategies

Behavior operating under the influence of positive and negative prediction error is referred to as an adaptive modal strategy or coping style. There are two general adaptive modal strategies: active and passive. Active modal strategies develop in association with reward incentives resulting from positive prediction error, whereas passive modal strategies develop in association with efforts aimed at avoiding negative prediction error. Adaptive modal strategies develop in the context of organizing and refining the expression of emotional command systems. For example, active modal strategies operating in association with the seeking system include forward movement, searching, exploring, experimenting, probing, discovering, risk taking, and so forth, whereas passive modal strategies consist of stopping or backing, hesitating, waiting, delaying, ritualizing, and so forth.

Active modal strategies are supported by reward incentives associated with positive prediction error, surprise, novelty, and enhanced arousal and excitement. As such, active modal strategies operate in accordance with what Gray (1990 and 1994) refers to as the behavioral approach system (BAS). Adaptive modal strategies incorporate and organize control modules, routines, and complex patterns of behavior. However, unlike control modules, which seek rewards that calm (reduce arousal) with comfort and safety, active modal strategies are motivated to discover and produce activity that results in better-than-expected outcomes (surprise). Passive modal strategies operate in close conformity with Gray's behavioral inhibition system (BIS), showing a heightened sensitivity for startle, and signals of loss and risk (punishment).

Control modules, operating under the combined influence of active and passive adaptive modal strategies, gradually become highly refined and reliable but thereby risk losing the ability to produce prediction error

and reward. Although valuable for purposes of culture building and survival, highly refined control modules are of little use for producing the excitement and surprise evoked by positive prediction error. By necessity, prediction error cannot be determined in advance; however, active modal strategies can incorporate control-module variations and novel actions to improve the likelihood of producing such error. Such modular variations and novel actions are referred to as *projects and ventures*. Ventures are distinguished from projects by the presence of an increased element of risk and potential for producing reward. As the result of the mutual and complementary influences of active and passive modal strategies, projects and ventures are gradually refined and fitted into the culture of modules, routines, and patterns of established behavior or they are extinguished. Consequently, it is not sufficient for a project merely to produce surprise in association with novelty (diverter), but the surprise must occur within a cultural context of established prediction-control expectancies; that is, it must be relevant to the existing culture and contribute to the process of adaptive optimization.

Dynamic Modal Relations, Affection, Play, and Bonding

Cynopraxic training theory postulates that prediction discrepancies between what a dog expects to occur and what in fact occurs while engaged in some purposive social activity result in emotional changes or establishing operations calibrated to optimize adaptive adjustments to the error. As such, social emotions are dependent on the formation of interactive prediction-control expectancies and interactive exchanges that result in outcomes that to some favorable or unfavorable extent mismatch or deviate from those expectations. Social exchanges that result in reciprocal emotional changes are referred to as *transactions*. Favorable transactions mediate mutual adaptations conducive to a polity of integrated social relations or, in the case of unfavorable transactions, exchanges result in mutual reactivity, antagonism, and social disintegration. For example, highly predictable and orderly social exchanges tend to produce formal relations, roles, and rule-based rituals of limited emotional and behavioral variability that are integrated into a rigid utilitarian hierarchy. Although a utilitarian polity of rigid dominant-subordinate relations and expectations can be productive in the context of a culture of well-established modules, routines, and patterns of interaction organized to perform some specific function, such hierarchical relations are relatively inflexible to change and lack the capacity to produce transactions conducive to positive prediction error and reward in support of affectionate bonding. Social transactions that are conducive to familial or guardian relations and roles are more flexible and mediate attachment, dependency, and feelings of comfort and safety (security). However, familial relations and roles tend to become progressively formal, rule based, and problematic with respect to emergent interactive conflict and tensions involving the ownership and control of group resources and sources of reward. The interactive conflict associated with familial hierarchies results in dispersal or the production of an ISS in response to punitive transactions.

The cynopraxic polity is formed in the context of resolving interactive conflict developing in association with conflictive familial relations and roles. Typically, interactive conflicts form around antagonistic control incentives, whereby the dog's interest in obtaining some reward object or activity is at variance with the owner's efforts to establish or maintain control over the dog's seeking impulses. Such situations become conflictive as the result of punitive efforts to block or suppress the dog's reward-seeking activity, but without subsequently leading the dog to obtain sought-after gratification via a reward deferment or delay of gratification (e.g., making the dog wait) or prompting a more acceptable substitute behavior (submissive ritual) and rewarding it with an alternative object or activity that provides a similar or greater amount of reward value to the dog than the one being forbidden. The punishment of appetitive and social seeking activities performed in the absence of alternative sources of gratification appears to set the stage for the development of an ISS. Interactive conflict is

gradually resolved by means of integrated compliance training (ICT), whereby forbidden activities and resources are systematically integrated as rewards for compliant behavior (see *Integrated Compliance Training*). In the process of resolving interactive conflict and tension by means of ICT, significant amounts of positive prediction error (rewarding surprise) are produced to mediate the expression of cooperative modal strategies. According to this view, competition is a necessary precondition and elemental aspect of all forms of social cooperation and happiness, that is, adaptive success. Without competition, there is no cooperation, without cooperation there is no happiness, and without happiness there is no joy. Competition is the foundation upon which a friendly relationship is built. As the result of ICT, interactive conflict is gradually resolved and replaced with interactive harmony and mutual appreciation.

With the emergence of interactive harmony, dynamic modal relations can be formed in the context of establishing affectionate and playful relations conducive to cynopraxic bonding. Dynamic modal relations consist of affectionate and playful give-and-take exchanges and creative social projects and ventures conducive to mutual reward (positive prediction error) and a joyful bond. Dynamic modal relations are liberated in the context of affectionate and playful transactions. Playful projects and ventures are an important source of variety and positive prediction error in support of friendly social relations, cooperation, and interactive harmony. Dynamic modal relations formed in association with play (reversing dominant-subordinate relations and role playing) mediate the transformation of competition into energetic, organized, and friendly cooperation. Play is an expression of freedom and represents a life symbol of adaptive success and harmonic social integration. Social play is possible only under the influence of a polity of mutually trusting relations. As such, play mediates social flexibility and cooperative-competitive dynamic modal relations and voluntary subordination strategies based on trust, mutual appreciation, interactive harmony, and joy.

Relations formed in association with affection and play cannot be forced, and they remain free from the influence of coercion, providing a basis of interaction conducive to a VSS Insofar as affection and play are freely given, freely received, and freely reciprocated, dynamic modal relations facilitate the integration of a harmonic social bond. Dynamic modal relations are *practiced* while giving and receiving affection and while engaging in experimental role playing and the mutual expression of flexible ascendant and descendant role reversals. In contrast to dominant-subordinate relations, dynamic modal relations and roles are fluidly and playfully expressed, exchanged, and reversed, with little more objective in mind than to maintain and intensify the relationship and its capacity to support transactions conducive to heightened feelings of mutual appreciation and trust, that is, to enjoy each other. Dynamic modal interaction becomes progressively spontaneous and free, with social transactions taking on a quality of joyful anticipation arising from the mutual anticipation of positive prediction error, thereby enlivening the relationship mutual appreciation and joy.

C-type and M-type Affinity for the Flight-Fight System

A history of friendly and supportive interaction provides an affiliative buffer and physiological calming effect, whereby the shock of exceptions to the rule or the new is absorbed by a schema-consistent bias toward reward, even though the interaction might signify a momentary setback or loss (e.g., taking a bone) or threat (e.g., unexpectedly grabbing the dog) at the sensory-input level or uncertainty (e.g., meeting a visitor at the door). Well-socialized and competent dogs learn to perceive and interpret the significance of interaction in terms of spatial, temporal, social, and contextual schemata built up in association with safe and supportive interaction with family members and others. Organizing behavioral activity in accordance with flexible prediction-control expectancies offers enormous advantages, enabling the dog to prepare in advance for impending events and to optimize its adaptive efforts to predict and control significant social exchanges (see *Functional Significance of Social Signals*). The over-

all effect of such social interaction is the integration of relations conducive to a VSS and a trust-based bond.

However, social environments lacking order may prevent a dog from establishing a coherent system of prediction-control expectancies, thereby impeding its ability to adjust effectively. Social interaction that lacks adequate predictability and controllability may cause modal activity to become progressively perturbed and reactive. Without an orderly and coherent foundation of standard or normal expectancies, the dog is not only deprived of the calming effects (secure mood) of somatic reward and enhanced comfort and safety, it is also barred from advancing to an organization of learning and adaptation conducive to cortical reward (e.g., surprise), and freedom, that is, behavior liberated from reactive adjustments. According to this hypothesis, uncontrollable reward and punishment, that is, aversive or appetitive events occurring independently of the dog's initiative or ability to control them, gradually leads the dog to become increasingly dependent, insecure, and incompetent. Instead of depending on its own initiative and ability, the dog may rely on the owner's daily vagaries and whims to obtain gratification for its comfort and safety needs. Since a dependent dog's needs for attention, comfort, and safety inevitably exceed the owner's ability or willingness to gratify them, an inherent state of dissatisfaction develops between the owner and the dog as the result of such interaction. A dependent and reactive dog is rarely content or secure with what it gets (it is invariably too little or too late), an insecure attachment and resentment (submission with insecurity and anger) seem to present in common with such problematic relationships.

As the result of nurturance (affection and caregiving) and punishment provided on a habitually noncontingent basis, the locus of control over significant attractive and aversive events may be externalized, that is, placed outside of a dog's voluntary initiative. For such dogs, the acquisition of comfort and safety may be integrated and experienced as something that happens to them, rather than perceived as something that they control and produce for themselves. Instead of learning to control such events by proactive means, they simply learn to receive or react to them. Just as the loss of control over aversive events is conducive to the debilitating effects of learned helplessness, the loss of control over appetitive ones can exert a similarly paralyzing effect on a dog's ability to adapt (Sonoda et al., 1991), perhaps a condition better referred to as *learned hopelessness* in the case of uncontrollable appetitive events. A persistent loss of control over significant events, whether appetitive or aversive, may render a dog progressively incompetent, emotionally undifferentiated, and straddled by a pervasive neediness (hopeless) and insecurity (helpless). Since what an overly dependent dog gets is provided or avoided on a relatively noncontingent and uncontrollable basis, it fails to obtain the confidence building and relaxing benefits of somatic (calming) and cortical (elating) reward. The inevitable uncertainty and insufficiency of such an arrangement may predictably lead to significant frustration and anxiety, perhaps helping to explain the increased irritability, intolerance, and resentment frequently shown by such dogs. Overly dependent and reactive dogs may possess a very impoverished set of control expectancies, operating primarily under a narrow range of motivations and behaviors dedicated to maintaining the dependent relationship. Lacking the ability to control significant social, appetitive, and aversive events by proactive means, such dogs may show signs of heightened vigilance for opportunities or threats and a boosted readiness to act impulsively, becoming increasingly insecure, needy, demanding, and obtrusive—characteristics of an ISS (see *Involuntary Subordination and Canine Domestic Aggression*).

In contrast to the rich and complex social schemata and organized scripting of well-adjusted and obedient dogs, overly dependent and reactive dogs appear to operate under a limited set of reactive expectancies biased with anticipatory anxiety, frustration, and a readiness to flee or confront benign threats and challenges with impulsive and disproportionate aggression or fear. Overly dependent and reactive dogs appear to be unable to integrate a trusting bond. Such dogs may become progressively insecure and intolerant of interference while engaged in comfort and safety-pro-

moting activities (e.g., resting and eating). They may resent and react to benign handling and changes in routine or habit. Such dogs appear to exhibit a negative cognitive bias and a selective attention for signals of punishment (loss and risk) and show a reactive affinity for FFS adjustments via anxiety (fear) and frustration (anger). Instead of responding to aversive or appetitive events in a measured and calibrated way, socially incompetent and reactive dogs may evidence varying degrees of impulsivity and a reactive coping style. Psychological stressors associated with adverse social interaction, especially uncontrollable or inescapable compulsion or punishment, may cause anxiety and frustration to shift motivationally in the direction of fear and anger, becoming progressively prominent, generalized, and reactive. The persistent frustration associated with a loss of control over significant events may result in an increasing readiness for social confrontation and aggression via an affinity with the anger-arousing branch of the FFS. The increased anxious vigilance and frustrative readiness associated with the reactive coping style are hypothesized to result in chronic stress and an increased risk of developing serious adjustment problems involving impulsive adjustments, including aggression.

As the result of individual differences, prenatal or postnatal stress, abusive or neglectful rearing practices, excessive interactive conflict and disorder, and chronic stress, pathways mediating anxiety and frustration may become sensitized and lose their capacity to adaptively regulate emotional arousal. These changes result in a spectrum of predispositions, behavioral threshold modifications, and adjustment characteristics consistent with Pavlov's choleric (c type) and the melancholic (m type) typology. The vast majority of dogs exhibiting reactive coping styles show a blend of behavioral characteristics evidencing both C and M elements or showing only moderate signs of BAS and BIS dysregulation and stress-related disorder. The c-type dog is highly motivated and prone to frustration-related reactivity and aggression (frustration intolerant). C-type dogs exhibit a reduced capacity for delay of gratification and passive-avoidance learning.

M-type dogs, on the other hand, may become progressively withdrawn, socially avoidant, and fearful, often showing a lack of interest in appetitive and social rewards, and consequently may be very difficult to train with rewards. M types show an increased capacity for delay of gratification and passive-avoidance learning, but may show striking deficiencies with respect to adjustments requiring active-avoidance learning. Although both c- and m-type dogs are reactive to punishment, c types show a heightened sensitivity or *readiness* to respond actively and offensively to threats of loss and frustration, evidencing a high degree of fearlessness, whereas m types show a heightened sensitivity or *vigilance* and a tendency to respond passively and defensively to threats of harm and anxiety, evidencing a high degree of fearfulness. Both c- and m-type dogs are oriented to signals of punishments (loss of gratification or threats of harm), resulting in global learning deficits, emotional disturbances, and adverse mood changes, in association with an inability to produce and sustain a state of comfort and safety (somatic rewards) as well as a failure to produce positive prediction error and surprise (cortical reward) via integrated active and passive modal activity.

C-type and m-type dogs tend to orient and engage the environment with a reactive coping style, vigilantly and selectively scanning for signals of punishment and exhibiting a behavioral affinity for the FFS. Depending on predisposing behavioral thresholds, c-type and m-type dogs tend to differentiate with increasing aggressive irritability (c type), fearful anxiousness (m type), or both, as in the case of panic-related aggression and separation distress. Also, c-type and m-type dogs are prone to show reactive aggression and escape behavior in response to conditioned triggers, making them vulnerable to CDA and phobias, respectively. The reactive dog's preoccupation with and scanning for signals of punishment is problematic and the source of escalating anxiety, fearfulness, and relative immunity to normal counterconditioning efforts—procedures requiring a sensitivity and responsiveness toward signals of reward and a capacity to form functional prediction-control

expectancies. Also, many of these m-type dogs show pronounced psychogenic anorexia that is refractory to food deprivation or the provision of highly appetizing food rewards. Finally, both c-type and m-type dogs show deficiencies with respect to their ability to initiate and sustain social play. To the extent that moderately unstable c-type and m-type dogs can be encouraged to play and to accept food and petting, a stabilization effect may be mobilized toward more adaptive coping styles.

In contrast to the reactive coping styles of c and m types, sanguine (s type) and phlegmatic (p type) dogs show distinctive adaptive coping styles. S types tend toward an active modal orientation (e.g., seeking and risk taking) with a BAS affinity, whereas m types tend toward a passive modal orientation (e.g., hesitating and risk avoidant), showing an adaptive response to anxiety and frustration. S types exhibit a selective attention and preference for signals of reward and playful modal activity. On the other hand, p types show a selective attention and preference for signals of successful avoidance, with a hesitation-sensitized affinity for the BIS (see Gray, 1990). S-type and p-type dogs may show defensive aggression and fear (attack and escape), but almost always only in response to unconditioned aversive stimuli that are otherwise uncontrollable. The vast majority of dogs incorporate a balance of s-type and p-type characteristics acquired in the process of coping and adjusting adaptively.

FILIAL AND SIBLING DOMINANCE-SUBMISSION RELATIONS

Dominance, leadership, and nurturing relations analogous to those exhibited by the wolf family/group appear to develop between people and dogs. The establishment of dominant-subordinate relations naturally emerges in the context of a puppy's relationship with the mother and by extension the dog owner. Puppies do not need to be made submissive but come readymade as obligate subordinates and, to the extent that they beg for nurturance (e.g., affection, food, and play), they are submissive. In contrast, the owner may fail to become a competent leader or misunderstand the significance of the puppy's persistent and intrusive active-submission behavior, perhaps interpreting it as a defiant threat to the household's social order. Instead of embracing the puppy's enthusiasm and keen motivation and using them to shape more appropriate behavior via contingencies of reward or rules, the owner may attempt to punish them or mechanically suppress them with excessive crate confinement. As a result, the incompetent leader and the puppy may gradually become wedded to a futile ritual of confusion and conflict involving convergent but antagonistic control incentives and relations. This general scenario of involuntary subordination is an all-too-common perversion of social dominance, in which submission and subordination occur in association with interactive conflict and stress. Instead of mediating friendly and mutually calming relations in association with adaptive coping styles, the owner and the puppy may become locked into a adversarial contest of wills.

Alternatively, owners may neglect to assert competent control and limit-setting actions. As a result, the puppy may become progressively intrusive and demanding in ways consistent with sibling competitive interactions, including playful sparring, harassment, and obtrusive interference. Family members who neglect to establish competent social limits may become the object of intrusive excesses (see *Competitive Social Excesses* in Chapter 6). To build a successful relationship and bond with the dog, the trainer must be both tolerant and able to set appropriate social limits constructively, as Schenkel (1967) nicely describes in the case of wolf social behavior:

> If the superior is tolerant but fails to display his superiority, the inferior may behave obtrusively. In case the superior is not tolerant, i.e., threatens or even attacks the inferior, the latter tries to escape and defend himself and shows signs of social stress … We may conclude that submission is a contribution by the inferior to harmonic social integration on the basis of social hierarchical differentiation. It does not elicit a stereotyped automatic response. Integration asks for a contribution by the superior also, that is, tolerance. The superior's contribution may even exceed submission in its competence to shape the social contact or relation. (325)

INVOLUNTARY SUBORDINATION AND CANINE DOMESTIC AGGRESSION

Whereas the differentiation of social relations and roles associated with filial submission appears to be based on obligate subordination (social polarity, active submission, and begging), the roles and relations associated with sibling competition involve a variable history of previous competitive successes and dominance-related behavior. Sibling competition appears to be organized in accordance with prediction-control expectancies and emotional establishing operations, giving rise to emergent adaptive (s type and p type) and reactive (c type and m type) strategies for coping with social conflict and tension, including (1) a VSS (affectionate submission, playfulness, confidence, flexibility, friendly, and appeasing) and (2) an ISS (obtrusive and interfering, adversarial and rigid, and reactive anger or fear).

The involuntary subordination theory of CDA suggests that dogs are socialized and trained from an early age to accept voluntary or involuntary subordinate roles with respect to family members who are conducive to an adaptive coping style (compromise and cooperation) or reactive coping style (conflict and flight-fight reactivity) that persists throughout a dog's life cycle. As a result of competent socialization, limit setting, and reward-based training (parenting style), a generally affectionate and submissive VSS is integrated into friendly and cooperative relations with family members. However, as the result of incompetent socialization and force-based training (dominating style), a dog may adopt an ISS, showing oppositional, conflictive, and reactive flight-fight behavior toward family members. Such dogs and households may fail to integrate relations conducive to the formation of a trusting bond. The ISS expresses itself in a broad spectrum of problem behaviors occurring within the household. Over the course of a dog's development, competitive tensions and reactive triggers evoking threat or overt aggression may develop around contested resources and privileges. As dogs reach maturity, interactive conflict and the potential for overt aggression may assume a more ominous significance, with dogs sometimes delivering serious attacks against the interference of family members (see *Filial and Sibling Dominance-Submission Relations*).

Whether aggression emerges or not in association with an ISS depends on biogenetic and ontogenetic influences, including the dog's relative excitability, behavioral thresholds controlling the activation of the FFS, and allostatic (stress) load. Allostatic load refers to the wider implications of stress, including biogenetic risk factors, early experience, lifestyle (nutrition, exercise, and play) and other quality-of-life influences, quality of social relations, and perceived control over stressors (McEwen, 2000). Too much or too little stress is problematic and potentially harmful. Dogs exposed to adverse prenatal or postnatal stress, abuse or neglect, or other sources of significant early stress may be particularly vulnerable to the disorganizing effects of psychological stress. Dogs showing heightened excitability with low anger/aggression (fight) thresholds (c type) tend toward offensive and impulsive aggression, whereas dogs showing a low fear/escape (flight) threshold combined with a medium-anger/aggression threshold (m type) are prone to show defensive and avoidance-related aggression. Excitable dogs showing low fear/escape and low anger/aggression thresholds are prone to conflict-related or panic-related aggression. Cynopraxic socialization and training conducive to a VSS exerts a protective influence against the development of household behavior problems by promoting a flirt-and-forbear coping style and consolidating an antistress, antifear, and antiaggression system, thereby offsetting adverse biogenetic and ontogenetic influences (see *Phylogenesis, Polymorphism, and Coping Styles* in Chapter 6).

Submission is mediated by establishing rights of ownership and setting limits around resources evoking seeking behavior. The valued resource or activity is then transformed into a reward by providing access to it in accordance with a rule and a submissive ritual (e.g., sit-stay), a change necessitating compro-

mise and delay of gratification. The object of appetitive seeking is subsequently provided to the dog in exchange for cooperative behaviors in the context of leader-follower activities incompatible with intrusions upon the social limit. Positive prediction error (surprise) occurring in association with the gratification of ensuing leader-follower activities promotes the consolidation of a VSS and the acquisition of interactive modules, routines, and patterns of behavior conducive to the resolution of interactive conflict and tensions. The vast majority of dogs exhibit a balanced admixture of emergent dominant-subordinate characteristics enabling them to respond adaptively to socially competitive situations. Social competition and cooperation are intimately linked, and the dog appears to be biogenetically engineered to respond to competitive situations by expressing cooperative adjustments (VSS), if only the human companion is competent and able to confidently take the lead. Cooperative activity appears to depend on a structure of hierarchical relations emerging in association with competitive transactions and play. As a result, adaptive coping styles develop to promote affectionate submission and tolerance and mutual reliance and appreciation (tend and befriend) (see *Adaptive Coping Styles: Play, Flirt, Forbear, and Nip* in Chapter 6). Under the influence of adaptive coping styles, competitive social behavior is gradually differentiated into a complex set of cooperative and friendly dynamic modal relations, roles, and mutual expectations conducive to interactive harmony and trust.

SOCIAL DOMINANCE: DISPOSITIONAL CAUSE OR ATTRIBUTIONAL ERROR

The social dominance hypothesis is frequently appealed to in one form or another to explain CDA. Although the dominance model has value for understanding certain types and aspects of domestic aggression in dogs, the hypothesis can also be used to justify faulty interpretations and misunderstandings, based on misleading linkages between dog aggression and social dominance (see *Concept of Social Dominance* in Volume 1, Chapter 8). As a result of bias and misinformation, attributing dispositional causes such as dominance to explain aggressive behavior is risky and prone to anthropomorphic error and the elaboration of explanatory fictions. The issues involved are complicated but deserve focused attention in advance of considering treatment protocols and procedures. Avoiding explanatory fictions is significant with respect to treatment programs because such errors adversely affect the way in which aggression problems are framed and approached, thereby influencing the selection of procedures used to address the problem. Historically, since dominance was viewed as something achieved by means of force and threats (Most, 1910/1955), the dominance hypothesis was and continues to be used in some quarters to justify inappropriate physical punishment and brutalization for the control of aggression problems. In addition to justifying inhumane methods, protocols and procedures that are based on phantom causes are doomed to produce chimerical cures. Social dominance is a significant and valid construct, but it requires careful definition and delimitation for practical use in the context of training and behavior therapy.

Dependent, Independent, and Intervening Variables

Observing and measuring behavioral changes as they occur in response to the presentation of highly controlled events or conditions is central to the experimental study of behavior. Most laboratory research involving animal behavior and learning involves a methodology in which antecedent and consequent events are rigorously defined and controlled. Behavior occurring under the influence of arranged antecedent and consequent events or conditions is referred to as *conditioned behavior*. The various controlled conditions or antecedent or consequent events are referred to as *independent variables*, whereas the observed changes in behavior that occur dependently in association with their presentation or omission are referred to as *dependent variables*. Independent variables are related to dependent variables as causes are related to effects. Many scientific theories also postulate another set of variables that, although not directly observable, are believed by inference to mediate or intervene between causes and effects. For example, in mechanical physics, the ability of one object to displace another is understood in terms of a variety of postulated intervening variables, such as gravity, mass, inertia, and momentum. No one has ever seen gravity, but the existence of gravity is inferred from the observable movements of objects and the effects they produce on the motion of other objects.

Intervening variables are often used to help explain how independent and dependent variables are related to one another, thereby rendering the relationship between them more predictable and controllable. For example, although the contingent presentation of food (independent variable) *can* increase the frequency of some target response (dependent variable), the presentation of food does not necessarily result in reinforcement; that is, the presentation of food does not necessary strengthen or increase the rate of responding. In order for food to function as reliable reinforcer, at minimum, a dog must be motivated to seek and eat food when it is presented; that is, the dog must be hungry. According to this interpretation, hunger is inferred as the intervening condition making the presentation of food more likely to result in reinforcement. Radical behaviorists reject intervening variables as being unnecessary for studying behavior. Instead of postulating hunger as an intervening variable, these researchers collect information about the animal's weight or the length of time that it has gone without eating—deprivation period. Theoretically, with the accumulation of data concerning the effects of deprivation on reinforcement, and holding all other independent variables constant, one would be able roughly to predict the probable size of the effect that reinforcement will have on the frequency of the target response based on the number of hours that the animal has been deprived of food.

Explanatory Fictions

Intervening variables such as hunger, thirst, and sleepiness are relatively harmless, providing a reasonable and useful, if not entirely reliable or scientifically framed, simplification for understanding the motivations underlying ordinary behavior. However, the use of intervening variables to understand the causes of complex social behavior is subject to several potential sources of error, including the promulgation of explanatory fictions. Explanatory fictions occur when an intervening variable is inferred as a cause mediating some behavioral effect where in fact no such causal relationship exists. The assignment of attitudinal attributions (e.g., "the dog is stubborn"), emergent dispositional attributes (e.g., attachment and social dominance), and appeal to emotional states as mediating causes are particularly prone to error and fictionalizing. Despite the risk of error, appeal to dispositional intervening variables is common in applied settings (e.g., boredom, conflict, stress, anxiety, frustration, or dominance). Since the identification and interpretation of dispositional causes are often an important aspect of behavioral diagnosis and treatment decisions, it is of utmost importance that such causes be carefully delineated; otherwise, treatment efforts may be inefficient or ineffective. In some cases, faulty dispositional inferences and explanatory fictions can be extremely harmful and represent significant obstacles to effective treatment. For example, owners commonly interpret their dogs' aggressive behavior as stemming from defiant belligerence. Responding under the influence of such an explanatory fiction, the owner may resort to severe punishment, thereby damaging their relationship with the dog and probably making the problem far worse and more difficult to resolve.

Fundamental Attributional Error

Explanatory fictions incorporating dispositional accounts are prone to develop when causal explanations require the consideration of events not immediately present or indicated by situational evidence. Dispositional causes are inferred from the situation, whereas the actual formative causes may not be present in the situation (e.g., adverse or inadequate socialization), but may be far removed from it and unavailable for consideration. Behavior observers tend to underestimate the causal significance of situational factors while overestimating the importance of dispositional factors in the control of behavior—a tendency known as the fundamental attributional error (Ross and Nisbett, 1991). The tendency to emphasize attitudinal or disposition factors (dispositionism) over situational ones appears to be most common in cases where immediate and remote causes (dependent variables) are ambiguous or unknown. In addition to being prone to error and misinterpretation, the assignment of attitudinal and dispositional causes tends to preclude or obscure the consideration of possibly more influential immediate and remote causes affecting a dog's behavior. In this regard, people tend to attribute situational causes to their own actions, while tending to attribute dispositional causes to the behavior of others, probably including other owners and their dogs (actor-observer discrepancy). For example, failing to meet a deadline, a person might explain their shortcoming by appealing to something that unexpectedly came up, whereas, if someone else fails to meet a deadline, there is a strong tendency for an observer to explain it by dispositional causes, such as laziness or the person is not interested in the project, rather than looking for proximal or remote situational causes. Finally, a significant motivation for attributing dispositional mediating causes to behavior is to provide a perception of enhanced predictability and control over it; even if in actuality the causes are fictitious and the treatment a placebo, nonetheless, one may feel more in control!

Dispositional versus Situational Causes

In comparison to the way in which the behavior of children is interpreted, dogs enjoy a significant *positive bias* in the direction of leniency and more favorable attributions (Rajecki et al., 1999). Attributional processes appear to be influenced by the sort of behavior involved. Observers tend to excuse dogs from antisocial behavior while crediting them with responsibility for prosocial behavior. Interestingly, whereas prosocial behavior is commonly attributed to internal and controllable dispositional causes, aggressive behavior is more likely to be attributed to external situational causes not under the dog's control.

Barring obvious limitations and provisos, dispositional attributions are not without value as a sort of predictive shorthand. In fact, emergent dispositional attributions resulting from careful observation are often highly predictive of future behavior. For example, a dog that has repeatedly submitted to owner limit-setting imperatives may rightly be called subordinate and submissive to human control, whereas a dog that consistently resists or defies owner control efforts may be rightly referred to as being competitive or oppositional. To what extent, though, are such post hoc descriptions consistent with the actual causes underlying the submissive and the opposition behavior; that is, to what extent is a dog's obedience to command attributable to submissiveness or disobedience attributable to the influence social dominance? In fact, dogs submit or compete as the result of a variety of causes. A pattern of apparent competition and unwillingness to submit may be due to a dog's temporary inability to exert inhibitory control over its behavior, despite its best efforts to submit to owner control efforts. In such cases, the dog's failure to obey and actively defer is not due to a disposition to compete and defy the owner's authority, but rather may be interpreted as the result of a temporary loss of inhibitory impulse control. Dispositional causes related to impulse-control deficits probably play a significant role in the competitive excesses of puppies. Impulse-control abilities in young puppies are developmentally limited, with dogs only gradually acquiring the neurobiological capacity to exert impulse control in a refined and reliable way. In the case of young dogs, impulse and action are tightly wedded. Efforts to suppress actions may serve only to potentiate and frustrate underlying impulses. The regulation of impulses is probably localized in prefrontal cortex, an area of the developing brain that may not be fully formed until late in the first year with the emergence of enhanced cognitive abilities (Gagnon and Dore, 1994) (see *Learning and Trainability* in Volume 1, Chapter 2).

Dispositional attributions not only affect the diagnosis of behavior problems, they also determine the likely course of treatment. Remembering that dispositional attributions are made in order to enhance control over a dog's behavior, it is logical that behavior believed to stem from defiant competitive motivations would be treated with procedures aimed at increasing a dog's submission to authority. Unfortunately, a dog's degree of submissiveness may be entirely irrelevant with respect to the actual causes underlying its inability to obey owner directives. Whereas physical restraint and punishment may enhance submission in cases where "defiance" is identified as the mediating dispositional cause of competitive behavior, such treatment would be entirely inappropriate in the case of impulsive behavior stemming from hyperactivity, attention or impulse deficits, or immaturity. Unfortunately, such distinctions are not consistently made, and dog behavior problems are often lumped together under the misleading rubric of dispositional causes, such as competitiveness or attention seeking, rather than ontogenetic or situational causes that may be more illuminating and useful. Dogs often seek attention with reference to objectives and needs other than the acquisition of social attention itself (e.g., they seek the owner's attention because they want food or because they want to go outside and so forth); likewise, dogs often compete and oppose owner directives as the result of situational incentives competing for the dog's interest—not as the result of a defiant disposition to resist owner control efforts. Outside of play, where competition may occur solely for the sake of interactive fun, competition is usually limited to situations in which the owner's control directives either thwart or interfere with a dog's enjoyment of some activity, object, place, or other valued resource, including the owner's presence. Other common dispositional causes attributed to competitive behavior may be self-serving to the extent that they are invoked to rationalize abusive training practices. For example, a dog's momentary unwillingness to obey an obedience command may be mistakenly interpreted as stemming from sullen defiance, whereas, in fact, the dog's disobedience and appearance of sullenness may be due to other causes (e.g., arthritic pain or emunctory distress), giving the appearance of resistance and unwillingness to obey. Without knowing the true causes of disobedience, the trainer may feel justified in using harsh compulsory measures to force the dog to perform.

Anthropomorphic Errors

Much harm is done to dogs as the result of attributing anthropomorphic dispositions and motivations to canine behavior. In general, cynopraxic counselors should resist temptations to unnecessarily attribute complex psychological causes to dog behavior in adherence to C. Lloyd Morgan's famous law of parsimony: "In no case may we interpret an action as the outcome of the exercise of a higher psychical faculty, if it can be interpreted as the outcome of the exercise of one which stands lower in the psychological scale" (Morgan, 1894:53). Nowhere is such restraint and self-discipline more necessary than when assessing the situational and dispositional causes underlying aggressive behavior, especially aggression directed toward family members.

Although most dogs are benignly subordinate and submissive toward their owners, some do appear to actively assert limits on their owner's behavior by way of threats and limited attack, suggesting that social dominance may play a dispositional role in the etiology of some forms of CDA. Domestic aggressors may threaten or bite if family members intrude upon a forbidden location, disturb them while resting or sleeping, threaten them with discipline, attempt to take something away from them, attempt to restrain them, and so forth. Of course, most dogs readily give up control over sleeping areas and chew objects, accept handling of all kinds, including punitive treatment, without ever resorting to threat displays or biting. Further, the environmental conditions are relatively constant between dogs that bite and those that do not bite. Why, then, does one dog passively submit while another one threatens or bites? According to the social dominance theory, the primary cause of

aggression in such situations is related to social status. The household aggressor either bites in response to a violation of its status or attacks with the goal of improving its social rank. This general theory is problematic on a number of grounds that have been explored in some detail in Volume 2. There are many potential causes standing lower than the defense or enhancement of status on Morgan's psychological scale to explain such behavior that should be systematically excluded when performing a behavioral assessment and diagnosis.

Dominance as a dispositional cause can be easily confused with other remote (e.g., ontogenetic), situational, and dispositional causes (e.g., irritability and frustration) that may be more directly relevant to behavior-therapy efforts. Although competitive conflicts may escalate into aggression, aggression is not necessarily the result of motivations associated with dominance, particularly not in sense of status and rank. For example, although dogs may become aggressively aroused when they are pulled away from sleeping or resting areas, the incentive to threaten or bite at such times may be borne out of a momentary autoprotective incentive to expediently control irritating or frustrating interference. Such domestic aggressors are not necessarily challenging family members for rank, but are simply responding reactively and incompetently to the handling and the momentary loss of comfort and safety. Dogs of this sort may lack the socialization and training necessary for them to respond in a more socially acceptable and cooperative way to intrusive and provocative handling. However, as the result of repeated offensive threats toward the owner, the dog may gradually assume a dominant relation toward the owner. This sort of CDA is most likely to result in ritualized threats and inhibited punitive biting, not severe and uninhibited bites that are commonly attributed to dominance.

Dogs that deliver hard and uninhibited bites often do so under the influence of varying degrees of panic and an apparent loss of impulse control—the antithesis of competent social dominance. The attacks of such dogs are often out of character, highly exaggerated, and disproportionate to the provoking stimulus. Such aggression frequently occurs under the influence of circumstances similar to that just described, but the attacks seem to differ with respect to the level of emotional arousal, the degree of competency and control over the action, and their severity. Panic-related aggression appears to occur in association with heightened autonomic arousal, behavioral rigidity, and a conflux of coactive emotional influences (e.g., anger, irritability, frustration, and fear) resulting in the catastrophic dysregulation of aggressive impulse. When punished, such dogs do not back down or retreat, giving them an appearance of fearlessness. Instead of submitting or fleeing when punished, panic aggressors tend to escalate their attacks rapidly under the excitatory influence of fear. In contrast to the impulsive character of panic-related attacks, competent control-related aggression is more likely to occur in accordance with prediction-control expectancies and a cost-benefit assessment, such that aggressive challenges or threats are rapidly abandoned if they prove too costly when they fail or offer little promise of benefit when they succeed.

Social Dominance as a Dispositional Cause of Aggression

Erringly identifying the causes of aggression as stemming from a dominance conflict may result in the initiation of training efforts designed to enhance owner dominance and control—efforts that may or may not be relevant to the actual causes underlying the problem. In other cases, the attribution of dominance may result in the use of highly intrusive and aversive procedures believed to alter canine social status.

The attribution of social dominance in the sense of rank or status as a primary cause of CDA is flawed and inconsistent with Morgan's law of parsimony. Most instances of CDA can be interpreted in terms of functional causes, including conditioned expectancies, adverse emotional influences, and conflict. Consequently, the term *control related* appears to more closely approximate and capture the intent and significance of such aggressive behavior. In any case, the term *dominance* is primarily used here in the sense of limit-setting actions, that contribute to social competency and foster the integration of a submissive bond. Domestic aggression most often reflects the influence of social confusion and a failure of the owner and the dog to interact in an organized and competent way with each other. As the result of past competitive successes involving aggression, attacks against family members may become more frequent and severe under the influence of conditioned aversive arousal (anxiety, frustration, irritability, or anger), stress-related disturbances, and the presence of inadequate social coping and communication skills.

ADVERSE ENVIRONMENTAL AND EMOTIONAL INFLUENCES AND CANINE DOMESTIC AGGRESSION

Most CDA currently attributed to dominance lacks a confident quality, making the diagnostic attribution of *dominance related* highly suspect in such cases (Guy et al., 2001). Such aggression appears to be more anxious and reactive than proactive and fearless. Impulsive aggression occurring under the influence of conflict might best be described as *autoprotective*. Instead of speculating and attributing excessive causal significance to rank and household dominance hierarchies, the causes of most CDA can be better understood and described in terms of distal polymorphic variances (individual differences) affecting excitability, fear and anger thresholds, and sociability; ontogenetic influences such as prenatal and postnatal stress, exposure to early adversity (abuse or neglect), socialization and habituation deficits, and toxic expectancies; the presence or absence of protective social nurturance and training; and proximal provoking situations and social triggers, reactive coping styles and ISSs, diminished capacity to regulate emotion and impulse, coactive establishing operations (e.g., anger, fear, excitability, irritability, frustration, and conflict), and allostatic load. Although threat displays can advertise relative social rank and status, these social signals can also reflect underlying coactive emotional and motivational states and a heightened readiness to act in particular ways to control a provocative situation (Figure 7.1), independently of standing dominant-subordinate relations. Aggression in association with owner control efforts typically involves varying degrees of elicited irritability, frustration, anger, or fear. Aggression in such cases is often triggered by owner interference or disturbance, conflicting with appetitive-seeking and comfort-seeking activities (control incentives or *vectors*). Gradually, as the result of actual or anticipated threats or losses, a dog may become progressively vigilant and irritable when approached, thereby gradually lowering aggression thresholds in association with owner intrusion or interference (comfort/safety violations). For example, approaching a dog with a history of object guarding and aggression while it is in possession of a bone evokes varying amounts of conditioned anger or irritability, emotional changes established in association with a history of owner intrusion and interference. Dogs prone to react aggressively to social signals associated with discipline (e.g., loud voice, direct stare, or abrupt reaching or leaning over actions) and restraint may also be responding under the influence of varying degrees of anxiety, frustration, or anger stemming from past experiences associated with positive or negative punishment (see *Anxiety, Frustration, and Aggression* in Volume 2, Chapter 8). These two general sources of aggressive arousal are respectively referred to as loss of comfort and loss of safety. *Comfort loss* refers to interference or intrusion upon activities and sources of stimulation that the dog would wish maintain or intensify. *Safety loss* refers to interference or intrusion that involves a threat or presentation of events that the dog would prefer to escape or avoid. Provocative comfort loss or safety loss are the two primary ways in which control-related aggression develops. The traumatic loss of comfort or safety may be especially problematic in dogs having formed close attachments with their owners (loss of trust), in dogs that have not learned how to cope competently with loss, in dogs exposed to provocative comfort and safety loss on a relatively unpredictable or uncontrollable basis (conflict), and in dogs operating under the influence of toxic expectancies resulting from a history of traumatic or abusive handling.

In addition to social causes, biogenetic and developmental influences appear to predispose some dogs to develop aggression problems. Dogs with reactive and excitable temperaments appear to be more prone to exhibit CDA (Dodman et al., 1995; Borchelt, 1986; Podberscek and Serpell, 1997; Luescher, 2000; Guy et al., 2001b). The combination of low fear and anger thresholds, presenting with a high degree of excitability, may strongly predispose dogs for developing CDA problems in association with impulse dyscontrol and panic. Panic-related aggression occurs under the influence of adverse emotional stressors and provocative conditioned and unconditioned triggers that overstrain a dog's ability to control aggressive impulses. Such dogs may bite, not as the result of control-related incentives or dominance, but rather because of an inability to cope competently with a provocative situation. Panic-related aggression occurs as the result of a momentary loss of control over aggressive impulse. In contrast, control-related aggression refers to competent (proactive) and incompetent (reactive/impulsive) efforts organized to assert control over aversive or intrusive social events portending a loss of security (threat to comfort or safety). Control-related aggression includes both offensive (anger-related) and defensive (fear-related) forms occurring under the pressure of autoprotective incentives. Whereas panic-related aggression appears to stem from an internal loss of control over arousal states anticipating rage, control-related aggression is triggered by an external loss of control over significant social exchanges that can present with competent proactive forms aimed at promoting adaptive optimization by taking advantage of favorable cost-to-benefit ratios or incompetent forms (reactive and impulsive aggression) operating under the adverse influence of social ambivalence (anxiety) and irritability. In any case, most forms of competent and incompetent aggression are expressed as means to ends in subservience to autoprotective interests and concerns rather than the pursuit of social dominance and rank. Rather than attempting to alter the dog's perception of rank, training efforts should be dedicated to restoring or developing a social bond based on trust in situations

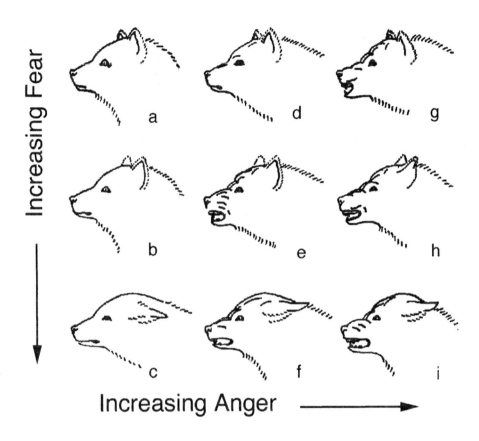

FIG. 7.1. Aggression occurs under the influence of varying admixtures of coactive emotional influences, such as anger and fear. These emotional states are reflected in a variety of postural and facial changes or signs that provide the receiver with information about the sender's probable course of future action, thereby enabling the receiver to better anticipate (predict) and adjust (control) to the impending situation. The facial expression in *drawing i* indicates signs of intense emotional arousal associated with the simultaneous provocation of high levels of fear and anger, a state of conflicted arousal that may overstrain executive impulse-control functions and result in explosive panic-related attacks in predisposed dogs. After Lorenz (1966).

that have provoked aggression in the past (Table 7.1).

SOCIAL COMMUNICATION AND THE REGULATION OF AGGRESSION

Functional Significance of Social Signals

Social communication provides a conduit of exchange and information about what affiliative partners are most likely to do in advance of them actually doing it (see *Communication and the Regulation of Social Behavior* in Volume 1, Chapter 10). In addition to signaling the sender's intent, communication serves to elicit preparatory emotional responses readying the receiver to act in certain ways. Depending on the sort of signal or display sent, the receiver is rendered more or less likely to greet, play, attack, submit, flee, and so forth; that is, the signal sets the occasion and elicits the emotional concomitants necessary for the emission of a certain class of behavior. As such, signals serve the dual function of discriminative stimuli and establishing operations. As discriminative stimuli, social signals announce a moment when a particular set or class of behaviors is most likely to result in reinforcement. As establishing operations, social signals momentarily alter a dog's motivational readiness to behave in ways that are in keeping with the discriminative significance of the social signal presented (see *Antecedent Control: Establishing Operations and Discriminative Stimuli* in Volume 1, Chapter 7).

In an important sense, effective social communication serves to make the behavior of the sender and the receiver more predictable and controllable to each other; that is, the exchange of orderly social signals helps to promote more trustworthy and reliable interaction. Under the influence of an orderly exchange of social signals and mutual adjustments consistent with those signals, social behavior is gradually shaped and refined in the direction of enhanced interactive harmony, whereas, on the other hand, social signals that lack a consistent and orderly significance and presentation tend to impede the development of interactive harmony, resulting in increased levels of social conflict, anxiety, and frustration. As a result of interaction lacking consistency and orderliness, varying degrees of unease, distrust, tension, and potential for disturbance are inexorably introduced and maintained under the influence of deranged reinforcement contingencies and classical conditioning. In the context of aversive emotional arousal occurring in association with aggressive behavior, a lack of quality predictive information may lower aggression

thresholds via anxiety, thereby increasing a dog's readiness to engage in disorganized defensive behavior.

Social signals involve both conditioned and unconditioned elements helping to make social interaction more predictable. Signals serving an establishing operation function are strongly influenced by feed-forward mechanisms that collect and appraise predictive information via the influence of classical conditioning (Domjan et al., 2000). Feed-forward information gives advance notice or warning of what is about to occur on the basis of what has occurred under similar circumstances in the past, thereby enhancing an animal's ability to control the impending occurrence by means of anticipatory adjustments that prepare it for appropriate action. Predictive social signals serve to make social interaction more effective and efficient, whereas unpredictive signals introduce escalating levels of anxiety and stress. Many common canine aggression problems appear to be under the control of Pavlovian feed-forward expectancies and instrumental contingencies of reinforcement. In addition, conditioned and unconditioned aversive and appetitive stimuli exert a direct excitatory or inhibitory effect on instrumental behavior, providing powerful means for modulating aggressive arousal and behavior (Dickinson and Pearce, 1977).

Dogs work to escape or avoid aversive social stimulation by means of behavioral adjustments that result in a reduction of the threat while simultaneously searching for safety from the danger. When the owner is

TABLE 7.1. Treatment of intra-familial aggression involves a multifaceted program consisting of at least eight elements

1. Exclude possible medical causes by veterinary examination and appropriate testing.

2. Obtain a thorough history and assess aggressive behavior.

3. Identify and reduce coactive emotional influences.

4. Systematically elevate pertinent aggression thresholds.

5. Improve the predictability and controllability of social interaction.

6. Promote interaction that is conducive to a restoration of trust between the family and dog.

7. Train the dog to respond more competently to situations involving appetitive loss or aversive threat.

8. Avoid unnecessary and provocative situations that may increase aggressive tensions or evoke actual attacks.

both the source of aversive stimulation as well as the dog's primary source of safety, a high degree of emotional conflict is likely to ensue with increasing levels of ambivalence, irritability, and intolerance. The traumatic disconfirmation of comfort and safety is hypothesized to evoke high levels of anger and fear, setting the emotional stage for reactive panic and aggression. Dogs that have formed close attachments with their owners may be energetically aroused by punishment, experiencing an unexpected discrepancy between a history of comfort and safety (security) conducive to trust and its rapid and traumatic loss. In cases where aversive stimulation is combined with an inescapable condition in which the owner ignores submissive signals and prevents the dog from getting away or otherwise controlling the punitive stimulation, biting to break free may be the dog's last resort. In the future when faced with situations portending similar treatment, the dog may preemptively threaten or bite the owner and flee to a hiding place in search of safety and protection. This is a very problematic state of affairs that frequently presents in close association with CDA problems. Such owners need to learn how to control their dogs more kindly and skillfully, while, on the other hand, such dogs need to learn how to respond more competently to social situations demanding obligatory subordination and cooperation. The dog's trust in the owner as a reliable source of comfort, safety, and consistency must also be restored—a change that is facilitated by cynopraxic training and therapy, attention and relaxation training, play, and a variety of predictable and controllable friendly interactions signifying comfort and safety to the dog. The cynopraxic process integrates owner relations with the dog consistent with a tend-and-befriend orientation, thereby activating a mutually beneficial antistress response, while mobilizing a VSS incompatible with flight-or-fight reactions.

Social Signals, Impulse Control, and Attention

Accurate prediction and control foster behavior that is appropriate to the circumstances in which it occurs—something that is commonly lacking in the case of CDA problems. Overstrain of attention and impulse-control faculties by adverse conflictive pressures originating from internal (e.g., emotional disturbances and stress) or external sources (e.g., unpredictable and uncontrollable events) may significantly impact upon a dog's ability to regulate its behavior, including aggressive impulses. Emotionally provocative stimulation occurring on a relatively frequent, unpredictable, and uncontrollable basis may be particularly problematic, inducing a high degree of conflict and stress. Dogs possessing unstable temperaments (choleric and melancholic types) may be more prone to exhibit various disorganized and maladaptive coping efforts when exposed to deranged environmental contingencies. Disturbances in attention and impulse control resulting from deficient prediction and control may also occur in situations where events are quite orderly but remain elusive to the dog because it has not yet learned how to apprehend them as such. Such difficulties may develop in association with inadequate socialization and training efforts. In such cases, remedial basic training may provide a therapeutic benefit by means of explicitly presenting significant events on a highly predictable and controllable basis—an influence conducive to enhanced social competence, confidence, and relaxation. Training activities also enhance both attention and impulse control, thereby improving human-dog communication and cooperation. Improved communication and cooperation promote interactive harmony and social trust between the dog and the owner, as well as helping to reduce physiological stress. Highly structured programs of ICT probably derive most of their aggression-reducing benefits from the enhancement of attention and impulse control rather then serving to alter the dog's social status. Finally, even though some dog-training authorities have overstated the importance of social dominance for regulating social interaction between people and dogs, the establishment of social order by limit-setting activities remains a necessary part of the training and socialization process.

SOCIAL COMPETITION, COOPERATION, CONFLICT, AND RESENTMENT

Social interaction integrating dominant and subordinate relations into cooperative activities by means of limit-setting actions, reward-based training, and play promotes emotional establishing operations and modal strategies conducive to social harmony. Under the ideal conditions of voluntary subordination, the filial/sibling subordinate defers to the leader/trainer's limit-setting actions with submission behavior. The leader/trainer nurtures active submission (affection and care seeking) with contingent rewards arranged to shape a cooperative pattern of interactive behavior. Essentially, cooperation is *gratified begging* organized to promote a friendly leader–follower bond.

Voluntary subordination is most likely to occur under conditions of minimal coercion, positive reinforcement, and play, whereby the subordinate's need for affectionate contact, nurturance, and protection are met by means of voluntary compliance to the trainer's leadership directives. The VSS is characterized by elevated mood (elation) associated with the success and safety obtained by cooperative compliance with a competent leader. Under the influence of adverse conditions in which subordination is coerced by means of punishment and maintained by threats, an ISS may develop in association with increased resentment and potential for CDA. The loss of effective social control and the ensuing conflict-related stress associated with ISS may result in depressed mood, increased irritability, and reduced tolerance for close contact and taction. The adverse effects of persistent involuntary subordination on emotional tone and mood have been theoretically implicated in the etiology of depressive illness in people (see Gardner, 1982; Price et al. 1994; Price and Gardner, 1995). In addition to social incompetence and intolerance, many offensive aggressors appear to be strongly affected by increased levels of anxiety and vigilance associated with involuntary subordination. Within the context of the family structure, these negative emotions may be selectively exhibited toward family members, depending on social considerations. During interaction with inferiors (e.g., children), the involuntary subordinate may exhibit heightened irritability and intolerance, whereas interaction with superiors (e.g., adults) may evoke vigilance and resentment. Interestingly, such dogs may show a particular fondness and tolerance toward children and adults incapacitated in various ways that prevent them from exerting a control threat to the dogs.

SPECIES-TYPICAL DEFENSIVE AND OFFENSIVE AGGRESSION

Generally speaking, aggression is a risky activity that operates within limits of cost-benefit expectancies, weighing the benefits of success set against the potential costs of failure (see *Cognition and Aggression* in Volume 2, Chapter 6). Aggressors attack under a risk that the target victim might fight back and, in doing so, perhaps injure or kill the aggressor. The threat of punitive retaliation exerts a significant inhibitory effect over animal social aggression (Clutton-Brock and Parker, 1995). Punitive retaliation against violence is a natural and virtually universal response, the assumed effectiveness of which is reflected in its ancient origins and continuous worldwide practice as a preferred means to inhibit aggressive behavior. Despite these natural and cultural precedents for the use of punishment to control aggression, punishment in the case of CDA is complicated and generally avoided except in the case of overt attacks. Even in the case of overt attacks, though, punishment poses serious challenges and risks. Punishing an adult dog while it is in the act of an overt attack risks producing a more dangerous situation via vicious-circle effects (Melvin, 1971) (see *Reactive Types* in Chapter 5). If the punitive effort is insufficient to produce immediate inhibition, the escalating attack may continue until the punitive effort is discontinued, often at the moment at which the dog succeeds in breaking free by biting. As a result of ensuing negative reinforcement occurring at such times, threats or attacks may rapidly escalate and morph into a much more dangerous form in response to future owner control efforts. In addition, preemptive attacks may begin to occur in response to benign body movements that resemble actions associated with the failed punitive effort (e.g., reaching or leaning over the dog). These adverse byproducts of punishment strongly militate against its use in the treatment of most forms of aggression.

Dogs respond to aversive events with a variety of species-typical defensive reactions (SSDRs), which provide rapid behavioral adjustments to threatening situations. SSDRs are highly stereotypic, phylogenetically significant, easily evoked, and rapidly learned as avoidance responses (see *Species-specific Defensive Reactions* in Volume 1, Chapter 8). In addition, dogs exhibit a variety of species-typical offensive reactions (STORs) that occur in response to socially provocative stimulation involving pain or frustration and the induction of anger. Antecedent social and contextual stimuli present at the time of provocative stimulation may be conditioned to control the preemptive expression of SSDRs and STORs. Not only is avoidance learning rapid, conditioning resulting in avoidance-related aggression is highly persistent and durable (see *A Cognitive Theory of Avoidance Learning* in Volume 1, Chapter 8; and *Conditioned Fear and Extinction* in Volume 2, Chapter 3). Whether a dog attacks or withdraws during punishment depends on biogenetic and developmental influences (temperament) affecting the functional thresholds controlling such behavior (see *Behavioral Thresholds and Aggression* in Volume 2, Chapter 8). Dogs possessing a low fear threshold and a high aggression threshold show a propensity to become fearful first, causing them to respond to aversive stimulation by various flight or freeze responses, such as running away or becoming rigid. At the other extreme, dogs with a low aggression threshold combined with a high fear threshold may rapidly transition into attack mode in response to minimal provocation.

Fearful dogs struggling to escape interactive punishment may eventually threaten or attack under the influence of escalating aversive arousal. Rather than flee or freeze in the future, these dogs may rapidly learn to threaten or bite preemptively in response to provocative social stimuli (see *Avoidance Learning and Aggression* in Volume 2, Chapter

6). Under the same interactive punishment, dogs exhibiting low aggression thresholds may eventually reach a fear threshold, causing them to freeze or flee or energizing their aggressive efforts under the excitatory influence of fear. Dogs exhibiting low behavioral thresholds for fear and aggression may be highly reactive and intolerant of provocative social stimulation. When exposed to physical punishment, such dogs may rapidly become enraged under the reciprocal excitatory influences of fear and anger on panic/rage circuits. Under the influence of sustained punishment, such dogs may become progressively violent (panic-related aggression). Dogs affected by elevated fear and aggression thresholds tend to exhibit tolerance for provocative social stimuli and enjoy a natural protection against the development of aggression problems.

Guy and colleagues (2001c) have questioned the relevance of dominance as an etiological factor in the development of CDA problems, arguing that aggression problems may be more closely related to the expression of temperament traits (e.g., excitability) and social anxiety/fear, perhaps more significantly so than social dominance. Such behavioral and emotional influences may be exacerbated by the use of punitive methods of control, perhaps further increasing the risk of aggression—practices that may be particularly problematic in the case of puppies showing low anger thresholds in combination with low or high fear thresholds. In such cases, physical punishment may trigger panic-related reactive aggression (low anger and low fear thresholds) or fearless attack (low anger/high fear thresholds) or cause aggressive behavior to rapidly escalate via avoidance learning and vicious-circle effects (Brown et al., 1964). Punishing reactive or fearless puppies may only serve to sensitize them to signals of punishment, however, instead of inhibiting the target behavior, punishment may actually increase aggression via vicious-circle effects, perhaps making the behavior more difficult to predict, control, and manage.

The use of interactive punishment for the control of aggression is problematic, but especially so when it is applied against threat displays (e.g., growling and snarling). The punishment of threat displays may cause dogs to withhold threats and possibly to learn to bite without warning. Growling and other threat displays provide a trainer with valuable information about a dog's emotional state as well as give advance warnings of impending attacks. As a result, threat displays provide a layer of safety to family members and others coming into contact with the dog—protection that may be removed by punishment. In addition to potentially suppressing valuable warnings, punishing a threat display risks triggering an escalation of aggressive tensions, especially in the case of excitable dogs, perhaps triggering an overt attack and breaking the ALL IMPORTANT inhibition controlling the first hard bite. After the first bite, subsequent biting becomes much easier for dogs. The power of the native canine inhibition against biting can never be duplicated by any amount of training and, once it is broken, can never be fully restored.

Instead of punishing aggressive threats, it is far better to reduce the frequency of threatening behavior by modifying the social and environmental causes controlling it. Growling and other threats should be viewed as useful diagnostic signs and protective warnings that should be monitored and reduced by displacing aversive arousal with incompatible emotional and behavioral responses conducive to friendly cooperation and play. One option for managing trigger situations is to avoid them whenever possible and practical. For example, in the case of dogs whose threats or attacks occur only in the context of control-related incentives associated with physical punishment, owners can be encouraged not to use such methods of training. Physical punishment is something that owners can easily learn to live without after learning how to control and train their dogs by less intrusive and provocative means. However, in cases involving critical and unavoidable interaction with dogs (e.g., approaching, touching, handling, grooming, or restraining), various behavior-therapy and training procedures should be introduced to help manage and reduce the risk of future aggression while shaping various behavioral changes incompatible with aggression and promoting interaction that supports enhanced safety and trust.

Finally, behavioral thresholds controlling fear and aggression are strongly influenced by experience. Puppies with low fear and low anger thresholds should be identified at an early age and provided with appropriate socialization and training. Although such puppies are at an increased risk of developing behavior problems associated with fear or aggression, owner counseling and early intervention appear to provide a protective influence.

LOSS OF SAFETY, DEPRESSION, PANIC, AND AGGRESSION

The formation of a close attachment between the owner and dog appears to be a necessary condition, but not a sufficient one, for the development of both reactive separation distress and CDA. A common link shared by these social behavior problems is the presence of conflict-related stress and panic occurring in association with the loss of comfort and safety (security). In the case of separation-distress syndrome, the loss of the attachment object at separation provokes varying degrees of distress under the coactive influences of anxiety, frustration, and panic, whereas, in the case of CDA, a loss of safety resulting from provocative stimulation at the hands of an attachment object may result in varying degrees of vulnerability and conflict under the coactive influences of anger, fear, panic, and rage (Figure 7.2). As an object of attachment, comfort, and safety, the owner may evoke significant conflict in the dog when delivering physical punishment producing high levels of pain and fear (see *Drive Systems, Aggression, and Behavior Problems* in Chapter 6), potentially resulting in a dramatic and permanent loss of security and trust. The potential for loss of trust and panic-related aggression is particularly high in situations involving abusive and inescapable punishment directed toward dogs with reactive temperaments (low fear/low anger threshold). As the result of traumatic stimulation and loss of trust, persistent toxic expectancies may form and mediate the expression of panic-related aggression in response to conditioned social stimuli present during the traumatic event. According to

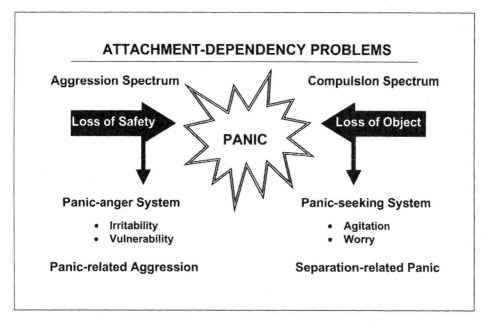

FIG. 7.2. Panic may play a pivotal role in the etiology of severe separation-related distress problems as well as certain presentations of owner-directed aggression, commonly described as dominance related. Both behavior problems appear to involve predisposing biogenetic, developmental, and experiential (e.g., toxic expectancies) influences that render a dog persistently vulnerable to attachment-related loss in association with owner separation (loss of object) or owner intrusions or interference (loss of comfort or safety). Following the emotional command system devised by Panksepp, separation-related distress may acquire an exaggerated and compulsive form as the result of panic-induced dysregulation affecting the seeking system (compulsive spectrum), whereas panic-related aggression may result in exaggerated and impulsive-episodic aggressive behavior (aggression spectrum) occurring as the result of panic-induced dysregulation of the anger-rage system. Both separation distress-panic and panic-related aggression tend to escalate dramatically under the excitatory influence of fear in contrast to the inhibitory effect that fear tends to produce on presentations of separation distress and owner-directed aggression not under the influence of panic.

the panic theory of CDA, provocative stimulation resulting in the loss of trust by a familiar social object may result in heightened autonomic arousal, the precipitous activation of anger-panic circuits, and the eduction of a momentary loss of control over aggressive impulses. Under the influence of panic, predisposed dogs may threaten or attack with bites of varying magnitude, but frequently resulting in grossly exaggerated and uninhibited bites. Many panic aggressors exhibit a distinctive red-glow or glazed-eye look in anticipation of an attack, indicating intense sympathetic arousal. In addition to heightened autonomic arousal, panic aggressors often appear fearless, belying the anger-induced nature of such attacks. Owners of panic aggressors often describe attacks as being out of character and inappropriate with respect to provoking stimulation.

Although an element of familiarity and affection (attachment) appears to be a necessary precondition for panic-related aggression to develop, many dogs form close attachments with balefully cruel owners and endure egregious violations of safety and loss of comfort without ever losing control and attacking their tormentors. In some cases, the dog may feel helpless and may simply passively absorb the abuse, perhaps redirecting it at some point with a vengeance toward an unsuspecting and innocent victim that comes into contact with the dog. In other cases, the tolerance exhibited by such dogs may be under the protection of biogenetic and developmental influences that promote elevated aggression thresholds (see *Phylogenesis, Polymorphism, and Coping Styles* in Chapter 6). Finally, the tolerance of some of these dogs for the loss of safety and comfort may be the result of a highly flexible bond structure that prevents the violation of trust as a result of threatening treatment (see *Cynopraxis, Antistress, and a Tend-and-Befriend System* in Chapter 6). These observations suggest the possibility that panic-related aggression may depend on an attachment that lacks a trust-forming or trust-protecting bond structure. The failure of such dogs to form flexible and tolerant relationships based on feelings of safety and trust may reflect the influence of inadequate or inappropriate socialization and training efforts (see *Drive Systems, Aggression, and Behavior Problems*). Such dogs may also be affected by biogenetic and developmental deficiencies that contribute to their inability to form viable and trusting bonds with their owners (see *Origin of Reactive versus Adaptive Coping Styles* in Chapter 4). In particular, dogs exhibiting low anger and fear thresholds from an early age may be especially prone to develop explosive panic-related aggression problems in adulthood (see *Behavioral Thresholds and Aggression* in Volume 2, Chapter 8).

Attacks associated with panic appear to be produced by an energetic synergy of anger and fear, perhaps resulting from a traumatic cross-association of anger and fear systems during a sensitive period of neurobiological development. The simultaneous elicitation of anger and fear is hypothesized to mobilize an all-out attack or rage response. Retaliatory punishment directed against impulsive aggression may release a more serious panic-driven attack. Instead of reducing the future risk of aggression, punishment may only worsen the situation by establishing conditioned triggers that cross-associate fear and anger circuits so that activating the one activates the other. The simultaneous elicitation of fear and anger by conditioned triggers may help to explain the exaggerated and disproportionate nature of such attacks.

Even innocuous interaction with family members may be highly stressful for such dogs. Under the influence of benign threats, anxiety may excite anger via cross-associations with fear circuits, which in turn may trigger more anxiety and set into motion a rapid escalation of aggressive arousal until a point of panic and dyscontrol is reached and a hard bite is delivered. In the case of proactive aggression, anger is an emotional establishing operation, recruiting a confrontational sequence. When adaptively aroused, anger is precisely calibrated and matched to the needs of the situation and adjusted in real time. This ability to monitor and adjust aggressive arousal and output depends on the presence of prediction-control expectancies and comparator-feedback networks assessing sensory input for prediction discrepancies. Under normal circumstances, worse-than-expected outcomes shift emotional establishing operations toward adjustments that increase agonistic risk or reduce it. These adjustments to negative prediction error are made under the influence of frustration (anger increasing) and anxiety (fear increasing). Under adaptive circumstances, frustration increases readiness for intensifying aggressive output (fight), whereas anxiety increases vigilance for threats and prepares a dog for fearful retreat (flight).

Under conflictive situations involving a collision of fight and flight vectors, a reactive response based on a slight shift of frustration or anxiety may cause a predisposed dog to attack or retreat, that is, result in a rapid and extreme *catastrophic* adjustment, not just making it more vigilant and ready. According to Zeeman's (1976) catastrophic model of canine aggression, a dog experiencing high levels of anger and fear has only two options available to it: fight or flight. However, such extreme adjustments to situations posing significant unknowns and risk would be adaptive only under circumstances where the cost (risk of injury or loss of social benefits) was significantly outweighed by the potential benefits of succeeding. Consequently, agonistic conflict situations brought on by escalating anger and fear may also be resolved by a third alternative: mutual forbearance and compromise. Instead of relying on catastrophic adjustments, the conflict situation is optimally resolved by mutually disengaging and cutting off animosities, compromising, and engaging in mutually reassuring and comforting reconciliation rituals. Such a strategy of mutual forbearance avoids the potential harm done if the conflict were allowed to escalate into an active fight or flight situation. Whether an agonistic conflict escalates into a reactive situation or not is often determined by the owner's capacity to lead, the quality and strength of the relationship, the social dynamics and stability of the family, the presence of trust, and an established history of the dyad resolving and reconciling differences amicably: "Every reconciled conflict is a choice against entropy" (De Waal, 1996:165). As the result of a tend-and-befriend leadership style and the competent management of conflict and reconciliation, the dog acquires emotional expectations and behavioral adjustment strategies that are incompatible with escalating anger or fearful arousal when exposed to social conflict (threats or challenges). Instead of confronting or retreating, the dog learns to flirt and forbear when experiencing anxiety or frustration in conflictive situations. If instead of encouraging compromise, forbearance, and reconciliation, the dog is severely punished and prevented by force from escaping at such times, it may attempt to break free by biting. In any case, the dog will lose its ability to trust the owner in proportion to the frequency, severity, and uncontrollability of such punishment. Instead of learning to inhibit aggression as the result of such treatment, the dog may attack more readily in the future under the influence of a cost-benefit assessment that now includes a self-preservation incentive; that is, the dog may struggle and fight as though its life depended on it.

Although Zeeman's catastrophe model may provide a useful set of predictions concerning reactive adjustments to conflictive situations involving escalating anger or fear, especially conflicts occurring between strangers exhibiting approximately the same anger and fear thresholds, the model does not offer much empirical or predictive value with respect to adaptive adjustments exhibited by dogs responding under the influence of divergent social dynamics (e.g., relative familiarity, affection, and trust) affecting their agonistic readiness to confront or retreat when aroused with anger or fear. In addition to not providing a cutoff option or an adaptive flirt-and-forbear strategy to cope with escalating anger and fear, Zeeman's model does not appear to predict the passive response of dogs expressing high anger and fear thresholds. Such dogs may neither attack nor retreat, but may instead respond to increasing anger and fear by becoming immobile (freeze) and wait for the aversive situation to change.

Similarly, depressed human patients frequently exhibit reduced positive affect together with episodic anger attacks that are frequently described as being uncharacteristic of their typical demeanor and out of accord with the provoking situation. Anger attacks occurring in association with depression resemble human panic attacks but without the prominent influence of fear and anxiety (Fava and Rosenbaum, 1998). Finally, perpetrators of domestic violence are often affected by a precipitous increase of autonomic arousal and loss of control occurring in association with violent attacks. The investigation of domestic violence reveals intriguing parallels with significant potential implications for understanding panic-related aggression in dogs (see *Autonomic Arousal, Heart Rate, and Aggression* in Chapter 6).

Both panic-related and avoidance-related types of aggression are often lumped together under the heading of dominance aggression. Although some superficial similarities exist, panic-related aggression and aggression associated with anxiety and avoidance differ from each other in several important respects. Panic-related aggression is most commonly directed against family members or others with whom the dog is closely familiar and otherwise affectionate toward, whereas avoidance-related or avoidance-*motivated* aggression is often directed against both family members and others with whom the dog is not familiar or on friendly terms (see *Avoidance Learning and Aggression* in Volume 2, Chapter 6). Panic-related aggression rapidly escalates under the excitatory influence of coactive anxiety and fear, to reflect a reactive loss of executive control over aggressive impulses. Avoidance-related aggression, on the other hand, is primarily of a defensive origin, but can be intensified under the secondary influence of anger and success, causing it to become progressively brave and preemptive. Panic-related aggression and avoidance-related aggression also differ in terms of the degree of control that a dog has over its aggressive impulses. Whereas panic-related aggression presents in ways that indicate compromised impulse control and a high level of autonomic arousal (e.g., fitlike attacks and red glow in the eyes), avoidance-related aggression usually occurs under the influence of significant impulse control, with avoidance threats and bites delivered under the influence of control-related incentives and expectancies. In contrast to the reactive and hard biting of panic aggressors, avoidance aggressors more often show well-targeted and inhibited bites, air snapping, and fang whacking, and much less frequently produce serious bites. Avoidance-related aggression is often associated with signs of conflict (threats), whereas panic-related aggression is more impulsive and often performed with little or no warning. Finally, unlike panic-related aggression, avoidance-related aggression is much more sensitive and responsive to the effects of reward and punishment. Consequently, whereas avoidance-related aggression falls under the category of control-related or proactive aggression, panic-related aggression is placed under the heading of impulsive or reactive aggression (see *Panic, Impulsivity, and Episodic Dyscontrol* in Chapter 8).

PART 2: ASSESSING AND TREATING CANINE DOMESTIC AGGRESSION

CANINE DOMESTIC AGGRESSION: ASSESSING THE THREAT

Dogs that bite family members defy simple characterization, exhibiting a wide spectrum of social traits and behavioral histories. Aggressive dogs may appear to be socially independent and aloof, serious-minded, depressed, or moody. However, depression

and lack of positive affect are not representative of all canine aggressors. In fact, many owners of biting dogs report that the dogs are genuinely affectionate and playful most of the time (Borchelt, 1983), but rapidly shift from an affectionate mode of interaction to become distant, irritable, and threatening. Many owners report that aggressors show contrition or signs of remorsefulness following an aggressive episode (Voith and Borchelt, 1982). Typically, the aggressor threatens or attacks only when it perceives a challenge or imminent threat to its control over some situation. Aggressive dogs may exhibit a variety of threatening displays, such as direct staring, growling, snarling, stiffening, raised hackles, air snapping, and inhibited biting, prior to actually delivering an overt attack. Some aggressors do not show any reliable signs or warnings at all in anticipation of an impending attack. Although aggressors sometimes bite hard and cause severe injuries, the majority of domestic dog bites are inhibited punitive snaps, aimed at controlling irritating, frustrating, or threatening stimulation.

Deciding to Accept a Case

Cases involving aggression directed toward family members involve many factors that should be carefully considered before accepting such cases. In addition to assessing the severity of the aggression problem, the cynopraxic counselor should evaluate the owner's attitude and the general family situation. Are children at risk in the household? How cognizant and responsible is the owner about the potential danger posed by the dog? Can the owner be realistically expected to carry out training procedures and follow through on a long-term basis? What are the odds of a lasting success and management of the problem? Unless the overall picture is one where benefits significantly outweigh hazards, the trainer should decline services and redirect the case back to the referring veterinarian.

If the case is accepted, the owner should be carefully informed of the risks involved, including the fact that long-term treatment outcomes are unknown and, although improvement should be expected and maintained, the risk of a future bite incident cannot be entirely eliminated despite the most conscientious and expert training. Currently, a wide range of treatment options exist, often containing conflicting rationales and recommendations with varying degrees of scientific legitimacy and therapeutic value. Voith and Borchelt (1982) observed early on the rather protean nature of the treatment process, stressing that no one technique is likely to work in all situations:

> There are, literally, an infinite number of variations on behavioral techniques for treating dominance aggression ... There are no specific techniques that work in all situations. In order to achieve a high rate of success, individual programs that require constant refinement should be designed for each case. There are no inflexible rules on how to respond in specific circumstances. (659)

These observations were written nearly 20 years ago but remain relevant today. At the outset of the training process, owners should be informed that none of the current behavioral protocols used for controlling and managing dominance-related aggression have been rigorously evaluated for efficacy. Despite the absence of definitive studies, preliminary work indicates that a variable therapeutic benefit is achievable in many cases. For example, Uchida and colleagues (1997) performed a follow-up study to evaluate the benefits of an 8-week program of nonconfrontational training on 20 dogs diagnosed with dominance aggression. The follow-up showed that 20% of the owners questioned believed that their dogs had been "cured," while another 30% of them indicated that a "marked improvement" had occurred as the result of the training process. Takeuchi and colleagues (2001) found that 51.2% of owners with dogs exhibiting dominance aggression (N = 82) reported that their dogs showed improvement as the result of behavioral treatment. Reisner and colleagues (1994) reported that 85% of owners with dogs diagnosed with dominance aggression observed some improvement in their dogs' behavior as the result of treatment. Similarly, Line and Voith (1986) found that 16 of 19 owners of dominance aggressors

observed improvement, with 13 of them indicating either very much or significant improvement. The extent to which these reports of improvement are attributable to actual changes in behavior due to behavioral training or due to various indeterminate factors such as placebo effect, a desire to please an authority figure, or denial has not been objectively assessed. Given the current state of the art, if pressed for a prognosis regarding a dog with a history of CDA, ethical counselors can only state with confidence that most cases of such aggression can be successfully treated with an expectation of stabilization and improvement, but there is no cure and the risk of future attacks cannot be entirely eliminated. Dog owners must be made acutely aware of these limitations and risks before training is begun.

Treatable versus Untreatable Aggression Problems

Canine domestic aggression presents with a high degree of variability with respect to targets, severity, location, and predictability of attacks. These variables need to be carefully assessed to evaluate the risk of serious injury or permanent scarring to family members (Table 7.2). The target and relative frequency, location, severity, and predictability of attacks determine the viability of behavioral intervention and likely prognosis. Intrafamilial attacks that occur on an unpredictable basis or with minimum provocation pose special difficulties. In cases where severe bites have occurred with little or no provocation or warning, professional training services should be withheld or only cautiously provided, and then primarily to advise the owners about the risks and instruct them on how to avoid eliciting circumstances and to introduce preventive management techniques. Because of the unpredictable nature of the attacks, it is difficult, if not impossible, to assess the benefits of training or to evaluate future risks safely without exposing family members and visitors to a potential bite, thus making such cases by definition "untreatable." Further, in the case of unpredictable aggression, the absence of aggression for some period is no reliable indi-

TABLE 7.2. Aggression ranked in accordance with predictability, frequency, severity, and location of threat or attack

1. Threatening stare and growling

2. Snarling and air snapping

3. Muzzle jabbing and fang whacking

4. Inhibited biting

5. Inhibited biting with bruising

6. Inhibited biting with slight puncture to extremities and torso

7. Inhibited biting with slight puncture to the head

8. Infrequent, but predictable, hard puncture biting delivered to the extremities

9. Infrequent, but predictable, hard puncture biting delivered to the torso

10. Infrequent, but predictable, hard puncture biting delivered to the head

11. Frequent, but predictable, hard puncture biting

12. Infrequent and unpredictable hard puncture biting

13. Frequent and unpredictable hard puncture biting

14. Puncture biting with head shaking and laceration

15. Sustained attacks involving multiple punctures and lacerations

cator that it will not unexpectedly recur at some point (see *Dead-dog Rule* in Volume 2, Chapter 2). Domestic aggression involving severe and unprovoked attacks is often tragically refractory and improvement notoriously transient and labile. Despite the most determined and conscientious training efforts, dogs that bite are at a significant risk for repeating the behavior—a fact that many dog owners eventually forget about over time with disastrous results. Consequently, given the obvious risk to public safety, one cannot rationally justify the treatment of dogs exhibiting severe uninhibited attacks or unpredictable aggression. Dogs exhibiting uninhibited or unpredictable hard biting should be referred to the family's veterinarian for medical evaluation and final disposition. In contrast, treatable CDA is associated with clear warning signals and precursor behaviors, such as direct staring, growling, snarling, and preparatory stiffening, with the dog biting only as a last resort when all else fails to control the situation. When the dog does bite, it is usually inhibited and causes minor trauma, if any. This form of CDA is much more responsive to management and behavior-therapy efforts and

has a better prognosis, but it remains technically incurable and its remission depends on a lifelong commitment to management and training.

The absence of a permanent cure and the tendency of aggression to recur may account for the routine euthanasia of dogs diagnosed with dominance aggression. Such a blanket euthanasia policy is inappropriate, however, since many dogs exhibiting CDA can be effectively trained and managed as the result of relatively brief interventions and owner education. In addition, some forms of CDA are significantly influenced by treatable medical conditions that should be excluded before euthanasia is considered. In the absence of medical causes, the decision to euthanize a dog should be based on a formula weighing the severity and location of bites, the frequency and predictability of the attacks, and the composition of household, especially the presence of young children at risk. In addition, a realistic assessment of the owner's ability to carry out training and management recommendations should be objectively considered when faced with such decisions. Unpredictable, frequent, severe bites directed toward the face or torso weigh strongly in the direction of euthanasia, whereas highly predictable, infrequent, inhibited bites directed to the hands weigh strongly in favor of treatment, at least in the case of homes not occupied by young children. The presence of young children significantly complicates matters, since children are often unable to follow instructions consistently to avoid interaction that might evoke aggression. In homes with young children, dogs exhibiting an established propensity for highly predictable and inhibited aggression toward children should be evaluated for rehoming. Most cases of aggression present with bite patterns that lie somewhere between the opposite extremes of severe, frequent, and unpredictable attacks and infrequent and predictable threats or inhibited bites, requiring objective assessment and evaluation on an individual basis to determine the viability of behavioral intervention.

The diagnosis of dominance aggression is problematic and lacks a universal and coherent set of inclusion and exclusion criteria, with considerable debate and controversy surrounding what is meant by the category. In general, what is referred to as dominance aggression in the literature seems to be deeply and insurmountably confused, representing a significant obstacle to research and the treatment of such problems. The notion of a dominance drive causing a dog to threaten or bite family members in order to achieve a superior rank is particularly problematic, since it is commonly used to justify interactive punishment—a training strategy that is tantamount to treating a burn with hot water. The spectrum of aggressive behaviors linked under the rubric of dominance aggression is more akin to involuntary subordination, social incompetence, reactive impulsivity, powerlessness, and panic rather than social dominance (see *Social Competition, Cooperation, Conflict, and Resentment*). The dominance hypothesis of CDA has not been established convincingly nor is it consistent with the generally obligatory subordinate and dependent nature of the relations between people and dogs. Identifying and controlling resources (e.g., food, affection, and play) of interest to a dog can more easily, rapidly, and safely produce active-submission behavior than force. Setting limits while methodically gratifying submissive behavior (begging) with the contingent delivery of rewards is conducive to the integration of leader-follower cooperation and friendly relations via competent dominance, leadership, and nurturance (see *Filial and Sibling Dominance-Submission Relations*).

Consequently, instead of placing undue and unjustifiable etiological emphasis on a dog's striving to achieve social dominance over the owner as a cause of aggression, cynopraxic treatment programs are better served by reinforcing active cooperation, reducing or removing adverse emotional influences known to lower or destabilize aggression thresholds, and avoiding provocative interaction that might trigger FFS arousal and reactive threats or attacks. Further, instead of emphasizing confrontational and coercive procedures aimed at suppressing aggression or reducing the dog's social rank by force and defeat, training efforts should be dedicated to increasing the dog's social competence by means of reward-based training, with the goal of improving attention and impulse control and shaping prosocial behavior under the influence of dependable prediction-control expectancies and emotional establishing operations incompatible with aggression. In addition to establishing useful control over the dog's behavior, such training efforts serve to mobilize an antistress response, helping to reduce irritability, intolerance, and reactivity, thereby improving the dog's ability to cope adaptively with stressful social interaction (see *Cynopraxis, Antistress, and a Tend-and-Befriend System* in Chapter 6).

AFFILIATIVE CONFLICTS AND THE RISE OF AGONISTIC COMPETITION

Owner Attitude and Personality, Spoiling, and Anthropomorphism

Owners lacking assertive and confident personalities have been implicated in the etiology of aggression problems. According to Beaver (1999), CDA problems often develop as the result of a mismatch of personality types between the owner and the dog, with timid owners being at a greater risk of falling victim to the aggression of a "dominant type" dog. Hart and Hart (1997) have expressed similar opinions, suggesting that puppies exhibiting signs of aggression should be "admonished or punished sufficiently so as to subdue the reaction, as long as the owners are safe from being bitten or injured" (1132). Hart and Hart (1985) have also suggested that pampering and spoiling activities play a significant role in the development of CDA problems. Voith and colleagues (1992) have disputed the role of spoiling activities and anthropomorphic attitudes in the etiology of aggression problems. For example, they found that behavior problems (including dominance aggression) appear to occur independently of spoiling activities (permitting a dog to sleep on the bed, giving it noncontingent treats, and sharing food from the table), anthropomorphism, and past obedience training (see *Excessive Indulgence* in Volume 2, Chapter 2):

> Taken together, the results of our analyses clearly and consistently failed to show any support for the notion that dogs that are "spoiled," treated like a person, or not obedience trained are more likely to engage in problem behaviors. In fact, the results … revealed that dogs taken on trips or that received shared snacks or food from the table were significantly less likely to engage in behavior problems. (270)

Although the data linking owner attitudes with the development of aggression problems are sparse and conflicting, some reports suggest that the amount of owner experience with dogs, emotional orientation, and the presence of anthropomorphic attitudes may affect the development and treatment of canine aggression problems (see *Psychological Factors* in Volume 2, Chapter 10). For example, in contrast to the aforementioned findings of Voith and colleagues, O'Farrell (1995) has suggested that owners exhibiting anthropomorphic emotional attachments toward their dogs may be at a greater risk of becoming the target of dominance-related aggression problems; unfortunately, O'Farrell's notion of *dominance* itself appears to be steeped in anthropomorphic assumptions and generalizations about the social functions of dominance and submission behavior. Jagoe and Serpell (1996) found that first-time dog owners are more likely to experience a variety of behavior

problems, including disobedience, excessive excitability, and a variety of dominance-related aggression problems. Similarly, Kobelt and colleagues (2003) have linked first-time ownership with reports of increased excitability and nervousness in dogs. Younger owners lacking breed knowledge and experience with dogs appear to be more likely to rear dogs showing aggression and other problems than are older, more knowledgeable, and experienced dog owners (Rugbjerg et al., 2003). Many owners may be fearful of their dog following an attack, making treatment difficult (Manteca, 1998). Some owners appear to be alternately angry or afraid of their aggressive dogs, often leading to disorganized and inappropriate training activities. Relevantly, Dodman and colleagues (1996a) found that thinking-type owners were more likely to succeed in treating dominance-related aggression than were feeling-type owners (see *Psychological Factors* in Volume 2, Chapter 10). Finally, Guy and colleagues (2001b) have suggested that allowing the puppy to sleep on the bed during the first couple months of ownership may be associated with an increased risk of aggression problems.

Dominance, Social Distance and Polarity, and Begging for Love

Among wolves living under natural conditions, the finding, ownership, and distribution of food are important prerogatives of dominance, with active submission representing little more than a food-begging ritual (Mech, 1999; Schenkel, 1967) (see *Wolf Model of Dominance and Submission*). Also, active-submission behaviors and begging for social contact and affection (attention-seeking behavior) are also forms of subordinate behavior, whereas receiving such behavior tolerantly and guiding it into socially constructive outlets is an expression of competent leadership. Submissive seeking is a natural concomitant of reward training and appears to play a significant role in the formation of dominant-subordinate relations resulting from ICT. Setting limits and providing rewards on the basis of a contingency or rule prevents seeking behavior from becoming obtrusive while at the same time facilitating a VSS. According to this interpretation, the dog is an obligate subordinate, and domestic aggression is most often due to social incompetence developing in association with an ISS, that is, a reactive coping style and preferential responsiveness to signals of punishment and loss. At bare minimum, simply requiring that dogs not become obtrusive while seeking gratification, and that they give their attention to family members by way of submissive "asking" behaviors before they are rewarded, appears be sufficient to maintain subordinate and friendly relations.

In cases where a long-standing history of indulgence and affectionate submission is directed toward the dog by family members (see *Dominance: Status or Control* in Volume 2, Chapter 8), a VSS based on submissive seeking and leadership may fail to develop or may develop in association with significant conflict. In the absence of appropriate social polarity and distance, the dog may show signs of increasing irritability, intolerance, and reactive biting (incompetence) in response to owner interference and intrusion (see *Social Distance and Polarity* in Volume 2, Chapter 8). The excessive affection, handling, and petting given to such a dog may activate nascent dominance dynamics, especially in cases where the dog is given such attention without actively seeking or welcoming it.

Affectionate contact is something that many owners crave and obtain from dogs by means of affectionate solicitation (sweet talk), handling (hugging and picking up), and petting. In an important sense, providing affectionate gratification to family members is a resource that a dog can own and limit access. When affectionate contact is not invited or welcomed, the dog may interpret the family's affectionate efforts as intrusive submissive care-seeking activity rather than care-giving activity; that is, the owner's affectionate contact may be viewed as submissive *begging for love*, to borrow Schenkel's terminology (Schenkel, 1967). This hypothetical reversal of roles associated with affection seeking and giving may generate intolerance, especially with regard to the unwelcome handling and petting provided by least-preferred family

members, perhaps triggering the dog's incompetent aggressive efforts to advertise ownership or to set limits on such interaction by threatening or biting them. Retaliation by the owner against such threats may subsequently set into motion an ISS, resentment, and heightened sensitivity to signals of punishment and loss. As the result of unwelcome familial affection-seeking behavior and subsequent punishment in response to the dog's threats, social polarity may be conflicted, with the dog exhibiting behavior toward family members consistent the classical signs of dominance-related aggression. Conflictive dynamics between dominance and submission may be further elaborated and integrated into the relationship by means of incompetent family control efforts (e.g., bribing, cajoling, crouching, repeating, and tricking). Instead of controlling the dog in a confident and friendly way, the owner's control efforts may take on a nervous and begging quality and significance for the dog. By bribing, cajoling, and entreating the dog to cooperate, the owner transfers the locus of control to the dog by allowing it to decide whether to comply. In such cases, the dog appears to reward the preferred owner's submissive asking behavior with compliant tolerance, but may show a lack of responsiveness to less-preferred family members despite their similar submissive strategies. However, regardless of preference, if a family member attempts to force the dog to comply with a stern voice or hand, the dog may actively resist, threaten, or bite hard.

Without identifying and substantially changing the interactive dynamics fostering the development of CDA, it is unlikely that contact aversion, resentment, and propensity for biting can be significantly modified. To promote submissive behavior and a VSS, the family must establish ownership and leadership with respect to significant resources, including the gratification associated with affectionate petting and handling. The key to treating such aggression problems is establishing social distance and systematically reversing social polarity, so that the dog is encouraged to seek affection, play, and rewards from family members while integrating friendly relations with everyone in the household. In addition to helping the owner understand the problem, an improved relationship based on a balance of dominance, leadership, and nurturance is facilitated by means of ICT. The cynopraxic process is carried out simultaneously on several levels with the goal of providing the owner support, knowledge, practical advice, and a model for more appropriate and friendly interaction with the dog (Table 7.3). Some owners appear to be so emotionally dependent and submissive toward their dogs for affectionate gratification that they accept the occasional bite in order to maintain the relationship. Such owners may also carefully avoid punishing the dog for fear of losing its affection. Such owners of aggressive dogs are also prone to engage in denial and magical thinking about the problem, requiring that the cynopraxist stay on guard for *subterfuge* (protecting the dog by not revealing vital information), *sabotage* (not carrying out the training recommendations), and *slippage* (reverting back to previous patterns of interaction with the dog).

To restore control, such dogs should be appropriately restrained to make them safe to interact with family members. At a minimum, dogs with a history of CDA should be kept on a collar and leash. The dog should be trained to orient on signal (e.g., smooch or squeak). As the dog shifts its attention (target arc), a click or "Good" is delivered and followed by a flick of the right hand to the side. Although, in general, small rewards are preferred, a larger and highly desirable food item can be given intermittently to the dog during the process of training it to approach. As the dog approaches the closed hand, the trainer says "Good" and opens it to reveal the reward. Initially, both the right and left hands are flicked out to the side. The sharp flicking movement of the hand is designed to attract the dog's attention while reducing reactive associations with fast-moving hands. Feeding the dog by hand is a viable way to restore confidence and reduce potential adverse associations associated with past rough handling or hitting. The hand should be flicked to the side, not toward the dog. In addition, a scented squeaker bulb can be held in the hand and gently squeezed (without squeaking) to deliver the dilute scent of orange or lavender just before the hand is opened. Tactile-target-arc training can be performed by getting the dog to orient to a gentle nonthreatening touch followed immediately by the conditioned odor alone or combined with the squeak or smooch sound. Such training appears to help integrate new sensory associations and input at the level of the sensory analyzer and gating channels leading to higher cognitive and emotional processing.

Gradually, the dog is required to look into the trainer's eyes for variable periods before the trainer says "OK" and flicks the right hand to the side, thereby causing the dog to break eye contact. The dog's name can be paired with the orienting signal and the vocal

TABLE 7.3. Elements of cynopraxic mediation and counseling

Respond sincerely and sympathetically to the owner's concerns about the dog's behavior.

Emphasize the positive aspects of the relationship and constructively frame the problem in the context of achievable goals.

Provide an authoritative and objective evaluation of the problem in both functional and interpersonal terms.

Discuss and clarify the dog's biobehavioral needs and provide practical ways of satisfying them.

Discuss possible social and environmental causes contributing to the problem.

Introduce scientifically sound behavioral principles for understanding and controlling or managing the problem behavior.

Demonstrate cynopraxic training procedures, stressing the importance of predictable and controllable training events to promote comfort, safety, and trust.

Provide the owner with a positive role model for interacting with the dog.

signal "Come" can be overlapped with the approach. These components are foundations that all family members can practice with the dog. Children are instructed to avoid directly approaching the dog, but may use the foregoing procedure in an abbreviated way (e.g., dog's name, smooch, flick the hand, "Good," and food reward) to encourage the dog to approach or follow them. Approximately half of the dog's daily ration should be fed by hand, with the dog approaching the child and the parent from various distances. The orienting, frontal approach, and sustained attending responses systematically integrate the social engagement system, serving to establish highly predictable and controllable interaction that is emotionally incompatible with aggression. As things progress, the dog will become more approachable and receptive to contact as the scripting of friendly roles and expectancies of reward are established. Training the dog to approach is an extremely useful procedure for changing the direction of attention and social polarity and managing potentially provocative situations. In situations where the dog shows signs of arousal, the trainer can back away and trigger the orienting response, bridge it, and perform the flick signal to bring about a friendly resolution of the conflict. Initiating cutoffs, integrating alternative behaviors incompatible with aggression, and performing a reconciliation ritual can be helpful in the management of many CDA problems (see *Loss of Safety, Depression, Panic, and Aggression*).

An adaptive coping style and VSS are further facilitated by means of shaping (see *Shaping: Training through Successive Approximations* in Volume 1, Chapter 7). The procedure offers many significant benefits in the training of dogs showing adjustment problems associated with social incompetence and a reactive coping style. Shaping procedures are highly beneficial in this regard because they explicitly shift the locus of control over significant events (reward and punishment) from the trainer's initiative and prompting to the voluntary initiative and experimentation of the dog. Excessive reliance on command-and-response training may foster an undesirable continuation of dependency on the owner for obtaining comfort and safety, perhaps merely complicating

the situation with another layer of behavioral entrapment and loss of freedom. Consequently, in addition to structured ICT and attention therapy, strong emphasis is placed on rewarding constructive initiative (offered behaviors) and active participation via shaping and play. Shaping is eminently compatible with cynopraxic training and therapy objectives (see *Prediction Dissonance and Shaping* in Chapter 10). During the shaping process, the dog's behavior is intensively differentiated and organized in accordance with the formation of instrumental prediction-control modules, calibrated appetitive and emotional establishing operations, and emergent adaptive modal strategies. As a result, shaping provides a potent source of somatic and cortical reward in the process of developing socially adaptive control modules and modal strategies. In addition to learning new behaviors, already established basic obedience modules and routines can be retrained by breaking them down into approximate components and steps for the dog to learn via the shaping. Offered responses need not precisely match the trained module or routine to warrant reward, but can be taken as a starting point for shaping. By waiting and giving the dog a fair chance to offer an appropriate behavior or learn to experiment without risk of punishment, the dog's sense of control, competence, and confidence is gradually improved and its trust enhanced. Patiently waiting and rewarding offered behavior or providing supportive guidance during the shaping process helps to improve the owner's leadership skills while increasing the owner's appreciation of the dog as learner.

Nothing in Life Is Free, Subordinate Postures, and Rank

During the 1970s, Voith (1977) explored the possibility of treating dominance-related CDA by means of a reward-based training protocol. Historically, this was a significant departure from earlier training methods based on the force-based concept of wolf and dog dominance hierarchies popularized in the writings of Lorenz (1955). Believing that CDA was primarily the result of dominance incentives operating within the household, she explored the possibility of altering the status of domestic aggressors by reinforcing subordinate postures (e.g., sit, lie down, and roll over) with food and a variety of everyday rewards (petting, play, opportunities to go outside, and so forth) in accordance with a "nothing in life is free" (NILIF) program. Once the dominance hierarchy was reversed by means of NILIF and graduated exposure to mildly provocative handling, owners were instructed to counteract growling and other threats by moving back and staring the dog down from a safe distance (Voith and Borchelt, 1982):

> Establishing the maxim that "nothing in life is free" is a means of subtly reversing a dominance hierarchy by requiring the dog to assume progressively more submissive postures before it gets anything it wants. If the dog indicates it wants to be petted, to go out, to come in, or to play, it must, for instance, sit before it is allowed to engage in the activity. Later, it may be requested to lie down, roll over, or gradually tolerate pressure on its back or muzzle before it is permitted access to what it wants. (659)

The NILIF program has been applied in various ways to treat dominance-related aggression and other common behavior problems. Despite its widespread use, scant research has been performed to test the hypothesis that positive reinforcement of submissive postures can help to reverse an established dominance hierarchy. Tortora (1980) reported some data obtained from a case study in which submissive behavior was selectively rewarded in an effort to reduce aggression in an 18-month-old bullmastiff. The dog exhibited a variety of aggressive behaviors toward family members and attacked several persons not belonging to the household, including a severe attack resulting in 11 stitches to one of the victims. The treatment program consisted of first reinforcing various submissive facial expressions and then shaping a progression of bodily postures leading to the dog rolling on its back and allowing the owners to put their hands around the dog's neck. Each facial expression and posture was prompted and paired with the vocal signal "Quiet." The rewards given to the dog consisted of attention and kibble. The submission training was carried out daily over the course

of 20 days, with the dog reportedly showing a dramatic reduction of threatening behavior. The improvement was still evident after a 6-month follow-up, despite inconsistent training efforts by the owners. Unfortunately, the significance of the foregoing case study is difficult to assess since the owners performed the procedures and collected the data. Further, given the severity of the problem and the owners' evident lack of behavioral experience, one cannot help being skeptical about the success reported. Such miraculous improvements are relatively rare in the process of working through serious aggression problems and, in any case, they are the exception rather than the rule. Whether it worked or not, conventional basic obedience procedures incorporate a similar but more systematic and controlled approach to prompting and rewarding compliance and submissive postures in the context of basic training. Combining reward-based training and various behavior-therapy procedures (response prevention, graduated interactive exposure, counterconditioning, TO, and so forth) with a modified NILIF program, integrated compliance training, directive prompting, mechanical manipulation (e.g., PFR training), escape/avoidance training, and play, selected and organized to match the needs of the dog, would seem to offer the needed flexibility and variability to respond to the individual differences and training requirements of the greatest number of dogs.

Other authors have questioned the ability of the NILIF program to reverse established dominance relations. Reisner (1997), for example, has expressed general doubts about the efficacy of behavioral efforts to reverse the household dominance hierarchy, but argues that "altering the dog's perception of rank order should be possible, if only in mild cases, so that conflicts are less likely to occur" (487). The idea that one might be able to alter a dog's perception of rank order without at the same time modifying its actual rank seems to be an extraordinary proposition. Logically, a hierarchical change in dominate-subordinate relations ought to occur before the dog's perception of rank order is modified, for what else other than such an actual change might sensibly explain the dog's altered perception of rank? Perhaps the statement refers more loosely to changes in interaction that alter the dog's perception of the social rank of family members without necessary changing its rank. In either case, the attribution of causal and therapeutic significance to hypothetical changes made to a dog's perception of rank order without changing its actual rank seems to exchange a difficult-to-prove dominant-rank hypothesis for an even more difficult-to-prove dominant-attitude or *perception-of-rank* hypothesis that is fraught with anthropomorphic pitfalls, potential for attributional error, and risk for pseudoscientific fictionalizing (see *Social Dominance: Dispositional Cause or Attributional Error*). Both of these social dominance notions contain etiological assumptions that are taken for granted as facts instead of unproven hypotheses or, worse yet, untestable beliefs.

In any case, Reisner contends that keeping the dog off furniture and not allowing it to jump up during greetings serve to modify its perception of rank order since "height inflates social rank" (488). The owner is also instructed to forbid the dog from entering the bedroom at night in order to prevent the dog from laying "claim to the owner's resting place" (488). The owner is warned to keep the dog away from the table and to feed it only after the family has eaten, apparently based on the assumption that the alpha eats first and so on. These various assumptions concerning dominance and the dog's perception of rank are problematic and difficult to defend. Interpreting human-dog interactions in terms of wolf social behavior is risky even when it is founded on accurate and complete ethological information. Although a dominant wolf may stand over a cowering subordinate (Van Hooff and Wensig, 1987; Mech, 1999), and such height differences may signify rank in the context of active threat and appeasement exchanges, to my knowledge there is no significant evidence supporting the idea that wolves or dogs advertise rank by claiming and defending elevated places or that they preferentially select such places for an advantage with respect to asserting control over group members. Many perfectly subordi-

nate dogs enjoy resting on furniture, sleeping on beds, taking treats from the table, and affectionately jumping up at greetings under the influence of attention-seeking and comfort-seeking incentives, without ever feeling an urge to threaten or bite family members. Such dogs may become obtrusive and irritating nuisances needful of training, but they rarely show aggression problems or become confused about their social rank. Voith and colleagues (1992) "clearly and consistently" failed to detect a relationship between allowing a dog to engage in the previously mentioned activities and an increased risk of developing behavior problems, including aggression toward family members. The suggestion that feeding the dog second may be helpful to reduce dominance-related problems also appears to be without support; in fact, such a change in feeding order may actually risk increasing aggressive behavior. Jagoe and Serpell (1996) found that deferring the dog's meal until after the family had eaten was positively correlated with an increased risk of territory-related aggression. Dogs that show threats when approached while on furniture or while occupying any other place in the house should be thoroughly desensitized to the owner's approach and trained to jump off furniture on signal and to refrain from getting back up unless invited up first. Also, dogs that have shown overt aggression while on beds should be repeatedly prompted to get on and off the bed until the response is performed fluently and without hesitation. All compliance training should be performed with positive reinforcement in conjunction with minimal leash prompting and brief TO, as needed to de-arouse the dog. Once trained, the dog should be permanently forbidden access to the bed, not because it might engender a misperception of the owner's rank, but simply because it reduces the risk of an aggressive event in the future. Since a significant correlation has been detected with respect to intrafamilial aggression and cosleeping during the first two months after coming into the home (Guy et al., 2001b), puppies should be prevented from sleeping on the bed during the first 2 or 3 months. Finally, as regards jumping up, such behavior is typically aimed at achieving close contact, intensifying tactile stimulation, and promoting friendly relations. Even when sociable dogs are greeted by crouching down, the owner does not risk losing rank, but rather invites affectionate licking, nudging, and pushing-in behavior and other active-submission behaviors. According to Schenkel (1967), among wolves such behavior may be interpreted as an "overwhelming offer of friendly affection" (324). When crouched down below the dog's eye level, few dogs will attempt to take advantage of the situation in order to advance their status; however, many may be prompted by the action to play, appearing to interpret the lowered posture as an invitation to play (see *Metacommunication and Play* in Volume 2, Chapter 8). Such interaction would be inappropriate and potentially dangerous in the case of an experienced aggressor simply because it places the trainer in a vulnerable position and exchanges an increased risk for a minimal potential benefit—not a wise training decision. Jumping up can become an obtrusive and unwelcome habit if appropriate limits are not set on it, but prompting a friendly dog to jump up is unlikely to adversely affect its perception of rank or promote aggressive behavior.

To further adjust the dog's perception of rank and increase owner control, Reisner (1997 and 1998) recommends an abrupt cessation of all affection and other sources of reward for 2 weeks, during which time family members are instructed not to speak to the dog, pet it, or show it affection. The dog is totally ignored except as necessary to meet its basic needs. During the next 2 weeks, attention and affection are partially restored, but only at the owner's initiative. All attention is given on a contingency basis, requiring that the dog first submit to an obedience command. The dog is only permitted to ask for attention after a month of social deprivation, and then attention is provided contingently on half of the occasions in which the dog solicits it from family members. All rewards are provided on a contingency basis, such that the dog must sit or lie down before being petted, given food and treats, taken for walks, let outdoors, and so forth. Finally, outdoor activ-

ities are severely curtailed by exercising the dog on leash, and ideally all off-leash romping in the yard is eliminated. The NILIF program, together with the previously mentioned prohibitions, is embedded into every significant social transaction for the remainder of the dog's life so that family members can dictate control over the dog's "daily decisions." The NILIF process, as described by Reisner, appears intended to externalize the locus of control and thereby undermine the dog's ability to initiate independent actions in search of reward. As such, the program appears to promote an increasing social dependency and powerlessness, whereby the owner dictates what the dog can do and when it can do it while frustrating the dog's ability to produce social reward on its own initiative.

Ironically, although extreme forms of positive punishment have been rightly repudiated, many of the same individuals who admonish dog owners not to use physical punishment show little compunction about hanging the dog out to dry. Whether intended as such or not, the withdraw of social reward is a highly stressful and anxiogenic form of punishment, indiscriminately targeting both desirable and undesirable social behaviors irrespective of what the dog does or does not do. Although both forms of extreme punishment are problematic and deserving of criticism, at least positive punishment is usually applied contingently against a specific target behavior. In contrast, the social-deprivation procedure punishes all social behavior with *inescapable* nonreward, disconfirming previously established prediction-control expectancies, and thereby generating considerable distress and confusion. If the social-deprivation procedure works to reduce aggression, it probably does so by inducing increased social anxiety and psychological stress via a variant form of learned helplessness induced by the abrupt and inescapable loss of control over social rewards (see *Learned Helplessness* in Volume 1, Chapter 9).

Abruptly depriving the dog of basic social and appetitive needs that had have routinely provided for in the past is a provocative shift of social and environmental expectations, potentially exerting a number of problematic side effects. Social isolation and restraint stress have been shown to increase anxiety and lower reactive thresholds among dogs and laboratory animals (see *Restraint, Unavoidable Aversive Stimulation, and Stress* in Chapter 10). Among rats, brief or acute restraint stress appears to exert an inhibitory effect on aggression, whereas exposure to chronic restraint stress causes rats to become significantly more threatening and hostile toward cagemates. Over the same period (14 to 21 days), nonstressed controls tended to form more friendly and stable relationships, showing significantly less aggressive behavior toward cagemates and no evidence of fighting by the end of the study period (Wood et al., 2003). While brief cold shouldering may pique a dog's interest in social rewards and increase its efforts to restore rewarding exchanges with family members, chronic social deprivation and confinement may risk activating dispersive tensions and entrapment dynamics, perhaps causing domestic aggressors to become increasingly unstable, incompetent, and confrontational around safe havens perceived as under threat.

The chronic stress associated with the social-deprivation procedure may generate a significant challenge to the dog's coping capacities and behavioral integrity, probably increasing its dependency while further reducing its ability to competently initiate and organize social behavior, impeding its ability to learn efficiently, and thwarting the *attentionis egens* mediating positive human-dog affiliation (Odendaal and Meintjes, 2003). The noncontingent loss of control over appetitive and social rewards, the disruption of daily social routines, changes in the demeanor and behavior of significant others, forced exclusion from significant family activities, increased interference and social thwarting around familiar places associated with comfort and safety, noncontingent rebuffing and snubbing of affection and contact seeking, increased social control and restraint, and entrapment (the dog cannot simply leave the situation) may exert significant depressive or aggression arousing and disorganizing cognitive, emotional, physiological effects, depending on individual differences expressed by the dogs treated with the social deprivation procedure. Although the procedure may temporarily reduce reactive aggression in some cases via increased anxiety and depressive inhibitory effects (m-type dogs), relatively fearless dogs with low-to-medium anger thresholds and intolerance for frustration (c-type dogs) may be more adversely affected by such stressful household changes.

As emphasized previously, the vast majority of intrafamilial aggressors appear to be socially incompetent and anxious dogs exhibiting a reactive coping style and ISS acquired in association with social interaction failing to support a secure and trusting bond. Social interaction lacking orderliness and consistency is productive of varying levels of anxiety, frustration, and conflict (see *Neurosis and Conflict* in Volume 1, Chapter 9). Instead of relating to family members in a proactive and adaptive way in anticipation of reward conducive to comfort and safety, the dog may become progressively vigilant for signals of punishment (loss of comfort and safety) and reactive. In addition to reducing the dog's ability to form a secure bond with family members, poorly organized interactive reward and punishment may disrupt the dog's ability to organize optimistic expectancies and active modal strategies needed to produce cortical rewards (positive prediction error). As a result, such dogs may exhibit a negative cognitive bias toward interaction with family members, appearing to expect the worst to occur as the result of social contact. These dogs appear on guard and vigilant for signals of punishment (anticipatory anxiety), often exhibiting an extreme intolerance for frustration or discomfort, and a heightened readiness to cope reactively by threatening (conflict) or attacking the owner in response to relatively innocuous social intrusion and interference.

In other cases, the social environment may be relatively orderly, but the dog may not be able to properly experience it as such. Many domestic aggressors appear to view the success or failure of their interaction with family members as something determined by external causes that are largely outside of their voluntary initiative to control. To borrow Rotter's terminology (Rotter, 1966), *externals* place the locus of control over events critical for their comfort and safety beyond their ability to produce or avoid them (see *Locus of Control and Self-efficacy* in Volume 2, Chapter 9). For example, overly dependent dogs may come to view rewarding interaction with family members as something that happens to them rather than something that they make happen for themselves as the result of cooperating successfully with others. As a result of acquired incompetence, such dogs may lack confidence and show high levels of social anxiety in situations that require independent initiative and choice. Externals tend to react to situations rather than adapt to them, and they may not learn very much of benefit from the consequences produced by their reactions. When exposed to increasing pressure, they tend toward extremes of increased motor impulsivity (c type) or immobility (m type). Such dogs may exhibit a number of serious aggression problems, the nature of which depends on reactive (anger and fear) thresholds and allostatic load. Reactive aggressors often show signs of an insecure attachment (neediness), often forming an overly exclusive attachment with a particular family member with whom they may feel relatively comfortable and safe or ambivalent but not aggressive. Such dogs are often diagnosed as dominance aggressors, but are probably better understood as socially incompetent aggressors operating under the influence of a reactive coping style and ISS (see *C-type and M-type Affinity for the Flight-Fight System*). Instead of viewing family members as sources of calming affiliation and reward, such dogs may experience social interaction as intrinsically stressful and productive of anticipatory anxiety and aversion (resentment). Such dogs may show significant conflict with regard to affectionate interactions, appearing to invite contact, but then turn and bite hard without provocation. The dog may allow a family member to pet its head or to rub its belly before the dog unexpectedly delivers a hard bite. Even during affectionate episodes of kissing, dogs have delivered severe and disfiguring bites to the face of loving victims. These dogs may

become progressively intolerant toward social contact, especially in certain areas (site-dependent attacks) associated with comfort and safety. When disturbed while in these locations, such aggressors may react to slightest interference as a provocative cost or threat to their island of security.

Canine polymorphic variations affecting anger and fear thresholds, ontogenetic adversity (e.g., prenatal and postnatal stress), problematic socialization and training, and a compromised capacity to experience reward may predispose dogs to acquire an ISS and exhibit aggression toward family members. However, the incompetent intrafamilial aggressor rarely develops without the abetment of an inexperienced or inept leader, lacking the necessary dog savvy, skill, or desire to properly socialize and guide the predisposed dog toward social competence and independence. Pushed to extremis by interactive conflict, mishandling, and entrapment, such dogs may become progressively insecure, reactive, and dangerous. Instead of punishing and further agitating the household aggressor with stressful deprivation procedures that will only serve to further externalize the locus of control, increase the dog's dependency, and perpetuate its incompetence, an opposite strategy is typically adopted whereby contingent reward opportunities are hugely increased in the process of organizing mutually gratifying and bond-enhancing interactions between the dog and family members. The goal of such training is to organize a proactive or adaptive coping style and to encourage interaction conducive to a friendly and cooperative VSS. According to this perspective, building a mutually rewarding and trusting relationship between family members and the dog is the best way to forestall intrafamilial aggression. An important step toward this goal is teaching the dog *how to competently operate family members* to produce somatic and cortical rewards, that is, helping the dog to internalize the locus of control over rewards and to patiently enhance its self-efficacy and mastery by means of cynopraxic training. In an important sense, the goal of such training is to increase the dog's competence, confidence, and independence, that is, to train it to become more dominant, relaxed, and effective with respect to the gratification of its needs.

In the process of organizing an adaptive coping style, an opioid-oxytocinergic anti-stress system may be activated to further support bond-enhancing neurobiological and physiological changes incompatible with aggression and anxiety. In addition to increasing affectionate interaction and reward availability, a quality-of-life assessment is performed to optimize exercise, playful interaction, household liberty, and so forth. Interactive conflict and tensions are traced to their sources and converted by means of ICT into situations of potential reward, providing a foundation for mutual appreciation and interactive harmony. A spirit of tolerance, fairness, and optimism should permeate the cynopraxic therapy process, with family members and the dog gradually *joining up* to interact more competently and confidently toward one another in accord with an emergent adaptive coping style, affectionate and playful dynamic modal relations, and the integration of harmonic social relations and roles via a VSS. Instead of perpetuating a heightened vigilance (anticipatory anxiety) for signals of punishment and a readiness for aggressive confrontation, cynopraxic therapy aims to increase the dog's alertness and preparedness for signals of reward by increasing leadership and interaction leading to enhanced comfort, safety, and relaxation (somatic reward) and better-than-expected outcomes (cortical rewards) in association with cooperative transactions. The integration of positive prediction error and surprise teaches the dog to anticipate something positive from the unexpected rather than bracing with anticipatory anxiety for something negative to occur. The cortical reward associated with positive prediction error appears to play a critical role in reorganizing prediction-control expectancies and modifying executive control over aggressive impulses. In general, rather than attempting to suppress aggression by means of physical or psychological domination tactics, the cynopraxic therapy process is carried out in conformity with the dead-dog rule

and is oriented toward forming a playful and friendly bond based on mutual trust, affection, and joy.

Limit-setting Actions, Basic Training, and Friendly Cooperation

Organizing functional boundaries between owners and aggressive dogs is based on setting social limits and systematically structuring rule-based interaction through ICT. Although the value of basic training for preventing aggression problems has been questioned (Voith et al., 1992), many authors have noted a beneficial effect on both the incidence of behavior problems and the quality of the human-dog bond following basic training (Blackshaw, 1991; Clark and Boyer, 1993; Jagoe and Serpell, 1996; Goodloe and Borchelt, 1998) (see *Role of Integrated Compliance and Obedience Training* in Volume 2, Chapter 6). Whether obedience training exerts a preventive benefit probably depends on the quality of the training provided and the reliability of the control established, with the dog's ability to follow commands being negatively correlated with the occurrence of behavior problems (Kobelt et al., 2003). Training the dog to defer to social limits and obey promotes a cooperative attitude conducive to effective communication and friendly social interaction. Most dogs exhibiting aggression problems benefit from the introduction of reward-based basic training and the shaping of cooperative behavior. It is not enough to explain to an owner what to do, but, more importantly, the owner must be shown how to do it. Establishing dominance is not just about setting limits, but rather, as J. H. Woolpy (1968) has well stated, "some as yet poorly understood personality factor seems to have the greatest sway" (46). Accomplished trainers not only instruct owners on procedural details, they personify the essential "personality factor" alluded to by Woolpy via subtle and gross body language, vocal expressions, personal presence, and sincerity of purpose. These nonverbal impressions are extremely useful for helping owners to establish an affectionate and healthy interactive relationship based on social limits, rules, and cooperative expectations. Presence and sincerity of purpose are the hallmarks of master trainers. Basically, such an attitude simply and confidently states without threat or doubt a presence of control. Social dominance is about establishing control, but more than anything else dominance depends on the projection of an attitude characterized by confidence and sincere purpose. Teaching owners how to succeed with their dogs and to avoid aggressive episodes improves their ability to project a confident attitude. Training and behavior-therapy efforts will yield little lasting benefit if the owner remains a victim in attitude toward the dog.

Problems associated with CDA do not emerge spontaneously like a fully armored Athena leaping from the head of Zeus, but gradually becomes serious over time (Takeuchi et al., 2001). CDA problems can often be traced to early ontogenetic influences involving affiliative conflicts. Adult dogs exhibiting domestic-aggression problems were frequently excitable, emotionally reactive, and difficult-to-control puppies (Guy et al., 2001b). Such puppies appear learn at an early age that their owners can be manipulated with threats, sharp teeth, and claws. In addition, puppies at risk are often hyperactive, aggressively possessive (growl and snarl) over food and toys, competitive and reactive to normal discipline, habitually steal and guard forbidden items, resist routine grooming and handling, engage in excessive and persistent mouthing, and may be reactive to physical restraint. Predisposed puppies may react aggressively to being placed into a down position or held there by force, but willingly lie down for a treat. As the result of a failure to establish appropriate limits and social distance (dominant-subordinate relations), the situation may become progressively unstable and rife for serious competitive contests. While this general competitive pattern is common, not all puppies exhibiting the foregoing behavior patterns go on to develop aggressive behavior as adults. Further, in some atypical cases, the aggressive dog may exhibit few or none of the aforementioned early indicators of risk.

Diversion and Interruption versus Punishment

Although punishment (e.g., time-out) can be effective in some situations involving control-related aggression, caution is advised whenever contemplating the use of physical punishment to handle growling and other threat displays. Recommending that a dog owner punish growling is highly questionable and makes little sense in the context of cynopraxic therapy efforts. Low-grade threat displays provide the trainer and others with a margin of safety and warning while interacting with the dog. Suppressing the growl is extremely easy to achieve, but nothing is gained by the effort since it is unlikely to alter the dog's motivation to bite in a way that fosters behavior incompatible with aggression. In managing aggressive dogs, threat behavior should be reduced by means of positive behavioral and emotional changes taking place as the result of establishing an adaptive coping style and reward-based training. The absence of threat displays should indicate the absence of aggressive arousal and intent, not the development of a far more dangerous situation in which the dog remains aggressively aroused but has learned to inhibit threat displays without reducing its propensity to bite (see Species-typical Defensive and Offensive Aggression). Consequently, instead of punishing the growling response, a better approach is to acknowledge the threat by moving away or by evoking a diversionary establishing operation aimed at encouraging behavior incompatible with aggression (see Establishing Operations in Chapter 1). The dog can be diverted from aggressive arousal by various means, including picking up a toy, going to a door and acting like a walk is in the offing, or tossing a treat, with the goal of evoking submissive seeking behavior for the activity or resource. The procedure follows the principle that active submission is established by evoking an appetitive- or social-seeking response that is subsequently rewarded in exchange for cooperative behavior and voluntary subordination (affectionate submission). Directly punishing threatening behavior is prone to produce aggressive reprisal or result in involuntary subordination with resentment and fear.

Moving away from the dog may reinforce the growling behavior, not an entirely desirable outcome, but one far better than suppressing it. Dogs encouraged to growl and threaten are probably at a reduced risk of biting without warning and, having learned that growling works with minimal risk of retaliation, such dogs may be more inclined to limit their aggressive control efforts to such threat displays rather than escalating to overt attacks when they become aroused. The second method (changing the motivational state) typically involves throwing the growling dog a highly prized food item, causing it to shift from a threat-producing mode to food-seeking mode. As the dog's attention turns to the food, it is more likely subsequently to offer behaviors incompatible with aggression, especially in cases where compliant behavior has been reinforced with food in the past. Habitually walking away from a growling dog to get some treats (situation change) and coming back to throw the dog a treat (motivational change) may help significantly to diffuse aggressive tensions associated with that specific trigger situation, especially if the dog is caused to beg and perform a simple exercise or two to obtain subsequent treats. In some cases, merely having the dog repeatedly orient to the sound of a squeaker or smooch followed by a click and the presentation of food can help to shift the dog rapidly from a threatening to a cooperative mode of interaction. The foregoing technique is most effective following several days of intensive preliminary attention training with sit, sit-stay, following, and recall training.

In contrast to the reinforcement that may follow if the trainer walks away from a growling dog, there is little likelihood of inadvertent reinforcement of aggressive behavior occurring as the result of giving the dog food as a diverter at such times, especially if rewards subsequent to the initial presentation (diversionary establishing operation) are made contingent on behavior incompatible with aggressive threats (orienting response, sit-stay, come, and so forth) (see *Interrupting Behavior* and *Diverters and Disrupters* in Chapter 1). Since the goal of threat behavior is the imposition of social or physical space between the owner and dog—not the acquisition of food—the introduction of food at such times is rather irrelevant with respect to the immediate goals of growling; however, in the unlikely event that the dog learns to growl as a way to get food, such growling is of an entirely different motivational significance and order. In such cases, growling for food is an innocuous trick performed under the influence of appetitive incentives and seeking behavior, which signifies something quite different from the growl advertising an imminent threat of overt attack. The appetitive activation of the seeking system appears to exert a potent inhibitory effect on the emotional command circuits mediating the expression of aggression (see *Drive Systems, Aggression, and Behavior Problems* in Chapter 6). In addition to tossing the dog a treat, a diversionary odor that has been previously conditioned with food or play (e.g., a scented squeaker or ball) or relaxation can be introduced at such times as a means to divert the dog's attention and to modulate aggressive arousal. A squeaker containing a wad of orange-scented cotton can be highly effective as a diversionary stimulus, especially if it has been previously conditioned and used as an orienting stimulus in the context of attention training.

ANGER, RESTRAINT, AND FRUSTRATION

Aggressive behavior is intimately associated with emotional antecedents that prepare dogs for aggressive action, especially anger and rage. Anger can be elicited by painful stimulation and physical restraint, but it is also associated with the anticipated loss of valued objects or activities via frustration (Dollard et al., 1939; Berkowitz, 1989). Dogs exhibit varying degrees of tolerance for pain and restraint, with the vast majority of well-socialized and habituated dogs appearing to cope extraordinarily well with mild pain and physical restraint, and rarely showing aggression in response to such stimulation except under circumstances of extreme duress and discomfort. However, some dogs are highly reactive to pain or the threat of painful stimulation, exhibiting a low threshold for discomfort and restraint. Under the influence of minimal restraint or discomfort, such dogs may struggle violently and attempt to bite in an effort break free. The way dogs respond to restraint and other forms of aversive stimulation depends on genetic and acquired influences affecting behavioral thresholds (Scott and Charles, 1954).

Prominent emotions associated with pain and restraint (loss of freedom) include fear, irritability, frustration, and anger. When pain and restraint are simultaneously produced, escalating fear and anger may be elicited and coalesce into a state of panic and rage, building dramatically and violently until the animal either breaks free or is exhausted. If biting and clawing are successful as the result of such struggle, such behavior will be more likely to occur under similar circumstances of painful restraint in the future. In addition, signals of punishment anticipating painful stimulation and restraint may become conditioned elicitors of fear and anger, resulting in preemptive efforts aimed at avoiding such stimulation. The simultaneous elicitation of conditioned fear and anger by the same social object that otherwise is associated with affiliative comfort and safety may represent a significant source of emotional conflict and anxiety. This general scenario is common in cases involving interactive punishment and reactive aggression.

Repeated exposure to restraint and inescapable aversive stimulation is highly stressful and productive of behavioral disturbance (see *Liddell: The Cornell Experiments* in Volume 1, Chapter 9). In addition, frustration associated with restraint (thwarting the freedom reflex) and loss of control over aversive or attractive events may activate anger/rage circuits. The function of anger is to motivationally intensify defensive behavior, preparing dogs to respond with aggression, if necessary, to successfully prevent the loss of some resource or to control (avoid or escape) an aversive event. As such, anger is adaptive and useful for controlling adverse environments. The evaluation of success and failure with regard to the control of attractive and aversive events entails the existence of significant cognitive processing, whereby the expected outcomes of actions can be compared with what actually occurs. Assessing outcomes and adjusting behavior to fit those assessments takes place at an executive level of organization, probably localized in the prefrontal cortex. The prefrontal area performs a variety of attention and impulse-control functions, modulating the expression of emotional behavior and mediating organized social behavior and learning. Prefrontal deficits are associated with a persistent failure to organize behavior appropriately in accordance with consequences. Under conditions resulting in the stressful habituation of the orienting and attending response (e.g., unpredictable and uncontrollable stimulation) (see *Locus of Neurotogenesis* in Volume 1, Chapter 9), a dog's ability to appraise behavioral output and organize behavior in an adaptive manner may be significantly disturbed. Actions associated with prefrontal disturbances are characterized by hyperactivity, impulsiveness, and immediate gratification. Prefrontal deficits may predispose dogs to exhibit intolerance for frustration and restraint and a resistance to inhibitory training, as well as showing an increased tendency to react to such stimulation with impulsive adjustments, including aggression.

Since the prefrontal area is highly sensitive to stress and prone to disturbances associated with stress, therapeutic efforts in such cases should involves steps to normalize function by reducing sources of environmental and social stress. In addition, various activities enhancing the dog's ability to cope with stress should be introduced and emphasized in advance of the implementation of more intrusive efforts (e.g., withdrawal of social attention). Areas of particular importance in this regard include exercise, play (as safe and appropriate), avoidance of aggression-provoking situations, graduated massage [posture-facilitated relaxation (PFR) training], reward-based training, and the avoidance of provocative punishment. Training a dog to orient and hold its attention on the trainer while performing various basic obedience exercises is a useful way to enhance impulse control and promote organized behavior. Linking the orienting and attending response to the occurrence of highly predictable and controllable events in association with basic training gradually serves to restore the appraisement and organizing functions of attention. In the case of highly stressed and reactive dogs, selective serotonin-reuptake inhibitors (e.g., fluoxetine or paroxetine) are commonly prescribed, perhaps producing a complementary effect on prefrontal executive normalization when given in conjunction with attention therapy (see *Pharmacological Control of Aggression* in Chapter 6).

BEHAVIOR THERAPY AND TRAINING PROCEDURES

Managing Aggressive Dogs

While the owner is most concerned about eliminating the threat of biting as quickly as possible, the trainer's goal should be to steer the owner's attention toward a better appreciation of the causal factors underlying the dog's biting problem and from there to develop an appropriate program of management, behavior therapy, and training. Effective management involves the introduction of various techniques for reducing adverse environmental stressors and emotional influences. Perhaps the most important goal of management is to teach the owner how to interact safely with the aggressive dog by taking precautions and using appropriate restraint strategies. The sort of management needed depends on the severity and frequency of the aggressive behavior. Dogs with a history of CDA should be kept on a leash whenever around family members at risk. In some cases, a muzzle or halter should be used for added protection, especially in the case of aggressors with a confirmed history of biting. The muzzle or muzzle-clamping halter should be introduced gradually with loads of positive reinforcement to encourage a relaxed acceptance of the restraint. Despite such preliminary efforts, some dogs may never relax while wearing such devices and may exhibit adverse side effects that limit their usefulness (Figure 7.3). The temptation to punish a dog while it is wearing a muzzle or muzzle-clamping halter should be avoided. Such treatment is highly problematic and probably does little or nothing to reduce the risk of aggression when the dog is not so

restrained, but may, in fact, make the dog more apprehensive and more determined than ever not to integrate friendly relations with the owner. Punishing a muzzled dog is contrary to the trust-building objectives of cynopraxic therapy and should be avoided. Instead of using the advantage of muzzling to punish the dog, the goal of such restraint is to enable to owner to safely interact in close quarters with the dog without risking an attack. Such restraint provides response prevention, thereby showing the dog that its aggressive behavior is not necessary. Every effort should be made to make the dog feel safe while it is muzzled or wearing a head halter. In some cases, aggressive dogs should be crate trained and learn to accept confinement in other places, as well, without making a disturbance (e.g., confinement in a locked bedroom when guests visit). All interaction with people should be carefully supervised, and persons at risk of making contact with the dog should be warned of the dog's propensity to bite. All social interaction should be managed and structured to promote safe and friendly exchanges. The control of CDA stresses training efforts designed to minimize the risk of an attack while improving human and dog social communication skills, increasing affection and playfulness, and enhancing the dog's willingness to defer and trust family members.

A detailed inventory should be compiled listing all situations in which the dog has either threatened to bite or has actually bitten. The owner is instructed to avoid these circumstances or any other provocative interaction that might lead to aggression. In addition to profiling past aggressive events, the owner should be encouraged to keep a daily journal keeping track of training activities and noting progress or setbacks. Threatening behavior or overt attempts to bite should be recorded with reference to the time, location, and the provoking situation precipitating the aggressive incident (Figure 7.4).

Social Withdrawal, Deprivation, and Cold Shouldering

Preliminary training efforts should focus on adjusting social polarity (see *Reversing Social*

Polarity and Establishing Leadership in Volume 2, Chapter 8), so that the owner becomes the object of increased attention and affection, with the goal of inspiring increased social cooperation and leadership. The owner should encourage the dog to seek attention, affection, and a variety of other rewards by making such things contingent on cooperative behaviors (sit, stand, down, come, stay, wait, and so forth) integrated into everyday activities. Some authorities recommend that a period of social deprivation and cold shouldering should precede NILIF training in order to enhance the dog's interest in social contact and motivation to seek owner affection. The necessity of such a deprivation procedure has not been clearly demonstrated; nonetheless, many anecdotal reports suggest that cold shouldering may pique a dog's interest in social contact and may be useful in some cases not otherwise responsive to reward-based training efforts. If a deprivation procedure is selected, the least amount of deprivation necessary to establish enhanced contact seeking should be used. A significant effect may be produced by as little as a half-day of cold shouldering to prompt a reorientation toward the owner. Typically, the direction of social polarity can be shifted by simply placing access to food, play, or petting on a contingent basis, that is, making the dog beg and work for it. Social deprivation procedures should be considered only in the case of dogs that do not show an active seeking response or willingness to work for the reward. The necessity of more lengthy periods of social deprivation and cold shouldering is questionable and should be avoided, at least until other less intrusive procedures have been tried without success.

Of course, in the case of dogs showing contact aversion with aggressive reactivity, petting and handling may be problematic (see *Contact Aversion and Aggression* in Volume 2, Chapter 8) and should be avoided, at least until progress is made that permits such interaction. In such cases, a brief withdrawal of petting and other forms of gratuitous affection may be beneficial as a starting point. However, the lengthy discontinuation of social contact and comfort giving functions as punishment and may serve only to introduce another element of stress into situation, perhaps making matters worse as a result. Petting and massage provide potential benefits by inducing relaxation and increased feelings of comfort and safety—emotional states incompatible with fear and aggression (see *Taction*

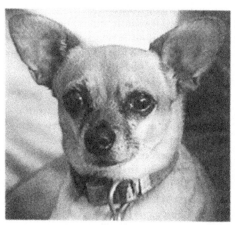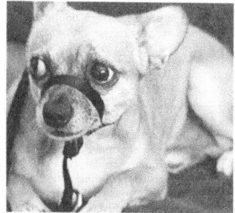

FIG. 7.3. Although most dogs eventually learn to accept halter or muzzle restraint by means of patient exposure and rewards, some may persistently react with an appearance of distress. In the case of this Chihuahua, his demeanor immediately and persistently changed as soon as the halter was fastened and thereafter he lost his appetite for treats, a side effect that severely limited counterconditioning efforts. The dog also refused to eliminate outdoors while walked on the halter, resulting in a brief house-training problem that was immediately resolve by again walking the dog on a leash and collar.

| DOG'S NAME: | | | | DATE: | |

RECORD OF AGGRESSIVE BEHAVIOR
(LIST MOST RECENT FIRST)

#	LOCATION	TIME OF DAY	ONGOING ACTIVITY / TRIGGER	TARGET	SEVERITY
1					

DESCRIBE EVENT:	CONSEQUENCES:

#	LOCATION	TIME OF DAY	ONGOING ACTIVITY / TRIGGER	TARGET	SEVERITY
2					

DESCRIBE EVENT:	CONSEQUENCES:

#	LOCATION	TIME OF DAY	ONGOING ACTIVITY / TRIGGER	TARGET	SEVERITY
3					

DESCRIBE EVENT:	CONSEQUENCES:

ADDITIONAL OBSERVATIONS:

FIG. 7.4. Chart for recording aggressive incidents.

and Posture-facilitated Relaxation in Chapter 6). Finally, in addition to lacking scientific justification, the lengthy withdrawal of social contact is highly intrusive and may violate the LIMA principle (see *Compliance* in Volume 2, Chapter 2). Asking a family to arbitrarily withdraw social attention and affection from a dog for long periods (e.g., 2 to 4 weeks) is a recommendation that is not likely to receive a high level of support and compliance. Abruptly withdrawing affection, play, and other forms of friendly interaction from the dog for weeks at a time is a punitive and stressful measure that may only serve to intensify interactive conflict and tensions between the dog and family members. Instead of asking the owner to withdraw affection and playful interaction from the dog, emphasis is better placed on helping the owner to discover ways to safely integrate affectionate and playful relations between the dog and family members in the process of building a trust-based bond incompatible with aggression (see *Integrated Compliance Training*). While short-term withdrawal of attention and affection may enhance the dog's willingness to beg for social rewards, there is little reason to assume that longer periods of social deprivation will produce a better effect. The benefits of social deprivation appear to be dose dependent, with relatively brief periods of social deprivation (e.g., time-out) enhancing submissive seeking and de-arousal, while longer periods of social deprivation and isolation may produce emotional withdrawal and depression. To my knowledge, no available scientific evidence supports the notion that long-term social withdrawal and tactile deprivation produces any benefit with respect to the reduction of CDA. However, some evidence does suggest that excessive social deprivation and cold shouldering may produce an adverse effect. For example, animals experimentally exposed to tactile deprivation tend to become more aggressively reactive when social contact with conspecifics is restored (see *Posture-facilitated Relaxation Training*).

Attention Therapy and Submissive Following Behavior

A less intrusive method that appears to be useful and more willingly adopted by owners involves an opposite strategy. Many dogs with a history of aggression may be already under the influence of a long period of social withdrawal and reduced affectionate interaction with the family. Social deprivation may naturally follow in the wake of CDA, as family members avoid making risky contact with the dog or withdraw affection from it as the result of a loss of trust, perhaps causing the problem to worsen over time. Instead of further adding to the dog's loss of social contact and other sources of reward, positive social interaction is deliberately intensified by increasing safe, affectionate, and rewarding interaction

between the dog and family members. The combination of somatic (comfort and safety) and cortical rewards (surprise) appears to promote an antistress response conducive to an adaptive coping style. Different types of appetitive and social rewards and toys are given to the dog in exchange for little more than orienting, approaching, following, attending, and waiting, that is, engaging in submissive modal activities.

Many dogs exhibiting increased aggressive reactivity may show evidence of attentional and impulse-control deficits. Such dogs may fail to *connect* or integrate an attentive orientation toward social signals, but may instead appear to actively ignore or resist efforts to establish an attentive interface. The dog may not be entirely oblivious to the trainer or unaware of important aspects of significance with respect to the signals given, but rather seem to respond to social signals in a rather narrow and parochial manner with respect to the more subtle cognitive and emotional significance of social communication. Since many aggression problems appear to involve a chronic failure between the dog and family members to competently communicate and adjust in ways that maintain a friendly field of social exchange, it is critical that a process of training aimed at improving cognitive and emotional regulation be initiated. The dog's ability to socially engage and connect with family members may be impeded by a state of anticipatory vigilance and heightened readiness to engage certain family members as threats, possibly stemming from a history of interactive conflict and disorder, mutual incompetence, or stress-related sensitization of FFS pathways. Whatever the original causes of social anxiety and frustration, the symptoms are treated by similar means involving highly predictable and controllable reward-based ICT. The goal of such training is to promote social competence, relaxation, and to reduce interactive conflict systematically. The enhanced comfort and safety produced by such training are incompatible with frustrative readiness and anticipatory anxiety. Further, the increasing competence and confidence associated with instrumental training promote relaxation and an increasing willingness to experiment and take risks toward the production of adaptive prediction error.

With the emergence of active-submission behavior (e.g., food, play, and affection seeking), a series of simple reward contingencies can be introduced to develop prediction-control expectancies and calibrated emotional establishing operations conducive to positive prediction error and surprise. For example, just as the dog orients in response to a squeaker or a smooch sound, the targeting arc is bridged with a click sound followed by a flick of a closed right hand (see *Target-arc Training* in Chapter 3). A vocal bridge is delivered just as the dog approaches the hand, and a reward is delivered by opening the hand. When taking food, the dog is discouraged from jumping up or grabbing at the food too forcefully. As the dog learns to orient to the sound of a squeaker, its name can be presented just in advance of the squeaker sound. The type and size of rewards are varied and presented in a manner that is conducive to positive prediction error and surprise (see *Prediction and Control Expectancies* in Chapter 1). A scented squeaker can also be used as an orienting stimulus or a conditioned diverter. In addition to orienting and bridge conditioning, preliminary training should include training the dog to make and hold friendly eye contact. With the dog standing or sitting, the trainer calls the dog's name or makes a smooch sound, followed by a bridge ("Good" or click) and the delivery of a food reward (see *Introductory Lessons* in Chapter 1). Training the dog to orient and hold sustained eye contact enhances the dog's ability to discriminate the trainer's actions and intent accurately and competently, thereby improving social communication and reducing the risk of aggression due to reactive adjustments. Squeakers can be placed on treat boxes and kept with leashes, toys, and other sources of attractive stimulation. The owner is instructed to sound the squeaker when coming into the house, especially at homecomings after a lengthy absence. The stimulus change is aimed at intensifying affectionate and appetitive attraction, precisely the opposite of the cold-shoulder procedure as described previously. The goal of these preliminary attention

and orienting procedures is to make the owner a source of focused attention and following behavior.

When taking food, the dog is discouraged from jumping up and encouraged to take the treat gently. Initial lessons should focus on training the dog to come from various place in the home. The squeaker can be used to get the dog's attention, followed by the word "Come" as the dog turns toward the trainer. The dog is rewarded upon coming and immediately released with "OK" and a clap. Once the dog learns to orient to the sound of squeaker, its name can be presented just in advance of the squeaker sound. After the dog has learned to come reliably, it is encouraged to follow along at the trainer's left side and is immediately rewarded as it approaches. Every few steps, the trainer rewards the dog so long as the dog remains close by on the left side. If the dog becomes distracted and moves away, the squeaker is squeezed and the orienting response is bridged with the clicker, as the trainer turns away from the dog and encourages the dog to follow along with friendly smacking, smooching, and sweet talking, whereupon it is rewarded by saying "Good," and the food reward is delivered from a closed hand. With the presentation of most food rewards, the dog is petted under the chin and other locations producing an affectionate response. Once the dog is coming and following the trainer, a sit response is introduced. With the dog following at the left side, the trainer clicks, stops, and waives the right hand over the dog's head. As the dog sits, the trainer says "Good" and rewards the sit action as it is completed. After staying for a brief period, the dog is rewarded again and periodically thereafter on a variable-duration schedule, but must continue sitting until it is released with an "OK" and clap signal. During the sit-stay, the dog should be encouraged to make and maintain eye contact with the trainer, especially at the beginning and at the end of the exercise. As the dog's abilities improve, variations are introduced and practiced with the purpose of increasing attention and impulse-control abilities. Voith's (1977) sit-stay program provides a systematic way of developing sit-stay and impulse-control abilities conducive to attention-therapy objectives (see Appendix A).

Integrated Compliance Training

The vast majority of domestic dog bites signify the presence of reactive incompetence in association with an ISS and a failure of the dog to integrate harmonious and trusting relations with family members. Restoring a trust-based bond incompatible with aggression depends on competence-enhancing ICT and the formation of affectionate and playful dynamic modal relations. An important function of ICT is to establish orderly cooperative relations between the dog and family members in association with everyday activities and sources of potential interactive conflict.

A significant aspect of social competency includes training the dog how to obtain and perpetuate gratifying experiences without resorting to aggression. In addition to relinquishing control over resting areas and possessions, the dog should learn when access to such things is permitted and how to go about getting such access. Similarly, the dog should learn to wait and make eye contact before entering or leaving the house. Social nuisances (e.g., barking and jumping up) can be brought under the control of vocal and gestural signals and then appropriately prompted and rewarded or discouraged as required by the particular situation. For example, during homecomings, the dog can learn to wait before being invited to jump up to say hello. Pawing dogs can be trained to give a paw on signal while pawing at other times is discouraged by the loss of reward. Rather than forbidding behavior, generally the best strategy is define occasions when such behavior is acceptable and productive of reward. Rather than reflecting dominance-related incentives, CDA most often involves a persistent failure of dogs to regulate aggressive impulses competently in the presence of social actions portending a loss of comfort or safety. Most dogs exhibiting domestic-aggression problems do not appear to be competing for rank or privileges of status, but are simply exhibiting socially inept and reactive behavior under the influence of autoprotective incentives. Aggres-

sion in such cases appears to stem from a history of inappropriate or inadequate owner control efforts and a failure to integrate friendly and playful dynamic modal relations and roles into a VSS for obtaining reward and avoiding punishment. According to the involuntary subordination hypothesis, reactive domestic aggression is prone to develop in the context of persistent interactive conflict and tensions, whereby interaction with the owner sensitizes the dog to social signals of punishment (loss of reward and nonreward).

Interactive conflict and tensions (intolerance and irritability) emerge in the context of antagonistic control incentives converging on points of common interest. Instead of the owner taking ownership of the resource and providing the dog access to it in accordance with a rule-based contingency promoting compromise and cooperation (VSS), the owner may interfere or compete with the dog by punishing reward-seeking activity or by preventing the dog from obtaining gratification (comfort and safety); that is, the owner comes between the dog and reward or physically denies the dog access to it, but without leading the dog to obtain the reward in a cooperative way. In such cases, ICT can be extremely useful for establishing a rule-based pattern of social interaction promoting enhanced cooperation and trust (see *Benefits of Cynopraxic Training* in Chapter 1). Sources of agitating interactive conflict are identified and objectified as potential sources of reward for mediating mutual appreciation and interactive harmony. Conflict is resolved by enhancing the owner's ability to take ownership of rewarding resources and to exert competent control by means of limit-setting actions and reward-based training, whereby subordinate compromise and cooperation are rewarded by access to previously barred activities and objects of reward. By such means, a VSS is mediated with the dog becoming progressively sensitive and alert for signals of social and appetitive reward while at the same time helping to mobilize oxytocinergic anti-stress and calming effects associated with the flirt-and-forbear coping style (see *Oxytocin-opioidergic Hypothesis* in Chapter 6). Instead of punishing aggressive tendencies, training is dedicated to instilling a heightened sense of trust and confidence in the owner as leader and friend. Emergent mutual competency and confidence between the dog and the owner naturally result in increased behavioral flexibility and relaxation. Rule-based social interaction facilitates cooperative behavior and prediction-control expectancies incompatible with reactive irritability and intolerance, educating the dog to form an affectionate, cooperative, and trusting orientation with respect to family members.

The effectiveness of ICT is enhanced when performed in conjunction with other training and therapy procedures. In addition to learning how to acquire rewards under an owner's control, a dog needs to learn how to cope with everyday provocative challenges via graduated exposure to directive control. Such training helps to restore a dog's sense of safety and control. By means of complementary behavior-therapy procedures, including graduated directive control and punishment (TO), nonprovocative restraint and taction therapy (PFR training), and avoidance training when appropriate, a dog in stages learns that it can control rewarding situations as well as provocative or mildly threatening ones without losing trust and resorting to aggression. In addition, behavior that is successfully brought under the control of appetitive and social rewards and avoidance training is steadily integrated and brought under the influence of ludic incentives by means of play training. Play antagonizes the emotional irritability and rigidity commonly present in dogs exhibiting CDA. Play is particularly valuable for integrating dynamic modal relations and promoting interactive harmony, tolerance, and trust. The success of an aggression-therapy program is based on the shaping of overt behavior incompatible with aggression, giving evidence of at least three areas of improvement: increased composure (competence and confidence), relaxation, and playfulness. Since aggressive threats may be rapidly suppressed by means of punishment, but without necessarily reducing the risk of overt aggression, the mere absence of aggression is not a useful measure of improvement. Evaluations based solely on the absence of aggres-

sion violate the dead-dog rule (see *Dead-dog Rule* in Volume 2, Chapter 2). Ultimately, the goal of dog behavior therapy, as well as preventive training, is to reduce the risk of CDA by taking appropriate safety precautions and promoting a more playful and trusting bond between the dog and family members.

Counterconditioning

Previously conditioned aversive and appetitive stimuli are subject to a variety of modifying influences, including extinction and counterconditioning. For example, if an conditioned stimulus (CS) is repeatedly presented independently of an unconditioned stimulus (US), the conditioned association between the CS and US will gradually degrade or extinguish, but it will not be permanently uncoupled. Contrary to a popular belief, extinction does not erase past learning. As a behavior-therapy procedure, extinction is notoriously inefficient and subject to "savings" that make its use problematic in the treatment of behavior problems (see *Spontaneous Recovery and Other Sources of Relapse* in Volume 1, Chapter 6). Counterconditioning provides a more effective and reliable means for altering conditioned aversive associations than punishment and extinction. Rather than passively discontinuing the contingency between the CS and US, counterconditioning actively establishes a new contingency and expectancy between the eliciting stimulus and the emotional arousal elicited by it. This change is produced by arranging the fear- or anger-eliciting stimulus to occur in close association with the elicitation of a stronger and incompatible response that overshadows and antagonizes aversive arousal.

Counterconditioning has many applications in dog training and behavior therapy, but is especially useful in cases involving problem behavior operating under the influence of specific conditioned aversive stimuli and evoking contexts (see *Counterconditioning* in Chapter 3). The process is based on the antagonizing effects that responses of opposite emotional and hedonic significance have on one another:

1. If two emotional responses of opposite motivational and hedonic significance are elicited at the same time, the stronger response will tend to overshadow and antagonize the weaker one.
2. If both emotional responses are of approximately equal strength, they will antagonize each other and produce varying degrees of emotional conflict.
3. If an aversive response is stronger than the antagonizing response, the latter will fail to restrain the former and may instead become associatively linked to it.

The risk of producing emotional conflict and stress or conditioning the antagonizing stimulus to elicit rather than restrain the aversive response underscores the importance of gradual exposure when applying a counterconditioning procedure and performing counterconditioning in conjunction with appropriate precautions and response-prevention procedures (see *Fear Reduction and Approach-Avoidance Induction* in Chapter 3). Counterconditioning usually involves the presentation of a series of graduated exposures in which provocative stimuli or situations are repeatedly presented to the dog in a progression of increasing strength and potential for eliciting aversive arousal while the dog is simultaneously presented with a stronger antagonizing stimulus that overshadows or restrains aversive arousal. After repeated trials in which the antagonizing stimulus successfully restrains aversive arousal, the provoking stimulus gradually becomes linked with the antagonizing stimulus and the emotional arousal produced by it. If the antagonizing and provoking responses are of approximately the same magnitude, stressful conflict may ensue adversely affecting counterconditioning efforts.

The provoking stimulus, as the result of newly formed associations with emotional arousal elicited by the antagonizing counterconditioning stimulus, gradually acquires new predictive and emotional associations that are incompatible with its previous significance. The power of counterconditioning to alter the significance of conditioned aversive stimuli makes it highly useful for the treat-

ment of many aggression problems. For example, presenting food (antagonizing stimulus) to a hungry dog that resents reaching and petting actions (provoking stimuli) may gradually alter the dog's response to such activity by the overshadowing effect of appetitive arousal. First tossing food to the dog from a distance, and then through progressive steps giving it to the dog by hand, may help to alter the dog's response to reaching and petting actions via the antagonizing effect of appetitive arousal. Over several trials, the dog may learn to welcome the previously provocative actions, now interpreting them as antecedents associated with getting food. A similar counterconditioning procedure can be used to alter aversive associations linked with being leaned over or stared at and so forth, thereby changing the dog's expectations regarding the significance of such actions. By repeatedly pairing provocative gestures and postures with the presentation of food (tossed to the dog), the dog is provided with new information with which to reinterpret and modify its expectations of such interaction.

The antagonizing effects of counterconditioning on aversive emotional arousal appear to benefit from the additive effects of multiple sources of antagonistic stimulation. Any conditioned or unconditioned stimulus can be used for counterconditioning purposes so long as it is capable of evoking a reliable incompatible emotional response from the dog. The selected stimulus can be used alone or in combination with other similarly effective stimuli. Food is the most commonly used antagonizing stimulus in routine training efforts, but affectionate petting and talking, massage, and play are also often used in combination or separately to antagonize aversive emotional arousal. The potency of food as a counterconditioning stimulus is dependent on the dog's level of hunger and its appetite for the food given to it. Increased appetitive counterconditioning effects can be produced either by increasing the dog's level of hunger or by increasing the appetitive value of the food reward. Although a 12- to 24-hour deprivation period is usually sufficient to pique an increased interest in food, some dogs with reduced appetites (not uncommon among stressed fearful or aggressive dogs) may require a reduced-calorie diet or medication in order to generate a more conducive level of motivation for appetitive counterconditioning. A significant enhancement of food as a antagonizing stimulus is achieved by varying the type and amount of food given to the dog from trial to trial. Odors that have been previously paired with relaxation induced by massage and PFR training work well in combination with other counterconditioning stimuli. The conditioned odor is delivered on the breath, hands, or body or by other various other unobtrusive means (e.g., squeaker bulb). Conditioned odors appear to help the dog relax, possibly restraining undesirable aversive arousal and thereby rendering the dog more receptive to other counterconditioning effects. The ultimate usefulness of ICT, counterconditioning, and other reward-based training efforts will hinge on the dog's willingness to integrate friendly relations with the target of aggression. Some dogs, despite the most conscientious and dedicated efforts, may continue to show a threatening attitude, remaining intolerant and reactive to the approach of certain family members. The subgroup of domestic aggressors that fail to show signs of integrating friendly and submissive relations in response to reward-based training and counterconditioning efforts, should be removed from the home. During all counterconditioning procedures, the dog should be appropriately restrained on leash, control post, halter, or muzzle, as necessary for safe exposure, handling, and response prevention.

Although counterconditioning appears to have several useful applications in dog training, there have been a number of laboratory studies that have questioned the efficacy of the procedure for modifying fears (see *Critical Evaluations of Counterconditioning* in Chapter 3) and aggression (see *Counterconditioning: Limitations and Precautions* in Chapter 8). Currently, the value of counterconditioning for controlling aggression remains unproven, however, sufficient anecdotal evidence and case reports exist to support the use of counterconditioning as a support tool in the context of canine behavior therapy, but perhaps

not as a stand alone classical conditioning procedure. Cynopraxic training theory emphasizes the unity of prediction-control expectancies, emotional establishing operations, and goal-directed action in the process of organizing adaptive behavior, making stand alone counterconditioning unnecessary. In general, the gradual disconfirmation of aggression-provoking expectancies by means of repeated instrumental exchanges around reactive points of conflict that result in mutual reward serves to integrate more competent and cooperative social behavior while naturally altering emotional establishing operations and control incentives in ways that are incompatible with aggression. Whatever benefits might be achieved by countercondtioning in isolation are achieved by cynopraxic training and therapy efforts in the process of shaping more competent prosocial and friendly behavior.

The effects of counterconditioning appear to be particularly problematic and variable in the treatment of impulsive, reactive, and trait aggression (see *Conflicts and Rituals Toward Novel Social Stimuli* in Chapter 8). For example, dogs possessing strong watchdog propensities may be genetically contraprepared to respond to counterconditioning efforts. In the absence of social familiarity and attraction, dogs expressing a rigid watchdog script may be unable to experience outsiders with the sort of trust needed to render food-sharing exchanges as safe–a precondition required to mediate the social benefits of counterconditioning. In addition, dogs expressing unstable temperaments and reactive coping styles may function under a persistent negativity bias for signals of punishment (loss and risk)—a bias that may overshadow and block counterconditioning effects. Counterconditioning may also prove problematical in the case of avoidance-related aggression problems (see *Response Prevention*) or aggression occurring in association with an ISS that has been partially suppressed by physical punishment. In the latter case, as fear is reduced by counterconditioning a transitional point may be reached that significantly increases the risk of aggression (see *Graded Exposure and Response Prevention* in Chapter 3).

Time-out

Although punishment can significantly complicate matters, if used properly and selectively, it can also provide a useful means for controlling certain forms of CDA. The primary function of punishment is to offset or minimize reinforcing consequences produced as the result of aggressive actions. Punitive measures incorporating disruptive startle or momentary social isolation are superior to procedures that depend on manual restraint and physical punishment. Ideally, punitive measures should meet at least two criteria: (1) punishment should not evoke more aggression, and (2) punishment should be motivationally relevant and antagonistic to the goals of aggression. A powerful punitive technique that meets both of these criteria is time-out (TO), which has been shown to suppress avoidance-motivated behavior (Nigro, 1966), competitive excesses in puppies (Polsky, 1989) and aggressive behavior in dogs (Nobbe et al., 1980) (see *Using Time-out to Modify Behavior* in Volume 1, Chapter 8). In addition to promoting rapid de-arousal, the brief period of isolation associated with TO serves to heighten subsequent interest in social contact and other rewards made available during time-in (Figure 7.5).

Besides being effective with minimal risk of side effects, TO avoids the hazards associated with physical punishment. Appropriate restraint and control of the dog is crucial for the effective use of TO. As deemed necessary to ensure safety, an aggressive dog should be kept on leash with a slip collar, halter, or muzzle at all times when it is in contact with people. If the dog lunges or snaps during exposure and counterconditioning efforts, the leash is pulled tight and the dog is rapidly hauled off to a separate room under continuous leash pressure (bridging stimulus). The entire procedure should make the dog experience a dramatic loss of control over the situation as the result of the aggressive action. When pulled forward by the leash, most dogs resist by pulling back, making forward attacks less likely, but such attacks do occur and may necessitate emergency defensive measures to counter. Dogs presenting such a risk should be kept on a muzzle-clamping halter or muzzle and slip collar. Rather than forcing the dog into the TO room or swinging it around, the trainer should enter the TO room (e.g., bedroom) and back out, leaving the dog on the other side. In cases where there is not enough room to turn around easily, the dog can be left outside of the room as the trainer enters and closes the door on the leash. A moment should be taken to make sure that the dog is clear of the door as it is slowly closed and then, when approximately 1 inch from being fully closed, the door is sharply shut for emphasis. The leash should be pinched in the doorjamb approximately 8 inches above the door handle, leaving only enough slack on the other side for the dog to stand or sit but not leaving room for it to move around or lay down. If the dog complains or scratches, the door can be opened a crack and an upward leash prompt can be delivered to discourage the behavior. After 30 to 60 seconds, the trainer should praise the dog as it is released from TO. The dog is immediately returned to the eliciting situation where an incompatible response is prompted and rewarded, thereby setting the stage for more positive and cooperative interaction. In the case of dogs that have received PFR training and olfactory conditioning, the odor used can be diffused into room to help facilitate relaxation and reduce aggressive tensions.

TO can be effectively used to control a variety of attention-seeking and competitive excesses that may also present with an aggression problem (see *Time-out, Response Prevention, and Overcorrection* in Chapter 5). After each TO, the dog is taken back to situation where the misbehavior occurred, and more appropriate behavior is prompted and rewarded. The TO procedure is repeated as needed until the undesirable response is suppressed or weakened sufficiently to allow for effective conditioning of alternative behavior. The suppressive effect of TO is cumulative and most common social excesses respond within three or four repetitions in close succession, given that an alternative behavior is encouraged at the same time. To be maximally effective, TO should be carried out in the context of a reward-dense training environment (see *Time-in Positive Reinforcement* in Volume 1, Chapter 8).

```
┌─ TIME-OUT ─┐                    ┌─ TIME-IN ─┐

PUNISHMENT                        REWARD
  • Loss of contact                 • Affection
  • Loss of reward                  • Food and toys
  • Loss of control                 • Enhanced control

DE-AROUSAL AND BRIEF              INCREASED SOCIAL
SOCIAL DEPRIVATION               REPSONSIVENESS
        ↓                                ↓
POTENTIAL INHIBITORY             PROMOTES PROSOCIAL
INFLUENCE ON AGGRESSION          AND COOPERATIVE
                                 BEHAVIOR INCOMPATIBLE
ESTABLISHING OPERATION           WITH AGGRESSION
ENHANCING SUBSEQUENT
REWARD TRAINING                  IMPROVES COMPETENCY
```

FIG. 7.5. Time-out (TO) is a highly effective punishment technique for the control of some forms of aggressive behavior. TO should be brief and performed within the context of reward-dense time-in (TI) training and counterconditioning efforts. The absence of a reward-dense TI situation significantly reduces the effectiveness and value of TO.

Response Prevention

Since many aggressive dogs appear to threaten or bite as the result of avoidance learning in association with the activation of the FFS, special problems may be encountered that necessitate the use of response-prevention techniques (see *Response Prevention and Directive Training* in Volume 1, Chapter 6, and *Graded Exposure and Response Prevention* in Chapter 3). Aggression operating under the influence of avoidance learning may persist despite conscientious counterconditioning and other positive training efforts. According to the Seligman-Johnston theory (Seligman and Johnston, 1973), once an avoidance response is established, the role of fear is gradually subordinated to reinforcement or extinction effects mediated by the confirmation or disconfirmation of expected outcomes occur-

ring in association with the avoidance response (see *Fear, Cognition, and Avoidance Learning* in Volume 2, Chapter 3). If the avoidance response preempts the aversive event, the controlling avoidance expectancy is confirmed and the response is reinforced, whereas, on the other hand, if the aversive event follows despite the occurrence of the avoidance response, the controlling avoidance expectancy is disconfirmed and the avoidance response is punished and undergoes extinction. The crucial issue here is that fear and its reduction are not directly relevant to the maintenance of a well-established avoidance response. Further, since reinforcement of the avoidance response is based on the preemptive nonoccurrence of the aversive event, the avoidance response may continue long after the aversive threat is removed. Consequently, despite intensive counterconditioning, an avoidance response may continue intact so long as the controlling expectancy is not disconfirmed or until an incompatible expectancy and response are formed.

There are two ways to disconfirm a faulty avoidance expectancy: (1) arrange for the avoidance response to fail (extinction-punishment), or (2) prevent the avoidance response from occurring in the presence of avoidance discriminative stimuli (response prevention). In the first instance, the aversive event is arranged to occur contingently upon the emission of the avoidance response (punishment), thereby disconfirming the controlling avoidance expectancy. As a result, the dog may experiment with other escape strategies until a response is found that succeeds. Consequently, the successful escape response will take the place of the disconfirmed avoidance response and continue so long as it successfully produces outcomes that confirm the modified avoidance expectancy. Although representing the most common procedure used to control avoidance aggression, the approach is problematic and fraught with risk. Under the influence of physical punishment, avoidance-related aggression may rapidly escalate and become significantly worse as the result of vicious-circle effects. In the second case, the avoidance response is prevented from occurring in the presence of avoidance-signaling discriminative stimuli, thereby compelling the dog to recognize that the avoidance response is no longer necessary. As a result of response prevention, the dog learns that the avoidance signals no longer predict an aversive event and that the avoidance contingency has been discontinued, thereby resulting in the extinction of the avoidance response. During exposure with response prevention, a new significance can be effectively linked with the defunct avoidance signals by means of counterconditioning. If a defunct avoidance signal is repeatedly paired with an attractive event (e.g., food, petting, or play), a new incompatible association and function are produced, whereby the previous avoidance expectancy is not only disconfirmed, but is gradually replaced by an antagonistic approach expectancy.

Similarly, in the case of avoidance-related aggression, a dog may continue to threaten or bite under the influence of a faulty avoidance expectancy, with the character of aggression becoming progressively confident and fearless as the result of a history of successful control, especially if it occurs in the absence of reprisals. The controlling avoidance expectancy may continue to maintain the aggressive response despite intensive counterconditioning and absence of aversive stimulation. The avoidance-related aggressive response is reinforced preemptively, requiring only that the original aversive event not follow the occurrence of an attack—an outcome that would disconfirm the controlling avoidance expectancy. As a result, avoidance-related aggression may continue to occur in the presence of certain social signals that are often benign and innocuous, until the aggressor discovers that the controlling avoidance expectancy is faulty and the aggressive avoidance response is unnecessary and defunct. Under normal circumstances, the avoidance aggressor may not discover that the avoidance contingency is no longer in effect, causing it to threaten or bite in the absence of actual threats and discomfort. By means of response-prevention procedures in which aggression is prevented by various means, including leash and halter restraint, crate confinement, and muzzling, the dog is compelled to learn that the avoidance threat or attack is unnecessary. Exposing a dog to innocuous and mildly provocative social stimuli, while at the same time blocking aggressive responses, gradually causes the dog to recognize that the aggressive response is unnecessary to protect its safety. Response-prevention procedures should be performed in a way that emphasizes safety from aversive stimulation. The presence of attractive and relaxing stimuli and a familiar location may help to reduce adverse emotional arousal associated with restraint and exposure. In addition, a graduated counterconditioning procedure is often used during response prevention in order to link provocative social signals with antagonistic emotional arousal incompatible with aggression, thereby replacing the defunct aggression-avoidance expectancy with an incompatible affiliative-approach expectancy. In some cases, especially those that are unresponsive to response prevention and graduated counterconditioning, punishment (TO) can be a viable means to disconfirm the controlling avoidance expectancy. Punishment in such cases works to the extent that it causes the aggressive avoidance response to fail while at the same evoking a response incompatible with aggression that permits reinforcement by the owner as a source of safety and comfort. However, inappropriate physical punishment may only cause the dog to fight back more violently under the combined excitatory influences of fear and anger, thereby resulting in a stronger and more dangerous response—a significant risk associated with punishment. Panic-related aggression may, in some cases, result from physical punishment inappropriately applied against avoidance-related aggression, thereby producing a much more dangerous and difficult-to-control problem.

Posture-facilitated Relaxation Training

Evidence of contact aversion and resentment of handling is frequently exhibited by aggressive dogs. Dogs may become averse to such interaction as the result of a history of unwelcome handling in the past (e.g., excessive picking up and hugging) or aversive-traumatic conditioning (e.g., physical punishment or traumatic restraint) (see *Contact Aversion and Aggression* in Volume 2, Chapter 8). Extremes involving too much (agitation) or too little (deprivation) tactile stimulation and handling may result in contact and handling aversion. Petting may be particularly annoying for dogs that lack a trusting bond with their owners. Whatever the cause, it is clear that tactile stimulation exerts a profound influence on a dog's emotional state, with the dog's relative receptivity to petting and other forms of handling reflecting various biogenetic and acquired differences affecting emotional reactivity, social attraction, and propensity for aggression (see *Taction and Posture-facilitated Relaxation* in Chapter 6).

Prescott (1971) has emphasized the role of tactile deprivation as a causative factor predisposing animals to overreact to social tactile stimulation. He has postulated the existence of a somatosensory-cerebellar pathway mediating increased excitability and stimulus-seeking behavior resulting from tactile deprivation. According to Prescott's hypothesis, stress associated with tactile deprivation promotes the development of a variety of emotional and behavioral disorders, including depressive reactions, stereotypies, hyperactivity, hyperexcitability, excessive seeking behavior, habituation disturbances, impaired pain sensitivity, and impulsive aggressive behavior (Prescott, 1971). Cairns (1972) also found that mice tend to become more reactive, irritable, and aggressive as the result of tactile deprivation. He tested this hypothesis by comparing the reactivity of social isolates to different sources of sensory stimulation, finding that isolates were much more emotionally reactive to tactile stimuli than to visual or auditory stimuli. Fuller (1967) found that isolated puppies were less fearful and reactive in an unfamiliar area if they were handled and stroked before and after exposure. Handling appeared to reduce arousal levels and stress-related reactions evoked by the situation. Persons with autism often show an aversion to tactile stimulation, causing them to stiffen, flinch, or attempt to pull away when touched. Autism is an emotionally insular condition of isolation and inability to relate empathetically with others. The autistic aversion to touch contact appears to be ameliorated by massage, an effect that may be facilitated by the highly predictable and rhythmic nature of the process (Field, 1995). Similarly, dogs exhibiting contact aversion toward human touch and handling often show a positive response to massage in the context of PFR training.

A central focus of PFR training is to form positive conditioned associations with handling and restraint via graduated exposure and massage, response prevention, counterconditioning, and the induction of progressive relaxation, with the net effect of antagonizing reactive emotional responses to such contact (see Appendix C). In addition to inducing relaxation, massage with PFR training, when performed in a highly repetitive and stereotypic manner, appears to produce significant benefits in most dogs by reducing stress, by promoting deference to manual control, and by reliably producing comfort and feelings of safety—behavioral and emotional effects that are highly beneficial in the context of behavior therapy. Nonthreatening manual restraint and postural shifts ranked in terms of a progressive loss of control and submission play an instrumental role in this process of progressive subordination and relaxation (see *Posture, Response Prevention, and Posture-facilitated Relaxation* in Chapter 6). PFR training facilitates a more organized psychophysiological response (parasympathetic dominance) by competing with the reactive and disorganizing influences of sympathetic arousal occurring in association with fear, anger, and frustration.

Dogs with a history of overt aggression should be handled with caution and always kept under appropriate restraint during PFR training. Dogs posing a significant risk of aggression should be leashed and muzzled during PFR training (Figure 7.6). In addition to reducing the risk of attack, the muzzle can provide a salutary response-prevention effect if properly introduced and used. As the risk of aggression is reduced, the level of restraint can be proportionately adjusted to match the risk presented by the dog. The provision of ambient music during PFR training may help to facilitate a relaxation response in some reactive dogs. Wells and colleagues (2002) have reported that classical music appears to exert a calming effect in dogs, as indicated by decreased barking and a greater amount of time spent resting in comparison to controls (no stimulation) living in a kennel environment. Each postural prompt and shift of position is paired with the word "Relax" or "Easy," vocal signals that may be gradually conditioned to predict safe handling and comfort. As the PFR cycle progresses, an olfactory stimulus can be introduced and paired with the deepening relaxation response (see *Olfactory Conditioning* in Chapter 6). After several cycles of PFR training, the odor can be presented at earlier points in the massage sequence, thereby acquiring conditioned properties associated with the induction of relaxation. Gradually, the odor itself can be use to produce a facilitatory effect on the induction and depth of the relaxation response. Certain odors may exert an intrinsic

calming effect that may make them more associable with massage-induced relaxation (see *Fear of Loud Noises and Household Sounds* in Chapter 3). For example, chamomile and lavender have been shown to reduce alpha 1 activity in association with subjective reports of increased feelings of comfort (Masago et al., 2000) and stress reduction (Motomura et al., 2001). The conditioned odor can be delivered by a squeaker or by hand or more generally by a mister or a pump diffuser. The conditioned odor is used in conjunction with other behavior-therapy procedures to help manage aversive states and promote relaxation during counterconditioning efforts.

Punishment

Punishment in the case of CDA should be viewed as a damage-limiting option rather than a routine aspect of the behavior-therapy process. Although harsh physical punishment is inappropriate and should be avoided, overt control-related aggression should be countered with disruptive startle or TO whenever possible, but only in situations were the punitive event can be safely performed and is unlikely to cause the dog to escalate aggressive efforts. Such punishment is primarily performed to offset inadvertent reinforcement that may be produced by overt aggression. Despite the risks involved (see *Species-typical Defensive and Offensive Aggression*), a limited use of punishment may be expedient in some cases, but only after basic control is established by means of reward-based training (Line and Voith, 1986). However, instead of focusing too much attention on punishment, the emphasis should be placed on avoiding provocative social interaction that poses a risk of triggering aggressive episodes while at the same time increasing the probability of evoking more friendly behavior. Finally, once reward-based control is established, mild punishment and avoidance training may be useful to further enhance competent coping skills. As the result of effective reward-based training and gradual exposure to inhibitory training, dogs learn how to regulate their responses to mildly provocative stimulation more adaptively and competently—influences that are highly beneficial

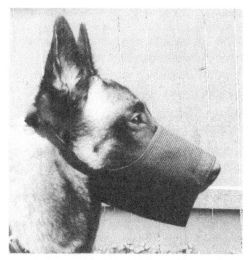

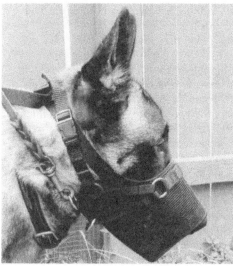

FIG. 7.6. A variety of muzzles are available, but perhaps the most comfortable are those made with a mesh fabric. The muzzle should be introduced gradually in association with highly attractive treats and other positive outcomes. Introducing muzzles too rapidly or roughly may cause dogs to react aggressively or refuse to let themselves be muzzled in the future. Muzzle and halter training requires significant experience and skill to avoid situations that might result in bites to the hands. In situations requiring a high degree of control while limiting the risk of biting, a halter and muzzle can be used in combination.

in the treatment of most forms of domestic aggression.

MANHANDLING AND PHYSICAL PUNISHMENT

Until relatively recent times, harsh physical punishment (e.g., beating) was commonly recommended as a preferred means for controlling aggression and other behavioral excesses (Most, 1910/1955; Lorenz, 1955). Although the measured use of physical force by leash and momentary manual imposition can be useful for enhancing control from time to time, manual methods that intentionally and routinely involve hitting, wrestling, and provocative manhandling directed against aggressive dogs have little (if any) redeeming value for long-term and generalized control of aggression and may make such problems potentially far worse than if nothing had been done at all. Even in cases where such methods succeed in intimidating the aggressor, there is little chance that the inhibition will generalize to other family members who are unable to defend themselves with such physically demanding and skill-dependent punitive actions. In situations where such punishment is used, children may be exposed to an increased risk of attack as the result of punitive agitation, unanticipated behavioral contrast effects (see *Behavioral Contrast and Momentum* in Volume 1, Chapter 7), and redirected attacks. Finally, severe physical punishment may succeed in suppressing threat displays, but without significantly modifying the dog's emotional propensity for aggressive behavior (see *Assessment and Treatment Priorities*). As a result, the roughed-up dog may gradually learn to bite without warning or bite preemptively when threatened by the owner with such treatment. In summary, there are three major problems associated with forceful manhandling and punishment:

- Manhandling places inexperienced dog owners at a significant and unnecessary risk of being bitten.
- Manhandling does little to change the causes of domestic aggression substantially and may actually cause the dog to escalate its aggressive efforts against the owner.
- Manhandling may rapidly suppress threat displays without reducing a dog's propen-

sity to bite, perhaps increasing the dog's aggressive propensity while at the same time making it less predictable and more dangerous.

The use of provocative striking, manhandling, and restraint techniques should be avoided except in the rare case of self-defense and the protection of others, where alternative means of emergency restraint are not available or prove inadequate. Trainers are under a professional obligation to perform training services with dogs under appropriate restraint and to avoid provocative circumstances that necessitate such methods of intimidation for self-defense. Mistakes can happen, and trainers should be skilled in a variety of restraint techniques for responding to such emergencies, but they should never be mistaken for training procedures.

Ramona Albert (1953) once sardonically observed that roughing up an aggressive dog made about as much sense as the old rhyme: "A woman, a dog, a walnut tree; the harder you beat them the better they be." Nothing could be more futile and wrongheaded than beating an aggressive dog, but with regard to beating a walnut tree, at least such activity might be edifying for those unable to see with open eyes and heart that nothing good has ever come of hitting dogs or women. Corporal punishment is a destructive act that risks losing a dog's trust and permanently damaging the human-dog bond. Cynopraxic trainers and applied dog behaviorists would do well to exemplify in word and action the embodiment of patience and forbearance, thereby avoiding the psychological and spiritual trap of manhandling and corporal punishment as a necessity of control, which it most assuredly is not. Given the current level of practice, there is no legitimate excuse for roughing up a dog to train it. The last of a series of principles enunciated by Skinner for his utopian society Walden Two included the following item apropos to the current discussion: "Regard no practice as immutable. Change and be ready to change again. Accept no eternal verity. Experiment" (Skinner, 1979:346). Once free of the option to hit and manhandle, the training process gradually becomes more thoughtful, creative, experimental, playful, friendly

and, most importantly, more successful and rewarding in terms of forming a trusting bond—an essential requirement for the control of domestic-aggression problems.

AGGRESSION AND DIET

Reduced Dietary Protein, Serotonin Production, and Aggression

Although the current evidence is equivocal with respect to the benefits of a diet containing reduced dietary protein for managing CDA, preliminary veterinary data suggest that some dogs exhibiting territorial aggression with fear may benefit from a low protein diet (Dodman et al., 1996b), especially when it is supplemented with tryptophan (De Napoli et al., 2000). De Napoli and colleagues have reported that dogs diagnosed with dominance aggression may also benefit from a low-protein diet or a high-protein diet enriched with tryptophan (see *Nutrition and Aggression* in Volume 2, Chapter 6). Salazar (2000) has proposed the hypothesis that increased insulin sensitivity to alpha-lipoic acid may influence circulating levels of tryptophan and thereby facilitate transport through the blood-brain barrier and increase its availability for serotonin synthesis (see *Diet and the Enhancement of Serotonin Production* in Volume 1, Chapter 3). Future studies using low-protein diets to modify serotonin production in dogs may want to consider the potential additive benefits of alpha-lipoic acid and dietary carbohydrates for improving tryptophan transport through the blood-brain barrier.

For various metabolic, physiological, and practical reasons, 5-hydroxytryptophan (5-HTP) may be more useful as a means for enhancing serotonin production than tryptophan. 5-HTP is the immediate precursor of serotonin and more easily crosses the blood-brain barrier than does tryptophan. Whereas the synthesis of 5-HT from tryptophan is dependent on an intermediate rate-limiting step and the availability of the enzyme tryptophan hydroxylase, 5-HTP is synthesized directly into 5-HT. Another important advantage of 5-HTP is availability. Unlike tryptophan, a product that is not currently available in a purified form over the counter, 5-HTP can be readily purchased. 5-HTP should be handled with respect, since accidental ingestion of it by dogs can result in severe toxicosis or death. Gwaltney-Brant and colleagues (2000), who investigated several reports of 5-HTP toxicosis in dogs, found that the minimum dose producing a toxic effect in dogs was 23.6 mg/kg, with a minimum lethal dose placed at 128 mg/kg. To put these findings into perspective, a 70-pound dog would need to ingest 749 mg (15 capsules containing 50 mg each) to become sick or 4.07 g (81 capsules containing 50 mg each) to reach a lethal dose. Of course, these doses are significantly higher than the amounts used therapeutically, but the report underscores the importance of keeping all medications out of a dog's reach and giving them only under the supervision of a veterinarian.

If a low-protein diet is used, in addition to reducing protein content to 15% to 18%, dietary levels of carbohydrate and fat should be adjusted and balanced to match a dog's energy needs. Supplementing the diet with vitamin C and E, alpha-lipoic acid, and a balanced spectrum of polyunsaturated fatty acids (especially omega-3) may provide additional benefit with respect to normalizing serotonin activity and reversing neuronal damage resulting from oxidative stress. Some special and senior diets are currently available with the appropriate levels of protein, but they may need to be supplemented with additional fat and carbohydrate. Cooked salmon (1 part), turkey (1 part), spinach (2 parts), and rice (6 parts) can be prepared on a weekly basis and shaped into the form of meal-sized balls and frozen. At feeding times, the rice balls are thawed by microwave and mashed into the low-protein senior diet. High-carbohydrate snacks and drinks can also be given (e.g., a rice cake, bagel, bread, or popcorn), especially as treats or a midday snack. Care should be taken not to exceed the dog's daily caloric needs. Whenever possible, a veterinary nutritionist should be consulted to help formulate the diet and provide advice concerning supplementation. In any event, the dog's veterinarian should be consulted in advance of implementing any dietary changes or supplementation in order to obtain appropriate dosages and other relevant information (e.g.,

potential side effects) and potential adverse interactions with other medications that the dog might be taking. For example, 5-HTP should never be given in conjunction with selective serotonin (5-HT) reuptake inhibitors or tricyclic antidepressants.

Diet Change and the Integrate-or-Disperse Hypothesis

Hennessey and colleagues (2002) have reported that a high-quality diet (HQD) with increased levels of protein (29%) and fat (20.5%) appears to produce a calming effect when combined with a social enrichment (SE) procedure, whereas a comparison diet (CD) (23.0% protein/10.1% fat) combined with SE produces a marked increase in behavioral reactivity. Pretest and posttest scores were obtained at week 1 and again at week 8. The behavioral tests consisted of the dog being left alone in a novel environment (arena), exposure to a motionless and moving stranger, the approach of a remote-controlled toy car, and the startling blast of an air horn while alone. Dogs receiving SE were given 20 minutes of dedicated attention in a friendly room 5 days per week. SE consisted of 3 minutes of moving about freely, 7 minutes of stroking and gentle efforts to make the dog lie down on a rug, and 10 minutes of training. Dogs not receiving SE remained in their kennels. The results of this study contain paradoxical and counterintuitive trends with respect to the effects of diet and SE on anxiety and fear thresholds and raise questions with respect to potential adverse effects of dietary change and SE efforts. Further, if the study reflects actual shifts in behavioral thresholds due to dietary change and SE (not an uncontrolled influence or artifact), it raises several intriguing hypotheses with respect to the effect of diet change on the dog's responsiveness to social rewards and provides experimental support for the necessity of improving the dog's quality of life as a necessary coactive factor to achieve the bond-enhancing objectives of cynopraxis (see *Quality-of-Life Matters* in Chapter 8).

The most interesting aspect of the study is the unexpected ways in which the dogs responded to SE under the influence of the different test diets. For example, when exposed to the previously described battery of behavioral tests, dogs fed the CD and given SE (CD/+) showed more escape attempts, panting, nervous social licking, and yawning than did counterparts fed the control diet but not given SE (CD/–). In contrast, dogs fed the HQD and given SE (HQD/+) showed significantly fewer escape attempts than did dogs fed the experimental diet but not given SE (HQD/–). Whereas the HQD/+ group panted less, produced fewer yawns, and gave fewer anxious social licks, the HQD/– group showed evidence of increased anxious arousal, producing more panting, yawning, and nervous social licking. Although the HQD/+ group showed a trend toward decreased reactivity and enhanced relaxation, the HQD/– group tended to become more anxious, but remained unchanged with respect to active reactivity measures (escape attempts). On the other hand, the CD groups showed an opposite trend of divergence with respect to the effect of SE. The CD/+ group exhibited a tendency to become more reactive and anxious, whereas the CD/– group appeared to show significantly less evidence of anxiety and reactivity. Oddly, the overall scores received by the CD/– group were comparable to the scores received by the HQD/+ group. The HQD/+ group scores were only marginally better than the CD/– group in the case of escape attempts.

These results seem to indicate that dogs fed a HQD need more social attention and care than dogs fed nutritionally adequate diets. In fact, one might surmise, that dogs fed an average diet while sheltered may be more likely to exhibit adverse behavioral and emotional changes when given more attention and care, whereas dogs fed a HQD may show increased signs of social anxiety when given less attention and care. In other words, the just-adequate diet appears to promote changes that alter a dog's response to friendly social interaction, making it subsequently more reactive and anxious to social and environmental stimuli. In contrast, the HQD appears to promote increased social anxiety in dogs that receive too little friendly interac-

tion, but yields a calming effect in the case of dogs receiving increased friendly social contact (e.g., stroking, massage, and training). As a result, one might speculate that the HQD/+ group would tend to form more rapid social attachments than the HQD/– group, whereas the latter might show a comparatively heightened reactivity to being left alone. On the other hand, the CD/– group might show a significantly decreased ability to form new social attachments, whereas the CD/+ group might be more prone to show increasing levels of social reactivity and anxiety with respect to social stimuli and situations involving close social contact. One might further speculate that decreasing the quality of the diet more in the case of the CD groups, while at the same time rapidly increasing the complexity and quantity of social interaction given to the CD/+ group, might substantially increase anxiety and frustration, perhaps producing additional social reactivity (e.g., anxious submissiveness and threats or resentment) and an increasing trend toward self-imposed isolation. How dogs react to such hypothetical changes in diet and social interaction would probably depend on individual differences, epigenetic adversity, and allostatic load. Relevantly, Kaplan and colleagues (1996) found that cynomolgus macaques exhibit significant changes in social affiliation and agonistic behavior when fed a low-fat/low-cholesterol diet. Monkeys fed the low-fat diet while living in an unstable social setting showed more overt aggression, but when living in a stable social setting with familiar conspecifics they showed both more aggression and submission behavior and spent much less time making close tactile contact with other monkeys. Kaplan and colleagues have argued that these results are consistent with the existence of a negative-feedback mechanism between dietary privation and the expression of appropriate behavioral adjustments.

Unfortunately, the study performed by Hennessey and colleagues lacks a control group for comparing the effects of the two diets and SE against a third diet (shelter diet) common to both experimental groups prior to the beginning of the study, making a comparison of contrast effects on behavior between the shelter diet, the CD, and HQD a matter of speculation. However, assuming that the CD was nutritionally inferior to the shelter diet and that the HQD was superior, then the changes in the dogs' behavior may be due in large measure to the contrast detected between the new diet and the accustomed one; that is, the new diets are either better or worse than the dogs are accustomed to eat. At some level, the brain may detect and respond to such discrepancies and mobilize one of two general phylogenetic survival modes (PSMs). According to the integrate-or-disperse hypothesis, if nutritional change is experienced physiologically as better than accustomed, dogs may mobilize a *social integration strategy* and exhibit a shift of priorities toward activities and exchanges leading to improved social relations and friendly proximity-seeking behavior. On the other hand, dogs experiencing the diet change as something worse than accustomed may fall under the influence of a *loner dispersal strategy*, causing friendly interaction to paradoxically lower anxiety and reactivity thresholds.

The integrate-or-disperse hypothesis postulates that dogs receiving better-than-accustomed diets tend to respond positively to close contact and cooperative interaction because such activities are consonant with the overarching integrative PSM to form friendly social relations, but such dogs may become increasingly anxious and reactive as the result of actions leading to social isolation or rejection. Conversely, the hypothesis predicts that dogs receiving worse-than-accustomed diets, resulting in the mobilization of a dispersing PSM, will tend to become increasingly anxious and reactive subsequent to actions leading to friendly social interaction, because such activity is dissonant with the dispersal PSM. Such dogs may become more relaxed and comfortable as they are ignored and left alone, that is, when engaged in activities that are consonant with the dispersal survival modes. Accordingly, actions that are dissonant with the operative integrating or dispersing PSM result in escalating anxiety, whereas actions that are consonant with the PSM result in increasing calm and relaxation. This hypothe-

sis points to the existence of a novel form of adaptive learning, which, if confirmed, may have powerful implications for understanding the development of emotional and behavioral disorders.

Under conditions of plenty, the most serious threat that the social animal faces is the loss of a place within the social group, that is, to be shunned or ostracized. As a result, during times of plenty, a persistent failure to experience increased social and friendly contact with others may stimulate significant uneasiness, feelings of vulnerability, and despair—a desperate plea for social attention (separation distress). Consequently, dogs operating under the influence of an integrative PSM may evidence increased social tolerance, enhanced mood, readiness to integrate new friendly relations, and calmness, developing in close association with social rewards and affectionate contact between the dog and family members. However, under the influence of diminished nutrition, physiological loss, and other quality-of-life deficiencies, priorities may turn inexorably toward self-interest and dispersion as a strategy of homeostasis and survival. In addition to a reduced ability to integrate friendly relations, the loner dispersal strategy may include increased object guarding, increased territoriality toward visitors, and intolerance toward intrusion around eating and resting places. The loner dog may tend toward activities that lead in the direction of increasing solitude (e.g., social avoidance, intolerance, and irritability). Instead of experiencing tactile stimulation and friendly interaction as being emotionally gratifying, the dog may instead become increasingly anxious and agitated by such treatment, insofar as the interaction conflicts with the mobilized dispersal survival mode. Instead of producing a physiologically calming effect, such dogs may react to petting as a stressor (see *Oxytocin-opioidergic Hypothesis* in Chapter 6). Like the reactive agonism of Kaplan's macaques fed a low-fat diet, dogs showing a loner dispersal strategy may also show increasing anxious submissiveness, aggressiveness, and intolerance (reactive agonism) in response to affectionate tactile stimulation given by family members. Whereas the social integration strategy mediates social engagement (e.g., frontal orientation, sustained eye contact, whining and howling, tolerance, increased proximity, and enjoyment of social tactile stimulation), the loner dispersal strategy mediates social disengagement (e.g., sideways orientation, refusal to make eye contact, growling, increased social distance, and increasing contact aversion). The dispersing loner may show an increasing intolerance or irritability toward family members. Under the influence of the loner dispersal strategy, the dog may become more and more prone to reactive conflict and withdrawal from social contact. If pressured for close contact or interaction, the dog may become increasingly anxious, irritable, depressed, and more aggressive—an angry loner. The angry-and-depressed coping style may be an extreme example of the loner dispersal strategy, perhaps helping to make sense of the reactive aggression shown by some dogs in response to the most benign and friendly handling by family members. For such dogs, operating under an actual or perceived state of privation, affectionate contact may be paradoxically anxiogenic and irritating. As circumstances become worse, the reaction to social comfort and contact may become more and more debilitating. In contrast, as the dog's circumstances or quality of life improves, its response to social contact and its willingness to integrate friendly relations should correspondingly make progress.

Interestingly, the integrate-or-disperse hypothesis may help to explain the temporary aggression-reducing value of the social-deprivation procedure previously discussed (see *Nothing in Life Is Free, Subordinate Postures, and Rank*). By withholding social contact from a dog operating under a loner-dispersal strategy, its anxiety and reactivity may be significantly reduced as it engages in activity consonant with the dispersal ESS. From this perspective, the procedure has little to do with the idea of changing a dog's perception of rank, but may mediate a calming effect by simply leaving the dog alone and preventing it from engaging in social activity dissonant with the dispersal ESS. However, if true, the procedure works with a severe cost with

respect to a dog's capacity to ultimately integrate friendly relations with the family, since it only serves to polarize the dog further. In contrast, instead of promoting social avoidance and withdrawal, the integrate-or-disperse hypothesis predicts that improving a dog's quality of life through diet, exercise, play, and minimized confinement may be sufficient to mobilize a social integration strategy, thereby reversing the dog's adverse response to social rewards and enabling it to integrate friendly social relations with family members without experiencing paradoxical anxiety.

The cynopraxic therapy process works only to the extent that both social and quality of life imperatives are satisfied, that is, the procedure used must both enhance the bond while improving the dog's quality of life. Provided that the integrate-or-disperse hypothesis is generally accurate, then gradually enhancing the quality of the dog's diet and the quality of other prominent aspects of its life would seem to be a logical and useful starting point in the treatment of CDA and other problems involving a failure of the dog to integrate friendly household relations. Even if the foregoing hypothesis concerning the precise causes turns out to be wrong, the value of improving the dog's diet and quality of life will remain a valid and useful way to initiate cynopraxic therapy.

Fat, Cholesterol, Fatty Acids, and Impulsive Aggression

In the experiment performed by Hennessey and colleagues, a significant aspect of the diet change was an alteration of fat content. The HQD contained twice as much fat as the CD together with a significant increase in protein. They found no evidence in support of the notion that a high-protein diet might promote aggressiveness or irritability. One possible alternative explanation for the benefits observed in dogs fed a reduced protein diet is the fat content of the diet. Dodman and colleagues (1996b) adjusted the energy density of their different diets by manipulating fat content. The fat content of the high (h), medium (m), and low (l) protein diets were adjusted in stepwise fashion from 27.5 (h) to

36.8 (m) to 44.8 (g/1000 kcal), respectively. Large adjustments in dietary fat content were carried out in the study performed by De Napoli and colleagues (2000). In this experiment, the low-protein diet contained five times as much fat as the high-protein diet. Although neither study controlled fat content as a potential therapeutic variable, dietary fat and cholesterol levels may exert a significant influence on serotonergic function and confound the modest behavioral effects attributed to increased tryptophan. The notion that a change in fat and cholesterol intake might influence reactivity and impulsive aggression has been a topic of considerable experimental interest, and numerous studies have shown evidence of a link between low cholesterol, reduced 5-HT activity, and various adverse impulse and mood (depression) effects, including an increased propensity for impulsive aggression (Buydens-Branchey et al., 2000; Golomb et al., 2000). As previously discussed, monkeys fed a low-fat and low-cholesterol diet are more aggressive and less friendly than monkeys fed a high-fat and high-cholesterol diet; such monkeys also have lower cerebrospinal fluid concentrations of the serotonin metabolite 5-hydroxyindoleacetic acid (5-HIAA) (Kaplan et al., 1994), suggesting a potential mechanism for the change in social agonism. Accumulating evidence appears to support the notion that low cholesterol is not merely of correlational interest, but may play a causative role in the process of producing serotonergic abnormalities (Brunner et al., 2002). The effect of fat and cholesterol on behavior and mood appears to be dose dependent, since excessively high cholesterol levels also appear to produce adverse effects on impulse control (Hilakivi-Clarke et al., 1996), suggesting that some optimal level is necessary for efficient serotonergic functioning and for producing preventive or therapeutic benefits (Hillbrand and Spitz, 1999).

Other lines of evidence suggest that low cholesterol may not be as critical a measure or predictor of impulsive aggression as low levels of omega-3 polyunsaturated fatty acids (PUFAs) (Hibbeln et al., 1998; Rogers, 2001). Omega-3 deficiencies have been identified in children exhibiting behavioral and cognitive deficits associated with attention-deficit hyperactivity disorder (e.g., learning difficulties, inattentiveness, and impulsivity) (Stevens et al., 1996), symptoms that are ameliorated by PUFA supplementation (Richardson and Puri, 2002). Omega-3 supplementation has also been shown to stabilize mood, reducing the severity of human depression and mania (Freeman, 2000). Finally, the oxidative depletion of essential fatty acids within the neuronal cell membrane has been implicated as a major factor in the progress of psychotic disorder, with supplemental PUFAs and antioxidants providing therapeutic benefits by helping to repair damage done to the cell membrane by oxidative stress (Mahadik et al., 2001). Interesting preliminary evidence suggests that supplementing the diet with PUFAs, especially omega-3 [eicosapentanoic acid (EPA) and docosahexanoic acid (DHA)] may enhance central serotonin function and reduce impulsive behavior, including aggression (Brunner et al., 2002). The clinical value of these dietary manipulations for dogs exhibiting CDA and other behavior problems has not been evaluated, but one double-blind, controlled trial has demonstrated mood-stabilizing efficacy in human bipolar patients (Stoll et al., 1999). A relatively high dose was used (omega-3 fatty acid: 6.2 g EPA and 3.4 g DHA divided in two daily doses). A recently reported trial involving briefer treatment and a lower dose of DHA alone (without EPA) proved ineffective for major depression. The foregoing data suggest strongly that cholesterol and/or PUFA plasma levels may represent a useful diagnostic marker and etiological factor in the development of CDA. Veterinary clinical investigation of cholesterol and PUFA levels in aggressive and nonaggressive dogs would seem justified.

Protective and Restorative Effects of Vitamins and Antioxidants

Dogs under chronic stress and increased metabolic strain may benefit from preventive measures taken to reduce neuronal damage due to oxidative stress. The brain may be particularly vulnerable to such damage as the result of increased metabolic activity associated with chronic stress and the maintenance of a reactive coping style. Diets enriched with antioxidants such as vitamins C and E and alpha-lipoic acid may exert significant neuroprotective effects (Packer et al., 1997) or reverse adverse cognitive changes associated with aging in dogs (Milgram et al., 2002) (see *Diet and Exercise* in Chapter 3). In addition to potent antioxidant effects, alpha-lipoic acid has been found to increase dopamine, norepinephrine, and serotonin activity in aging rats (Arivazhagan and Panneerselvam, 2002), perhaps helping to explain some of the cognitive benefits observed in older dogs fed diets containing increased levels of the substance (Milgram et al., 2002). Vitamin C and vitamin E perform complementary water-soluble and fat-soluble antioxidant functions. Normally, a dog's need for vitamin C is at least minimally satisfied by endogenous synthesis; however, as the result elevated allostatic load, the requirement for vitamin C may increase. Also, dietary supplementation of vitamin E and PUFAs may produce an increased demand for vitamin C. Vitamin C may influence vitamin-E potency and help prevent the propagation free radicals (Mahadik et al., 2001; Milgram et al., 2002). Interestingly, vitamin C is rapidly absorbed after ingestion, suggesting that dogs may have an active intestinal transport mechanism to increase the absorption of vitamin C (Wang et al., 2001). Dogs have evolved the ability to taste furaneol, a sweet flavor associated with fruits (see *Gustation* in Volume 1, Chapter 4). The ability to efficiently absorb vitamin C combined with the presence of gustatory receptors dedicated to the taste of fruity flavors suggests that vitamin C may possess an underappreciated physiological significance for dogs.

EXERCISE

Some data suggest that exercise may exert a significant modulatory effect over biological stress as well as influence the activity of various neurotransmitter systems (see *Exercise and the Neuroeconomy of Stress* in Volume 1, Chapter 3). These general physiological effects of exercise may help to account for the lower incidence of dominance- and possession-related aggression occurring in dogs obtained for the purpose of exercise (Jagoe and Serpell, 1996). Putting a dog outside in a fenced yard or on a run line is not enough to ensure adequate exercise (Delude, 1991). To produce a benefit, the owner must become directly involved in the exercise activity, ensuring that the exercise (walking, running, jumping, fetching, and so forth) is done in way that produces physiological and psychological benefit.

BRIEF PROTOCOLS FOR CANINE DOMESTIC AGGRESSION

Assessing and modifying aggression in adult dogs is complicated by a dearth of reliable scientific and technical information with which to construct rational treatment protocols. Most of the current literature is composed of clinical impressions, case histories, anecdotes, and statistical analyses of questionnaires. Such methodology is subject to many confounding influences, not the least of which are the investigator's personal biases and beliefs. Although such information may offer promising insights from time to time, it is also prone to an opposite effect: the perpetuation of unfounded opinions and "cherished preconceptions." Few of the contemporary treatment protocols used to control or manage CDA have been subjected to rigorous clinical evaluation and validation. Clearly, much more needs to be done by way of basic and clinical research to advance our knowledge about how to best treat dog aggression problems. In any case, there are no cookbook procedures for controlling aggression, and effective intervention depends on both theoretical and applied knowledge together with competent skills and practical experience acquired as the result of treating such problems.

Assessment and Treatment Priorities

All provocative situations and control incentives that have been associated with aggressive threats or attacks in the past should be identified and evaluated (see *Assessment and Identification* in Volume 2, Chapter 8) (Table 7.4). Many domestic aggressors threaten or bite in more than one situation. In addition to identifying the situations where aggression occurs, potential motivational factors should be explored, including emotional establishing operations (e.g., fear, anxiety, frustration, irritability, or anger). In many cases, these various emotional influences are coactive and present in varying proportions and admixtures. Frequently, domestic aggressors show evidence of fear just before or after biting, leading to a widely held belief that all such attacks are motivated by fear. Although fear appears to play an active motivational role in triggering or escalating some forms of CDA, it also exerts a strong inhibitory effect over many forms of aggression. Fear occurring just before an attack in association with threat displays may serve to stop or reduce the severity of the resulting bite, whereas fear occurring during an attack may either serve to limit the attack or cause it to rapidly escalate, as is prone to occur in response to inappropriate punishment. An aggressive dog's reliance on threat displays belies a significant amount of fear and conflict; otherwise, the dog would not hesitate and threaten before launching into an attack. The fearlessness associated with some forms of panic-related aggression may be responsible for the lack of threat and warning before a dog launches into a hard, uninhibited attack. In such cases, efforts to instill fear may worsen the aggressive response. The presence of fear in association with threats may help to explain the greater sensitivity and responsiveness of the threat sequence to the inhibitory effects of punishment. Although punishment may be more likely to interrupt and prevent an aggressive episode at the threat sequence, it does so at the risk of suppressing the threat display without reducing the dog's propensity to attack. In cases involving dogs that are aggressively reactive to fear-eliciting stimulation, such treatment also runs the risk of triggering an overt attack that might not have occurred without the punitive stimulation.

The role of fear in aggression is complicated. Fear reduction should be primarily the result of increased feelings of safety and trust occurring in association with enhanced inter-

action between the dog and the owner. Placing too much emphasis on fear reduction by means of situational counterconditioning efforts or medication may not significantly improve the overall situation and long-term prognosis, but may inadvertently make things worse, perhaps even more dangerous (see *Pharmacological Control of Anxiety and Fear* in Chapter 3). For example, tranquilization appears to cause wolves to become more aggressive and more likely to attack without giving threat displays (Woolpy and Ginsburg, 1967). In addition to evaluating control incentives, trainers should carefully assess and address coactive emotional factors, such as anger, frustration, irritability, and panic (loss of control). The role of fear in aggression varies significantly under influence of different control incentives and coactive emotional influences. Dogs showing fear while exhibiting aggression in the context of object guarding represent a significantly different diagnostic picture than dogs showing fear and aggression while their paws are handled. Although graduated counterconditioning is effective and can be used to reduce specific fears, behavior therapy of aggression problems occurring in associated with control-related incentives should stress training activities that teach the dog and owner how to cope more competently and confidently with provocative situations. Without such a broad-based cynopraxic approach to such problems, the dog may learn not to bite in the specific situation treated with counterconditioning, but still harbor a control-related propensity to threaten or bite the owner in other provocative situations involving other control incentives.

Many situations leading to CDA are associated with a loss of safety or comfort. Under circumstances resulting in the loss of safety or comfort, predisposed dogs may threaten or attack under varying coactive emotional influences, including irritability, anger, frustration, and fear. Both control-related aggression and panic-related aggression occur under the influence of such provocative stimulation. Dogs exhibiting control-related aggression most often present threats and inhibited punitive attacks. In contrast, dogs exhibiting

TABLE 7.4. Common situations and triggers provoking aggression in dogs

When the dog is approached while in close proximity or in possession of toys, food or food bowls, and other prized objects (possessive aggression)

When the dog is approached while occupying a resting place

When a person enters a certain room while occupied by the dog

When a person is putting a collar on the dog or grabbing the collar

When the dog's leash is yanked

When the dog threatens some person or dog but turns the attack toward someone else who is closer or attempts to restrain it (redirected aggression)

When the dog is shouted at loudly

When the dog is being forced into its crate

When the dog is physically displaced from the bed or favorite pieces of furniture

When the dog is approached while resting or sleeping in or near doorways

When the owner is leaving the home

When the dog is approached directly, reached for, or stepped over

When the dog is near a particular family member

When the dog is being picked up, manually restrained, or physically threatened

When the dog is touched in a particular place (e.g., top of head, shoulder, belly, feet, or hindquarters)

When the dog is given unwelcome affection or petting

When the dog is being groomed (brushing, trimming nails, cleaning ears, or bathing)

---

panic-related aggression show a significant degree of dyscontrol over aggressive impulses, representing a significantly more dangerous problem. Panic aggressors often appear to attack incompetently and impulsively, reacting in the most violent and uninhibited ways to the most innocuous and trifling intrusions or interferences disturbing their comfort or safety. Such dogs seem to lack a normal degree of social flexibility and tolerance. Panic-related attacks frequently occur under the prompting of heightened autonomic reactivity, anger, fear, rigidity, and the momentarily loss of impulse control. In contrast to control-related and avoidance-related aggression, panic related aggression appears to occur as the result of an incompetent loss of impulse control. Physical punishment in such cases serves only to further heighten aggressive arousal, perhaps because of a fear-mediated excitatory influence on anger/rage circuits.

Domestic aggressors often show affection toward their victims, but appear to tolerate innocuous intrusion, interference, or loss. Without the formation of an affectionate bond based on trust, the daily interaction between the owner and the dog may be vulnerable to the adverse effects of interactive conflict and stress. The resulting stress-related autonomic and behavioral changes may contribute to the development of CDA. Some domestic aggressors show a persistent intolerance to the affectionate and playful overtures of certain family members while tolerantly accepting the affection from others. In addition to showing intolerance and increased irritability, these dogs may show varying levels of resentment toward physical handling and control, increased emotional reactivity and vigilance, rigidity, and a lack of responsiveness to play. Such dogs appear to actively resist the rejected family member's efforts to establish a close connection and may deliver a hard bite while being hugged or petted affectionately. In the absence of affectionate trust or willingness to form an affectionate relationship, petting, handling, and invitations to play might naturally become sources of resentment and irritation and, in some cases, set the occasion for aggressive reprisals (see *Loss of Safety, Depression, Panic, and Aggression*).

Aggression Associated with Disturbances While Resting

Dogs exhibiting aggressive tensions, threats, or overt biting when approached while in certain locations, such as doorways, near feeding areas, or beds, should be trained to leave such areas by vocal and hand signal, rather than reaching for them or attempting to displace them manually. Cooperative compliance at such times is appropriately rewarded with affectionate vocal encouragement and food rewards or by providing the dog with activities that it enjoys (e.g., going for a walk or play). Eventually, the dog acquires a something-positive-is-about-to-happen-to-me expectation whenever the owner approaches. Training a dog to orient in response to its name and to hold its attention briefly on the owner is an important aspect of this training process. The orienting and attending response is repeated frequently from different directions and while approaching the dog in different ways. The dog gradually learns to orient and make sustained eye contact with the owner before being rewarded. Various types of approaches including slow, normal, and fast movements toward the dog are associated with the sequence of calling its name, holding its attention, and tossing it a treat. In some cases, a squeaker containing an odor previously paired with PFR training is used as an orienting stimulus—a procedure that is especially useful while working with a dog at close quarters or when prompting it from a hypnagogic or sleeping state. The odor provides contextual and associative information stemming from PFR training that may compete with or restrain aggressive arousal. Alternatively, during approach and attention therapy, the odor can be put on hands and clothing or sprayed into the air by a plant mister or a modified carbon-dioxide (CO_2) pump. At times when the dog must be awakened, its name is called or the squeaker is used. Orient-

ing and attending training helps to condition a positive anticipatory response in association with being awakened or disturbed. The orderly presentation of training events associated with attention therapy serves to enhance executive control over impulse. Attention therapy also improves the likelihood that a dog is orienting and attending to training events and getting the most from counterconditioning and other behavioral procedures.

Dogs that threaten or bite if they are disturbed or moved while resting or sleeping should also be trained to defer to command in situations where they have exhibited aggression in the past. Frequently, these locations involve furniture or a bed, but it can be any place where the dog habitually rests, including the owner's lap. In addition to preliminaries already discussed, such dogs should be trained to surrender defended areas on the command ("Off") and do so without hesitation or resistance. Such training is performed with the dog kept on leash and collar or halter to make handling and control more safe and effective. The dog is trained to both jump onto ("Hup") and off furniture in various locations around the house. The on-off ritual is repeated until the dog's performance is fluid and brought under the control of both voice command and hand signal. Initially, the dog is prompted to leave furniture by gesture or by tossing a treat some distance away, requiring that it get up to retrieve the food. Tossing a ball or some other valued toy can also be used to prompt the off action. The hand movement used to toss the treat is incorporated as a hand signal by gradually fading the treat. As the dog takes its reward for getting off, it is called back and prompted by gesture to jump back up on the furniture and rewarded again. Other resting places associated with previous threats or attacks should be identified and treated in a similar way. If the dog shows overt aggressive actions, it is appropriately directed off the furniture by leash and hauled off to TO. Once a dog is trained to jump on and off furniture, the owner should allow the dog to get up on furniture only after it sits and waits for an invitation to jump up. Dogs that have seriously threatened or have bitten while on a bed should be restricted from such access and learn to sleep on the floor or in a crate, if necessary.

Aggression Associated with Social Signals and Intrusive Movements

In addition to training the dog to perform various cooperative behaviors incompatible with aggression, the predictive and emotional significance of social signals are modified by linking them with prosocial exchanges incompatible with aggression. Social signals provide the dog with predictive information about what is most likely to occur in the immediate future, thereby motivationally preparing it to cope effectively with the impending social situation (see *Social Communication and the Regulation of Aggression*). For example, some dogs by virtue of severe or repeated noncontingent punishment in the past, may become aggressively aroused when exposed to social and contextual stimuli that resemble those present at the time of event. A wide variety of social signals occurring immediately before the event may acquire provocative significance via classical conditioning, including loud voices, staring, the smell of anger, standing over, raised hand, quick movement, reaching actions, grabbing, or touching, and patting. Many of these social signals (e.g., loud voices, fast movements, and smells of anger) may be biologically prepared for rapid conditioning and the formation of associative linkages with anger and fear. As a result of such conditioning, subtle and benign movements may provoke aggressive arousal, especially when they occur under the influence of contextual cues similar to those present at the time of the original provocative event. In addition to external contextual stimuli, internal contextual stimuli consisting of mood and emotional changes also contribute to setting occasions in which aggression is most likely to occur. Together with external and internal contextual cues, the dog's activity and body posture at the time of the event may have been strongly associated with the traumatic event. After identifying these various provoking social and contextual stimuli, they are hierarchically organized in accordance with

their provocative potential. The preparatory aversive arousal associated with these various stimuli and contextual settings is gradually modified by a pattern of rewarding and safe exchanges that promotes social expectancies and emotional establishing operations incompatible with reactive arousal and aggression.

Aggression Associated with Guarding and Possessiveness

Possessive guarding of food and toys is a common dog aggression problem. From the results of a large survey (N = 3226), Guy and colleagues (2001a) found that approximately 20% of dogs either growled or snapped while in possession of toys, food, or other objects. Dogs are often highly selective about the sort of items that they defend, and removing those items from the house can be a helpful preventive measure. Object guarding and possessiveness are not necessarily indicators of dominance, even though superficially the behavior appears to be motivated by dominance-related incentives. Among wolves, there is little correspondence between object guarding and dominance, with wolves of all ranks exhibiting heightened possessiveness over objects located within their ownership zone around the mouth. In addition, all wolves, regardless of rank, will attempt to steal food from other wolves irrespective of dominance (Mech, 1999). Competition between the owner and the dog over the control of forbidden objects appears to magnify the perceived value of the objects and to promote guarding incentives. A history of chasing, cornering, capturing, restraining, punishing, and the forceful extraction of objects from the dog's mouth may stimulate a problematic control incentive associated with possessions, especially involving objects possessing significant appetitive value for the dog. The appetitive motivations associated with guarding behavior suggest that the behavior is not under a strong influence of fear, but is primarily associated with comfort-loss incentive under the coactive influences of anxiety, frustration, and anger. Dogs affected by low anger/rage thresholds and high excitability levels are particularly prone to serious aggression problems occurring in association with object guarding.

Dogs that grab, run off, and guard objects frequently exhibit aggression problems involving hard bites to family members, and these problems require significant retraining and owner education to resolve. Such dogs should not be chased or challenged when they possess objects. The best method for the treatment of such problems is prevention. A high correlation seems to exist between the activity of grabbing forbidden objects and provoking a chase-and-evade game with the owner and the later development of object-related aggression. Puppies and dogs that engage in this sort of behavior should be encouraged to bring such items back to the owner in exchange for a treats and other rewards. Dogs that refuse to exchange an object for a treat can often be enticed to come by ringing a doorbell, shaking a set of car keys, or picking up a leash. Once the object is retrieved, the dog is put on a leash as necessary for added control and safety, and the forbidden object is placed on the floor with the voice signal "Leave it." If the dog approaches the object, the trainer says "Leave it" in a firm voice and, if necessary, prompts the dog with the leash to leave the object. If the dog turns away from the object, it is rewarded with praise, food, and an alternative item that is both acceptable for chewing purposes and attractive for fetching. This general procedure is repeated until the dog avoids the object in a variety of situations. The subsequent steps in this process are described in Chapter 2 (see *Controlling Inappropriate Chewing Activities*).

Dogs that show a guarding response while eating represent a significant threat to family members, especially young children who may not be appropriately respectful of the dog's need for space while eating. Again, prevention is the key to avoiding such problems. The common practice of repeatedly taking a puppy's food bowl away while it is eating does not appear to be useful and may actually make matters worse. The best strategy is to train the puppy to expect that it will get something, rather than lose something, when it is approached while eating. Feeding each meal in several small portions appears to help

reduce negative tensions around the food bowl. Feeding with two bowls can also be used in a similar way, allowing the owner to place food unobtrusively into one of the bowls while the dog is eating from the other one. Changing the type of food fed, the type of bowls used, and the schedule and location of feeding may help to reduce stimulus and contextual cues associated with possessive reactivity. In some cases, decreasing the appetitive value and palatability of the food may help to reduce the dog's incentive to guard it. The trainer can restrain the dog on leash or tie-out and use a probe stick or broom handle to move the food bowl away from the dog, thereby getting some indication of the dog's level of reactivity. The absence of an aggressive response to such intrusion is not necessarily a reliable indicator of safety from a potential attack, however. Dogs showing food-guarding reactivity should receive intensive basic training and exposure to various object-guarding techniques and restraint measures as needed to reduce reactivity occurring in association with intrusions while eating. At a minimum, such dogs should be kept on leash and trained to wait in a sit-stay before being released on cue to eat. They should also learn to leave the bowl on voice command and wait at a distance as an attractive food item is put into the bowl, whereupon they are released to take it. When approaching a dog while it is eating, the practice of tossing food items of varying value near or into the food bowl can also be helpful. Food guarding should be treated with a high-degree concern and with many of the same precautions and techniques described for object-guarding behavior. Although many of these dogs limit their agitation to becoming uncomfortable, stiff, and vigilant around the bowl, some excitable and highly food-motivated dogs have delivered severe and unexpected attacks following a history of low-grade threats and snaps. Dogs that are given training before they reach the stage of hard biting appear to be significantly less likely to escalate their aggressive efforts around food. Food guarding can be managed by simply avoiding contact and not interfering with the dog while it is eating, except as required for counterconditioning efforts. Dogs that show a high level of agitation while eating should be fed in a separate room from people or other dogs or crated as a further precaution and safety measure.

Object guarding is a common source of dangerous control-related aggression. Attacks associated with possessive aggression present with a great range of potential danger and variety, requiring careful assessment and evaluation that take into account the risk of future attacks against family members. Object guarding and possessive aggression are particularly problematic in busy households with children and visitors who may inadvertently come into contact with the possessive aggressor while it is in possession of a protected object. Severe object-guarding threats and biting sometimes occur without much warning in response to minor intrusive threats. Other dogs attack with inhibited snaps or bites only after a significant amount of intrusive interference has transpired around the protected object in the presence of various threats and warnings by the dog. Dogs exhibiting the first pattern of object guarding in association with hard biting present a guarded prognosis and should be removed from homes with children. The second group of dogs are generally more responsive to training efforts, but may still represent a significant threat to children or others coming into contact with them under adverse circumstances. Although such dogs may pose a risk, it is often one that can be managed with common sense, conscientious precautions, and a lifelong commitment to the dog's training. Hard decisions sometimes need to be made regarding object-guarding dogs, and those decisions should error on the side of safety, especially in the case of children. Object-guarding aggression has resulted in severe and disfiguring facial bites suffered by children while they were innocuously reaching toward, leaning over, snuggling, or playing tug with an object-guarding dog. A dog that has delivered an uninhibited hard bite in the context of food or object guarding should be considered prima facie at risk of biting under similar circumstances in the future; no matter what treatment is used to control the behavior and no matter how successful it appears to be, the risk may continue permanently despite the appearance of improvement.

Object guarding can be divided into five stages of escalating threat and propensity for attack: conflict, challenge, critical point, crisis, and panic. These stages are exhibited in varying degrees by food- and object-guarding dogs. Approaching an object-possessive dog while it is occupied with a prized object often causes the dog to slightly or greatly stiffen with anticipation of interference—the first overt sign of aggressive tension. The stiffening response reflects conflict-related autonomic change elicited by an expectancy of impending loss. Conflict associated with anticipated loss is followed by the dog picking up the object and evading the owner or remaining near the object, possibly under the influence of a mounting control incentive as the owner gets closer. As the owner approaches beyond the conflict point, dogs prone to guard and defend objects show an increasing anticipatory vigilance and readiness to resist or challenge the owner. If the owner advances closer and reaches toward the dog, the challenge is brought to a critical point with the dog making a rapid choice to allow the owner to intrude safely or to intensify the rising threat, sometimes leading to a sidelong preemptive snap or loss of nerve and retreat with the object. If the dog intensifies the threat, what occurs next depends on how the owner responds. If the owner backs off, the dog's guarding response may be reinforced, thereby strengthening guarding and other behaviors operating under similar control-related incentives in the future. If the owner persists and intrudes further or attempts to take the object, the dog may deliver a protective snap or bite. In the case of highly reactive and incompetent dogs, a panic point may be rapidly reached that causes the dog to dramatically intensify its threat or compels the release of a hard and uninhibited bite. From the critical point forward, the situation becomes progressively problematic, finally becoming a no-win situation. Punishment at any of these points may result in a rapid escalation and worsening of the problem. Following punishment, the protective response may occur at an earlier point in the sequence (e.g., conflict or challenge) or else cause the dog to inhibit threats until a crisis or panic level of arousal is reached, thereby possibly making the attack more dangerous and difficult to anticipate. Instead of excessive reliance on confrontational procedures, various behavior-therapy techniques can be used to reduce guarding behavior by means of counterconditioning, response prevention, and training the dog to relinquish objects under a positive expectancy of gain by way of reward rather than loss.

Dogs that persistently guard objects may require intensive preliminary basic training and behavior therapy to establish a reliable willingness to relinquish guarded objects. At minimum, the dog should receive several sessions of attention conditioning, sit-stay and down-stay and back and wait training, and be trained to take, fetch, and release toys that have not been protected in the past. A major focus of therapy is to facilitate a bond of trust that is incompatible with autoprotective incentives. The object-guarding dog is kept on leash and limited-slip collar or muzzle-clamping halter during all training procedures. Dogs exhibiting a serious potential risk for aggression should be restrained on a tie-out or active-control line during graduated challenges. An active-control line is made by hooking a carabiner to a loop of nylon that has been fastened to some immovable object (see *Walking Stand-Stay and Distance Exercises* in Chapter 1). Alternatively, a heavy eyehook can be screwed into sturdy molding. Depending on need, a 6-foot leash or a 15-foot long line is passed through the eyehook and attached to the dog's collar or halter, thus securing active control over the dog while performing object-guarding procedures. By pulling back on the line, the dog is turned away from the object and forced toward the anchored eyehook. An additional safety consideration is to attach a length of light rope to objects before presenting them to the dog (object line), thereby preserving a means to take objects away from the dog with less risk of getting bitten in the process.

Training is initiated with attention therapy and reward-based ICT. With a foundation of enhanced attention and impulse control, the object-guarding dog is first trained to take and then release various objects in exchange for a treat. Objects are introduced in accordance with their potential for provoking a guarding response. Training the dog to release objects should begin with objects that the dog is least likely to guard and then gradually moving to items that it is more likely to guard. Slowly progressing through these items without evoking threats makes the process safer and more likely to succeed. The first step is to train the dog to take ("Take it") and release a neutral item (e.g., a toy) to the hand ("Out") or to the floor ("Drop it"). With the object in the dog's mouth, the trainer says "Out" as a closed hand with a treat in it is presented to the dog. As the result of preliminary basic training, most dogs will release the object in order to obtain the treat. The size and type of food reward should be varied, but all treats used during such training should be highly attractive to the dog. After eating the treat, the object is given back to the dog after it sits on command and waits for a variable length of time. In cases involving a greater threat, the dog is trained to back away from the object after dropping it and to sit or lie down before it is rewarded. With the dog in the sit-stay (a response that should be well conditioned in the context of preliminary attention training), the trainer picks up the object, rewards the dog with a treat, and then returns the object to the dog.

The backing, sit or down, and waiting responses are facilitated by attention-controlling prompts delivered by means of the control line. These various responses should be brought under appropriate vocal and hand signal control (e.g., "Back," "Stay," "Wait," and "Take it"). The next step is to prompt the dog to remain in a sit or down-stay by saying "Stay" as the valued object is tossed out of its reach. If the dog moves toward the object, the action is abruptly blocked with the control line, and a confident vocal command "Stay" is delivered. During the brief waiting period, the dog is prompted to turn its attention toward the trainer in response to a smooch or squeaker sound, followed by a click, flick of the right hand, and the delivery of a food reward. Finally, the trainer retrieves the object and gives it back to the dog as a reward for its cooperation. The dog is also trained to pick up objects, drop them, and back away from them or, if the dog refuses to pick up objects, it is trained to back away from a tossed object, whereupon the trainer retrieves it and gives it to the dog. Whenever safe to do so, the dog should be trained to play a tug-and-fetch game with a variety of items, thereby helping to reduce competitive tensions while increasing cooperation and trust. After the item is dropped, the trainer signals the dog to "Back" and repeatedly tugs into the control line to prompt the backing response. If the dog refuses to drop the object after picking it up, it is pulled gently from its mouth by the object line. As the object is released, the dog is rewarded and then prompted to back away. If the dog refuses to release the object, the control line is pulled back as the object line is pulled harder, as necessary to compel the dog to release the object. The dog is always rewarded after releasing the object, often by allowing it to approach and take the object on signal or by tossing the object for the dog to fetch. This general procedure is repeated until the dog releases the item without objection or hesitation and backs away under vocal command and hand signal. Delayed prompting and fading of the control line together with various startle-type tools and strategies, as needed, are used to gradually achieve the backing and stay response. To be effective, these procedures require a high degree of diligence and daily practice and a strong foundation of basic training. Owners not likely to follow through with the dedication needed to succeed or lacking the necessary aptitude should not be encouraged to pursue it in the first place.

As the dog's response improves, progressively more natural circumstances can be introduced until it readily drops and backs away from objects on command. In cases where risk permits, daily object play involving tug-and-fetch games and variations on the release, sit-stay or down-stay, attention, wait, back, and fetch modules and routines should be practiced in the context of nonthreatening retrieve games with objects that the dog is unlikely to defend.

In some cases, once preliminary training has been successful, remote training (electrical and spray devices) can be used to establish a higher level of compliance over the dropping, backing, and the stay responses. Such training should involve a competent introduction of remote training in advance of using electrical stimulation to control possessive behavior (see *Electronic Training and Problem Solving*, Chapter 9). Remote electronic training can help to enhance impulse control while appearing to produce beneficial secondary effects conducive to the enhancement of relaxation and safety (Tortora, 1983) and to enforce compliance once behavioral control has been established via reward training (Borchelt and Voith, 1996). A significant advantage of electrical training for managing aggression problems is that it can be used to capture a dog's attention and reliably prompt behavioral adjustments at a distance and without necessitating that the trainer make risky direct contact with the dog. Radio-activated electronic devices can deliver a controlled motivational state conducive to inhibition, but without associating the event with the trainer as the source, something not possible in the case of interactive punishment. Also, the stimulus remains consistent, steady throughout, and inescapable by means of aggressive reprisals, thereby minimizing the risk of reinforcing undesirable behavior.

The dog first learns how to escape a low-level electrical stimulus and then to avoid stimulation by performing various responses in accord with vocal commands, hand signals, and prompts (see *Remote Electronic Training* in Chapter 9). Special emphasis is placed on attention training, stay, recall, and the enhancement of emergency exercises (e.g., quick-sit and instant-down). With every successful escape or avoidance response, petting and massage are given to overlap with relief and safety from the electrical stimulus. In addition to relief and safety, the discontinuation of the electrical stimulus results in a progressive state of increasing relaxation, an opportune source of stimulation conducive to social-contact tolerance. As the result of orderly electrical training, a dog gradually learns that it can predict and control the aversive electrical event by responding cooperatively to the trainer's signals and prompts. These various skills promote increased social competence, confidence, and relaxation in the dog, thereby helping it to learn how to cope in a more constructive and organized way when faced with other forms of provocative social stimulation involving threats of comfort or safety loss. Electrical stimulation can also be used in the context of back, wait, and halt-stay training. With such preliminary training in place, the electrical stimulus can be introduced into the context of object guarding, as a means to compel the dog to drop, back away, and stay at a distance from guarded objects until it is released by the trainer. With the offset of stimulation, an immediate relief response is followed by a slower and progressive relaxation response. During the course of relief/relaxation, the trainer provides the dog with vocal reassurance, petting, and massage, as can be safely performed. An olfactory safety signal can be presented at such times for the purpose of capturing and generalizing the safety-relaxation effect to other situations in which such a conditioned modulatory effect might helpful. The odor is further conditioned in association with PFR training and used in the context of graduated counterconditioning efforts. Of course, appropriate restraint (e.g., limit-slip or muzzling-type halter) and other safety precautions need to be taken at all times when working with a potentially dangerous dog (secure tie-out or active-control line). Electrical training in the context of managing aggressive behavior should be performed in the spirit of opening a window of opportunity for additional reward-based training activities aimed at conditioning behavior incompatible with aggression. The foregoing is a brief overview of steps used to manage one form of control-related aggression involving refractory object guarding. As a last resort, such training may produce a significant benefit when applied in conjunction with complementary behavior-therapy techniques. The procedure requires a high degree of skill and experience with dog aggression and electronic training and should be attempted only under the supervision of a highly skilled applied dog behaviorist or cyno-

praxic trainer well versed in such training procedures.

PART 3: CHILDREN AND DOG AGGRESSION

Infants and Dogs: Toward the Prevention of Problems

Dogs exhibiting active aggression problems represent a significant risk to children living in the household. Whenever possible, dogs exhibiting an excitable and reactive temperament with a demonstrated propensity to bite should be removed from homes with children. These dogs often do well in homes with adult owners, and rehoming should always be explored before more drastic measures are considered (see *Evaluating the Risk* in Volume 2, Chapter 6). Although such dogs represent an unacceptable threat to children, the majority of dogs are friendly and gentle companions for children. Even so, precautions should be taken to prevent interaction between children and dogs that may lead to an increased risk of biting or injury associated with inappropriate intrusiveness or overactivity.

Trainers are often consulted for advice regarding the best ways to introduce an infant to the family dog. The key to making this critical transition a successful one is careful preparation in advance of the infant's arrival. These preparations include selection, socialization, basic training and behavior management, counterconditioning and desensitization, exposure-habituation, and establishing a daily routine consistent with the way things will be when the baby comes home.

Selection

Advanced preparation begins with the selection of the dog. Thoughtful breed and breeder selection can help to reduce the risk of problems by increasing the likelihood that the dog is successfully matched to the owner's level of dog savvy and the needs of the household. Selective breeding has resulted in significant alterations in behavioral thresholds and temperament traits. In addition to breed-specific characteristics, individual differences predispose dogs toward behavior conducive to interaction with children or not. Obviously, highly excitable dogs bred for wariness and guarding behavior, or those exhibiting reactive fear, aggression, or a strong predatory drive, represent a much greater risk of showing problem behavior toward children than dogs exhibiting a more calm, playful, and friendly temperament (see *Evaluating the Risk* in Volume 2, Chapter 6).

Socialization

Perhaps the most important single factor influencing an adult dog's positive reaction to a baby or child is a history of positive socialization with children. Couples who plan to have children should make an effort to socialize the young dog with children of various ages. Allowing children to pet quietly and gently or give the puppy food can be very helpful. However, allowing a wild group of screaming kids to mob the puppy is certain to have an opposite effect on the puppy's expectations and future response to such contact, possibly causing it to become fearful of children. Another way to socialize a puppy with children is for the owner to baby-sit, thereby allowing the puppy to interact with children in the context of the home. Socialization experiences of this sort probably benefit the children as well, especially if they do not have a dog of their own, since previous noneventful contact with dogs appears to exert a preventive influence on the development of a fear of dogs by older children and adults (Doogan and Thomas, 1992).

Basic Training and Management

The importance of appropriate obedience training cannot be overemphasized. Basic training is essential, especially in the case of dogs exhibiting impulsive or hyperactive behavior. Dogs showing excitable tendencies should be exposed to intensive attention therapy, recall to front-and-finish, starting exercise, following, controlled walking and quick-sit, off, leave it, back, wait, go-lie-down, and down-stay training. All of these modules and routines should be practiced to a high degree of proficiency in advance of the baby coming

into the home. The dog's overexuberance during greetings and full-tilt rampages through the house and garden represent a considerable risk of injury for a baby or toddler.

Managing an overactive dog includes the provision of adequate daily exercise (including walks, jogging, and ball play), basic training, and necessary restraint and confinement (see *Hyperactivity and Social Excesses* in Chapter 5). The skills learned during basic training provide the owner with the means to control the overactive dog effectively in everyday situations. Whether it is done privately or in class, training should be initiated long before the baby's arrival and should continue for several weeks thereafter. Training should include practicing basic exercises while the owner is engaged in activities that mimic actions and situations that are likely to occur with the baby in the home. For example, the owner should have the dog perform exercises such as sit-stay while the owner is holding a doll wrapped in a towel or while rehearsing a diaper change. Also, the dog should be trained to walk next to a stroller until it becomes comfortable with its sound and movement. This should be done before the baby is actually placed inside of it. Practice should include exiting and entering the home, getting into and out of the car, and other likely situations that will regularly occur with the baby and dog in tow. An extremely useful way to enhance control during walks is a hip-hitch with a control lead and fixed-action halter collar. If halter use is planned in the context of introducing the dog to the baby, it should be slowly introduced in association with reward-based training.

A high chair should be set up, with food, bibs, towels, and other items placed upon it that might be present when the baby is being fed. The dog should be trained to avoid jumping up on the high chair in the owner's presence and absence, thus probably requiring some form of appropriate booby trap. Further, the dog should learn not to jump up on people or furniture (bed, sofa, chairs, etc.) without permission, thus preventing potential incidents involving the dog stepping on the infant while he or she is in the mother's charge being fed or changed. An overly active dog should be routinely constrained to wait outside of the kitchen until released to enter on the owner's signal. If necessary, gates or crate training may be introduced to facilitate a safer transition.

Competition around passageways should be systematically discouraged by training the dog to defer to the owner's entitlement to enter first or to move ahead only if prompted to do so. Similar practice efforts should be carried out around the front door and back door, with bolting being vigorously suppressed with appropriate leash training. The active dog should received focused training around indoor and outdoor steps, learning to wait or to move ahead of the owner on signal, but never charging ahead without the owner's consent. Again, such training efforts as just described should be introduced long before the baby comes into the home.

Exposure, Counterconditioning, and Habituation

Fearful dogs should receive intensive behavioral training and conditioning aimed at increasing their confidence and tolerance toward children and their actions. A fearful dog, appropriately restrained on leash and collar or halter, should be exposed to structured social encounters with children of all ages. During such counterconditioning efforts, the dog is prompted to sit and relax by giving it food and petting while in close proximity with children (see *Social Fears and Inhibitions* in Chapter 3). The owner can also mimic some of the sounds and awkward movements of the baby or toddler. For example, the dog should be exposed to having its ears, tail, and other parts of its anatomy grabbed and gently pulled, thereby simulating the touch and handling of a curious child. Such handling exposure should be performed in association with appetitive counterconditioning or with the dog in a relaxed state induced by PFR training. The fearful dog is gradually exposed to a wide variety of situations involving children both in the home and away from home. Again, babysitting an infant would give the dog a chance to learn about babies, thereby possibly helping to mit-

igate problems later on. Fearful dogs exhibiting a demonstrated propensity to snap or bite rather than retreat from children should be removed from the home.

Habituating a dog to new sounds and smells associated with a new baby in the home may also be useful (see Appendix C). This ought to include "pretend" activities in which the expectant mother holds a doll wrapped in a blanket while changing it, applying various oils and powders. It is useful to play tape recordings of an infant crying and other sounds occurring during such activities in order to make the situation more realistic. Items imbued with the baby's odor (e.g., clothing or blankets) should be brought home from the hospital in order to allow the dog to habituate gradually to the various olfactory stimuli associated with the infant's presence.

PFR training is a central part of the dog's preparation for the baby's homecoming. The PFR cycle can be carried out with small amounts of the various odors (oils and powders) scenting the owner's hands. As the massage progresses from day to day, the recorded sounds of a baby crying can be played at progressively increasing volumes, emanating from different parts of the house. A conditioned odor [e.g., dilute (1:30–50) orange, lavender, or chamomile] can also be introduced in association with PFR, first introduced as an olfactory signature at the end of the cycle and then using it to help consolidate the relaxation response by presenting it at progressively earlier steps in the PFR process. The massage should result in deep relaxation, at which point the right hand is gently cupped over the dog's nose for a brief moment, causing it to sniff the odor. The dog is petted over its entire body, carefully following the lay of the coat, and, at last, released with a quiet clap of the hands and "Okay." With the baby's arrival, blankets and clothing imbued with the child's scent can be brought home and paired in a similar way with deep relaxation and feelings of comfort.

The dog should be familiarized with the baby's room and permitted to investigate freely, but access to the room should never be allowed in the owner's absence. Booby-trapping the doorway of the baby's room may provide additional inhibition about entering the room without supervision. Otherwise, the room should always be gated or closed. In general, a baby should never be left alone with a dog.

Establishing a Routine

The owner should establish a daily routine of activities prior to the baby's arrival that reflects realistic estimates of time available to dedicate to the dog when the baby comes home. To ensure a successful transition, this allotment of time should not be significantly changed. The daily schedule should include sufficient time for training, exercise (at least 20 minutes twice a day), and affectionate attention. Daily walks are a good postparturient activity for the new mother as well as a positive activity for the infant and dog. Perhaps even more important than the amount of time given to the dog, the quality of interaction should not be compromised or become superficial. There is a natural tendency to turn affectionate contact away from the dog and to redirect it toward the infant. The ensuing neglect of the dog's social needs for daily affectionate contact may stimulate insecurity and prompt intrusive efforts to gain contact and attention by undesirable means.

INTRODUCING BABY AND DOG

First impressions are lasting. It is imperative, therefore, that the first meeting between the dog and the baby occur without incident. Many techniques are available to help ensure an uneventful introduction. The usual method involves having the mother enter the home *without the child* in her arms. After the initial excitement has dissipated, the dog can be familiarized with various items containing the baby's odor while being fed treats and affectionately petted. After a brief period, the leashed dog can be permitted to sniff the blanket covering the baby while continuing to receive treats.

Whenever possible, however, the baby should be introduced while the dog is preoccupied on a walk away from the property

together with the mother and a helper holding the baby. This procedure minimizes a number of natural tensions that are prone to occur if the baby is taken directly into the house, especially in cases involving a dog that is unfamiliar with infants. The most common reaction by far is curiosity, but sometimes the dog is alarmed by the "strange creature," resulting in nervous growling or barking. This is definitely a result that one would wish to avoid. Going for a walk serves to distract the dog from the baby's presence, which is overshadowed by the excitement of being outdoors. Under such conditions, the dog's curiosity and potential anxiety are reduced to a more manageable level. If the dog becomes overly excited, it should be prompted to sit and thereupon rewarded by the owner with affection and food. After the dog has calmed down and settled into the walk, the mother can take the child herself and hand over control of the dog to her helper for the remainder of the walk.

Upon returning to the house, the dog is required to wait before entering, allowing the mother and baby to enter first, followed momentarily by the helper and dog. The leashed dog is permitted to smell the covered child and given numerous treats and vocal encouragement so long as it remains lowkeyed and calm. With things going well, the dog may be engaged in normal play and affectionate activities, first with the helper and then with the mother. Lastly, the dog is fed while the mother attends to the baby nearby as though nothing very remarkable has taken place. The leash and collar should remain on the dog during the next few days for added control and safety.

Although every effort should be made to make the transition a positive one, limits should be immediately and clearly set, if necessary, especially in cases were the dog becomes overly pushy or demanding. If necessary, such dogs should be kept on a fixed-action halter for added control and safety. Repeated and brief TO (30 to 45 seconds) with intensive time-in reward training (orienting, attending, sit and down, and stay) can be used to help reduce arousal and impulsiveness. Behavior to be particularly on guard about involves excessive efforts to poke and smell, jump up, or to grab at the baby's blanket. Such behavior can be discouraged with a split-second hiss with a modified CO_2 pump dry-loaded with a dilute conditioned odor (e.g., cedarwood-eucalyptus). The conditioned odor is delivered with stealth (e.g., under the jaw or from behind) and at pressure appropriate to the dog's response to the hiss-type startle (see *Olfactory Conditioning and Excessive Biting* in Chapter 6). The conditioned odor and modified CO_2 pump can be used to help set limits around undesirable household behavior requiring mild inhibitory conditioning to control. If a modified CO_2 pump is used, it should be introduced in advance of bringing the baby home, giving the dog a chance to become familiar with the treatment strategy.

In some cases, an overly excitable dog can be restrained on a tie-out or active-control line while being introduced to the baby. The mother and child are seated on the floor some distance away while the helper gives the dog treats as the two gradually inch forward in progressive steps toward the dog until they are situated just in front, where the dog receives food and affection from the mother and is permitted to smell the baby's clothing (see *Graded Interactive Exposure* in Chapter 3). An alternative method involves giving the dog a hollow rubber toy stuffed with a piece of bread smeared with peanut butter. During such graduated exposures, the helper can initiate a cycle of massage and introduce odors previously association with PFR training, thereby helping to recruit a relaxation response in association with petting and massage. The conditioned odor can be delivered by means of scented tissue or a squeaker bulb with the squeak valve removed. As the dog calms down, the child's hand can be placed in the middle of the mother's hand and held in front of the dog's nose, allowing it to sniff in association with reassuring talk and petting. This procedure is repeated several times and then as needed to relax the dog when it becomes overly excited.

Another strategy involves having the dog live somewhere else temporarily and then to habituate it slowly to the presence of the child over the course of 2 or 3 days. Initially, the owner can spend time with the dog alone, reviewing obedience work with a doll wrapped in the baby's clothing, either carrying the doll or pushing a stroller. These practice sessions can be followed by controlled meetings between the dog and the baby, at first outdoors and then inside the home. A conscientious effort should be made to establish positive associations with the baby's presence, including the provision of affection, treats, toys, and other sources of pleasure for the dog. Ideally, the dog should learn to anticipate attractive and pleasurable outcomes whenever the baby is brought into its presence. Although temporarily housing the dog elsewhere is sometimes very useful, it is far better not to remove the dog from the home situation, but to make the necessary arrangements and efforts to work things out while the dog remains in the home.

THE TODDLER AND INCREASED RISK

As the child becomes ambulatory and begins to explore the dog with clumsy hands and awkward movements, new opportunities for disaster inevitably follow. Naturally, with the advent of such increased interaction, a greater risk presents itself that the dog will resent such contact or become progressively intolerant of it, possibly resulting in aggressive threats or snaps. Dogs that are possessive toward food, toys, or places are particularly dangerous around toddlers. Not surprisingly, toddlers are a common target of aggressive attacks, with boys being bitten much more often than girls (Harris et al. 1974; Wright, 1991). This difference may be attributable to the male child's greater tendency to engage in risk-taking behavior (Ginsburg and Miller, 1982). Another possible explanation is that boys may simply spend more time interacting with dogs than girls do (Lehman, 1928). Dogs exhibiting irritable or possessive aggression toward the child should be removed from the home.

The most significant threats at this age are generated by the child's failure to recognize and respect the dog's needs for space and gentle handling. Although children exhibit increasing evidence of empathy by years 3 and 4 (Love and Overall, 2001), the display of these sensitivities is not particularly evident in the relentless teasing and torment that a young child can inflict upon the family dog. Children aged 2 to 3 appear to exhibit the highest frequency of provocative behavior toward dogs, making close supervision of child-dog interaction especially critical during this age period. Children aged 4 to 5 exhibit less provocative interaction and make more comforting-giving tactile contact with the dog (Millot and Filiatre, 1986). In any case, allowing the child to taunt, grab, pull, pinch, step on, chase, throw things at, hit, kick, stomp, or fall upon the dog is a sure way to increase irritability and reduce tolerance for close social contact with the child. Every normal dog has a breaking point that is sooner or later reached, and the child is finally punished for his or her lack of consideration and sensitivity.

Many problems can be avoided by making sure that the young child is allowed to interact with the dog only while an adult is present to supervise, at least until the child demonstrates an adequate ability to treat the dog with care and respect. During such periods of supervised interaction, the child's behavior is carefully monitored, with appropriate behavior being reinforced with affection and other suitable rewards, while inappropriate behavior is consistently discouraged. The child should be taught that interacting with the dog is a privilege based on good behavior. One strategy for promoting this learning involves giving the child merits for appropriate interaction and demerits for inappropriate behavior toward the dog. The accumulation of three demerits causes the child to lose the privilege of interacting with the dog for some set period. The child can avoid this consequence by working off demerits by earning merits based on appropriate behavior. In other words, demerits can be canceled by earning merits based on giving the dog appropriate care and respect. In addition, after earning three merits, the child may be given a token (e.g., a star) that he or she can save and exchange for various rewards or desirable activities.

CHILD-INITIATED AGGRESSION AND SIBLING RIVALRY

Within the context of family dynamics, emergent canine behavioral characteristics (individual differences) are differentiated and expressed, giving rise to an extraordinary variety of social behavior and coping styles. In large families, preferred affiliative relations may form that produce conflict and competition between children for a dog's attention. Some of these attachments and affiliations appear to promote distinctions resembling social rank. The dog may show favoritism toward certain family members and become progressively intolerant of interaction with others. Much of this organizing process is based on the quality of the exchanges and transactions between the dog and different family members. Transactions conducive to enhanced comfort and safety are preferred to transactions producing discomfort and threats. The obligatory subordinate status of dogs is dependent on leadership (see *Dominance, Social Distance and Polarity, and Begging for Love*), that is, structured interaction that results in enhanced comfort and safety (nurturance). In relation to other obligate household subordinates (dogs and children), the dog may form dominant-subordinate sibling relations. The nature of these sibling relations and dynamics may be in part due to competition for the same social resource, that is, the nurturance and security provided by the parent. As a result of combined needs that exceed the parent's ability or willingness to fulfill, a potential source of conflict between the dog and children may develop and result in sibling rivalry. This natural sibling tension may be intensified significantly in cases where the parent shows an evident preference toward the dog by the quality of attention and care given to it versus the child. The added attention given to the dog may inadvertantly establish a problematic alliance between the parent and the dog, perhaps activating species-typical agonistic scripts and competition between the dog and children.

Typically, dogs are enormously tolerant of child-initiated interactions, most often ignoring or reciprocating in kind (especially with regard to friendly and comfort-giving behaviors), or retreating in response to aversive or aggressive behaviors. Millot and colleagues (1988) found that the aggressive behavior initiated by a child toward a dog was most likely followed by retreating or avoiding behaviors. The most likely child behaviors to produce biting or attempts to bite were pulling the dog's tail, fur, or paws. Dogs were found to be surprisingly tolerant toward threatening, hitting, or object-throwing behavior. Interestingly, dogs exhibited no aggression toward children interfering with them while in possession of objects, but were most likely to give the object up or retreat. The researchers suggest that much of the child's aggressive behavior toward the dog *could be* of a redirected nature. Such child-initiated aggression toward the family dog may reflect a more general failure of the child to integrate friendly and cooperative social relations with peers and adults. Thus, the dog may represent to some children a relatively safe object for discharging frustration and passing on aggression received from other children or adults (see *Sources of Conflict and Tension Between Children and Dogs* in Volume 2, Chapter 6). Children suspected of showing such behavior need to learn how to cope more effectively with social stressors and how to redirect their aggressive impulses into more constructive outlets. A small percentage of children who are persistently provocative and cruel toward the family dog and other animals may be affected by disturbances impeding their ability to regulate emotion and aggressive impulses. Approximately 2% to 9% of children in the United States are affected by conduct disorder. Some authorities estimate that 25% of these children show cruelty toward animals and that animal abuse is often the earliest sign of the disorder (Miller, 2001). Inculcating a caring and humane attitude toward dogs and other animals should be a central part of childhood education and socialization.

Interspecific sibling rivalry and competition for parental attention and care may also represent a significant source of agonistic tension between children and dogs. How children respond to sharing the home and parental attention with the dog depends on a wide range of emotional, behavioral, and developmental variables. Children may show a highly ambivalent and conflictive attitude toward the dog. Young children often show inconsistent social interaction toward the dog, including elements of affection, intrusive interference, and exploitive mischief. In many cases, these behaviors appear to be calculated to obtain or to divert parental attention and resources away from the dog. For emotionally secure children, the dog may mediate a more mature and cooperative relationship with the parent and other siblings. Such children may take an active role in training and caring for the dog; that is, they help to parent it. Other children may show a variable lack of interest or an apparent aversion toward it (e.g., an inordinate disgust toward its saliva). Such children may form a relationship with the dog only to please the parent, but secretly hold the dog at a distance emotionally. Some children may be highly critical of the dog's habits and intelligence, refusing to form a relationship with it and rejecting efforts to help bridge the gap. Finally, a small minority of children may exhibit an overt and habitual pattern of insensitivity, cruelty, and stimulation-seeking activities that may include agitating or tormenting the dog.

Dogs shown preferential treatment by adults in the household may become increasingly confident and bold with respect to sibling subordinates. Instead of fleeing to avoid the interference of children, they may simply confront and threaten them fearlessly. Such dogs may show a high degree of social competence and purposefulness in the process of setting limits on the intrusive behavior of children. They may show a welcoming tolerance for interaction that is gentle and respectful, but rapidly respond to mishandling or uninvited intrusions by stiffening, growling, snarling, snapping, or biting the child to impress their point. Mishandling and interference with the dog while it is eating, resting, or chewing on toys may significantly decrease the dog's tolerance for contact and lower aggression thresholds. Clumsy and painful efforts to pick up the dog as a puppy may also play a prominent role in the development of preemptive threats and attacks to hugs and grabbing movements. Such dogs may show little sign of anxiety or active aversion toward the child, but instead seem to use aggression in a proactive way to limit unwanted social behavior and rewarding appropriate behavior with affectionate tolerance.

The selectiveness, purposefulness, cool-headed, and limited nature of these confrontations and limit-setting actions is consistent with a social-training interpretation, insofar as social training is defined as a process whereby limit-setting actions serve to open a social space within which appropriate behavior is encouraged by reward. The adaptive and measured nature of such attacks warrants the term proactive aggression. In some cases, however, successful control of one family member with threats or force may lead to dynamic changes in a dog's interaction with other family members belonging to the subordinate-sibling group (see Chase et al., 2002). Other family members observing these educational transactions may exhibit an increased sensitivity and avoidance of exchanges that might agitate the dog, thereby learning from the demonstration and reinforcing the dog's trainer role. Smaller breeds expressing medium anger and high fear thresholds may be particularly prone to exercise social power of questionable competence by means of threats and inhibited bites directed against intrusive children. Although the danger of such behavior would naturally rise to an entirely different level of significance and concern in the case of larger dogs or dogs showing impulsive aggression, the diminutive aggressor may enjoy a special status and alliance with a parent, who may grant "training" privileges to the dog with respect to an unruly child. To prevent the escalation or transition of the "trainer" script into the despot script and interaction that poses a much greater risk to the child's safety, it is imperative that dogs and children learn from parents how to respectfully interact one another.

In addition to procedures used to organize the social engagement system (orienting, approaching, and attending) (see *Dominance, Social Distance and Polarity, and Begging for Love*), preliminary testing suggests that the model/rival method may be useful in certain cases to help integrate more friendly interaction (see *Rapid Complex Social Learning* in Chapter 10). By allowing dogs to observe highly formalized and friendly exchanges between a parent and child (model/rival dyad) with exchanges focused on an object of significant interest to the dog, some dogs appear to rapidly encode the general significance of the observed interaction and show immediate behavior remarkably consistent with it. While observing such brief social encounters, dogs may internalize the emotional significance of the interaction, appearing to prepare them to respond to the object and the model/rival demonstration in a script-consistent way. Dogs appear to be highly sensitive to the significance of social interaction between a social superior and inferior (rival) in the process of obtaining reward or punishment in the context of controlling a valued object. The full value of the method remains to be explored, but preliminary indicators suggest that the effect produced is robust and useful as an adjuvant procedure for priming emotional arousal and rapidly integrating social scripts. In addition to modeling affectionate behavior and cooperative behavior, the procedure may have usefulness for treating object-guarding problems and for helping to mediate the integration of more tolerant and friendly behavior toward visitors.

REFERENCES

Albert RC (1953). *Living Your Dog's Life*. New York: Harper and Brothers.

Arivazhagan P and Panneerselvam C (2002). Neurochemical changes related to ageing in the rat brain and the effect of DL-alpha-lipoic acid. *Exp Gerontol*, 37:1489–1494.

Beaver BV (1999). *Canine Behavior: A Guide for Veterinarians*. Philadelphia: WB Saunders.

Berkowitz L (1989). Frustration-aggression hypothesis: Examination and reformulation. *Psychol Bull*, 106:59–73.

Blackshaw JK (1991). An overview of types of aggressive behaviour in dogs and methods of treatment. *Appl Anim Behav Sci*, 30:351–361.

Borchelt PL (1983). Aggressive behavior of dogs kept as companion animals: Classification and influence of sex, reproductive status, and breed. *Appl Anim Ethol*, 10:45–61.

Borchelt PL (1986). Dominance aggression tempered by fear: A case study. *Anim Behav Consult Newsl*, 3(1).

Borchelt PL and Voith VL (1996). Dominance aggression in dogs. In VL Voith and PL Borchelt (Eds), *Readings in Companion Animal Behavior*. Trenton, NJ: Veterinary Learning Systems.

Brown JS, Martin RC, and Morrow MW (1964). Self-punitive behavior in the rat: Facilitative effects of punishment on resistance to extinction. *J Comp Physiol Psychol*, 57:127–133.

Brunner J, Parhofer KG, Schwandt P, and Bronisch T (2002). Cholesterol, essential fatty acids, and suicide. *Pharmacopsychiatry*, 35:1–5.

Buydens-Branchey L, Branchey M, Hudson J, and Fergeson P (2000). Low HDL cholesterol, aggression and altered central serotonergic activity. *Psychiatry Res*, 93:93–102.

Cairns RB (1972). Fighting and punishment from a developmental perspective. In JK Cole and DD Jensen (Eds), *Nebraska Symposium on Motivation*. New York: University of Nebraska Press

Calhoun JB (1962). Population density and social pathology. *Sci Am*, 206:139–148.

Calhoun JB (1963). *The Ecology and Sociology of the Norway Rat.*

DHHS Publication no. 1008. Washington, DC: U.S. Government Printing Office.

Chase ID, Tovey C, Spangler-Martin D, and Manfredonia M (2002). Individual differences versus social dynamics in the formation of animal dominance hierarchies. *Proc Natl Acad Sci USA*, 99:5744–5749.

Clark GI and Boyer WN (1993). The effects of dog obedience training and behavioural counselling upon the human-canine relationship. *Appl Anim Behav Sci*, 37:147–159.

Clutton-Brock TH and Parker GA (1995). Punishment in animal societies. *Nature*, 373:209–216.

Delude LA (1991). Spontaneous exercise of dogs under three methods of constraint. *Vet Res Commun*, 15:285–289.

De Napoli JS, Dodman NH, Shuster L, et al. (2000). Effect of dietary protein content and tryptophan supplementation on dominance aggression, territorial aggression, and hyperactivity in dogs. *JAVMA*, 217:504–508.

De Waal F (1996). *Good Natured: The Origins of Right and Wrong in Humans and Other Animals.* Cambridge: Harvard University Press.

Derix R, Van Hoof J, De Vries H, Wensing J (1993). Male and female mating competition in wolves: Female suppression vs male intervention. *Behaviour*, 127:141–171.

Dickinson A and Pearce JM (1977). Inhibitory interactions between appetitive and aversive stimuli. *Psychol Bull*, 84:690–711.

Dodman NH, Mertens PA, and Aronson LP (1995). Two dogs were evaluated because of aggression. *JAVMA*, 207:1168–1171.

Dodman NH, Moon R, and Zelin M (1996a). Influence of owner personality type on expression and treatment outcome of dominance aggression in dogs. *JAVMA*, 209:1107–1109.

Dodman NH, Reisner I, Shuster L, et al. (1996b). Effect of dietary protein content on behavior in dogs. *JAVMA*, 208:376–379.

Dollard J, Miller NE, Doob LW, et al. (1939). *Frustration and Aggression.* New Haven: Yale University Press.

Domjan M, Cusato B, and Villarreal R (2000). Pavlovian feed-forward mechanisms in the control of social behavior. *Behav Brain Sci*, 23:235–282.

Doogan S and Thomas GV (1992). Origins of fear of dogs in adults and children: The role of conditioning processes and prior familiarity with dogs. *Behav Res Ther* 30:387–394.

Drews C (1993). The concept and definition of dominance in animal behaviour. *Behaviour*, 125:283–313.

Fava M and Rosenbaum JF (1998). Anger attacks in depression. *Depress Anxiety*, 8(Suppl 1):59–63.

Field T (1995). Massage therapy for infants and children. *Dev Behav Pediatr*, 16:105–111.

Freeman MP (2000). Omega-3 fatty acids in psychiatry: A review. *Ann Clin Psychiatry*, 12:159–165.

Fuller JL (1967). Experiential deprivation and later behavior. *Science*, 158:1645–1652.

Gagnon S and Dore FY (1994). Cross-sectional study of object permanence in domestic puppies (*Canis familiaris*). *J Comp Psychol*, 108:220–232.

Gardner R (1982). Mechanisms in manic-depressive disorder: An evolutionary model. *Arch Gen Psychiatry*, 39:1436–1441.

Ginsburg HJ and Miller SM (1982). Sex differences in children's risk-taking behavior. *Child Dev*, 53:426–428.

Golomb BA, Stattin H, and Mednick S (2000). Low cholesterol and violent crime. *J Psychiatr Res*, 34:301–309.

Goodloe LP and Borchelt PL (1998). Companion dog temperament traits. *J Appl Anim Welfare Sci*, 1:303–338.

Gray JA (1990). Brain systems that mediate both emotion and cognition. *Cognition Emotion*, 4:269–288.

Gray JA (1994). Framework for a taxonomy of psychiatric disorder. In SHM van Goozen, NE van de Poll, and JA Sergeant (Eds), *Emotions: Essays on Emotion Theory*. Hillsdale, NJ: Lawrence Erlbaum.

Guy NC, Luescher UA, Dohoo SE, et al. (2001a). Demographic and aggressive characteristics of dogs in a general veterinary caseload. *Appl Anim Behav Sci*, 74:15–28.

Guy NC, Luescher UA, Dohoo SE, et al. (2001b). Risk factors for dog bites to owners in a general veterinary caseload. *Appl Anim Behav Sci*, 74:29–42.

Guy NC, Luescher UA, Dohoo SE, et al. (2001c). A case series of biting dogs: Characteristics of the dogs, their behaviour, and their victims. *Appl Anim Behav Sci*, 74:43–57.

Gwaltney-Brant SM, Albretsen JC, and Khan SA (2000). 5-Hydroxytryptophan toxicosis in dogs: 21 cases (1989–1999). *JAVMA*, 216:1937–1940.

Harris D, Imperato PJ, and Oken B (1974). Dog bites: An unrecognized epidemic. *Bull NY Acad Med*, 50:981–1000.

Hart BL and Hart LA (1985). *Canine and Feline Behavioral Therapy*. Philadelphia: Lea and Febiger.

Hart BL and Hart LA (1997). Selecting, raising, and caring for dogs to avoid problem aggression. *JAVMA*, 210:1129–1134.

Hennessy MB, Voith VL, Travis L, et al. (2002). Exploring human interaction and diet effects on the behavior of dogs in public animals shelter. *J Appl Anim Welfare Sci*, 5:253–273.

Hibbeln JR, Umhau JC, Linnoila M, et al. (1998). A replication study of violent and nonviolent subjects: Cerebrospinal fluid metabolites of serotonin and dopamine are predicted by plasma essential fatty acids. *Biol Psychiatry*, 44:243–249.

Hilakivi-Clarke L, Cho E, and Onojafe I (1996). High-fat diet induces aggressive behavior in male mice and rats. *Life Sci*, 58:1653–1660.

Hillbrand M and Spitz RT (1999). Cholesterol and aggression. *Aggression Violent Behav*, 4:359–370.

Jagoe JA and Serpell JA (1996). Owner characteristics and interactions and the prevalence of canine behaviour problems. *Appl Anim Behav Sci*, 47:31–42.

Kaplan JR, Fontenot MB, Manuck SB, and Muldoon MF (1996). Influence of dietary lipids on agonistic and affiliative behavior in *Macaca fascicularis*. *Am J Primatol*, 38:333–347.

Kaplan JR, Shively CA, Fontenot MB, et al. (1994). Demonstration of an association

among dietary cholesterol, central serotonergic activity, and social behavior in monkeys. *Psychosom Med*, 56:479–484.

Kobelt AJ, Hemsworth PH, Barnett JL, and Coleman GJ (2003). A survey of dog ownership in suburban Australia: Conditions and behavior problems. *Appl Anim Behav Sci*, 82:137–148.

Lehman HC (1928). Child's attitude toward the dog versus the cat. *J Genet Psychol*, 35:67–72.

Line S and Voith VL (1986). Dominance aggression of dogs towards people: Behavior profile and response to treatment. *Appl Anim Behav Sci*, 16:77–83.

Lorenz K (1955). *Man Meets Dog*. Boston: Houghton Mifflin.

Lorenz K (1966). *On Aggression*. New York: Harcourt Brace Jovanovich.

Love M and Overall KL (2001). How anticipating relationships between dogs and children can help prevent disasters. *JAVMA*, 291:446–453.

Luescher AU (2000). A dog was examined because of aggression toward household members. *JAVMA*, 217:1143–1145.

MacDonald K (1983). Stability of individual differences in behavior in a litter of wolf cubs (*Canis lupus*). *J Comp Psychol*, 97:99–106.

MacDonald K (1987). Development and stability of personality characteristics in pre-pubertal wolves: Implications for pack organization and behavior. In H Frank (Ed), *Man and Wolf*. Dordrecht, The Netherlands: Dr W Junk.

Mahadik SD, Evans D, and Lal H (2001). Oxidative stress and role of antioxidant and omega-3 essential fatty acid supplementation in schizophrenia. *Prog Neuropsychopharmacol Biol Psychiatry*, 25:463–493.

Manteca X (1998). A dog was evaluated because of severe aggression. *JAVMA*, 213:616–618.

Masago R, Matsuda T, Kikuchi Y, et al. (2000). Effects of inhalation of essential oils on EEG activity and sensory evaluation. *J Physiol Anthropol*, 19:35–42.

McEwen B (2000). Allostasis and allostatic load: Implications for neuropharmacology. *Neuropsychopharmacology*, 22:108–124.

Mech LD (1999). Alpha status, dominance, and division of labor in wolf packs. *Can J Zool* 77:1196–1203.

Mech LD (2000). Leadership in wolf, *Canis lupus*, packs. *Can Field-Nat*, 114:259–263.

Miller C (2001). Childhood animal cruelty and interpersonal violence. *Clin Psychol Rev*, 21:735–749.

Melvin K (1971). Vicious circle behavior. In HD Kimmel (Ed),

Experimental Psychopathology: Recent Research and Theory. New York: Academic.

Milgram NW, Zicker SC, Head E, et al. (2002). Dietary enrichment counteracts age-associated cognitive dysfunction in canines. *Neurobiol Aging*, 23:737–745.

Millot JL and Filiatre JC (1986). The behavioural sequences in the communication system between the child and his pet dog. *Appl Anim Behav Sci*, 16:383–390.

Millot JL, Filiatre AC, Gagnon A, et al. (1988). Children and their pet dogs: How they communicate. *Behav Proc*, 17:1–15.

Monks of New Skete (1978). *How to Be Your Dog's Best Friend.* Boston: Little, Brown.

Morgan CL (1894). *Introduction to Comparative Psychology.* London: Methuen.

Most K (1910/1955). *Training Dogs.* New York: Coward-McCann (reprint).

Motomura N, Sakurai A, and Yotsuya Y (2001). Reduction of mental stress with lavender odorant. *Percept Mot Skills*, 93:713–718.

Nigro MR (1966). Punishment of an extinguishing shock-avoidance response by time-out from positive reinforcement. *J Exp Anal Behav*, 9:53–62.

Nobbe DE, Niebuhr BR, Levinson M, and Tiller JE (1980). Use of time-out as punishment for aggressive behavior. In B Hart (Ed), *Canine Behavior.* Santa Barbara, CA: Veterinary Practice.

Odendaal JSJ and Meintjes RA (2003). Neurophysiological correlates of affiliative behaviour between humans and dogs. *Vet J*, 165:296–301.

O'Farrell V (1995). The effect of owner attitudes on behaviour. In J Serpell (Ed), *The Domestic Dog.* New York: Cambridge University Press.

Packer L, Tritschler HJ, and Wessel K (1997). Neuroprotection by the metabolic antioxidant alpha-lipoic acid. *Free Radic Biol Med*, 22:359–378.

Penturk S and Yalcin E (2003). Hypocholesterolaemia in dogs with dominance aggression. *J Vet Med A Physiol Pathol Clin Med*, 50:339–342.

Podberscek AL and Serpell JA (1997). Environmental influences on the expression of aggressive behaviour in English cocker spaniels. *Appl Anim Behav Sci*, 52:215–227.

Polsky RH (1989). Techniques of behavioral modification: "Time-out"—An underemployed punishment technique. *Bull Companion Anim Behav* (Newsl), 3:4.

Prescott JW (1971). Early somatosensory deprivation as an ontogenetic process in the abnormal development of the brain and behavior. In

EI Goldstein and J Mody-Janokowski (Eds), *Proceedings of the Second Conference on Experimental Medicine and Surgery.* Basel: Karger.

Price J and Gardner R (1995). The paradoxical power of the depressed patient: A problem for the ranking theory of depression. *Br J Med Psychol*, 68:193–206.

Price J, Sloman L, Gardner R, et al. (1994). The social competition hypothesis of depression. *Br J Psychiatry*, 164:309–315.

Rajecki DW, Rasmussen JL, Sanders CR, et al. (1999). Good dog: Aspects of humans' causal attributions for a companion animal's social behavior. *Soc Anim*, 7(1). http://www.psyeta.org/sa/sa7.1/rajecki.html

Reisner IR (1997). Assessment, management, and prognosis of canine dominance-related aggression. *Vet Clin North Am Prog Companion Anim Behav*, 27:479–495.

Reisner IR (1998). Canine aggression: Neurobiology, behavior, and management. In *1998 Friskies Symposium on Behavior.* http://www.vet-show.com/friskies/cani.htm.

Reisner IR, Erb HN, and Houpt KA (1994). Risk factors for behavior-related euthanasia among dominant-aggressive dogs: 110 cases (1989–1992). *JAVMA*, 205:855–863.

Richardson AJ and Puri BK (2002). A randomized double-blind, placebo-controlled study of the effects of supplementation with highly unsaturated fatty acids on ADHD-related symptoms in children with specific learning difficulties. *Prog Neuropsychopharmacol Biol Psychiatry*, 26:233–239.

Rogers PJ (2001). A healthy body, a healthy mind: Long-term impact of diet on mood and cognitive function. *Proc Nutr Soc*, 60:135–143.

Ross L and Nisbett RE (1991). *The Person and the Situation: Perspectives of Social Psychology.* Philadelphia: Temple University Press.

Rotter JB (1966). Generalized expectancies for internal versus external control of reinforcement. *Psychol Monogr (Gen Appl)*, 80:1–28.

Rowell TE (1974). The concept of social dominance. *Behav Biol*, 11:131–154.

Rugbjerg H, Proschowsky HF, Ersboll AK, and Lund JD (2003). Risk factors associated with interdog aggression and shooting phobias among purebred dogs in Denmark. *Prevent Vet Med*, 1773:1–16.

Salazar MR (2000). Alpha lipoic acid: A novel treatment for depression. *Med Hypotheses*, 55:510–512.

Schenkel R (1967). Submission: Its features and function in the wolf and dog. *Am Zool*, 7:319–329.

Scott JP and Charles MS (1954). Genetic differences in dogs: A case of magnification by thresholds and by habit formation. *J Gen Psychol*, 84:175–188.

Seligman MEP and Johnston JC (1973). A cognitive theory of avoidance learning. In FJ McGuigan and DB Lumsden (Eds), *Contemporary Approaches to Conditioning and Learning*. Washington, DC: Winston-Wiley.

Skinner BF (1979). *The Shaping of a Behaviorist: Part Two of an Autobiography*. New York: Alfred A. Knopf.

Sonoda A, Okayasu T, and Hirai H (1991). Loss of controllability in appetitive situations interferes with subsequent learning in aversive situations. *Anim Learn Behav*, 19:270–275.

Stevens LJ, Zentall SS, Abate ML, et al. (1996). Omega-3 fatty acids in boys with behavior, learning, and health problems. *Physiol Behav*, 59:915–920.

Stoll AL, Severus WE, Freeman MP, et al. (1999). Omega 3 fatty acids in bipolar disorder: A preliminary double-blind, placebo-controlled trial. *Arch Gen Psychiatry*, 56:407–412.

Takeuchi Y, Ogata N, Houpt KA, and Scarlett JM (2001). Differences in background and outcome of three behavior problems of dogs. *Appl Anim Behav Sci*, 70:297–308.

Tortora DF (1980). Applied animal psychology: The practical implications of comparative analysis. In MR Denny (Ed), *Comparative Psychology: An Evolutionary Analysis of Animal Behavior*. New York: John Wiley and Sons.

Tortora DF (1983). Safety training: The elimination of avoidance-motivated aggression in dog. *J Exp Psychol*, 112:176–214.

Uchida Y, Dodman N, De Napoli J, and Aronson L (1997). Characterization and treatment of 20 canine dominance aggression cases. *J Vet Med Sci*, 59:397–399.

Van Hooff JARAM and Wensing J (1987). Dominance and its behavioral measures in a captive wolf pack. In H Frank (Ed), *Man and Wolf*. Dordrecht, The Netherlands: Dr W Junk.

Voith VL (1977). Aggressive behavior and dominance. *Canine Pract*, 4:11–15.

Voith VL and Borchelt PL (1982). Diagnosis and treatment of dominance aggression in dogs. *Clin North Am Small Anim Pract*, 12:655–663.

Voith VL, Wright JC, Danneman PJ, et al. (1992). Is there a relationship between canine behavior problems and spoiling activities, anthropomorphism, and obedience training? *Appl Anim Behav Sci*, 34:263–272.

Wang S, Berge GE, Hoem NO, and Sund RB (2001). Pharmacokinetics in dogs after oral administration of two different forms of ascorbic acid. *Res Vet Sci*, 71:27–32.

Wells DL, Graham L, and Hepper PG (2002). The influence of auditory stimulation on the behaviour of dogs housed in a rescue shelter. *Anim Welfare*, 11:385–393.

Wood GE, Young LT, Reagan LP, and McEwen BS (2003). Acute and chronic restraint stress alter the incidence of social conflict in male rats. *Horm Behav*, 43:205–213.

Woolpy JH (1968). The social organization of wolves. *Nat Hist*, 77:46–55.

Woolpy JH and Ginsburg BE (1967). Wolf socialization: A study of temperament in a wild social species. *Am Zool*, 7:357–363.

Wright JC (1991). Canine aggression toward people: Bite scenarios and prevention. *Vet Clin North Am Adv Companion Anim Behav*, 21:299–314.

Zeeman EC (1976). Catastrophe theory. *Sci Am*, 234:65–83.

8

Impulsive, Extrafamilial, and Intraspecific Aggression

PART 1: INTRAFAMILIAL AND EXTRAFAMILIAL AGGRESSION

The care and training received by dogs with aggression problems is frequently not much different from the treatment received by dogs that do not develop aggression problems. Why one dog is friendly and another dog aggressive when both grow up in the same household is only an enigma to the extent that one assumes that the needs of the two dogs are the same. This underappreciation of the diversity of canine individual differences and needs for individualized socialization and training has led to considerable confusion and mismanagement of dogs. The interactive and environmental needs of dogs vary considerably, not just between breeds, but also between individuals of the same breed. What for one dog may promote a secure attachment, for another may represent an intolerable situation facilitating ambivalent social and place attachments. The obvious implication with regard to the prevention and treatment of aggression problems is that dogs require socialization, training, and quality-of-life enhancements that are tailored to meet the dog's particular needs.

As argued in Chapter 7 and expanded upon below, the social dominance hypothesis does not appear to have much value for understanding and treating most intrafamilial and extrafamilial aggression problems. Several features of canine domestic aggression (CDA) conflict with the dominance hypothesis, including the incompetent and insecure nature of attacks; the antecedent activities and situational peculiarities leading up to attacks; the panicogenic, catastrophic, and paroxysmal nature of arousal associated with attacks; the reactive negativity bias shown toward ambiguous social signals given by persons intimately familiar to the dog; and the terrified appearance of aggressors at the flash point of attack. Diagnosing such behavior as dominance aggression seems akin to tossing a pig in the air and claiming that pigs can fly. Although dominance relations in the organization of dog behavior are not entirely trivial, especially as regards interdog relationships and the setting of social limits on undesirable behavior, dominance as a proximal cause of reactive and impulsive aggression appears to be little more than a narrative account with little substantive value as a causal concept. The dominance diagnosis appears to be more relevant to how humans cope with dog bites and canine misbehavior in general than to the etiology and rational treatment of aggression problems.

Anthropic dominance ideation converts intrafamilial and extrafamilial CDA into a form that absolves the victim from responsibility while demonizing the canine aggressor with despotic social or territorial intent, thereby justifying abusive appetitive and emotional deprivation, stressful isolation tactics, and physical maltreatment in the name of canine behavior therapy aimed at changing the dog's dominant attitude (see Bugental et al., 1997 and 1999; also see *Anthropic Dominance Ideation, Perceived Power, and Control Styles* in Chapter 10). Far from the confident picture that one might expect from a dominant dog, many of these so-called dominance aggressors appear to be socially incompetent, insecure, and reactive in their dealings with people. In severe cases, just before attacking, impulsive aggressors appear to be overwhelmed by intense sympathetic arousal that seems foreign to the dog and inappropriate to the evoking stimulation. Although impulsive aggression has been linked to seizure activity (see *Epilepsy* in Volume 1, Chapter 3, and *Assessment and Identification* in Volume 2, Chapter 8), most authorities currently downplay the seizure hypothesis. Although limbic seizure and a host of other biogenetic and neurobiological factors (e.g., serotonergic/dopaminergic imbalance) appear to contribute in various ways to the expression of aggression, very little clinical or experimental evidence points to any single variable or set of variables as a cause of aggression.

Autoprotective aggression can occasionally be traced to specific abusive or traumatic experiences. In one such case, a woman with a psychotic condition obtained a puppy as a companion after her release from a state psychiatric hospital, where she had apparently resided for several years. According to reliable witnesses, the woman came outside at various times during the day to sit on the stoop and affectionately stroke the puppy and fuss over it with sweet talk. For unknown reasons, the woman periodically became enraged and would turn without warning and slap the puppy forcefully along the side of its head, whereupon she would appear to be very sorry for the action and attempt to comfort the puppy with petting and other expressions of affection and comfort giving. As the puppy calmed down, the woman would again, for no apparent reason, turn and forcefully hit the puppy, causing it to yelp in distress. This ritual was observed on several occasions and prompted neighbors to take action to rescue the puppy. It was adopted and raised successfully without notable adverse signs of the abuse from its experience until approaching adulthood, when it began to bite visitors in a very odd way. During greetings, the dog showed very friendly behavior and quickly warmed up to visitors and accepted their petting without any sign of resentment or fear. But suddenly, and without warning or provocation, the dog's demeanor would rapidly change from affection to rage and, in an instant, it delivered hard bites to hands as it was petted about the head. The aggression was limited to visitors with whom the dog had formed some degree of affectionate contact, and the attacks occurred only while the dog was being petted. The dog had an affectionate and nonaggressive relationship with a caring and protective owner. The bizarre attacks were otherwise inconsistent with the dog's temperament and by observation could not be guessed from any behavioral signs. The etiology of this bizarre and dangerous aggression appears to have stemmed from the abusive unpredictable and uncontrollable handling that the dog was exposed to as puppy, perhaps resulting in the formation of toxic expectancies in association with petting. While initially accepting the visitors' petting, as the interaction continued an apparent internal conflict emerged that rapidly escalated into a fearless panic-type attack. One is tempted to interpret the aggression exhibited by the dog in terms of a collision of affection, a toxic expectancy formed in puppyhood, and a sudden loss of safety and trust, resulting in the release of an angry hard bite. The owner may have been protected from such attacks by having formed a trust-based bond with the dog reinforced by a history of safety in the context of affection (see *Contact Aversion and Aggression* in Volume 2, Chapter 8).

In addition to etiologies associated with abuse, aggression problems appear to be related to less obvious biogenetic and epigenetic causes (e.g., exposure to prenatal stress) that are incubated by social exchanges promoting a negative coping style. According to cynopraxic theory, neurobiological systems are malleable and adapt in response to both positive and negative adjustment pressures, making selective attention and behavior the axial conduit for the mediation of both disturbance and therapeutic change. The neural plasticity resulting from cynopraxic attention and behavior training serves to entrain compensatory neural and physiological changes in the process of integrating social skills, adaptive coping style, and secure attachments. These neurobiological changes are hypothesized to promote autonomic, cognitive, and emotional regulation conducive to enhanced attention, impulse control, and calming. More specifically, with respect CDA, cynopraxic therapy facilitates the acquisition of cognitive and behavioral skills incompatible with aggression by arranging conditioned and unconditioned stimuli, social exchanges, and environmental enhancements to promote autonomic attunement and affectionate play. As such, the executive attention and impulse-control deficits, emotional distress, and autonomic disturbances associated with a reactive coping style and aggression are interpreted as flowing from social interaction and home environments promoting ambivalent (nervous/insecure) attachments. The integration of secure social and place attachments via cynopraxic therapy promotes social trust and autoattunement, enabling dogs to form social bonds and to explore new social relations competently and novel environments under the regulatory control of enhanced sympathovagal balance.

CLASSIFYING AGGRESSION

In general, proactive control-related or instrumental (offensive and defensive) aggression is organized to achieve specific goals not otherwise achievable, showing the following characteristics: (1) a relatively consistent ensemble of sequential events and junctures (i.e., transitional points leading to escalation or de-escalation of hostility based on control-related outcomes) that move predictably from agonistic arousal, precursor intention movements, ritualized threats, and formalized interaction (e.g., exchanges and transactions) conducive to conflict resolution and subsequent reconciliation or, in the absence of alternative options, conclude with a moment of menacing suspense and overt confrontation/attack; (2) a demonstrated ability to escalate, de-escalate, or cancel agonistic processing at any juncture in the formal sequence of events; (3) a concordance or context appropriateness between the provoking situation, the trigger, and the magnitude of arousal and attack (i.e., severity and duration); (5) a functional significance [e.g., an offensive response to promote control interests (i.e., get-and-keep incentive) or a defensive response to aversive stimulation or an imminent threat of same (i.e., bite-or-die incentive) and responsiveness to outcomes (e.g., suppression by defeat); and (6) rarity (see Smith, 1977). Instrumental attacks may take a more confrontational and direct form (without much warning) in the context of social code violations (e.g., threatening to take a prized item and disturbing a sleeping dog), but such attacks (nips and snaps) remain inhibited and appropriate to the evoking situation.

In contrast, reactive or impulsive autoprotective aggression shows a lack of competent sequential organization, with antagonistic arousal rapidly transitioning into a default attack mode that is often severe, uninhibited, out of character, and disproportionate to the provoking social context. Impulsive attacks tend to increase in frequency and severity over time, suggesting a process of progressive disinhibition influencing the expression of such behavior. Twelve prominent independent variables appear to play important roles in the etiology of reactive/impulsive autoprotective aggression: (1) genetic predisposition; (2) developmental adversity (prenatal, perinatal, and postnatal stress and insults); (3) interactive disturbances impairing executive attention and impulse control; (4) lack of competent social coping skills and play; (5) persistent interactive conflict; (6) social ambivalence (distrust and unfairness) in association with growing anxiety, irritability, and intolerance; (7) a history of mismanaged competition and proactive aggression; (8) a reactive trigger formed in association with loss or risk; (9) the presence of nervous/insecure social and place attachments; (10) loss of trust and autonomic attunement; (11) deprivational environmental conditions; and (12) entrapment.

An aggressive dog's appearance of aloofness, inattention to social signals, insular resistance to owner control efforts, reduced playfulness, and arbitrary threats and attacks are frequently viewed through the distorted and pseudoscientific image of the "alpha wolf" and other prominent ethological myths. According to cynopraxic theory, the social withdrawal and tuning out of an ambivalent attachment object is not indicative of dominance, but rather represents a gradual process of social and attentional disengagement in anticipation of reduced impulse control and increasing social repulsion and intolerance. Under the inescapable conditions of domestic life, dogs are compelled to cope and adjust to the social and environmental circumstances that they find, since leaving the situation is not a viable option. Domestic situations lacking sufficient fairness, order, and resources to meet basic canine social and biological needs pose special challenges. Dogs cope with adverse and inescapable household conditions in three principal ways, depending on perceived controllability and fairness: (1) Households and interaction perceived as being relatively uncontrollable and deprivational promote a reactive coping style and autonomic regulation conducive to nervous attachments. (2) Households and interaction perceived as being relatively controllable and providing for basic needs, but unfair and enabling or coercing dependency by means of indulgence and/or subjugation, tend to promote insecure attachments. (3) Households perceived as being relatively uncontrollable, deprivational, and unfair facilitate autonomic shifts and dys-

regulation, making the ambivalent attachment object a target for reactive or impulsive autoprotective aggression.

In addition to conditioned aversive associations stemming from interactive conflict, a major source of anxiety and anger is related to the motivated disengagement of attention and social resources from an ambivalent attachment object. As such, the *anxious anger* of social ambivalence is an amalgam of anxiety and anger fused under the escalating tensions of entrapment and autoprotective motivations evoked by interaction perceived as inconsistent, unfair, and inescapable. Social ambivalence and entrapment dynamics are hypothesized to promote reactive and impulsive behavior flowing from the gradual or precipitous disengagement of attentional and social resources in the process of degrading impulse control and autonomic/emotional regulation. Increased anxiety and reduced impulse control are the natural corollaries of diminished selective and sustained attention. The anxiety component of social ambivalence is hypothesized to infuse ambivalent exchanges with distrust, whereas the anger component of social ambivalence, flowing principally from the retraction of the social engagement system in response to anxious and unfair exchanges, generates social repulsion, irritability, and intolerance.

The net effect of social ambivalence and entrapment is to install a preemptive negativity bias consisting of distrust and intolerance, altering the way the dog perceives, interprets, and responds to exchanges with the ambivalent attachment object. Autoprotective or exploitative (antisocial) behavior shown in response to ambiguous actions and unexpected change reflect a negativity bias and autonomic misattunement, whereas prosocial behavior in response to ambiguous actions and unexpected change reflects a positivity bias and autonomic attunement. Whereas incompetent reactive or impulsive dogs may respond to ambiguous social exchanges as signifying a threat of loss or risk, dogs operating competently under the regulation of secure attachments tend to approach ambiguous situations confidently with an anticipation of fair exchange and reward.

ANTIPREDATORY STRATEGY AND AUTOPROTECTION VERSUS DOMINANCE

Dogs that fail to attract, attach, and please human companions prove too expensive or inconvenient, or otherwise become undesirable or unwanted as pets are at risk of being relinquished, concentrated in shelters, and destroyed if no one takes an interest in forming an attachment with them. The millions of dogs killed every year is stark evidence of the human appetite for the pleasures of canine companionship and the default lethality awaiting dogs that fail to provide it. Among the Romans, unwanted infants were often left to die in a public place unless a passerby happened along to rescue them, a practice that frequently resulted in the children becoming slaves. The foregoing practice of infant exposure seems to roughly prefigure the modern-day function of the shelter whereby dogs that are no longer wanted are relinquished, put on public display, and subsequently killed if they fail to inspire sufficient attraction or pity to integrate an attachment. The act of relinquishment allows owners to seek a more gratifying pet while separating themselves from the unpleasantness of disposing of the unwanted one. The subsequent killing of the unwanted dog makes room for more dogs, thereby perpetuating the cycle of extracting affection and submission from the canine attachment object and destroying those that fail to provide it. The pattern of taking an infant puppy away from its biological family, subjugating it by force and restraint, abandoning or relinquishing it, and destroying the dog when it is no longer wanted represents a pattern of exploitation that infuses the human-dog relationship with an inherent paradox (Tuan, 1984; see *Yi-Fu Tuan* in Volume 1, Chapter 10). The predatory exploitation of the dog for its fur and flesh is sublimated and institutionalized into a less obvious predatory preoccupation with the exploitation of its capacity to provide affection, submission, and utility. As such, the dog is transformed into a prey object whose ability to gratify human needs depends on it staying healthy and alive, at least during times of plenty. These predatory pressures centering on the human

appetite for affectionate companionship and dominion have selected for traits compatible with taming, social submission, and training, while simultaneously suppressing canine predatory propensities and behaviors.

As an object of human attachment and domination, a dog is spared from the knife and fork but not from cruelty and death if it fails to yield the social resources for which it is spared and upon which its protected status depends. Under these sorts of life-and-death pressures, it is reasonable to expect that dogs might have evolved various complementary antistress and antipredatory coping strategies to reduce the risk of human exploitative appetites and abuses. Dogs appear to have evolved an ability to integrate secure attachments that mediate autonomic regulatory changes in their human keepers. The dependency and insecure attachment produced by indulgence and domination is hypothesized to combine with affectionate submission and begging to facilitate parental-like care and protectiveness, the secure feelings of unconditional acceptance, and, potentially, the joy of affectionate play. These emotional and behavioral effects of autonomic attunement may help to ensure that keepers will not decide to abuse, eat, abandon, or kill their dogs. The dog's neotenous appearance, soft fur and appreciation of petting, and the giving of unconditional acceptance to the keeper may be important positive antipredatory adaptations that further enhance attachment-mediated autonomic control. However, in response to ambivalent attachments and entrapment, negative antipredatory survival modes may be activated in the process of lowering autoprotective flight-fight thresholds. Historically, at times of dearth, dogs may have lost their protected status, just as today dogs are at an increased risk of relinquishment and death if they become inconvenient or too costly to maintain. As a result, indicators of reduced parental investment (social attention and care) and resource availability appear to activate additional antipredatory survival modes that increase avoidance and dispersive tensions. The dog's apparent sensitivity to social and environmental quality-of-life changes, as indexed by changes of affiliative receptivity, dispersive tensions, and altered flight-fight thresholds, is consistent with the activation of encoded survival modes responsive to changes likely to anticipate a change in predatory risk.

Despite the evolution of a specialized anti-stress system for coping with ambiguous, novel, and unexpected events, dogs appear to be especially vulnerable to show reactive behavior at times when selective attention is disengaged. For example, disturbing a dog while it is asleep has been associated with fierce attacks that have confirmed the wisdom of the proverb "Let sleeping dogs lie" countless times (see *Aggression Associated with Disturbances While Resting* in Chapter 7). The dog's love of sleeping in close company with humans, especially on the bed, and the immense enjoyment that many people derive from sleeping in close quarters with a dog may point to an important adaptation having ancient origins, perhaps helping to keep many dogs out of the communal pot. Sleeping with dogs may have provided ancient dog keepers with feelings of enhanced security and comfort (see *The Dingo: A Prototypical Dog* in Volume 1, Chapter 1). These comfort-enhancing benefits may have been especially important resources for the young, sick, frail, or elderly, perhaps providing an interesting account for the evolution of traits conducive to a natural sense of compassion and gentleness. Instead of preying on the weakness of such people, dogs often show them special treatment— behavior that is commonly extended to young children, as well. During the dog's evolution, it has shed most of its predatory instincts, in the process acquiring traits conducive to forming a symbiotic mutualism with human guardians. Essentially, the domesticating process has transformed the canine predator into a predatory object dependent on the sub-jugating predator for care and protection. Within the context of these evolutionary developments and trends, the notion that dogs might have evolved a set of complementary or antithetical antisocial and antipreda-tory tactics to cope with the uncertainties and risks associated with living with a predator represents a plausible hypothesis. The reactive and impulsive nature of CDA seems to have far more in common with an antipredatory

coping strategy (Kavaliers and Choleris, 2001) than it shares with the idea that dogs attack people to enhance their social status or defend their territory, something that they may do with conspecifics but not with human subju-gators. Just as a prey animal may seek to avoid predators by reducing activity and limiting the time it spends in open spaces, the auto-protective orientation shown by many dogs may stem from an analogous antipredatory strategy activated in the context of home situations perceived as unsafe and unsatisfying.

Dogs appear to survive under domestic conditions by means of forming attachments facilitated by affectionate play. According to this hypothesis, affectionate play transactions integrate an autonomic attunement in humans that is conducive to a state favorable to alloprotection and caregiving, perhaps off-setting human predatory interests and power-dominance motivations toward the canine attachment object. The autonomic attune-ment associated with reciprocal affectionate play exchanges between the dog and human predator promotes social trust and bonding in support of the continuation of affectionate playfulness and the integration of harmonious social relations and mutual appreciation. In addition to secure attachments and the auto-nomic attunement facilitated by affectionate play, the human-dog bond appears to depend on predictable and controllable exchanges giv-ing mutual advantage via enhanced comfort and safety (security). Canine social trust appears to depend on a fair balance of advan-tages given and advantages taken in the process of obtaining comfort and safety. An appreciation of fairness appears to emerge in the context of play, since, in the absence of parity, play stops or becomes increasingly exploitative and cruel. Affection is motiva-tionally incompatible with cruelty and, in combination with play, promotes fairness and harmony in human-dog relations. Insecure attachments based on relatively consistent but unfair interaction promote social dynamics conducive to a loss of trust and increased reactivity toward ambiguous social exchanges and unexpected change. Social exchanges that give excessive advantages to the dog, or unfairly force the dog to yield advantages to the human controller, mobilize disruptive social dynamics that impair affectionate play and bonding. For example, dogs that unfairly receive advantages by indulgent treatment may become increasing dependent and form an expectancy of interaction that is narrowly focused on receiving rather than yielding advantages. In contrast, dogs from which unfair advantages are taken may become increasingly unwilling to yield to exploitative control efforts. In both cases, the dog's ability to trust is reduced, along with social attraction and its ability to play, thereby setting the stage for social repulsion, irritability, and contact intolerance, and activating antipredatory coping strategies and autoprotective behavior in response to human exchanges perceived as posing a predatory threat. In contrast to the playful and cooperative response to human control efforts by dogs expressing secure attachments, dogs expressing insecure attachments show increasing rigidity in response to human control efforts. Similarly, nervous attachments formed in association with exploitative play and inconsistent and manipulative exchanges that evoke anxiety (lack of security) and anger (lack of attraction) keep the social engagement system off-line while mobilizing a variety of antipredatory autoprotective behaviors in response to human control efforts.

The intolerance for physical handling, restraint, and interference that reactive and impulsive aggressors show is consistent with an antipredatory function. These dogs may show tolerance for close proximity and petting but deliver severe and uninhibited bites if picked up. Many dogs reach the flash point of no return only after struggling unsuccessfully to break free from restraint or coping with abusive punishment. Under the influence of inescapable social anxiety and irritability stemming from interactive conflict and ambivalence, the home or areas within it may become more generally associated with entrapment and frustrated dispersive tensions evoking highly motivated autoprotective behavior toward family members. Reactive dogs frequently show aggressive behavior in response to unwelcome grooming, under the influence of an obvious autoprotective incen-

tive. Such dogs may snap if their paws are touched, and become particularly reactive and dangerous if the owner attempts to trim the nails. Again, consistent with the antipredatory hypothesis, some dogs will bite only if grabbed or reached for after fleeing to cover behind a sofa, inside a crate, or under a bed or table, appearing to attack after an intensification of aggressive arousal triggered by entrapment and autoprotective panic. The relative amount of reactive arousal shown by dogs toward ambiguous or threatening social stimuli under such circumstances appears to index social attraction and trust rather than social status or a perception of rank.

Ambiguous activities, such as abruptly crouching down and kissing or caressing a sleeping dog around its muzzle, may stimulate sensations interpreted by the dog as an attack. Attacks at such times are often severe and damaging, followed by pronounced signs of emotional distress consistent with remorse. Dogs may be particularly vulnerable to such attacks when falling asleep (hypnagogic) or awaking (hypnopompic). The vibrissae provide autoprotective sensory information relevant to the detection of objects coming in contact with the face. For example, brushing the canine vibrissae evokes nonhabituating defensive blinking. Also, when making an angry pucker, the vibrissae are turned out and forward. These reflexive effects suggest the possibility that vibrissal stimulation around the face may trigger autoprotective sensations or threatening hallucinations (preemptive processing) when other sensory and attentional resources are off-line. Dogs dream, and these dreams often have sequences that involve apparent efforts to run away or attack an adversary. When startled from sleep, the imaginal content of these dreams may continue during hypnopompic transitions while a dog is awakening. The nature of dream images and their emotional significance may distort how the dog perceives and interprets the owner's actions. Further, during hypnagogic transitions between wakefulness and sleep, dogs may be vulnerable to disinhibited attacks in association with reduced attentional resources and impulse control.

Among human subjects, vague feelings of someone in the room or hallucinations of being attacked or experiencing terror (e.g., falling into an abyss or being caught in a fire) while transitioning in or out of sleep have been reported (Ohayon, 2000). In an urban population, violence in association with sleep and hypnagogic and hypnopompic hallucinations were found to be more prevalent among persons diagnosed with post-traumatic stress disorder (PTSD) than subjects not diagnosed with PTSD (Ohayon and Shapiro, 2000). Consequently, the possibility of a history of abuse or trauma should be evaluated in dogs exhibiting reactive explosive behavior when disturbed while sleeping or resting (hypnagogic). Reactive behavior in response to minimal provocation may be associated with the hair-trigger activation of dysregulated sympathetic circuits. The signal triggering the event may be arrhythmias or the abrupt withdrawal of vagal tone (e.g., when the dog is disturbed while resting) and the provocation of a potent sympathetic surge (see *Autonomic Arousal, Heart Rate, and Aggression* in Chapter 6). Such sudden surges of arousal may induce widespread disinhibition. Ascending signals may kindle stress-sensitized amygdalar or hippocampal circuits, perhaps resulting in reactive attacks (Pontius and LeMay, 2003). The canine amygdala is highly sensitive to kindling effects, resulting in pronounced cardiovascular changes as well as neck and jaw movements (Thompson and Galosy, 1983). In many of these cases, dogs also show autoprotective behavior in response to interference while in havens of comfort and safety while fully awake. Autoprotective behavior at such times may only rise to the level of crankiness and low-grade threats; in other cases, however, it might rapidly transition into a strong threat or attack. These variations in magnitude and severity suggest that trait anger may contribute to an increased propensity for such reactive behavior. A possibility exists that autoprotective aggression in association with sleeping and resting areas may stem from reactive arousal originally evoked in association with being awakened and then subsequently contextualized to the situation and associatively linked to the person. This could

help to account for some cases involving inappropriate and explosive aggression near resting places in response to minimal provocation. It is interesting to speculate that during periods of increased social and environmental stress the dog's sleep may be agitated and susceptible to reactive adjustments in response to being awakened. The aversive emotional arousal and reactive behavior evoked at such times might facilitate conditioned social and place associations that may increase the dog's reactivity in the future when disturbed while in such resting places. The liability to develop this behavior may be especially problematic for dogs that have not had time to form competing expectancies incompatible with aggression. These observations may have relevance for understanding the odd finding reported by Guy and colleagues that suggests that puppies allowed to sleep on beds during the first 2 months had an increased risk of developing an aggression problem. In addition, given the disruptive influence of rehoming on previously established attachments and autonomic attunement, puppies may be vulnerable to integrate insecure attachments when allowed to sleep in the bed during the first few weeks.

Whether autoprotection takes a defensive or offensive (confrontational) form is determined by the presence or absence of anxiety/fear (defensive) and anger/frustration (offensive) (see *Species-typical Defensive and Offensive Aggression* in Chapter 7). According to the antipredatory hypothesis, the defensive form of autoprotective aggression is shown reactively toward familiar and unfamiliar targets in response to interaction perceived as posing an inescapable threat. In contrast, the offensive form of autoprotective aggression is impulsively directed toward familiar targets perceived as posing an unappeasable or uncontrollable challenge. Whereas autoprotective defensive arousal is activated by the uncertainty evoked by social novelty or unexpected change, familiar persons and household members with whom the dog has formed nervous attachments via interaction lacking consistency may evoke conditioned autoprotective arousal in conjunction with the disengagement of attention (anxiety), dispersive tensions, and entrapment. In the absence of attachment relations, vigilance may represent a tactic used by reactive dogs to regulate autonomic tone to establish a state of readiness while simultaneously postponing action. In the case of nervous attachment objects, the withdrawal of attention by the reactive dog is hypothesized to occur primarily as the result of a perceived lack of predictability or relevance informing the object's exchanges. Attentional disengagement from a nervous attachment object is believed to increase social anxiety and decrease impulse control via the withdrawal of parasympathetic tone. Autoprotective offensive behavior, on the other hand, appears to develop in association with insecure attachments or secure attachments that have been disconfirmed and disrupted by a loss of trust and the autonomic dysregulation resulting from social disengagement (anger), motivated inattentiveness (anxiety), social ambivalence, and entrapment. Whereas autoprotective defensive behavior is primarily dedicated to reactive coping with risk, autoprotective offensive behavior is primarily dedicated to impulsive coping with loss. Finally, autoprotective panic—a catastrophic or explosive state of aggressive arousal—is triggered by social interaction simultaneously evoking both loss (anger) and risk (anxiety) occurring in the context of reactive adjustments to social challenges or threats.

Entrapment appears to switch the dog motivationally from a flight mode to an autoprotective fight mode. Punishing the dog beyond the first sign of appeasement, or pursuing it into safe refuges and denying it the ability to obtain comfort and safety (entrapment), represent critical interactive changes that escalate autonomic and emotional arousal and cause the dog to shift the motivational direction of autoprotective behavior away from flight to turn and confront the threat with aggression. The autonomic and emotional regulation and arousal profile concurrent with the relaxation phase of escape to safety appears to be qualitatively similar to the autonomic and emotion arousal evoked by safe havens (e.g., resting on a sofa or bed). Safe refuges and havens (secure place attachments) evoke autonomic relaxation and feelings of enhanced security (comfort and safety). The antipredator hypothesis of canine domestic aggression postulates that the primary causes of aggression are related to social triggers that threaten (defensive) or challenge (offensive) the dog's ability to optimize survival security (comfort + safety) and well-being by (1) thwarting the dog's ability to escape to safety when threatened with danger, (2) interrupting the relief or relaxation phase of safety by invading the safe refuge, (3) intrusion or forcible theft of a valued comfort activity or object, (4) interruption of a survival activity conducive to comfort (e.g., eating or sleeping) (5) conditioned stimuli acquired in association with items 1 to 4 and the integration of ambivalent (nervous/insecure) social and place attachments, and (6) acquired triggers that activate autonomic preparatory arousal and sympathetic tensions conducive to the activation of the antipredator mode. Whether a dog adopts a defensive or offensive tactic depends on the incentive operating at the moment of arousal (fear or anger) and history of consequences resulting from past autoprotective actions (see *Species-typical Defensive and Offensive Aggression* in Chapter 7).

The ability to sneak off with food objects left unattended or discarded may have been an important source of nutrition in the dog's evolutionary past. With the loss of predatory modal behavior, dogs may have integrated scavenging and pilfering survival skills to enhance their ability to survive as they became increasingly dependent on human resources for survival. Dogs that succeeded in getting away with such pilfery probably enjoyed a higher likelihood of survival, but stealing food may have exacted a heavy penalty if the dog was caught in the act, perhaps exerting selection pressures that gradually encoded relevant sensory, cognitive, and emotional propensities improving the dog's ability to interpret and anticipate human deictic (pointing) signals and threats (e.g., finger and gaze directional commands) and attentional states (see *Deictic Signals and Directional Cues* in Chapter 10). These survival skills may have included defensive strategies to evade capture or to escape, if caught (nip), perhaps learned in the context of certain play activities. Many of these enhanced adaptations and phylogenetic survival skills appear to be patched into canine play via augmented capacities for forming complex social attachments and coping with social ambiguity and uncertainty—critical paedomorphic changes that shadow decreasing predatory self-sufficiency and reduced fear of humans in the process of promoting a lifelong dependency on humans. These paedomorphic changes enhancing the dog's ability to form affectionate and playful relationships enable the dog to integrate the phylogenetic survival skills and coping abilities needed to adjust to domestic life.

Taking a forbidden item, evading capture, and then escaping to a safe refuge with the prize are part of a highly prepared sequential pattern that is rapidly learned by dogs. Mishandling of such exchanges may integrate problematic autoprotective dynamics, perhaps facilitating overt antipredator defenses in adulthood toward family members. For example, punishing a dog after forcing it out of a safe refuge, grabbing a leg or tail and dragging the dog into the open, chasing and cornering it with the help of other family members (particularly boisterous children), or prying objects out of the dog's mouth appear to be correlated with adult aggression problems. Similarly, punitive handling associated with safe havens, such as repeatedly grabbing a dog by its collar or scruff and pulling or throwing it off furniture, may promote increased vigilance and readiness to bite when approached under similar circumstances, especially in cases where reactive exchanges are a prominent part of a general pattern of daily conflictive interaction and ineffectual discipline. Most canine reactive behavior is the mirror reflection of incompetent human control efforts. The antipredatory mode appears to mobilize stress-sensitized flight-fight-freeze networks formed in association with inescapable interactive conflict. Reactive autoprotective behavior is distinguished by the presence of a preemptive negativity bias and automatic adjustments in response to ambiguous or ambivalent social stimuli. In contrast, proactive interaction and training activities

integrate a positive preemptive social orientation and bias toward social uncertainty via structured exchanges conducive to an adaptive coping style. In addition to the mutual autonomic attunement and balance mediated by structured training, cynopraxic procedures serve to activate flirt-play, forbear-nip, and forgive-reconcile antistress and antiaggression systems (see *Phylogenesis, Polymorphism, and Coping Styles* in Chapter 6)—changes conducive to an enhanced capacity to cope with ambiguity, ambivalence, and novelty. Affection and playfulness are the reflection of preemptive emotional and behavioral biases that govern an adaptive coping style organized in association with the integration of secure social and place attachments and a trusting bond—changes incompatible with the dispersive tensions and dynamics that coalesce in the expression of impulsive or reactive autoprotective attacks.

The binding of attentional functions to chronic social ambivalence and entrapment dynamics diverts adaptive resources away from social engagement, cooperation, and reward-seeking activities. This shift of attentional focus is not only correlated with aggression but is hypothesized to represent a significant proximate factor mobilizing the autonomic misattunement and emotional distress conducive to ambivalent attachments, a reactive coping style, and the activation of an antipredatory mode of social interaction. The notion of an autoprotective phenotype activated in response to social conflict and entrapment appears to offer a far more useful way for studying the motivational and social etiology of aggression problems than does the social dominance narrative. According to cynopraxic theory, the interaction between friendly familiars consists of transactions that evoke feelings of comfort and safety and mutual autonomic attunement while promoting secure attachments. The refinement of social adjustments and changes conducive to mutual autonomic attunement and secure attachments is mediated by an adaptive coping style emerging in association with autoinitiated control incentives, prediction-control expectancies, and calibrated emotional establishing operations in the context of mutually beneficial cooperative exchanges and fair-play compromise. In contrast, social interaction lacking sufficient consistency to promote an adaptive coping style and secure attachments promotes nervous attachments, dispersive tensions, and autoprotective behavior arising in association with social ambivalence (apprehension and resentment) in response to inescapable coercion, exploitation, and domination. Under the influence of coercion and inconsistency, social behavior becomes increasingly alloinitiated, dependent, and reactive. Dogs showing a reactive coping style may lack the ability to competently autoinitiate behavior based on proactive control incentives. In addition, such dogs appear to lack the requisite autonomic and emotional regulation needed to integrate and refine secure social and place attachments. According to cynopraxic training theory, the autonomy of interactive exchanges is a critical factor mediating adaptive social behavior and secure attachments. Social interaction lacking sufficient order (predictability and controllability) and variety to support autoinitiated behavior and an adaptive coping style will exert an intrinsically disorganizing influence on attachment behavior via social ambivalence, dispersive tensions, autonomic misattunement, and the integration of a reactive coping style. These observations emphasize that freedom and choice are critical aspects of social interaction conducive to the integration of an adaptive coping style and behavior incompatible with autoprotective behavior.

The motivated diversion of attentional and social resources away from the proactive processing of social exchanges appears to figure prominently in the etiology of reactive and impulsive social behavior and the activation of a antipredatory mode. Whereas attentional disengagement results in increased social anxiety and decreased selective attention and impulse control, social disengagement results in repulsion (irritability and intolerance) and withdrawal of the autonomic attunement that mediates attachment behavior. With the retraction of attentional and social engagement, family members may become increasingly alien and threatening (estrangement) to dogs. As a result of these autonomic, cogni-

tive, and emotional changes, antipredator strategies become increasingly reactive, taking an active (flight-fight) or passive (freeze-helplessness) motivational direction, depending on the dog's temperament and the relative predominance of state versus trait anger and anxiety. The associated behavioral inhibition, withdrawal, and reactive irritability shown by such dogs may profoundly impair their ability to engage in competent social behavior. Such dogs may meet unwelcome approach and proximity with autoprotective conflict or attack. In other cases, perhaps where severe punishment has been used to suppress threat autoprotective threats, the dog may simply withdraw inwardly, becoming rigid and unresponsive to human contact. In contrast to nervous attachments, which reflect insufficient autonomic and emotional regulation to support impulse control and an adaptive coping style, insecure social attachments develop in association with an excessive and exclusive dependency on particular persons and places for autonomic and emotional regulation. Under the influence of social ambivalence and entrapment, insecure attachments may be focused on specific persons (e.g., adult parent) and places within the home (e.g., crate, sofa, or bed). Family members not included may be treated as threats insofar as their interference disturbs the comfort and safety obtained by the dog from being in close contact with the preferred attachment object or place. The loss of trust (disconfirmation of a safety expectancy) and the gradual or rapid withdrawal of attentional and social resources from an insecure attachment object may generate an increasing vulnerability for panicogenic arousal and explosive behavior in response to ambiguous interaction or handling perceived as threatening. For example, punitive efforts aimed at suppressing low-grade threats and growls shown by such dogs—displays that essentially signify inhibition and uneasiness about launching into an attack—may disrupt the dog's ability to process (inhibit and disinhibit) threat displays sequentially. In response to such mismanagement, the dog might learn to block low-grade threats by internalizing attentional resources and by coping passively until a flash point of no return might be reached and an inappropriate attack is released under the exigency of blind panic.

In addition to the effects of social and attentional disengagement on a heightened risk of impulsivity, overly vigilant and apprehensive dogs may show cognitive deficiencies that impair their ability to shift attention selectively and to adjust emotional arousal in a phase-flexible way in response to ambiguous or novel social stimuli. Ambiguous signals may pose particularly onerous interpretive challenges for such dogs. Dog owners showing power-dominance conflicts and uncertainty about their ability to control social exchanges perceived as challenging their authority or showing signs of incipient household aggression may probe the dog with intentional and unintentional ambiguous signals to test its propensities, but in so doing only further agitate the dog and aggravate the problem. Low-grade reactive threats or growling prompted by ambiguous probes may cause the owner to punish the dog and thereby confirm the threat significance of ambiguous signals and increase the dog's reactivity and potential for releasing forceful autoprotective attacks toward similar social signals in the future. The repeated evocation and punishment of low-grade threats may systematically reduce the social trust (benefit of doubt) that normally inhibits reactive adjustments to ambiguous signals, causing the dog to become increasingly autoprotective and reactive when in doubt about the significance of social exchanges.

ONTOGENY AND REACTIVE BEHAVIOR

The process of autonomic attunement and behavioral integration appears to emerge early in life and is strongly influenced by a puppy's experiences prior to entering the home.

Antistress Neurobiology, Maternal Care, and Coping Style

Maternal care exerts several prominent effects on an offspring's ability to cope with social and environmental stressors in adulthood.

These behavioral effects are reflected in numerous neurobiological changes that facilitate antistress capacities. For example, maternal responsiveness, nursing position, grooming, and licking behavior are closely tied to the density of oxytocin receptors expressed in brain areas mediating social and maternal behavior (e.g., the lateral septum and medial preoptic area). Rodent mothers providing high levels of grooming and licking also show significantly higher oxytocin-receptor densities in areas of the brain that mediate alarm and reactive behavior (e.g., the central nucleus of the amygdala and the bed nucleus of the stria terminalis) (Champagne et al., 2001). Most interestingly, however, is the finding that the mother's pattern of grooming and licking appears to stimulate the expression of a similar pattern of oxytocin-receptor densities in her daughters, thereby programming a maternal style resembling her own. In addition to being better mothers, the offspring of competent mothers are significantly less fearful of novelty than are offspring cared for by mothers that provide less grooming and licking care (Caldji et al., 1998). These less reactive offspring show increased gamma-aminobutyric acid/benzodiazepine (GABA/BZ)-receptor densities in the lateral, basolateral, and central nuclei of the amygdala. In addition, offspring receiving quality maternal care show decreased corticotropin-releasing factor (CRF)-receptor expression in the locus coeruleus together with increased α_2-adrenoceptor densities, changes consistent with reduced emotional reactivity.

Mothers may also transmit antistress effects to their young via lactation. Offspring of mothers given water tainted with corticosterone show a significant reduction in serotonin (5-hydroxytryptamine or 5-HT) subtype 1A receptors in the hippocampus (Meerlo et al., 2001). The offspring appeared to cope with stressors in a more passive manner than did controls, a change that reflected reduced reactivity rather than inhibition due to anxiety. Although chronic exposure to excessive corticosterone is harmful, moderate levels of the hormone ingested during lactation appear to produce beneficial effects on an offspring's ability to cope with stress in adulthood. Affected animals show improved learning abilities, reduced fearfulness, and a higher density of glucocorticoid receptors in the hippocampus—a change consistent with enhanced hypothalamic-pituitary-adrenal (HPA)-system regulation (Catalani et al., 2000). These various findings support the hypothesis that maternal care may *program* emotional and behavioral responses to environmental and psychological stressors that alter an offspring's coping style, perhaps by modifying thresholds controlling the activation of the flight-fight system.

The distribution of 5-HT and glucocorticoid receptors traced out during infancy appears to play a profound role in determining a dog's relative ability to cope with social stressors in adulthood. Postnatal handling has been shown to reduce significantly the density of 5-HT$_2$ receptors expressed in the frontal cortex and the hippocampus of adult animals, while 5-HT turnover and the density of glucocorticoid receptors in the amygdala and hypothalamus are left unaffected (Smythe et al., 1994). The reduced expression of frontal 5-HT$_2$ receptors may have relevance with regard to the etiology of impulsive aggression in dogs. Recent neuroimaging studies performed by Peremans and colleagues (2003) have found that dogs showing impulsive aggression exhibit increased 5-HT$_{2A}$ receptor-binding potential localized in frontal cortical areas in comparison to nonaggressive dogs. They found no difference in the binding potential of 5-HT$_{2A}$ receptors expressed in subcortical areas between aggressive and nonaggressive dogs (see Stress, 5-HT$_{2A}$ Receptor Upregulation, and Aggression in Chapter 10). Also of interest are findings showing a close relationship between 5-HT and thyroid activity and infant stimulation. Meaney and colleagues (1987) showed that the distribution of 5-HT receptors fostered by neonatal handling depends on the activation of the pituitary-thyroid system and the release of triiodothyronine (T3). T3 stimulates the raphe bodies to release 5-HT into the ascending serotonergic system. 5-HT networks appear to guide the expression of cortical and hippocampal glucocorticoid receptors (Meaney et al., 2000). The early functional relationship

between thyroid and 5-HT in organizing the stress-management system underscores the important role that 5-HT plays in mediating allostasis. The close linkage between 5-HT and thyroid in the organization of stress circuits gives some credence to the combined use of serotonergic antidepressants with low-dose thyroid in the treatment of certain aggression problems (see *Stress, Thyroid Deficiency, Hypocortisolism, and Aggression*).

Parent-Offspring Conflict and Interactive Conflict

Trivers (1972) proposed that an inherent conflict between parents and offspring revolves around the giving and receiving of care and nurturance. The theory postulates that mothers are selected to provide enough care to ensure the survival of their young but without impairing their ability to reproduce and care for more offspring in the future, striking a balance referred to as *parental investment* (PI). In contrast, the offspring appear to be governed by an exploitative incentive to inveigle the mother into giving more care than she can provide without endangering her ability to produce and care for more young. The parent-offspring conflict is hypothesized to exert a potent and dynamic influence on the development of social behavior, prompting a variety of psychological and behavioral strategies for manipulating the mother into giving more care than her PI allows:

> How is the offspring to compete effectively with its parent? An offspring cannot fling its mother to the ground at will and nurse. Throughout the period of parental investment the offspring competes at a disadvantage. The offspring is smaller and less experienced than its parent, and its parent controls the resources at issue. Given this competitive disadvantage the offspring is expected to employ psychological rather than physical tactics ... It should attempt to induce more investment than the parent wishes to give. (Trivers, 1974:257)

The striving to induce the mother to give more care then her PI permits may be organized into analogous efforts to obtain from nature and others more than they are willing or able to give, as well. In fact, the dynamic related to the parent-offspring conflict may be embedded in many motivational processes driving the optimization of control over significant social and environmental events and resources. According to this hypothesis, the core active incentives—exploitation and power—governing purposive behavior are balanced and tempered by submissive ritualization that may originate in the appeasement and begging strategies shown toward the mother to squeeze more attention and care from her. These core incentives may be further tamed in the context of play with siblings and the acquisition of social codes based on fair play. Perhaps, even what the dog values as a reward and abhors as punishment can be traced to the mother's contingent provisioning or withholding of nurturance (e.g., social proximity, tactile stimulation, and appetitive gratification).

The manner in which the mother copes with the conflict and manages the manipulative efforts of her offspring to exploit her may exert a lasting effect on the way the puppy copes with limits and social conflict situations in adulthood. The hypothesis being posited here is that the conflictive dynamics between the puppy and mother may contribute to the mobilization of either an adaptive or a reactive coping style, depending on how the mother responds to the puppy's care-seeking behavior. Accordingly, strategies developed to cope with the threat of maternal punishment and the delay or denial of anticipated care (frustration) may anticipate the organization of passive modal strategies (e.g., hesitating and delaying). In addition, the dynamic balance of activity success and failure associated with parent-offspring conflict may play a prominent role in regulation of autonomic tone mediating the organization of secure, nervous, and insecure social and place attachments. The relative balance of success versus failure in a puppy's efforts to attain comfort and safety or to exploit the mother might impact significantly on how well the puppy copes with anxiety and frustration associated with interactive conflict within the home, potentially exerting a profound influence on the organization of impulsive and reactive behavior. Mothers that are excessively respon-

sive or unresponsive, punitive, or unpredictable in response to their offspring's care-seeking behavior may produce lasting developmental changes in canine personality development and capacity to integrate an adaptive coping style and concept of fairness. The good mother sets limits and manages conflict with her young in a constructive way, fostering a flirt-and-forbear/forgive (reconcile) orientation toward social conflict. Cognitive and emotional processing associated with parent-offspring conflict may contribute significantly to social engagement and shape tendencies toward a fair, exploitative, despotic, or an avoidant orientation toward others. Ideally, the transition from nursing and an exploitative dependency on the mother to a relationship based on affectionate submission, respect for limit, and ability to compromise sets the stage for the integration of harmonious relations in the home.

Maternal Mistreatment

Canine mothers exhibit significant variability in the way they cope with puppy care-seeking excesses. How the mother responds to demands for care depends on a huge array of variables, including allostatic load, available nutrition, the size of the litter, maternal experience, quality of maternal instincts, individual differences expressed in the behavior of the offspring, and the way the mother was cared for by her own mother. In addition to regurgitating for the puppies and providing them with solid food, the mother may cope with offspring care seeking by evading or shortening nursing or by leaving her young alone for longer periods. The mother may also assume ownership of the activity and set limits on it by means of a variety of overt tactics, including punishment. Highly competent canine mothers appear to make a deliberate effort to calm tensions and reduce conflict by means of gentle and slow movements. Rather than punishing her young, such mothers may block, nudge, or delicately muzzle her offspring to discourage unwelcome nursing while encouraging compromise. The mother appears to persuade her young to comply with a mild and affectionate approach rather than resorting to intimidation and coercion, but the most patient and competent mother is not above applying a sharp rebuke against an overly obtrusive offspring.

In contrast to the competent maternal behavior just described, Rheingold (1963) found that canine mothers showed a wide spectrum of species-typical agonistic behavior toward their offspring (e.g., growling; barking; baring teeth; inhibited biting around the head, neck, or muzzle; brief shaking; or using a paw to hold the puppy down or pouncing at it) to which the puppies reciprocated various passive-submission displays (e.g., yelping, backing, lowering and submitting, rolling over, or scampering away). Of the five mothers and litters studied, two mothers habitually punished their offspring: a brown sheltie and a cocker spaniel. These mothers were observed continuously from shortly after birth of the litters to week 9. From the period immediately preceding the onset of weaning and extending to week 9, maternal agonism was frequent and severe in these mothers. A beagle and a black sheltie were never observed to punish their offspring, perhaps only because observations of those dogs were stopped at days 29 and 19, respectively. A merle sheltie was observed to begin punishing her puppies shortly before being removed from the study at day 42, a time coinciding with the peak of punishing activities exhibited by the brown sheltie and the cocker. The brown sheltie was often found in the whelping box from which vantage she would threaten her puppies if they attempted to enter. The cocker made normal life impossible for her offspring, attacking them whenever they attempted to eat from wet mash pans, when they approached her, or even when facing in her direction while she ate. Both the brown sheltie and cocker spaniel were observed to punish their puppies several times during most of the 15-minute observation periods. In addition to being frequent and severe, the punishment was delivered on an inconsistent basis, perhaps inoculating their offspring with an emotionally reactive orientation to social limitations, a tendency toward forming nervous or insecure attachments, and a reactive autonomic tone and HPA-system

response to stress. Despite the harsh treatment received by the puppies, they continued to approach their intolerant mothers throughout the duration of the study:

> The pups persisted in trying to nurse, to make contact and to play with the mother. A cocker pup might flee from the mother's punishment, yelping and dragging its rear as though in pain, then, shortly, return to the activity. On the last day of observation [day 66], pups were still being punished upon approaching the mother, but they no longer tried to suckle.

> The pups' persistence should be weighed against the inconsistency of punishment, for the same act would be followed with punishment one moment but not the next. At times mothers seemed distracted by outside noises; at times they dozed. Then, especially, the brown Sheltie pups would try to enter the whelping box from the side or in back of the mother. Sometimes individual pups were indulged; the brown Sheltie, for example, occasionally permitted the runt of the litter to sleep in the box with her while the other pups were kept outside. (Rheingold, 1963:188)

Adverse stressors and insults taking place during exposure to an inconsistent, intolerant, and inimical mother, as in the case of these mothers, would likely install autonomic changes conducive to a coping style similar to her own and inoculate them with a tendency to form nervous or insecure attachments. Relevantly, Rheingold described the play behavior of these puppies as a "low frequency" activity. Play appears to serve a significant role in integrating secure social and place attachments and promoting autonomic balance (calm). Calcagnetti and Schechter (1992) found that rats given access to a play partner while in a place that they previously avoided showed a significant conditioned place preference toward that area as a result of playing there, spending nearly 200% more time in the area than before. Wilsson (1984) reported that puppies exposed to excessive inhibited biting in association with weaning were less willing to approach a passive handler. Also, the amount of growling received by the puppy was significantly correlated with a reduced willingness to fetch a ball, perhaps stemming from autonomic changes reducing its ability to play. After the aggressive mother was taken away at week 8, her offspring were described as "noisy and violent" (112), consistent with the possibility that conflictive interaction may have installed a reactive autonomic tone. The coincidence of weaning with dramatic autonomic shifts, as indexed by heart-rate changes (see *Play and Autonomic Attunement*), suggests that during this period the puppy may be especially vulnerable to integrate autonomic disturbances via maternal mistreatment, perhaps damaging the offspring's ability to form secure attachments and predisposing it to express a reactive coping style. The quality and quantity of play during this period may represent a useful marker or indicator of risk for reactive problems, since competent coping in response to agonistic challenges appears to depend on the autonomic attunement that play appears to provide (Van den Berg et al., 1999) (see *Play, Social Engagement, and Fair Play*).

Audience effects and observational learning might further contribute harm by inculcating social schemata consistent with an aggressive or avoidant social orientation (see *Maternal Influences on Secondary Socialization* in Volume 1, Chapter 2). According to this hypothesis, the mother's behavior toward sibling rivals in association with conflicts over significant objects, resources, or locations may rapidly organize schemata and behavioral scripts matched to the scenes enacted between the mother and rivals. During demonstrations, bystanders observing the interaction might be assumed to acquire social information derived from watching, listening, and processing the proxemic exchanges between the mother and rival siblings. These demonstrations between the mother and sibling rivals should be of considerable interest to bystanders. Combining the direct emotional experience of previous maternal punishment (conditioned arousal component), coupled with observations of siblings receiving maternal punishment, a variety of complex emotional and behavioral propensities may be schematically etched into the puppy's memory and organized into prepared behaviors ready for rapid acquisition later on in life. In adulthood, these prepared behaviors and propensities may

be enacted in response to situations resonating with emotional memories integrated in association with maternal punishment (see *Model/Rival Theory, Fair Play, and Sibling Hierarchy*).

Natal Environment and Autonomic Attunement

Subtle changes to rearing conditions may produce pronounced short-term and long-term modifications in a dog's capacity to cope with stress. For example, Wilsson and Sundgren (1998) found that changing the flooring material of the whelping box from cardboard to a soft piled blanket exerted a lasting effect on both puppy and adult temperament test scores, pointing to the important role of quality-of-life influences for mobilizing pronounced changes in behavior. The mere presence of a soft comfort object appears to contribute a positive regulatory influence on the development of autonomic tone. Puppies given a soft stuffed animal through week 4 showed less distress when they were left alone in a strange place with the comfort object than did puppies not provided such preexposure to the object (Marr, 1960). Marr (1964) also demonstrated that tactile, kinesthetic, and visual stimulation early in life alters the way puppies cope with emotionally provocative situations. As the result of being repeatedly petted, rocked back and forth, or exposed to a flashing light while facing a circular shape, 3-week-old puppies subsequently spent more time in close proximity with the shape and showed less emotional distress when tested alone with the shape at week 4 in comparison to nonstimulated controls. The stimulated puppies appear to have connected the circular shape with autonomic regulation incompatible with reactive emotional arousal. Marr's finding emphasizes the lasting subtle effects of early stimulation on the integration of sympathovagal tone with place attachments.

Appleby and colleagues (2002) have suggested an apparent linkage between natal environmental conditions and adult aggression and avoidance behavior in dogs. Questionnaire data provided by dog owners appear to indicate that puppies obtained from non-domestic sources (e.g., commercial kennel) may be more prone to exhibit certain forms of aggression and avoidance behavior than are puppies obtained from a home environment (e.g., backyard breeder). Dogs acquired from nondomestic sources appear to be at an increased risk of showing aggression toward unfamiliar persons, especially while at home. These dogs also showed more aggression while receiving veterinary examinations. A possible explanation for such a linkage may be an increased sensitivity among puppies reared under nondomestic conditions to aversive stimulation and restraint by a strange person in an unfamiliar place. No relationship was extracted between the type of natal environment and intrafamilial aggression, suggesting that the combination of social and environmental familiarity may reduce the risk of reactive behavior associated with adverse developmental influences, whereas a lack of social familiarity or nervous attachments may increase the risk of such behavior. Puppies obtained from nondomestic sources at week 8 or later showed significantly more fear-related behavior than did puppies obtained prior to week 8.

These findings are consistent with the notion that vulnerability for reactive behavior is organized early in life (before week 8), and that subsequent experiences may augment or diminish reactive tendencies. First impressions are lasting, especially so for puppies between weeks 8 and 10 (see *Learning and Trainability* in Volume 1, Chapter 3), a time when many young dogs are taken to the veterinary hospital for the first time. Early aversive or frightening experiences may establish lasting anxiety-evoking associations with the hospital environment. Stanford (1981) found that 60% of dogs entering a veterinary hospital showed signs of fear and urinated. When restrained, many of dogs (18%) were classified as "fear-biting." These dogs showed reactive vocalization, efforts to escape, and aggression; 17% of the dogs were described as showing a willing entrance and controllable demeanor, but still urinated. Remarkably, only 5% of the dogs were observed to enter willingly and did not urinate (N = 462).

These findings, combined with those of Appleby and colleagues, recommend that efforts be made to minimize young puppies' exposure to discomfort or frightening restraint (e.g., wobbly or noisy exam tables and scales) during veterinary visits, especially during the first few appointments. Puppies that show reactive tendencies during routine examinations should prompt appropriate counseling and referral to a cynopraxic therapist or trainer for supportive behavioral care.

HOUSEHOLD STRESS AND AGGRESSION

The adoption transition is often highly stressful for young puppies (see *Adoption and Stress* in Chapter 4)—stress that may be magnified by mishandling, manhandling, and excessive or inappropriate isolation and confinement (see *Dangers of Excessive Crate Confinement* in Chapter 2). Gantt (1944) observed that when dogs were moved from a farm or home environment to the increased confinement and reduced quality of life associated with the laboratory, they often underwent dramatic and persistent behavioral and emotional changes in the opposite directions of depression or hyperactivity, depending on their temperament and the balance of excitatory and inhibitory tendencies expressed. Excessive confinement within the home environment may increase behavioral reactivity in predisposed puppies. Although the effects of crate training and lengthy crate confinement and isolation on puppies within the home environment have not been studied, the preponderance of experimental evidence seems to suggest that stressful restraint, confinement, and isolation exert a problematic influence on a young animal's ability to cope with stress. Rats, for example, exposed for 21 days to 6 hours of daily restraint in a narrow wire-mesh tube in their home environment show significant changes in stress-related aggressive behavior toward cagemates (Wood et al., 2003). The experimenters found that the initial exposure to restraint had a sharply inhibitory effect on aggressive behavior toward cagemates; however, a trend toward increasing irritability and aggression became evident over the next several days and significant by day 14. Aggressiveness continued to increase through day 21. Over this same period, the unrestrained controls showed less aggressive behavior toward cagemates. Excessive confinement and isolation may increase allostatic load while decreasing a dog's ability to cope with stress constructively, impair its ability to cope with novelty and uncertainty, impede its ability to form secure attachments with family members and the home, and promote reactive behavior. Aside from the potential emotional harm and welfare concerns associated with excessive crate confinement and isolation, dogs that are confined in zinc-galvanized wire crates may ingest potentially toxic levels of zinc by chewing or licking the crate (Goicoa et al., 2002). Both the zinc coating as well as "white rust" are apparently toxic (Howard, 1992). Dogs exhibiting serious impulsive aggression have been found to show significantly higher concentrations of plasma zinc (1.69 ± 0.49 µg/ml) in comparison to nonaggressive dogs (0.76 ± 0.16 µg/ml) (Juhr et al., 2003).

There is a natural attraction that inclines dogs to follow human leaders, to engage in give-and-take exchanges, and to participate in cooperative projects. Such relationships are associated with emergent affection, trust, playfulness, and the integration of secure social attachments. Under the influences of leadership and nurturance, the dog copes with human control efforts by integrating a voluntary subordination strategy (VSS) and cooperative relations with the human leader; whereas, in situations in which subordination is displaced by subjugation and coercion, the dog may cope by mobilizing an involuntary subordination strategy (ISS), giving rise to significant interactive conflict and adversarial fallout (e.g., anxiety, irritability, intolerance, and resentment) (see *Involuntary Subordination and Canine Domestic Aggression* in Chapter 7). Secure attachments and an adaptive coping style are necessary for dogs to construct a belief or *illusion* that the world is safe, orderly, and responsive to autoinitiated control efforts. Conflictive attachment dynamics, perhaps originating in the mother-offspring relationship and perpetuated by domestic

social ambivalence and entrapment, may promote ambivalent (insecure/nervous) social and place attachments, incompetence, and a reactive coping style. These influences may diminish or eclipse the developing dog's ability to form a bias of safety to buffer nerves when exposed to sudden change or social novelty and to provide the confidence needed to organize competent social behavior under such adverse circumstances. Just as the mother's licking, nibbling, nudging, and affectionate attention toward her offspring appear to mediate an autonomic capacity to form secure social and place attachments in adulthood, supportive family interactions with the puppy may provide a protective influence against adverse developmental stressors, while helping to mobilize an affectionate and playful orientation toward social novelty, ambiguity, and unexpected change that is incompatible with reactive behavior.

LIVING SPACE, PROXEMIC RELATIONS, INATTENTIVENESS, AND AUTOPROTECTIVENESS

Just as the ideal canine mother exhibits a high degree of forbearance and consistency in the management of her offspring and their appetites, the human parent should set limits in the context of reward-based leadership and training. By emulating the mother's use of the least force and threat necessary to discourage obtrusive behavior, the cynopraxic trainer works to deflect and redirect competitive tensions into alternative outlets and avoids placing undue emphasis on punishment. Play and safe exposure to varied social and environmental stimuli at a young age are critical aspects of training dogs to respond confidently to unfamiliarity and uncertainty in adulthood. During interactive exposure, habituation and latent learning processes are constantly at work shaping competent sensorimotor gating and orienting functions. Habituation and latent learning provide a foundation for the organization of an adaptive coping style. Preventive-exposure training (PET) (see *Habituation, Sensitization, and Preventive-exposure Training* in Chapter 3) serves to transform the home and neighborhood into places perceived as safe and coherent while concurrent integrated compliance training (ICT) helps to transform sources of interactive conflict into opportunities for reward and play.

Interactive conflict typically develops around activities that are intrinsically gratifying to the dog but that are incompatible with domestic control interests. Social and environmental conditions perceived as punishing (unrewarding) or unsafe, coupled with interactive conflict, stress (i.e., state anxiety and anger), and inescapability, may serve to transform the security of the home into a place of anxiety, anger, and entrapment. The resulting interactive conflict and stress may trigger various reactive and coercive strategies by the owner to prevent or suppress the unwanted behavior. Most of these efforts are aimed at depriving the dog of freedom or forbidding it access to the house. Depriving the dog of freedom of movement and access to the home and interaction with family members by excessive restraint or abusive training practices may temporarily empower the frustrated owner with an illusion of mastery but may actually do significant harm to the bond and degrade the dog's quality of life, as well as set the stage for more serious adjustment problems. Instead of learning how to predict and control significant events competently while learning to adapt and cope, the socially antagonized and entrapped dog may withdraw, become marginalized, and establish trigger *safe* areas within the home reserved for itself and preferred others, but that are defended aggressively against the intrusion of unwelcome others.

According to the foregoing hypothesis, many forms of intrafamilial aggression may be better understood and treated as originating from proxemic autoprotective incentives rather then hierarchical challenges or threats to the dog's perception of rank. Such aggressive episodes frequently occur without apparent provocation while the dog is resting in a favorite place or while in a location associated with or containing a prized object. Some of these dogs may also show strong threat behavior toward certain family members when the dogs are approached while inside a crate. The

victim's mere presence or intrusion into a certain location may disturb the dog's mood and trigger impulsive autoprotective adjustments. According to a proxemic analysis, such attacks may be provoked by the victim's unwelcome intrusion into an intimate zone of comfort and safety in the absence of appropriate social affiliation or attraction. In some cases, dogs may threaten or attack in response to violations of social codes associated with interference while sleeping or resting or when in possession of objects (e.g., rights of first possession). In other cases, the dog's attachment to the place may be stronger than its attachment to the family member; in other cases, the family member may actively *repulse* the dog. While ensconced in such trigger areas, such dogs may permit access to certain family members with whom they appear to be strongly attached, while threatening or attacking other family members with little warning if they engage in intimate proxemic behaviors (e.g., pet, hug, cuddle, or pick up). The occurrence of aggression around locations providing the dog with emotional regulation conducive to comfort and safety (insecure place attachments), together with a state of reduced attention and unwelcome proxemic interactions, set the stage for a rapid vagal shift from inhibitory to excitatory arousal. However, instead of shifting back to a parasympathetic mode of relaxation, the impulsive aggressor may rapidly escalate into a catastrophic surge of sympathetic arousal and the phasic disinhibition of aggressive impulse. These observations suggest that impulsive aggression of this type may stem from regulatory attention and impulse-control disturbances affecting vagal tone. In general, dogs fitting this description rarely go out of their way to bite and typically bite only when approached or disturbed while in specific places associated with comfort and safety.

Although a subgroup of these dogs appears to be selective with respect to preferred targets and tends to focus attacks on family members, the notion that such dogs attack only household members is dubious, since many of these dogs will also attack nonfamilial visitors who violate defended trigger areas. Gershman and colleagues (1994) found that dogs with a history of nipping or biting directed against family members were just as likely to attack nonfamily members. The tolerance that visitors and persons away from home appear to obtain, at least temporarily, is hypothesized to stem from the increased attention and interest that social novelty evokes in such dogs. Focused attention and social exploratory behavior is hypothesized to increase vagal tone, making catastrophic or explosive shifts of sympathetic arousal less likely to occur toward unfamiliar persons. The attentional disengagement and tuning out that impair impulse control and reduce sympathovagal tone appear to develop in association with three patterns of social interaction. Under the constraints of entrapment, dogs may cope with inescapable social anxiety and ambivalence produced by particular family members by actively ignoring them, a phenomenon referred to as *defensive inattentiveness*. The dog may also withdraw attention from family members that pay it little or no attention, a process of disengagement referred to as *reactive inattentiveness*. Defensive and reactive inattentiveness are closely associated with the withdrawal of social engagement, depersonalization, and the establishment of rigid social relations and roles.

Attentional and impulse-control processes are also adversely affected by social interaction that lacks consistency and relevance, causing the dog to actively disengage attentional resources from family members whose communicative behavior is irrelevant to the occurrence or nonoccurrence of significant events. Dogs also appear to withdraw attention and tune out from persons lacking competent leadership qualities. Family members who seek to establish control over the dog but who are unsure of their ability and proceed haphazardly or coercively (incompetently) may project ambiguity and mixed messages that are difficult for the dog to sort out and match with appropriate emotional establishing operations and response selections. Such ambiguity in the communication style of insecure leaders plays a prominent role in the development of social ambivalence and may help to explain the dog's aggressive response to seemingly benign signals. Proxemic signals given

by an insecure or insincere leader may communicate a negative message despite a facade of friendly intent, perhaps expressing the powerless family member's underlying disappointment and resentment at failing to integrate secure affiliative power relations with the dog. The disengagement of attention resources from family members may impair socialization or reverse the effects of socialization, causing the dog to view family members as being increasingly unfamiliar via a process of depersonalization. According to cynopraxic theory, attention and impulse control are interdependent constructs that are closely integrated and attuned with autonomic processing. Orienting, attending, exploring, and playing activities serve to mediate enhanced familiarity, augmented sympathovagal regulation, and impulse control. In contrast, attentional disengagement and social avoidance result in decreased sympathovagal regulation, increased emotional reactivity, and lowered flight-fight thresholds. As the result of attentional disengagement, the approach of family members may trigger conditioned sympathoexcitatory shifts in autonomic arousal associated with interference and interactive conflict that have resulted in loss and risk in the past. The dog's efforts to ignore or tune out the person may serve only to relinquish impulse control and impair vagal control, perhaps via the activation of GABAergic neurons by arginine vasopressin (AVP) circuits at the level of the brainstem (Wang et al., 2002), resulting in the reduction of parasympathetic tone and generating a permissive state conducive to rapid sympathetic arousal and catastrophic autoprotective responses. Social ambivalence and entrapment dynamics may cause such dogs to defend the trigger area as an escape-to-safety refuge and default point of no return.

SOCIAL SPACES, FRAMES, AND ZONES

The living space or home range refers to the places routinely occupied or used by the dog and shared with others in the pursuit of everyday interests and reward. The living space of the home and surroundings consists of local and global frames, spaces, and zones defined by individual attraction-repulsion dynamics and proxemic relations extending from the intimate safe center and moving outward to the unfamiliar and uncertain edge. Within the context of the home range itself, artificial global (e.g., walls and fences) and local (e.g. windows, doors, gates, and crates) frames define the spatial and physical contexts that set the stage for scripted social *scenes* or avoiding them (e.g., hiding behavior). The living space is framed into several social spaces distinguished by functional significance with respect to the sort of proxemic exchanges that the dog enjoys, tolerates, or might forbid depending on attraction, familiarity, and trust. Doors and walls artificially frame the home, thereby setting off intimate and safe spaces exclusive for use by family members to hide, rest, and obtain comfort (familial space), whereas fences globally frame the property and define an open and familiar space used to explore, play, and meet others (familiar space). The leash may be conceived of as framing a free-floating *intimate zone* between the handler and the dog and extending into the surroundings, representing variable degrees of familiarity and safety (transitional space). A satellite space containing the free-floating intimate zone is established wherever the handler and dog interact with each other. Finally, a training space is formed as the result of establishing a default hierarchy and leader-follower bond in association with limits set on pulling into the leash, jumping up, and biting on hands and clothing.

Most family dogs appear to treat visitors either as absentee pack members (insiders) deserving affectionate recognition or as intruding strangers (outsiders) warranting alarm and suspicion. Dogs that treat guests as part of an extended family-pack are typically highly demonstrative, exhibiting a high degree of social excitement and eagerness to make contact with people and other dogs; such dogs show minimal differentiation with respect to social space definition and represent a low risk of intrafamilial or extrafamilial aggression. On the other hand, dogs viewing visitors as outsiders often continue to exhibit a significant amount of wariness and aggres-

sive readiness even after becoming thoroughly familiar with a visitor. Such a dog may accept and reciprocate friendly contact with familiar outsiders while in the yard but become reactive if they attempt to enter the house (violation of the familial space), especially if they are unattended by a family member. Also, such a dog may tolerate the approach of unfamiliar outsiders when away from home with a family member, but become strongly aroused if an unfamiliar outsider enters the yard unannounced (violation of the familiar space). Dogs combining a reactive vigilance for social novelty and sudden change (stimulation-seeking deficit), a propensity to discriminate aggressively between outsiders and insiders irrespective of familiarity, and a relatively low-fight threshold (trait anger) appear to be most prone to express a rigid watchdog script and extrafamilial aggression (see *Flexible versus Rigid Watchdog Scripts*).

NOVELTY, SUDDEN CHANGE, AND REACTIVE ADJUSTMENTS

Escape to Safety versus Escape from Danger

Under natural conditions, the activation of phylogenetic survival modes mobilize drives that educe (not elicit) adaptive behavior, causing animals to strive against adversity and to take risks likely to improve their ability to survive and reproduce. For many animals, the neophobic stress evoked by unfamiliar stimuli and situations is overcome by forming a base of familiar and secure place and social attachments from where they can venture into unfamiliar surroundings by means of furtive sallies or more adventuresome journeys, depending on their ability to cope with uncertainty and risk. Knowing that they can scurry back into a hole or climb up a tree or fly away appears to increase the confidence of many animals to approach and explore promising novel objects. In any case, most animals appear to treat the exploration of novel objects and unfamiliar places as a source of risk and only take such risks to obtain a biologically significant advantage or reward. In nature, however, danger is at every turn and one cannot escape from its ubiquity; there are two primary solutions: (1) escape to the security of the familiar and safe place or (2) confront the threat. Under threatening conditions perceived as inescapable with no hope of reaching safety, autoprotective panic or tonic immobility (behavioral helplessness) may ensue. Both of these reactive strategies to inescapable stressors are biologically organized to mediate adjustments to catastrophic situations where an escape to safety is blocked, leaving the animal vulnerable to extreme danger.

When startled and caused to flee, animals *escape to safety*; they do not merely *escape from danger*. This distinction is vital for understanding avoidance learning and how dogs learn to cope with novelty and danger. The fleeing animal is not stressed by the novel or fear-evoking stimulus per se but becomes distressed only if its ability to detect the threat is obstructed (i.e., reduced predictability) or its escape to safety is impeded or blocked (i.e., reduced controllability). If an animal can successfully dodge danger and escape to a secure and familiar place, it may slowly recover and return to the spot it had fled, taking significant predatory risks for the sake of increased food intake (Arenz and Leger, 1999). The validity of this notion of trade-off and flight to safety can be observed in the persistent escape and approach behavior of squirrels exploiting a birdfeeder; despite being repeatedly chased away by a dog and only narrowly escaping its teeth, a persistent squirrel does not appear to be rapidly deterred by the danger from returning to the feeder, nor does it show much evidence of fear while there. In fact, with every successful escape, the squirrel's confidence appears to grow, causing it to linger longer at the feeder before dashing off. The squirrel may even increase the frequency of its visits to the feeder, perhaps under the synergistic effects of appetitive reward and the reward of successful escape/avoidance. However, if the accustomed escape route is changed or blocked, forcing it to delay or take a detour, the squirrel will show a significant change in behavior as the result of the hindrance slowing its escape to safety. Subsequent to such events, the squirrel appears to take more time before returning to the feeder (if returning at all), becomes more vigilant

while at the feeder (stopping to look and listen more often), and wastes no time in getting away from the feeder as soon as it detects the dog heading its way. Young squirrels appear to show far less vigilance than adult squirrels, evident from birdfeeder observations and also in the sluggish way in which they respond to other threats (e.g., cars). Arenz and Leger (2000) found that vigilance levels appear to be closely related to appetitive motivation and physical state, with squirrels fed a high-energy food (HEF) showing more vigilance than those fed a low-energy food (LEF). As the HEF squirrels matured, they showed greater body mass and were more vigilant than the LEF squirrels, suggesting that the malnourished and smaller LEFs were willing to take greater risks by reducing antipredator vigilance for the sake of increased food intake. Since vigilance is incompatible with eating, as the squirrel becomes increasingly vigilant and uncertain of its ability to escape the feeder location successfully, the tradeoff ought to become less attractive, with the squirrel gradually showing an escape-from-danger strategy and avoidance of the birdfeeder rather than an escape-to-safety strategy and approach to the birdfeeder.

The escape and avoidance behavior of squirrels appears to agree with experimental findings showing that safety functions as a reward in the acquisition of avoidance learning (see *Safety Signal Hypothesis* in Volume 1, Chapter 8). The acquisition of avoidance behavior varies proportionately to the relative length of time that an animal is exposed to danger and safety (Cándido et al., 2002). Under conditions in which the danger period is held constant, avoidance learning is slower when successful responses are followed by brief safety and more rapid when avoidance responses are followed by a longer period of safety (Cándido et al., 1989). If avoidance was acquired primarily as the result of escape from danger, then the relative duration spent in safety should be of little importance to the speed of acquisition, since the primary reinforcing event occurs at the moment of escape. As such, the safe situation need only confirm that a successful escape or avoidance response had occurred—information that should be of greatest value at the moment the animal enters the safety box. An additional experiment varied the length of the danger period while keeping the length of the safety period constant. The results indicated that the acquisition of avoidance was accelerated if exposure to a dangerous situation was brief before the warning signal and shock were delivered, whereas acquisition slowed down if the time spent in danger was increased, causing a delay in the warning and shock. If escape from danger was the primary incentive underlying such avoidance learning, one would expect an opposite relation to prevail; that is, the longer the animal remained in danger, its motivation to escape should increase and thereby accelerate avoidance learning.

The pattern of avoidance learning just described is consistent with the notion that danger may function as a discriminative stimulus for an escape-to-safety response, whereas exposure to a lengthier period in the danger box may facilitate habituation and reduce the associative linkage between the box context and the postponed aversive event; that is, the danger box gradually becomes a safe box. The foregoing findings are consistent with an opposite extrapolation concerning the extinction of avoidance learning; namely, brief exposure to preevent danger followed by brief exposure to safety may exert a stronger influence on the disconfirmation of avoidance learning and the integration of abolishing operations than do lengthier periods of preevent danger followed by long periods of safety. According to this hypothesis, massed trials (brief danger > no aversive event > brief safety) should be transiently more effective than spaced trials (lengthy danger > no aversive event > lengthy safety) for mediating extinction, whereas, brief exposure to danger in anticipation of the aversive event followed by lengthy exposure to safety should produce the strongest avoidance learning. Consequently, repeated and massed exposure trials should work better to extinguish active-avoidance behavior, at least initially, whereas longer exposures to the danger situation followed by lengthy periods of subsequent safety appear to help habituate aversive contextual associations while consolidating incompatible expectancies

predicting safety from the aversive event. Recent experimental work by Cain and colleagues (2003) supports the hypothesis that massed trials of extinction followed by spaced trials of consolidation training represent a more effective strategy for reducing fearful associations and avoidance than the converse strategy, but also see Martasian and Smith (1993) for variations affecting lengthy exposure versus distributed trials of response prevention.

Coping with Novelty and the Escape-to-Safety Hypothesis

The way in which mice cope with novelty also appears to support the escape-to-safety hypothesis. Mice are often described as being neophobic, but Misslin and Cigrang (1986) have reported that anxiety or fearfulness in response to novelty depends on how the novel object is presented. In comparison to mice that are physically placed into a novel situation and prevented from escaping to a familiar place, mice that are allowed to regulate how and when they approach and explore a novel situation from the vantage of a familiar place show little evidence of autonomic distress. Similarly, piglets cope with novelty by scampering as a group between familiar and unfamiliar areas, suggesting that the behavior may be a form of group play organized to enable the animals to explore novel areas and objects (Wood-Gush and Vestergaard, 1991). MacDonald (1987) found that wolf pups show significant individual differences in the way they enter into and explore an unfamiliar place. Among the pups studied, one showed a high level of confidence and willingness to enter an unfamiliar arena and explore novel objects (novelty seeking), while the others showed variable amounts of hesitation or reluctance (harm avoidance). The confident or leader pup appeared to facilitate other less confident pups to follow and approach novel objects, while fearful pups remained inside the start area. The way piglets and wolf pups explore and cope with novelty may reflect species-typical differences in the organization and function of their respective social hierarchies and the strategies that they use to hunt and exploit environmental resources (Brown, 1966). For example, among field mice living in a natural habitat, social rank is closely correlated with differences affecting home-range exploratory behavior. Dominant mice range farther and explore the home range with greater confidence than subordinate mice. Subordinate mice were observed to stay out of the way of dominant mice and suspend object explorations if the dominant mouse was nearby. Among puppies, inappropriate punishment associated with house training may significantly alter their exploratory behavior and ability to cope with novel situations. In comparison to puppies trained with petting and food, puppies trained by blowing a puff of air into their ear or by rapping them with a rubber hose showed longer latencies to enter an unfamiliar area and explored by covering shorter distances at a time, suggesting increased tentativeness and anxiety (Matysiak et al., 1973).

In MacDonald's study, the leader pup was found to be the most successful of the group in its ability to control the bone in free-for-all dominance tests. The leader pup also exhibited the greatest confidence in response to the approach of a threatening familiar person opening and closing an umbrella. Pups that showed the greatest fearfulness toward the unfamiliar situation, refusing to enter the arena on their own or with the leader pup, exhibited the least fear toward a human stranger, whereas the leader pup showed the greatest fear toward the stranger. These findings suggest that there exist complicated relationships between social attraction and fear, nonsocial novelty seeking and harm avoidance, and dominance. In particular, an inverse relationship appears to exits between a fear of unfamiliar settings and things and a fear of unfamiliar persons. The relationship between social dominance and leadership in coping with unfamiliar situations and novel objects underscores the importance of leadership for facilitating exploration and learning. The follower/submissive traits mediating social subordination appear to be relatively independent, with the following being related to a fear of novelty and high social attraction and relative fearlessness, whereas submission is related

to an inability to compete successfully over prized objects, perhaps as the result of being handicapped by a fear of unfamiliar circumstances. Wright (1980) reported a similar independence between competitive success and social dominance among German shepherd puppies. Like wolf pups, competitive success in the bone test is strongly associated with novelty seeking, but successful control over the bone does not necessarily predict social dominance (i.e., the ability to assert control over the behavior of littermates). Success in competition appears to reflect differences in motivation to possess and control the object (e.g., low-reward and high-reward incentive) and an ability to cope effectively under unfamiliar circumstances. One might extrapolate and predict that dogs exhibiting a high-reward incentive and history of competitive success, a low fear of unfamiliar places and novel objects, a high attraction toward familiar persons, and a high reactivity toward strangers would tend toward complete dominance, whereas dogs exhibiting a low-reward incentive and history of competitive loss, a high fear of novelty, and a high attraction toward unfamiliar and familiar persons would tend toward complete submission and dependency. Further, a history of competitive success, novelty seeking, and a reactive orientation toward strangers may predispose dogs toward social integration and extrafamilial aggression, whereas dogs with a history of competitive success, harm avoidance (bias for signals of punishment), dependency, and an attraction for strangers may be predisposed toward intrafamilial aggression and dispersal.

COLLICULAR-PERIAQUEDUCTAL GRAY PATHWAYS AND REACTIVE ADJUSTMENTS

A subcortical pathway that might mediate sympathoexcitatory arousal in response to sensory input may originate in preattentive nonhabituating or slow-to-habituate collicular-periaqueductal gray (PAG) circuits. The superior colliculus (SC), an ancient midbrain structure located near the PAG, plays a central role in numerous integrative sensorimotor functions (e.g., prepulse inhibition) associated with orienting behavior and rapid preemptive adjustments to expected and unexpected sensory events (*see Orienting, Preattentive Sensory Processing, and Visual Acuity*). Within the SC, multimodal cells responsive to visual, auditory, and tactile stimuli serve to map auditory and tactile inputs into a visuospatial coordinate system. The sensory maps represented in the SC are linked with motor maps that control involuntary eye movements and rapid preparatory motor adjustments (Dean et al., 1989). Under the influence of highly stimulating and disorderly environments, these sensorimotor processing functions may become sensitized, disorganized, and reactive. Pathways sensitized at the level of the deep SC and PAG appear to be of a nonhabituating type, perhaps due to inaccessibility by regulatory cortical networks needed to exert inhibitory control (King, 1999).

Inescapable events occurring unpredictably may be particularly prone to produce such reactive nonhabituating elaborations (e.g., noncontingent punishment), since they establish connections independent of predictive control expectancies and are perceived as inescapable. The unexpected occurrence of inescapable multisensory events involving visual, auditory, and tactile stimuli may trigger a summative effect that entrains nonhabituating reactions to the evoking stimuli present in the multisensory traumatic event. As a result of inescapability, the threat-arousing event may escalate to a defensive attack or panic, thereby integrating a deep subcortical nonhabituating circuit mediating reactive arousal and aggression. Consistent with the collicular-PAG hypothesis, the deep layers of the SC have been implicated in the expression of audiogenic "wild running" seizures resembling panic (Faingold and Randall, 1999), nonhabituating escape reactivity in response to repeated stimulation of the SC (King, 1999), and defensive behavior (Dean et al., 1989; Dringenberg et al., 2003). Stimulation of the SC via the optic nerve appears to mediate a rapid increase in blood pressure and heart rate (Cheng et al., 2001). More significantly, such stimulation also inhibits postevent vagal bradycardia—a state of sympathetic arousal consistent with the sustained

activation of the flight-fight system. The SC probably contains phylogenetically conserved fields or submaps that mediate a preference for sudden change (e.g., sudden movement, looming overhead movement, loud noise, or striking/restraining actions against the body) and evoke phylogenetically prepared emergency adjustments to threatening stimuli (Westby et al., 1990). Studies investigating the electrical and chemical stimulation of the SC suggest that the area may initiate emergency motor activity and defensive behavior, perhaps involving the participation of the PAG (see Dringenberg et al., 2003). Interestingly, serotonin (5-HT) appears to exert a generalized inhibitory effect over the SC and PAG, suggesting that serotonergic medications may be particularly helpful in the treatment of reactive behavior stemming from dysregulation at the level of the SC and the PAG. Since the SC appears to play an important role in the mediation of prepulse inhibition of auditory startle (Fendt et al., 2001), dogs exhibiting reactive problems organized at the level of the collicular-PAG pathway may show sensorimotor-gating disturbances reducing prepulse inhibition to visual, auditory, and tactile startle events. Prepulse inhibition tests may be useful for identifying and differentiating such problems.

ORIENTING, PREATTENTIVE SENSORY PROCESSING, AND VISUAL ACUITY

The way dogs respond to fast-moving objects is probably strongly influenced by cognitive and preattentive negativity/positivity biases. The functional differentiation of cortical and subcortical processing of visual input may have significant implications with regard to how a dog responds to highly salient visual input associated with rapid movement and sudden change. Visual signals projecting from motion-sensitive receptor ganglions organized in the peripheral retina are relayed by dedicated pathways to the SC, where they undergo excitatory and inhibitory processing in preparation for the production of an orienting response or inhibition (habituation). Saccadic eye movements precede the orienting response via a *target arc* formed between the sensory event and the frontal eye field located in the prefrontal cortex. Both the prefrontal cortex and the SC establish connections with premotor and motor nuclei in brainstem, which produce the motor signals that generate reflexive eye movements and orienting responses in anticipation of more complex behavioral adjustments.

Salient sensory input capturing attention is processed competitively based on species-typical significance and attractive/aversive (hedonic) value, with the vast majority of potential sensory events passing without notice. Out of the chaotic multitude of potential stimuli, the evocation of an orienting response signifies a selective organizing process narrowing possibility down to one orienting event and action at a time. Consequently, a sensory event may produce a saccadic alert, cause an orienting response, evoke a flinch, or release complex behavioral adjustments associated with surprise and startle (e.g., approach or avoidance). The process of selecting an appropriate response and suppressing all other responses to novelty (surprise) and sudden change (startle) is an important function of competent sensorimotor processing localized at the level of the SC and closely allied structures. As such, the SC appears to play an integrative role in organizing selective attention and sensorimotor-gating functions (e.g., prepulse inhibition) (Fendt et al., 2001), as well as mediating the expression of behavior operating under the influence of prediction-control expectancies. The SC encodes visual, auditory, and tactile sensations into multisensory maps in accordance with a visuospatial coordinate system. The resulting multisensory relations and fields are coordinated with motor reference points that initiate and guide orienting movement or complex adjustments toward sources of stimulation via the inhibitory and excitatory influences of the basal ganglia and the cerebellum (Niemi-Junkola and Westby, 2000).

In addition to conspicuous attractive and aversive events, positive and negative prediction error may increase eye movements and attentional focus on stimuli relevant to the refinement of prediction-control expectancies

and the calibration of emotional establishing operations (Ikeda and Hikosaka, 2003). Prediction mismatches resulting in disappointment, threat, startle, or surprise intensify attention, evoke autonomic changes and shifts in cardiovascular activity, generate anxiety and frustration in association with behavioral conflict, and other emotional changes (e.g., anger and fear) congruent with the significance and the degree of deviation from the expected norm. These attention-activating signals enable dogs to adjust proactively and preemptively to predicted events. In reactive dogs, a preemptive and nonhabituating vigilance and anxiety bias may overshadow the acquisition of more positive expectancies toward social novelty and sudden change. Hypervigilant scanning appears to be preferentially dedicated to the detection of social objects, which are preemptively represented as potential threats (anxiety/threat bias). Vigilant scanning for social objects under an anxiety bias may essentially blind the dog to the recognition of safe social objects, thereby blocking learning that might enable it to discriminate nonthreatening social objects from threatening ones.

The dog's reactivity toward fast-moving and still objects may be linked to individual differences affecting visual acuity and discrimination ability. In addition to the influence of retinal variations on vision (e.g., size and complexity of the visual streak and central area) (see *Retina* in Volume 1, Chapter 4), dogs vary considerably in their ability to process visual information due to other causes. For example, to see clearly, the object image must be focused on the retina—not behind or in front of it, as in farsightedness and nearsightedness. One study examining the eyesight of German shepherds and Rottweilers found that more than half of the dogs tested were nearsighted (Murphy et al., 1992). Nearsightedness impairs a dog's ability to see objects detected at the *alert distance*, perhaps predisposing such dogs to respond to such events as intrinsically ambiguous and uncertain. With respect to objects that are located nearby within the *startle distance*, a dog's ability to form accurate retinal images rapidly decreases as the object moves within 20 to 13 inches away from the retina; objects (e.g., a child's face) viewed at a point closer than this focusing range may be blurred and require other senses to facilitate recognition (e.g., olfaction, hearing, and touch) (Miller and Murphy, 1995). Dogs expressing a sparsely enervated central area may be especially impaired in their ability to recognize nearby faces. Dogs with poor vision may rely on established expectancy biases to process the uncertain events, resulting in friendly acceptance or possibly a bite in the face. Casual tests (e.g., dropping small treats on the ground, throwing a ball, or tossing a toy or treat for the dog to catch) can give the trainer a rough idea of visual function; however, a veterinary ophthalmic examination should be performed in dogs suspected of exhibiting a possible visual impairment in association with reactive behavior.

SOCIAL ENGAGEMENT AND ATTUNEMENT

According to Porges (2001), the visual communicative facial and head movements that are exchanged during social engagement are mediated by a network of cranial nerves operating under the regulatory control of corticobulbar pathways and special visceral efferents originating in the ventral vagal complex (VVC). The VVC is a relatively recent mammalian adaptation, enabling social animals to match autonomic arousal levels to complex social exchanges and transactions. The VVC consists of the myelinated vagus nerve, the nucleus ambiguous, and the source nuclei of the social engagement system (SES). Prosocial interaction perceived as safe appears to activate the mammalian SES, producing a lowered heart rate and a general calming effect, whereas threatening or challenging social exchanges result in the retraction of the SES and the activation of disengagement or confrontational systems.

Whereas wiggle dancing and animated tail wagging are indicative of social confidence and friendliness, a lowered tail held stiffly between the legs indicates a state of apprehension and reserve. Similarly, an elevated head position is indicative of an excited and bright mood, whereas a lowered head position or *hangdog* look is associated with a dark mood (dysthymia). These sorts of kinesic indicators of emotion and mood combine in almost endless ways to communicate a wide range of social messages while mediating autonomic attunement or misattunement. The differential showing and concealment of the white of the eyes and teeth appears to be used by dogs to convey a wide range of signals while modulating social stress (see DeVries, 2003). Many of these signals are extremely subtle and brief and may pass unnoticed (e.g., winking) but may nevertheless exert variable antistress and autonomic attunement effects. For example, cow-eyed gazing in which the white of the eye is slightly shown in association with bright glistening eyes appears to signify contented and focused affection, whereas exposure of large portions of white with anxious staring and nose licking appears to reflect a highly stressful state. Fang flashing (a quick and subtle expression of social anxiety in which a fang is briefly bared) usually anticipates uneventful and nonthreatening *cutoff* transitions, whereas baring of the teeth into a steady agonistic pucker obviously conveys a significantly different message. Numerous subtle licks and slurps, grunts and sighs, or chomping or clacking noises, especially at the conclusion of certain yawns, appear to signify frustration at waiting or other delays. The steady expiration that occurs when a dog growls may exert a vagal braking effect on autonomic arousal that permits the target to move away safely, whereas the extended expirations associated with howling or whining may stabilize autonomic arousal and enable the dog to cope with confinement or restraint preventing it from gaining access to the attachment object while signaling the attachment object to come to its rescue.

Many of these social behaviors and displays appear to be used in coping with domestic interactive stress with the apparent goal of integrating social relations and attachments conducive to autonomic regulation. In contrast to constructive social exchanges, dogs showing social signals signifying a serious intent to attack, thereby precluding or terminating attachment relations, show a loss of facial expressiveness and warmth, exhibiting a deadpan look of utter seriousness and determined resolve, backed by a steady and unflinching stare that locks on the target in an utter readiness to attack (Figure 8.1). In contrast to the flat, expressionless appearance of dogs preparing to attack, dogs prepared to engage in friendly social behavior express their intent with an invigorated and sustained attention (e.g., eye contact and social head tilt), intensified social engagement (e.g., jumping up), or displays aimed at evoking play (e.g., play bow and face). These various social behaviors are mediated in association with preemptive and preparatory arousal that reflects varying degrees of sympathovagal balance or imbalance and allostatic load resulting from attachment dynamics.

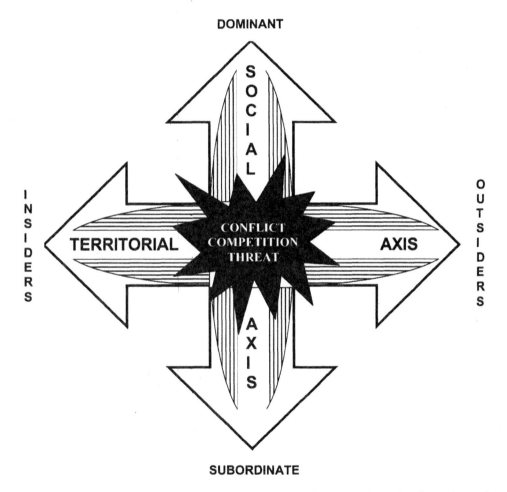

FIG. 8.1. Dominance hierarchy and territory serve complementary functions with regard to the regulation of aggression between conspecifics. The social distance between group members is achieved by means of vertical, hierarchical spacing via the establishment of social rank. Territory, on the other hand, defines the horizontal, physical space existing between competing groups. Whereas the dominance hierarchy is concerned with the regulation of aggression between group members, territory limits hostilities between members of competing groups. As a result, social dominance and territorial imperatives appear to share a common functional axis based on the need to establish cooperative group activity and to promote peaceful coexistence between neighboring conspecific groups.

The social head tilt is a distinctive canine social display of considerable interest. The social head tilt most often occurs in situations involving anticipatory excitement and intensified interest in the significance of the owner's vocalizations. Socially apprehensive and reactive dogs do not appear to exhibit the head-tilt response to human vocalization and generally show reduced capacities for sustained eye contact and other activities requiring social attention skills. Francis Barraud's famous painting, *His Master's Voice*, Nipper the dog is captured with his head cocked to the side in a rapt moment of looking intently into the horn of a phonograph. The action of tilting the head appears to be integrated at the level of source nuclei in the nucleus ambiguus that control the muscles of the middle ear and various expressive facial and head movements used to initiate and sustain social engagement (Porges, 2001). The middle-ear muscles are hypothesized to aid in extracting useful acoustic information from complex sources of auditory stimulation. The neural control of the middle-ear muscles is also linked with the regulation of facial expression, gaze, and vocalization. When the dog tilts its head, it may be attempting to concentrate on vocal sounds to identify familiar words and intonations associated with some anticipated activity. Gazing and talking to a dog in a manner that evokes a head tilt exerts a strong activating effect on the canine SES. The head-tilting behavior appears to be most robust in cases where the dog shows excitement and anticipation about something being said, suggesting the possibility that the head tilt may serve to help modulate arousal in situations of building anticipation and excitement. Sustained attention and evocation of head tilting, social gazing, talking, and other expressive movements of the face and head may exert a highly desirable invigorating effect on the SES while enhancing parasympathetic regulation over impulsive arousal. The intensified social gaze and attention associated with the head-tilt response should receive careful study as a conduit for social learning and the integration of secure attachments and autonomic attunement.

OXYTOCIN, ARGININE VASOPRESSIN, AND AUTONOMIC ATTUNEMENT

Consistent with the autonomic regulatory function of social communication and engagement, oxytocin and AVP appear to play important roles in assessing the relative safety or danger posed by social situations. The social recognition and calming effects mediated by oxytocin probably play a central role in activating the VVC, promoting social engagement and attachment, and supporting group cohesiveness. Conversely, AVP may promote a bias of social anxiety and danger, especially when its release is triggered by ambiguous or uncertain situations in association with CRF while social repulsion or nervous social attachments are being mediated. A study involving humans is interesting with respect to a possible role of AVP in the discrimination of ambivalent social facial expressions (Thompson et al., 2004). Experimental and control subjects showed little change in their attentional or autonomic responses when shown photographs of neutral, happy, or angry facial expressions; however, subjects given nasal AVP showed a significant change in the activity of the corrugator muscle in response to neutral facial expressions. The corrugator muscle, located above the brow, is involved in the expression of anger. The authors suggest that the increased corrugator activity may indicate that AVP mediates an aggressive bias in response to neutral and ambiguous social facial expressions. In contrast, oxytocin appears to mediate an antistress bias of anticipated comfort and safety when exposed to social ambiguity and uncertainty (Windle et al., 1997; Uvnäs-Moberg, 1998).

AVP and oxytocin play important regulatory roles in the adaptive attunement of cardiovascular function to environmental and social threats and challenges. Central oxytocin mediates a slowing of the heart rate by increasing vagal tone via projections to the dorsal motor nucleus of the vagus (DMV), whereas AVP increases heart rate via projections to the nucleus of the solitary tract (NTS), probably via inhibitory pathways targeting GABAergic parasympathetic neurons (Wang et al., 2002). Whereas oxytocin appears to produce a calming antistress effect via repeated exposure to social stimuli producing comfort and safety, AVP appears to mediate a self-protective vigilance in response to repeated exposure to social threat and loss. Oxytocin appears to switch on the SES as the result of interaction perceived as safe (Porges, 2001), whereas AVP appears to toggle off the SES and switch on the sympathetic-adrenomedullary system (SAM) in response to social challenges and threats (see Sewards and Sewards, 2003). The SAM system is phylogenetically older than the social engagement system. The passive response to defeat appears to be mediated by the dorsoventral vagal complex (DVC), which is described by Porges as a vestigial immobilization system and regarded as the most ancient of the mammalian arousal control systems. The DVC probably plays a prominent role in learned helplessness. The dynamic influences of AVP and oxytocin on cognitive, emotional, and social activity suggest that the neuropeptides perform integrative roles in the organization of behavior, perhaps via the activation of survival modes and modal strategies (see *Survival Modes and Allostasis*). AVP has been demonstrated to play a prominent role in the expression of territorial marking and aggression in hamsters (see *Arginine Vasopressin and Aggression* in Volume 1, Chapter 3), but its effects vary considerably from species to species, even closely related ones. For example, whereas AVP increases both intermale aggression and affiliative behavior in monogamous and nonterritorial prairie voles, it does not produce these effects in nonmonogamous and territorial montane voles (Young, 1999).

ARGININE VASOPRESSIN, HYPERKINESIS, AND AGGRESSION

Although an overactive HPA system (allostatic hyperdrive and high cortisol) may mediate a disorganizing effect on a dog's ability to cope adaptively with social stressors, playing a major role in the elaboration of reactive aggression, other lines of research suggest that an underactive HPA system (allostatic hypodrive and low cortisol) may increase the individual's vulnerability to show impulsive

aggression (see *Stress, Low Cortisol, and Aggression* in Chapter 6). Hypocortisolism may diminish adrenal feedback restraint over central AVP and CRF and trigger a variety of endocrine disturbances and behavioral changes associated with impulsivity (see *Stress, Low Cortisol, and Aggression* in Chapter 6). Children with attention-deficit hyperactivity disorder (ADHD) in combination with comorbid oppositional defiant disorder (ODD) exhibit reduced salivary cortisol levels in comparison with children not affected by ADHD (Kariyawasam et al., 2002). The difference, however, was only significant among a subgroup of ADHD children not taking stimulant medications, suggesting that stimulants may serve to normalize HPA-system tone. Among dogs, low plasma cortisol has been shown to elevate AVP and CRF (Papanek and Raff, 1994), perhaps representing a significant link between low-cortisol activity and autoprotective aggression (see *Arginine Vasopressin, Testosterone, and Serotonin* in Chapter 6). Sewards and Sewards (2003) formulated a model of defensive behavior and aggression based on the activating effects of CRF and AVP. Whereas central and peripheral CRF concentrations are postulated to trigger the defensive autoprotective mode, the central concentration of AVP is proposed as the primary trigger entraining the offensive autoprotective mode. A significant correlation between AVP and a life history of aggression has been established in humans (Coccaro et al., 1998), suggesting the possibility that a similar correlation may exist in dogs. Elevated CRF augments norepinephrine (NE) activity via the stimulatory action of CRF at the locus coeruleus (LC), leading to increased vigilance and sympathetic arousal. Dogs stimulated to induce anger show an increase in adrenal NE, whereas fearful dogs show a relative increase in adrenal epinephrine release (Verrier and Dickerson, 1991). Chronically blunted HPA activity may also gradually disrupt endogenous opioid restraint over CRF activity (Valentino and Van Bockstaele, 2001) or diminish 5-HT$_2$-mediated modulation of NE neurons (Done and Sharp, 1994). In addition to mediating an increased release of proinflammatory cytokines, reduced cortisol levels have been linked with decreased heart-rate variability (HRV) in response to mild stress (Kunz-Ebrecht et al., 2003)—a diagnostic indicator of sympathovagal imbalance.

Increased AVP appears to elevate baroceptor set points significantly while reducing vagal tone (Michelini, 1994), a permissive cardiovascular background compatible with impulsivity and a reactive coping style. Corson and colleagues (1980) found that hyperkinetic dogs show various signs of *visceral turmoil*, including increased AVP release, rapid heart rate, panting, profuse salivation, and stimulant-responsive forms of impulsive aggression. This pattern of hyperexcitability and impulsivity in dogs was first observed and described by Pavlov (1928). He found that certain dogs exhibited spontaneous and constant salivation while restrained in the experimental harness. In addition, these dogs exhibited persistent efforts to escape and showed learning and appetitive disturbances—behaviors that Pavlov attributed to the frustration of an overresponsive freedom reflex:

> The conditioned reflex formed slowly, remained weak, and always fluctuated. The spontaneous salivary secretion continued, and gradually increased with each experimental séance. Also the animal constantly moved, struggling in every possible way in the stand, scratching the floor, and pulling and biting at the frame, etc. This was accompanied by dyspnea, always increasing toward the end of the experiment. (283)

Impulsive aggression associated with AVP-mediated antidiuresis and hyperkinesis has been successfully treated with stimulants (see *Two Case Histories* in Volume 2, Chapter 5, and *Pharmacological Control of Hyperkinesis* in this volume, Chapter 5). Stimulant therapy may be particularly useful in the treatment of impulsive aggression in association with severe socialization and habituation deficits (Corson et al., 1980).

STRESS, THYROID DEFICIENCY, HYPOCORTISOLISM, AND AGGRESSION

The chronic stress associated with social ambivalence and entrapment may profoundly affect neurophysiological substrates mediating the organization of canine coping styles. Stress-related modifications of 5-HT, dopamine (DA), and NE systems can exert pervasive effects on mood, attachment, and impulse control. In addition, the dysregulation of the HPA system may predispose dogs to develop a variety of behavioral and immunological disturbances (Padgett and Glaser, 2003). Changes affecting the immune system appear to be sensitive markers of stress. For example, salivary immunoglobulin A (IgA) levels have been shown to be an accurate indicator of acute stress reactivity in dogs (Kikkawa et al., 2003), with low IgA levels indicating a stressful state of arousal (e.g., exposure to the sound of vacuum cleaner), whereas elevated IgA levels may be indicative of a confident and adaptive orientation to novelty (Skandakumar et al., 1995). Another potentially useful physiological marker associated with immunological impairment (Muldoon et al., 1997), psychological distress (Chen et al., 2001), and impulsivity is cholesterol level (see *Fat, Cholesterol, Fatty Acids, and Impulsive Aggression* in Chapter 7). Penturk and Yalcin (2003) have reported that dogs with serious aggression problems show significantly lower total cholesterol and triglyceride levels than do nonaggressive controls. In combination with other diagnostic tools, IgA and cholesterol panels may provide useful indicators for exploring etiologies of stress-related behavior problems and refining treatment protocols.

Stressful conditions also appear to exert a dysregulatory effect over thyroid activity. In addition to metabolic regulatory functions, the thyroid appears to exert far-reaching influences on development and behavior (Meaney et al., 1987; Anderson, 2001). Subclinical disturbances in thyroid function have been linked to the etiology of a number of canine behavior problems, including impulsive aggression (Reinhard, 1978; Dodds, 1992; Fatjó et al., 2002). In addition to the adverse effects of chronic and acute stress, thyroid levels may be blunted by environmental contaminants, diet, and age (Reimers et al., 1990; Crockford, 2003). Strong evidence suggests the possibility that thyroid function may be adversely affected by immune reactions produced by vaccinations (Scott-Moncrieff et al., 2002). After receiving vaccinations, antithyroglobulin antibodies are elevated, with some dogs showing concentrations comparable to the range observed in autoimmune thyroiditis. Whether these antibodies induce thyroiditis and damage thyroid function has not been demonstrated, but such an iatrogenic effect may be a real risk in susceptible dogs (Dodds, 2001). Hypothyroidism is the most commonly diagnosed canine endocrine disease, with at least half of all cases attributed to autoimmune thyroiditis (Scott-Moncrieff et al., 2002).

Impulsive aggression with subclinical hypothyroidism appears to occur most commonly with indicators of cognitive disturbance and may affect older dogs that were previously nonaggressive. Such dogs may show a heightened aggressive reactivity in response to unwelcome social interaction having an ambiguous character or seem to bite out of the blue. Among rats, antidepressant drugs have been found to increase thyroid concentrations selectively in the amygdala (myelin fraction), in contrast to other brain areas, which showed no significant change (Pinna et al., 2003). These findings suggest the possibility that the critical target site for the action of thyroid on behavior may be through the amygdala, a hypothesis consistent with certain types of attacks against familial persons in which the dog may fail to recognize the victim or misinterpret the significance of the person's actions. For example, the role of the amygdala in face recognition and the decoding of the emotional significance of facial expressions is consistent with the tendency of some of these dogs to snap at the face of familiar persons. Chronic stress putting the HPA system into allostatic hyperdrive and resulting in elevated plasma glucocorticoid levels may blunt thyroid activity, perhaps via glucocorticoid receptors expressed by thyroid-releasing hormone (TRH) cells in the hypothalamus (Swaab et al., 2000). On the other hand, hypocortisolism and allostatic hypodrive may also blunt thyroid function via autoimmune disease and thyroiditis (Tsigos and Chrousos, 2002). A possible linkage

between hypocortisolism and hypothyroidism has been reported in Leonbergers (Smallwood and Barsanti, 1995). In addition, the incidence of hypoadrenocorticism (Addison's disease) appears to be relatively high in bearded collies (Sells, 1996; Oberbauer et al., 2002), a breed that shows a broad spectrum of behavior problems in association with thyroid deficiency and hypothyroidism, including aggression (Hamilton-Andrews et al., 1999). Although hypoadrenocorticism is regarded as a rare canine endocrinopathy (Peterson et al., 1996), subclinical hypocortisolism may be more common than commonly assumed. Plechner (1976 and 2003) has suggested that hypocortisolism is underdiagnosed and that dogs are afflicted by an incompletely understood polyglandular endocrine disorder that results in a chronic cortisol and thyroid insufficiency. In addition to producing too little cortisol, the adrenal cortex of affected dogs may release excessive sex prohormones in response to dysregulated adrenocorticotropic hormone (ACTH) levels. According to Plechner's hypothesis, plasma estrogens synthesized from these adrenocortical prohormones in turn bind with circulating thyroid (T3/T4) to further augment a health-threatening endocrine imbalance. Plechner claims to have treated 50,000 dogs and cats with a low-dose regime of glucocorticoid and thyroid replacement therapy but provides little documented evidence in support of his hypothesis. Nevertheless, given the apparent role of low cortisol and thyroid in the etiology of certain forms of impulsive aggression, more routine testing of thyroid, cortisol, and immunoglobulin levels (IgA, IgG, and IgM) should be performed in aggressive dogs.

A number of commonly used drugs (e.g., aspirin, diazepam, phenobarbital, and prednisone) have been reported to blunt thyroid activity in dogs (Ferguson, 1984; Daminet and Ferguson, 2003). Thyroid disturbances have also been linked to phenothiazines (e.g., chlorpromazine) and psychotropic drugs (Sauvage et al., 1998). Tricyclic antidepressants (e.g., amitriptyline and clomipramine) appear to produce a significant blunting effect on thyroid activity. A recent study found that clomipramine reduced T4 levels by 35% in dogs over a 4-month treatment period (Gulik-ers and Panciera, 2003). The behavioral effects of such a reduction in thyroid activity are unclear, but they may be potentially prob-lematic in dogs already showing compromised thyroid function or in dogs being treated for behavior problems with the antidepressant drug. Dogs exposed to long-term clomipramine treatment may be at an increased risk of developing thyroid-related anomalies, perhaps recommending that thy-roid levels be monitored and appropriate actions taken to prevent thyroid-related prob-lems from occurring secondary to clomipramine therapy (e.g., thyroid supple-mentation).

Diminished thyroid activity may reduce the efficacy of antidepressant drugs for con-trolling behavior problems in dogs, a prob-lematic effect observed in human patients treated for depression (Henley and Koehnle, 1997; Cole et al., 2002). Several reports have noted the beneficial effects of combining thy-roid with antidepressants to augment their effect. Interestingly, the tricyclic antidepres-sant imipramine, when given in conjunction with T3, exerts a significant down-regulating effect on the 5-HT_{2A} receptors (Moreau et al., 2001). According to Henley and Koehnle (1997), the low dosages of thyroid used to augment antidepressant effects in humans do not pose a significant risk of inducing a state of hypermetabolism. These observations sug-gest that CDA nonresponders to antidepres-sant therapy may benefit from a treatment program that includes low-dose thyroid. Given the apparent side effects of clomipramine therapy on thyroid function, together with the potential synergistic effects of giving the two medications together, it seems like a natural combination in the treat-ment of certain behavior problems.

ACTIVITY SUCCESS AND FAILURE, PAVLOVIAN TYPOLOGY, AND COPING STYLES

Activity success in obtaining nurturance dur-ing early development may predispose pup-pies toward extraversion and fearlessness, active modal strategies (seeking and explor-ing), excitability, curiosity, playfulness, confi-dence, and social dominance, whereas social interaction resulting in activity failure may predispose the puppies toward introversion and fearfulness, passive modal strategies (wait-ing and hesitation), inhibition, insecurity, and social subordination. Both extraversion and introversion mediate adaptive social coping styles comparable to Pavlov's sanguine (s) and phlegmatic (p) types. The stability of these types depends on the support of secure social and place attachments (autonomic attune-ment) formed by social exchanges promoting comfort and safety (somatic reward) and the avoidance of loss and risk (p type), together with sufficient variability, flexibility, and nov-elty to support surprise via cortical reward (s type). The association of behavioral success with surprise, cortical reward, and increased active modal activity is consistent with Brace's (1962) notion that the differentiation of dog behavior is mediated by two primary behav-ioral traits—*activity success* and *general activity*—which can be conveniently collapsed into a single supertrait referred to as *activity-success seeking* (extraversion). Svartberg and Forkman (2002) have reported evidence that seems to support such a temperament-organ-izing supertrait associated with activity success and closely resembling extraversion. Accord-ing to cynopraxic training theory, the invigor-ation of active modal strategies (e.g., seeking, investigating, exploring, and risk taking) via cortical reward (surprise) evokes elation and increased modal activity (extraversion dimen-sion), whereas somatic reward (comfort or safety) and the emergence of passive modal strategies (e.g., waiting, hesitating, ritualizing, and risk-avoiding behavior) mediate calming, inhibition, and decreased activity levels (intro-version dimension). The adaptive canine per-sonality consists of a balance of s-type and p-type characteristics organized in the process of integrating autonomic attunement and secure social and place attachments. Social interac-tion conducive to autonomic attunement depends on an adaptive coping style shaped in accord with a principle of fairness and mutual activity success.

Broadly speaking, these observations sug-gest that the differentiation of s-type and p-type characteristics is the result of changes flowing from social interaction promoting a perception that significant events are controllable by means of cooperation and that cooperative social exchanges are fair, whereas reactive dogs, corresponding to Pavlov's choleric (c) and melancholic (m) types, are differentiated by social exchanges that result in a perception that significant events are uncontrollable and that social exchanges are unfair. Reactive dogs are hypothesized to express two general reactive coping styles in response to social and environmental novelty and sudden change: (1) c-type dogs (unstable extraverts) combine a bold (fearless) bias toward novelty (neophilia) with risk taking, (2) m-type dogs (unstable introverts) combine a shy (fearful) bias toward novelty (neophobia) with risk avoidance (see *C-type and M-type Affinity for the Flight-Fight System* in Chapter 7).

C types are further differentiated into socially obtrusive and exploitative dogs driven by impulsive social and environmental seeking activities (exploiters), on the one hand, and socially impulsive and reactive dogs operating under the influence of autoprotective power-dominance motivations (despots), on the other. The lack of autonomic attunement resulting from social exchanges and transactions perceived as fair is an important source of impairment for reactive dogs. The autonomic attunement promotes selective and sustained attention, emotional autoregulation, and impulse control. Without the autonomic attunement afforded by the integration of secure attachment, a dog's ability to regulate impulsivity and reactive behavior competently is significantly degraded. Instead of hesitating and responding in accord with control modules and adaptive modal strategies, bold c types appear to perceive social novelty and sudden change as signals to prepare for uncontrollable appetitive or challenging events, causing them to orient in a state of preemptive readiness to exploit or confront under the invigoration of state anger (anticipatory frustration/irritability). Whereas exploiters are driven to get more, despots are driven to get and keep what they take. The presence of trait anger, reduced fear, and avidity for risk taking make c-type despots poten-

tially dangerous (see *Flexible versus Rigid Watchdog Scripts*). M types are differentiated into socially hesitant and insecure dogs that are anxious and avoidant of social contact and emotionally withdrawn, depressed, or helpless. Whereas c-type dogs are driven to get and keep under the preemptive influence of exploitative motivations and autoprotective power-dominance motivations (trait anger), m-type dogs are driven to escape and avoid harm under the preemptive influence of autoprotective vigilance and readiness to flee (trait anxiety). Dogs expressing nervous attachments (autonomic dysregulation) show variable amounts of c-type and m-type behavior, with specific attributions based on the presence of trait anger (c type) and trait anxiety (m type) and behavioral threshold shifts resulting from social interaction producing state anxiety or anger. Under the influence of social interaction inducing anxiety (attention disengagement), c-type dogs may integrate m-type characteristics conducive to panicogenic arousal and impulsive aggression; on the other hand, m-type dogs may integrate c-type characteristics under the panicogenic influence of state anger (social disengagement) triggering catastrophic arousal and reactive aggression.

Activity success is capable of significantly altering general activity levels via the effects of cortical (elating) and somatic (calming) reward. In a sense, these two prominent types of reward can be characterized as expressing energy-expending and energy-conserving coping styles, orientations that may shift in accordance with social or environmental changes that favor expending energy to obtain an advantage at some risk or conserving energy to maintain known resources and avoiding disadvantages as the result of loss or risk. Finally, puppies showing s-type temperaments tend to be playful and independent, whereas those showing a p-type temperament tend to be affectionate and dependent. The significance of independence for developing puppies is linked with the formation of prediction-control expectancies and learning to adjust behavior in accordance with positive and negative prediction error, fair-play exchange, and autoattunement rather than merely seeking and receiving comfort and safety from a surrogate maternal object. The s-type orientation toward social independence, playfulness, exploratory curiosity, and spontaneity is probably strongly influenced by the quality of maternal care and the formation of secure attachments. The p-type orientation involving reduced playfulness, greater social dependency, increased affection and contact seeking, avoidance of risk, and reactivity toward ambiguous social stimuli reflects social and cognitive adjustments associated with the integration of insecure attachments. The vast majority of dogs express and merge both s-type and p-type characteristics while adapting to the social demands of domestic life. These changes are mediated via the differential inhibitory and excitatory influences of adaptive anxiety and frustration on behavior. An important goal of cynopraxic therapy is to balance and integrate s-type and p-type traits systematically. The canine personality is perfected by social interaction that promotes fairness while facilitating secure attachments (autonomic attunement), affectionate playfulness, mutual appreciation, and interactive harmony.

PROACTIVE VERSUS PREEMPTIVE PROCESSING AND CYNOPRAXIS

Dogs operating under the influence of a reactive coping style respond preemptively and incompetently to social novelty and unexpected change as representing relatively uncontrollable opportunities, challenges (loss), or threats (risk), whereas dogs exhibiting an adaptive coping style tend to respond to similar circumstances under a preemptive bias of confidence and alertness for signals of reward. As the result of a history of activity success, adaptive dogs appear to acquire a buffer of tolerance or *adaptive optimism* that enables them to cope more effectively with uncertainty. Both strategies are subject to error, but whereas adaptive dogs tend to adjust to error in a proactive way, reactive dogs tend merely to react to error without learning from it. To borrow Rotter's terminology (see *Locus of Control and Self-efficacy* in Volume 1, Chapter 9), reactive dogs are external-type learners that respond impulsively, helplessly, or fearfully to perceived opportunities, challenges, and threats

under a bias of event uncontrollability and uncertainty/danger, whereas adaptive dogs are internal-type learners that cope with change and novelty under a bias of event controllability and safety via the organization of prediction-control expectancies, calibrated establishing operations, and adaptive modal strategies.

The approach of a stranger appears to set off a three-way race between seeking-mode processing, flight/fight-mode processing, and stop-mode processing (Band and Van Boxtel, 1999). What a dog ultimately does is largely determined by the system that finishes processing operations first. If reactive processing is completed before stop-mode processing is finished, the flash point of no return may be reached, causing the flight or fight adjustment to escape from inhibitory control. The decision to exploit, attack, hold ground (engage in conflict behavior), or retreat is determined by reactive behavioral thresholds, ongoing arousal, and inhibitory coping skills. With increasing appetitive arousal the dog is likely to approach and exploit the object; with increasing fear the dog is likely to feel threatened and try to escape; whereas with increasing provocation the dog is more likely to confront the unfamiliar person. On the other hand, if the inhibitory stop processing is completed first, the reactive flight/fight-mode processing may be brought to a halt (all-stop signal) or after interrupting flight-fight processing an incompatible approach response may be produced (stop-change signal). Since the reactive response becomes progressively more difficult to cancel as reactive processing nears the point of no return, it is critical that stop-change processing be initiated at the earliest stage in the race.

Unfortunately, reactive dogs are problematic in this regard, since subcortical flight-fight processing networks may be maintained in a tonic state of preparatory arousal (vigilance and readiness to react) under the influence of reactive sympathovagal deregulation (sympathetic dominance), priming preattentive auditory, visual, and motor systems to process and respond to novel and ambiguous social signals with a negativity bias that causes the dog to perceive the developing situation as an signifying an uncontrollable challenge or threat. Preemptive amygdalar activation (autoprotective anticipatory anxiety) stemming from aversive and traumatic emotional learning resulting from threatening events perceived as inescapable may support a chronic state of autonomic disturbance and nervous attachments that are incompatible with effective inhibitory stop or stop-change processing and social engagement. The preattentive and preemptive nature of reactive adjustments serves to support a tonic state of autonomic deregulation in support of a heightened state of vigilance and reactive readiness—changes that may require specialized cynopraxic procedures (e.g., target-arc training) to reboot and restore competent preattentive functions. A central goal of cynopraxic therapy is to integrate secure social and place attachments and autonomic attunement incompatible with reactive behavior. Together with the emergence of secure attachments and attunement that enable the dog to independently autoregulate sympathovagal tone conducive to an adaptive coping style, a number of bond-promoting quality-of-life changes are simultaneously introduced to activate survival modes conducive to social exploration and play. However, insofar as interactive conflict persists in the household, the amygdalar autoprotective circuits previously mentioned will remain active. Consequently, an important part of the cynopraxic process is ICT, with the goal of identifying sources of conflict, building a training space around them, and converting conflictive reward interests into shared opportunities for mutual reward based on fair-play cooperation and compromise, thereby systematically reducing social ambivalence and entrapment dynamics while increasing mutual appreciation and interactive harmony.

With the emergence of autonomic attunement, the dog transitions out of impulsive gratification to seeking activities organized to produce somatic reward, that is, outcomes promoting comfort and safety. The refinement of autonomic attunement is critically important for the experience of both somatic reward and cortical reward. Initially, surprise promotes exploitative modal activity that rapidly spirals into disappointment and loss. Within the context of an adaptive coping

style, disappointment depresses modal excess (mania) and integrates passive modal strategies such as hesitation and delay of gratification, which, in turn, set the stage for better-than-expected outcomes and active modal activity that becomes increasingly focused, investigative, and experimental. These changes in active and passive modal behavior reflect a further refinement of autonomic balance, the organization of which moves the dog from manic excitement to elation. A similar shift toward stability occurs in passive modal adjustments, with the dog learning to process disappointments as information obtained while optimizing discovery, instead of reactively responding to them as threatening obstacles. Passive modal strategies enable the dog to seek, explore, and investigate without unduly sacrificing or risking loss of comfort and safety. Affectionate transactions and play gradually become the primary focus of cynopraxic therapy as a foundation of secure attachments is established. The balancing effects of affection and play on autonomic functions are profound and appear to open a healing space from where human-dog companionship facilitates a heightened state of well-being and mutual appreciation referred to as *cynopraxic joy*. As autonomic attunement becomes clarified and precise, human-canine interaction appears to become increasingly spontaneous, playful, and creative: liberated. The elation of discovery may now slowly or precipitously transition into the joy of becoming—a transition marked by a playful acceptance and rejoicement in the aleatory nature of life—and herald the opening of a paradoxical play space. Instead of seeking reward in prediction error or optimized control, the direct experience of ambiguity and uncertainty becomes the object of appreciation infusing everyday activities with a quiet sense of affectionate playfulness and freedom—a state of innocence that radiates from the heart of the dog as beacon for human betterment.

BARKING, MOTOR DISPLAYS, AND AUTONOMIC AROUSAL

Whereas threat barking and piloerection may be used to advertise threats at a distance, the growl is usually reserved for making threats at close quarters (Bleicher, 1963). Alarm and threat barking appears to be performed to affect the behavior of the intruder at a distance as well as to alert group members and to draw their attention to the situation (see *Behavioral Effects of Domestication* in Volume 1, Chapter 1). In addition to performing a coordinated defense function by alerting and arousing group members to a potential threat, barking may ward off intruders, perhaps causing them to avoid the area in the future. Alarm and threat barking may be rewarded by attracting the attention of family members or by stimulating the barking of other dogs (social contagion effect). Threat barking may also be rewarded by its ability to cause the intruder to withdraw from the defended area. Alarm and nuisance barking may be stimulating and intrinsically rewarding for some dogs. Motor displays are coordinated with barking threats, perhaps with the goal of disambiguating the dog's intent and strengthening the overall impression. The dog may thrust its front feet into the ground, giving the impression that it is straining to hold itself back, perform lateral shunts over a wide expanse of turf, intermittently charge forward and turn sharply about to snap angrily at the tail, and show a variety of threatening and shifting signs of intent indicative of reactive arousal. However, the most serious threat is a hard-to-describe but unmistakable "sick with repugnance look" that may present with some threat barking or other more subtle signs of aggressive intent.

The acoustics of barking vary according to context, type of provoking stimulation and arousal, and developmental factors (Bleicher, 1963). When responding to disturbances provoking alarm and aggressive arousal, individual barks are lower pitched, last longer, and are more rapidly repeated than barks associated with isolation and play (Yin, 2002). Alterations in respiration associated with different vocalization patterns may exert signature vagal effects on arousal levels via sinus arrhythmias. During inspiration, heart rate tends to increase whereas with expiration heart rate tends to decrease. These sinus arrhythmias are most evident while the dog is resting and reflect influence of breathing on vagal tone. The repetitive action of barking may modulate defensive arousal via afferent vagal feedback on forebrain and midbrain areas. The pressure and forceful cadence of threatening barking rhythms may contribute to the maintenance of a high level of state arousal and readiness, whereas the steady diaphragmatic pressure associated with whining and howling may serve to moderate or reduce emotional distress. This hypothesis suggests that canine vocalizations not only serve a communication function, but may also modulate the signaler's emotional state via a vagal mechanism. For instance, the squeak or yelp in response to unexpected discomfort may circumvent a reflexive aggressive response via rapid vagal feedback on aggression-mediating pathways. As such, the yelp appears to represent a bidirectional inhibitory stop signal, acting both internally and externally on the social source of aversive stimulation. Instead of attacking the source of discomfort, the well-socialized dog tends to respond to such events by yelping, thus appearing to give the doer of the aversive action the benefit of doubt.

The confrontational intent of the aggressive dog is accented by direct eye contact and pupillary dilation. Intent may be signaled at intermediate distance by a stiff gate and erect posture augmented by a bristling of hackles on the neck and along the back. Piloerection is mediated by sympathetic enervation of smooth muscles (arrector pili) attached to hair follicles. The contraction of arrector pili causes the hair shaft to stand up. Hackles make a dog look bigger and more formidable, perhaps increasing the dog's resource-holding potential and serving to intimidate a potential adversary. Unlike pupil size changes, which are under the combined influence of both sympathetic and parasympathetic control, piloerection is under the exclusive control of the sympathetic nervous system (SNS). Skeletal muscle tone and plantar sweating (indicated by sweat marks left on flooring) are useful markers of sympathetic arousal in dogs.

Dogs appear to organize a schema of safe and familiar expectancies that determines whether they initiate friendly social engagements. In addition to barking at the approach of people and other dogs, dogs bark in response to unexpected stimulus change or mismatches between the usual or safe schema and an unexpected change (Adams and Johnson, 1995). The various mismatches between social and environmental stimuli and the accustomed safe and familiar expectancies of them produce varying levels of uncertainty, producing alarm, uncertainty, threat, and challenge. Alarm in response to environmental or social novelty and uncertainty may increase progressively or catastrophically, to borrow Zeeman's (1976) term, depending on the size and suddenness of the mismatch between the event and the familiar schema. Further, alarm barking may be evoked by the startle of sudden change or as a threat in response to a perceived challenge posed by the approach of an unfamiliar person. Threat barking is probably associated with an approach-avoidance conflict triggered by the approach of a stranger or the occurrence of a sudden change (e.g., strange sound or bell ringing). Many barking styles appear to reflect uncertainty and conflict of incompatible emotional and behavioral tendencies evoked by the approach of an unfamiliar person. Conflictive barking activity may allow the dog to hold ground, secure the stranger's attention, and keep the intruder at a safe distance, but without necessarily wanting to drive them away. As such, the barking response may delay social decisions about engagement, disengagement, or confrontation long enough to assess the relative safety and significance of the situation. Still other dogs will bark and continue to threaten persons with whom they are familiar but who are viewed as outsiders. Such dogs may tolerate a guest if the guest remains in the yard (the familiar space) but threaten a guest who comes in the house (the familial space). Finally, not all dogs bark to give alarm or threaten people, and many will bark just because they are intoxicated with the excitement of someone visiting the house. In fact, most barking by dogs in response to visitors to the home appears to be related to nonspecific excitement—not aggressive intent.

VARIABLES AFFECTING EXTRAFAMILIAL AGGRESSION

Under the influence of confinement and restraint (e.g., when inside a car, crated, or chained) territory-like aggression may be invigorated (see *Variables Influencing Territorial Aggression* in Volume 2, Chapter 7). Children appear to be at an increased risk of serious attacks by chained dogs or by dogs that have broken free of chain restraint. Although keeping a dog continuously on a chain appears to exert a potent agitating effect—as Shaw (1906) says, "The chain makes a dog savage"—the results of a study performed by Le Boeuf (1967) in which dogs were periodically staked out and exposed to the approach of free-moving male and female dogs do not support the notion that chaining per se makes dogs more aggressive. Occasional and brief tethering outdoors is unlikely to produce adverse welfare effects or alter aggression levels, but the quality-of-life degradation, agitation, frustration, lack of gratifying social contact, and entrapment associated with excessive and routine chaining and penning of dogs outdoors may significantly increase a dog's aggressive propensities. A major source of increased risk associated with chaining is simply the result of increasing the public's exposure to an aggressive dog. Whereas a fence provides a protective, albeit imperfect, barrier, a dog on a chain is much more accessible to the approach of a stranger or an innocent child. Excessive confinement of a dog appears to reflect a failure of the family to integrate the dog effectively into the home.

Based on opinions that continuous tethering can be inhumane, the U.S. Department of Agriculture (USDA) has banned the practice of tethering in facilities that fall under its jurisdiction (Animal and Plant Health Inspection Service, USDA, 1997). To test the hypothesis that penning might be better for the dog than tethering, Yeon and colleagues (2001) performed a study that evaluated the behavioral effects of tethering and penning on Alaskan sled dogs. The study failed to show a significant welfare advantage from penning in comparison to tethering: "Our findings provide no evidence that tethering was any more or less detrimental to dog welfare than being housed in pens (as recommended by the USDA)" (2001:268–269). These preliminary findings appear to suggest that both forms of confinement can be equally problematic when used to restrain dogs continuously. The report appears to raise significant welfare issues about the use of continuous pen confinement, as well as continuous tethering. Consequently, if tethering and penning are equally stressful, then alternative means of laboratory housing may need to be explored and recommendations made based on scientific findings rather than good intentions. Ultimately, however, as the result of the dog's special needs for human companionship, its highly developed social cognitive abilities, and its adaptation to domestic life, there may not be any practical way to house dogs under laboratory conditions that one can truly call *humane*, or honestly say that it serves a dog's best interests and welfare, without at the same time appearing painfully ignorant of the dog's nature and devoid of anything approaching sincerity with respect to laudable aspirations pertaining to animal welfare.

Social facilitation and inhibition appear to exert a significant effect on extrafamilial aggression. Two dogs aroused by the same provocative target may stimulate aggressive arousal in each other that exceeds what either of them would do if alone. The facilitative effect in such cases is often so strong that a third entity appears to emerge from the two, an effect reminiscent of the ferocious three-headed Cerberus, the mythical guard dog of Hades (Figure 8.2). The connection suggests a nice term for the social facilitation of extrafamilial aggression toward unfamiliar outsiders: the *Cerberus effect*. Dogs may also exert a significant, but less recognized, inhibitory effect on the barking behavior of other dogs. Scott (1983), for example, described an interesting situation illustrating the effects of social inhibition on territory-like behavior. He observed that when shelties and beagles were housed together, the shelties consistently became controlling over the beagles. Both shelties and beagles exhibit a very strong tendency to bark at strangers, but when reared together the more controlling shelties kept the yielding beagles from barking, resulting in "barkless beagles" (8). In other cases, social facilitation

and inhibition might interact dynamically in the context of complex activities, such as predatory behavior. Dogs that might not otherwise be tempted into chasing or harming another animal may be caused to engage in such activity by the example of an aggressive model. For example, Christiansen and colleagues (2001) found that when a dog that did not chase sheep was paired up with a dog that did, the nonchaser invariably chased sheep. However, they also found that the presence of the nonchasing companion had an inhibitory effect on the severity of the attacks made by dogs that chase sheep when alone.

CONFLICTS AND RITUALS TOWARD NOVEL SOCIAL STIMULI

Ritualized activities such as barking, lateral pacing, and turning about often develop in association with the conflictive arousal and opponent behavioral dynamics evoked by the presence of an unfamiliar person or dog. The bark and motor responses may help modulate arousal (sympathovagal tone) and prevent a dog from reacting to the intruder prematurely or inappropriately. Instead of simply attacking, retreating, exploiting, or accepting the intruder's presence, the barking ritual may serve a number of adaptive coping functions by enabling the dog to hold ground, to *take time* to evaluate the situation, or to *kill time* to let the situation develop and become better defined before deciding what to do next. The ritual activates and maintains a state of general excitement and readiness conducive to several possible courses of action: emergency (flight-fight), acceptance (flirt-forbear), or exploitation. Whereas unstable and reactive dogs are prone to confront intruders or run away in accord with a negative expectancy bias toward unfamiliar persons, dogs operating under an adaptive coping style are more likely to respond to intruders in accord with a positive expectancy bias and response toward novelty (see *Expectancy Bias* in Volume 2, Chapter 3). Impulsive dogs operating under the influence of behavioral disinhibition may bark wildly and then exploit a visitor for anything they can get. Dogs operating under a reactive coping style tend to perceive social

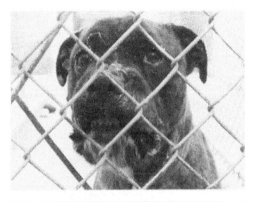

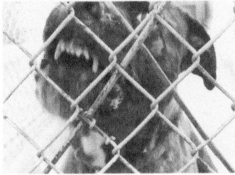

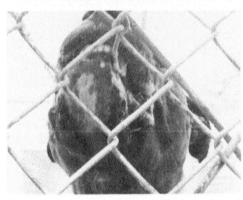

FIG. 8.2. Territorial aggression can represent a serious threat of injury, especially when occurring under the influence of offensive incentives. This dog became aggressively aroused when approached and undeterred by the presentation of food, which he would eat and immediately return, threaten, and bite at the fence. As a puppy, he was removed from its litter shortly after birth and raised in a shelter environment until he was 2 months old, when he was adopted. The dog was returned to the shelter at 8 months after attacking and pinning his owner to the ground. The owner received several bites to her hands and arms. Over the course of the 2 years in the shelter, the dog became progressively reactive and could not be safely approached by anyone, despite efforts to socialize and train him.

novelty and sudden change as intrinsically threatening and respond to outsiders with preemptive preparations for social confrontation or disengagement via the activation of the flight-fight system.

Dogs showing a reactive coping style operate under the precarious influence of an unstable equilibrium between attacking and avoiding visitors that may rapidly and precipitously shift in the direction of one extreme or the other. Although such dogs may exhibit relatively stable behavior while under the influence of familiar circumstances and optimal levels of arousal and stimulation, they can rapidly transition into a fearful, irritable, or confrontational orientation when responding to an unfamiliar person perceived as posing a threat or challenge. Such dogs seem to jump from a "Who's that?" or "What's that?" orienting phase (e.g., sound of a doorbell or person standing up) to an impulsive reactive phase. Cognizant of the potential danger, the owner may attempt to comfort and reassure the dog in hopes of facilitating more friendly behavior or at least to prevent the dog from launching into an attack or retreating from the situation. However, like a double-edged dagger held upright on its tip by the support of a finger keeping it steady, the unstable equilibrium shown by such dogs can be immediately lost as the owner withdraws support or lets down his or her guard. The inflexible pattern of repetitive aggressive threats that such dogs sometimes show toward visitors holds more in common with a compulsion than an adaptive behavior operating in accordance with functional prediction-control expectancies and calibrated emotional establishing operations. To refer to such behavior as protective or territorial is rather misleading, especially since the behavior occurs independently of any apparent threat to family or property. In most cases, such aggressive behavior is probably better understood as an autoprotective response to the uncertainty evoked by the unexpected appearance and approach of an unfamiliar person. Conversely, an adaptive dog's positive orientation toward uncertainty via the formation of viable expectancies and competence may facilitate more friendly social engagement. For such dogs, the alarm-barking ritual gives way to a control incentive urging the dog forward to seek reward by initiating social exchanges with the visitor. In an important sense, adaptive dogs are oriented toward the conditional significance of events in order to optimize reward opportunities and avoid punishment (i.e., loss of comfort or safety), whereas reactive dogs are more concerned with the here-and-now unconditional significance of appetitive and aversive events.

The unexpected appearance of the stranger or outsider sets the stage for interactive scenes between the dog and visitor that take place under the influence of a reactive bias of uncertainty and suspicion. Dogs showing deficiencies in their ability to habituate or cope with social novelty and strangeness often show a highly reactive orienting response that may become progressively vigilant and dedicated to a rigid watchdog script. Affected dogs appear to combine a sustained suspicion or suspense toward strangers, indicating an inability to habituate and to activate the social engagement system (SES), which may remain in a state of phasic retraction so long as the dog perceives the situation or the person as unsafe (i.e., strange). Without sufficient social attraction to offset repulsion toward visitors, the dog may take food from them but not integrate social relations incompatible with aggression toward them; in fact, some such dogs, especially those expressing trait aggression, may become increasingly dangerous as their fear is reduced by food. Just as prey animals can eat while remaining vigilant for predators, dogs in a persistent autoprotective mode will take food but remain ever vigilant and ready to launch an attack against any unexpected changes or movements perceived as a threat. The person giving food remains an outsider and continues to be perceived as a significant threat. As a result, even though the dog's level of fear may be reduced, the SES may remain off-line, so to speak, and prevent the integration of friendly relations. Many of the foregoing characteristics point to the possible involvement of vagal deregulation, whereby the detection of social novelty and unexpected change mediates heart-rate changes conducive to a rigidly defensive orientation that impair a dog's ability to process

benign social events and respond with appropriately regulated behavior. Instead of responding with heart-rate deceleration when orienting and exploring a visitor, reactive dogs may fail to fully habituate but instead maintain a state of attentional vigilance and readiness characteristic of sympathetic arousal. Such dogs may have diminished HRV, reflecting reduced vagal tone and predisposing them to overreact to the slightest change in a visitor's behavior after they have apparently calmed down.

WATCHDOG BEHAVIOR

Aggression always occurs within a sociospatial frame of reference, but the reasons dogs show aggression are not always explicitly or obviously motivated by alloprotective or territorial incentives, although such incentives appear to exist in certain dogs. In many cases, aggression appears to be motivated by autoprotective incentives or merely represents an impulsive reaction to social novelty or sudden change without reference to redeeming territorial or social purposes; that is, the mere uncertainty presented by a stranger may trigger a preemptive wariness or evoke aggression in a predisposed dog. Alarm barking and threat barking are normal and useful when expressed appropriately, but under the influence of inadequate socialization or improper training, social novelty or unexpected change may generate a catastrophic shift in autoprotective arousal that sets off reactive adjustments that are impulsive and difficult to control.

Alarm at Uncertainty: Discriminating the Familiar and the Unfamiliar

The tendency of dogs to become wary and alarmed by the approach of strangers prompted Heraclitus to remark, "Dogs bark at the man they do not know" (Nahm, 1964:75). This rather prosaic observation, as characteristic of the Dark One of Ephesus, probably held a deeper significance for the cryptic philosopher than the obviously false notion that dogs bark only at people they do not know (see *Barking, Motor Displays, and Autonomic Arousal*). Plato also considers the significance of knowing and not knowing as it relates to watchdog behavior in *The Republic* (Jowett, 1941). The subject is raised in the context of a philosophical discussion pertaining to the relationship between beliefs and actions. Socrates held that effective action depends on one's ability to discriminate between what is known and what is not known and then to act in accord with the former and to avoid the latter. In a dialogue between Socrates and Glaucon, the philosopher notes that these discriminative abilities are traits shown by a good watchdog:

> Many animals, I replied, furnish examples of them; our friend the dog is a very good one: you know that well-bred dogs are perfectly gentle to their familiars and acquaintances, and the reverse to strangers.
>
> Yes, I know.
>
> Then there is nothing impossible or out of the order of nature in our finding a guardian who has a similar combination of qualities?
>
> Certainly not.
>
> Would not he who is fitted to be a guardian, besides the spirited nature, need to have the qualities of a philosopher?
>
> I do not apprehend your meaning.
>
> The trait of which I am speaking, I replied, may be also seen in the dog, and is remarkable in the animal.
>
> What trait?
>
> Why, a dog, whenever he sees a stranger, is angry; when an acquaintance, he welcomes him, although the one has never done him any harm, nor the other any good. Did this never strike you as curious?
>
> The matter never struck me before; but I quite recognize the truth of your remark.
>
> And surely this instinct of the dog is very charming; your dog is a true philosopher.
>
> Why?
>
> Why, because he distinguishes the face of a friend and of an enemy only by the criterion of knowing and not knowing. And must not an animal be a lover of learning who determines what he likes and dislikes by the test of knowledge and ignorance. (375a–e)

According to the Socratic ideal, a good watchdog is the result of selective breeding for the mental and physical abilities that enable it to discriminate friend from foe and to act effectively upon that knowledge, traits that apply equally well to the selection and training of guardian rulers of the city-state. A watchdog must be vigilant for intruders and bold in its readiness to confront them. Such dogs must possess a physical size, strength, and fleetness sufficient to chase and subdue an intruder, while always treating those familiar to them with affection and gentleness. The tendency of dogs to show friendliness toward familiar people but hostility toward strangers was interpreted by Socrates as evidence of rational conduct. The dog's ability to discriminate friend from foe on the basis of relative familiarity and unfamiliarity, and then to act in accord with such knowledge, won the philosopher's admiration. The Socratic oath "by the dog of Egypt" is an apparent tribute to the dog's sagacity and ability to make fine social judgments based on the discrimination of what is known (recognized) and unknown (uncertain) about a person. The reference to Anubis, the dog god of Egypt, may allude to a canine power to search a person's heart and discern secret intent. Just as the judgment of Anubis served to grant or deny a deceased person access to the Fields of Peace in Egyptian mythology, the dog appears to play at least a symbolic role in determining whether a visitor is admitted into the home or turned away at the threshold.

Although it is certainly true in everyday life, as Heraclitus observed, that dogs often bark at strangers, some do not bark at strangers, and still others bark at persons they know well or just bark because they are excited by the approach of someone that they love. Further, although dogs are usually friendly toward people they know, many are also exceedingly outgoing and obtrusive toward people they do not know—the antithesis of Socrates's watchdog ideal. Finally, mere familiarity with a dog does not ensure friendliness, nor does it necessarily constrain the dog's animus. In fact, some dogs may even attack a familiar person without any provocation, perhaps only because the person intruded upon a forbidden social space or engaged in exchanges reserved for affiliated others. Nevertheless, the basic pattern described by Socrates appears to be generally faithful to the behavior exhibited by a great many dogs showing extrafamilial aggression:

whereas familiar people are recognized as safe and treated in a friendly way, unfamiliar people are regarded as a potential threat and treated with alarm and suspicion, even though the latter may offer the dog food and other rewards to reassure it of a friendly intent. Aggression targeting unfamiliar persons may occur with significant conflict and barking, or it may be triggered with no apparent conflict or barking. In such cases, as soon as the dog spots the intruder, it may fiercely rush the target and attempt to bite. Still other dogs may attack visitors only after appearing to have slowly accepted them. Dogs showing such behavior require lifelong supervision and appropriate physical restraint to avoid future attacks when exposed to unfamiliar persons or familiar outsiders.

Flexible versus Rigid Watchdog Scripts

Normally, social novelty and sudden change (e.g., unfamiliar persons in association with the ringing of a doorbell) evoke excitement and approach-avoidance conflict causing dogs to bark, followed by friendly resolution and approach, social investigation, and the initiation of reward-seeking behavior toward visitors. This familiar pattern of friendly proactive and prosocial behavior is disrupted in extrafamilial aggressors. Instead of merely hesitating and barking (ritualizing) before approaching and initiating prosocial introductory and exploratory behavior, the aggressor shifts instantly from alarm arousal evoked by sudden change or social novelty to a confrontational orientation, transforming a visitor into an object for the discharge of aggressive tensions and threats. Whereas most reactive dogs appear to warm up slowly to visitors (flexible watchdog script) and accept their approach and contact, other dogs (rigid watchdog script) may resist such accommodation and remain persistently on guard, even after repeated uneventful visits. Some of these dogs may appear to warm up to a visitor but then suddenly become aggressively aroused and threatening toward the visitor. The tendency of dogs that show a flexible or *habituating* watchdog script to warm up slowly to visitors and to show tolerance or initiate

friendly behavior is consistent with the social novelty hypothesis. Such dogs rapidly and competently habituate to the novelty of an unfamiliar person and show an ability to initiate or reciprocate friendly social contact based on expectancies derived from the behavior of the visitor. The appearance of friendly tolerance can be deceptive, however, especially with dogs showing a rigid or *nonhabituating* watchdog script. Such dogs not only preemptively react to the strangeness of a visitor but also appear to discriminate between persons perceived as belonging to the household (insiders) and all others not belonging to the household (outsiders). Even as a dog becomes familiar with the visitor, it may refuse to integrate friendly relations with the outsider (see *Variables Affecting Extrafamilial Aggression*). In many cases, defensive and offensive components appear to conjugate in peculiar ways in such aggressors, whereby dogs operating under the influence of conflict and a rigid watchdog script may readily accept food and even tolerate petting from visitors but then shift back into an aggressive mode and threaten or bite them as they stop or attack from behind as a guest gets up to leave the house. Such aggressive behavior in response to an upturn of activity and sudden change appear to implicate a sympathovagal mechanism. The tendency of such dogs to threaten or bite visitors as they get up, when they approach the owner, or when they prepare to leave the house may be related to rapid shifts in autonomic arousal. Special precautions need to be taken and maintained until such aggressors show unambiguous signs of friendly acceptance toward the visitor.

Most dog owners appear to welcome a moderate amount of alarm barking and household protection as an added benefit of dog ownership. In some cases, wariness toward strangers is not only appreciated and encouraged, but the dog may gain a special status as the family's protector as the result of its territorial prowess. Unfortunately, aggressive propensities in the absence of proper training are often misdirected and turned haphazardly against family members or innocent persons visiting the home rather than against criminals (see *Incidence and Targets of*

Aggression in Volume 2, Chapter 6). Children are the most frequent targets of such bites, followed by passing adults, neighbors, and innocent visitors to the home (Blackshaw, 1991). Despite the dangers represented by untrained dogs, with appropriate training and socialization, the rigid watchdog type can be of tremendous value for personal protection and working purposes. In the hands of unskilled owners or busy households, though, such dogs represent a significant risk. In contrast to a reactive aggressor, a properly trained protection dog is a marvel of behavioral control and interspecies cooperation. As the result of effective training, the dog's aggressive impulses are systematically augmented and educated while inhibitory control is enhanced. Interestingly, dogs that have been skillfully trained in protection work are rarely presented with problems related to aggression. From a training theory perspective, integrating the aggressive impulse into a functional activity organized in accord with adaptive control expectancies and calibrated establishing operations represents a potentially valuable way to convert the conflictive or reactive impulse to threaten or attack into a proactive pattern of highly controlled protection behaviors. Such training appears to enable dogs to autoregulate impulses that previously operated under loose executive control. Systematic obedience and protection training shapes and integrates aggressive impulse into a proactive pattern of alert, threat, attack/attack-stop, bite/bite-release, guard, and denouement sequences. As an adjunct strategy, the goal of such training is not to make an extrafamilial aggressor into a protection dog, but to incorporate protection-training methodologies as a means to convert impulsive and reactive aggression into a more proactive form, making it responsive to contingent outcomes and inhibitory control. By bringing the aggressive impulse under instrumental control, an adaptive platform for subsequent behavior-therapy efforts may be established.

Although the combination of obedience and protection training may be a reasonable approach in certain cases, in the author's experience, the sort of commitment, dog sense, and experience needed to make such

training a success is rarely found in average households. Further, improper handling and incompetent protection training may only serve to make a dog more dangerous and difficult to handle. Many legal and practical factors need to be carefully considered before recommending such a strategy, but with highly dedicated and responsible dog owners such training might be explored as an option in the treatment of dogs living under the right set of circumstances that justify the risks involved. Select dogs and owners that might benefit from such training are most likely to receive responsible guidance and competent instruction from trainers working in association with established schutzhund organizations.

ATTENTION AND AUTONOMIC REGULATION

Attentional processing of significant events is divided into four steps—target arc, orienting, sustained attention, and attention termination—that simultaneously coordinate autonomic and cognitive adjustments and the expression of changes to cardiovascular activity. In addition, attentional behavior is strongly influenced by the autonomic effects of interference (distracter stimuli) and interruption (diverter or disrupter stimuli). The detection of the target stimulus produces a rapid parasympathetic effect that is observable within the first beat after the stimulus is detected (Berntson et al., 1992) roughly corresponding to the temporal relation between the flinch-alert response produced by the S1 (squeak) and S2 (click) in target-arc training (TAT). In contrast to the rapid parasympathetic changes, sympathetic effects on the canine heart are more sluggish and may take 2 to 3 seconds or longer to develop (Berntson et al., 1992). The sympathetic phase corresponds to the flick, treat, and pet sequence in TAT (see *Attention and Play Therapy*). These findings indicate that autonomic processing is temporally partitioned in a way that favors the antecedent activation of parasympathetic circuits in advance of sympathetic ones in the process of organizing a controlled response to unexpected events producing surprise or startle. In addition to autonomic partitioning, a dog's response to significant attractive or aversive events evoking surprise or startle appears to be moderated by the coincidence of nonevocative stimuli that occur in a close forward contiguity with the evocative event. In the case of startling stimuli, these antecedent neutral stimuli serve to attenuate fear responses evoked by the unexpected startle, an effect referred to as *prepulse inhibition* (see *Interrupting Behavior* in Chapter 1). As a result of the buffering effect on withdrawal behavior mediated by the antecedent stimulus, the previously neutral antecedent stimulus may enable a dog to cope more effectively with such sources of startle in the future, appearing to play an important role in the integration of passive modal strategies and proactive avoidance behavior. One might imagine that a similar effect is produced by antecedent stimuli linked with attractive stimuli producing surprise, but instead of reducing arousal associated with surprise, as in the case of startle, such antecedent stimuli linked preattentively with surprise may serve to amplify seeking incentives in association with the mobilization of active modal strategies.

These behavior-modulating capacities are reflected in preattentive bias and searching behavior, causing the dog to show a preferential alertness or vigilance for the detection of antecedent stimuli evocative of excitement or apprehension, thereby facilitating and setting the stage for an orienting or defensive response. Such preattentive biases are probably preferentially linked with neutral stimuli via a filtering process that excludes stimuli that are already associatively valenced with attractive or aversive bias, thereby preventing the cross-association of opposing arousal states. Such a filtering process would be necessary to guard against the confusion that would flow from an antecedent stimulus that evoked both excitement and apprehension at once or evoked inappropriately high levels of excitement or apprehension toward an event or stimulus warranting only minor attention, causing the dog to search inappropriately, unnecessarily, or persistently for significant events and impairing its ability to orient or engage selective attention capacities effectively.

These rapid preattentive gating and information-handling processes serve to invigorate attentional systems and tune autonomic motor systems for impending action. The adaptive changes configured in preattentive processing appear to profoundly influence a dog's capacity to hesitate (to "wait and see") and to selectively orient and attend to social and environmental stimuli and to extract significance from their occurrence for the optimization of prediction-control expectancies. In less time than it takes for the heart to beat, the eye to blink, or the puppy to yelp, autonomic circuits integrate a critical shift in arousal while mediating adaptive adjustments to environmental change. In contrast to the rapid deceleration effects of automatic targeting responses, the orienting response is associated with a slower inhibitory or excitatory effect on heart rate, reflecting the interaction of parasympathetic (vagal) and sympathetic influences on canine cardiovascular activity (Billman and Dujardin, 1990; Little et al., 1999). The orienting response is associated with a discrimination process, resulting in the differentiation of stimuli warranting immediate attention from those that do not, with the latter stimuli undergoing a process of habituation. Stimuli evoking attention activate cortical processing for evaluating an event's prediction-control significance and to stimulate an appropriate level of emotional arousal while selecting a measured and appropriate response. During periods of sustained attention, autonomic changes result in the stimulation, inhibition, and disinhibition of cardiovascular activity via gross and subtle changes mediated by sympathetic and parasympathetic divisions of the autonomic nervous system (ANS) on vagal tone. The various effects of cognitive and emotional processing on autonomic arousal and heart activity may index attentional effort and emotional establishing operations while matching arousal to behavioral needs. Among humans, sustained attention has a profound influence on vagal tone, which Porges (1992) has compared to partial atropine blockade, resulting in a phasic reduction in HRV. He found that children with attention and impulse-control deficits show disturbances in their ability to appropriately adjust vagal tone while engaged in activities requiring sustained attention. In comparison to children not exhibiting ADHD, children diagnosed with ADHD exhibit increased phasic HRV, a difference that is removed by medication with the psychostimulant methylphenidate. The HRV during sustained attention shown by children with ADHD appears to reflect reduced mental effort in comparison to controls without ADHD, implicating an executive frontal role in the phasic modulation of vagal tone during sustained attention (Borger et al., 1999).

Attentive and preattentive functions play a profoundly influential role in the organization of adaptive and reactive coping styles. The critical interface between the external and internal environment is mediated by attention and the modulatory effects it has on autonomic arousal. External and internal environmental conditions exert a number of limitations on attentional resources that may lead to disturbances affecting a dog's impulse control, mood, and ability to cope with stress. According to cynopraxic theory, the aversive states of arousal associated with anxiety, frustration, anger, boredom, and depression are the acute (phasic) and chronic (tonic) correlates of attentional disturbances and autonomic deregulation impairing a dog's ability to achieve adaptive attunement and harmony via behavioral initiative. The quality of life (QOL) index is broadly correlated with the relative social and environmental order and variety, with extremes in either direction resulting in attentional disengagement, autonomic deregulation, and increased impulsivity resulting from anxiety (harm avoidance) and boredom (lack of stimulation or novelty seeking). Cynopraxic theory postulates that anxiety and boredom are the result of environmental conditions that lack sufficient order or variety to support attentional engagement. Accordingly, anxiety is the autonomic correlate of social and environmental conditions that lack sufficient order (consistency and predictability) to *support* attentional engagement, whereas boredom is the autonomic correlate of environmental conditions that lack sufficient variety (novelty and uncertainty) to *sustain* attentional engagement. In both cases,

attentional disengagement results in reduced impulse control and behavioral changes tending toward depressive or compulsive disorder.

In addition to external social and environmental influences, internal drive conditions originating in overactive subcortical networks may overstrain attentional functions, causing them to develop an opposite pattern of incapacitation associated with an inability to flexibly disengage attention, to habituate to irrelevant stimuli, or to shift attentional focus selectively in accord with prediction-control expectancies. Reactive dogs appear to approach the environment in a rigid and one-dimensional way, showing a high degree of vigilance and readiness to act, depending on preattentive biases (positive or negative), preemptive arousal, and the behavioral system involved. Reactive dogs express four general patterns of hyperexcitability in association with an *inability to disengage* attentional processing: excessive seeking, exploiting, avoiding, and fighting. In contrast to reactive dogs, impulsive dogs are saddled with an opposite attentional burden resulting from social interaction that lacks sufficient consistency or clarity to form reliable prediction-control expectancies and calibrated establishing operations. Instead of being unable to disengage attention and relax, impulsive dogs appear to be motivationally disengaged from social stimuli. Operating under the influence of social ambivalence and loner/dispersive tensions, impulsive dogs may automatically disengage attentional resources, perhaps as a measure to protect cognitive processing from the adverse influence of information inadequate or inimical to the formation of predictive correlations. Dogs that respond to social proximity and contact with motivated efforts to disengage attention tread a perilous tightrope, because withdrawal of attentional resources is anxiogenic and tantamount to relinquishing control over impulse. The reactive or intentional disengagement of attention is hypothesized to result in blunted prefrontal activity and the deregulation of parasympathetic tone, a state of instability that is further amplified and complicated by the loss of social attraction. The retraction of the SES incurs the loss of emotional regulation and vagal stability afforded by attunement with attachment objects, as well as mediating anger—the motivational state mediating social repulsion. As the result of the social and attentional disengagement, a dog may become increasingly vulnerable toward ambiguous or conflictive social signals, causing the momentary arrest of parasympathetic outflow and promoting a preparatory state of catastrophic arousal. The sympathovagal imbalance associated with the disengagement of attentional and social resources not only mediates generalized anxiety, the lack of autonomic stability exhibited by such dogs appears to contribute to increased moodiness, impulsivity, and changes in general activity levels.

Dogs with flexible attention skills can form and test prediction-control expectancies and adjust their behavior accordingly, thereby enabling them to anticipate events and to prepare emotionally in advance to behave in ways that are most likely to succeed. In contrast to the rigid adjustment styles of reactive and impulsive dogs, dogs expressing an adaptive coping style can rapidly shift expectancies and emotional arousal in order to keep pace with changing circumstances and, in doing so, optimize their ability to respond competently to significant events.

PLAY AND AUTONOMIC ATTUNEMENT

The propensity to play is not equal among dogs. Dogs evidencing emotional and behavioral disturbances associated with anxiety, fear, and anger often show significant impairments in their abilities to sustain playful interaction with other dogs and people. Reduced exploratory behavior and playfulness may impair a dog's ability to cope adaptively with unfamiliar or uncertain situations, as well as diminish its ability to initiate or reciprocate competent exchanges needed for social engagement and integration of secure attachments with family members. A reduced alertness for signals of reward is characteristic of a reactive coping style, perhaps, by default, forcing such dogs to rely on signals of punishment and unconditioned sources of gratification. The emotional states associated with a

reactive coping style (anxiety, anger, irritability, intolerance, and withdrawal) may simply reflect the mood changes that occur when a dog cannot effectively process and experience the rewards necessary to play and to actively learn.

The ability to play is probably organized at an early age. Among wolves, play fighting emerges as a prominent mode of social interaction in advance of fighting in earnest and the establishment of sibling hierarchy relations. In contrast, less sociable canids (e.g., coyotes, jackals, and red foxes) show more aggressive behavior and less play as infants than do wolves and dogs (Bekoff, 1977). Individual and breed differences affect a dog's propensity to fight. For example, Frank and Frank (1982) found that malamute puppies show "unrestrained fighting" (513) starting at week 2 and do not exhibit play fighting until weeks 4 to 5. Wolf pups exhibit an opposite pattern, with play fighting appearing during week 2, followed by a brief period of serious fighting between weeks 4 and 6. The malamute's adult predilection for intermale fighting may be attributable to permanent epigenetic changes affecting sympathovagal tone that stem from the ontogenetic timing and order of agonistic contests in relation to the emergence of play. Developmentally antecedent play may integrate an autonomic tone that enables dogs to cope less reactively with agonistic exchanges later on, whereas developmentally antecedent fighting or the absence of coemergent play may adversely sensitize and permanently bias dogs with a more reactive orientation toward social agonism. Highly sociable dog breeds appear to show more playfulness and less overt fighting than breeds prone to excessive interspecific aggression in adulthood. As a result, some dog breeds appear to be far more aggressive than wolves, whereas others are much less aggressive, reflecting breed differences and the effects of selective breeding pressures on aggressive propensities (Scott and Fuller, 1965).

Lund and Vestergaard (1998) found that the levels of play versus social agonism shown by dogs between weeks 6 and 8 is negatively correlated with the levels of play and social agonism present at week 3 and weeks 3 to 4, respectively. In other words, puppies that played less at 3 weeks of age tended to play more later on, whereas puppies that fought more during weeks 3 to 4 fought less later on. Conversely, puppies that play less early on play more later on, whereas puppies that fight less early on fight more later on. These changes are attributed to compensatory rebound effects, but may just as likely reflect developmental processes and neurodevelopmental shifts mediating the expression of different temperament types. The developmental timing of play fighting and social agonism appears to exert a lasting influence on sympathovagal tone. A period of parasympathetic dominance emerging at around week 3 is followed by a brief sympathetic rebound between weeks 5 and 7, gradually moving toward progressive autonomic equilibrium through week 16 [see *Primary Socialization (3 to 5 Weeks)* in Volume 1, Chapter 2]. The autonomic fluctuations and behavioral rebound effects during these early weeks of development are reflected in significant heart-rate changes (Scott and Fuller, 1965), which are strongly correlated with changing emotional propensities that differentially enhance social attraction and play (parasympathetic dominance) or facilitate emergent social agonism and fear (sympathetic dominance). The physiological integration of mechanisms that facilitate neonatal thermoregulation may foreshadow the organization of regulatory systems dedicated to the control of sympathovagal arousal and flight-fight adjustments, suggesting the need for studies to track and correlate temperature variations with autonomic changes occurring during this period of development. Temperature changes in response to social stressors may provide revealing information and help to detect sympathovagal disturbances at an early age.

An improved ability to regulate sympathetic arousal is hypothesized to emerge during this integrative period of neurodevelopment, together with emergent social skills facilitating competent social interaction, engagement and bonding, disengagement and separation, and confrontation and defense. Accordingly, social attraction and the timing of play and fighting during these early weeks may exert lasting effects on the functional integration and relative equilibrium or disequilibrium of autonomic activity, thereby predisposing a dog at an early age toward sympathovagal balance or imbalance and the integration of an adaptive (proactive) or a reactive coping style in adulthood. Tendencies toward a reactive coping style may develop in association with autonomic imbalance resulting in either potentiation (allostatic hyperdrive) or blunting (allostatic hypodrive) of the HPA system, whereas an adaptive coping style appears to help integrate an adaptogenic response to stressors (allostatic normodrive). Finally, the energetic tactile stimulation associated with social play may contribute to the activation of an oxytocin-mediated antistress system. The canine flirt-and-forbear system is hypothesized to enable dogs to cope more effectively with stressors associated with social ambivalence and antagonism. Conversely, serious fighting between littermates may sensitize the AVP/CRF flight-or-fight system, perhaps reducing the ability of such dogs to form friendly and playful relations as adults. Competent social skills and trust appear to develop in the context of play, perhaps via adaptive parasympathetic attunement and vagal control developing in association with play activities.

Evidence supporting the hypothesis that autonomic tone is integrated at an early age and that it might exert a persistent influence predisposing dogs to integrate a reactive or adaptive coping style has been reported by Clark (1994), who studied the cardiac acceleration and deceleration responses of puppies exposed to brief restraint, elevation stress, and pain or startle elicited by tactile, auditory, and visual stimuli. Baseline heart-rate measures were obtained and compared with heart-rate recovery patterns. Puppies that showed emotionally reactive (anxious) temperaments, as indicated by owner reports and temperament tests, tended to return to baseline heart rates more slowly than puppies that exhibited less emotionally reactive temperaments. The study found breed and individual differences linking lengthier heart-rate recovery periods with heightened emotional reactivity, whereas socially confident dogs tended to show briefer heart-rate recovery periods consistent with competent sympathovagal tone. These findings suggest that heart-rate and poststimulation recovery patterns may offer predictive or diagnostic markers for identifying puppies prone to integrate reactive coping styles, recommending the routine collection of heart-rate data as part of puppy testing.

Play in the absence of a principle of fairness and empathy degrades into cruelty and exploitation via a composite motivational influence of lust, greed, and power when unilateral advantages are sought without concern for the loss or pain suffered by the coplayer. The excitement of taking an advantage at the expense of the play partner appears to be an important motivational aspect of exploitative play, perhaps explaining why play sometimes slips into serious competition and overt fighting. A serious form of impulsive aggression exemplifies this tendency that may be shown by certain outgoing dogs bred for enhanced fighting propensities and expressing intrusive exploitative and power-dominance motivations toward unfamiliar persons. Up until the flash point, the dog may wear a "happy clown" face and only show evidence of a growing threat by an unmistakable attitude shift and increasing roughness, often matched with a deceptively charming "pretty boy" look and constant eye contact, seeming to lure the player in for more fun. Should the handler attempt to shift the play toward an advantage or abruptly stop, the intensity of the exchanges may torque up and suddenly turn into an all-out attack. The foregoing is one example of many types of situations where pseudoludic interaction may set the stage for aggression. Usually, play with such dogs is held off until a foundation of familiarity, cooperation, and trust is established. When play is initiated with a potentially aggressive dog, keeping the dog on tie-out and directing its play energy into an object is a useful precaution. Learning to trust ones "gut" is critical for avoiding dangerous situations such as the one just described. Knowing when to play or not is something that a trainer learns only with experience, close calls, and sometimes the wisdom born of hard knocks.

ATTENTION AND PLAY THERAPY

Dogs functioning under a reactive coping style appear to harbor negative biases that predispose them to process social uncertainty and sudden change as a threat or challenge rather than a potential source of reward. Affected dogs may be unable to habituate to the perceived threat of an outsider or may do so very slowly and only after many safe encounters. Reactive dogs of this type pose a significant risk of snapping or biting strangers or familiar outsiders who approach or attempt to interact with them too soon in the social familiarization process or approach them in unexpected ways. Such dogs may be particularly dangerous in unfamiliar situations perceived as unsafe and previously associated with loss, discomfort, or risk. Most behavior problems are shaped while a dog copes with aversive affects stemming from a history of interactive conflict and a failure to produce reward or to avoid punishment (activity failure). The Stoic philosopher, Epictetus (Internet Classics Archive, 2000), speaks to these distressful affects in his *Discourses*: "An affect is produced in no other way than by a failing to obtain that which a man desires or a falling into that which a man would wish to avoid ... and by these causes we are unable even to listen to the precepts of reason" (3.2). Cynopraxic training and therapy efforts are organized with the goal of reducing the distressing affects of *failing and falling* and the consequent reactive adjustments to loss and risk by educating, in the words of Epictetus, the "faculty of pursuing an object and avoiding it, and the faculty of desire and aversion, and, in a word, the faculty of using the appearances of things" (1.1). Learning successfully to predict and control the environment serves to integrate an adaptive coping style, competence, playfulness, a bias of safety, and spontaneity, that is, the ability to autoinitiate prosocial behavior conducive to interactive harmony.

Attention Disturbances, Dissociation, and Orienting/Target-arc Training

The theory underlying the efficacy of orienting/TAT supposes that preattentive arousal and submerged attentional functions mediating reactive adjustments are gradually linked and integrated into a network of cortical prediction-control expectancies and calibrated establishing operations in the process of mediating functional attention and impulse control. The process appears to reboot executive functions while enlivening the SES. A critical factor in this process is training the attention to orient selectively toward the flow of events with the purpose of detecting and appraising the significance of prediction error occurring in the context of purposeful behavioral projects and ventures, and appropriately adjusting behavioral output to accord with a preference for surprise (positive prediction error) and an aversion for disappointment (negative prediction error). Essentially, prediction error occurs when an anticipated outcome is better than expected or worse than expected, thereby mobilizing adaptive modal strategies aimed at producing more surprise (e.g., increased searching and exploration) while avoiding disappointment (e.g., hesitating and waiting). The systematic juxtaposing of a standard expectancy against appetitive events that variably result in verification or positive (surprise) and negative (disappointment) prediction error serves to enliven cortical learning functions and facilitate the organization of prediction-control expectancies and calibrated establishing operations (control modules). Prediction error results in hedonic as well as cognitive and behavior changes compatible with the optimization of activity success and the integration of an adaptive coping style.

Orienting/TAT appears to facilitate the integration of a selective-attention interface that enables dogs to sort out relevant from trivial input competing for attention during training. In the case of reactive dogs, the functional gating capacities that orienting/TAT appears to invigorate seem to help a more adaptive way to cope with novelty and sudden change. Once conditioned, the target-arc stimulus can be presented in anticipation of persistently evocative stimuli to modulate emotional and cognitive overload and prevent the default mobilization of reactive flight-fight adjustments. Orienting/TAT may facilitate the activation or normalization

of pathways communicating between parallel preattentive subcortical circuits and attentive cortical networks mediating adaptive behavior in accordance with organized expectancies and calibrated establishing operations. Although these parallel cortical and subcortical systems appear to operate with a high degree of functional autonomy, they share a common autonomic axis that enables dogs to process sensory input and behavioral output in a motivationally coherent way. This organizing axis appears to be activated and modulated by orienting and attending behaviors. The attentional interface brings the demands and pressures operating within and without dogs into directional (drive) and functional alignment and tunes autonomic arousal to accord with changing needs. Adaptive orienting and attending result in increased parasympathetic tone (relaxation), whereas reactive orienting and defensive vigilance result in sympathovagal imbalance (muscular tension and a persistent readiness to act), as reflected in heart-rate changes and indexed by HRV(Billman and Dujardin, 1990; Porges, 1992).

Many of the therapeutic benefits of attention and play therapy are probably mediated through classical conditioning of sympathovagal tone. However, instrumental control over significant events plays a critical role in the way dogs respond to predictive signals. Whereas signals anticipating unconditioned aversive or appetitive events that are perceived as uncontrollable result in sympathetic tone shifts that promote reactive (escaping and confronting) and impulsive (seeking and subduing) adjustments, signals anticipating unconditioned aversive or appetitive events perceived as controllable result in parasympathetic tone shifts that are conducive to proactive adjustments and calming effects. Both appetitive conditioning (Hunt and Campbell, 1997) and aversive discrimination training (Billman and Randall, 1981) produce autonomic changes, evoked by conditioned stimuli, that are consistent with the requirements of an adaptive coping style.

According to cynopraxic training theory, the integration of prediction-control modules results in autonomic attunement and the adaptive optimization of behavior. In combination, cynopraxic procedures refine selective attention and executive impulse control, increase adaptive modal activity (e.g., social and environmental exploratory behavior), foster optimistic expectancies to social ambiguity and uncertainty, integrate secure social and place attachment, and promote autonomic attunement and autoregulation.

The orienting/TAT procedure can be used to modify preattentive priming effects that negatively bias dogs to respond reactively to visual and tactile stimuli (e.g., sudden change, gestures, body movement, touching, handling, and restraining). To reduce preemptive and reactive processing, evocative stimuli are cross-associated with the auditory target-arc stimulus. The auditory target-arc response is linked with the earliest alert-intention movements shown by the dog in response to the visual signal. For example, in the case of preemptive reactivity to sudden hand movements, the target-arc stimulus (e.g., smooch) is presented just as the dog turns its attention toward the hand movement, followed rapidly by a click, right-hand flick, and delivery of a highly valued reward enclosed in the right hand. The presentation of the well-timed target-arc stimulus and reward immediately following the sudden movement serves to integrate the visual event into a positive network of preemptive associations and expectancies previously established during orienting/TAT. Additional confidence and attraction to the hands is promoted by using the hand as a target stimulus to guide the dog into various postures or movements before delivering the reward. As reactive processing is replaced by improved executive attention and impulse control, controlled exposure is more likely to succeed in organizing adjustments consistent with stable emotional equilibrium and social competence.

Reward: Standard Expectancy and Surprise

The orienting/TAT procedure appears to gradually integrate an attention-axial interface between cortical inhibitory networks and subcortical excitatory loops processing surprise

and mobilizing exploitative seeking behavior via the repeated presentation of sequentially ordered events that provide a high level of predictability, controllability, and potential for producing surprise. Cortical surprise is hypothesized to require the existence of a previously established control expectancy, a calibrated establishing operation, and an action, collectively referred to as a *control module*, against which response-produced outcomes are compared, mismatches detected, and the new information integrated into the flexible control module to optimize the dog's future control efforts (see *Prediction Error and Adaptation* in Chapter 10). Orienting/TAT is initiated with a food reward of the least value and smallest size necessary to maintain an orienting/approach response (control module) while conditioning the bridge signal. This reward is referred to as the *standard expectancy* (SE). The SE provides an informational backdrop for comparing the relative value of outcomes produced and for detecting mismatches or positive prediction errors signifying better-than-expected outcomes and surprises. Food rewards of variable sizes, types, and presentations are randomly interspersed among rewards matching the SE value. Whereas orienting stimuli and the food reward are varied, the conditioned reinforcer (e.g., click/"Good") remains constant. The procedure is designed to enhance incentive, promote autonomic attunement, and invigorate attentional functions with cortical reward (surprise). The vocal bridge signal "Good," spoken in a chirped form, is paired with the rapid opening of the hand (visual target arc) and the delivery of the food reward and petting. The vocal bridge signal is also used to support eye contact and sustained attending behavior. Once an attending response (briefly sustained eye contact) is established with the dog's name/smooching and the vocal bridge "Good," talking to the dog, winking, smiling, and head tilting appear to further stimulate the canine SES. A useful technique for transitioning into play is to incorporate directional cues (e.g., gazing, pointing, leaning, and orienting) toward play objects in advance of walking and running toward them. Pointing or looking toward some spot before throwing the play object in that direction can also help to stimulate interest and coordinated engagement. Directional cues are further integrated as signals by using them to help a dog solve problems (e.g., helping a dog to find a hidden food item). Training a dog to turn right and left, to back up and move forward, and to move in a wide circle so that it is facing away before signaling it to orient can enhance attention control while providing useful preliminary training.

Eventually, the orienting response is integrated into other training objectives (e.g., come, sit-front, eye contact, and following routines) by delaying the bridge until the target behavior is emitted or prompted, whereupon the bridge signal and terminal reward are delivered. As previously discussed, the surprise and active modal strategies emerging in association with orienting/TAT are hypothesized to mediate a cortical/subcortical attention interface or *operant/respondent axis* comprised of instrumental and classical elements (see *Defining Insolvable Conflict* in Volume 1, Chapter 9). As a result of the repeated evocation of surprise associated with the target-arc response (flinch alert), a network of cortical synapses are gradually interwoven into submerged attentional functions, thereby bringing preattentive arousal and reactivity under the modulatory and normalizing influence of executive control. As this critical conduit of information exchange between these parallel neural processing systems is strengthened in the context of orienting/TAT and other cynopraxic therapy efforts, a backbone of order and variety appears to form that enables the dog to engage in greater spontaneity and to show an increased capacity for play and social engagement. The efficiency of orienting/TAT for increasing social spontaneity, play, and social engagement is often nothing short of extraordinary, making it one of the most powerful tools currently available for moderating reactive behavior and integrating an adaptive coping style. To describe the effect of orienting/TAT most succinctly, the dog simply appears to wake up. To attain the multiple cortical and SES benefits of orienting/TAT, the target-arc alert/flinch response may need to be evoked and rewarded several hundred times. When performed properly, preliminary orienting/TAT provides a useful platform for all subsequent reward-based training and cynopraxic therapy efforts. The orienting signals used during orienting/TAT gradually become potent stop-change countermand signals, while the conditioned click and flick bridging signals are enhanced by the attention-focusing influence of such training. The simple shaping procedures used to promote attending and following behavior target and encourage autoinitiated behaviors that improve a dog's sense of control over significant events.

The repeated presentation of contingent rewards (e.g., food and petting) in accord with a standard expectancy, periodic surprise, and occasional disappointment contributes to the organization of an adaptive coping style, biasing the dog to search for signals of reward rather than signals of punishment. Along with surprise-seeking adaptive modal strategies, passive modal strategies are organized by such training toward the adaptive goals of securing reward gains at a minimal risk (i.e., avoiding unnecessary risk taking) and learning to cope with inevitable delays and setbacks (delay-of-gratification skills). Finally, the repeated activation of appetitive and social reward pathways in association with orienting/TAT may mobilize the oxytocinergic antistress system, contributing to feelings of comfort and safety, calm, and well-being (see *Adaptive Coping Styles: Play, Flirt, Forbear, and Nip* in Chapter 6). Orienting/TAT and social engagement therapy also include frontal approach, attending behavior (making and holding eye contact), and submissive ritualizing (sit-stay and down-stay) brought under the control of hand and vocal signals. Reciprocal frontal orientation and mutual gazing appear to initiate a communicative orientation unique to the human-dog relationship, thereby laying the foundation for following, cooperative problem solving, mutual appreciation, and interactive harmony.

The orienting/TAT procedure appears to provide significant benefits for the treatment of a variety of canine behavior problems stemming from attention and impulse-control impairments (see *Locus of Neurotogenesis* in

Volume 1, Chapter 9). The obvious similarities between some of these problems and human psychiatric disorders suggest the possibility that orienting/TAT or similarly organized procedures may have therapeutic value in the treatment of certain of these disorders. Also, many of the social engagement and learning deficits associated with autism are consistent with an axial dissolution between cortical regulatory networks and various subcortical attentional loops necessary for initiating and sustaining social cognition, communication, and engagement. Whether intensive orienting/TAT might provide similar benefits in such cases is unknown; nevertheless, the procedure appears to offer exciting possibilities and novel applications that warrant future investigation.

Attention Therapy, Orienting/TAT Procedures, and Play

1. Target Arc, Orienting, and Approach

A squeak or smooch (S1) sound is followed immediately by a click (S2) and a flick of closed right hand (S3) as the dog orients toward the trainer. The duration of the target arc is approximately 200 to 300 msec, a very rapid succession of events. Although the S1 is presented in various ways from a soft to loud squeak, the timing of S2 is kept constant. The flick and reward combination is variably delayed to occur 1 to 5 seconds after the dog orients.

Orienting and approach to the closed right hand is rewarded by the bridge "Good" spoken just before the hand is opened to reveal the treat.

The SE is established with the smallest effective reward needed to maintain orienting and approach behavior.

Better-than-usual rewards consisting of changes of type, size, context, and delivery are periodically given to produce positive prediction error and incentive shifts (Flaherty, 1996). The cortical reward (surprise) associated with positive prediction error is a critical factor in cynopraxic therapy. In addition to reorienting the dog to reward signals, cortical reward generates active modal strategies that enliven social behavior and promote play.

Forward movement activates the seeking system and is an instrumental part of orienting/TAT. Signaling the dog to orient and thereby to break off the direction of forward movement and to turn toward the trainer has the effect of making the trainer the object of seeking. The effects of this simple stop-change procedure on cognitive function and social engagement are profound and pervasive (see *Attention and Impulse Control* in Chapter 1). The procedure appears to access preattentive cognitive processing, organizes stop-change inhibitory processes, intensifies associative conditioning of the click-and-flick bridging signals, serves to promote feelings of comfort and safety, and activates the SES. In a sense, the squeak and click stimuli result in a series of activating and organizing effects that are analogous to the effect of turning a key to start a car. The simple action of turning the key produces a number of automatically coordinated events that lead to the engine starting and the car working under the guidance of the driver.

2. Frontal Orientation and Coming

As the dog orients and starts moving toward the trainer, the vocal signal "Come" is spoken just before flicking the right hand out to the side.

3. Attending and Submissive Rituals (Sit-Stay Training)

The dog is periodically prompted to sit-front after coming and to make eye contact in response to its name or smooch sound before the bridge "Good" and reward are delivered. The dog is released with the release signal "Okay" and a flick of the right hand, followed by the delivery of a food reward or play. Sit-stay is gradually introduced in the context of enhancing the attending response.

4. Gaze Orienting and Directional Cuing

As the dog orients to come, the trainer points directly over a treat or ball lying on the ground and then places the right hand over it as the dog approaches. The treat is given or the ball tossed as the dog approaches the spot. Numerous variations are used to encourage the dog to make eye contact and follow gaze and other deictic (pointing) signals.

5. Parallel Orientation and Following

Food or toys can be hidden and the dog supported in its search efforts by periodically getting eye contact and then gazing, pointing, and walking in the direction of the cached item. Found rewards are conducive to significant surprise, and such interaction strongly supports following behavior and cooperation. Coordinated movements shaped with reward serve to integrate behavioral approach and social engagement while promoting cooperation, mutual appreciation, and interactive harmony.

The dog is encouraged to follow near the trainer's side by clicking and prompting it to sit with the right hand, saying "Good" as the dog begins to sit and delivering the treat and petting as the action is completed. The dog is released from the position with "Okay" and prompted to follow along or sent to chase a ball.

6. Dynamic Modal Activities and Play

Various play activities are introduced in accordance with the dog's ability to reciprocate. Intensive orienting/TAT (squeak), cortical reward (click-flick-surprise), attending (frontal orientation and eye contact), and following naturally promote dynamic modal activities and play. The emergence of play during social engagement therapy is an extremely valuable asset in the treatment of behavior problems. Training a dog to play tug, fetch, and catch games can promote joy and enhanced bonding. Retrieve games can be also be used to promote valuable go/no-go inhibitory conditioning effects and to encourage recall habits. Play adds complexity and refinement to the attentional nexus and improves a dog's ability to synchronize behavioral sequences so that they stay in temporal register with the behavioral sequences of the co-player. Competitive play activities, such as tug-and-fetch games, appear to fuse attention onto a point of common interest that promotes friendly exchange, rather than contest, via the differentiation of distinct roles that are equally necessary to initiate and continue the activity. Play continues only so long as it is rewarding for both players—a criterion that serves to promote mutual appreciation (empathy) and fair play, since to take advantage of the other or to neglect the other's needs might result in a loss of play momentum and cause the activity to grind to a halt. Nothing is more revealing of human character and canine temperament than their respective abilities and styles of play. Dogs exhibiting behavior problems invariably exhibit disturbances in their ability to play.

Many features of ball play recommend its use when organizing an adaptive coping style and cooperation. Russell (1936) long ago recognized the value of ball play for organizing adaptive behavior, listing six characteristics of special importance (paraphrased):

1. Chasing a ball involves the whole dog in relation to an object-activity outside of itself.
2. The dog's activity is attentively focused and coordinated with the course of action being pursued.
3. The activity is directed toward a particular goal, that is, picking up and returning with the ball.
4. The goal-directed activity shows a persistence of purpose as evidenced by the dog's willingness to search repeatedly over likely ground for a misplaced ball.
5. The activity is governed by the result produced by it; if the ball is not found, the searching sequence continues for a variable period or until the ball is found, whereupon the search stops.
6. The activity shows evidence of social cooperation and adaptive flexibility, as indicated by the dog's ability to shift from an unproductive search to turn to the trainer for help to find a misplaced ball.

Ball play mediates an intensely focused orientation on an object that the dog would wish to possess but must relinquish to produce the activity that engenders the object with its reward value. Likewise, the trainer shares an interest in the ball as a means to control the dog's searching and retrieving behavior, entailing that the ball be received and thrown to generate the object-activity valued by the dog. As a result, the dog obtains the object-activity that it graves but sacrifices control of the object to the trainer to maintain the mutually rewarding exchange. For the ball game to continue, both the dog and trainer must give and take advantages with respect to the ball. If the dog grabs the ball and runs off with it, the object of interest is obtained, but the activity that makes it interesting is lost. The ball can be kept in play only by compromise and cooperation in accord with a principle of fairness. As a result of the give-and-take nature of ball play, a sense of fair play and trust (i.e., comfort with social uncertainty) appears to emerge. Tug games integrated into the ball game exemplify the competitive and possessive conflict underlying the activity, that is, the necessity of giving up the object in order to get the valued activity. The relinquishment of the ball to the trainer represents a submissive act of trust based on a belief that the trainer won't selfishly walk off with the object, but will toss it again, thereby meeting the obligation incurred by *accepting* the dog's trust (taking another's trust always involves obligations and responsibilities) and proving oneself as a leader fit to follow. The chase-and-retrieve sequences reflect a cooperative resolution of competitive conflict via the mutual reward resulting from sharing, fair play, and compromise. In contrast, a dog that gets the ball and runs off with it primarily obtains reward via the gratification of selfish and possessive interests stimulated by the owner's pleading for the ball (submissive begging) or by evading attempts by the owner to chase it down, thereby promoting competitive exchanges with little hope for a cooperative resolution. Such play results in interactive conflict, whereby reward is obtained by depriving the other of reward; that is, either the dog or the owner will win or lose. Whatever the outcome, the victory is achieved at the expense of the other and the integration of conflictive tensions and distrust. Under the influence of social attraction mediated by play, such unfair advantages promote social ambivalence by evoking frustration and anger. In the context of cynopraxic theory, tug and ball play, when performed in accord with a principle of fairness and compromise, mediates mutual appreciation (i.e., an attentiveness and responsive to the emotions and covert intent of the play partner) and trust, key transitions in the process of promoting interactive harmony and the integration of a friendly bond.

Finally, in addition to orienting/TAT and play, petting helps to promote a physiological state incompatible with both aggression and fear, providing a viable strategy for decreasing sympathetic arousal in some reactive dogs. Along with play, social rewards (petting and praise) should be integrated into training activities as a major source of reward for all basic obedience work. Not only does petting provide a potent calming and bond-enhancing effect, but excessive reliance on food-related incentives may adversely impact social attachment and affection levels by persistently overshadowing social attraction. Seeking food serves a useful function in basic training and many behavior-therapy efforts, but ultimately appetitive-seeking behaviors should be subordinated to seeking for social acceptance and affirmation while forming an affectionate and playful bond. In dogs showing a deficiency of social attraction, excessive reliance on food rewards may produce a relationship based more on food-getting incentives than on social attraction—a very undesirable outcome. Food-getting incentives are not intrinsically incompatible with social attraction, but appetitive training alone does not necessarily facilitate social attraction. The widespread belief that social rewards do not possess reward value in the absence of primary reinforcement is an operant-conditioning myth contrary to a number of scientific studies (see *Tactile Stimulation and Adaptation* and *Taction and Posture-facilitated Relaxation* in Chapter 6). McIntire and Colley (1967) found that the performance of experienced working dogs (military scout dogs) and naive dogs learning new basic obedience skills (sit, down, come, stay, and heel) showed a reliable decrease in response-latency scores as the result of petting and increased response-latency scores when petting was withdrawn.

In a related study, the researchers found that dogs trained by means of directive control and compulsion in combination with food reinforcement showed increased response-latency scores when the food reward was withdrawn. Interestingly, with regard to the value of social rewards, if the food reward was replaced with petting, the extinction-related latency effects were avoided. Maintaining a balance between petting, play, and food rewards is particularly important in integrating an affectionate bond with puppies.

Insufficient social attraction and appreciation of tactile stimulation appears to play a significant role in the etiology of certain forms of canine intrafamilial aggression (see *Posture-facilitated Relaxation Training* in Chapter 7). Among human adolescents, massage therapy has been shown to reduce aggression, perhaps by decreasing dopamine levels while increasing serotonin activity (Field, 2002). The guided restraint and focused tactile stimulation produced by posture-facilitated relaxation (PFR) training can be use to induce a potent relaxation response in dogs (see *Taction and Posture-facilitated Relaxation* in Chapter 6). The combination of nonthreatening controls, prompts, postural shifts, and restraint serves to promote measured shifts in parasympathetic and sympathetic activation while facilitating autonomic attunement in association with the induction of enhanced comfort and safety. PFR training programs a regulated response correlated with a positive set of expectations in association with a loss of control and increasing vulnerability in association with physical restraint, postural shifting and pressure, and regional manipulations. Rhythmic massage and petting help to further refine the attunement process and set the stage for the dog to transition into a deep relaxation. Repetitive petting appears to exert an adaptogenic effect on HPA drive and may help to integrate antistress and antiaggression effects via the activation of the oxytocinergic system (see *Oxytocin-opioidergic Hypothesis* in Chapter 6). In addition to stimulating changes in major neurotransmitter systems, posture-facilitated relaxation with massage may promote beneficial effects on vagal tone. A dilute odor (e.g., chamomile, lavender,

ylang-ylang, or orange) that has been repeatedly paired with posture- and touch-induced relaxation appears to promote arousal conducive to calming and social engagement, perhaps by promoting an ambience of safety and conditioned relaxation. The autonomic attunement mediated by PFR training is bidirectional, with both the person providing the relaxation training and the dog receiving it benefiting from the enhanced sympathovagal balance and calming brought about by the experience.

QUALITY-OF-LIFE MATTERS
Survival Modes and Allostasis

In addition to providing modal direction to species-typical behavior and mediating epigenetic adaptations appropriate to age and survival needs, specialized phylogenetic survival modes (PSMs) appear to be conserved from the dog's evolutionary past and activated by changing social or environmental conditions. PSMs are expressed cyclically throughout the canine life cycle in a relatively orderly way in the process of coordinating biobehavioral adjustments conducive to adaptation and survival. Benign PSMs promote adjustments conducive to dynamic autonomic equilibrium (sympathovagal balance) and long-term survivability. According to the survival-mode hypothesis, epigenetically programmed survival modes are variably activated and deactivated by environmental changes determined to be better or worse than ordinary, as indexed by the activation and tone of the HPA system, autonomic attunement/misattunement, and the mobilization of allostasis, that is, the coordinated adjustments needed to maintain biological integrity and stability in the context of change (Wingfield, 2003). The activation of a PSM is variably intrusive and compelling, ranging from a condition of motivational transparency overlaying everyday activities (appetites and preferences) to intrusive motivational imperatives (modal drives) that cannot be ignored without enduring significant agitation or distress. Autonomic networks probably coordinate the expression of modal drives that subserve PSMs activated or deactivated in association with social exchanges (attunement/misattunement), QOL shifts, and allostatic changes associated with the switching on and off of the HPA system. The PSM defines in advance the class of behavior that will produce reward; it also determines whether a particular outcome will be satisfying.

The survival-mode hypothesis postulates that adaptation is relative and dependent on an organism's ability to cope by staying in step with the PSMs active at any given moment via the organization of appropriate control modules and adaptive modal strategies. Since the survival mode appears to determine in advance the class of behavior and outcomes that will produce reward, the activated mode exerts a global organizing effect on behavior, giving it motivational direction via modal drive. By these means, *instinct* exerts a profound influence on behavior without usurping executive functions. In the context of modal shifting or switching, reactive or rigid (compulsive/impulsive) adjustments to changes in motivational direction promote autonomic imbalance and negative mood, whereas flexible adjustments in harmony with modal change promote autonomic balance and positive mood. From a human perspective, obtaining gratification in harmony with modal drive and PSMs might be akin to obtaining meaning and contentment from behavioral efforts, whereas gratification obtained in conflict with modal drive and PSMs might produce subjective feelings of ennui, meaninglessness, and despair. These observations emphasize the relative independence of the cognitive and emotional effects produced by gratification and reward. According to cynopraxic theory, adaptive success is achieved by maintaining a dynamically stable state (allostasis) in the process of integrating secure social and place attachments via the optimization of comfort and safety (security) and the mobilization of adaptive modal strategies that are in harmony with survival modes and drive.

The activation and deactivation of PSMs is the coordinated outcome of countless neural networks and neurotransmitter systems, but DA, 5-HT, and NE systems appear to play prominent roles in the process. The present

hypothesis speculates that oxytocin and AVP act as cofactors or moderators of DA, 5-HT, and NE activity in the process of activating, modulating, and deactivating PSMs in response to social and environmental stressors. Under worse-than-ordinary conditions (adversity), DA, 5-HT, and NE systems may be configured into survival modes aimed at avoiding danger and harm (autoprotective or loner mode), causing a dog to respond with increased anxiety, irritability, impulsivity, and aversion in response to social novelty and sudden or unexpected change; whereas, under the influence of better-than-ordinary circumstances, neural activity and traffic may be rerouted to produce modal changes conducive to calming, social integration, invigorated autonomic tone, and an adaptive coping style.

5-HT is hypothesized to contribute to the maintenance of stability over time against which backdrop modal changes weave in and out of sync and phase. The stability of biobehavioral systems is expressed in the form of biological rhythms that give rise to consistent adjustments having a cyclical or waveform shape and regularity (e.g., sleep/wake cycles) and expressed in the daily patterns of activity and rest, vigilance and foraging, hunger and satiation, and social comfort seeking and giving, as well as in various functional and dysfunctional adjustments to social and environmental stressors. In coping with adverse conditions, the serotonergic system may undergo harmful modifications via allostatic load and overload, impairing its ability to maintain a condition of flexible stability over time, perhaps causing behavior to become increasingly rigid (compulsive or impulsive). The increased $5-HT_{2A}$-receptor binding potential shown by dogs exhibiting impulsive aggression (Peremans et al., 2003) may represent the cumulative allostatic load resulting from the serotonergic management of stress adjustments stemming from chronic HPA or SAM hyperdrive.

PSMs integrated under the influence of optimal developmental conditions are behaviorally invigorative and unifying, switching on and off at appropriate times and durations to enhance behavioral adaptation. However, with dogs exposed to adverse developmental stress,

PSMs may become stress sensitized and reactive, turning on impetuously to minimal triggers or switching off sluggishly or remaining chronically active or inactive. The activation of flight-or-fight survival modes and drive by conditioned and unconditioned stimuli anticipating imminent harm is adaptive, but many reactive dogs appear to remain persistently aroused to a state of vigilant readiness under the influence of a dysfunctional flight-or-fight mode. The resulting reactive coping style and allostatic load/overload may severely impair a dog's ability to adjust competently to household stressors. Although dysfunctional survival modes may remain relatively quiescent under auspicious environmental conditions that place few demands on the dog, they may be activated in response to social conflict and stress or as the result of integrating the PSM into social behavior emerging epigenetically at the time of puberty and early adulthood. Functional PSMs that ordinarily mediate adaptive adjustments may become dysfunctional (hyperreactive or hyporeactive) as the result of developmental stress. Instead of mediating adaptive behavior, the dysfunctional PSMs may be variably modified and integrated into a persistent state of sympathovagal imbalance producing a vulnerability to express generalized anxiety, depression, impulsivity, compulsivity, hyperactivity, separation distress, and aggressive reactivity. Under conditions of social ambivalence and entrapment, the dysfunctional PSM may lower reactive thresholds and predispose the dog to panicogenic impulsive or reactive aggression and numerous other adjustment problems. Once toggled on by stress or epigenetic triggers, the dysfunctional PSM may profoundly disrupt normal processing and impair the dog's ability to toggle off the malignant PSM. As a result, the dysfunctional mode may become progressively autonomous, perseverant or cyclic, and maladaptive in the process of degrading or abolishing executive control and fostering a reactive state of autonomic instability.

Quality-of-Life Index

Among dogs, the activation of survival modes is indexed by the release of circulating hormones and the activation of modal drives giving motivational direction to behavior. These chemical signals are hypothesized to configure into molecular keys that switch on and off potent PSMs affecting mood and behavior, including courtship, pair bonding, reproduction, social organization, maternal care, and territorial behavior. In addition to PSMs regulating the expression sex-related behaviors, survival modes are expressed in association with the release of chemical signals indexing stress-related changes. The diversified functions of AVP and oxytocin are consistent with the routing of modal shifts conducive to social integration or a loner-dispersal strategy (see *Diet Change and the Integrate-or-Disperse Hypothesis* in Chapter 7).

According to the integrate-or-disperse hypothesis, oxytocin facilitates social bonding, integration, and calming under the influence of environments perceived as safe and biologically optimal (adaptogenic), whereas, under the influence of environments perceived as unsafe or biologically suboptimal (stressogenic), AVP/CRF may cause the SES to retract and to promote dispersal and entrapment tensions, agitation, irritability, intolerance, and withdrawal (depression). Under the influence of social and environmental stressors that stimulate increased SAM activity, the HPA-system activity of susceptible dogs may be cranked up into a state of HPA hyperdrive, thereby mobilizing an allostatic state conducive to a reactive coping style that may be expressed in association with a defensive autoprotective mode or a defeat mode, depending on the allostatic vulnerabilities and traits expressed by the dog. The defeat mode promotes generalized anxiety, impassivity, and social withdrawal, whereas the autoprotective mode is associated with heightened anticipatory anxiety, sensory vigilance, and reactive readiness. By contrast, in addition to promoting antistress and calming effects via the activation of the flirt-and-forbear antistress system, oxytocinergic-opioid interactions with other neuropeptides and neurotransmitters may configure an intricate neuroregulatory network that promotes allostatic normodrive, social engagement, play and activity success, and modal strategies conducive to the organization of an adaptive coping style.

A dog's ability to integrate harmonic relations with people and other dogs inside and outside of the home depends on the presence of secure social and place attachments. The quality of social attachments is positively correlated with a variety of QOL factors, including diet, exercise, somatic and cortical reward, perceived safety, play, freedom of movement, exploration, and access to diverse social and place experiences. A high QOL index is hypothesized to promote social attraction and drive consistent with secure attachments and play, whereas a low QOL index tends to promote social repulsion and withdrawal, dispersive tensions, and autoprotectiveness. According to the integrate-or-disperse hypothesis, moving from an adequate QOL index to a higher QOL index tends to promote tolerance for social novelty and sudden change, but only insofar as QOL enhancements are linked with an increase in affiliative exchange. Improving a dog's diet or increasing exercise (e.g., putting the dog outdoors) without simultaneously increasing positive social interaction [e.g., tactile stimulation (petting and massage), socialization, and reward-based training activities] may increase its vulnerability for reactive behavior in response to social novelty and unexpected change. In contrast, dogs transitioned from an adequate QOL index to a suboptimal QOL index may respond in an opposite way to increased proxemic exchange (e.g., close contact, handling, and tactile stimulation) by showing signs of social avoidance and withdrawal or decreased exploration of novel situations. Augmenting a dog's QOL index without supplemental social interaction and training or degrading its QOL while simultaneously increasing demands for exchanges with unfamiliar persons or exploring novel environment and things may promote counterproductive autonomic misattunement dynamics (see *Diet Change and the Integrate-or-Disperse Hypothesis* in Chapter 7).

Cynopraxic training procedures typically embody both QOL enhancements and intensified social exchange with the goal of promoting mutual appreciation and interactive

harmony. As such, play is an ideal cynopraxic procedure because it incorporates QOL enhancements associated with physical exercise and the activation of a variety of drive systems while simultaneously increasing the quantity and variety of affiliative exchanges. As such, increased social and object play should promote enhanced responsiveness to social novelty and sudden change, whereas decreased social play appears to increase the risk of reactive arousal to ambiguous or uncertain social exchanges between the dog and the nervous or insecure attachment object and increase latency or reduce the amount of exploratory behavior in response to novel objects or places. An opposite set of effects should flow from training procedures that systematically decrease social and appetitive stimulation (withholding of affectionate interaction, play, food, tactile stimulation, and access to toys) while increasing social isolation, physical restraint, and confinement—practices that are generally referred to as emotional and deprivational abuse by the pediatric community (Golden et al., 2003) but are commonly used as therapy to treat canine separation-distress and dominance-aggression problems on the basis of compelling the dog to detach or coerce a change of attitude with respect to perceived social rank by compelling detachment from insecure social and place attachments. Such procedures seem counterintuitive and contrary to the basic tenets and goals of cynopraxis. In the case of dogs showing intrafamilial autoprotective aggression in association with unfairness and incompetence and a loss of trust, the use of social, emotional, and appetitive deprivation procedures should only increase social ambivalence, dispersive tensions, and entrapment dynamics in the process of elevating the dog's irritability and reactivity in response to ambiguous social exchanges. These collective changes in response to deprivational establishing operations may actually increase the risk of impulsive aggression rather than helping to reduce it. Attempting to coerce an indulgently dependent and reactively incompetent dog into submission by abruptly extracting insecure attachment relations or refusing access to attachment objects and places associated with comfort and safety may only serve to exchange dependency by indulgence for dependency by domination; nothing has essentially changed, except that the interaction has now become dramatically more volatile and imbalanced in an opposite direction.

Environmental improvements and degradations affecting a dog's QOL appear to mobilize distinct survival modes conducive to enhanced social integration or dispersal (entrapment). Social interaction incompatible with the educed mode appears to result in social anxiety and aversion. This general hypothesis is central to cynopraxic theory, whereby interactive changes conducive to enhanced bonding are coordinated with environmental changes conducive to an improved QOL, thereby simultaneously integrating secure social and place attachments while promoting autonomic attunement (calming), social bonding and trust, and emotional and drive propensities (i.e., affectionate playfulness) incompatible with aggression. Attempting to improve interaction and integrating consistent, fair, and structured interaction via ICT without simultaneously improving a dog's QOL is problematic and may only increase insecure attachments or serve to activate autoprotective dispersal/loner tensions, whereas improving a dog's QOL without integrating social interaction and affiliation based on a principle of fairness may actually heighten social insecurity and dependency rather than helping to reduce it. Even slight modifications of diet may exert pronounced changes in a dog's social behavior (see *Fat, Cholesterol, Fatty Acids, and Impulsive Aggression* in Chapter 7). For example, supplementing the diet with fat or polyunsaturated fatty acids (PUFAs), especially omega-3 [eicosapentanoic acid (EPA) and docosahexanoic acid (DHA)] may enhance a dog's ability to cope with emotional stressors and reduce impulsive behavior, perhaps via the improvement of serotonergic transmission (Buydens-Branchey et al., 2000). However, McCreary and Handley (2000) could not produce any change in $5\text{-}HT_{1A}$- or $5\text{-}HT_{2A}$-mediated behaviors in rats treated with a cholesterol-reducing drug for nearly 2 months, suggesting that the

adverse effects of low cholesterol on stress-related behavior and impulsivity may be mediated by another system. Another possible target of omega-3 therapy may be stress-related proinflammatory cytokines that are produced in association with allostatic hypodrive and linked with depression and irritability. A recent report lends some support to the hypothesis that low cholesterol levels (hypocholesterolemia) may play a role in the etiology of certain forms of autoprotective impulsive and reactive aggression. The researchers found that dogs diagnosed with dominance aggression showed low total cholesterol, low serum triglycerides, and low high-density lipoprotein cholesterol (HDL-C) in comparison with nonaggressive controls (Penturk and Yalcin, 2003).

In addition to dietary and social considerations, QOL enhancements should focus on exercise, play, grooming, activity success and freedom of movement, and varied environmental activities contributing to a state of canine well-being. Recording the amount of time that a dog spends crated or otherwise socially isolated during the day and night provides a useful QOL and social attachment indicator. Excessive crate or outdoor confinement is contrary to cynopraxic goals and typically points to significant interactive conflict and dispersive tensions between a dog and household. Cynopraxic training and QOL improvements are organized to address these disruptive influences comprehensively.

OPENING THE TRAINING SPACE

In comparison with animals trained under the constraints of the laboratory, a typical family dog is exposed to a far greater diversity of arousing stimuli, extraneous reinforcement opportunities, and adjustment demands, some of which are potentially harmful to it or to others with whom the dog comes into contact. Unable to restrict a dog's access to these opportunities or to block entirely the undesirable behaviors that dogs are apt to show, cynopraxic trainers are compelled to construct a behavioral analogue to the physical restrictions and controls found in the laboratory setting via the agency of inhibitory conditioning

(McIntire, 1968). Establishing inhibitory control is particularly important for dogs exhibiting attention and impulse-control deficiencies affecting their ability to accept social limits, to delay gratification, to regulate emotion, and to control aggressive behavior. To address such issues properly, a training space is configured at three points of interaction: pulling, jumping up, and biting. The training space is established to provide a social context of interaction conducive to reward-based training and play.

The first step in this critical process focuses on the inhibition of pulling into the leash. Instead of physically holding the dog back and causing it to strain into the leash, the impulsive dog learns to regulate its behavior within the limits set by the leash in the context of controlled and slack-leash walking. Deliberately allowing such dogs to pull into a dead leash is misguided and potentially harmful (see *Walking on Leash* in Chapter 1). Not only is the persistence and novelty seeking of such dogs virtually inexhaustible, the frustration produced by such efforts will only cause impulsive dogs to pull harder in the process of activating and conditioning oppositional reflexes. Although the passive restraint afforded by a muzzle-clamping halter may be more effective and less prone to the foregoing effects, such restraint is not without significant potential problems. Impulsive dogs often show considerable arousal and distress when first exposed to halter restraint. Many of these dogs struggle persistently and violently to escape by scraping at the halter with the front paws; by twisting, flailing about, falling down to rub their head against the ground; or by pulling back and shaking their head violently back and forth in an effort to break free of the collar (see *Aggressive Barking, Lunging, and Chasing*). The latter maneuver, however, results in a severe and persistent clamping action across the muzzle. After repeated exposures of this kind, the dog may finally recognize that its efforts to escape are futile and simply give up, appearing to adopt an attitude of resignation and surrender to the owner's domination. Halter training of this sort does not appear to translate into avoidance and inhibitory conditioning of the sort needed to facilitate improved attention, impulse control, and autonomic regulation. As a result of such

mishandling and improper exposure to halter restraint, the dog, discovering that the aversive restraint is inescapable, may move from an active state of hyperarousal into a passive state of behavioral inhibition and hypoarousal resembling learned helplessness—and both states reflect autonomic dysregulation but from opposite extremes.

Introducing dogs to halter restraint with a nonclamping halter in the context of reward-based training can mitigate many of these problems. The nonclamping halter is designed to prevent the clamping action that occurs when dogs attempt to back out of muzzle-clamping halters. When introducing the muzzle-type halter to impulsive or reactive dogs, it is most safely and humanely accomplished with two leashes: one attached to the muzzle-clamping loop and the other attached to a flat-buckle collar or limited-slip collar. The arrangement allows a dog gradually to accommodate the unfamiliar and potentially threatening feel of the halter-clamp action seizing its muzzle, thereby avoiding a potent aversive event that may needlessly link the device with fear, pain, and panic. First impressions are powerful and lasting, especially in the case of things that trigger threat arousal and sustained pain, or impose a condition of inescapable aversive stimulation, while simultaneously disabling a dog's primary means of defense and blocking its means to flee—psychologically nothing could be more traumatic for reactive dogs. A similar state of affairs and helplessness effects appear to ensue as the result of improper crate training, whereby a dog is forced into a condition of inescapable restraint and social isolation, and then left to cope with escalating separation distress and emotional dysregulation. In both cases, the novelty of the events and the loss of control over threatening situations result in intense and persistent sympathetic hyperarousal and finally activate the immobilization system (helplessness) as the stimulation is perceived as inescapable. Since crates and halters are readily available to novice owners with little or no significant instruction, great potential harm is done to impulsive or reactive dogs by such instruments of restraint. It is distressing to consider the miserable state of a young energetic dog that spends 16 to 18 hours a day *stored* in a crate barely big enough for it to lie down, and whose only respite from the drudgery and tyranny of such confinement is to be taken outdoors periodically on a muzzle-clamping halter to eliminate. As a result of these welfare concerns, pains are taken to introduce the crate and halter in uneventful stages and to use such mechanical suppressors of behavior in the least intrusive and minimally aversive ways necessary to achieve training objectives in a timely and humane manner and then to fade their use as these training goals are met.

Despite the potential for abuse and misuse, if properly introduced and used in the context of reward-based training, the muzzle-clamping halter can help to provide head and jaw control that makes handling aggressive dogs safer for both the trainer and others coming into the dog's vicinity. For dogs with a history of aggressive behavior toward visitors, the muzzle-type halter gives the handler an effective means to restrain a dog that might become aggressive unexpectedly during training. Consequently, despite valid concerns, the potential benefits of muzzle-clamping halters for managing and controlling aggressive dogs appear to outweigh the manageable risks. A reactive dog should be kept on a muzzling halter and leash or a muzzle for the sake of added head control and restraint, but other collars are typically selected for inhibitory training purposes. For example, the often-maligned and misused prong collar can be used to rapidly establish active limits on pulling excesses with little risk of harm to the dog, thereby opening a viable training space and allowing the trainer to focus more exclusively on other behavior-therapy objectives. Although giving the appearance of a medieval torture device, the prong collar is a sophisticated training device with a number of obvious and not-so-obvious features that make it extremely versatile and useful in the context of controlling highly motivated and impulsive behavior and in developing effective go/no-go and all-stop inhibitory control.

INHIBITORY CONDITIONING

The selection of a training collar and the techniques used for inhibitory training is guided by a dog's particular temperament, sensitivity, history of training, and its owner's ability and commitment to learn the skills necessary to use the equipment properly (see *Training Tools* in Chapter 1). A tool of considerable value in this regard is the limited-action slip collar with or without a fixed-action halter. This training collar gives skilled trainers the means to deliver a precise level of stimulation, ranging from gentle pulsing and directive prompts to a *dead-halt saccade*. The term *saccade* is borrowed from horse training and refers to a sharp action applied to the reins. The word also refers to the sudden and forceful movement of a violin bow that causes the sound of two or more strings being struck sharply at once. In any case, the function of the saccadic prompt is to inhibit impulsive behavior rapidly without inducing disorganizing anxiety and fear. The saccade is always associated with an abrupt release of leash slack immediately before stepping back and anchoring the leash with both hands in front of the torso, just above the center of gravity, before shifting back and tensing as the dog hits the end of the leash. The sequence establishes a close forward association between the release of leash slack and the saccadic event. Yanking against a taut (dead) leash is not a saccade, and such uses of the leash should be avoided. Allowing a dog to pull into a dead leash is virtually always counterproductive and indicative of incompetent dog-handling skills. The saccade is followed by vocal reassurance and sustained petting around the underside of the neck and continues widely over the dog's body, followed by massage on the back of neck and shoulders to further facilitate calming and autonomic attunement. The saccade often produces a one-trial learning effect, whereby the dog learns to rapidly stop whatever it is doing at the moment the leash slack is dropped (all-stop response) or to turn its attention toward the trainer (stop-change response), thereby reentering the training space.

The directive saccade reduces stress while establishing inhibitory control and entraining parasympathetic tone incompatible with reactive arousal. The systematic entrainment of parasympathetic tone while mediating an adaptive coping style promotes emotional states incompatible with impulsive and reactive adjustments. The autonomic effects mediated by directive training are key to understanding how such procedures help to increase the confidence of shy dogs and reduce the aggressiveness of bold dogs. Contrary to erudite opinion to the otherwise, such procedures do, in fact, promote beneficial change and do so without increasing reactive emotion or behavior. However, aversive events that lack predictability or controllability are stressful to dogs and should be avoided. Inhibitory training is typically carried out with the dog outdoors while it is engaged in energetic and non-specific seeking of drive-activating stimulation.

The changes in parasympathetic tone by means of leash prompts and saccades may be mediated by pressure stimulation of arterial baroreceptors located in a dog's neck. When placed correctly on the neck, the training collar closes over the carotid sinus, the brief compression of which may result in the generation of an electrical signal that causes the heart to slow down (Seagard et al., 1999). Afferent vagal signals also leave the heart and communicate the change in cardiac rhythm to the brainstem, which may in turn activate cortical and limbic regulatory centers in the process of tuning sympathovagal state arousal to enable the dog to cope proactively with the abrupt and surprising change. Although changes in heart rate following carotid stimulation quickly abort, the afferent vagal signals returning to the brain may shift autonomic balance to match the physiological requirements needed to facilitate improved orienting, maintain the all-stop response, or promote sustained attention—changes that are often directly reflected in a general calming and improved attention and impulse control that immediately follow such training events. According to cynopraxic training theory, the directive prompt evokes an emotional establishing operation conducive to the expression of behavior that enabled the dog to control similar events successfully in the past.

The autonomic changes produced by the directive event are associatively linked with various antecedent stimuli (e.g., dropping the leash slack, smooch sound, and all-stop signals) that are arranged to occur immediately prior to the directive prompt or saccade. As a result, these conditioned stimuli acquire the capacity to shift parasympathetic tone in the absence of the unconditioned vagal reflex evoked by the leash prompt. The petting and vocal comforting that follow directive events may amplify or sustain vagal tone and actively oppose sympathetic activation, thereby helping to promote sustained attention and calmness. The power of traditional dog-training techniques to calm overly reactive and impulsive dogs appears to be related to these potent and complementary effects of the directive leash prompt and tactile stimulation for tuning sympathovagal tone. As such, the leash prompt is a corrective event insofar as it *corrects* autonomic tone that facilitates reactive behavior. The combination of leash prompting followed by petting and praise serves to facilitate autonomic tone conducive to adaptive behavior, calming, and a secure *connection* mediated by autonomic attunement. Dogs appear to have evolved an autonomic nervous system designed to cope with such training, exhibiting significantly increased parasympathetic tone than found in humans (Little et al., 1999) and wild canids (Fox, 1978). The brief pressure of a leash prompt stimulating baroreceptors located in the carotid sinus appears to produce a significant parasympathetic response while promoting enhanced attention and impulse control, whereas steady pulling (horizontal hanging) or forceful yanking into a dead leash appears to agitate the dog and to further disturb executive control functions.

An impulsive dog is generally walked in a controlled position at the handler's left side, with the dog's hip aligned with the handler's left leg. The handler holds the leash in the left hand as described in Chapter 1 (see *Leash Handling*). The dog is prompted to orient while on leash with a smooch or squeak sound and later with its name. As the dog gives a flinch alert to the orienting signal, a click is delivered, followed by a right-handed flick and delivery of the reward by tossing it to the dog. The reward is given to the dog while the trainer maintains forward movement or after stopping and prompting a sit response. If the dog becomes distracted or moves out of position, the orienting signal is given, an abrupt stop or right turn-away from the distraction is performed, or the dog is prompted back into the proper starting position (scc *Walking on Leash* in Chapter 1), as required by the circumstances. The standard reward is periodically interspersed with a highly valued food reward (surprise) and petting. Surprises are frequently timed to occur in association with antecedent praise and petting. In addition to varying the size and type of the reward, sustained rewards with several small treats can be highly effective, especially with respect to shaping introductory attention (eye contact) and stay training. Surprise can also be generated by the introduction of periodic bouts of ball play or other forms of play as appropriate for a particular dog. Go/no-go inhibitory training can be effectively introduced in the context of periodically saying "Wait," stopping, and prompting the dog to stop with a wave of the right hand and gentle leash prompting if necessary before continuing on. Go/no-go training can be mastered at the door before going for a walk, before coming inside after a walk, before going up and down steps, before allowing a dog to take its meals, and on numerous other situations in a manner consistent with ICT. Go/no-go countermand signals can also be developed in the context of ball play. Once a strong ball drive and routine are established, the dog can be taught to delay gratification and wait (no-go) before it is prompted to chase the ball. "Wait" functions as a cancellation signal countermanding the impulse to chase the ball while imposing a no-go condition that eventually results in the reinstatement of the original impulse via the go signal "Take it," releasing the dog to fetch the ball.

COUNTERCONDITIONING: LIMITATIONS AND PRECAUTIONS

When performed by skilled trainers, appetitive counterconditioning, reward-based training, and play can integrate a significant amount of behavioral control, but only within the context of a reliable training space formed by setting limits on reactive/impulsive behav-iors. Typically, the modification of impulsive behavior incorporates a combination of strategies, depending on its severity, including pre-emptive prompts (e.g., diverters and dis-rupters), stop-change conditioning (e.g., orienting/TAT), go/no-go (e.g., "Wait"), all-stop conditioning, and intensive basic training. All of these elements are critical for establishing a viable platform for graduated counterconditioning within the home environment. Technically, counterconditioning is a classical conditioning procedure, but, in practice, classical and instrumental procedures are inextricably intertwined and wedded. An effective counterconditioning stimulus not only serves to evoke emotional arousal incompatible with reactive emotional conflict, but it may also reinforce instrumental behavior incompatible with aggressive behavior. Generally, counterconditioning procedures are useful in three ways, reflecting the complementary effects of classical and instrumental conditioning: (1) counterconditioning stimuli elicit appetitive and emotional responses that are incompatible with or overshadow competing negative reactions elicited by the target, (2) counterconditioning stimuli (e.g., food, taction, and play) can function as appetitive and emotional establishing operations, and (3) counterconditioning stimuli can be used as rewards to shape prosocial behavior.

Pavlov (1928) tested the efficacy of graduated exposure, appetitive counterconditioning, and instrumental training for controlling reactive guarding behavior in dogs housed under laboratory conditions. The two dogs treated by Pavlov showed reactive aggression toward any person, other then the experimenter, who approached them while they were restrained in an experimental harness. When out of the harness and walking freely about the experimental room, the dogs tolerated the approach of strangers. When away from the experimental setting, the dogs were friendly and showed no signs of aggressive behavior. At such times, they showed a social indifference toward the experimenter and would allow others to approach and even strike the experimenter without showing any sign of resentment toward the action. Interestingly, Pavlov found that the level of aggression exhibited by the dogs was strongly influenced by the character of the experimenter. When in the company of an experimenter who displayed a commanding control style with positive and negative aspects, the dogs showed a significant increase in aggression toward people entering the experimental room in comparison to the aggression levels shown when the dogs were in the company of a more reserved experimenter who displayed a more circumspect control style. In the latter case, strangers could enter the room without evoking aggression, so long as they did not make any sudden movements, whereas, in the former case, the dogs were stimulated into a "furious rage" when approached.

The different control styles exhibited by the two experimenters described by Pavlov is consistent with the low-power and high-power autonomic/cognitive profiles described by Bugental and colleagues (1993 and 1997). The increased aggressive reactivity while restrained in company with the reactive experimenter may be due to autonomic changes resulting from inescapable exchanges with an emotionally labile (low power) and ambivalent attachment object, whereas the reduced aggressive reactivity expressed while entrapped with the reserved experimenter may reflect the autonomic effects of inescapable exchanges with an emotionally stable (high power) and ambivalent attachment object—findings that may be of significant value for evaluating the effects of person on intrafamilial and extrafamilial aggression. In short, the highly specific nature of the provoking situation (restraint in an experimental harness) suggests the possibility that the inescapable exchanges with the two experimenters served to differentially modulate the aggressive reactivity shown by the dogs via different stimulatory on autonomic tone. These observations raise the possibility that entrapment with an ambivalent attachment object may facilitate the expression of different types of extrafamilial aggression, dependent on their control style and autonomic tone, perhaps giving clues to the etiology of dogs that express habituating versus nonhabituating watchdog scripts.

Pavlov tested two counterconditioning procedures for potential efficacy in reducing the reactive guarding behavior of these dogs. One procedure used appetitive counterconditioning to condition stimuli emanating from his person (e.g., shape, odor, and voice) with food to cause his presence to evoke arousal incompatible with aggression. A second dog was trained in similar fashion with the addition of an instrumental response not trained in the first dog. The training process was performed by Pavlov himself and lasted for 2 months, concluding with several days of testing to evaluate the effects of the procedures. Training was initiated by feeding the dogs by hand in a minimally provocative situation, the main hall, where both dogs were friendly with people. Feeding by hand was performed to bring the scent of the experimenter into the composite conditioned stimulus (CS). One of the dogs, Usatch, was trained to respond to the word "sausage." Conditioning was performed by saying "Sausage, Usatch," and then reaching into a pocket, removing a glass case, opening the case, and selecting a piece of food that was delivered by hand or dropped on the floor. Next, Pavlov developed a discrimination procedure, whereby he stood among a group of people before calling to the dog and rewarding him. To foster contextual generalization, the dogs were called from unusual locations with a variable tone of voice, thereby invigorating the auditory component of the composite CS. The second dog, Calm, was given similar training, except that he was required to sit and to give a paw with the command "Sit down; give your paw" before obtaining the food reward.

Contrary to anticipated results, the restrained dog launched into a fierce attack mode as the trainer entered the room, just as it had done with any stranger entering the room in the past. Counterconditioning by pairing food with the person CS proved inadequate and failed to compete with aggressive arousal. Additional control (e.g., interrupting the barking response) was evoked by commanding Calm to sit and to give its paw or by calling Usatch by name, but the strength of these CSs and command components to restrain aggressive arousal were fragile and rapidly diminished as the trainer attempted to approach closer to the dog and experimenter, whereupon the dog again became aggressive. However, if the trainer reached into the pocket usually containing food, the dog could be persuaded to allow a slight additional advance, followed by more if the trainer withdrew the *empty* glass container previously associated with food. A full approach to Calm could be achieved only by showing the dog the glass case containing food as the trainer moved forward. If the dog was fed from the trainer's hand, it allowed him to threaten and to strike the experimenter lightly, actions that would have previously led to uninhibited attack.

Pavlov's investigation appears to draw into question the viability of counterconditioning and sit-stay training as stand-alone procedures in the treatment of aggression problems. The study strongly recommends that these procedures, as used in many contemporary applied animal behavior systems, should receive experimental and controlled clinical investigation for efficacy. Despite their widespread use and virtually unquestioned acceptance, neither procedure has been proven to reduce aggression. Although counterconditioning may palliate or antagonize the arousal elicited by aversive stimuli and facilitate the disconfirmation of previously acquired conditioned threat expectancies, preattentive biases in association with trait anger and anxiety may nevertheless persist or be rapidly reinstated despite the most conscientious counterconditioning efforts. The acquisition of food may momentarily quell aggressive arousal, but the nonfamilial status of a visitor may persistently evoke distrust, suspicion, and potential for animosity. Dogs expressing a rigid watchdog script may be genetically programmed to resist counterconditioning effects actively (see *Flexible versus Rigid Watchdog Scripts*). Counterconditioning applied to reduce state anxiety associated with extrafamilial aggression may rapidly decrease signs of defensive behavior but may not reduce the dog's distrust or propensity for offensive behavior, operating under the motivational influence of trait anxiety and anger. Problematically, state anxiety and anger (agitation) associated with reactive conflict appear to be more rapidly decreased with counterconditioning than are trait-anger

propensities causing the dog to confront the intruding stranger. Further, the mere reduction in agitation does not automatically increase social attraction and the dog's ability to integrate friendly relations with a visitor. Furthermore, despite the reduction in overt reactive behavior, conditioned autonomic responses may persist or worsen over time via schizokinetic and autokinetic mechanisms (Gantt, 1944; Dykman and Gantt, 1997). As a result, even though a dog appears to be more relaxed, it may still remain under the influence of an unstable sympathovagal equilibrium that can unexpectedly shift and trigger aggressive behavior.

Many reactive and impulsive dogs appear to be affected by disturbances of their ability to engage and disengage attentional resources and to shift flexibly in and out of motivational states necessary to explore and habituate competently to novelty, learn to relax in the presence of unfamiliar persons and places, and respond in a neutral or positively biased way to unexpected or sudden changes. These deficits appear to develop in association with chronic defensive arousal (anticipatory anxiety) and stress. The allostatic load associated with being constantly on guard and at the ready for the worse to occur may result in the disengagement of critical social and attentional resources that are needed to regulate and attune autonomic tone to changing circumstances, perhaps causing the dog to rely on subcortical systems for the processing of social novelty and for mediating autonomic adjustments via the activation of the flight-fight system. Consistent with such a hypothesis, extrafamilial aggressors often show a persistent inability to habituate and relax. Overly vigilant and reactive dogs cannot disengage attention from the novel aspects of an unfamiliar person to turn attention toward more positive and familiar associations that might serve to activate the social engagement system—a system that remains inactive so long as the dog remains apprehensive. In the absence of active social attraction, the persistent vigilance exhibited by such dogs is shadowed by a preemptive readiness to attack (see *Collicular-Periaqueductal Gray Pathways and Reactive Adjustments*). Bottom line, despite the most dedicated counterconditioning efforts, aggressive dogs may continue to harbor a negative bias toward nonfamilial persons and respond to them as potential threats.

A related stumbling block impeding the effectiveness of counterconditioning is associated with the timing of incompatible appetitive stimuli. Aggressive arousal elicited prior to the presentation of the orienting stimulus or incompatible diverter (e.g., food, petting, or play) may shield sensorimotor gating, orienting responses, and aggressive intention movements against beneficial counterconditioning effects. The key to avoiding such problems is to evoke preemptive establishing operations, establish effective orienting and attention control, and develop reliable instrumental control. Targeting preattentive processing and the preemptive emotional arousal resulting from it figures prominently in integrating an adaptive coping style and reducing reactive behavior. However, habitually presenting diverters and disrupters after a dog has already reached the point of showing overt agonistic intent is contrary to effective behavior therapy. Orienting/TAT appears to be useful for limiting the adverse effects of reactive preattentive processing and, together with inhibitory conditioning, should be an important part of preliminary training efforts. Essentially, the conditioned target-arc stimulus (e.g., squeak, smooch, or whistle) serves to establish preemptive processing and arousal incompatible with aversion, making it easier to integrate more positive associations.

PRECAUTIONS FOR SAFER CONTACT

Working with dogs that show an established propensity for extrafamilial aggression requires that the counselor-trainer take appropriate precautions to minimize risk of personal injury. Since such aggressive behavior occurs under the influence of territorial incentives and triggers, territorial aggressors are best initially approached away from the home. Approaching a dog that is sensitive and reactive to territorial intrusion by directly entering the house is a very risky practice that should be avoided for several reasons. Not only is the trainer vulnerable to an attack if the owner loses control of the dog, but it is likely that a lasting negative impression will be produced, further reinforcing adverse expectations associated with the arrival of guests and making future training efforts more difficult. First impressions for dogs (and owners) are influential and lasting. In addition to optimizing first impressions and reducing the risk of precipitating an aggressive episode, the gradual approach allows the trainer to perform a variety of procedural probes and tension-reducing procedures to evaluate safely the dog's level of reactivity and to initiate a pattern of interaction conducive to acceptance by the dog. The trainer should mentally rehearse a plan of control or escape if the owner fails to follow instructions or loses control of the dog. Although one should prepare for the unexpected and possess the means and skills to defend oneself against attack and minimize any resulting injuries, mastery is primarily concerned with the acquisition of skills and knowledge to avoid such situations in the first place. The risk of serious attack is an occupational hazard of professional dog training that cannot be entirely prevented; nevertheless, much can be done toward preventing bite-related injuries by taking common-sense precautions, exercising appropriate respect toward the dog, minimizing the use of confrontational procedures, heeding the wisdom of fear, and learning from past mistakes.

The procedure for approaching dogs showing aggression toward strangers and visitors involves several steps. The owner is instructed in advance to have the dog on leash with a slip collar attached in tandem with a muzzle-clamping halter, as appropriate for safety. Instead of directly entering the house, the trainer should knock at the door and walk away from the house while laying a trail of treats dropped at varying distances. The sole of one shoe can be smeared with a small amount of a fragrant odor (e.g., orange, lavender, or chamomile), thereby forming a scented link between the treats. The selected odor can also be put inside a squeaker and dispensed just before tossing the dog a treat. The owner is instructed to direct the dog's attention to the treats or to pick them up by hand and feed them to the dog. During this introductory phase, the dog should be kept at a safe distance, approximately 10 to 15 feet behind the trainer. Going for a walk is a rewarding activity for most dogs that is made even more so by finding easy treats along the way. As the walk proceeds, the trainer can step off to the side and allow the owner and dog to pass by, and then follow them from behind at a nonthreatening distance. Throughout the process, the trainer and owner should converse, with the owner periodically calling the dog by name, prompting it to sit (if previously trained to do so), and rewarding nonthreatening behavior with affection and treats. The trainer gradually moves in closer, calls the dog's name, uses the squeaker, and tosses the dog a treat. For dogs that remain defensive, the trainer can walk out in front and drop a few more treats for the dog to find. Periodically, the trainer should stop and let the owner and dog pass by, before walking in the opposite direction and signaling the owner to turn and follow along from behind. The approach, follow, and turn procedure is repeated several times. Throughout the process, the owner and trainer should maintain a friendly dialogue.

As the dog's willingness to accept the trainer's presence improves, the trainer can take the leash in hand. With large or potentially dangerous dogs, the trainer can take control of a second leash. The two-leash arrangement provides added control and safety, but should not be used for the sake of gaining an advantage from which to punish the dog. Although the equipment can be effectively used to restrain the dog, if needed to prevent or block an attack, no significant advantage is achieved by punishing a dog while it is restrained or muzzled. The idea is to use the added safety and control of the arrangement to foster trust and help the dog to learn that aggression is not necessary to control the situation. Although some dogs may become reactive as the trainer takes control of the leash, they are easier to calm and typically less aggressive than would be the case if approached or handled while inside the house. The outcome of the introductory

process is typically peaceful and serves to provide a useful step toward establishing a working rapport with the dog and the owner. The owner should be encouraged to introduce guests and visiting dogs in a similar way or, at minimum, allow the dog to become familiar with the person before entering the house. The foregoing method of introduction allows the dog to interact away from reactive associations linked to the door. Taking a walk together may allow an outsider to become at least superficially accepted into the family group. During such introductions, the owner and the visitor can perform a number of friendly model/rival exchanges in association with a favorite toy or food item. The visitor is encouraged to toss treats rather than attempt to feed the dog by hand. Feeding a potentially aggressive dog by hand is dangerous and could result in a severe bite, especially at times when the dog is highly excited and distressed. Throughout the introduction and visit in the home, the dog should be appropriately restrained on leash and collar, halter, or muzzle, as needed to prevent an aggressive episode.

AGGRESSIVE BARKING AND THREATS TOWARD VISITORS

A complete history of aggressive episodes, including target, location, and severity, should be obtained. Extrafamilial aggression occurring in specific contexts with predictive threats is much more easily treated than is highly generalized or unpredictable aggression. Dogs involved in territorial attacks producing serious injuries should only be cautiously accepted for behavioral training. Similarly, dogs delivering bites unpredictably without warning are by definition untreatable (see *Control and Management of Behavior Problems versus Cure* in Volume 2, Chapter 2). The sorts of judgment needed to assess risks safely and provide appropriate behavioral training come from knowledge-based experience, and only the most knowledgeable and experienced trainers should work with dogs exhibiting extrafamilial aggression.

Dogs showing threats or aggressive behavior during greetings should receive intensive basic and integrated compliance training focusing on attention, controlled walking, sit-stay, and down-stay modules and routines. The dog's training should be performed throughout the house, yard, and immediate neighborhood, but efforts should be especially focused and intensive around doorways and other territorial frames associated with aggressive arousal (e.g., windows, fence lines, and gates). The starting exercise should be practiced to a high degree of proficiency, with the dog going to the handler's left side without hesitation. The sit-stay routine should be trained to a high degree of reliability up to a 1-minute duration and down-stay up to a 10-minute duration. During the early phases of down-stay training, the handler should frequently return to the dog with rewards, gradually decreasing the reward frequency as the dog's ability to stay improves. The dog's greeting routine should be brought to a high degree of refinement via repeated rehearsal prior to using it in the context of behavior therapy and staging actual greetings with visitors. In addition to practicing the starting exercise and stay training, a quick-sit module should be brought to a high degree of proficiency and practiced under a variety of increasingly difficult conditions. The dog should sit rapidly and remain in the sit position. The training process should set clear limits on impulsive behavior within the context of reward-based training efforts, whereby the foregoing control modules and routines are shaped with food rewards, affection, play, and various everyday rewards (e.g., opportunities to go for a walk). In addition to basic training, PFR training should be performed in locations near doorways (see *Appendix C*). An odor is paired with the induction of relaxation and used during greetings to support social exposure and habituation efforts. Interactive play activities are initiated in association with ringing of the doorbell. Various pieces of equipment, treats, toys, and so forth, should be kept conveniently within reach near the door. A leash should be permanently kept looped over the door handle together with a sign on the door to remind family members not to open the door until the dog is properly restrained or confined.

In some cases involving persistent alarm or threat barking, a remote-activated doorbell can be installed, allowing the handler to activate the sound of the bell while rehearsing the greeting routine. Initially, the bell mechanism may need to be muffled to enable a more gradual exposure and counterconditioning process. Counterconditioning the dog's response to the bell is performed in different parts of the house and at variable times of day. The bell can be used to announce mealtimes and opportunities to go for a walk. Family members can ring the doorbell before entering the house and again as they leave. The combined effect of such conditioning is to integrate new associations with the sudden change associated with the sound of the bell, giving it a broader significance than just announcing the arrival of a visitor. In cases where the dog is highly reactive to the bell, it can be disconnected, or visitors might be encouraged to knock on the door instead. Training dogs that become agitated during greetings to bark on cue may be useful to shift their alarm-barking behavior slowly from conflictive motivations toward a more appetitive incentive. Naturally, this approach is most effective with dogs that have strong appetites. Perhaps the most important training needed to improve control during greetings involves attention training and establishing basic leash control, especially focusing on controlled and slack-leash walking. Orienting/TAT that incorporates periodic positive prediction error (surprise) is a highly effective preliminary strategy for establishing control over excessive barking and reduced impulse control. In cases where the dog becomes highly aroused to the sound of the bell, a family member [familial intermediary (FI)] can go outside and bring the guest inside the house. A rival/model procedure can be used at such times, whereby the guest is given a highly desirable food item or toy by the FI. The guest should show interest and gratitude but return the item to the FI, who in turn gives the item to the dog. Afterward, the guest and FI can exit the house, followed shortly thereafter by the dog and handler. Perhaps the best way for the dog to habituate to the novelty of an unfamiliar visitor is by going for walks. For highly reactive dogs, such familiarization efforts should be performed in advance of counterconditioning. The familiarization process appears to be largely mediated by habituation. A great deal of behavior therapy is involved in facilitating familiarity on a number of sensory levels. Repeated and noneventful exposure gradually helps to reduce aggressive reactivity in many dogs, but not all.

During the enactment of staged greetings, aggressive dogs should be kept on a muzzle-type halter hooked via a closed-loop leash to a limited-slip or prong collar. In the case of owners uncertain of their ability to control the dog, the dog should be muzzled or crated during greetings. The dog can also be kept on the same leash-and-collar arrangement while outdoors (see *Halter Collars* in Chapter 1). Dogs expressing a rigid watchdog attitude or an established history of serious aggression toward visitors are best kept on leash and muzzle or crated during visits.

Ideally, in anticipation of a visit, the owner should practice ringing the doorbell and pairing the event with a treat tossed against the door and repeatedly rehearsing the dog's role, using both reward-based and directive means to establish reliable control. Whenever possible, asking visitors to call a few minutes before their arrival can help time such preliminary preparation and training. In the case of highly reactive dogs, the owner and dog can meet the visitor outdoors and take a walk. At such times, the visitor is instructed to walk 15 or 20 feet out in front, and the dog is walked in the controlled position on the left side. Pulling is consistently countered with appropriate leash prompts and directive control efforts. The visitor can be instructed to fade back by slowing down and staying safely to the left or right of the owner and then to go back in front again. The visitor can also be instructed to turn about and approach the owner and dog frontally following a wide arc first away from them and then toward them. Gradually, more direct frontal approaches can be practiced. The trainer usually plays the visitor's role, at least initially. If the dog shows signs of habituating, a greeting at the door may be staged. As the doorbell rings, the handler tosses a highly valued treat against the

door, taking advantage of the click as it glances off the door, and draws the dog's attention to it. The idea is to link the doorbell with surprise of sufficient strength to antagonize aggression-instigating associations established with the bell sound. The dog is prompted away from the door and drawn to the handler's left side (starting exercise), where it is prompted to sit. In some cases, a large and highly attractive food item is left outside for the visitor to find and give to the dog. As the item is placed on the floor and the handler releases the dog to take it, the guest should not attempt to directly interact with the dog. Subsequent rewards are delivered in accordance with a differential reinforcement of other behavior (DRO) schedule, whereby the dog is given a food reward of variable value after a brief period, regardless of ongoing behavior, provided that no threats or barking occur during the DRO period. When the DRO criterion is satisfied, a smooch or squeak previously conditioned in the context of orienting/TAT is delivered to cause the dog to orient, followed by a click or "Good" as the dog makes eye contact with the handler. A flick of the right hand is used to deliver the reward. If the dog fails to orient within a 1-second limited-hold period, the reward is lost and the dog is prompted to turn about by taking two or three steps back, whereupon it is guided into the starting position and rewarded. As the dog is focused, it is released and the DRO schedule is reset.

During this phase of training, a pattern of control and reward is established that encourages more cooperative behavior and a perception of safety. The repeated activation of an orienting response appears to produce a significant calming effect (see *Autonomic Arousal, Heart Rate, Aggression* in Chapter 6). The handler should give the dog treats until it begins to relax, whereupon the guest is invited to make the squeak or smooch sound as the handler continues to deliver the click and food rewards, gradually encouraging the dog to make eye contact. Eventually, the guest is given treats to toss on the floor for the dog to take. After brief preliminary training, most dogs can rapidly learn to accept the presence of a visitor on limited terms. However, some dogs may persist in threat barking and other displays that strongly recommend inhibitory measures for control. During exposure procedures, any aggressive lunging is countered with a directive leash prompt with the dog taken to time-out (TO). The combined punitive and dearousing effects of TO can be highly useful for controlling such agonistic excesses (see *Time-out* in Chapter 7). TO is initiated with a firm tone of voice ("Enough, Time-out"), whereupon the dog is abruptly hauled through the front door. The door is then shut on the leash, giving the dog just enough room to stand and sit on the other side. Provided that the dog is not barking, after 30 seconds it is brought back inside with a squeak, orienting response, click, and food reward. A food reward is delivered according to a brief DRO schedule (3 to 5 seconds), provided that the dog does not show threatening behavior. If the dog begins to bark again, the TO is repeated in a similar way, and additional TOs are applied as needed. Repeated TOs appear to mobilize passive modal strategies, which can be complemented by using a modified DRO schedule as previously described. Not only do such rewards help to reinforce prosocial behavior, they also serve to produce a calming effect by evoking emotional arousal incompatible with anger and fear. Most importantly, however, surprise generates active modal strategies in association with the activation of the seeking system—arousal and behavior incompatible with an aversion for social novelty. Whenever possible, massed trials are staged at the door until the dog appears to welcome the entry of the guest (e.g., the trainer). The preliminary exposure and habituation process combined with staged greetings helps to process the integration of scripted roles and social rituals in accordance with safe expectations, thereby building a foundation of trust and an anchor of continuity extending to future encounters with the same people or other unfamiliar people visiting the house.

A cycle of PFR training can also be performed in the presence of a visitor, but usually only after preliminary control has been established. Before attempting to perform the PFR procedure in the presence of a visitor, the dog should receive several cycles of PFR training and olfactory-signature conditioning (see *Appendix C*). After staging a greeting, as previously described, the guest is brought into the house and situated at a nonintrusive distance away from the dog and instructed to inch forward slightly at each step of the PFR cycle. The gradual approach is continued until the dog is in the lateral-control position. The visitor should not continue the gradual approach if it disturbs the dog and should not come closer than 6 feet of the dog. Any efforts by the dog to get up should be blocked and the PFR process resumed. A previously conditioned dilute odor (olfactory signature) can be used to initiate the massage cycle to facilitate the relaxation response. Each step in the cycle should produce a relaxation response before proceeding to the next. If necessary, the dog can be muzzled during the massage, but at minimum it should be kept on a muzzle-clamping halter attached in a closed-loop fashion to a limited-slip collar (see *Halter Collars* in Chapter 1). Before the dog is released from the last step of the PFR procedure, the visitor is instructed to move back slowly to a safe distance. When the dog is released, the visitor is instructed to make a smooch sound, whereupon the handler should quickly click, reward the dog, and then continue to give variable food rewards on a DRO schedule, providing the visitor with treats to toss (not give) to the dog. The olfactory signature can be dispensed from a scented squeaker, a compressed-air pump, or by other nonobtrusive means. For example, a tissue can be scented and placed in the handler's pocket. When needed, the tissue can be rubbed between the fingers and the odor presented to the dog. The scent can also be passively delivered by putting a small amount of it on the doorknob or entry mat. Another passive method used to transfer the scent is by handshake. The goal of the conditioned odor is to modulate reactive emotional arousal and make the dog more receptive to social engagement and calming efforts.

Precautions in the management of potentially aggressive dogs should lean heavily on the side of safety to fully protect the guest from an attack, as well as to protect the dog from the consequences of biting. Again, depending on risk and circumstances, the dog may need to be muzzled, confined in a crate, or locked in a bedroom. If restrained in a bedroom, the door must be locked. Visitors have been attacked as the result of accidentally entering a bedroom while searching for a bathroom, for example. Finally, great care should be taken when releasing a dog from such confinement before the visitor has left the home. Many dogs after a period of restraint or confinement can lull owners into believing that they have accepted a visitor's presence. Instead, upon being released from confinement, such dogs may simply trot straight to the visitor and without hesitation attack them. Dogs that have bitten or attempted to bite visitors in the past should not be permitted to take food from a guest's hand, even though it may appear safe to do so. In the early stages of the training process, the guest should be discouraged from making eye contact with the dog; however, once some trust has been gained, progressively more natural social exchanges can be explored in association with orienting and attention training. The dog should be kept on leash and maintained under close control during the entire visit, perhaps kept in a down-stay at the handler's side and provided with periodic massage to support a relaxation response.

An alternative to crate confinement or isolation is the tie-out station, which consists of a length of quarter-inch nylon rope or a vinyl-coated steel cable for dogs at risk of chewing through the line. The line is fitted with a bolt-swivel snap and securely attached to an eyebolt fastened to a wooden beam in the wall. The length of the tie-out cable should not exceed the length of the dog's body plus a half. The tie-out location should be situated in such a way that there is no risk of the visitor coming into too close proximity with the dog. While on the tie-out, the dog should also be kept on leash, with the handler applying appropriate leash prompts to prevent straining, lunging, or rearing up. A tie-out arrangement is useful with particularly aggressive dogs. The tie-out station also gives the handler more freedom to handle the various training paraphernalia without worrying about losing control of the dog. In some cases, an active-control line can be used in combination with a tie-out. The active-control line enables the trainer to exert directive control over the dog while at the same time giving it more freedom to move about. An active-control line is a good compromise between the secure restraint of the tie-out station and the reduced control provided by a leash alone.

As previously mentioned, some extrafamilial aggressors are particularly dangerous at times when guests get up to move around the house or when preparing to leave. Many people have been seriously bitten while reaching down to offer the dog an unwelcome farewell pet. Others have been bitten as they stop petting and say "Good-bye" to the owner. The gradual appearance of acceptance shown by a dog toward a guest during a visit with lots of rewards may lead the owner into a false estimation of the risk. Since highly impulsive dogs (rigid watchdog type) may react aggressively to the increased activity and excitement associated with departures, at such times the dog can be maintained in the starting position or prompted to maintain a sit-stay or down-stay as the visitor gets up and prepares to leave the house. This procedure can be repeated in massed trials, so that the guest getting up comes to be associatively linked with the sitting or lying-down response. In some cases, a PFR cycle can be initiated to precede the guest's getting up and preparing to leave the house and continued a minute or so after the guest has left the house. During PFR training, the dog should be appropriately restrained on leash by means of a muzzle-clamping halter or muzzle, as necessary to ensure safety. Otherwise, the handler should restrain the dog and take appropriate precautions as the visitor prepares to leave the house. As the visitor steps through the doorway, he or she can toss the dog a highly valued food item or toy before closing the door. Careful management, restraint, and safe exposure are crucial for the successful control of such problems.

AGGRESSIVE BARKING, LUNGING, AND CHASING

On walks, many precautions need to be taken to head off problems. Both children and adults enjoy meeting and petting strange dogs on the street. Some extrafamilial aggressors can be surprisingly tolerant of social contact when away from home, whereas others may be more aggressive or unpredictable toward people approaching them when in unfamiliar places. Even with dogs that have a history of aggression toward visitors but appear to be friendly under such circumstances away from home, a difficult-to-assess risk may be present that advises against allowing the dog to have casual contact with the public. As a result, the handler should forewarn anyone attempting to approach the dog about the potential danger and even physically block contact, if necessary, especially if the dog is not wearing a protective muzzle. A muzzle-clamping halter does not protect against such close-quarter attacks and may actually worsen the severity of the bite by causing the dog's jaws to clamp down and hold as the dog is yanked back or the victim attempts to pull away. Many extrafamilial aggressors are particularly reactive in the car, and care should be taken to keep windows rolled up to prevent foolhardy fingers from being injured or lost. Dogs that threaten or lunge at passersby need to be handled assertively to discourage such behavior in the future. Consequently, it is critical that dogs exhibiting such problems learn to walk on leash without pulling. The inhibitory control established in the context of leash training has a generally beneficial effect on a dog's ability to control reactive behavior in response to social and nonsocial change.

Fast-moving objects, especially rapidly accelerating ones in the dog's immediate vicinity, may stimulate a chase-and-grab sequence. Running children, bicyclists, or joggers suddenly appearing and moving rapidly through the dog's home space or along a driveway or property line may instigate intense aggressive arousal in certain dogs. The acquisition of a reactive response to stimuli combining novelty, sudden change, and rapid movement may be highly prepared in predisposed dogs and organized at an early age. Puppies showing signs of reactive behavior in response to the approach of strangers or sudden change should be gradually exposed to provoking stimuli in order to promote habitu-

ation, to develop new associations, and to improve impulse control via appropriate control efforts. Many dogs appear to enjoy the invigoration and control associated with the chase-and-threat sequence (see *Drive Systems, Aggression, and Behavior Problems* in Chapter 6). Less confident dogs may be emboldened under the influence of handler reassurance, food, and forward movement. In addition, aggressive threats may be reinforced by a perception that they succeed. Even in cases where the target is not actually influenced by the dog's threats, it may appear from the dog's perspective that its threats caused the intruder to go away; passersby may seem to flee in response to the dog's barking and threats. As the result of barking and running fence lines in response to the approach of passersby, such dogs may become progressively frustrated and annoyed. If they finally succeed in breaking through the barrier or the target attempts to approach them, a serious attack may follow.

The allure of chasing moving objects can be so potent that dogs will often continue to engage in the behavior even after being hit and seriously injured. One particular dog comes to mind that had developed the peculiar habit of chasing and biting the tires of service trucks on a university campus. While lunging and poking around a rear tire, he managed to get his head stuck under the wheel. The dog suffered multiple facial fractures as his head was pushed into soft ground that probably prevented more severe, or fatal, injuries. The dog remained conscious, presumably fully aware of the entire ordeal, and fully recovered, but to the chagrin and amazement of the owner, almost as soon as the dog was well enough to play on the campus lot again, he resumed the same pattern of chasing and worrying the service vehicles that nearly killed him a few weeks before. The dog's passion in life was focused on barking and biting at the tires of slow-moving vehicles. Such dogs require preventive management, alternative outlets, intensive attention therapy, leash training, halt-stay and recall training, and inhibitory conditioning. Although significant progress can be obtained via reward-based training and play therapy, the competing reward associated with the periodic opportunity to chase may be potent enough to maintain the problem behavior. When performed in the context of reward-based training, electronic training can be highly effective in controlling such problems (see *Electrical Stimulation and Chasing Behavior* in Chapter 9).

When in contact with the public, dogs with an established propensity to threaten or bite people should be appropriately restrained by a muzzle or a muzzle-type halter. Since such dogs can easily back out of certain halter designs if they are put on too loosely, the halter should be hooked in tandem with an oversized slip collar (see *Conventional Slip Collars* in Chapter 1) or used in combination with a limited-slip or prong collar via a closed-loop or two-leash arrangement. The slip collar provides a source of added security and backup control if the halter fails. For example, dogs can escape by struggling vigorously against a halter and backing out of it. These canine escape artists can shift the muzzle loop forward by pulling against the leash and sharply wiggling in such a way to cause the loop to slip over the nose, thereby making the halter come off their head. A dog can also break free when an owner nervously attempts to hold the dog back by grabbing the neck strap of the halter and in the process inadvertently squeezes the side-release buckle, releasing the dog. Flimsy plastic buckles should be replaced with metal fasteners. Occasionally, a collar may come apart due to defective sewing or hardware; consequently, every new halter or collar should be carefully inspected and tested for strength before it is used. The author once found that a brand new halter was held together at a critical juncture by only two loose threads. The halter was being fitted on a large and extremely aggressive dog—the extra time spent to inspect the halter narrowly averted disaster. Finally, moleskin can be attached to the underside of the muzzle loop to prevent chaffing and friction sores in the case of highly reactive dogs prone to struggle against the halter. To avoid these problems, the halter needs to be properly fitted and introduced. Unfortunately, novice owners with aggressive or reactive dogs may unwisely attempt to use such devices without hands-on instruction appropriate to the dog's individual needs—a formula for a potential disaster (see *Opening the Training Space*).

Dogs exhibiting an established pattern of extrafamilial aggression away from home should receive thorough orienting/TAT, intensive basic obedience training, graduated interactive exposure with response blocking, and inhibitory conditioning, aimed at enhancing attention and impulse control. Preliminary training should include *reliable* leash-control and stay behaviors. Training a dog to orient away from a target and to make eye contact or to sit or lie down without hesitation on signal and to stay there until released are essential training objectives. The dog gradually learns to cope with the approach of a target by increasing impulse control and turning its attention toward the handler. Interactive exposure with response blocking and reward of behavior incompatible with the chase or threat sequence may help to reduce reactive arousal contributing to the behavior (see *Social Fears and Inhibitions* in Chapter 3). Response blocking or diversion and differential reinforcement of other (DRO) or incompatible (DRI) behavior offers many potential benefits once adequate inhibitory control over impulsivity is in place. Without opening a viable training space via preliminary inhibitory conditioning, most reward-based behavior-therapy efforts are unlikely to succeed and might actually make matters significantly worse. To proceed efficiently with interactive exposure procedures, all evocative situations need to be identified and ranked so that a hierarchy of exposure stimuli is obtained, ranging from least evocative to most evocative. For example, dogs that chase cars might first be exposed to a parked car and then to a slow-moving car, a moving and stopping car, a normally moving car, and so forth. At each stage, barking and lunging behaviors are interrupted or blocked by means of a stop-change or all-stop inhibitory procedure, followed by appropriate reward (e.g., petting and massage) as the dog defers to the limit set on its impulsive actions. In addition to DRO/DRI training using food, ball play can often be introduced in such situations as a substitute source of stimulation and reward. From behind the safety of a fence, ball tug and fetch and flying-disc play offer the dog a substitute outlet to chase and grab, as the impulse to chase forbidden things is suppressed.

A solid recall and halt-stay response should be established on leash and long line and honed to a high level of proficiency. A long line with a limited-slip collar tied into it can be highly useful for establishing an all-stop response. The long line requires skill to use safely and effectively (see *Leash and Long Line* and sections on stay and recall training in Chapter 1). Preliminary training (e.g., attention, following, recall, and halt-stay) and practice with the long line is begun in a fenced backyard or similar area. When using the long line to discourage impulsive charging, a length of rope is laid out and stepped on firmly at a point that gives the dog enough slack to generate a running speed and momentum that will generate a significant and lasting impression as it is brought to a dead halt. The length of rope set off for the procedure is determined by the specific needs of the dog and should be adjusted to prevent excessive or unnecessary force. A temporary handle is tied into the long line approximately 6 feet beyond the point selected and held with both hands as previously described for holding the leash in Chapter 1. The long line is held as a backup and to turn the dog about or prompt it to come, if necessary. The halt-stay procedure is performed with the dog on leash and long line. Once an impulsive response reaches the point of no return (all-go response) and slips out of inhibitory control, directive or saccadic prompts of sufficient force to counter the dog's forward momentum and turn it about are frequently necessary to regain control (all-stop response). As the dog pulls toward the target, the leash is dropped and the trainer shouts firmly "Stay!" or "Stop!" and braces by shifting weight over the foot standing on the long line and firmly grips the line with both hands. As the dog is brought to an abrupt halt, the trainer approaches the dog or calls it back and, after a brief recovery period, the dog is again exposed to the target with attention and DRO/DRI training. Most dogs show a marked all-stop response to the vocal counter-

mand after one to three exposures to the foregoing procedure. Additional control over the all-stop response can be established by means of practice with throwaway objects (see *Stay Training* in Chapter 1).

In addition to all-stop training (dead halt and stay), stop-change and go/no-go inhibitory training is intensively practiced. The orienting response is repeatedly bridged and rewarded with food to capture and focus the dog's attention on the trainer and to evoke an appetitive establishing operation. As the target is spotted at a nonprovocative distance away, the orienting stimulus is delivered, and a hand and vocal signal is used to prompt the dog to hold a stand or sit. Any efforts made by the dog to move forward or to get up while sitting are preemptively countermanded by appropriate vocal, physical, or leash prompts. As the dog begins to sit, the bridging stimulus (click) is delivered and followed by a food reward of variable value together with relaxing petting and massage aimed at calming and soothing the dog. The dog is periodically called by name and/or a smooch or tongue click sound to make eye contact and is rewarded. So long as the dog orients and makes brief eye contact, a food reward is delivered. If the dog fails to orient and make eye contact or becomes agitated, it is turned about and moved away from the target before being turned around at a less provocative distance for the procedure to be repeated. As the dog's tolerance for contact improves, down-stay and PFR training (e.g., collar, stand, sit, and down controls) is introduced to enhance inhibitory control further.

Effective counterconditioning depends on gradual, nonthreatening exposure to unfamiliar places and provocative target stimuli in combination with appetitive and emotional stimulation (e.g., food, touch, and play) that is incompatible with aggression and fear. The counterconditioning process moves from the least provocative to the most provocative situation. A variety of motivational, contextual, and proximity factors impinge on the efficacy of counterconditioning efforts (see *Stimulus Dimensions Influencing Fearful Arousal* in Chapter 3). Several counterconditioning variations are used, depending on the dog and problem. The least provocative technique involves walking the dog toward the target and having the dog sit every few steps. A more provocative variation involves having the dog sit and stay as the target gradually moves toward the dog. Here, the target takes several steps toward the dog and stops, whereupon the handler provides the dog with appropriate appetitive or tactile stimulation to offset aversive arousal. In either case, if the dog becomes overly aroused, it is abruptly turned away from the target and walked back to a less provocative distance and the process started over again. Another method involves having the dog follow the target person, who is instructed to drop treats every few feet while moving away from the dog. This procedure can be modified to initiate a searching game, whereby the dog is encouraged to follow a trail of treats laid down by the unfamiliar person. In the beginning of the trail, treats are laid down evenly and frequently (e.g., every 10 feet), but gradually the trail of treats is more randomly spaced requiring that the dog search for clues, including the person's body odor or an odor applied to the person's shoes. Changing the size, frequency, or type of food laid on the track can generate cortical reward and facilitate the process. The combination of the olfactory incentive system, forward movement, and seeking activity may exert a positive effect on the dog's response to the signature odor of the person, perhaps facilitating social familiarity and counterconditioning efforts. Whatever method is used, the objective is gradually to replace reactive arousal elicited by the approach of strangers or persons not belonging to the household with appetitive anticipatory arousal and positive social expectancies conducive to social attraction and friendly behavior. Other variations used during graduated exposure include the approach of groups, situations involving loud noises or boisterous activity, exposure at different times of day (some dogs appear to be more aggressive at night), and varying the speed and naturalness (oddity factor) of the approaching target. Another possibility involves having the target walk back and forth on the horizon line, forming an arc that progressively opens toward the dog, causing the target to come closer and

then recede. On succeeding trials, the curve of arc becomes increasing steep as the distance traveled on the horizon line is narrowed. Each variation of exposure to change and novelty should be arranged along a continuum of evocativeness to prevent reactive responses.

Dogs that become reactive during exposure procedures can be dearoused by means of TO. Ideally, the outdoor TO is performed at a tie-out station set up in the open or behind a blind. The tie-out line is wrapped at least twice around a sturdy post and then fixed in place with a carabiner hooked into the handle and snapped onto the line. The tie-out line is positioned on the post to give the dog enough room to stand comfortably or to sit but not lie down. A bolt-swivel snap is used to fasten the tie-out line to the dog's collar. A blind is constructed from two 5-foot by 1-inch PCV tubes that are cut at a sharp angle so that they can be easily pushed or pounded into the ground. For a medium-sized dog, a piece of light cloth material is cut into a 4-foot by 7-foot rectangle, and both ends are folded over and sewn (or stapled) into sleeves large enough for the support poles to be inserted. A center post can be inserted to pull the blind and form an inverted V shape. The blind is rolled up on one of the support poles, making it easy to unfurl and set up. During time-out, the trainer sits in front of the blind while holding a leash attached to a muzzle-clamping halter. In addition to TO, the blind can be very useful for controlling and varying exposures to the target during counterconditioning.

The TO procedure is initiated by saying "Enough, time-out" and then assertively hauling the dog to tie-out post. After 30 to 60 seconds or when the dog has been quiet for at least 10 seconds, the trainer signals approval ("Good boy/girl") and returns to the dog, releases it, and initiates attention and DRO/DRI training at a previously nonprovocative distance from the target. Additional TOs are repeated as needed to control arousal levels and discourage overt aggression. Under conditions that allow it, the TO procedure can include a walk-away consequence, whereby the trainer leaves the dog and waits in a concealed location. Persistent barking excesses associated with TO can be discouraged by means of a leash attached to a muzzle-clamping halter or by pairing an all-stop vocal signal (e.g., "Enough") with a conditioned odor and compressed-air startle or the sound of a shaker can delivered from behind the dog. As the barking ceases, the trainer returns to the dog and initiates attention and DRO/DRI training to maintain quiet behavior. Bark-contingent muzzling may be useful in some cases of persistent barking, but long periods of muzzling should be avoided, especially in warm weather when unimpeded panting is needed for thermoregulation. In refractory cases, a remote-activated training collar can be effectively used to facilitate the rapid inhibition of barking behavior.

PART 2: INTRASPECIFIC AGGRESSION

With the exception of certain breeds developed for an exaggerated propensity to fight, the dog's domestication has generally resulted in an elevation of the reactive thresholds controlling intraspecific flight-or-fight behavior while selecting for traits conducive to social affiliation and play. Unlike the animosity typically shown by wolves toward unfamiliar conspecifics, the majority of dogs are far more likely to exhibit friendly interest and affiliative behavior toward unfamiliar dogs. Aggression between dogs is under the motivational influence of a variety of social factors (e.g., relative familiarity, playfulness, and tolerance for close interaction and contact) and emotional tensions (e.g., fear, anger, frustration, and irritability). When functioning properly, ritualized agonistic exchanges and transactions may serve to reduce overt fighting; however, as the result of genetic predisposition, developmental stress, socialization deficits, or traumatic learning (e.g., being attacked by another dog), a dog's ability to send, receive, or reciprocate agonistic signals appropriately may be disrupted.

HIERARCHY, TERRITORY, AND THE REGULATION OF AGGRESSION

Among wolves, cooperative order within the family/pack appears to develop in the context of an emergent leader-follower bond established in association with a natural tendency for the young to follow the breeding pair. Social dominance and leadership are expressed in a division of labor between the male and female, whereby the male defends the living space against intruders and leads hunting activity aimed at procuring food for the mother and offspring, and the female defends the den and immediate core surroundings and leads activity dedicated to offspring care and protection (Mech, 1999). Active submission and greeting behavior appears to develop in association with food begging, whereas passive-submission training carried out by adults appears to constrain obtrusive behavior. Regurgitation and the cooperative provision of other stores of food by the wolf parents sets the stage for sibling social differentiation (sibling dominance hierarchy) based on their relative abilities to compete successfully for limited food rations. With the introduction of solid food and an increasing unwillingness of the mother wolf to nurse, a process of weaning slowly transitions the pup from a completely dependent status to a progressively independent relation with the parents. Wolf behavioral ontogeny transitions through several developmental stages from complete vulnerability and dependency to a state of self-reliance, independence, and dispersal to form a separate family and home range.

Among wolves, dominance is most predominantly correlated with the procurement, ownership, and distribution of food, scent-marking behavior, and the defense of territory. Territorial claims are secured by means of residency, advertisement (e.g., scent marking and vocalization), mutual recognition and avoidance of the territorial claims of others, and the capacity to eject intruders (see *How Territory Is Established and Defended* in Volume 2, Chapter 7). Scent marking is the prerogative of the breeding pair or more rarely subordinates ascending in rank (Mech, 1999; Peterson et al., 2002). The breeding pair often engages in double marking, especially during the breeding season (Asa et al., 1985; Mertl-Millhollen, 1986). The double-marking ritual may help to establish a strong pair bond prior to estrus. Coyotes living in packs exhibit a similar pattern of scent-marking behavior (Gese and Ruff, 1997). Scent marking appears to be well suited for the demarcation of territorial boundaries. Odor signals do not depend on the immediate presence of the signaler to be effective, they can be deposited in small amounts over a large area, and they persist for a long time after being deposited. The distribution of scent marks provides a spatial and temporal record of the signaler's past activities and likely whereabouts, thus improving the ability of neighboring conspecifics to avoid contact and potential animosities (Peters and Mech, 1975). At closer distances, vocal indicators of presence (howling) (Harrington and Mech, 1979) and barking threats (Mech, 2000) may advertise residency and warn intruders of trespass. Actual attacks on conspecific intruders are initiated and led by the breeding male (Mech, 1970).

Whether dogs use urine to demarcate territory remains controversial (see *Urine Marking and Territory* in Volume 2, Chapter 7) and, although a communication function appears to be involved (Bekoff, 1979a and b), the precise nature of the message and its function remains enigmatic. Bekoff (2001a) collected data regarding a dog's sniffing and urine-marking habits over 5 years. The dog marked somewhat more frequently over the urine of other males than females and only infrequently urinated over its own urine spots. These findings support previous work indicating that the trigger for urine marking is the scent of another male or female dog (see *Eliminatory Behavior* in Volume 2, Chapter 9). Pal (2003) has reported that free-ranging dogs are more likely to mark after observing another dog mark, suggesting that the leg-lifting action may perform a visual releaser function. Raised-leg displays (RLDs) (leg lifting without urinating) were found to occur frequently after competitive interactions involving territory and courtship, indicating that such behavior might serve an agonistic function. Similarly, Bekoff (1979b) reported that RLDs occurred most frequently while another dog was present. Among free-ranging dogs, urine marking is more frequent during the breeding season in areas associated with courtship and territorial boundaries (Pal,

2003). Also, dog mothers scent mark more frequently near the den site, perhaps with the intent of warding off intruders, but there is little evidence that dogs avoid areas scented with urine. Increased scent marking by male dogs appears to occur in association with the trespass of territorial boundaries and in response to finding unfamiliar objects within the territory. High-ranking male dogs appear to mark over urine deposits left by estrus females, suggesting to Pal that such marking may perform an ownership function. Pal also observed that dogs urinated on garbage and food left over after eating, and speculated that such marking might help dogs to find the food when they returned to the area. Pal refers to the work of Henry (1977) in support of the foregoing hypothesis. Henry, however, demonstrated that foxes urinated on inedible food items and substrates scented with traces of food so that such items and locations could be ignored when come upon in the future, thereby making scavenging activities more efficient. A similar *bookkeeping* function of urine marking has been reported in coyotes and wolves, providing further support for Henry's bookkeeping hypothesis; that is, cache marking is probably performed by canids and other species (Devenport et al., 1999) to help them to discriminate the absence of edible food (Harrington, 1981; Gese and Ruff, 1997). In the case of wolves, Harrington observed that, after emptying a cache, urine was deposited into the hole presumably to mark the cache as empty.

Dogs take an avid interest in the urine deposits of females, regardless of their reproductive status, suggesting the possibility that such investigation and urine marking may serve a similar reproductive bookkeeping function. After observing a female urinate, the intact male often goes to the spot, investigates the urine with its nose or licks it, and then deposits a splash of urine nearby or directly on it. According to the bookkeeping hypothesis, the dog's interest in the female's urine may serve the purpose of collecting and appraising olfactory and pheromone information indicative of her reproductive status. The increased interest shown by males toward the urine of females in estrus may also be organized to detect pheromone signals (e.g., methyl *p*-hydroxybenzoate) that are shed in association with the onset of ovulation (see *Vomeronasal Organ* in Volume 1, Chapter 4). The subsequent scent mark may not denote possession, but rather serve to let the marker know that the spot had been previously checked. Dunbar and Buehler (1980) have suggested that dogs might urinate over female scent marks in order disguise or mask them, ostensibly with the goal of throwing other males off the female's scent. Urine marking by male dogs preceding a fight may transmit identifying olfactory information that is associatively linked with the outcome of the agonistic encounter. According to this hypothesis, urine deposited by the winner may not only serve to weakly conceal the female's scent, as proposed by Dunbar and Buehler, but, more significantly, the winner's urine may evoke active avoidance of marked spots, thereby deterring closer scrutiny and discovery of the female's reproductive status.

Another plausible function of urine marking is related to *securing* an unfamiliar place or object by rendering it familiar with the dog's urine scent (Kleiman, 1966) (see *Behavioral Effects of Domestication* in Volume 1, Chapter 1). According to this hypothesis, urine deposits may at least indicate to a dog that it is on ground that had been safe in the past. Urine deposits may also provide information about the shared use of an area (Eisenberg and Kleiman, 1972), performing something akin to a public bulletin-board function (see *Urine Marking* in Volume 2, Chapter 9). Observing the urine marking of other dogs may prompt close investigation of the spot, followed by double marking, a ritual that frequently anticipates sexual play and the integration of friendly relations between male dogs not sharing the same household. In some cases, however, dogs may urinate in close association with hostile arousal and intent, perhaps performing the display as part of a preliminary ritual in anticipation of a fight (Ralls, 1971), whereas others may be more likely to mark under the influence of conflictive arousal and uncertainty. In both cases, urine marking might represent a nerve-steadying ritual, engendering confidence and

place security, and briefly killing time before deciding on a course of action. Urine marking may also serve a cutoff function, occurring subsequent to the exchange of intense threats that are broken off before escalating into an actual fight. For example, Lorenz (1955) describes an agonistic encounter between two evenly matched dogs that concluded with the competitors slowly disengaging and saving face by mutually standing down and walking away in opposite directions, whereupon both eyed the other and simultaneously squirted urine against separate posts and left the scene without further incident. Ground scratching frequently follows urine marking. Bekoff (1979a) has observed that dogs performing the display may be avoided by other dogs during the activity and for a short time afterward, but they do not subsequently avoid the urine deposit and scratch marks.

The ancient phylogenetic origins of urine marking have probably resulted in a number of polymorphisms influencing the form and function of the rituals and displays associated with it. The significance of urine marking, like that of barking, probably depends on the survival mode active at the time and the context in which it occurs. A genetic factor appears to affect the urinating behavior of purebred and mixed-breed dogs, with purebred male dogs urinating more frequently than mixed-breed counterparts (Reid et al., 1984). The evident hypertrophy of marking behavior in purebred dogs may be a secondary characteristic resulting from the selection of dogs that readily and enthusiastically perform siring functions—a highly desirable and valuable trait in stud dogs. Purebred dogs are also most frequently implicated in household fighting—behavior that is sometimes also associated with household marking problems (Sherman et al. 1996). Sherman and colleagues interpret urinating/marking as a way that such dogs assert dominance and mark territorial boundaries, suggesting that such dogs should be prevented from performing the "alpha wolf behavior of marking territorial boundaries during walks" (107). Aside from practical considerations regarding how one might achieve such an intrusive prohibition without risk to desirable urination habits and various other potential problems associated with the proposed treatment procedure (see *Urine Marking and Intermale Aggression* in Volume 2, Chapter 7), the underlying assumption that urine marking serves a territorial function in dogs remains to be convincingly demonstrated (see *Evidence for a Territorial Function of Urine-marking Behavior* in Volume 2, Chapter 7). The danger of placing undue emphasis on a threat-signaling function of urine marking was a concern of Eisenberg and Kleiman (1972), who admonished researchers to avoid thinking of scent marking as performing a territorial defense function:

> Thus, we must divorce ourselves from considering scent marks as a means of territorial defense; rather, we should think of scent as a means of exchanging information, orienting the movements of individuals, and integrating social and reproductive behavior. (24)

Furthermore, even if urine marking did deter territorial trespass, evidence of avoidance alone would not necessarily support the notion that the marking activity was performed with an agonistic or territorial intent:

> The thesis that scent marking in mammals arose from autonomic responses and evolved into a means of familiarizing the animal with its environment and reassuring it in unknown situations is very useful. It certainly does not exclude the numerous social functions which scent marking has gained during the evolution of the behavior, but it does imply that they evolved secondarily. This thesis also suggests that scent marking is not used as an agonistic display for territorial defense even though the behaviour is effective in maintaining a territory. Its efficiency simply lies in the avoidance responses which are shown by the intruding individual. (Kleiman, 1966:176)

FRAMING THE CONCEPT OF HIERARCHY AND TERRITORY

Wolf Family Life, Hierarchy and Territory, and Feral Dogs

The closely interwoven and complementary functions of hierarchy and territory cannot be arbitrarily separated and studied in isolation without losing significance. Just as the boundaries of a country are defended to protect cultural and political interests as well as economic assets, territory serves multiple social, reproductive, and ecological functions conducive to the viability of the group to survive and reproduce successfully. Among wolves family/pack defense is the prerogative of the breeding pair, with the breeding male leading attacks against territorial intrusions, while the breeding female appears to take the most active role in the defense of the den (Mech, 2000). Governance by hierarchy and territory appears to subserve reproductive goals and family survival functions by promoting the equitable distribution of family resources and by facilitating cooperative hunting and sundry other group activities conducive to reproductive success, group stability, and the survival of offspring (Mech, 1999). The reproductive significance of governance becomes strikingly evident if the breeding male dies. With the loss of the breeding male, subordinate members of the family/pack appear to be much less concerned by the intrusion by outsider males and may rapidly integrate social relations with them. At such times, territorial intolerance and animosities toward outsiders are dramatically relaxed, thereby giving dispersed males an opportunity to enter the home range and fill the vacancy as pack leader (Stahler et al., 2002). The cooperative governance, stable pair bonding, family organization, and cooperative care for offspring shown by wolves are not evident in feral dogs, suggesting the possibility that a functional system of governance by hierarchy and territory may not exist in dogs or is expressed in a significantly variable and modified form. Although a socially integrated group of feral dogs has been observed to show territorial aggression around the edges of shifting core areas where they spend most of their time in close association with food resources, resting and retreat sites, and dens (Boitani et al., 1995), they do not appear to exhibit the coherent social organization that is evident in the governance of the wolf family. Finally, in addition to the social function of territory, territoriality serves a valuable ecological function by spreading competing groups over a geographical region, thereby preventing overhunting and the depletion of local resources while opening up new areas for exploitation. The territorial separation of small family/pack groups may also serve an important epidemiological function by slowing the spread of contagious disease that might risk decimating larger groups living in close proximity.

Social Attraction and Repulsion, Governance, and Canine Proxemics

Whereas territory moderates conflict by means of physical spacing, hierarchy moderates conflict by means of social spacing. Together, territory and hierarchy form a unified sociospatial complementarity in the regulation of conflict (Figure 8.3). The attraction and repulsion dynamics and sociospatial relations formed while organizing a default hierarchy is referred to as a *social space* (see *Horizontal and Vertical Organization of Social Space* in Volume 2, Chapter 7). Typically, interactive conflict is triggered by dyadic-control vectors converging on some point of common interest that can support only one interactant at a time (e.g., possession of a bone, resting spot, or mate). The mutual agonism and affiliation associated with the formation of sociospatial relations is expressed in attraction-repulsion fields that radiate out from the point of common interest or conflict along a gradient of decreasing conflict and repulsion. *Axipetal forces* consisting of appetitive and social attraction draw the repulsed subordinate back toward the point of common interest and the center of social space, whereas *axifugal forces* consisting of social repulsion produce dispersal dynamics that cause the subordinate to withdraw and stay away. These forces of appetitive and social attraction and repulsion are reflected in canine-proxemic relations (see Hall, 1963 and 1968), affecting the various ways dogs use and regulate close social space and tactile contact in the process of attuning (coregulating) to one another and human companions. Essentially, sociospatial relations are the result of the expansion and contraction of social space in association with the establishment of hierarchy and territory. As such, hierarchy and territory represent the warp

and weft of a single cloth of integrated social and environmental regulation referred to as *governance*.

Under circumstances in which a high level of appetitive and social attraction counters the repulsion generated during the establishment of sociospatial relations, the subordinate may be drawn back to offer sincere conciliatory-submission displays, seek acceptance from the dominant, and beg for nurturance and protection. If the dominant possesses sufficient social attraction to accept the subordinate's submissive efforts, collectively referred to as a *voluntary subordination strategy* (VSS), then a cooperative and harmonious relationship may develop between them via the formation of a leader-follower bond and interaction organized in accord with a principle of fairness, the mutual adherence to social codes, and the emergence of pluralistic ascendant and descendant relations. The development of ascendant and descendant relations within a shared social

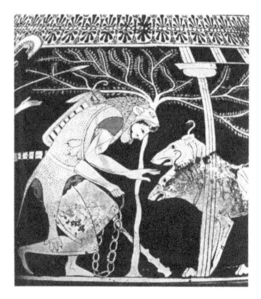

FIG. 8.3. Attic red-figure vase by Andocides, ca. 510 B.C. Territorial aggression can be significantly escalated by social facilitation. Two dogs aroused by a common target appear to become a third entity in their union of animosity—a transformation reminiscent of the three-headed Cerberus, the monstrous dog guarding the portals to Hades in Greek mythology.

space provides several significant benefits for both the subordinate and the dominant members of the group (see *Unilateral, Bilateral, and Pluralistic Relations*). Whereas submission with attraction toward the dominant appears to generate affection, loyalty, and respect (i.e., secure social attachment), submission without attraction results in social ambivalence (anxiety, resentment, and contempt) in association with an *involuntary subordination strategy* (ISS) and entrapment. Under the influence of social ambivalence and entrapment, conflictive dynamics and tensions infiltrate the social space in the process of mobilizing dispersive dynamics and autoprotective behavior.

The dynamic axipetal and axifugal forces resulting from mutual attraction and repulsion produce a state of social equilibrium and integration (s and p types) or social disequilibrium and dispersal (c and m types). In addition to agonistic tensions, the organization and maintenance of social relationships is subject to stress-related modal switching that requires flexible coping skills and an ability to shift in accord with the activation and deactivation of survival modes. Attraction is a composite force consisting of appetitive and social incentives; as such, social attraction in the absence of appetitive security is not sufficient to maintain secure attachments, just as appetitive gratification in the absence of social affirmation and affection is also insufficient. Under the influence of insecure attachments and a reactive coping style, proxemic relations may become increasingly unstable under the disorganizing influence of social anxiety and contact aversion. Building secure attachments is a central focus of cynopraxic therapy, which places equal emphasis on bond-enhancing training and QOL enhancements—the yin and yang of cynopraxic therapy. Training without QOL enhancements or vice versa is not conducive to the attainment of cynopraxic objectives. The dynamic effects of survival-mode switching on the regulation of social attraction and repulsion represent a potentially valuable area for future study into the relationships between QOL, canine proxemics, and aggression.

Avoidance Learning and Despotic Hierarchies

According to the avoidance model of hierarchy, the establishment of hierarchical relations consists of an *escape phase* and an *avoidance phase*. During the escape phase, the dominant displaces the subordinate by severe threat or the infliction of pain or injury (if necessary) and thereby eliminates the conflict and takes control of the contested resource. The subordinate is doubly punished by the physical pain and injury resulting from the attack and the immediate and perpetual loss of control over the contested resource. Repeated defeat may cause the subordinate to experience increased social anxiety and depressed mood—psychological effects of defeat that may reduce testosterone and growth hormone levels, decrease immune functions, and thereby adversely affect the animal's fitness. Under similar circumstances, at least in the short term, the subordinate will fear and avoid the dominant and the places it occupies. In addition, the subordinate in the future may now respond to threatening intention movements (e.g., piloerection, direct stare, stiff frontal approach, and snarl) as discriminative stimuli controlling avoidance behavior (e.g., turning away and hesitation). Also, behaviors associated with the reduction or termination of attack (e.g., dorsal recumbency) may be used to interrupt the attack sequence. If these avoidance responses are successful, the subordinate may experience some degree of relief and relaxation—emotional sources of intrinsic reward that may support subordinate avoidance and antagonize fear. To the extent that subordinate avoidance responses work in this way, they will tend to promote feelings of safety. The subordinate's heightened responsiveness to the slightest tension in the dominant's gaze may cause the latter to feel securely in control, thereby reinforcing the threat sequence and perhaps reducing the likelihood of an actual attack. Threat gazing may be used to regulate subordinate behavior or prompt retreat, whereas averting eye contact by the subordinate may signal its prompt intent to move in a direction away from the conflictive encounter.

The threat of the dominant is an expression of anger held in check by competent emotional regulation and confidence that the subordinate will not fight back. While the threat display expresses an angry intent to attack held in check, the antithreat display of the subordinate is an antithetical intention movement geared toward immobility or flight that is matched to the perceived strength of the threat. When directed toward a subordinate, the dominant threat elicits fear. In contrast, agonism between two dominant individuals results in rapidly escalating threat exchanges based on mutual anger. In the case of equally dominant dogs, threats are reciprocated by counterthreats measured to accord with the perceived readiness of the other dog to attack until a flash point of no return is reached. Accordingly, threat displays induce anger in the dominant dog receiving them. The agonism between the dominant and subordinate dyad is kept in equilibrium by confirmative transactions consistent with anger/fear expectations formed as the result of past encounters. If the antithreat display given by the subordinate is delayed or insufficient (disconfirmed), the discrepancy between the expected antithreat display and the actual antithreat display may escalate threat tensions, that is, increase fear and anger. Under the influence of elevated anger, the dominant may intensify its threats, causing it to become increasingly angry and, if sufficiently provoked, launch into an attack. Alternatively, the subordinate, recognizing that the antithreat display given not only failed to reduce the threat but, in fact, increased it, may respond to the discrepancy by becoming more fearful, causing it to increase the intensity of the antithreat display, thus making it commensurate to the escalating threat of attack. In both cases, social signaling is exchanged under the modulatory influence of social feedback on control incentives, anger/fear-establishing operations, and prediction-control expectancies. The gestural conversation between the competitors is adjusted in accordance with discrepancies between the size of the threat given and the latency/size of the antithreat display reciprocated. Antithreat displays that match the expectations of the dominant result in a de-escalation of threat tensions, whereas mismatches result in the escalation of threat tensions, perhaps followed by an attack and defeat while reinforcing the dominant-subordinate relationship and increasing the subordinate's future readiness to show antithreat displays when challenged.

Consequent to a successful attack, the dominant is doubly rewarded by the emotional elation of enhanced power and the control established over the contested resource. As the result of similarly successful attacks on other group members, the aggressor systematically consolidates power and exploitative control over the group's resources. Group subordinates may similarly compete among themselves until a hierarchy of power relations is established. As a general rule, more extraverted and fearless (bold) group members tend to dominate and exploit more introverted and fearful (shy) members. As the result of receiving the most attacks from other group members, individuals at the bottom of the nipping order may be most adversely affected physiologically and psychologically by formation of a rigid hierarchy. However, a despotic dominator also stands to lose out and may not ultimately reap the benefit of its power exploits. The power gained by the dominant is won at the cost of bond-enhancing interaction with subordinate group members—a factor that may influence its a ability to function effectively within the group. The increasing success of the dominant to intimidate and exploit other group members promotes social avoidance and the gradual degradation of social attraction and attachments. The loss of social ties with group members may mobilize dispersal dynamics that marginalize the dominant (ostracism) and gradually cause its expulsion from the natal group (see Bekoff, 1977). As a result, the despotic hierarchy appears to be in the long-term advantage of middle-ranking individuals, who can interact on a friendlier basis with one another and thereby form stronger group ties.

Among dogs, submission rituals appear to serve important social modulatory functions that offset the adverse effects of hierarchy formation by helping to decrease social distance and facilitate reconciliation by paradoxically increasing social attraction in response to dominator threats and attacks. The formation of hierarchy is not merely the outcome of avoidance learning but also involves the molding of social attachments via submission and reconciliation rituals. These affiliative rituals mediate enhanced attachment by establishing exchanges and relations that regulate aversive emotional arousal produced in association with agonistic threats or fights. Consequently, the formation of dominant-subordinate relations in the absence of social attraction, submission, and reconciliation promotes dominant intolerance/irritability or *contact aversion* and subordinate anxiety, resentment, and avoidance. Accordingly, dominants that fail to attract affectionate submission displays or fail to accept and reconcile with subordinates subsequent to agonistic conflicts may weaken social attachments and reduce the ability of the competitors to form social attachments in the future, thereby increasing the risk of setting into motion dispersive tensions. The lowest-ranking member (omega) faces a similar risk of dispersal in situations where social avoidance replaces submission and reconciliation rituals in the process of constructing a nipping order. Whereas all group members may be compelled to avoid the increasingly intolerant and irritable dominant, the omega may be compelled to avoid all other group members and enter into a similar condition of social marginalization but on the opposite end of the hierarchy. As a result of reduced social attraction and affiliation, both the despot and the omega may fail to form social relations conducive to secure attachments. In social situations that bar dispersal, the marginalized dominant and omega may become increasingly irritable, intolerant, and reactive toward interference by other group members.

UNILATERAL, BILATERAL, AND PLURALISTIC RELATIONS

The foregoing inherent limitations affecting the despotic model of governance appear to be addressed by evolution of a pluralistic form of social governance based on the primacy of social attraction, social codes, and fair play. In contrast to the unilateral avoidance relations making up the despotic hierarchy, the pluralistic model of social organization differentiates between unilateral avoidance relations and bilateral ascendant-descendant relations organized in accordance with a principle of fairness. Within a pluralist system, a default hierarchy informs the structure of the relationship, but hierarchy relations do not define the sociospatial and dynamic content of the relationship. In pluralistic systems, dyadic attraction and repulsion dynamics appear to shape social attunement strategies organized to establish stable and harmonious group relations. Whether two dogs fight over a common object of interest depends on default-hierarchy relations, mutual-need tensions, control vectors and incentives, relevant social codes, relative social attraction or repulsion dynamics, and competency to coregulate each other without fighting. Although the more aggressive and dominant member of the dyad might choose to displace the more inhibited and submissive member in accordance with the default hierarchy, such activities require energy and are performed with some degree of risk that the subordinate might fight back, especially in situations involving highly valued items. Such fighting might also result in a loss of interactive contact with the defeated subordinate and increased dispersive tensions. These factors appear to add a component of "politics" to the formation and maintenance of power relations. Consequently, in situations where the subordinate might indicate a strong interest in some resource or activity that might be of only moderate or passing interest to the dominant, relinquishing control to the subordinate may be in the dominant's best interest.

The emergence of bilateral ascendant and descendant social relations organized in accordance with individual control incentives and the dominant's consent appears to reduce interactive conflict over resources of little value to the dominant but still leaves open a significant risk for disruptive competition to break out over resources of high value to both dominant and subordinate members. In addition to the formation of rigid hierarchy relations around the point of common interest, some of these conflict situations may be reduced by mutual adherence to emergent social codes (e.g., rule of first possession). Adherence to social codes and rules of fair play appears to help promote friendly relations, harmony, and trust-based bonding. The safe center of the home or living space is defined by secure social and place attachments mediated by mutual attraction and desire to affiliate (affection) in accordance with social codes, fair play, and trust. The safe center is conducive to social engagement, play, mutual appreciation, and interactive harmony. These social codes acknowledge the rights of other group members to comfort and safety and to own and defend personal space and the objects contained within that space conducive to comfort and safety. Group members often (but not always) respect the rights of first possession, especially as regards highly prized items. Social codes appear to develop in the context of give-and-take negotiations and play fighting. For example, puppies learn early on that if they bite too hard or in the wrong place, the play partner will either quit or attack in retaliation. Puppies lacking sufficient play experiences with other puppies often show poor bite inhibition and reactive incompetence toward other dogs and people in adulthood. Interestingly, most socialized puppies show evidence of code-consistent behavior with respect to the site of playful biting directed toward people. Puppies that avidly and persistently bite hands will often switch to licking if presented with the human face. This shift from biting hands to licking the cheek occurs independently of training and appears to represent a canine polymorphic variation conducive to human-dog affectionate bonding. Other puppies show a highly problematic and persistent pattern of periodically jumping at the face and nipping at the nose or around the eyes, perhaps representing a canine polymorphic variation that impedes human-dog affectionate bonding. Face-licking-type and face-nipping puppies appear to express coping styles associated with social dynamics and tensions that tend toward the integration of voluntary and involuntary subordination strategies, respectively.

In contrast to the despotism, involuntary subordination, and dispersive tensions that develop in the context of unilateral power-dominance relations, social interaction guided by pluralistic ascendant and descendent relations tends to promote flexible social relations and voluntary subordination. Bilateral relations and sharing of group resources facilitate cooperative projects and ventures, whereby leader (ascendant) and follower (descendent) roles are determined in accordance with natural talent and skill to accomplish some group-beneficial objective. For example, among wolves, the mother wolf takes the lead in the care and protection of offspring, whereas the father wolf leads hunting and territorial activities. In practical terms, the notion of a *working dog team* is based on a similar balance of bilateral leadership relations and the functional specialization of cooperative roles based on talent and skill. Each member of the working dog team plays obligatory leader or follower roles depending on the needs of the mission and the practical tasks for which the team has been trained. The performance of mission-consistent tasks is called work but is really disciplined play. The process of training integrates a balanced organization of handler-dog ascendant and descendent relations and roles shaped in conformity with the work performed by the team. The handler needs the dog's olfactory sagacity and skill to locate the hidden object of common interest and must defer to the dog's lead in finding it. The dog needs the handler's guidance to ensure that the work succeeds and concludes in play. Only the trainer knows the practical significance of the mission; for the dog, the mission is aimed at securing a common point of interest that denotes activity success and prompts the handler to initiate a bout of vigorous social affirmation and play. The working dog team works to affirm one another's expectations and to celebrate their mutual success by engaging in play.

Social Attraction, Submission, and Pluralistic Agreements

Social dominance is not always and consistently unilateral, but may involve considerable variation especially among dogs that share a strong mutual attraction, playfulness, and a common set of secure attachments. Instead of forming a unilateral dominant-subordinate relationship, such familial canine dyads may establish complex ascendant or descendant pluralistic relations with one another, depending on the situation involved, individual-need tensions, and control incentives associated with the resource (see *Unilateral, Bilateral, and Pluralistic Relations*). Most dogs sharing a household appear to integrate bilateral pluralistic relations with respect to access to valued resources and group activities, whether a default-hierarchy relationship between them exists or not. The establishment of bilateral ascendant and descendant relations depends on shared expectations and trust that the other will adhere to a code of play fair. According to the pluralistic hypothesis of social organization between canine familial dyads, the agonism between evenly matched competitors is held in check by pragmatic self-interest and trust-related expectancies mediated by give-and-take exchanges and adherence to a principle of fair play. Highly playful and affectionate young dogs establishing attraction-based dyads appear to form relationships that are primarily of a pluralistic nature, since neither of them are willing or are unable to compel the other to submit. In the absence of a default-hierarchy relationship, such dyads may be at an increased risk of certain competitive problems as they grow into adulthood. The most stable social relationship forms in the context of high levels of social attraction and playfulness in which one partner compels the other one, at least once, to yield submission and in turn accepts the submission of the subordinate, reconciles, and forms a harmonious default hierarchy around which to integrate fluid and pluralistic relations.

Interactive conflict around points of common interest varies in accordance with individual-need tensions, control vectors, and control incentives. For some dogs, getting close proximity and attention from the handler is a resource worth seeking, whereas others may be more likely to seek food or other tangible items that they prize. As a result of such motivational differences, control interests converging on social and appetitive resources in the home produce different competitive tensions and potential for striking up aggressive conflict. Pluralistic dynamics between dogs shift depending on the value placed on the convergent point of interest, with one dog taking an ascendant priority of access relative to the other, depending on motivational differences and incentives to control the object or situation. When conflicts emerge in such situations, it is not so much about asserting or testing dominance as it is about laying claim to valued resources and transmitting information about the value that particular resource holds for them. Whereas a resource possessing a high value is reflected in a willingness to invest a significant amount of energy and to take risks to secure it, less valued resources tend to attract a minimal investment of energy or risk taking. In conflict situations over valued resources, dyad members bring different energy-investing and risk-taking strategies (control incentives) to the conflicted situation. The pluralistic hypothesis predicts that there is a greater likelihood that a dog willing to invest only a little energy or take minimal risks to control a resource (dog A) will relinquish control over it to a competitor with whom it has established a default-hierarchy relation and who shows an established willingness to invest more energy and take greater risks to control it (dog B). As a result of such pluralistic competition, dog A will yield ascendant priority to dog B when faced with similar conflict situations in the future, provided that need tensions and control vectors are held approximately constant. The resulting pluralistic agreement serves to reduce interactive conflict around the particular resource, but without affecting the default-hierarchy relationship holding between dog A and dog B; that is, dog A remains dominant and dog B subordinate, even though dog A yields by agreement an ascendant priority of access to the resource held by dog B. The pluralistic strategy is not only conducive to the formation of affiliative ties and loyalty, but provides a way for the dominant to maximize group control over living-space resources in a way that favors those group members that integrate subordinate relations with it.

Among closely bonded dogs, the avoidance of interactive conflict may also be influenced by a social incentive to optimize affectionate and playful interaction or to preserve cooperative relations and trust by adhering to a principle of fairness. The formation of pluralistic relations allows dogs to compete in relatively peaceful and give-and-take ways over resources that are not unilaterally controlled by the dominant dyad member. The reduction of interactive conflict over resources that are highly valued by both dogs is provided by a unilateral default-hierarchy relation defining a rigid rule of priority to such resources, thereby reducing the risk of fighting in association with scampering contests, for example. Such competition is also controlled by mutual adherence to the rule of first possession. By adhering to the rule of first possession, many potentially competitive situations involving highly valued reward items are effectively decided in advance; that is, the dog that possesses the resource assumes an ascendant priority or claim to the resource that is respected by the other dog, even though the latter has a unilateral claim to the resource. The owner may leverage social control over both dogs by defining occasions (e.g., discriminative stimuli) and rules of access (contingencies of reinforcement) to highly valued social and appetitive resources that are otherwise unavailable for the dogs to compete over. The resulting ascendant and descendant relations between the dogs is managed by the owner to make their interaction and access to owner-controlled resources more orderly, cooperative, and harmonious.

Although pluralistic relations appear to reduce interactive conflict, such flexible agreements of privilege and access priority are vulnerable to changing motivational conditions and cheating. For example, although dog A may ordinarily acknowledge the ascendant priority of dog B to food items, dog A—if sufficiently hungry or attention needy—may cheat dog B by getting to the food item first or by butting in front of dog B for owner attention and claiming rights of first possession—a maneuver that may be perceived as

unfair and provocative by dog B. Such events may disrupt the ordinary stability holding between the dogs and precipitate uncertainty or instigate overt animosities and potentially dissolve dyadic hierarchy relations by reducing social attraction and trust and integrating a despotic hierarchy based on fear and avoidance (see *Avoidance Learning and Despotic Hierarchies*). According to this hypothesis, hierarchy relations dissolve when social attraction and trust are insufficient to facilitate (1) submission by the subordinate, (2) acceptance of submission by the dominant, and (3) reconciliation. Assertions of dominance in the absence of social attraction and trust destabilize dyadic relations to heighten interactive conflict, to promote social ambivalence (anger and fear) and avoidance, to instigate dispersive tensions, and, in inescapable domestic situations, to mobilize entrapment dynamics and survival modes conducive to the integration of a reactive coping style and autoprotective adjustments. The necessity of social attraction for facilitating hierarchy relations may ensure that those individuals that enter into the hierarchy bond with the dominant are affectionate and trusting toward the dominant and are received as objects of fondness by the dominant, thereby establishing an organization based on affection and trust conducive to mutual appreciation and harmony, but while serving the self-interests of all involved.

Scrambling Competition

The probability of overt fighting is related to the strength of competing vector momentums set against the relative social competence, mutual affection, and trust exhibited by the dogs. Under conditions of heightened excitability and sudden or unexpected change, the momentum of control vectors may be significantly increased and doubly so for rare or highly valued resources. Although the social codes associated with the rule of first possession are generally conducive to reducing competitive conflict over objects in possession, the rule may also increase control vectors and incentives to reach the object first. Scrambling competition may be particularly problematic in situations where a highly motivated and quick subordinate may be able to get to objects of interest first that are ordinarily held exclusively by a slower but more aggressive and dominant dog. Under such circumstances, both dogs may escalate competitive tensions under a perceived violation of their right of access and privilege to the item. For example, if two dogs have formed unilateral dominant-subordinate relations with respect to food access, the subordinate is obligated under circumstances of conflict to defer to the dominator, except when the subordinate is in possession of the object or location first. Unlike the relative hierarchy formed in the context of pluralistic relations, unilateral relations promote a rigid dominance hierarchy with respect to certain resources. The rule of first possession conflicts with this rigid determination of access priority and privilege by giving the subordinate special rights in association with items already in its possession, thereby making strategies of first access of adaptive value to subordinates and giving them loop holes for securing control over highly valued items held exclusively by the dominant member. The successful scrambler may also take advantage of owner support, whereby aggressive threats exhibited by the dominant member in association with scrambling contests may be punished by the owner, thereby giving the subordinate an unfair advantage.

ONTOGENY OF PLAY AND FIGHTING AMONG DOGS

Competition between littermates first emerges in the context of relatively symmetrical need tensions blindly propelling them toward the mother's teats. These passive (at first) control vectors enable the puppies to fully exploit the nutritive resources controlled by the mother. Access to the resource (e.g., the most readily available teat) is spatially and temporally determined in such a way that it can accommodate only one puppy body and mouth at a time. Initially, competitive success depends on scrambling success, that is, the ability to get to the teat first. Since the resource cannot be shared, it becomes, at least for the moment,

the exclusive possession of the puppy that reaches it first, perhaps prefiguring the rule of first possession. Unlike piglets (Hafez et al., 1962) and kittens (Rosenblatt and Schneirla, 1962), which establish fairly rigid teat orders, puppies do not appear to show such orderly teat preferences but instead persistently "battle for a nipple" (Rheingold, 1963:176). Puppies with the strongest appetitive need tensions are likely to generate the strongest scrambling efforts, thereby enabling them to reach teats first and to stay on them once attached. As a result, these successful scramblers may derive nutritive benefits that support growth and other potential fitness advantages, including an enhanced ability to compete.

Dependency relations between the mother and puppy during the first week or so of life primarily revolve around the regulation of alimentary functions via nursing and tactile stimulation, whereas dependency relations among littermates primarily consist of thermoregulation, mutual orientation toward the mother, and the collective initiation of nursing bouts and sleeping. As a puppy develops, it shows increasing autonomy with respect to its dependency on the mother and littermates. The emergence of social dynamics reflects this developing trend toward autonomy. With increasing autonomy, a puppy learns to relate to the other as a separate entity and forms relations and attachments. The autoregulation of emotional states and impulses is a crucial aspect of the organization of social relations, an adaptive coping style, and secure attachments. In addition to learning how to regulate emotional states and impulses, active rivalry for maternal care and other resources appears to enable rivals to learn how to alloregulate one another through the exchange of various social threat and appeasement displays. However, under adverse conditions, persistent conflict and power-dominance tensions may gradually cause mutual repulsion to exceed social attraction between rivals. Under the strain of competitive tension, where the attraction for local resources exceeds the social attraction between competitors, a pattern of increasing intolerance and agonism may emerge (loner-dispersal mode), whereby the subordinate is unable to yield submission displays and the dominant (despot) is unable to accept such displays even if they should occur. The result of such interaction is increasing intolerance and avoidance leading to social disintegration. In contrast, under conditions of comfort and safety, social attraction and playfulness will tend to exceed social repulsion gradually transforming competition into cooperation, fear into affectionate submission, avoidance into reconciliation, and despotism into the integration of harmonious pluralistic relations based on fairness and the stabilizing influence of a default hierarchy (see *Unilateral, Bilateral, and Pluralistic Relations*) and a VSS.

Exploitative Competition, Sibling Rivalry, and Emergent Fair Play

The emergence of play fighting between competitors in accordance with a principle of fairness may originate as a secondary adaptation to parent-offspring conflict. Without fair play, competitors would remain conflicted over the sharing of resources and would be constantly in search of taking advantage and getting more at the expense of others via the integration of despotic hierarchy relations. Play serves to transmute competition into cooperation. According to this hypothesis, the gratification associated with play fighting may trace back to the mother-offspring conflict and the associated social attraction/competition conflict emerging between sibling rivals struggling to maximize their share of maternal care. As such, the emergence of play fighting may contribute to the resolution of these primal sources of conflict. Play is a bridge between social attraction and competition mediated by an emergent principle of fairness. According to this hypothesis, the drive to exploit the mother is incorporated into dynamic modal relations consisting of playful exploitative exchanges between sibling rivals (see *Play, Social Engagement, and Fair Play*). The exploitative incentives and advantages taken, given, or denied during play bring the puppies together to play fight arouse precocious sexual, predatory, and fighting sequences that are kept in check by an emer-

gent give-and-take sense of fair play and a shared desire to keep the play activity going. Adhering to fair-play rules and codes enables play partners to get the most out of their mutual exploitation.

Play, Social Engagement, and Fair Play

Competent social engagement skills and tolerance appear to be developmentally dependent on the activation of age-appropriate play activities and the integration of social codes based on fair play. During playful sparring activities, fair-play codes of conduct appear to emerge in the context of give-and-take exchanges controlling aggressive behavior. Puppies learn during bouts of play fighting that, if they exceed a certain limit in how hard they bite or bite in the wrong place, the partner will either yelp and quit playing or retaliate by attacking them. Such give-and-take dynamics appear to have long-term effects on a dog's ability to moderate aggressive behavior and impulsivity in adulthood as well as helping to facilitate the organization of social behavior based on a principle of cooperative fair play. Lund and Vestergaard (1998) traced the appearance of social investigation, play, and agonistic behavior in four litters of dogs consisting of Siberian huskies, English springer spaniels, and mixed breeds. They found that play interactions were closely associated with agonistic behavior, observing that the number of play interactions initiated was closely correlated with the number of agonistic interactions received and, conversely, the number of playful interactions received was closely correlated with the number of agonistic interactions initiated. These findings are consistent with the fair-play hypothesis, whereby playful and agonistic interactions facilitate give-and-take exchanges and the modification of social behavior in accord with a principle of fairness.

During development, the ability to play without fighting gradually results in the integration of stable friendly relations, whereas individuals that cannot play without fighting gradually disperse. The notion that infant social contact and play might help to mediate behavioral changes conducive to social integration and the moderation of adult impulsivity and aggressiveness has been studied in farm animals and laboratory rodents. For example, Price and Wallach (1990) found that if hand-reared Hereford bulls were denied access to other calves in infancy, in adulthood the bulls showed increased impulsivity and aggressiveness, making them dangerous for caretakers to handle. In contrast, hand-reared bulls that had been allowed to remain in close contact with other calves appeared to learn from an early age to inhibit aggressive impulses in order to avoid the retaliation of others. Similarly, rats deprived of social contact and play early in life exhibit a variety of deficits in their abilities to cope with social challenges (Van den Berg et al., 1999). In particular, rats deprived of early play with conspecifics show a significant impairment in their ability to submit when attacked and to prevent additional attacks by remaining immobile. After social defeat, play-deprived rats appear to go into a disorganizing state of allostatic hyperdrive, showing a higher level of corticosterone and NE than controls. The increased reactivity to social stressors exhibited by play-deprived rat appears to impede their ability to effectively initiate and maintain inhibitory control. Play-deprived rats also appear to be more susceptible to irritability and reactive aggression, showing an increased frequency and magnitude of attacks delivered to cagemates in response to aversive stimulation (Potegal and Einon, 1989).

Model/Rival Theory, Fair Play, and Sibling Hierarchy

The establishment of sibling hierarchy relations appears to be strongly influenced by bystander effects and model/rival dynamics. Observing the relative fighting abilities of littermates may change a bystander's estimation of the rivals' resource-holding potential (Dugatkin, 2001), thereby making it more or less likely for the observer to challenge or defer to the competitors in the future, based on the outcome of the fight. Watching siblings compete over valued objects may play an important role in the way complex hierarchies are formed and social codes inculcated, per-

haps serving to reduce the amount of actual fighting needed to stabilize competitive tensions among group members. In addition to bystander effects, some puppies may adopt controlling or yielding roles by modeling the behavior of sibling rivals competing over attractive resources, that is, scripting hierarchy-relevant roles without ever actually competing themselves. Observing that certain interactive scenes regularly trigger overt fighting between littermates may transmit code-relevant information to a bystander that is conducive to fair play and cooperative interaction. For example, the bystander might observe that many fights develop in the context of rights of first possession, perhaps causing it to be less competitive over objects already in a rival's possession in the future. The dog's capacity to incorporate social codes and scripts via model/rival learning appears to be highly developed, and such learning may represent a social cognitive adaptation that has a close functional relationship to social play and the evolution of fairness.

The model/rival hypothesis also predicts that, after observing a fight in earnest between sibling rivals in which a winner and a loser outcome occurs, more inhibited puppies (trait-anxious introverts) will tend to identify with the loser (rival) and adopt loser-scripted roles with respect to the winner and other puppies in the group similarly perceived as possessing a high resource-holding potential. On the other hand, puppies operating under a more confident social orientation (trait-aggressive extraverts) will tend to identify with the winner and adopt winner-scripted roles with respect to the loser and other puppies perceived as subordinate in the group. As the result of model/rival learning, clever and exploitative extraverts might increase social rank and resource control by merely putting on a confident display of winner-scripted role playing, essentially mimicking the attitude and mannerisms of the dominant model. This role-playing strategy might work to obtain significant advantage and social power, at least so long as the actor avoids a competitive scene and contest with the dominant model and thereby risks revealing to bystanders its true resource-holding potential. Interestingly, the ascendant role player may inherit a default leadership role in situations where an overly aggressive dominator fails to obtain the friendly acceptance of the group. The ability to use dominant signals to achieve rank without fighting and social codes of fair play to maintain social harmony and peace is likely correlated with a high level of intelligence and social adaptability.

FAIR PLAY, EMERGENT SOCIAL CODES, AND CYNOPRAXIS

Species-typical social codes and rules of fair play appear to emerge in the context of play, and some of these canine social codes may not develop in the absence of social or object-mediated play. Social codes and fair-play rules help to regulate potentially disruptive behavior around objects (e.g., rights of first possession) and define how, when, and where coplayers can bite one another. In addition to bite inhibition and rights of first possession, social codes based on a principle of fairness appear to impart numerous other subtle proxemic restrictions on what is allowed and not allowed in play (e.g., ambushing or biting a coplayer that is sleeping). These fair-play codes of social behavior exert a significant influence on how dogs cope with conflict in association with close social interaction and tactile stimulation while organizing and regulating proxemic relations among themselves and people. In general, obvious exploitative or unfair advantages obtained by one partner at the involuntary expense of the other result in the cessation of play or a rapid transition into overt threats or fighting. Whereas survival modes exert broad motivational regulatory control over behavior and mood by altering the significance and reward value of events, social codes appear to regulate complex exchanges and transactions between individuals via the intrinsic reward produced by code-consistent behavior. According to this hypothesis, *code-consistent behavior* facilitates social integration and cooperation, whereas *code-violating behavior* results in social disintegration, competition, and dispersal. Not only play but also many other social behaviors dependent on cooperation appear to be per-

formed in a code-consistent manner. Since the intrinsic reward value of play appears to depend on a mutual adherence to a principle of fairness, emergent code-consistent interaction may also be acquired and maintained via the intrinsic reward associated with the give-and-take exchanges that occur during fair play. The foregoing hypothesis has many interesting implications with regard to the organization of social behavior and the evolution of cooperation. In addition to providing insight into how friendly cooperation and mutual appreciation might develop and contribute to feelings of social comfort and safety, the approach might prove useful with respect to conceptualizing some significant causes of aggressive behavior. The violation of fair-play codes (e.g., cheating or ambush) may trigger a catastrophic loss of trust and a sense of betrayal, and prompt aggressive reprisal or retribution, perhaps in search of something akin to natural justice.

Fair-play Dynamics

Canine social engagement and play depend on the presence of a safe and comfortable environment. The presence of fear or anger rapidly suppresses play and dynamic modal relations (see *Dynamic Modal Relations, Affection, Play, and Bonding* in Chapter 7). The sensitivity of play and social engagement to anxiety suggests that similar cortical pathways probably mediate both play and social engagement. During play activity, facial, motor, and vocal sequences are expressed that superficially resemble flight-or-fight behavior but independently of aggressive or fearful arousal or intent, and instead produce a joyful release of social inhibition. The social exploration and curiosity needed to confidently engage unfamiliar social and environmental stimuli appear to be strongly influenced by social attraction, fearlessness, and an ability to play. A dog's capacity to produce surprise and reward while exploring or playing is coupled with an increased behavioral flexibility to cope with the risk and uncertainty associated with such activities (see Spinka et al., 2001).

Constraints on play activity appear to promote social attentiveness, empathetic appreciation, and compromise. The continuation of play fighting depends on the ability and willingness of play partners to regulate exploitative and power-dominance impulses in accord with a principle of fairness (Bekoff, 2001b) and to participate in a way that keeps the activity fun. To play fairly entails that a dog devote attention to the effects that its actions have on the play behavior of the partner and to adjust its actions in a give-and-take manner to accord with the changes observed. To play well, a dog must possess a rudimentary appreciation of the emotion and covert intent of the play partner and a belief that its actions will affect what the play partner does in return, suggesting the possibility that the dog might possess a rudimentary theory of mind (Horowitz, 2002). During play, dogs take turns in the exchange of gambits and play off one another's actions in kind, thereby setting into action play-mediated pressures conducive to a do-unto-others principle of reciprocation and fairness. Offenses to fair play and slight injuries incurred during play are more likely to incur conciliatory gestures, and such efforts are more likely to be accepted than might be the case following a serious fight. As a result, play may help to mediate tolerance and help to facilitate social skills necessary to reconcile following more serious offenses or injuries.

Although play exchanges and transactions gradually result in a shared construct of fair play, the course of play activities is only loosely determined, and some exchanges will result in mismatches relative to what the individual players might consider fair. Exchanges perceived as more than fair result in an advantage to the player taking them and a disadvantage to the player giving them, whereas exchanges perceived as less than fair result in advantages to the player making them and disadvantages to the player forced to accept them. Imbalances resulting from advantage and disadvantage during play are translated into social attraction and repulsion dynamics and proxemic relations. Learning to give advantages in order to receive advantages or to avoid disadvantages in the context of fair play is hypothesized to prefigure the development of pluralistic ascendant and descendant relations. In general, play exchanges and

transactions that are perceived as more than fair are play enhancing (promoting social attraction), but only to the extent that the receiving play partner reciprocates in some way in accord with the principle of fairness. However, if the reciprocation given by the coplayer is not forthcoming or perceived as being less than fair or as selfish, the ultimate effect of the original more-than-fair action will be play diminishing (promoting social repulsion), unless the generous player is strategizing for the sake of some future advantage unknown to the selfish player taking the favors but not returning them. An overly generous player that continues to play despite repeated and unreciprocated sacrifices may gradually become an object of exploitation and aggression. As a rule, both overly generous and overly selfish players introduce discord and hazard into play activity via violations of fair-play codes.

Play and Learning to Cope with Social Uncertainty

Playful transactions involve a considerable element of uncertainty, requiring that coplayers form flexible and friendly expectancies about the other's play behavior and intent. As a result, play appears to promote learning that enables dogs to optimistically appraise and respond to social uncertainty by giving a default benefit of doubt to others. As such, play can be viewed as learning to trust while interacting with others in accord with a principle of fairness, as opposed to the selfish and self-limiting advantages obtained by means of power-dominance struggles. Just as learning to trust entails that one accept and cope with a certain degree of risk and uncertainty, the goal of play is not merely to interact fairly, but to interact in ways that enable coplayers to optimize social advantages gained at the expense of the other in the context of fair-play exchanges. Play appears to enable dogs to confidently navigate through uncertain and unfamiliar social situations under the heightened social attraction and reward afforded by trust. The reward associated with play is hypothesized to serve a cortical training function, enabling dogs to cope better with unexpected and uncontrollable stressors associated with domestic life (e.g., startle, strangeness, and uncontrollable events). Consequently, play in combination with the canine antistress system may improve a dog's ability to maintain an adaptive coping style while experiencing social circumstances that might otherwise promote reactive behavior.

Play not only enables dogs to cope with social uncertainty, it may also instruct them on how to use uncertainty purposefully in the context of benign deception strategies. A variety of faking-out, teasing, and deceiving tactics and exchanges are performed in the context of friendly play. Players appear to learn to take advantage of one another by means of teasing and enticing the coplayer rather than by coercing and threatening it. Players increase the momentum of play when they are getting more advantages from the play partner than they expected to receive (surprise) and hesitate or inhibit play when they get fewer advantages than expected (disappointment). Play becomes merely boring when it is just equal or entirely devoid of competitive tension and risk. Despite the momentary ups and downs, the net accumulation of advantages taken and disadvantages incurred during friendly play is generally fair, but with a variance that may slightly favor one of the players at the expense of the other. If the inequities during play are perceived as being too great (unfair), the disad-vantaged player may quit or play may precipitously slip into a fighting-in-earnest mode. To avoid some of the pitfalls associated with play fighting, mature players may instruct younger coplayers on how to play fairly by engaging them in object play (e.g., running about holding a long stick in common). If one of the partners pulls too hard, the stick is dislodged from the other's mouth and the fun ends. Tug games may serve a similar instructive function. In addition to object play, a sense of fairness appears to motivate adults and large powerful dogs to handicap themselves to better sustain play with younger or smaller coplayers.

Play, Fairness, and Social Leadership

A dog's propensity to engage, disengage, or confront strange dogs appears to be strongly influenced by social attraction and repulsion, social engagement skills, individual emotional differences affecting reactive thresholds, and cognitive abilities to process subtle social signals. Most dogs show more social attraction than repulsion toward unfamiliar dogs and rapidly approach one another up to a point where repulsion dynamics may cause them to hesitate (conflict distance) and engage in more circumspect and reciprocal social investigations that eventually transition into play. Unlike the extreme behavior of fearlessly obtrusive or power-seeking dogs, most dogs require an introductory phase of mutual investigation before proceeding to more playful or agonistic interaction or disengagement (cutoff). The introductory phase between unfamiliar but friendly dogs is mutually flirtatious and exploratory, consisting of genital investigation and licking. In addition, dogs appear actively and, at times provocatively, to probe one another with sudden fits and starts of activity together with metasignals (e.g., play bow and play face), perhaps to uncover the other's intent, level of irritability, and willingness to play. The play of friendly but unfamiliar dogs is often of a sexual nature. Playful chase-and-evade games, feigned stalk-and-charge sequences, and sparring activities are also frequent and sustained. The playful care seeking and caregiving, competition, sexual exploration, and predatory components may enable dogs to rapidly explore one another and to get on familiar and friendly terms, while stimulating a variety of reward systems conducive to social engagement. Playful sexual behavior may mediate effects akin to pair bonding, whereas caregiving and care-receiving sequences may stimulate maternal/offspring-like bonding processes via the release of oxytocin and prolactin. Predatory-like sequences and reversals may stimulate reward via the activation of the seeking or behavioral approach system (BAS), while play fighting might promote feelings of affiliation and trust. The proxemic scenes and behavioral topographies exhibited by dogs engaged in play may reflect transient states of emotional arousal relevant to the functional system activated by the play activity (e.g., sexual, predatory, and agonistic or power dominance).

When performed in conformity with a principle of fairness and mutual appreciation, these emotional states may synergistically interact to produce a state of joy. However, when activated in the absence of social attraction and fairness, these systems may produce an opposite set of synergistic effects promoting behavior akin to cruelty. Consequently, play in the absence of social attraction and a principle of fairness may quickly transition into exploitation or fighting, resulting in social repulsion and dispersive tensions.

Affectionate proximity seeking and gestures of a friendly nature are common between playful dogs when they are not engaged in play (e.g., gentle facial investigation, sniffing, and licking of the ears). As dogs become familiar and start to integrate friendly relations, they may mutually assert limits on one another, often by the most patient and gentle means, including, if necessary, by direct stare, fang flashing, baring teeth, inhibited nips, and nonbiting snaps or lunge barks. Gradually, a friendly leader-follower bond emerges with the most socially competent, physically active, and confident dogs usually taking a leadership role. Such leaders often show an extraordinary *play drive* and appetite for friendly social interaction. Leaders establish harmony by means of example and adherence to social codes, which includes a fastidious caution with respect to the first law of canine etiquette: the right of first possession. Leaders of this type appear to inspire a subtle form of imitation, submission, and the integration of a voluntary subordination strategy. In contrast, a socially exploitative dog responds to the approach of an familiar dog with a rapid transition to obtrusive play, whereas a socially despotic trait aggressor may stridently approach an unfamiliar dog and compel it to fight. Both of these types violate the principle of fairness necessary for friendly cooperation and play.

INTRASPECIFIC STATE AND TRAIT AGGRESSION

Dogs exhibiting a power-dominance orientation toward unfamiliar males may deliver vigorous and unprovoked attacks based solely on gender and unfamiliarity. As youngsters of 4 to 9 months of age, or occasionally younger, such dogs may suddenly become aggressive and intolerant of close proximity with other dogs—an intolerance that may persist throughout their lives despite intensive positive socialization efforts. The propensity to fight shown by such dogs does not appear to be aimed at integrating hierarchical relations, since trait aggressors will seek a fight with the same dog that the day before was thoroughly intimidated. Many of these dogs appear to operate under the influence of a persistent motivation or drive to fight. A useful term for this sort of agonism is *intraspecific trait aggression*, emphasizing a strong genetic influence predisposing certain dogs to fight. Trait aggression reflects a persistent disposition or temperament trait to experience other dogs as objects to attack. In contrast, dogs exhibiting state aggression fight only to escape or avoid an unconditioned social stimulus evoking frustration or irritation. Whereas state anger is highly emotional and intrinsically aversive, trait anger appears to mediate fighting under the influence of quiet attack and power-dominance motivations (reward incentive). The notion of trait aggression suggests an enduring predisposition to seek out and confront other dogs for the purpose of picking fights, whereas state aggressors fight back or retaliate, exhibiting an unwillingness to submit in response to provocative stimulation (low-fight/high-fear thresholds). Trait aggressors appear to derive reward from fighting, whereas state aggressors obtain reward by avoiding fights (threat display) or fight to escape the fight-evoking situation. The notion that aggression might be rewarding has been recently demonstrated among mice trained to perform an instrumental nose-poke task for the opportunity to attack an intruder for 12 seconds (Fish et al., 2002). These findings suggest that the reward associated with trait aggression may be largely derived from the positive emotions (elation) associated with trait anger and the activation of the BAS (Harmon-Jones, 2003).

Consistent with the intrinsic-reward hypothesis, trait aggressors may develop various strategies to improve the likelihood of getting an opportunity to fight, and show a preference for locations of past fights. On walks, such dogs may lag behind or, if permitted off leash, they may take advantage of turns or intersections with an apparent hope of putting themselves in a better position to encounter another dog. The trait aggressor may urine mark to attract the marking activity of potential rivals and thereby track their general activity and whereabouts. Urine marks are carefully examined and licked, and surface earth is sometimes slightly upturned while inspecting them. Repeated exposure to the urine odor of a potential target may exert a potent instigating effect on trait aggression. When entering into areas associated with past fighting, trait aggressors often urinate or defecate and then cut deep signature marks into the ground by forceful scratching. Some of these dogs become very stealthy and deceptive, appearing to minimize signs of arousal and intent in order to put the owner at ease before breaking free to attack or lunging and grabbing the other dog and refusing to let go. Trait aggressors live to fight and habitually provoke aggressive interaction with other dogs, irrespective of apparent territorial incentives, appearing to seek aggressive encounters as something akin to a sport activity. Trait aggressors often approach other dogs excitedly with unwavering eye contact and present an inflexible and propped-up appearance that may be misinterpreted as an excited prelude to play. The carriage of the tail expresses social confidence and determination, and trait aggressors usually hold their tails in a stiffly erect position that may quiver and twitch with anticipation. If ignored or not reciprocated with complete submission and obsequiousness, these displays are followed by rapidly escalating threats, including intrusive proximity and contact posturing, an agonistic T orientation, mouthing or nervously licking at the scruff, rising up and mounting actions, and a point of no return. Some trait aggressors show a wide-eyed look of glee (clown face) and an excited tight tail wag just before launching into an attack. Experienced trait aggressors may decide to attack while at considerable distance from the target. In such cases, the aggressor may skip *foreplay* niceties

and execute a frontal charge and crash directly into the target, thereby securing an immediate and perhaps devastating advantage. Trait aggressors fight vigorously but appear to maintain emotional composure and often do not bark before attacking.

Many of these dogs seem to be governed by something akin to a chivalrous code that seems to obligate them to fight with other adult male dogs of approximately the same size or larger, whereas they show extremely friendly behavior, bordering on fawning, toward females, with whom they often enact playful courtships. Such dogs appear to fight as though their honor and self-respect depended on it. Trait aggressors are usually gentle and paternal in attitude toward puppies, but are not above serving out harsh punishment to obtrusive juveniles. Although neutered dogs are not immune to attack, in some cases experienced trait aggressors appear to treat them differently, almost as though they did not exist. Some trait aggressors may perceive neutered dogs as being neither male nor female and consequently treat them as nonentities—a feature that suggests a possible gender-specific olfactory trigger or modulatory mechanism controlling such behavior. As they age, trait aggressors typically become less aggressive toward other dogs and seem to retire from fighting altogether in old age. Unlike male aggressors, female aggressors are often equally aggressive toward males and females (see *Virago Syndrome* in Volume 2, Chapter 7). Female aggressors appear to be motivated to fight by different incentives than males (trait/state motivations), showing greater contact intolerance toward other dogs, and, unlike male counterparts, female trait aggressors do not appear to derive the same amount of intrinsic reward from the fighting activity and probably fight for different reasons. Whereas male trait aggressors might be described as fighting for the thrill, female trait aggressors appear to fight for the kill, but are usually satisfied with merely getting rid of the other female. The severity of fighting between females appears to exceed that of comparable males, especially in fighting between dogs sharing the same household. Severe and persistent fighting between females living in the same home is often motivated by social repulsion and dispersal incentives.

CONTROLLING INTRASPECIFIC AGGRESSION TOWARD NONFAMILIAL TARGETS

Unfortunately, owners of dogs that like to fight are often under the influence of denial, refusing to appreciate fully the danger posed by their dog's appetite for fighting. Such owners are prone to offer capricious interpretations and rationalizations to lessen the seriousness of the behavior or to find excuses for it. Many owners appear to treat dog fighting as a normal canine nuisance behavior and are reluctant to seek professional help to control it (Baranyiova et al., 2003). Occasionally, owners may get a vicarious thrill from the dog's eagerness to fight. Such owners may allow a serious problem to develop or intentionally facilitate a dog's propensity to fight. Many owners of aggressive dogs are strikingly irresponsible and permissive with regard to the lackadaisical effort they put into keeping their aggressive dogs under control while in public. Some continue to give their aggressors the liberty to attack other dogs on multiple occasions while in public places. Roll and Unshelm (1997) found that 31% of dogs that fight do so with other dogs known to be targets by the owner in advance of the fight.

All intraspecific aggressors should undergo intensive basic training to tame their aggressive impulses. The goal of remedial training is to promote inhibitory control and introduce countermand signals that reliably interrupt attack-sequence processing and integrate more appropriate ways to cope with the presence of another dog nearby. Large powerful breeds should be exercised on muzzling-type halters attached in combination with a slip collar or a prong and closed-loop leash arrangement, as previously described. As with other cases involving aggression, graduated and massed-trial exposure, response blocking, and inhibitory conditioning can help to reduce reactive behavior and make the dog more immediately responsive to owner command. The following set of procedures assumes that the dog has received intensive preliminary ori-

enting/TAT, thorough basic obedience training, and preliminary inhibitory conditioning.

Aggressive Tensions Around Fence Lines

A common focal point of aggression is fence fighting, which can be a serious problem and cause neighboring dogs to become increasingly agitated and aggressive toward one another. The impulse to fight appears to be intensified by daily instigative exposure to the odor and sight of agonistic targets. Laboratory animals exposed to the sight and smell of opponents but not permitted to fight show a significant increase in aggressive threats and attacks when they are finally free to fight (de Almeida and Miczek, 2002). Whenever possible, fighting dogs that share adjoining yards should be prevented from seeing one another through a fence. Stockade fencing backed with chain-link fencing buried in the ground can be helpful. With aggressive dogs that need to be kenneled in adjoining runs, it is a good idea to divide runs with a 3-foot walkway between enclosures or to separate runs with opaque dividers. Kenneled dogs sometimes break off canines while fence fighting, a significant problem with working dogs whose teeth are needed in working order. Setting up a schedule with neighbors for putting the dogs out separately can be a helpful way to avoid unsupervised encounters between the dogs. Since some dogs appear to develop increased tolerance as the result of graduated exposure, arranging to go for walks with the neighbor and dog can help to reduce tensions. During walks, the dogs should be appropriately restrained and kept far enough apart to minimize aggressive tensions. Both dogs should be discouraged from pulling into the leash and prompted to orient and sit at the least sign of building tensions. Strong emphasis is placed on positive reinforcement, with both dogs receiving vocal encouragement, petting/massage, and food rewards so long as they mind their own business. After returning home, the dogs can be walked along the shared fence line at a nonprovocative distance. Every few steps, both dogs should be prompted to sit or lie down and stay followed by appropriate rewards. If everything goes well, the owners can initiate object-oriented play activities with the dogs on long lines. When in the yard, performing attention and recall training and playing tug and fetch can help to focus a dog's attention on activities more gratifying than fence fighting. To break up the habit of exiting the house to immediately search for the other dog or scramble to the fence, the dog should receive appropriate inhibitory training around such occasions. Taking the dog outdoors periodically during the day and engaging it in ball play and other basic-training activities can also be helpful.

Dogs showing excessive and persistent aggressive behavior toward other dogs along fence lines should receive intensive recall and halt-stay training, enabling the owner to interrupt the behavior reliably (see *Aggressive Barking, Lunging, and Chasing*). Once a high level of command and countermand control is established, the use of various behavior- and remote-activated devices can be considered, as needed, to enhance inhibitory control over barking excesses and charging at the fence line. The toss of a scented shaker can or jangle of throw rings can be highly effective for interrupting and deterring some fence-related problem behavior, especially in situations where alternative behavior is prompted and rewarded consequent to the startle event. Some electronic devices currently available incorporate both remote and bark-activated capabilities that can be extremely effective when properly introduced. Although electronic training tools are of significant value in such situations, they can also produce significant harm if used improperly. As things progress, various behavior-activated and remote techniques can be applied as appropriate and needed to bring the behavior under more reliable control. For example, in persistent cases, a spray deterrent or electronic containment device might be used to keep the dog away from the fence line.

Attention Control and Gradual Exposure Techniques

Since preattentive processing anticipates the mobilization of arousal leading to aggression, preemptive control is established in advance of a dog showing overt signs of aggressive intent or behavior in order to promote an autonomic state and emotional establishing operations conducive to behavior incompatible with aggression. A conditioned orienting stimulus or a diverter/disrupter may be used to evoke the necessary motivational changes. Diversion with the orienting stimulus or food can be highly effective, if followed by efforts to shape incompatible behavior. If the dog is diverted with food, it is required to perform at least five simple responses (e.g., repeated orienting and eye contact, approach and sit, stand-stay, and so forth) before being allowed to turn back toward the target. Alternatively, a DRO schedule can be implemented whereby the dog is given a reward after some brief period has passed (3 to 5 seconds), provided that it does not show aggression toward the other dog. The delivery of periodic surprise consisting of a highly valued food item (e.g., chunks of chicken, beef, or fish) appears to help integrate new expectancies and to mobilize active modal strategies incompatible with aggression. Access to a rubber toy containing the reward can be very useful in support of DRI and DRO training and for producing a sustained interruption of aggressive arousal and activating appetitive-establishing operations that may antagonize provocative arousal and set the stage to advance the exposure process. The rubber toy is attached to a 6-foot piece of rope with a handle so that toy can be pulled around and the dog enticed to follow and grab it. The dog is permitted to keep the item for a variable length of time to (e.g., 10 seconds to 2 minutes) before it is required to release it to the handler. If the dog barks aggressively or lunges during a DRO cycle, the object is taken from the dog, followed by a right-turn maneuver and directive leash prompt sufficient to secure the dog's attention and to ease the escalating tension, whereupon the dog is hauled off to a post or tree previously set up as a tie-out station. The tie-out should give the dog enough room to stand and sit comfortably but prevent it from lying down during the 30- to 60-second time-out.

In some cases, forced backing can be used in combination with the forward pattern to counteract aggressive arousal. The dog is trained to walk backward in response to leash prompting and the vocal signal "Back" in a training setting without a target dog. For example, a backing-and-waiting routine can be incorporated into a ritual used when preparing to exit the house for a walk. At such times, if the dog charges impulsively through the door, the leash can be pulled short and pinched in the door jamb, leaving the dog in TO for 30 seconds before trying again. In situations where the dog shows aggressive arousal, it is prompted to back away five steps or so from the target before its attention is diverted with the orienting stimulus and a cycle of DRI or DRO training is initiated. A thoroughly conditioned sit-stay response and orienting/attending response can be extremely useful in such cases. After the dog is prompted to sit, it is periodically prompted with a smooch to make eye contact, followed by the vocal bridge "Good" and a variable or sustained reward. Sustained rewards are provided to the dog by means of sustained petting or massage and several small pieces of food. As the dog shows signs of relaxing, it is walked 5 feet closer to the target and rewarded. If the dog becomes aroused again, though, it is backed off once more from the target, but perhaps more forcefully than before. Whereas forward locomotion is associated with the activation of the seeking system and reward, backward locomotion is mildly aversive and associated with inhibition and retreat. The combination of orienting/TAT, DRI-DRO training, forward-exposure, and backward-exposure procedures with appetitive surprise, and sustained reward, appears to provide complementary modulatory influences over arousal shifts.

Another gradual approach strategy incorporates the starting exercise and basic obedience modules that are first trained to a high level of proficiency, with the dog going to the trainer's left side, sitting, standing, lying down, and staying put until released by the handler (see *Stay Training* in Chapter 1). The dog is started at a nonprovocative distance and turned about to face the target and prompted to sit, rewarded, and released. The starting exercise is repeated over and over again until the dog turns away from the other

target, goes to the handler's left side, and sits squarely without hesitation. The dog is then prompted to stand by the handler taking one step forward on the left foot, and again the dog's attention is prompted by means of its name or orienting stimulus (e.g., smooch, squeak, or whistle). Orienting prompts are repeated as the dog is walked at a slow pace toward the target, with the orienting stimulus and click sequence occurring every three to five steps followed by the SE and high-value surprises delivered periodically by hand or tossed to the dog. At the first point in the forward progression in which the dog refuses to yield its attention to the trainer, the handler takes two or three steps back while signaling the dog to the starting position. If dog fails to sit squarely, the handler again steps back and guides the dog into the position. After a moment, the dog is prompted to stand and then to sit, followed by another stand and then prompted to sit and lie down once more. This pattern, consisting of the sit, stand, sit, down, and stand cycle is repeated, with each module of the routine taking 5 seconds to complete, with sustained reward (vocal reassurance, petting, and food), until the distance walked backward is regained in an inchworm fashion. When the original point is reached, the dog is release with an "Okay" and engaged in tug-and-fetch play on leash. If the dog turns from the toy toward the other dog, it is prompted to the starting position by taking two or three steps back and guiding it around. The starting routine is repeated with variations (e.g., left and right approach, interrupting the automatic sit, heeling the dog out of the starting position, and leaving the dog in a sit-stay). Interrupting the dog's attention at the earliest sign of shifting arousal is preferred, but, if arousal escalates at any time into an overt threat (e.g., barking or lunge), a directive prompt or saccade (all-stop procedure) and right-about turn is carried out, whereupon the dog is repositioned at a less provocative distance from the target where the starting exercise with orienting stimulus, bridge, and social and appetitive reward are repeated.

Prompting the dog to orient and repeatedly guiding it into the starting position until it goes to the position and sits without hesitation can be helpful for integrating inhibitory stop-change control. As the dog begins to sit, the vocal bridging stimulus is delivered, followed by relaxing petting, the presentation of a food reward of significant value, and massage as the dog continues to remain compliant. Inhibitory conditioning is focused on the sit-stay routine rather than punishing overt lunging and threat behavior. In some cases, scented compressed air can be delivered silently, followed by a countermand (e.g., "Stop!" or "Out!") and a brief burst from the modified air pump can effectively grab the dog's attention and generate rapid inhibition without risk of damaging the dog's ears or the ears of bystanders, as might occur with a nautical horn used at close quarters. Exposure to other dogs is carried out under varying conditions and degrees of interactive exposure and risk, as determined to be appropriate, safe, and most likely to succeed. Exposure is best mediated in the context of practicing a variety of basic obedience exercises on a 6-foot leash and later graduating to long-line control. Muzzling should be considered for the sake of public safety in the case of a dog that represents a significant threat to other dogs and people, at least until the handler has acquired the necessary skills and experience to interrupt and reliably control the dog's aggressive behavior whenever and wherever it occurs.

Since many aggressors appear to derive significant gratification from the opportunity to fight, appetitive counterconditioning and reward-based shaping procedures are of limited value, especially for dogs that would place the opportunity to fight above the acquisition of social attention, food, and play. Persistent aggression toward other dogs not belonging to the household can also be brought under stimulus control by training the dog to turn on and turn off aggressive arousal and threat displays. This particular procedure is especially useful with trait aggressors. However, before implementing such a procedure, serious consideration needs to be given to the owner's dog sense and dedication, because the approach, if improperly implemented without appropriate inhibitory con-

trol, may only make the problem worse. Controlling trait aggression depends on rapid decisions and actions in response to the earliest signs of aggression. For effective control, directive and saccadic prompts need to be delivered with sufficient conviction and strength to bring the developing attack sequence to a dead halt. The application of preemptive prompts in anticipation of aggressive arousal can be highly effective for establishing inhibitory control. These general control requirements can be expedited by electronic training (see *Electronic Training and Problem Solving* in Chapter 9). The electronic collar is introduced in the context of reward-based training and only after basic modules and routines have been well conditioned. Enhanced attention control, recall, halt-stay, and sit-stay and down-stay training are emphasized. The dog is gradually exposed to other dogs in incremental steps, and sequences similar to the procedures and variations are used to stage exposure, as previously described (see *Aggressive Barking, Lunging, and Chasing*). The exposure procedure can be highly effective when performed in association with electronic training for mediating avoidance control over aggressive impulses. In addition to mediating avoidance learning and improving inhibitory control, the electrical stimulus may help to offset intrinsic reward derived from the dog fighting activity.

FIGHTING BETWEEN DOGS SHARING THE SAME HOUSEHOLD

Preliminary Considerations

Assessing and controlling fighting between resident dogs is multifaceted (see *Aggression Between Dogs Sharing the Same Household* in Volume 2, Chapter 7). The first step in the process is to assess the frequency and severity of past incidents. In addition to obtaining detailed information about the specifics (e.g., eliciting triggers and situations), a summary of injuries to the dogs should be obtained as well as injuries to people that resulted from redirected aggression or accidental bites that occurred while fighting dogs were being separated. Since interdog aggression may occasionally stem from increased irritability and mood changes resulting from an undiagnosed medical condition, it is important to collect information about the dog's health and recommend that a veterinary examination be performed to exclude such potential factors. In cases involving damaging fights that have resulted in significant injury, various strategies for keeping the dogs apart should be discussed and implemented, including the possibility of rehoming one of the dogs. Sturdy gates, tie-out stations, and crates can be useful in the management and training of such dogs. The trainer should thoroughly explore the risks involved to the dogs, as well as risks of injury to family members that can stem from redirected attacks, or accidental bites that might occur if someone attempts to separate the dogs while fighting. Finally, in some cases, what appears to be fighting to a novice owner is actually just play (Figure 8.4).

Ability and Readiness to Fight

Dogs appear to rapidly appraise each other's relative ability and readiness to fight, referred to as *resource-holding potential*. Resource-holding potential is often correlated with size but is also strongly influenced by need tensions and control incentives, that is, the individual's determination to establish control over a contested resource or place. A small but highly motivated dog can defend a valued object against a much larger but less motivated challenger. The effects of past victories and defeats appear to influence significantly the dog's readiness to fight, perhaps by switching on or off neuroendocrine modes conducive to confrontation or retreat behavior. Perhaps the most important considerations affecting resource-holding potential are prior residency and age. Age and prior residence appear to confer special advantages and expectations with respect to privilege and governance rights. Newly introduced young dogs appear to defer as obligatory subordi-

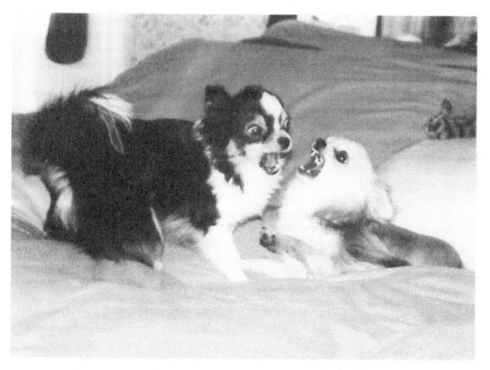

FIG. 8.4. From appearances, these dogs look as though they are fighting with some degree of seriousness, but actually they are playing and have never fought in earnest to inflict or defend against injury.

nates to the most original resident of the home or living space, which is often the oldest dog in the group. The implication of age in the organization of hierarchy may stem from increased experience and prior use of the home range. Established residency appears to imply ownership and control over the entire living space, at least as regards canine interests.

To form secure social and place attachments, the newcomer must enter into pluralistic relations with the resident, but, to achieve this level of social integration, the resident and the newcomer must share mutual social attraction that is sufficient to integrate dyadic hierarchy relations. As such, social attraction and repulsion are the most primary modes of social grouping or dispersion. The ease with which males and females integrate social relations and tolerate the introduction of a nonrelated puppy is probably based on attractive preferences shown toward the opposite sex and a readiness to integrate young animals into the familiar social structure. In addition to residency, social status is broadcast by a dog's attitude, with the most conspicuous and consistently reliable indicator of relative dominance represented in the way in which the dog carries itself—not its size or physical strength. A feisty 10-pound dynamo with *attitude* can challenge and roundly subordinate other dogs many times its size as though it were perfectly natural and correct, especially if it is older and holds privileges of prior residency. However, the ultimate determinants of dominant or subordinate status are closely related to temperament differences, especially relative fearlessness, excitability, and aggression thresholds. Holding other variables constant, dogs that are relatively shy and inhibited are typically more likely to avoid confrontation and to back down if confronted, whereas dogs that are relatively bold, excitable, possessive, and prone to aggressive impulsivity are more likely to confront other dogs and fight if confronted.

Stake-and-Circle Test

If uncertain about an adult dog's propensity for fighting, a potentially useful way to evaluate relative dominance and social tolerance is a modified stake-and-circle test, which is based on a procedure devised by Le Boeuf (1967) to evaluate interindividual relations between dogs. The test situation used by Le Boeuf consisted of a stake and 5-foot chain and harness attached to one dog and a large arena that allowed the other dog to rove about freely. Approach behavior was quantified by counting the number of times that the roving dogs made contact with tethered ones and the amount of time they spent in close proximity (i.e., remained within the circle defined by the chain). Dogs did not appear to become more aggressive when tethered; in fact, roving male dogs initiated most of the aggressive encounters, with the tethered dogs fighting back or submitting. Agonistic encounters between the most aggressive dogs usually ended before escalating into overt fighting, with neither of the dogs submitting or reducing their animosity or willingness to fight in the future. Interestingly, the dogs that spent the most time visiting tethered dogs were also least likely to receive visits from other dogs when they were tethered. The dogs making the most frequent approaches to tethered dogs were typically more outgoing, fearless, and aggressive. These more socially outgoing and aggressive dogs appeared to establish friendly alliances and cohort relationships with certain submissive dogs toward which they showed little or no aggression. The most aggressive males initiated more visits to other dogs irrespective of past encounters. In contrast, males rarely approached other dogs that had previously defeated them. Whenever the most aggressive and fearless dogs came together, they consistently showed mutual hostility. More aggressive dogs appear to approach other dogs more frequently because the former are less fearful. The relative fearlessness or boldness of such dogs may account for their inability to establish dominance over one another. These results suggest that the stake-and-circle test might reveal individual differences associated with extraversion and social dominance.

A variation of the stake-and-circle test is performed by alternately tethering one dog (T) on a 5-foot line or cable and allowing the other dog (R) to rove about on a 30-foot long line that is tied off at a point that allows R to reach within 2 feet of T. Roving dogs with a bold disposition will tend to approach tethered dogs rapidly, irrespective of their relative boldness or shyness, whereas dogs with a more shy disposition will tend to avoid approaching other dogs perceived as a threat. Dogs showing aggression in association with autoprotective incentives may show preemptive threats toward the approach of a roving dog but avoid the same dog when it is tethered. The basic test is performed with the owner at the midway point between the roving dog and tethered dog. In addition, two subtests are used to evaluate the influence of the owner's presence on aggression tensions. Subtest 1 is performed with the owner positioned to the right or left of the tethered dog at a point that is just out of reach of both the roving and tethered dogs. Subtest 2 is performed with the owner positioned within the reach of the tethered dog and making an excited and affectionate fuss over it as the roving dog is released. Subtest 3 is the same as subtest 2 except that, as soon as the roving dog is released, the owner immediately withdraws from the tethered dog and approaches the roving dog and makes an excited show of affectionate attention just out of the tethered dog's reach. After 30 seconds, the owner abruptly stops and returns to the tethered dog. Relatively fearful and submissive dogs may be emboldened by the presence of the owner to approach closer than they normally would, perhaps triggering animosities, whereas more aggressive and socially intolerant dogs may show heightened animosity when approached in close association with the owner.

SOURCES OF CONFLICT BETWEEN A NEWCOMER PUPPY AND A RESIDENT DOG

When bringing a new puppy into the home, many dog owners are apprehensive about how the resident dog will react to the newcomer. Although the pattern of coping is variable, most dogs gradually learn to accept and enjoy the new addition to the household. Adult dogs rarely attack a puppy to injure it, but may set limits with a severity and force that may seem excessive and inappropriate to the dog owner. Canine behavior toward puppies appears to be governed by a social code that forbids injurious bites or life-threatening attacks. Dogs that violate this social code are truly abnormal and should not be in the same household with a young puppy.

Although serious attacks are rare, irritability and intolerance toward a puppy are common. The way a dog copes with a puppy is determined by numerous developmental, experiential, and health variables. For example, due to age-related differences affecting playfulness or physical condition, older dogs are often less engaging and tolerant than are younger dogs. Highly active and intrusive puppies can be a source of significant distress for elderly dogs. Typically, a socially competent dog will rapidly establish appropriate limits and integrate social relations with the puppy that develop into a secure attachment and mutual attunement. Inhibited or insecure dogs may allow the puppy to violate normal canine boundaries with impunity and, instead of punishing it, may do everything possible to avoid it. As a result of persistent exposure to an inescapable puppy, insecure dogs may resort to compulsive barking or other rituals whenever forced into intimate contact with the newcomer. In such cases, nothing that the puppy can do will change the situation or make the insecure dog more accepting. Initially, owners may misinterpret the obtrusive play behavior of the puppy and the apparent acceptance shown by the insecure dog as an indicator of forbearance and gentleness, but the withholding of social punishment (limit-setting actions) in such cases is more often a sign that the dog has refused to accept the puppy, perhaps refusing to acknowledge its existence by passively disengaging. Further, puppy play unconstrained by fair-play limits may rapidly degrade into exploitative cruelty, whereas indiscriminate punishment of friendly social engagement and play by an overly reactive dog promotes social repulsion, dispersive tensions, and a nervous attachment. In contrast, nervous dogs may punish a puppy whenever it comes too close. Punishment, as delivered by nervous dogs, is not aimed at educing submission or integrating hierarchical relations—its only purpose is to keep the puppy at a distance. Allowing a bold puppy to take advantage of an overly tolerant and insecure dog, or allowing the puppy to fall victim repeatedly to the threats and snaps of an intolerant and nervous one, may permanently prime social exchanges with reactive dynamics and expectancies. All of these problematic responses to the introduction of a puppy are related to a common denominator: insufficient autonomic balance and social attraction to initiate and sustain friendly interaction.

How a dog responds is strongly determined by the nature of already established social and place attachments. Whereas dogs under the autonomic attunement of secure place and social attachments tend to show an adaptive coping style that promotes attentive and calibrated emotional engagement (inquisitive boldness), dogs expressing nervous or insecure attachments exhibit various deficits and deficiencies that impair their ability to cope with the social demands posed by a puppy. Whereas the nervous dog lacks sufficient stability to establish social relations, the insecure dog lacks sufficient flexibility to integrate new social relations. The reactive instability and rigidity of nervous and insecure types represent significant challenges when a new puppy is introduced.

The critical issue at stake when introducing a puppy is to provide social and environmental incentives that promote mutual attraction and attachment. Outdoor activities, involving walks, play, and reward-based training activities, may serve to link the puppy with a positive QOL-index shift, thereby helping to activate survival modes conducive to social integration. The perception of an improved QOL index can be amplified by increasing the number and variety of appetitive and social rewards given to the dog during the day, both in the puppy's presence and at other times. Improving the quality the dog's diet by making small changes (adding favorite food items), or just allowing the dog to eat a small portion of puppy food at every feeding, can make a difference in how the dog

perceives the new situation. In contrast, however, isolating the dog or reducing its access to valued rewards may have an adverse effect on its ability to integrate affectionate relations.

In general, the relationship between the puppy and the dog is one of imbalance on practically every level. Significantly, a puppy is far more interested in attaining the regulation provided by attachment than a dog is in giving it. From the dog's perspective, the puppy is a disruptive influence over well-established relations and attachments between the dog and the household. The owner should be encouraged not to become overly involved or attempt to micromanage the transition. Ultimately, the goal is to facilitate and foster interaction rather than attempt to dictate a relationship that depends on the owner's constant supervision to work. Generally, giving the resident dog support and the benefit of doubt in its efforts to curb the youngster's excessive behavior is beneficial. Owners who side with the puppy risk establishing a highly undesirable alliance and misperception that can exert long-term destabilizing effects. Instead of forming bonds with each other, such dogs may establish triangulated relations via the meddling owner. As a result, the puppy may become increasingly obtrusive toward the dog when in the owner's presence, with the latter becoming increasingly insecure, irritated, and intolerant of contact with the puppy.

Since social attraction is a necessary precondition for a dog to accept a puppy, owner interference may effectively block the integration of hierarchical relations. The primacy of social attraction, reconciliation rituals, and social engagement for organizing harmonious relations cannot be overemphasized. A dog that continues to avoid the puppy and treats it as a source of loss, irritation, and intolerance may become increasingly repulsed by its approach, showing a rigid and reactive pattern of avoidance and threats. As the puppy matures, it may become increasing bold and reckless in its interactions with the reactive dog. As a result of owner efforts to splice together a relationship in the absence of social attraction, the dogs may become increasingly defensive and autoprotective whenever in the presence of the owner, until they cannot be in the same room together without restraint. Attempting to integrate dyadic relations between dogs lacking social attraction is difficult, but integrating such relations between dogs that are mutually repulsed and intolerant is often impractical and raises many QOL and welfare questions.

INTRODUCING A NEW ADULT DOG INTO THE HOUSEHOLD

Whenever introducing adult dogs, efforts should be taken to set things up for success and not to take unnecessary risks and shortcuts that might result in a fight. A fight during the introduction leaves a very durable and, perhaps, insurmountable first impression. Consequently, great care should be taken to ensure that the first encounter is as positive and uneventful as possible. Organizing the first meeting to take place in a transitional location where the resident dog is accustomed to meet strange dogs and has been exposed to a history of playful interaction with them is a useful starting point. Alternatively, arranging to take the dogs on a long walk together can be a relatively nonprovocative way to break the ice. If tensions erupt, various reward-based attention-control techniques can be helpful. Taking turns with each dog to play ball while the other looks on seems to reduce tensions while priming the dogs with arousal more conducive to positive social interaction. If animosities emerge despite precautions, an appropriate assertion of control at the instant they begin to percolate can prevent escalation and reduce the risk of reaching a flash point of no return. If necessary, a directive leash prompt is used to restore control and order before continuing the walk as though nothing had occurred. Evenhanded and decisive interruption of argumentative exchanges can help to deflate competitive tensions and make it easier for the dogs to engage in less provocative exchanges and to promote conversations conducive to mutual tolerance and eventually acceptance. The goal of the introduction is to mediate increasing familiarity to set the stage to allow sufficient social attraction to develop between the dogs to generate play. Without

adequate preliminary safe interaction to mediate familiarity, an atmosphere of mutual uncertainty may block the emergence of social attraction and increase the risk of a fight breaking out instead of play. Fighting between unfamiliar dogs is not conducive to the integration of dominant-subordinate relations based on submission, but instead results in social polarization, mutual intolerance, or persistent aggressive tensions. Between strangers, the exchange of threats will either increase mutual anger and trigger fighting or increase fear in one of the competitors, thereby setting the stage for flight and persistent avoidance.

Unfortunately, due to hesitation or lack of appropriate control over the dogs, inexperienced dog owners may hesitate at the critical moment and allow the tensions to escalate and erupt into a serious fight. The owner may subsequently become increasing uneasy and nervous with the dogs interacting nearby, especially at times and places associated with increased excitement (e.g., homecomings, preparations for walks, and feeding times) and previous fighting. These various times and places may acquire conditioned associations that trigger preparatory arousal and lead to an increased risk of fighting whenever the dogs encounter each other under those evocative circumstances. These exciting situations appear to simultaneously disinhibit the dogs in anticipation of a rewarding activity with them together, but, as they interact in the close vicinity of the owner, the exciting arousal drawing them together may dissipate as overshadowed fear and anger gradually take front stage. Under these circumstances, owner anxiety may add an additional element of uncertainty to further destabilize the rapidly escalating conflict. Dogs probably do not process owner anxiety egocentrically, but are more likely to associate the changes in the owner's behavior allocentrically, that is, attribute its cause to the other dog. As a result, a possibility exists that both dogs may cross-attribute the owner's anxiety to each other. Determining specifically how different human mood states influence dog behavior is an important area of basic research that remains to be worked out in detail, but anxiety-related changes to the owner's olfactory signature may play a role. Whereas negative owner mood states under such situations are probably processed allocentrically, positive changes in owner mood states are probably processed egocentrically. Thus, maintaining a positive and confident mood may result in helping both dogs to relax and become less ambivalent or reactive toward each other while in the owner's presence. Conversely, a worried owner may cause the dogs to interpret the situation as unsafe as the result of causes due to the other dog, thereby increasing mutual vigilance, agitation, intolerance, and the readiness for the dogs to fight. Although the precise details of the signaling system mediating these changes remain to be studied, the composite of conditioned stimuli, contextual cues, and owner anticipatory-anxiety signals may establish a hierarchy of trigger events that lead to increasing reactive arousal and set the occasion for fighting. Unquestionably, owner inexperience and lack of dog sense and training skill in such matters is a significant factor in the development of interdog aggression (see Rugbjerg et al., 2003).

Aggression between such dogs is not likely the result of dominance, as it is a conditioned behavior mediated by history of fighting and owner mismanagement. Under the influence of repeated and ineffectual interference, the resident dog may gradually turn on the newcomer at the least provocation. What began as relatively infrequent and innocuous scraps may develop into a frequent and serious pattern of injurious fighting (Figure 8.5). It is interesting to note that such dogs may not fight when left alone, but this cannot be relied on in every case, especially where a high degree of interactive tension and rejection is present and where damaging fights have occurred in the past. Further, once fighting has escalated to include damaging bouts, then the option to allow the dogs to fight is neither effective nor humane. To reiterate, once tensions have graduated beyond the level of ritual contests, staging tournaments between the dogs in order that one of them might finally win decisively and become dominant over the other is not a viable treatment option and could result in one of the dogs being severely injured or killed. Dogs operating under strong

repulsion incentives and entrapment are not fighting to integrate hierarchy relations but instead may only be satisfied after the other is gone or dead.

In an important sense, submission is a social distance-decreasing activity occurring within the vertical hierarchy dimension. This is interesting because hierarchy is based on the formation of social distance-increasing relations. Submission appears to ease vertical social tensions, reflecting the involvement of social attraction in integrating harmonious

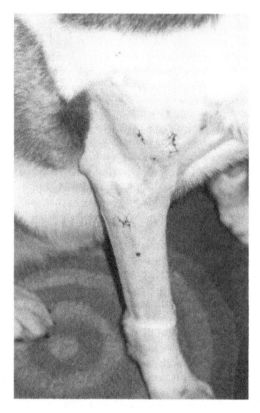

Fig. 8.5. Fighting between dogs sharing the same household can be serious, with females showing a greater risk for such problems than males. Breed-specific tendencies may exert a predisposing influence. Even after several years of tolerant interaction, increased tension, flare-ups, and overt fights may break out. The injuries can be significant and costly. The Akita pictured lived with another female with whom she shared the house for several years. Both dogs sustained numerous lacerations and punctures to front legs, shoulders, and the neck.

social relations. Submission by the newcomer and reciprocated tolerance shown by the resident dog is a form of social reconciliation and fairness enabling the dogs to build a friendly relationship. Submission rituals, social attraction, and trust based on fair play appear to give rise to pluralistic ascendant and descendant relations organized around a default dominant-subordinate relationship formed between the resident dog and the newcomer. In the case of puppies and young dogs, friendly dynamics and trust are facilitated by the concentrated exchange of numerous playful transactions in accord with a principle of fairness. The number of transactions taking place during a play bout may correlate with a mutual motivation to integrate friendly relations, that is, provide a social attraction-repulsion index. During an average play bout, dozens of fair-play exchanges may take place in comparison to a mere handful of fair exchanges that might take place during the course of an average day. According to this hypothesis, what might be achieved in terms of social integration following one or two bouts of play might take weeks or months to achieve in the absence of play, if at all. The surprises and joy generated by energetic interaction with a fair coplayer may be cathected to the coplayer as an object of affection and pleasure, thereby increasing attraction and antagonizing social emotions incompatible with social integration. In addition, object-mediated play between the handler and the dogs can be used to facilitate improved inhibitory control via the command and countermand regulation (e.g., go/no go and all-stop inhibitory exercises) over object-chase sequences involving prized toys and throwaway items.

INTERDOG AGGRESSION WITHIN THE HOUSEHOLD

Because of the obvious dangers involved, dogs sharing the same home that fight are frequently isolated from one another. Although separation is an important precaution to take when the dogs are left alone, constant isolation in different parts of the home is not a solution and does not appear to improve their

chances of restoring trust. Social isolation is often convenient and may be a useful measure to prevent fights for the short term, but as a long-term arrangement separating the dogs may only serve to increase estrangement, torque up aggressive tensions, and generally worsen the situation. Eventually, someone will forget or lose track of their whereabouts and allow the dogs to get together. If a decision is made to keep such dogs in the household—which is not always practical or wise—then both dogs should receive intensive basic obedience training, graduated exposure and response blocking, counterconditioning, and appropriate inhibitory conditioning (e.g., go/no-go, stop-change, and all-stop procedures) to reduce aggressive tensions and improve the owner's ability to interrupt escalating tensions before they reach the flash point of no return. Fighting that breaks out at times of increased excitement (e.g., owner homecomings, feeding times, and before opportunities to go outside) often benefit from intensive wait (go/no-go) and delay-of-gratification training. Building a virtue around waiting and taking turns to obtain attention, affection, and other rewards by following rules can be very helpful.

Training Recommendations

The assumption that dogs fight because of a failure to form a dominance hierarchy has led to a widespread practice of treating such problems by having the owner leverage one dog into a dominant role and the other into a subordinate role by means of owner-controlled rewards and preferential alliances. Whether such brokering strategies exert a significant effect on dominance relations has not been demonstrated in dogs; one might assume, however, that such recommendations are not likely to provide much help with dogs lacking social attraction. In the absence of social attraction, it is unlikely that dogs can submit (subordinate) or to accept submission (dominant) while forming conciliatory proxemic relations. Further, despite the appearance of being ethologically sensible, the hypothesis requires a considerable leap of faith to assume that coherent and stable dominant-subordinate relations might be telegraphed by means of owner leveraging and refereeing. Stable dominance relations appear to be dyadic in nature, requiring that one dog, the dominant, assert dominance and, in turn, accept submission from another dog, the subordinate, in order for them to integrate a friendly relationship. If the dominant dog fails to compel the subordinate to submit or is unwilling to accept the subordinate's offer of submission, there is no hierarchy relationship integrated between them. Training procedures aimed at integrating a social hierarchy by means of proxy seem especially problematic and ill-fated for dogs operating under the influence of mutual repulsion and dispersive tensions. In general, attempting to integrate power and hierarchy relations in the absence of mutual attraction results in social ambivalence (anxiety and distrust) and an ISS, whereas the integration of hierarchy relations under the influence of mutual attraction promotes affection, trust, and a VSS. According to this perspective, it is not only futile to establish hierarchy relations between dogs that are repulsed by one another, such efforts may actually worsen the situation. Instead of worry about which dog is dominant or not, the focus of training should be to leverage owner control over both dogs in a way that facilitates voluntary subordination and engenders confidence that the owner has the situation in hand. A strong and evenhanded owner presence provides a sense of security that may help the dogs to relax and feel safe, and thereby facilitates the activation of the SES.

To enhance owner control, both dogs are kept on leash at all times when under supervision. In all potentially provocative situations, efforts are taken to mediate nonprovocative access and sharing of appetitive and social rewards in a pluralistic way that supports cooperation and acknowledges social codes based on fair play, mutual attraction, and adherence to owner rules. The right of first possession is especially important with regard to competitive situations developing around attention-seeking behavior toward the owner, especially in situations where fighting has broken out in association with such activities in the past. Socially intolerant dogs that engage

in excited jostling for proximity with the owner during greeting frenzies may incidentally enter proxemic zones inappropriate to their level of social attraction and as a result trigger a rapid escalation of arousal, possibly setting off an all-out fight. To prevent such situations in the future, precautions need to be taken to prevent close contact between the dogs during greetings, at least until they have integrated more friendly relations. During greetings, and at other times as well, interaction between the owner and dogs is formalized with rules of access that the owner dictates without respect to the rank of the dogs. Both dogs are discouraged from crowding and jostling with each other for owner attention. The owner should become a source of social control and order rather than attempt to broker dominant status or play the role of a referee between the dogs.

When left alone, such dogs should be separated, perhaps by keeping them in crates. Upon entering the house, the owner should give the dogs a few minutes to calm down before greeting them one by one. During such homecoming activities, the dogs are both put through a series of basic obedience modules and routines until attention and impulse control are fully established. The focus of work is directed toward establishing limits on pulling and stay/wait training. If warranted for safety purposes, the first dog is restrained at a tie-out station, while the second dog is leashed and greeted in a similar fashion. Dogs that exhibit tensions around feeding should be fed in separate rooms or crates. During food preparations, the dogs can be placed in separate rooms, crates, or tethered, where they should remain until both have finished eating and the food bowls have been taken up. When going outdoors for walks or coming back inside the house, the owner should determine the order of egress. Since squabbles and fights often develop around transition points involving excitement, the rules and rights of egression should be the focus of significant training and inhibitory conditioning until both dogs have learned to "Wait" and "Back" on signal. When giving treats or toys, the owner should determine which dog gets its share first, not based on a perception of rank but based on compliance to command. If aggression tensions have occurred on furniture or beds, both dogs should be trained to stay off such items, unless invited up, and to obey rapidly when prompted to get off.

Dogs with fighting problems should receive intensive attention and impulse-control training, ICT, and inhibitory conditioning using the procedures previously described in Part 1, with both dogs learning to defer without hesitation to owner demands and directives. When agonistic tensions escalate and necessitate intervention, the owner should establish control without taking sides or worrying too much about which dog is dominant or how the limit-setting actions in the present might affect dominance relations between the dogs later. Social dominance is of little consequence in the beginning and, in any case, hierarchy relations will naturally take shape as social attraction and trust build between the dogs. If the dogs cannot tolerate being in the same room with each other, dominance relations are moot. In the long run, the social status of the dogs is far less important than preventing fights and providing a social space for promoting social attraction. Dogs given a sufficient number of safe opportunities to interact with each other may gradually acquire the necessary social attraction, confidence, and trust needed to integrate friendly relations. However, dogs that are pressured to integrate hierarchical relations in the absence of social attraction will only become progressively avoidant, intolerant, and reactive. When dogs possess adequate social attraction to give and accept submission, the establishment of default hierarchy relations naturally follows without much consequence. Only when the relationship is conflicted with repulsion and entrapment dynamics does dominance become a central point of concern and tension.

A social space conducive to social attraction and friendly interaction is established by setting limits on intrusive behavior and provocative exchanges. The training of an effective all-stop inhibitory response is of immense utility for controlling dogs in such situations. Both dogs are required to defer to the same basic imperative: fighting is not an option. Since fighting will only serve to sharpen animosities and promote social repulsion, when a fight is in the suspense phase every effort is applied to exert decisive inhibitory control, leaving no doubt or wiggle room concerning the handler's position on the matter. Nagging reprimands, ineffectual leash grabbing, fussing, and bribing will only ripen the problem, whereas an appropriately firm reprimand originating from the belly and delivered with force, a directive or saccadic leash prompt, or a brief electrical pulse can effectively interrupt and discourage the escalation of such behavior. Electrical training procedures can be useful for interrupting the preparatory phase, but once a fight has commenced, the use of electrical stimulation may only intensify reactive arousal and potentially worsen the problem. The goal is to take control and prevent the fight, not to referee or direct the ongoing drama and suspense between the dogs. The idea is to end fighting, not to explore dominance theories. Since the owner is more likely to possess sufficient social attraction to integrate a dyadic hierarchy with the dogs, it is the owner's dominance that most needs clarification in the process of establishing limits and order conducive to friendly relations between the dogs. A strong and fair owner presence appears to go a long way toward decreasing agonistic tensions between dogs, perhaps by helping them to feel safer while in the owner's presence and by using their attraction toward the owner to integrate submissive behavior and enhanced impulse control.

Transitional situations that stimulate a high level of excitement (e.g., going through doors) are particularly risky. In addition to taking steps to reduce excitement at such times, basic training and inhibitory conditioning are performed to establish and enforce appropriate rules and behaviors to reduce competitive tensions and to keep the dogs apart. Both dogs need to regulate interactive exchanges around valued resources and activities in accordance with a "first come, first serve" rule, to actively defer to the owner's directive authority, and to exercise preemptive restraint over aggressive impulses. Along with reward-based procedures, time-out offers a means both to discourage inappropriate behavior and to reduce autonomic arousal and excitability. Anticipatory agonistic arousal and intention behaviors should be carefully monitored and diverted or disrupted before they intensify into overt threats. Prompting competitors to perform basic obedience modules and routines while in the presence of each other may be beneficial. Such activities provide a structure of rewards and owner approval conducive to cooperative interaction and fairness that may help to reduce agonistic tensions. The interactive benefits of such training may be especially beneficial if the response of the worker results in a reward matching the standard expectancy (SE) while the observer is given a reward that exceeds the SE for merely being present and not interfering. Alternatively, having the worker perform some basic exercise, but giving the immediate reward matching the SE to the observer and then giving the worker a reward exceeding the SE (surprise), may also promote constructive dynamics. Variations on this plan include surprises for the observer that result from interaction between the owner and the worker. For example, after prompting the newcomer to sit or lie down, the observer is prompted to orient by smooch or squeak, whereupon the orienting response is immediately bridged and the dog tossed a reward. Every so often, a surprise (high-quality reward or toy) is delivered, perhaps in association with showing added attention to the worker in the context of object-mediated play. The observer should be tethered in the beginning but can become increasing involved by means of an active-control line.

Organizing training activities so that surprise is arranged to occur as the result of cooperative interaction in various social situations can help to facilitate social exploratory behavior and mutual tolerance and possibly set the stage for play. The goal is to teach the dogs to take turns and to cooperate in order to avoid inappropriate contact and aggressive arousal. Training both dogs to walk on leash without pulling promotes a number of significant benefits mediating positive change. For example, walking appears to exert a potent stress-reducing and counterconditioning effect, in addition to stimulating beneficial allelomimetic associations that may create a sense of pack affiliation. Walks, especially those in which the owner imposes effective limits on pulling, a rule that is fastidiously enforced, may enhance the dogs' perception of the owner as a source of control and order. Initially, the dogs may need to be controlled by separate handlers, but as things progress the owner should be able to walk the dogs in brace (not coupled), as appropriate and safe. During controlled walks, orienting responses, quick-sits, and sit-stays or down-stays should be frequently practiced and rewarded.

Preventing and Breaking Up a Dogfight

Breaking up dogfights is fraught with dangers. The catastrophic arousal supporting combative behavior is the result of an avalanche of neurobiological events that may precipitously lower aggression thresholds in response to interference and restraint, causing fighting dogs to redirect hard snaps toward anyone that may foolishly attempt to stand between them. Owners enacting a referee role toward evenly matched dogs seem to be particularly prone to this error in judgment during a fight, perhaps stemming in part from a perceived loss of authority that they may feel obliged to regain or as the result of a fear that the dogs will seriously injure one another. However, going up against claws and sharp teeth with soft human skin and bravado is not an action that either dog would likely expect from the brightest member of the pack. It is especially risky to reach for the head or neck of fighting dogs, since such sites are typically active targets for biting. The bites received by owners as the result of interfering are often severe. Hitting or kicking dogs while they are fighting may only serve to inflame animosities or result in a bite to hand or foot or possibly cause an unintentional injury to one of the dogs. Although dogs rarely kill one another, letting dogs fight until one subdues the other may result in a rapid and uncontrollable escalation of aggression, perhaps causing serious injuries and expensive veterinary treatments. The danger is increased when unevenly matched or strange dogs are let alone to fight it out. The majority of dog fights are rather noisy and unskilled affairs that are more about getting out of the fight than winning it, making it fairly easy for an assertive person to break them up. In contrast, serious fights between experienced combatants are often much more quiet and focused on conserving energy and acquiring favorable bite holds. Dogs with a propensity to fight should be kept under appropriate muzzle or leash control at all times when they are around other dogs in order to help prevent fights and to provide safe means to separate them should a fight break out. When potentially aggressive dogs are left alone, they should either be crated or confined to separate rooms.

Some experts have suggested that shouting reprimands or yelling obedience commands like "Sit!" might stop dogfights. In practice, such vocal demands will likely go unheeded and may actually inflame the situation, especially if the fight is well under way. An assertive reprimand, startling noise, or sharp leash jerk might be sufficient to interrupt a fight before it begins, but once the fight is under way yelling loud commands typically does little good. Although an experienced trainer can often succeed in breaking up a fight by force of will and intimidation without being bitten or causing more harm, the average dog owner or handler is more likely to be bitten and should be discouraged from getting between fighting dogs or attempting to jerk them apart, a procedure that might cause more serious injuries to the dogs. Since restraining one dog while the other one is free to attack at will puts the restrained combatant at a significant disadvantage and increases its risk of sustaining injuries, whenever possible two people should work together to separate fighting dogs. Pulling the dogs steadily apart by leash without jerking them is frequently effective. When outdoors, a large bucket of water and hose should be kept ready for emergencies. When fighting breaks out, the bucket of water is splashed on the combatants, thereby often (but not always) dousing their enthusiasm for the fight. A hose delivering a forceful stream of water typically works better. Indoors, a large bath towel can be soaked in water and kept in a plastic bag for

emergency use. The towel is thrown over the dogs, whereupon they can be more easily separated by leash. In addition, quart-sized plastic bottles containing club soda can be strategically placed around the house. Another method uses a modified carbon-dioxide pump to spray a disruptive blast of compressed air at the rear end or belly of the attacking dog to disrupt the fighting impulse.

As a serious fight develops, experienced fighters may take mutual bite holds where they periodically shake their heads to set deep puncture wounds or grind into the flesh of the other dog and refuse to let go. Assuming that both dogs are leashed, in some cases squirting club soda in the mouth and face of fighters can cause them to break their bite holds. In other cases a foamy shaving cream can be sprayed liberally on the nose and mouth of aggressors to help loosen bites before pulling them apart by leash. A highly effective alternative employs two or three aromatic ammonia inhalers that are taped to the handle of a leash. After the inhalers are broken, they can be tangled near the nose of fighting dogs as they are pulled apart. The number of ammonia inhalers broken is determined by need, with the majority of dogs requiring that only one ampoule be crushed. Ammonia inhalers should not be presented by hand, because a dog may rapidly break its hold only to transfer the bite to the hand holding the ammonia inhaler.

When dogs fight off leash, separating them is considerably more complicated and risky. Despite opinions to the contrary, lifting a dog by its tail or hind legs does not reliably inhibit aggression or stop fighting. Grabbing fighting dogs by their rear legs or the base of their tails can work, but these are dangerous practices with large and highly aggressive dogs that risks evoking a redirected attack. The method requires two experienced handlers possessing sufficient strength to control the dogs properly after breaking up the fight to avert being bitten on the rebound. Also, dogs handled in such a way may twist and flail about and snap to break free only to race back and attack the other dog again. A better approach involves passing a leash around the dog's waist and then hooking the bolt snap over the leash to form a noose. The noose is cinched up snugly and steady pressure is applied, lifting up and the pulling back until they let go. An alternative method used to set a waist noose involves passing the bolt snap through the handle of the leash. If a leash is not handy, a strong belt can be used instead. The foregoing method can be modified in situations where only one handler is available. A waist noose is applied to the more aggressive of two dogs, and both dogs are dragged to a place where the restrained dog can be safely tied off. A waist noose can now be applied to the second dog while various techniques are used to break the aggressor's bite (e.g., ammonia inhaler, club soda, shaving cream, compressed air, or breaking stick in the case of some fighting breeds) while the second dog is steadily pulled away. All bite wounds received by dogs during fights should receive veterinary treatment to prevent infection.

Repulsing the Approach of Threatening Dogs

Highly aggressive dogs should be muzzled or restrained on a muzzle-clamping halter when in public places. When performing exposure procedures in public, a risk always exists that another dog wandering around without supervision will approach the handler and dog. Every effort should be made to avoid such encounters and places where such situations might develop. Allowing an established aggressor to negotiate with a strange dog of unknown aggressive propensities poses a significant risk that might be penalized by the instigation of a fight and a significant setback in the dog's training. The approach of a potentially aggressive dog requires handler intervention to maintain a safe space between the approaching dog and the dog on leash. Preparation is crucial for effective prevention and control. When approached by a threatening dog, the handler should take account of all possible alternatives to direct confrontation, but given that the encounter is likely to occur, immediate precautions and preparations for decisive action should be taken. Keeping the dogs apart is usually far easier than breaking up a fight. The first step is to

reinforce control over the dog by firmly grasping the leash with the left hand and setting a brake (see *Leash Handling* in Chapter 1). The remaining portion of the leash and handle is then tossed back over the right shoulder. The right hand should grasp the standing end of the leash just in front of the shoulder in preparation to swing the leash handle down forcefully, if necessary, to strike the approaching dog with enough force to turn it away.

In the case of an approaching dog that represents a limited menace, throwing a handful of treats in its direction can give the handler and his or her dog time to escape the situation. If the procedure works, it might need to be repeated several times to keep the other dog at a distance. In the case of a more persistent dog, a threatening step or two in the dog's direction, combined with a direct stare and shout ("Go Away!"), is often enough to cut short the adventure and cause the dog to veer away or to remain at a safe distance. If the dog ignores the warning and continues to approach with a threatening attitude, the handler might need to assert more forceful measures to deter its approach. Depending on the urgency of the situation, the handler might have enough time to first cast a forceful swing of the leash across the dog's path. This strategy, while kindhearted to the intruding dog, might complicate the situation and make it more difficult to ultimately control if the dog turns out to be looking for a fight. The deterrence of the warning flick may stop the dog from moving straight in, but not keep it from circling around to the rear or rushing in at the flank. Many dogs that get within close range can be deterred by a blast of compressed air. For ordinary purposes, a walking stick provides the best general defense against the threat of unsupervised dogs. The stick is used to jab at the aggressor in order to keep it at bay, not to pummel it.

SEX HORMONES AND INTRASPECIFIC AGGRESSION

Perinatal Distress, Androgenization, and Intrauterine Position Effects

Perinatal distress in association with obstetric complications has been shown to blunt prefrontal DA inhibitory transmission while at the same time increasing excitatory mesolimbic DA activity (Brake et al., 2000). Diminished medial prefrontal cortex (mPFC) activity appears to reduce an animal's ability to competently regulate subcortical activity, to optimize adaptive coping efforts, and to selectively focus attention and impulse control. Trauma during this critical period of biobehavioral integration may lay the groundwork for the development of various aberrant forms of impulsive behavior in predisposed dogs. The attention and impulse-control deficits, distractibility, and hyperactivity associated with birth-related distress may offer useful clues relevant to the etiology of canine hyperkinesis and other developmental behavior problems in dogs associated with exploitative obtrusiveness and social impulsivity.

A significant gender-related influence affecting the integration and attunement of autonomic control may stem from sexually dimorphic maturation rates. Among rats, DA fibers begin reaching prefrontal destinations earlier in the gestation period than 5-HT and NE fibers and continue to develop and proliferate later than them as well (Berger-Sweeney and Hohmann, 1997). Due to the influence of gonadal hormones, DA afferent pathways targeting executive control areas in the mPFC develop more rapidly in females than in males. These gender differences in the development of prefrontal DA pathways agree with developmental findings (Wilsson and Sundgren, 1998). At week 8, male and female puppies show clear maturational differences. Females are more active, spend more time exploring and less time in close proximity with the experimenter, and are more interested in objects than are male puppies. The delayed maturation of prefrontal DA pathways and mesocortical organization may confer an added vulnerability to environmental or social insults (Brake et al., 2000), perhaps adversely affecting the male puppy's ability to regulate emotion and impulse in adulthood. The canine PFC does not appear to reach full functional capacity until the end of the first year, marked by the emergence of object-permanence abilities and mature working memory (Gagnon and Dore, 1994).

Shortly before and after birth, a surge of gonadal testosterone enters the brain of male puppies, where it undergoes enzymatic conversion into hormonal derivatives that bind to androgen and estrogen receptors expressed in various target areas of the brain. The perinatal action of sex steroids on the brain predisposes dogs to express gender-appropriate social and reproductive behavior at puberty and adulthood. Among most animals, sex steroids play an active role in the organization of social hierarchy and territory via the development of species-typical patterns of agonistic and reproductive behavior. Sex hormones mediate numerous physiological, structural, and connectivity changes to serotonergic and other neural pathways that contribute to the regulation of mood, emotional reactivity, and aggression thresholds. Adverse prenatal and perinatal conditions may disturb the organization of androgen- and estrogen-responsive pathways, perhaps predisposing susceptible dogs to show lower reactive thresholds and impulsivity toward provocative social stressors in adulthood. The higher incidence of fighting problems among male dogs may be linked to perinatal androgenizing influences affecting the serotonergic system. For example, blockade of $5-HT_{1A}$ receptors during week 2 postpartum increases offensive aggression in adult intact rats, but a similar antagonist treatment failed to increase offensive aggression in female rats or male rats castrated on day 1 (Albonetti et al., 1996). In spontaneously hypertensive rats, an animal model of ADHD, early testosterone treatment has been shown to integrate a persistent HPA-axis dysfunction resulting in high ACTH levels and a blunted adrenocortical response (King et al., 2000)—a state of allostatic hypodrive that may dysregulate the SAM system.

In addition to the behavioral effects of perinatal testosterone on the central nervous system of male dogs, in utero exposure to testosterone may alter reactive thresholds in adult female dogs (see *Perinatal Androgenization* in Volume 2, Chapter 7). Female fetuses may be androgenized in a number of physiological, morphological, and behavioral ways by the transfer of testosterone from males to adjacent females situated between them.

Intrauterine position effects have not been definitively demonstrated in dogs, but have been shown to exert a significant influence on aggressive behavior in a number of other species (Ryan and Vandenbergh, 2002). For example, female mice and pig fetuses situated between males initiate more fights than females situated between other females. Interestingly, males situated between other males appear to be more sensitive to the effects of testosterone at maturity. These findings may account for some of the individual differences shown by dogs in response to elevated pubertal testosterone activity and response to castration. Females situated between other females may be more adversely affected by prenatal stress, suggesting that intrauterine exposure to testosterone may have a protective effect. Exposure to excessive stress or lack of appropriate stimulation during this perinatal period may exert lasting changes in the organization of aggression-mediating circuits.

Castration and Hormonal Therapy

Since a hormonal factor is believed to play a role in the development of intermale aggression, castration is frequently recommended (see *Hormonal Influences* in Volume 2, Chapter 7). Surprisingly, the effects of castration on dog fighting have not been carefully studied or documented (see *Effects of Castration on Aggressive Behavior* in Volume 2, Chapter 6). Existent studies are confounded by methodological shortcomings and suffer from inadequate sample sizes from which to derive therapeutic conclusions. The most commonly cited study estimates that approximately 40% to 60% of intermale aggressors show a combination of short-term improvement (within 2 weeks) and long-term improvement (after 6 months) following surgery (Hopkins et al., 1976). What this improvement exactly means is not clarified. Unfortunately, the potential beneficial effects of castration are often exaggerated, causing great dissatisfaction when the procedure fails to produce the hoped-for relief. Even where significant change is evident, it is rarely dramatic and almost never complete, especially when an experienced dog fighter is involved.

Clearly, the effects of castration are variable, with some dogs experiencing little or no discernible benefit. The author's impression is that very few adult dogs give up fighting as the result of castration. A few owners have reported that their dog's fighting activity actually worsened after castration. A frequently overlooked benefit of neutering is the effect it appears to have on other dogs. The most commonly observed consequence of neutering is a decline in the frequency of challenges and attacks directed against the castrated dog by intact males. Intact dogs may find castrated or prepubertal dogs less attractive to fight or, perhaps, such dogs may simply transmit fewer provocative signals. At any rate, despite limitations and questionable efficacy, neutering should be considered in the case of serious fighting problems or in young dogs showing a heightened propensity for interdog aggression. Among rodents, castration appears to reduce 5-HT_{2A}-receptor densities in the frontal cortex and ventromedial hypothalamus (Zhang et al., 1999; Sumner and Fink, 2000). Although gonadal testosterone is entirely eliminated from a dog's bloodstream within the first 24 hours after surgery, the physiological and psychological benefits associated with neutering may take several weeks to months to develop fully. The effects of castration are sometimes augmented by the administration of progestins (see *Sex Hormones: Estrogen, Testosterone, and Progesterone* in Volume 2, Chapter 6), a problematic option that is occasionally used in cases unresponsive to castration alone (Hart and Eckstein, 1998). Male dogs treated with progestins may produce a confusing olfactory signature that short-circuits the aggressor's interests, perhaps making treated dogs less attractive as targets for attack. Also, dogs treated with progestins appear to be less interested in fighting. Progestin therapy is associated with several potential side effects that should be evaluated by the supervising veterinarian and carefully monitored.

Testosterone, Serotonin Therapy, and Intraspecific Aggression

Although the use of serotonergic medications for the control of interdog aggression is needful of clinical evaluation and controlled trials, some preclinical evidence suggests that circulating testosterone might provide a permissive or facilitatory effect on serotonin therapy. For example, the aggression inhibiting effects of 5-HT_{1A}- and 5-HT_{1B}-receptor agonists appear to depend on the permissive influence of androgens (Cologer-Clifford et al., 1999), suggesting the possibility that the therapeutic benefits of serotonergic agents for the treatment of dog fighting may be facilitated by the presence of circulating testosterone. Support for this hypothesis is provided by a study in vervet monkeys that evaluated the behavioral effects of three medications known to increase 5-HT activity by different mechanisms (Raleigh et al., 1985). Fluoxetine, quipazine (a $5\text{-HT}_{1/2}$-receptor agonist), and tryptophan were given to dominant and subordinate monkeys. The researchers found that dominant individuals respond to 5-HT-enhancing therapies in a more robust manner than did subordinates. An increase in several prosocial behaviors attributed to the effects of enhanced 5-HT activity was also correlated with social dominance, including increased social approach, grooming, resting, eating, and huddling. Increased huddling was found to be a behavior produced only by fluoxetine. Dominant individuals also showed a greater reduction in negative behaviors, such as social avoidance, vigilance, and solitariness. The various 5-HT treatment regimens promoted a general calming effect and increased sociability—an effect that was especially prominent in dominant monkeys. Dominant individuals often exhibit higher levels of circulating testosterone, as well as other status-linked hormonal differences associated with HPA-system tone and gender-related agonistic behavior. For example, AVP appears to play a major role in forming hierarchical relations and territory (Ferris et al., 1986) and mobilizing power-dominance motivations (Sewards and Sewards, 2003). AVP-mediated aggressive behavior among hamsters is testosterone dependent (Delville et al., 1996). Ferris and colleagues (1997) found that fluoxetine inhibits gender-related offensive aggression in hamsters by antagonizing the action of AVP in the hypothalamus via 5-HT_{1A} receptors.

These reports emphasize the close interaction among AVP, testosterone, and 5-HT in the regulation of agonistic behavior. Most dogs showing serious intraspecific aggression problems are routinely castrated prior to drug-therapy initiation. Given the aforementioned findings, the absence of circulating testosterone might reduce the efficacy of selective serotonin (5-HT) reuptake inhibitor (SSRI) medications such as fluoxetine for controlling gender-related intraspecific aggression. The foregoing data also suggest that aggressive dogs left intact during fluoxetine therapy might respond better to treatment. For previously castrated dogs, combination treatments incorporating dehydroepiandrosterone (DHEA), the adrenocortical precursor to testosterone and estrogen, with a compatible SSRI might prove useful (Wolkowitz et al., 1999).

AGGRESSION TOWARD CATS IN THE HOUSEHOLD

A common aggression problem involves dogs that chase or attack cats living in the same household. Once established, the urge to stalk and chase or attack cats can be highly resistant to behavioral change. Dogs that show a propensity to attack and injure or kill cats represent a significant risk, and they (or the cats) should be removed from the home. In other cases, dogs that lack appropriate training and socialization with cats may engage in playful chase escapades that cause the target cat significant distress. Often cats exposed to an aggressive or playful dog may remain in a part of the house that is inaccessible to the dog and only occasionally come out of hiding. Dogs prone to chase cats should be exposed to remedial socialization, reward-based integrated compliance training, and appropriate inhibitory all-stop conditioning aimed at suppressing the chase impulse. Most cases involving such behavior can be managed successfully by using a combined approach of exposure-habituation, response prevention, and graduated counterconditioning.

Getting the dog accustomed to being around the cat without evoking a chase response is best achieved by habituating the cat to a wire carrier. Attempting to restrain a cat by leashing it with a harness or collar is highly problematic and can result in serious scratch and bite injuries to the handler. Carrier confinement allows the dog to approach the cat safely while minimizing undesirable behavior. The cat and dog are exposed to graduated counterconditioning under diverse circumstances. The leashed dog is progressively moved toward the confined cat while being fed a highly valued food item. One technique involves coating a wooden spoon with peanut butter and allowing the dog to lick from it as it approaches the cat in stages without becoming reactive. The cat should also be fed a highly prized treat (e.g., puréed tuna) through the carrier by a helper. A muzzle-clamping halter or muzzle can be used to help discourage lunging and barking. Incorporating brief exclusionary TO with DRO training can also reduce such behavior. In cases not sufficiently responsive to the foregoing training efforts, remote electronic training can be used to entrain potent inhibitory control over chasing behavior. Internal electronic containment can be used to reinforce such training, but such devices are far from foolproof, and under the excitement of the chase the dog may run through the field and attack the cat. Dogs with a history of chasing cats should either be crated or be confined to a safe room when left alone. A device that could be helpful for controlling undesirable canine behavior around cats would involve a small medallion worn by the cat. If the cat is approached within a certain critical distance, a receiver device worn by the dog is activated that delivers an appropriate warning and aversive stimulus of sufficient strength to cause the dog to avoid the cat.

REFERENCES

Adams GJ and Johnson KG (1995). Guard dogs: Sleep, work and behavioural responses to people and other stimuli. *Appl Anim Behav Sci*, 46:103–115.

Albonetti E, Gonzalez MI, Siddiqui A, et al. (1996). Involvement of the 5-HT$_{1A}$ subtype receptor in the neonatal organization of agonistic behaviour in the rat. *Pharmacol Biochem Behav*, 54:189–193.

Anderson GW (2001). Thyroid hormones and the brain. *Front Neuroendocrinol*, 22:1–17.

Animal and Plant Health Inspection Service, USDA (1997). Humane treatment of dogs: Tethering. *Federal Register*, 62:43272–43275.

Appleby DL, Bradshaw JW, and Casey RA (2002). Relationship between aggressive and avoidance behaviour by dogs and their experience in the first six months of life. *Vet Rec*, 150:434–438.

Arenz CL and Leger DW (1999). Thirteen-lined ground squirrel (Sciuridae: *Spermophilus tridecemlineatus*) antipredator vigilance decreases as vigilance cost increases. *Anim Behav*, 57:97–103.

Arenz CL and Leger DW (2000). Antipredator vigilance of juvenile and adult thirteen-lined ground squirrels and the role of nutritional need. *Anim Behav*, 59:535–541.

Asa C, Mech LD, and Seal US (1985). The use of urine, faeces, and anal-gland secretions in scent-marking by a captive wolf (*Canis lupus*) pack. *Anim Behav*, 33:1034–1036.

Band GP and Van Boxtel GJ (1999). Inhibitory motor control in stop paradigms: Review and reinterpretation of neural mechanisms. *Acta Psychol*, 101:179–211.

Baranyiova E, Holub M, Martinikova M, et al. (2003). Epidemiology of intraspecies bite wounds in dogs in the Czech Republic. *Acta Vet Brno*, 72:55–62.

Bekoff M (1977). Mammalian dispersal and the ontogeny of individual behavioral phenotypes. *Am Nat*, 111:715–732.

Bekoff M (1979a). Ground scratching by male domestic dogs: A composite signal. *J Mammal*, 60:847–848.

Bekoff M (1979b). Scent-marking by free-ranging domestic dogs: Olfactory and visual components. *Biol Behav*, 4:123–139.

Bekoff M (2001a). Observations of scent-marking and discriminating self from others by a domestic dog (*Canis familiaris*): Tales of displaced yellow snow. *Behav Processes*, 55:75–79.

Bekoff M (2001b). Social play behaviour: Cooperation, fairness, trust, and the evolution of morality. *J Consciousness Stud*, 8:81–90.

Berger-Sweeney J and Hohmann CF (1997). Behavioral consequences of abnormal cortical development: Insights into developmental disabilities. *Behav Brain Res*, 86:121–142.

Berntson GG, Boysen ST, and Caciopppo JT (1992). Cardiac orienting and defensive responses: Potential origins in autonomic space. In BA Campbell, H Hayne, and R Richardson (Eds), *Attention and Information Processing in Infants and Adults*. Hillsdale, NJ: Lawrence Erlbaum.

Billman GE and Dujardin JP (1990). Dynamic changes in cardiac vagal tone as measured by time-series analysis. *Am J Physiol*, 258:896–902.

Blackshaw JK (1991). An overview of types of aggressive behaviour in dogs and methods of treatment. *Appl Anim Behav Sci*, 30:351–361.

Bleicher N (1963). Physical and behavioral analysis of dog vocalizations. *Am J Vet Res*, 24:415–427.

Boitani L, Francisci F, and Ciucci P (1995). Population biology and ecology of feral dogs in central Italy. In J Serpell (Ed), *The Domestic Dog: Its Evolution, Behaviour, and Interaction with People*. New York: Cambridge University Press.

Borger N, Van der Meere J, Ronner A, et al. (1999). Heart rate variability and sustained attention in ADHD children. *J Abnorm Child Psychol*, 27:25–33.

Brace CL (1962). Physique, physiology, and behavior: An attempt to analyze a part of their roles in the canine biogram [PhD dissertation (Introduction and Summary)]. Boston: Harvard University Press.

Brake WG, Sullivan RM, and Gratton A (2000). Perinatal distress leads to lateralized medial prefrontal cortical dopamine hypofunction in adult rats. *J Neurosci*, 20:5538-5543.

Brown LE (1966). Home range and movement of small mammals. *Symp Zool Soc Lond*, 18:111–142.

Bugental DB, Blue J, Cortez V, et al. (1993). Social cognitions as organizers of autonomic and affective responses to social challenge. *J Pers Soc Psychol*, 64:94–103.

Bugental DB, Lyon JE, Krantz J, and Cortez V (1997). Who's the boss? Differential accessibility of dominance ideation in parent-child relationships. *J Pers Soc Psychol*, 72:1297–1309.

Bugental DB, Lyon JE, Lin EK, et al. (1999). Children "tune out" in response to the ambiguous communication style of powerless adults. *Child Dev*, 70:214–230.

Buydens-Branchey L, Branchey M, Hudson J, and Fergeson P (2000). Low HDL cholesterol, aggression and altered central serotonergic activity. *Psychiatry Res*, 93:93–102.

Cain CK, Blouin AM, and Barad M (2003). Temporally massed CS presentations generate more fear extinction than spaced presentations. *J Exp Psychol Anim Behav Processes*, 29:323-333.

Calcagnetti DJ and Schechter MD (1992). Place conditioning reveals the rewarding aspect of social interaction in juvenile rats. *Physiol Behav*, 51:667–672.

Caldji C, Tannenbaum B, Sharma S, et al. (1998). Maternal care during infancy regulates the development of neural systems mediating the expression of fearfulness in the rat. *Proc Natl Acad Sci USA*, 95:5335–5340.

Cándido A, Maldonado A, Rodriguez A, and Morales A (2002). Successive positive contrast in one-way avoidance learning. *Q J Exp Psychol [B]*, 55:171–184.

Cándido A, Maldonado A, and Vila J (1989). Relative time in dangerous and safe places influences one-way avoidance learning in the rat. *Q J Exp Psychol [B]*, 41:181–199.

Catalani A, Casolini P, Scaccianoce S, et al. (2000). Maternal corticosterone during lactation permanently affects brain corticosteroid receptors, stress response and behaviour in rat progeny. *Neuroscience*, 100:319–325.

Champagne F, Diorio J, Sharma S, and Meaney MJ (2001). Naturally occurring variations in maternal behavior in the rat are associated with differences in estrogen-inducible central oxytocin receptors. *Proc Natl Acad Sci U S A*, 98:12736-12741.

Chen CC, Lu FH, Wu JS, and Chang CJ (2001). Correlation between serum lipid concentrations and psychological distress. *Psychiatry Res*, 102:153–162.

Cheng ZB, Kobayashi M, and Nosaka S (2001). Effects of optic tract stimulation on baroreflex vagal bradycardia in rats. *Clin Exp Pharmacol Physiol*, 28:721–728.

Christiansen FO, Bakken M, and Braastad BO (2001). Social facilitation of predatory, sheep-chasing behaviour in Norwegian elkhounds, grey. *Appl Anim Behav Sci*, 72:105–114.

Clark GI (1994). The relationship between emotionality and temperament in young puppies [PhD dissertation]. Fort Collins: Colorado State University.

Coccaro EF, Kavoussi RJ, Hauger RL, et al. (1998). Cerebrospinal fluid vasopressin levels: Correlates with aggression and serotonin function in personality-disordered subjects. *Arch Gen Psychiatry*, 55:708–714.

Cole DP, Thase ME, Mallinger AG, et al. (2002). Slower treatment response in bipolar depression predicted by lower pretreatment thyroid function. *Am J Psychiatry*, 159:116–121.

Cologer-Clifford A, Simon NG, Richter ML, et al. (1999). Androgens and estrogens modulate 5-HT_{1A} and 5-HT_{1B} agonist effects on aggression. *Physiol Behav*, 65:823–828.

Corson SA, Corson E, Beckler RE, et al. (1980). Interaction of genetics and separation in canine hyperkinesis and in differential responses to amphetamines. *Pavlov J Biol Sci*, 15:5–11.

Crockford SJ (2003). Thyroid rhythm phenotypes and hominid evolution: A new paradigm implicates pulsatile hormone secretion in speciation and adaptation changes. *Comp Biochem Physiol A Mol Integr Physiol*, 135:105–129.

Daminet S and Ferguson DC (2003). Influence of drugs on thyroid function in dogs. *J Vet Intern Med*, 17:463–472.

De Almeida RM and Miczek KA (2002). Aggression escalated by social instigation or by discontinuation of reinforcement ("frustration") in mice: Inhibition by anpirtoline—a 5-HT$_{1B}$ receptor agonist. *Neuropsychopharmacology*, 27:171–181.

Dean P, Redgrave P, and Westby GW (1989). Event or emergency? Two response systems in the mammalian superior colliculus. *Trends Neurosci*, 12:137–147.

Delville Y, Mansour KM, and Ferris CF (1996). Testosterone facilitates aggression by modulating vasopressin receptors in the hypothalamus. *Physiol Behav*, 60:25–29.

Devenport L, Devenport J, and Kokesh C (1999). The role of urine-marking in the foraging behaviour of least chipmunks. *Anim Behav*, 57:557–563.

DeVries AC, Glasper ER, and Detillion CE (2003). Social modulation of stress responses. *Physiol Behav*, 79:399–407.

Dodds WJ (1992). Thyroid can alter behavior: Bizarre behavioral changes? Check your dog hypothyroidism. *Dog World*, Oct:40–42.

Dodds WJ (2001). Vaccine protocols for dogs predisposed to vaccine reactions. *Am Anim Hosp Assoc*, 37:1–4.

Done CJ and Sharp T (1994). Biochemical evidence for the regulation of central noradrenergic activity by 5-HT$_{1A}$ and 5-HT$_2$ receptors: Microdialysis studies in the awake and anaesthetized rat. *Neuropharmacology*, 33:411–421.

Dringenberg HC, Dennis KE, Tomaszek S, and Martin J (2003). Orienting and defensive behaviors elicited by superior colliculus stimulation in rats: Effects of 5-HT depletion, uptake inhibition, and direct midbrain or frontal cortex application. *Behav Brain Res*, 144:95–103.

Dugatkin LE (2001). Bystander effects and the structure of dominance hierarchies. *Behav Ecol*, 12:348–352.

Dunbar I and Buehler M (1980). A masking effect of urine from male dogs. *Appl Anim Ethol*, 6:297–301.

Dykman RA and Gantt WH (1997). Experimental psychogenic hypertension: Blood pressure changes conditioned to painful stimuli (schizokinesis). *Integr Physiol Behav Sci*, 32:272–287 [originally published by the *Bulletin of the Johns Hopkins Hospital*, Aug 1960, Vol 107].

Eisenberg JF and Kleiman DG (1972). Olfactory communication in mammals. *Annu Rev Ecol Syst*, 3:1–32.

Faingold CL and Randall ME (1999). Neurons in the deep layers of superior colliculus play a critical role in the neuronal network for audiogenic seizures: Mechanisms for production of wild running behavior. *Brain Res*, 815:250–258.

Fatjó J, Stub C, and Manteca X (2002). Four cases of aggression and hypothyroidism in dogs. *Vet Rec*, 151:547–548.

Fendt M, Li L, and Yeomans JS (2001). Brain stem circuits mediating prepulse inhibition of the startle reflex. *Psychopharmacology*, 156:216–224.

Ferguson DC (1984). Thyroid function tests in the dog: Recent concepts. *Vet Clin North Am Small Anim Pract*, 14:783–808.

Ferris CF, Meenan DM, Axelson JF, and Albers HE (1986). A vasopressin antagonist can reverse dominant/subordinate behavior in hamsters. *Physiol Behav*, 38:135–138.

Ferris CF, Melloni RH Jr, Koppel G, et al. (1997). Vasopressin/serotonin interactions in the anterior hypothalamus control aggressive behavior in golden hamsters. *J Neurosci*, 17:4331–4340.

Field T (2002). Violence and touch deprivation in adolescents. *Adolescence*, 37:735–749.

Fish W, De Bold JF, and Miczek KA (2002). Aggressive behavior as a reinforcer in mice: Activation by allopregnanolone. *Psychopharmacology*, 163:459–466.

Flaherty CF (1996). *Incentive Relativity*. Cambridge: Cambridge University Press.

Fox MW (1978). *The Dog: Its Domestication and Behavior*. Malabar, FL: Krieger.

Frank H and Frank MG (1982). On the effects of domestication on canine social development and behavior. *Appl Anim Ethol*, 8:507–525.

Gagnon S and Dore FY (1994). Cross-sectional study of object permanence in domestic puppies (*Canis familiaris*). *J Comp Psychol*, 108:220–232.

Gantt WH (1944). *Experimental Basis for Neurotic Behavior: Origin and Development of Artificially Produced Disturbances of Behavior in Dogs*. New York: Paul B Hoeber.

Gese EM and Ruff RL (1997). Scent-marking by coyotes, *Canis latrans*: The influence of social and ecological factors. *Anim Behav*, 54:1155–1166.

Goicoa A, Fidalgo LE, Suarez ML, et al. (2002). Zinc poisoning associated with separation anxiety in an Argentinean bulldog. *Vet Hum Toxicol,* 44:14–16.

Gershman KA, Sacks JJ, and Wright JC (1994). Which dogs bite? A case-control study of risk factors. *Pediatrics,* 93:913–917.

Golden MH, Samuels MP, and Southall DP (2003). How to distinguish between neglect and deprivational abuse. *Arch Dis Child,* 88:105–107.

Guidotti A, Dong E, Matsumoto K, et al. (2001). The socially-isolated mouse: A model to study the putative role of allopregnanolone and 5alpha-dihydroprogesterone in psychiatric disorders. *Brain Res Brain Res Rev,* 37:110–115.

Gulikers KP and Panciera DL (2003). Evaluation of the effects of clomipramine on canine thyroid function tests. *J Vet Intern Med,* 17:44–49.

Hafez ESE, Sumption LJ, and Jakway JS (1962). The behaviour of swine. In ESC Hafez (Ed), *The Behaviour of Domestic Animals.* Baltimore: Williams and Wilkins.

Hall ET (1963). A system for the notation of proxemic behavior. *Am Anthropol,* 65:1003–1026.

Hall ET (1968). Proxemics. *Curr Anthropol,* 9:83–108.

Hamilton-Andrews S, McBride EA, and Brown I (1999). Hypothyroidism and aberrant behaviours in the bearded collie. In *Proceedings Mondial Vet Lyon 99* (cd), Sep 23–26. Lyon: World Veterynary Association.

Harmon-Jones E (2003). Anger and the behavioral approach system. *Pers Individ Differ,* 35:995–1005.

Harrington FH (1981). Urine-marking and caching behavior in the wolf. *Behaviour,* 76:280–288.

Harrington FH and Mech DL (1979). Wolf howling and its role in territory maintenance. *Behaviour,* 68:207–249.

Hart BL and Eckstein RA (1998). Progestins: Indications for male-typical problem behaviors. In NH Dodman and L Shuster (Eds), *Psychopharmacology of Animal Behavior Disorders.* Malden, MA: Blackwell Science.

Henley WN and Koehnle TJ (1997). Thyroid hormones and the treatment of depression: An examination of basic hormonal actions in the mature mammalian brain. *Synapse,* 27: 36–44.

Henry JD (1977). The use of urine marking in the scavenging behavior of the red fox (*Vulpes vulpes*). *Behaviour,* 61:82–105.

Hopkins SG, Schubert TA, and Hart BL (1976). Castration of adult male dogs: Effects on roaming, aggression, urine marking, and mounting. *JAVMA,* 168:1108–1110.

Horowitz AC (2002). The behaviors of theories of mind, and a case study of dogs at play [PhD dissertation]. San Diego: University of California.

Howard BR (1992). Health risks of housing small psittacines in galvanized wire mesh cages. *JAVMA,* 200:1667–1674.

Hunt PS and Campbell BA (1997). Autonomic and behavioral correlates of appetitive conditioning in rats. *Behav Neurosci,* 111:494–502.

Ikeda T and Hikosaka O (2003). Reward-dependent gain and bias of visual responses in primate superior colliculus. *Neuron,* 39:693–700.

Internet Classics Archives (2000). Epictetus: The Discourses. http://classics.mit.edu/Epictetus/discourses.html.

Jowett B (1941). *Plato's* The Republic. New York: Modern Library.

Juhr NC, Brand U, and Behne D (2003). Impact of zinc-metabolism on canine aggression? [Abstract]. *Berl Munch Tierarztl Wochenschr,* 116:265–268.

Kariyawasam SH, Zaw F, and Handley SL (2002). Reduced salivary cortisol in children with comorbid attention deficit hyperactivity disorder and oppositional defiant disorder. *Neuroendocrinol Lett,* 23:45–58.

Kavaliers M and Choleris E (2001). Antipredator responses and defensive behavior: Ecological and ethological approaches for the neurosciences. *Neurosci Biobehav Rev,* 25:577–586.

Kikkawa A, Uchida Y, Nakade T, and Taguchi K (2003). Salivary secretory IgA concentrations in beagle dogs. *J Vet Med Sci,* 65:689–693.

King SM (1999). Escape-related behaviours in an unstable, elevated and exposed environment. II. Long-term sensitization after repetitive electrical stimulation of the rodent midbrain defence system. *Behav Brain Res,* 98:127–142.

King JA, Barkley RA, Delville Y, and Ferris CF (2000). Early androgen treatment decreases cognitive function and catecholamine innervation in an animal model of ADHD. *Behav Brain Res,* 107:35–43.

Kleiman D (1966). Scent marking in the Canidae. *Symp Zool Soc Lond,* 18:167–177.

Kunz-Ebrecht SR, Mohamed-Ali V, Feldman PJ, et al. (2003). Cortisol responses to mild psychological stress are inversely associated with proinflammatory cytokines. *Brain Behav Immun,* 17:373–383.

Le Boeuf BJ (1967). Interindividual associations in dogs. *Behaviour,* 29:268–295.

Little CJ, Julu PO, Hansen S, and Reid SW (1999). Real-time measurement of cardiac vagal tone in conscious dogs. *Am J Physiol*, 276:758–765.

Lorenz K (1955). *Man Meets Dog*. Boston: Houghton Mifflin.

Lund JD and Vestergaard KS (1998). Development of social behaviour in four litters of dogs (*Canis familiaris*). *Acta Vet Scand*, 39:183–193.

MacDonald K (1987). Development and stability of personality characteristics in pre-pubertal wolves: Implications for pack organization and behavior. In H Frank (Ed), *Man and Wolf*. Dordrecht, The Netherlands: Dr W Junk.

Marr JN (1960). The influence of soft body-contact on the development of canine affection. Alma: Michigan Academy of Science, Arts, and Letters. [Reported in Marr, 1964.]

Marr JN (1964). Varying stimulation and imprinting in dogs. *J Genet Psychol*, 104:351–364.

Martasian PJ and Smith NF (1993). A preliminary resolution of the retention of distributed vs massed response prevention in rats. *Psychol Rep*, 72:1367–1377.

Matysiak J, Jankowski K, Knoll E, and Maszkiewicz K (1973). The effect of the kind of reinforcement during toilet training on dogs' behavior in novel situation [Abstract]. *Przegl Psychol*, 16:19–28.

McCreary AC and Handley SL (2000). Chronic administration of the cholesterol reducing drug gemfibrozil fails to alter 5-HT$_{1A}$ and 5-HT$_{2A}$ mediated receptor behaviours in rats. *J Psychopharmacol*, 14:280–283.

McIntire RW (1968). Dog training, reinforcement, and behavior in unrestricted environments. *Am Psychol*, 23:830–831.

McIntire RW and Colley TA (1967). Social reinforcement in the dog. *Psychol Rep*, 20:843–846.

Meaney MJ, Aitken DH, and Sapolsky RM (1987). Thyroid hormones influence the development of hippocampal glucocorticoid receptors in the rat: A mechanism for the effects of postnatal handling on the development of the adrenocortical stress response. *Neuroendocrinology*, 45:278–283.

Meaney MJ, Diorio J, Francis D, et al. (2000). Postnatal handling increases the expression of cAMP-inducible transcription factors in the rat hippocampus: The effects of thyroid hormones and serotonin. *J Neurosci*, 20:3926–3935.

Mech LD (1970). *The Wolf: The Ecology and Behavior of an Endangered Species*. Minneapolis: University of Minnesota Press.

Mech LD (1999). Alpha status, dominance, and division of labor in wolf packs. *Can J Zool*, 77:1196–1203.

Mech LD (2000). Leadership in wolf, *Canis lupus*, packs. *Can Field-Nat*, 114:259–263.

Meerlo P, Horvath KM, Luiten PG, et al. (2001). Increased maternal corticosterone levels in rats: Effects on brain 5-HT$_{1A}$ receptors and behavioral coping with stress in adult offspring. *Behav Neurosci*, 115:1111–1117.

Mertl-Millhollen AS, Goodmann PA, and Klinghammer E (1986). Wolf scent marking with raised-leg urination. *Zoo Biol*, 5:7–20.

Michelini LC (1994). Vasopressin in the nucleus tractus solitarius: A modulator of baroreceptor reflex control of heart rate. *Braz J Med Biol Res*, 27:1017–1032.

Miller PE and Murphy CJ (1995). Vision in dogs. *JAVMA*, 207:1623–1634.

Misslin R and Cigrang M (1986). Does neophobia necessarily imply fear or anxiety? *Behav Processes*, 12:45–50.

Moreau X, Jeanningros R, and Mazzola-Pomietto P (2001). Chronic effects of triiodothyronine in combination with imipramine on 5-HT transporter, 5-HT(1A) and 5-HT(2A) receptors in adult rat brain. *Neuropsychopharmacology*, 24:652–662.

Muldoon MF, Marsland A, Flory JD, et al. (1997). Immune system differences in men with hypo- or hypercholesterolemia. *Clin Immunol Immunopathol*, 84:145–149.

Murphy CJ, Zadnik K, and Mannis MJ (1992). Myopia and refractive error in dogs. *Invest Ophthalmol Vis Sci*, 33:2459–2463.

Nahm MC (1964). *Selections from Early Greek Philosophy*. New York: Appleton-Century-Crofts.

Naylor AM, Ruwe WD, and Veale WL (1986). Thermoregulatory actions of centrally-administered vasopressin in the rat. *Neuropharmacology* 25:787–794.

Niemi-Junkola UJ, Westby GW (2000). Cerebellar output exerts spatially organized influence on neural responses in the rat superior colliculus. *Neuroscience*, 97:565–573.

Oberbauer AM, Benemann KS, Belanger JM, et al. (2002). Inheritance of hypoadrenocorticism in bearded collies. *Am J Vet Res*, 63:643–647.

Ohayon MM (2000). Prevalence of hallucinations and their pathological associations in the general population. *Psychiatry Res*, 97:153–164.

Ohayon MM and Shapiro CM (2000). Sleep disturbances and psychiatric disorders associated with posttraumatic stress disorder in the general population. *Compr Psychiatry*, 41:469–478.

Oluyomi AO and Hart SL (1992). Antinociceptive and thermoregulatory actions of vasopressin are sensitive to a V1-receptor antagonist. *Neuropeptides*, 23:137–142.

Padgett DA and Glaser R (2003). How stress influences the immune response. *Trends Immunol*, 24:444–448.

Pal SK (2003). Urine marking by free-ranging dogs (*Canis familiaris*) in relation to sex, season, place, and posture. *Appl Anim Behav Sci*, 80:45–59.

Papanek PE and Raff H (1994). Physiological increases in cortisol inhibit basal vasopressin release in conscious dogs. *Am J Physiol*, 266:1744–1751.

Pavlov IP (1928). *Lectures on Conditioned Reinforcement, Vol. 1.* W H Gantt (Trans), New York: International Publishers.

Penturk S and Yalcin E (2003). Hypocholesterolaemia in dogs with dominance aggression. *J Vet Med [A]*, 50:339–342.

Peremans K, Audenaert K, Coopman F, et al. (2003). Estimates of regional cerebral blood flow and 5-HT$_{2A}$ receptor density in impulsive, aggressive dogs with (99m)Tc-ECD and (123)I-5-I-R91150. *Eur J Nucl Med Mol Imaging*, 30:1538–1546.

Peters RP and Mech DL (1975). Scent-marking in wolves. *Am Sci*, 63:628–637.

Peterson ME, Kintzer PP, and Kass PH (1996). Pretreatment clinical and laboratory findings in dogs with hypoadrenocorticism: 225 cases (1979–1993). *JAVMA*, 208:85–91.

Peterson RO, Jacobs AK, Drummer TD, et al. (2002). Leadership behavior in relation to dominance and reproductive status in gray wolves, *Canis lupus. Can J Zool*, 80:1405–1412.

Pinna G, Broedel O, Eravci M, et al. (2003). Thyroid hormones in the rat amygdala as common targets for antidepressant drugs, mood stabilizers, and sleep deprivation. *Biol Psychiatry*, 54:1049–1059.

Plechner AJ (1976). Canine immune complex diseases. *Mod Vet Pract*, 57:917–921.

Plechner AJ (2003). An effective veterinary model may offer therapeutic promise for human conditions: Roles of cortisol and thyroid hormones. *Med Hypotheses*, 60:309–314.

Pontius AA and LeMay MJ (2003). Aggression in temporal lobe epilepsy and limbic psychotic trigger reaction implicating vagus kindling of hippocampus/amygdala (in sinus abnormalities on MRIs). *Aggression Violent Behav*, 8:245–257.

Porges, SW (1992). Autonomic regulation and attention. In BA Campbell, H Hayne, and R Richardson (Eds), *Attention and Information Processing in Infants and Adults.* Hillsdale, NJ: Lawrence Erlbaum.

Porges SW (2001). The polyvagal theory: Phylogenetic substrates of a social nervous system. *Int J Psychophysiol*, 42:123–146.

Potegal M and Einon D (1989). Aggressive behaviors in adult rats deprived of playfighting experience as juveniles. *Dev Psychobiol*, 22:159–172.

Price EO and Wallach SJR (1990). Physical isolation of hand-reared Hereford bulls increases their aggressiveness toward humans. *Appl Anim Behav Sci*, 27:263–267.

Raleigh MJ, Brammer GL, McGuire MT, and Yuwiler A (1985). Dominant social status facilitates the behavioral effects of serotonergic agonists. *Brain Res*, 348:274–282.

Ralls K (1971). Mammalian scent marking. *Science*, 171:443–449.

Reid JB, Chantrey DF, and Davie C (1984). Eliminatory behaviour of domestic dogs in an urban environment. *Appl Anim Behav Sci*, 12:279–287.

Reimers TJ, Lawler DF, Sutaria PM, et al., (1990). Effects of age, sex, and body size on serum concentrations of thyroid and adrenocortical hormones in dogs. *Am J Vet Res*, 51:454-457.

Reinhard (1978). Aggressive behavior associated with hypothyroidism. *Can Pract*, 5:69–70.

Rheingold HL (1963). Maternal behavior in the dog. In HL Rheingold (Ed), *Maternal Behavior in Mammals.* New York: John Wiley and Sons.

Roll A and Unshelm J (1997). Aggressive conflicts amongst dogs and factors affecting them. *Appl Anim Behav Sci*, 52:229–242.

Rosenblatt JS and Schneirla TC (1962). The behaviour of cats. In ESC Hafez (Ed), *The Behaviour of Domestic Animals.* Baltimore: Williams and Wilkins.

Rugbjerg H, Proschowsky HF, Ersboll AK, and Lund JD (2003). Risk factors associated with interdog aggression and shooting phobias among purebred dogs in Denmark. *Prev Vet Med*, 58:85–100.

Russell ES (1936). Playing with a dog. *Q Rev Biol*, 2:1–15.

Ryan BC and Vandenbergh JG (2002). Intrauterine position effects. *Neurosci Biobehav Rev*, 26:665–678.

Sauvage MF, Marquet P, Rousseau A, et al. (1998). Relationship between psychotropic drugs and thyroid function: A review. *Toxicol Appl Pharmacol*, 149:127–135.

Scott J P and Fuller JL (1965). *Genetics and the Social Behavior of the Dog.* Chicago, IL: University of Chicago Press.

Scott JP (1983). A systems approach to research on aggressive behavior. In EC Simmel, ME Hahn, and JK Walters (Eds), *Aggressive Behavior: Genetic and Neural Approaches*. New York: Lawrence Erlbaum.

Scott-Moncrieff JC, Azcona-Olivera J, Glickman NW, et al. (2002). Evaluation of antithyroglobulin antibodies after routine vaccination in pet and research dogs. *JAVMA*, 221:515–521.

Seagard JL, Dean C, and Hopp FA (1999). Role of glutamate receptors in transmission of vagal cardiac input to neurones in the nucleus tractus solitarii in dogs. *J Physiol*, 520(Pt 1):243–253.

Sells E (1996). Report on the autoimmune endocrine health survey. Bearded Collie Club of America. http://www.beaconforhealth.org/Nov97SurveyReportBulletin.htm.

Sewards TV, Sewards MA (2003). Fear and power-dominance motivation: Proposed contributions of peptide hormones present in cerebrospinal fluid and plasma. *Neurosci Biobehav Rev*, 27:247–267.

Shaw B (1906) Preface to *Major Barbara*: First aid to critics. http://eserver.org/drama/major-barbara/essay-to-critics.html.

Sherman CK, Reisner IR, Taliaferro LA, and Houpt KA (1996). Characteristics, treatment, and outcome of 99 cases of aggression between dogs. *Appl Anim Behav Sci*, 47:91–108.

Simpson JW (1998). Diet and large intestinal disease in dogs and cats. *J Nutr*, 128(Suppl 12):2717S–2722S.

Skandakumar S, Stodulski G, and Hau J (1995). Salivary IgA: A possible stress marker in dogs. *Anim Welfare*, 4:339–350.

Smallwood LJ and Barsanti JA (1995). Hypoadrenocorticism in a family of leonbergers. *J Am Anim Hosp Assoc*, 31:301–355.

Smith WJ (1977). *The Behavior of Communicating: An Ethological Approach*. Cambridge: Harvard University Press.

Smythe JW, Rowe WB, and Meaney MJ (1994). Neonatal handling alters serotonin (5-HT) turnover and 5-HT$_2$ receptor binding in selected brain regions: Relationship to the handling effect on glucocorticoid receptor expression. *Brain Res Dev Brain Res*, 80:183–189.

Spinka M, Newberry RC, and Bekoff M (2001). Mammalian play: Training for the unexpected. *Q Rev Biol*, 76:141–168.

Stahler DH, Smith DW, and Landis R (2002). The acceptance of a new breeding male into a wild wolf pack. *Can J Zool*, 80:360–365.

Stanford TL (1981). Behavior of dogs entering a veterinary clinic. *Appl Anim Ethol*, 7:272–279.

Sumner BE and Fink G (1998). Testosterone as well as estrogen increases serotonin2A receptor mRNA and binding site densities in the male rat brain. *Brain Res Mol Brain Res*, 59:205–214.

Svartberg K and Forkman B (2002). Personality traits in the domestic dog (*Canis familiaris*). *Appl Anim Behav Sci*, 79:133–155.

Swaab DF, Fliers E, Hoogendijk WJ, et al. (2000). Interaction of prefrontal cortical and hypothalamic systems in the pathogenesis of depression. *Prog Brain Res*, 126:369–396.

Thompson ME and Galosy RA (1983). Electrical brain activity and cardiovascular function during amygdaloid kindling in the dog. *Exp Neurol*, 82:505–520.

Thompson R, Gupta S, Miller K, et al. (2004). The effects of vasopressin on human facial responses related to social communication. *Psychoneuroendocrinology*, 29:35–48.

Trivers RL (1972). Parental investment and sexual selection. In B Campbell (Ed), *Sexual Selection and the Descent of Man*. Chicago: Aldine.

Trivers RL (1974). Parent-offspring conflict. *Am Zool*, 14:249–264.

Tsigos C and Chrousos GP (2002). Hypothalamic-pituitary-adrenal axis, neuroendocrine factors and stress. *J Psychosom Res*, 53:865–871.

Tuan Yi-Fu (1984). *Dominance and Affection: The Making of Pets*. New Haven: Yale University Press.

Uvnäs-Moberg K (1998). Oxytocin may mediate the benefits of positive social interaction and emotions. *Psychoneuroendocrinology*, 23:819–835.

Valentino RJ and Van Bockstaele E (2001). Opposing regulation of the locus coeruleus by corticotropin-releasing factor and opioids: Potential for reciprocal interactions between stress and opioid sensitivity. *Psychopharmacology*, 158:331–342.

Van den Berg CL, Hol T, Van Ree JM, et al. (1999). Play is indispensable for an adequate development of coping with social challenges in the rat. *Dev Psychobiol*, 34:129–138.

Verrier RL and Dickerson LW (1991). Autonomic nervous system and coronary blood flow changes related to emotional activation and sleep. *Circulation*, 83(Suppl 4):81–89.

Wang J, Irnaten M, Venkatesan P, et al. (2002). Arginine vasopressin enhances GABAergic inhibition of cardiac parasympathetic neurons in the nucleus ambiguus. *Neuroscience*, 111:699–705.

Westby GW, Keay KA, Redgrave P, et al. (1990). Output pathways from the rat superior colliculus mediating approach and avoidance have different sensory properties. *Exp Brain Res,* 81:626–638.

Wilsson E (1984). The social interaction between mother and offspring during weaning in German Shepherd dogs: Individual differences between mothers and their effects on offspring. *Appl Anim Behav Sci,* 13:101–112.

Wilsson E and Sundgren PE (1998). Behavioral test for eight-week old puppies: Heritabilities of tested behaviour traits and its correspondence to later behaviour. *Appl Anim Behav Sci,* 58:151–162.

Windle RJ, Shanks N, Lightman SL, and Ingram CD (1997). Central oxytocin administration reduces stress-induced corticosterone release and anxiety behavior in rats. *Endocrinology,* 138:2829–2834.

Wingfield JC (2003). Control of behavioural strategies for capricious environments. *Anim Behav,* 66:807–816.

Wolkowitz OM, Reus VI, Keebler A, et al. (1999). Double-blind treatment of major depression with dehydroepiandrosterone. *Am J Psychiatry,* 156:646–649.

Wood GE, Young LT, Reagan LP, and McEwen BS (2003). Acute and chronic restraint stress alter the incidence of social conflict in male rats. *Horm Behav,* 43:205–213.

Wood-Gush DGM and Vestergaard K (1991). The seeking of novelty and its relation to play. *Anim Behav,* 42:599–606.

Wright JC (1980). The development of social structure during the primary socialization period in German Shepherds. *Dev Psychobiol,* 13:17–24.

Yeon SC, Golden G, Sung W, et al. (2001). A comparison of tethering and pen confinement of dogs. *J Appl Anim Welfare Sci,* 4:257–270.

Yin S (2002). A new perspective on barking in dogs (*Canis familiaris*). *J Comp Psychol,* 116:189–193.

Young LJ (1999). Oxytocin and vasopressin receptors and species-typical social behaviors. *Horm Behav,* 36:212–221.

Zeeman EC (1976). Catastrophe theory. *Sci Am,* 234:65–83.

Zhang L, Ma W, Barker JL, and Rubinow DR (1999). Sex differences in expression of serotonin receptors (subtypes 1A and 2A) in rat brain: A possible role of testosterone. *Neuroscience,* 94:251–259.

9

Biobehavioral Monitoring and Electronic Control of Behavior

PART 1: MONITORING AUTONOMIC AND EMOTIONAL STATES

STRESS, TEMPERATURE, AND BEHAVIOR

In addition to preparing dogs for physical exertion and emergency action, the sympathetic nervous system mediates physiological changes associated with thermoregulatory control that closely parallel the preparatory arousal associated with fear and anger. Thermoregulatory adaptations for coping with thermogenic changes appear to have been recruited and incorporated into systems evolved to cope with emotional stressors (e.g., decreased/increased activity, vascular dilation/constriction, panting, sweating, shivering, and piloerection). The close relationship between physiological changes associated with thermoregulation and sympathetic arousal suggests an interesting potential relationship between reactive emotional states and increased thermogenesis. The persistent panting and excessive salivation exhibited by some separation-reactive and separation-distressed hyperactive dogs may reflect a shift in energy metabolism and thermogenesis resulting from reactive states triggered by the loss of social contact or control over significant events. The reactive relationship between separation distress and increased thermoregulatory activity suggests an interesting developmental hypothesis; namely, the contact dynamics between neonatal puppies while mediating mutual thermoregulation may orchestrate the expression of neurobiological substrates that anticipate the later emergence of social attraction and attachment behavior, and the integration of competent regulation of sympathovagal arousal and impulse control. According to this hypothesis, early stressors and insults affecting canine thermoregulatory capacity may exert far-reaching effects on the organization of sympathetic regulatory networks needed to competently modulate reactive thresholds controlling separation distress and flight-fight behavior. These reactive propensities may be partially revealed by the size of differences between basal body temperatures and temperatures obtained after exposing the dog to

provocative stimulation. In addition to early developmental insults, thermogenesis and compensatory thermoregulatory changes appear to be strongly influenced by individual genetic differences. Corson and colleagues (1973), for example, found that dogs differentiate along two general lines in the way they cope with exposure to uncontrollable aversive stimulation. The first group, referred to as *anti-diuretic* types, shows a quintet of reactive physiological changes: tachycardia, persistent hyperpnea, excessive salivation, and increased secretion of vasopressin. The researchers hypothesized that these sympathetic changes were a reactive pattern of compensatory thermoregulation in response to a reactive increase in energy metabolism and thermogenesis. Other dogs, referred to as *diuretic* types, responded to the same uncontrollable stimulation in a less global and reactive way, showing a greater capacity to adapt, consistent with a well-developed flirt-and-forbear anti-stress system. These findings suggest the possibility that temperament differences affecting a dog's relative ability to cope with provocative stimuli may be revealed and indexed by the size of temperature changes evoked by uncontrollable threats and challenges.

Although the significance of core temperature to temperament in dogs remains to be worked out in detail, body temperature appears to provide a sensitive index of psychological distress and stress in laboratory rodents. Stress-induced hyperthermia is associated with anticipatory anxiety and increased glucocorticoid activity (Groenink et al., 1994). Exposure to social conflict can produce durable changes in daily temperature patterns, depending on whether the animal accepts defeat or fights back (see Meerlo et al., 1996 and 1999). Other research has shown that temperature changes are particularly sensitive to psychological stressors as opposed to physical ones. Long-term temperature changes can occur in association with the psychological distress from being in the same compartment with conspecifics receiving daily sessions of shock delivered every 60 seconds for an hour over 12 weeks. Distressed bystander rats showed a long-term elevation in temperature, with a 0.20°C elevation in temperature after a 2- to 3-month rest period (Endo and Shiraki, 2000). Among rats, temperature change appears to index contextual fear conditioning, perhaps warranting validation in dogs (see Godsil et al., 2000). These findings suggest that tracking temperature changes might be a useful noninvasive tool for assessing psychological distress in dogs.

Functional Lateralization and Tympanic Temperature

Some lines of research have formed around the significance of tympanic temperature differences between the ears as measured by infrared tympanic thermometers. These temperature differences may be due to lateralized cortical functions, with right-side prefrontal asymmetries associated with the behavioral inhibition system (BIS), negative emotion, inhibition, hesitation, stress regulation, defensive behavior, anxious arousal, and passive modal strategies, whereas left-side prefrontal asymmetries appear to be associated with the behavioral approach system (BAS), positive emotion and arousal, curiosity, surprise, joy, exploration, offensive behavior and trait anger (Harmon-Jones and Sigelman, 2001), and active modal strategies. Anger generating positive affect, arousal, confidence, struggle, conquest, and power appears to be integrated by the BAS (see Harmon-Jones, 2003), whereas the BIS integrates negative affect, anxiety, disappointment, resentment, defeat, and failure. According to this hypothesis, both the BAS and the BIS play a role in representing different functional and motivational aspects of anger and anxiety.

In conjunction with executive functions, the prefrontal cortex (PFC) appears to index and modulate allostatic load via hypothalamic-pituitary-adrenal (HPA)-system regulation (Diorio et al., 1993)—a function performed chiefly by the right medial PFC (Sullivan and Gratton, 1999). The frontal area via the anterior cingulate cortex (ACC) also figures prominently in the integration of attention shifting, emotional processing, and the corticovisceral regulation of sympathovagal tone (Thayer and Lane, 2000). Consistent with the lateralization of cognitive functions,

the orienting response of a dog to a click or the presentation of food following a conditioned stimulus evokes increased electroencephalogram (EEG) activity in the left cerebral hemisphere, whereas once the orienting response to the click is extinguished, the click stimulus tends to increase activity in the right hemisphere (Simonov et al., 1995). While processing novel auditory and visual stimuli, left lateralization appears to predominate, but, as the conditioned response is well established, asymmetry is either absent or shifts to the right hemisphere (Preobrazhenskaia, 2000).

In general, right hemisphere specializations are organized to cope with defensive demands and threats evoking withdrawal and behavioral inhibition, whereas left lateral hemisphere adaptations are closely tied to approach, behavioral activation, challenging situations, and heightened appetitive drive states. The right hemisphere appears to promote withdrawal, anxious arousal, and activation of the HPA system (Wittling and Pfluger, 1990). When the provocative event is uncontrollable, cortisol levels may dramatically increase along with a heighten risk for defensive or reactive aggression in predisposed dogs. In contrast, increased left frontal activity tends to be associated with positively valenced states of arousal promoting approach, power, and potential for offensive or impulsive aggression. In contrast to the increased cortisol levels observed in association with right hemisphere stimulation, left hemisphere activation in response to emotionally aversive stimuli tends to suppress salivary cortisol secretion (Wittling and Pfluger, 1990), a finding consistent with a hypothesized linkage between low cortisol levels and impulsive aggression.

Lateral shifting of cortical activity appears to anticipate changes in brain metabolism rates and vascular flow to the left and right sides of the brain, depending on the processing being performed. These metabolic and vascular changes appear to be reflected in rapid changes in temperature. Among chimpanzees, for example, observing a video recording of severe aggression results in elevated right-ear tympanic temperature, whereas observing neutral images or images of playful activity does not alter baseline temperatures (Parr and Hopkins, 2000). When engaged in visual cognitive tasks, chimpanzees show an opposite pattern of neurothermal lateralization, with left-ear temperatures increasing and right-ear temperatures decreasing (Hopkins and Fowler, 1998). Several studies have shown that human impulsive aggressors exhibit increased subcortical arousal, together with reduced right and left prefrontal activity (see Raine et al., 1997 and 1998), suggesting that impulsive aggression may be associated with reduced executive function and regulatory control over subcortical emotional states and aggressive impulses. Children with intractable partial epilepsy presenting comorbidly with impulsive aggression show temporal and bilateral medial PFC (mPFC) hypometabolism (Juhasz et al., 2001). Maximal differences in cerebral glucose metabolism were found in the right and left middle temporal gyrus in comparison to nonaggressive children with epilepsy. The foregoing is consistent with the notion that the right hemisphere might play a predominant role in the representation and modulation of excitatory sympathetic arousal mediating rapid behavioral adjustments to emotionally provocative threats and uncertainty (Wittling, 1990; Wittling et al., 1998b), whereas the left hemisphere is more directly involved in the modulation of parasympathetic pathways in association with emotional arousal mediating social coping and control strategies (Wittling et al, 1998a). In combination, left and right hemispheres exercise profound autonomic attunement and integrative influences over blood pressure, heart rate, and HPA-system activity.

Paw Preference, Laterality, and Tympanic Thermal Asymmetry

Tan (1987) has reported that more dogs exhibit a right-paw preference (57.1%) than a left-paw preference (17.9%), with 25% being ambidextrous (N = 28, 19 females and 9 males). Wells (2003) has shown that the lateralized preference for paw use is probably gender related in dogs, with females appearing to show a right-paw preference and male dogs tending to show a left-paw preference. However, Wells' findings concerning paw preference are possibly confounded by an uncontrolled influence of previous training, at least with respect to one of the tasks used to evaluate handedness (i.e., giving a paw). More recently, though, Quaranta and colleagues (2004) have reported additional data concerning the lateralization of paw preference that appears to support Wells' gender hypothesis. They also report evidence suggesting that paw-use lateralization is correlated with various immune functions; however, these immune differences are not correlated with gender. Since dogs show evidence of cerebral asymmetry, with the right hemisphere tending to be significantly heavier and larger than the left in most dogs (Tan and Caliskan, 1987a and b), one might suppose that paw preference is related to morphological asymmetry, but Tan could not establish a correlation between brain morphology and a specific paw preference in dogs. The larger mass and area comprising the right hemisphere suggests that the right side of the brain should be associated with increased metabolic activity and blood flow in association with right cerebral dominance. Research on paw preference in rodents introduces an interesting dimension to this hypothesis. As in dogs, the right hemisphere of rats tends to be larger than the left. In addition, rats exhibit a pattern of neurothermal asymmetry that is correlated with paw-use preference (Klimenko, 2000), but the temperature gradient between left and right hemispheres is most conspicuous in left-handed rats and least so in right-handed rats; ambidextrous rats show an intermediate thermal gradient. These various differences affecting interhemisphere thermal gradients appear to be ontogenetically stable (Klimenko, 2001). Temperature kinetics on the surface of the cerebrum that have been imaged in rats (Shevelev et al., 1986) indicate relatively rapid left-right and right-left hemispheric asymmetries and crossover patterns of movement and equilibrium. The stability of interhemisphere thermal gradients from an early age raises the possibility that tympanic temperature might be of value in identifying temperament traits and coping styles early in life. Further, given the findings reported by Quaranta and colleagues in dogs and numerous studies in rodents linking behavioral lateralization and neural asymmetries to immune reactivity (Fu et al., 2003) and HPA-system activation (Neveu and Moya, 1997), both aspects of adaptation may be correlated with tympanic thermal asymmetries and changes in bodily temperature associated with stress and sickness. Rodents showing a right-paw preference appear to be more vulnerable to physical and behavioral stressors (Neveu et al., 1998), whereas those exhibiting a left-paw preference may be more prone to immune disorders (Fu et al., 2003). Consequently, it would be of interest to learn whether the basal intertympanic thermal gradient is a good predictor of paw-use preferences in dogs.

Measuring Tympanic Temperature

Thermal scanners can be used to rapidly (in 1 second) and accurately measure tympanic temperatures from a dog's ear. Whenever possible, at least three readings from each ear should be taken and a mean score assigned. Tympanic thermal asymmetries may possess value as novel endophenotypes identifying temperament traits and coping styles, as appears to be the case among children (Boyce et al., 2002) and various animal species. Tomaz and colleagues (2003), for example, have reported that marmosets exhibit asymmetrical tympanic temperature shifts consistent with a right brain specialization for coping with capture/restraint stress and fear. Monkeys that have been repeatedly captured show a significant reduction in tympanic temperatures on the right side. A similar effect appears to occur in some dogs. For example, temperature readings from a nonaggressive but emotionally reactive Labrador retriever (5-year-old neutered male), which responded with vigorous escape arousal associated with restraint, initially showed a left-right asymmetry (left ear, 102.1°F; and right ear, 100.6°F). However, after the struggling ceased, a slightly opposite right-left asymmetry (left ear, 101.5°F; and right ear, 102.0°F) emerged that was followed by a gradual temperature

decrease and left-right equilibrium in association with comforting talk and massage (left ear, 100.6°F; and right ear, 100.3°F).

Some preliminary data suggest that dogs exhibiting canine impulsive aggression may show lateralized tympanic temperature variations consistent with the foregoing hypothesis. For example, a male Wheaton terrier (neutered 3-year-old) with a history of threatening and biting strangers and familiar visitors showed an initial increase in temperature in the left ear in association with the ringing of a doorbell plus greeting (left ear, 99.1°F; and right ear, 98.0°F). A follow-up reading taken after the trainer had been in the house for approximately 1 hour showed that the temperature range had not significantly changed but that the asymmetry had shifted from the left to the right ear (left ear, 98.7°F; and right ear, 99.4°F). The initial higher left-ear temperature may reflect an increase in glucose metabolism or a change in regional blood flow to the left side of the brain in response to the sudden change and the excitement triggered by the unexpected visit. The relatively low temperatures in response to the doorbell is a bit surprising, however, since the dog was highly agitated and aggressive (e.g., strong threat barking, lunging, and vigilant readiness)—behavior that one might expect to elevate temperature. The presence of a low basal cortical temperature is consistent with increased regional blood flow. Cerebral blood flow in dogs appears to be autoregulated by means of metabolic signals, consistent with the idea that the lower temperature may reflect a rapid increase in arterial flow of blood to the left or right side of the brain.

In another case, a female Saint Bernard (spayed 1-year-old) that showed hyperactivity and extreme delay-of-gratification deficits, intrafamilial agonism, and social control/frustration intolerance from an early age onward toward one particular male family member exhibited an unusual pattern of tympanic asymmetries and temperature fluctuations consistent with decreased cerebral metabolic activity or pronounced cerebral blood-flow changes. In contrast to the pattern of impulsivity exhibited by the aforementioned Wheaton, the Saint Bernard exhibited a pattern of intrusive hyperexcitability and exploitive behavior toward visitors. Tympanic temperatures taken 15 to 20 minutes after arriving at the home indicated a right-left asymmetry (left ear, 100.4°F; and right ear, 102.0°F). After a long walk, tympanic temperatures were taken again. Interestingly, as the family member who was the prime target of aggression approached to help restrain the dog during the scanning procedure, the dog's temperature plunged bilaterally (left ear, 95.2°F; and right ear, 95.3°F). Since these measurements seemed oddly low, a second measurement was taken that confirmed a significant hypothermic event (left ear, 96.6°F; and right ear, 97.1°F). The dog's tympanic temperatures continued to move in the direction of normothermia and an opposite left-right asymmetry as it calmed (left ear, 101.4°F; and right ear, 100.3°F).

CARDIOVASCULAR ACTIVITY AND EMOTIONAL BEHAVIOR

Early factor analyses found that various cardiovascular patterns loaded with certain emotional variables and temperament traits in dogs (Royce, 1955; Brace, 1962; Scott and Fuller, 1965; Cattell and Korth, 1973). Royce's work, in particular, points intriguingly toward a potential link between temperament, heart rate, vagal tone, and emotional tendencies predisposing a dog toward reactive behavior. For example, he found that heart-rate changes in response to divergent social stimuli, including potent vagal braking effects in response to both calming and threatening vocal control efforts, loaded with an increased tendency toward behavioral reactivity. Royce describes an aggression factor that occurs with impulsiveness and a deceleration in heart rate in response to electric shock. Vagal braking in response to both shock and a threatening voice is also associated with an unidentified trait consisting of attraction, dominance, and temperature variables. Royce also found that dogs showing an increased propensity for behavioral reactivity exhibit a rapid sympathetic acceleration in heart rate in response to muzzling restraint, but showed no change in heart rate when administered an electric shock.

Heart Rate

Among laboratory dogs, Beerda and colleagues (1998) reported a nonspecific increase in heart rate in response to both social and nonsocial stressors, concluding that "heart rate increases should best be regarded as general responses to possibly meaningful events, irrespective of whether these are appreciated as positive or negative" (378). Although these researchers could not demonstrate the existence of discriminative heart-rate changes in response to acute social and nonsocial stressors, they did show differences in the HPA activity of dogs exposed to nonsocial stressors (e.g., loud sound, electric shocks, and a falling bag) versus dogs exposed to social restraint and startle delivered by a social object. Whereas nonsocial fear-eliciting stimuli increased cortisol release, startling events (repeatedly opening an umbrella in the dog's direction) and mechanically forcing the dog down to the floor by pulling up on a rope passed under a bar fixed to the floor or by shoving it down by hand and holding it there for 20 seconds (restraint) did not increase cortisol release. The steady pulling and manhandling procedure was performed twice with a 20-second interval between each trial. All of the social procedures were performed with the experimenter wearing a mask, hat, and coat scented with an unfamiliar odor. Despite the directive challenge, risk, and novelty of such stimulation, no significant increase in cortisol activity was observed. The absence of stress in response to restraint (defeat) is opposite to the robust and long-lasting effects that novelty and social defeat have on other species tested under laboratory conditions (see Koolhaas et al., 1997). The increased submissive precursor behaviors exhibited by challenged dogs (e.g., oral activities, paw lifting, slightly lower body posture, changes in ear position, and other signs of submission) appear to reflect a standing readiness to submit mediated by an effect of person. This hypothesis is consistent with a specialized flirt-and-forbear antistress system and enhanced parasympathetic capacities that enable dogs to cope with challenges and risks in a nonstressful manner, whereby the HPA system remains relatively unperturbed even though a dog shows various submissive precursors. In the absence of the flirt-and-forbear antistress system (e.g., socialized wolves), similar social challenges and threats would likely cause stressful flight-or-fight reactions and the activation of HPA system.

Recently, King and colleagues (2003) have suggested that heart rate might be a more practical and sensitive measure of a dog's reactivity to novelty and fear than are cortisol levels. Other researchers have found that a reactive pattern of cardiac acceleration and deceleration in response to social and environmental stressors appears to correlate with an increased vulnerability to reactive social behavior and stress proneness (Vincent and Michell, 1996; Vincent and Leahy, 1997) (see *Autonomic Arousal, Heart Rate, and Aggression* in Chapter 6). Blood-pressure and heart-rate changes appear to be highly sensitive to traumatic events, and conditioned cardiovascular changes may persist (schizokinesis) or worsen (autokinesis) long after the overt escape/avoidance behavior has ceased (Dykman and Gantt, 1997).

The evolution of specialized flirt-and-forbear antistress capacities has given dogs relatively sophisticated capacities for maintaining sympathovagal balance and HPA-system stability via the integration of an adaptive coping style in the context of forming secure attachments. The integrated and refined attention and impulse control resulting from adaptive learning and the vagal-mediated attunement of autonomic control systems reguates increases or decreases of heart rate in anticipation of expected needs, motivational changes that enable dogs to cope with social challenges and risks without becoming overly stressed by them. The failure of earlier work (Beerda et al., 1998) to detect a differentiation of heart rate in response to different stressors might be understood within the context of these adaptive specializations evolved by dogs to cope with domestic life. Accordingly, companion or service dogs (see Vincent and Leahy, 1997) reared under the influence of consistent and enriched home or training environments may express autonomic elaborations and complex attunement dynamics while integrating an adaptive coping style that dogs living under the more austere and impoverished conditions of the laboratory do not acquire. In addition, rewarding exchanges that occur within the home setting appear to be necessary precursors for the activation of the social engagement system (SES), which, in turn, facilitates vagal-mediated secure social and place attachments.

Heart-rate Variability

Cardiac markers of sympathetic or parasympathetic tone may be useful for detecting disturbances affecting the SES. For example, sympathetically reactive wild rats exhibit dramatically more arrhythmic ventricular events (premature beats) and less parasympathetic rebound after defeat than do Wistar rats, a strain that is more sociable and less reactive to novel social stimuli and showing increased heart-rate variability and marked vagal recruitment following defeat stress (Sgoifa et al., 1998). In another study, Sgoifa and colleagues (1999) found that wild rats also exhibit significant differences in the way they respond to social versus nonsocial stressors, with wild rats showing more ventricular arrhythmias and sympathetic dominance after social stress than after nonsocial stress (restraint).

Dogs appear to produce a comparatively greater parasympathetic inhibition over cardiovascular activity than do humans (Little et al., 1999). When orienting toward novel stimuli, dogs show a rapid decrease in heart rate that continues while engaged in sustained attention or exploratory activities. A lower heart rate is also produced by a wide range of evoking social stimuli, including petting, muzzle holding, pinning, and holding in the arms, suggesting that parasympathetic motor systems may play an integral role in the integration of submission behaviors (Fox, 1978) and hierarchic relations (Sgoifa et al., 2001). Scott and Fuller (1965) observed that respiratory sinus arrhythmia (RSA) and heart rate are closely related among dogs, in that a slow heart rate is typically arrhythmic, whereas a fast heart rate is usually more regular and indicative of increased sympathetic tone. While lying down and resting, heart activity is prominently under the control of parasympathetic tone, whereas, when standing, heart rate is a composite of sympathetic and parasympathetic components (Palazzolo et al., 1998). During emotionally exciting events, parasympathetic control is withdrawn, causing the heart rate to increase, whereas the reinstatement of parasympathetic control (vagal braking) by vocal reassurance or petting decreases heart rate while increasing heart-rate rhythm variability. As a result, measures of *heart-rate variability* (HRV)—that is, beat-to-beat changes in heart rate—appears to reflect the state of autonomic systems mediating behavioral adjustments and may be useful for evaluating the effects of stress on sympathovagal tone and reactive/impulsive adjustment (Pagani et al., 1986; Billman and Dujardin, 1990).

Hypothetically, dogs expressing relatively high tonic HRV measures might be expected to be more adaptable and to habituate more rapidly to social and environmental novelty and unexpected change, whereas dogs expressing reduced tonic HRV should tend to be more reactive and exhibit a nonhabituating orientation toward novelty and unexpected change. The normally reduced heart rate in response to environmental and social exploration may be diminished or unstable in such dogs, especially when exposed to unfamiliar situations or novel social targets. In addition, dogs exhibiting reactive arousal show variable amounts of plasma adrenal epinephrine and norepinephrine, depending on the relative contributions of anger and fear comprising the reactive state (Verrier and Dickerson, 1991), with epinephrine (fear) and norepinephrine (anger) representing potentially useful markers for assessing arousal and aggression risk. Dogs affected by anticipatory social anxiety may exhibit signs of persistent (nonhabituating) anxious or conflictive arousal in association with hypervigilance and readiness for defensive autoprotective behavior, changes that are correlated with heart rate, HRV, and other indicators of autonomic activation. Autonomic states associated with past anger or predisposing a dog to anger may be correlated with signature changes expressed in cardiovascular activity (see Kovach et al., 2001). As a result, cardiovascular data may provide

valuable information relevant to a better understanding of the etiology and treatment of behavior problems associated with impulsivity and a reactive coping style.

As a result of social ambivalence, dispersive tensions, and chronic inhibitory strain, dogs may show signs of autonomic dysregulation in response to ambiguous or uncontrollable social stimuli or physical challenges. The relative stability of sympathovagal tone may be reflected in changes to heart rate and indexed by HRV following sensory and physical challenges (e.g., novelty, unexpected change, demands requiring sustained attention, exposure to provocative stimuli, unwelcome approach while in safe refuges, and pulling the dog by leash from a resting area). Conflict and emotional distress may contribute to the disruption of attention functions gradually impairing a dog's ability to competently engage and disengage selective attention. Social and attentional disengagement facilitate the loss of autonomic attunement, thereby significantly reducing the dog's ability to adjust arousal and to cope adaptively with changing environmental and social demands. Basic training appears to exert a beneficial influence on sympathovagal balance by improving vagal regulation over sympathetic shifts in response to novelty, handling, and restraint. Heart-rate deceleration is reliably evoked by petting dogs that respond to social tactile stimulation as a reward (Fonberg et al., 1981), perhaps contributing to the evident cognitive and emotional attunement that is brought about by the training and socialization process. Conditioned appetitive stimuli and behaviors trained in association with food reinforcement tend to promote parasympathetic balance and calming effects, as well.

The potent parasympathetic effects of stimuli anticipating the presentation of food on arousal was a central finding of Pavlov's work, with salivation being closely regulated by the parasympathetic branch of the autonomic nervous system. Among young horses, those having received training tend to be less emotionally reactive, showing a lower nonmotor heart rate and greater HRV than untrained horses (Visser et al., 2002). The adaptogenic benefits of basic training appear to depend more on an ability to freely choose and act upon events that are relatively predictable and controllable rather than the motivational direction of the incentives prompting behavioral change (see Stichnoth, 2002). When a dog is physically immobilized, aversive events may be perceived as more threatening and conducive to the activation of autoprotective adjustments, whereas a dog that can move about freely may feel more in control, perhaps perceiving the event as being at least escapable, if not fully predictable or controllable.

Effects of Restraint and Immobilization

Many studies with diverse taxa have shown that inescapable physical restraint or the induction of cataleptiform immobility results in bradycardia, even cardiac arrest and sudden death in some cases. Richter (1957) found that wild rats held until they stopped struggling rapidly succumbed when placed into a vat of water, unlike nonstressed wild rats that continued swimming for 2 days or more. With a highly unstable dog, the mere presence of a person may trigger intense vagal braking and severe bradycardia. For example, Gantt and colleagues (1966) described a dog restrained in a Pavlovian harness whose heart rate moved from 140 to 180 bpm to as low as 20 bpm when exposed to a person standing nearby, and on several occasions this dog went into cardiac arrest for 6 to 8 seconds when petted.

A study by Reese and colleagues (1982) on the effects of physical restraint and petting on nervous and normal pointer dogs revealed intriguing behavioral and heart-rate differences in the way dogs cope with physical restraint. The dogs were restrained by turning them on their backs in a sling-restraint device. Once in the restraint sling, the dogs were calmed with stoking on the belly (1 stroke/second for a minute). After the induction phase, the dogs were left alone in the sling-restraining device during a 2-minute observation phase and watched from a separate room through a one-way mirror. Nervous pointers showed persistent cataleptiform immobility with bradycardia throughout the induction and observation phase and remained in the sling until they were tipped out of it. During a 5-minute postrestraint observation period, the nervous dogs showed a significant postrestraint sympathetic increase in heart-rate activity. In contrast, normal pointers show an initial tachycardia associated the induction phase, followed by postural and muscular relaxation, and a sustained postrestraint bradycardia as they move about after freeing themselves from the sling or upon being tipped out of the device. The normal dogs that remained in the sling after the induction period appeared relaxed and showed no head or neck immobility, and one of them even wagged its tail at the end of the 2-minute observation period. All of the nervous dogs had to be tipped out of the sling, whereupon they reflexively righted themselves and remained in an upright frozen posture during the 5-minute postrestraint period. Normal dogs that freed themselves from the sling during the 2-minute observation period exhibited more pronounced bradycardia scores (105 to 87 bpm) in comparison to normal dogs that remained in the sling (106 to 99 bpm) during the same period. The lower heart rates of the normal pointers that freed themselves may reflect parasympathetic relief associated with successful escape to freedom, whereas the sustained tachycardia of the nervous pointers may reflect increased anxious arousal associated with an escape from danger (see *Escape to Safety versus Escape from Danger* in Chapter 8).

Williams and colleagues (2003) have studied the effects of inescapable immobilization on the heart rate and HRV of a Great Dane. The dog was immobilized inside a wooden box that allowed it to stand with its head protruding from an opening in the front. Immobilization was achieved by filling the box with triple-cleaned oats until the dog's body was fully covered, allowing only its head to move about freely. To control head and neck movements, a short leash was attached to a flat collar and fastened to the front of the box. The dog was also fitted with a muzzle-clamping halter to control its head and jaws. Heart-rate and HRV data were collected by means of an ambulatory monitoring device. During a pretest-baseline procedure, the dog was exposed to an unknown target dog to instigate aggressive arousal and establish baseline reactivity. The leashed dog showed strong reactive behavior (e.g., lunging, jumping, growling, and barking) and an elevated heart rate (160 bpm) toward the unknown dog in comparison to its response to a familiar dog (135 bpm) and no dog (111 bpm). Pretest HRVs in response to both the unknown and known dog were identical. After an hour of immobilization, the dog showed a significant decrease in heart rate (91 bpm) and an increase in HRV indicative of parasympathetic activation. During an exposure procedure in which the unknown dog was presented to the immobilized dog, first at 15 meters away and then gradually moved incrementally closer over 31 minutes, aggressive behavior was suppressed. During the postimmobilization tests, the dog "was not as reactive" toward the unknown dog and showed a decrease in heart rate together with a slight increase in HRV in comparison to preimmobilization scores. The reduced heart rate and slight increase in HRV at the end of the experiment toward the approach of an unknown dog might reflect parasympathetic relief associated with getting out of the box—a state of arousal incompatible with aggression.

Since bradycardia and alterations in HRV in dogs can be produced by a variety of procedures (e.g., petting and massage, pinning restraint, and tonic immobilization) producing a high or low level of physiological stress, future investigations should include other relevant autonomic arousal markers (e.g. catecholamine and cortisol levels) to help determine whether the immobilization procedure works by relaxing dogs or as the result of some other mechanism triggered by immobilization, fear, or loss of control (see *Stress-related Potentiation of the Flight-Fight System* in Chapter 6). In particular, many features of the procedure seem consistent with the learned-helplessness paradigm. Exposure to inescapable aversive stimulation while fully immobilized is a central feature of the learned-helplessness protocol (see *Stress, Traumatic Avoidance, and Laboratory Experiments with Shock*). Exposing a reactive dog to the slow approach of an unfamiliar dog (a social stimulus eliciting intense defensive arousal) in the manner described reminds one of being buried up to the neck in sand and then forced to watch the tide slowly come in without any means of defending oneself or escaping the encroaching threat. The induction of learned helplessness has been shown to reduce escape and avoidance behaviors and to exert potent antiaggression effects in dogs (Seligman, 1975) and rats (Maier et al., 1972), perhaps explaining the effect that the immobilization procedure is believed to have on defensive aggression in dogs (Williams and Borchelt, 2002).

The authors speculate that immobilizing restraint combined with "tactile pressure" might explain the observed changes in heart rate, HRV, and reduced aggression exhibited by the immobilized dog. They compare the immobilization procedure that they use with Grandin's squeeze machine (see *Taction and Posture-facilitated Relaxation* in Chapter 6) but overlook an essential difference: the person in the squeeze machine is not exposed to a threat slowly moving in their direction from which they cannot escape. While immobilization and "loss of control" procedures may temporarily reduce aggression, they may also adversely impact more desirable social behaviors and learning capacities that depend on voluntary initiative. Finally, in the case of highly reactive and unstable dogs or dogs with heart disorders, the stressful induction of pronounced fluctuations in heart rate by means of rapid exposure to an inescapable threat educing high levels of fear or anger under immobilizing restraint may pose a significant cardiovascular risk (Kovach et al., 2001; see Kamarck and Jennings, 1991).

DEVICES USED TO MONITOR AUTONOMIC AND STRESS-RELATED CHANGES

Although HRV may ultimately provide the most useful diagnostic information with respect to linking behavior problems with autonomic tone and sympathovagal imbalance, such equipment is relatively expensive and complicated to use. The dog's heart rate is an extremely sensitive indicator of autonomic tone, often shifting dramatically in response to sympathetic arousal and showing varying degrees of receptiveness to countervailing parasympathetic influences indicative of autonomic balance. Suggestive autonomic information providing a rough index of sympathovagal tone may be derived by tracking cardiac recovery patterns in response to startling or provocative events and the modulation afforded by the delivery of arousing and calming stimuli. In addition to monitoring the dog's autonomic changes in response to petting and other rewards, various changes associated with orienting and attending, leash prompts and saccades, training modules and routines (e.g., sit-stay and down-stay training), and relaxation effects mediated by PFR can be monitored and tracked over time.

The author has found that a variety of inexpensive and readily available heart monitors can be useful for tracking autonomic shifts during training and the behavior-therapy process (see Vincent and Leahy, 1997; Stichnoth, 2002; King et al., 2003). Sports monitors provide a useful real-time window for observing and quantifying a dog's response to various training and counterconditioning procedures. These relatively inexpensive radiotelemetry devices can be attached to a harness to prevent the elastic band from shifting off the heartbeat signal. The effective use of such devices through dog hair requires that an electrode gel be applied on the skin to establish a viable signal. The monitor is attached to the top of the harness, making easy viewing possible. In addition to sports heart monitors that are fitted around the chest of a dog for recording real-time heart-rate changes, wrist-type heart-rate and blood-pressure monitors are available. Reasonably priced cuff-type monitors together with recording and graphing capability are also available and useful, especially for tracking changes in the relaxation response during PFR training. Various tympanic thermometers are readily available for measuring changes in temperature, including one device designed for dogs. Pill-sized telemetry devices are also available for tracking temperature. These pill thermometers are designed to be

ingested and to transmit core temperature data. Pill thermometers offer a nonintrusive way to monitor and record real-time temperature changes (O'Brien et al., 1998), perhaps having unique applications for following stress-related changes associated with canine behavior problems. Real-time temperature information might be particularly revealing, perhaps providing a biological marker useful for the diagnosis as well as tracking the outcome of treatment efforts. Given the apparent close relationship between emotional regulation and thermoregulation, sympathovagal disturbances affecting a dog's ability to regulate fear and anger may be expressed in the form of temperature changes. In addition to temperature, other pill-sized sensors might be developed to measure stomach acid content (a stress measure) and other relevant biochemical changes affecting the gut in association with stress. Movement and general activity levels can be tracked and quantified by pedometers.

However, what is really needed is the ability to monitor simultaneously the activity of several relevant physiological parameters to establish a signature profile or configuration of specific physiological arousal states that are unique correlates of the target problem behavior. In addition to heart rate, devices measuring activity levels, respiration rates, skin potential, changes in muscle tone, and temperature, perhaps incorporated into a collar worn by the dog and receiving signals directly from the neck and from a vest containing ambulatory monitoring equipment, might be designed to track prominent autonomic changes in anticipation of aggression. In the case of dogs that give little or no advanced warning before reaching a flash point of no return, such devices might help to identify specific markers that regularly precede aggressive episodes and help to facilitate behavior-therapy efforts. Canine biofeedback collars might be programmed to automatically deliver various sensory stimuli to interrupt the aggressive sequence at an early and flexible stage or to provide the trainer with radio-controlled means to activate stimulation, perhaps involving attention-stimulating auditory stimuli, the delivery of odors that can increase parasympathetic tone at the critical moment, and various other stimuli able to interrupt the aggression sequence and to induce behavioral inhibition. Electronic training collars incorporating biofeedback capabilities might be useful in the treatment of numerous behavior problems.

AUTOSHAPING AND AUTOMATED TRAINING

The full-body restraint and passive-exposure apparatus and techniques described by Williams and colleagues (2003) require little involvement of the owner or behavior therapist. The dog is simply put in a box, covered completely in a material that prevents movement and slowly exposed to the approach of a target or person. It is easy to imagine how such a technique might be further automated. Electronic products of various kinds are reportedly being developed with the goal of getting dogs to train themselves. Dunbar (2000) has dubbed the methodology *autoshaping*, borrowing the term from an experimental procedure in which laboratory animals are trained to manipulate levers and switches to obtain food reinforcement without the experimenter's aid. Dunbar predicts that autoshaping will revolutionize the way dogs are trained: "Electronics can train a dog by a flick of a switch overnight. The autoshaping revolution will be mind boggling" (transcribed). In addition to electronic collars emitting low-level electrical pulses, devices that Dunbar calls *tickling collars* and other electronic control devices designed to distract dogs in various ways will be programmed to interrupt and shape behavior automatically, presumably with the aid of a programmable food-delivery mechanism. Although autoshaping procedures and environmental programming may eventually offer significant applications for the control and management of certain behavior problems, in principle such procedures and goals are problematic with respect to the objectives of cynopraxic training and therapy. Certainly, owners lacking sufficient time or incentive to train their own dogs will be attracted by quick-fix devices offering effortless overnight gratification; however, nothing can ultimately take the place of the interactive and shared experience of training. Ironically, even designers of robotic pets have recognized the importance of interactive training to make entertainment robots seem more natural, gratifying, and pleasant (Kaplan et al., 2002):

> One of the challenges and pleasures in keeping a real pet, like a dog, is that the owner has to train it. A dog owner is proud when he has the impression that his pet changes its own behavior according to his teaching. We believe this is also a way for an interesting relationship to emerge between an entertainment robot and its owner.... This paper focuses on a method for teaching actions to an animal-like entertainment robot. Of course, the simplest way would be to allow the owner to program directly new actions for the robot. But for the purpose of entertainment robotics it would be much more interesting if this teaching would take place only through interactions, as it does with real pets. (197)

According to the authors, programming robotic dogs to behave in predetermined ways, without giving the user the ability to change a robot's behavior through training, significantly diminishes the potential fun and gratification derived from interacting with such pet toys. If automatic control is not satisfying for the users of robotic toys, how much less gratifying would autoshaping techniques be for the owners of sentient dog companions. By excluding the owner from the training process, autoshaping risks causing the dog to become progressively mechanized and detached from the owner as a source of predictability and control. Instead of enhancing the bond and the dog's quality of life, such products and techniques may serve only to reduce and constrict the human-dog bond while further alienating the dog from the home and family. Indeed, as a dog becomes an automated household accessory, one may gradually need devices to record and evaluate the dog's progress and emotional state. One such device, called a *Bowlingual* (Takara Corporation), may already be here (Tham, 2002). If it lives up to its maker's claims, the device would nicely fit into the futuristic autoshaping scheme. The collar device is equipped with a wireless microphone to pick up and transmit vocalizations to a receiver that interprets the bark, howl, whine, yelp, and so forth into a literal translation of how the dog feels and projects it on a small terminal screen (e.g., "I'm sad"). In addition, the device can record vocalizations when the owner is not at home, providing a summary of the dog's emotional state and mood during the day.

Numerous electronic devices are currently available for monitoring and interfacing with dog behavior via various means of radio- and behavior-activated stimulation. Inexpensive noise-activated recorders and movement-sensitive video cameras provide extremely useful baseline and treatment-tracking information. Many of these devices have been previously discussed in the context of controlling destructive behavior (see Chapter 2). The most frequently used deterrent interface typically involves noise stimulation via booby traps and alarms activated by infrared or movement/vibration detectors. Such devices can be highly effective for controlling many nuisance problems, but the suppressive effect of loud noise for many dogs is problematic, especially with respect to the control of highly motivated behavior. Although initial exposure to a loud noise stimulus evokes pronounced startle, repeated exposure typically results in gradual habituation and loss of aversion. Further, dogs possessing high-startle thresholds may require noise stimulation at a level of intensity that potentially risks doing physiological harm to the ear (e.g., a nautical horn) (see Campbell and Bloom, 1965).

PART 2: ELECTRONIC TRAINING

Note: Throughout the following discussion, the terms used to describe electronic training collars (e-collars) and electrical stimulation (ES) are self-explanatory or specifically defined, as needed. However, one terminological decision requires some explanation to head off potential confusion. Specifically, the term *electrical stimulus* or *e-stimulus* has been selected to replace the word *shock*. The term *e-signal* is used in cases where a dog has learned to respond to the e-stimulus as an avoidance cue. There are several reasons for

this decision. First, at low levels, the term shock is hardly fitting to describe the effects produced by electronic training collars, since there is virtually no effect beyond a pulsing tingling or tickling sensation on the surface of the skin. Second, the word shock is loaded with biased connotations, images of convulsive spasms and burns, and implications associated with extreme physical pain, emotional trauma, physiological collapse, and laboratory abuses. Third, the e-stimulus or signal generated by most modern devices is highly controlled and presented to produce a specific set of behavioral and motivational responses to it. In general, the terms e-stimulus, e-signal, and ES have been decided on for the sake of neutrality and because they more accurately describe the low to medium electrical events produced by radio-controlled and behavior-activated e-collars. In most cases where historical research has referred to ES as shock, the original terminological convention is maintained.

Currently, the most common aversive interface and deterrent used in dog training is ES. The use of electronic training devices is the subject of significant controversy and the propagation of misinformation and exaggeration on both sides of the debate. Historically, dog trainers working with hunting dogs were the primary end users of commercial electronic training collars. These early collars reputedly generated a harsh shock, causing significant pain and distress to dogs. In addition to producing a highly aversive shock, these early devices were prone to significant reliability problems, such as discharging in response to extraneous radio signals. In contrast, the safety and reliability of most modern electronic training and behavior-control devices have been significantly improved. Most current devices deliver a highly controlled e-stimulus, ranging from low levels of stimulation (imperceptible or just barely perceptible to human touch) to higher levels capable of causing significant startle and discomfort. High-quality contemporary devices enable trainers to select stimulation levels that precisely match a dog's needs, tolerance for ES, and training objectives, thereby preventing excessively painful stimulation and unnecessary distress.

The combined advantages of immediate and reliable radio-controlled delivery of precisely regulated ES make electronic training a viable and humane alternative to many traditional techniques for applying negative reinforcement and punishment. Traditional techniques can be effective when skillfully used, but they are often encumbered by undesirable side effects associated with interactive punishment, poorly regulated force, and retroactive timing. Finally, although potentially capable of producing significant psychological distress and harm when used improperly, electronic training devices are relatively safe and humane when used competently and selectively. Recently, the Delta Society, in cooperation with dozens of nationally recognized dog-behavior and welfare experts, has produced a document outlining professional humane standards for the dog-training profession. Both radio-controlled and behavior-activated electronic devices have been recognized as effective and humane training equipment when used properly and in accordance with humane principles (Delta Society, 2001). Given the potential benefits of radio-controlled electronic training and the relatively safe nature of ES, professional dog trainers are well advised to master the basic technical knowledge and behavioral skills needed to use such tools effectively and humanely.

Today, a variety of products are available over the counter for purchase and use by ordinary dog owners possessing little behavioral knowledge or understanding of the benefits or potential harm that can result from the improper use of electronic training equipment. Obviously, for proper and humane use, electronic training devices require support instruction and knowledge of basic-training principles; nonetheless, large numbers of radio-controlled e-collars are sold in pet stores to relatively naive and inexperienced dog owners without much in the way of appropriate instruction regarding their use, misuse, and potential for abuse. Unfortunately, the instructional material typically packaged with these powerful training tools is woefully inadequate. This neglect poses a significant welfare concern that should be addressed by responsible manufacturers and distributors of these products. Without proper instruction and guidance, electronic training collars cannot be used competently and humanely, and, in the hands of misinformed or incompetent users, e-collars can all too easily become instruments of abuse and cruelty. Of course, a similar criticism can be made concerning many other training collars and tools commonly used in dog training. Nevertheless, the radio-controlled and push-button operation of electronic devices poses special problems that justify additional concern with respect to misuse and potential for abuse. Furthermore, with promises of rapid control and instant gratification, impatient and unknowledgeable dog owners may resort to electronic training as a push-button panacea, without first giving conventional reward-based training methods a chance to succeed. Lastly, since there is considerable variation in the ES produced by e-collars, manufacturers should freely disclose critical information concerning the output of their collars, including open-circuit voltage, closed-circuit voltage, current and power, and pulse and waveform characteristics (pulse duration and pulse repetition rates), together with explanations regarding the significance of such specification in order to help consumers and professionals select devices best suited to their needs. Sadly, most of the manufacturers that the author contacted for information concerning output specifications either did not reply or were strangely evasive and uncooperative, arguing that such data were of a proprietary nature. Of course, all the needed electrical output and waveform information needed can be obtained with an oscilloscope. Further, reasonably accurate output comparisons can be obtained with a true RMS multimeter. Many of the details regarding circuit design and output specifics can also be obtained by consulting patent claims.

Although low-level electrical stimulation (LLES) is humane and highly effective, electronic training devices should not be used in the absence of reward-based training, nor should they become a crutch or a way of life. Success in electronic training is achieved when it is completely replaced by reward-based training efforts. As a humane process, cynopraxic training strives to enhance affection, mutual appreciation, and trust between people and dogs, steering the relationship toward the ideals of interspecies cooperation and interactive harmony. Training is a lifelong process of befriending the dog—a process of mutual understanding and care that is most fully and satisfyingly achieved through gentle and considerate means. Excessive reliance on aversive procedures for controlling a dog undermines the attainment of these goals and risks damaging the relationship. Ultimately, the value of electronic training is measured by its ability to limit or extinguish itself, while at the same time liberating the dog from unacceptable behavior impeding a more enriched and rewarding life experience with people. Unfortunately, just as electronic training offers many significant benefits, it is fraught with significant risks of abuse and misuse. Instead of being used as a humane tool for enhancing the human-dog bond and improving a dog's quality of life, electrical control may be abused to enslave a dog by means of fear and pain. Using electrical control procedures to dominate a dog for the sheer sake of domination and exploitation is offensive and violates human sensibilities and the goals of cynopraxic training. Of course, similar concerns and considerations should guide the use of all aversive techniques used in dog training and behavior therapy.

Technical Considerations

Electrical Potential, Current, and Power

The relative potential of ES to produce pain or distress depends on a number of variables that are often ignored or underappreciated. Putting aside individual differences and psychological factors (e.g., the predictability and controllability of the event), parameters such as intensity, frequency of application, duration, and location of ES figure prominently into the sort of experience that bioelectrical stimulation produces (Price and Tursky, 1975; Sang et al., 2003). The e-stimulus is focused on a circumscribed area of skin tissue located immediately beneath and between the electrodes, referred to as the *electrode-skin inter-*

face. Because e-collars are designed to limit arcing, both electrodes of the stimulator need to make close contact with the skin to establish a closed circuit. Separation of electrodes from a dog's skin by thick hair or air of a distance greater than 1 millimeter will result in an open circuit. The high-voltage arcing of modern e-collars is minimal and may require magnification and darkened surroundings to view.

When discussing the effects of ES, some care should be exercised not to confuse electrical categories or phenomena. A common error is to equate voltage with current. Electrical potential or *voltage* is relative and depends on the electromotive difference between two points, whereas *current* refers to the amount of electrical charge or amperes flowing between those points over some period. The electrical quantity of a current is measured in coulombs (C), whereby 1 ampere (A) equals a flow of 1 C per second. A Van de Graff generator produces in excess of 300,000 volts (V) of electrical potential (the equivalent of a stun gun) but is relatively harmless to touch. On the other hand, as little as 25 V can be lethal to a person. The critical factor is the amount of energy (joules) or power that flows through the body. When one scuffs along on a carpet, the body accumulates a charge of several thousand volts, and voltage levels may rise to 3000 V or more when getting out of a car. Nevertheless, the energy released is miniscule, something on the order of 0.005 joules (J). The output of an e-collar tested by the New Zealand Department of Scientific and Industrial Research (Dix, 1991) was found to produce 3000 times less electrical energy than that allowed by standards for electrical fences, six times less electrical energy than that produced by the static discharge produced by walking on a carpet, and 50 times less than what is considered necessary to reach pain thresholds. Although the collar was estimated to produce a peak open-circuit amplitude of 961 V, when a current was passed through a 500-ohm load (simulating the electrode-skin circuit), a peak voltage of 58 V was found to drive a current of 116 milliamperes (mA) for 0.78 milliseconds (msec). When converted into energy values, the foregoing output current at peak amplitude and duration was determined to be on the order of 1.2 millijoules (mJ). Kouwenhoven and Milnor (1958) demonstrated that extremely brief low-energy (0.0001 to 2.4 J) high-voltage shocks of 40,000 V in anesthetized dogs could not induce ventricular fibrillation, cardiac arrest, or "any other untoward effect" (45).

The following analogy may help to clarify some important distinctions between voltage, current, and resistance. Imagine a scenario involving subway train and two conductors. The first conductor forces passengers (electrons) into a train car while his twin pulls them off again as quickly as they board. The force that the first conductor uses to push the passengers on board will depend on the size of the entryway and any obstructions blocking the flow of passengers within the train itself. Similarly, the force used to pull the out passengers again will depend on internal resistance and the size of the exit (out-circuit impedance). To the extent that both conductors push and pull the passengers (electrons) in and out of the train, a current or flow of charge is established between them, without either of the conductors actually entering the train themselves. As such, voltage can be described as the pressure or force needed to cause a current of electrons to flow between two points of a closed circuit; *voltage* always implies difference and distance, whereas *current* implies movement and time. A current of electricity is conducted through the electrode-skin circuit at a certain rate or amperage depending on the combined resistance and capacitance (impedance) of the conducting circuit. The various relationships between voltage (E), resistance (R), and amperage (I) are derivable from Ohm's law: $E = IR$. For example, provided that one knows the amperage and resistance of a circuit, one can then calculate the voltage by multiplying the values together. For example, a 20-mA current requires 14 V of electromotive force to move through a circuit having a 700-ohm resistance. Similarly, by dividing the known voltage by the circuit resistance or load ($I = E/R$), the amperage can be obtained. The amount of electrical energy used by a circuit as a current passes through it is described in terms of tem-

poral and heat units (e.g., amperes, watts, and joules).

When authors make statements about radio-controlled stimulators delivering shocks at a level of 3000 V, the reader may picture an event quite different than what actually occurs. The practice is doubly problematic when open-circuit and closed-circuit categories and measures are mixed together. The voltage between two electrodes of an open circuit may equal several thousand volts, and e-collars may generate open-circuit voltages of 3000 to 10,000 V, but one cannot sense the open-circuit voltage even though an electrical field radiates between the two electrodes of an activated e-collar. The open-circuit voltage is expressed as the difference in charge, electrical potential, or electromotive force between the electrodes. Without knowing other variables, however, such as the total impedance of the electrode-skin circuit, the amperage of the current, and the duration of the electrical event, the open-circuit voltage of the collar is not very meaningful information with respect to estimating the intensity of the e-stimulus reaching a dog. Referencing the open-circuit voltage may lead to unjustified connotations of severity. Christiansen and colleagues (2001a), for example, have claimed that the e-collar they used to suppress predatory behavior delivered an astounding 3000-V shock at 0.4 A. The notion that electronic training collars generate a 3000-V shock at 400 mA is misleading and must be wrong, since doing so for a 1-second period, as reported, would generate an astounding 1200 J of electrical energy—enough energy to light twelve 100-watt (W) light bulbs for 1 second. The authors appear to confuse the electrical potential between electrodes of an open circuit with the voltage between electrodes establishing a closed circuit—only a closed circuit can produce a flow of current capable of producing electrical power. With the current density localized around the small-diameter steel electrodes, such levels of shock as described by Christiansen and colleagues would likely seriously damage the skin. Finally, even though a particular e-collar may generates an open-circuit electrical potential of 3000 V, the actual operational voltage driving current through the electrode-skin circuit is far less. According to Ohm's law, an e-collar set to produce a current of 12.8 mA through a 100-ohm load would require a voltage of 1.28 V. The same current flowing through a 1000-ohm load requires 12.8 V. These predictions obtained from Ohm's law are closely reflected in actual measurements obtained with a true RMS digital multimeter (Extech 22-811). The voltage output or amplitude of a popular e-collar driving the aforementioned current value (12.8 mA) through 100-ohm and 1000-ohm loads was measured at 1.27 V and 10.3 V, respectively.

To avoid some of the confusion that occurs when the output specifications of collar devices are reported in the scientific literature, it would make sense to report such information in terms of closed-circuit values based on some load constant (e.g., 700 ohms) or in terms of a power-output formula (Forbes and Bernstein, 1935). Power or watts is the rate of energy dissipated over some period. In a closed circuit, the amount of electrical energy produced is based on volts, current, and time (t): energy = $t(EI)$, and 1 W is equal to the use of 1 J of energy per second. Consequently, power (P) is derived from the collar's voltage (E) times its amperage (I), or P = EI, making it a potentially useful value with respect to estimating the stimulation effect of an e-collar's output. In addition to quantitative parameters (e.g., current density and power), the subjective sensation produced by the e-stimulus is strongly affected by its waveform. The pulse duration and pulse repetition rate (frequency) are major determinants of the relative aversiveness or intensity of a current at a given amplitude flowing through the electrode-skin circuit. Keeping current and impedance constant, the subjective effect of the e-stimulus can be strongly affected by changes made to the pulse duration and pulse repetition rate (frequency), with longer pulse durations and increasing repetition rates producing more aversive effects (Kaczmarek et al., 1991). Many e-collars appear to shift intensity levels by altering the pulse duration or repetition rate while keeping the output current and voltage relatively constant, depending on the electrode-skin load. In such

devices, the pulse amplitude (voltage) is less important with respect to the actual intensity of the e-stimulus produced. Although an oscilloscope is needed to graphically display the various changes in pulse amplitude, duration, and repetition rates, a multimeter can be used to get a general idea of the relative pulse duration at different levels of intensity via frequency and duty-cycle readings. The *duty cycle* represents the ratio of the pulse duration to the pulse period expressed as a percentage.

Electrode-Skin Interface: Resistance and Capacitance Factors

The combined resistance and capacitance of the electrode-skin circuit is referred to as its *impedance*. The impedance determines the amount of voltage needed to cause a current of electrical charge to flow through it; the higher the impedance is, the more voltage is needed to establish a flow of current. The voltage output of many e-collars appears to shift up or down in response to changes in fur and skin resistance, with an upper output limit set to prevent excessive discharge and heat-generative arcing. In addition, a current limiter is built into these devices to reduce the risk of malfunction and delivery of dangerous shock. These bioelectrical design features enable the device to compensate safely for individual impedance, thereby ensuring that a highly discrete and measured dose of ES is delivered, depending on the individual characteristics and needs of a particular dog. Brief doses (momentary), as commonly used to support avoidance training, typically require higher-amplitude stimulation to reach threshold values, whereas longer-duration (continuous) doses of ES appear to establish a circuit at a lower amplitude via ionic microenvironment changes localized around the electrodes, vascular dilation (Greenblatt and Tursky, 1969), and other changes conducive to reduced impedance (Sang et al., 2003). Continuous stimulation techniques enable a trainer to apply LLES effectively at levels that do not exceed the threshold values of A-beta sensory pathways (tickle and tingle effects).

The condition of a dog's coat and the outer layers of the skin (stratum corneum) are the primary sources of cutaneous impedance. An important impedance factor is the skin's level of hydration, with dry and oily skin requiring more voltage than moist skin. Although skin moisture may improve its conductivity and increase the flow of current between electrodes (Chesney, 1995), external wetness may actually shunt current away from the electrode-skin interface and decrease current flow. Insulating the exposed sides of the electrodes with rubberizing paint may help to reduce current diversion due to wetness. Skin resistance varies between 10,000 to 100,000 ohms (or more depending on location) for dry skin and 1,000 ohms for skin that is well hydrated (Klein, 2000). The e-collar used by Tortora (1983) was reported to produce a pulse train having a 255-Hz repetition rate (50% duty cycle) with a peak voltage, measured across a 100,000-ohm load, estimated to be 1134 V. The high voltage of e-collars is designed to jump small gaps (1 millimeter) and pierce resistance barriers caused by bits of fur lying between the electrodes and the skin. Electrical arcing occurs when the electrode loses contact with the skin and the circuit is slightly opened. Relatively high voltage is needed to generate an arc between the electrode and a dog's skin. After the cutaneous resistance is transited by a brief high-magnitude pulse, skin impedance drops to a mean of 700 ohms (Kouwenhoven and Milnor, 1958). Measurements taken between internal and external electrodes have determined that the out-circuit impedance for dogs ranges from between 100 and 5000 ohms (Niwano et al., 2001). Subcutaneous resistance was measured to range between 95 and 225 ohms, whereas skin impedance at 10-V pacing showed significant variability, ranging from 460 to 16,600 ohms, depending on the size of the electrode used.

The impedance of the electrode-skin interface is also strongly influenced by the electrode diameter (Kaczmarek et al., 1991). Narrow-diameter electrodes require significantly more electrical potential to generate a charge that will pass through the skin (Forbes and Bernstein, 1935). In addition, since the current density concentrates at the out edge of the electrode, narrow-diameter electrodes, as used in e-collars, produce a highly localized and focused effect. The disadvantage of high-voltage ES is that the current density is established immediately beneath the electrode, which is prone to produce a pricking effect at levels just above detection thresholds (Kaczmarek et al., 1991; Poletto and Van Doren, 1999), perhaps in association with microscopic arcing around the outer rounded edge of the electrode, requiring great care to avoid eliciting pain when increasing stimulation amplitudes. In contrast, larger electrodes, as used in transcutaneous and neuromuscular electrostimulators, produce stronger ES intensity levels at lower pulse amplitudes and current levels.

The impedance load of the electrode-skin interface decreases as current increases, requiring less voltage at higher amperage levels, a principle applied to the design of transcutaneous electrostimulators. The cutaneous load also appears to be affected by the frequency of the pulse train (Rosell et al., 1988), with high-frequency pulses passing through the skin-impedance barrier more freely than low-frequency pulses. As pulse duration and pulse repetition rate are increased, the subjective magnitude of the e-stimulus is intensified. A major advantage of constant current devices is that they can shift the level of ES by altering the pulse duration or repetition rate rather than relying on changes to the pulse amplitude, thereby reducing the risk of discomfort generated by increased voltage in association with narrow-diameter electrodes. Many modern e-collars appear to hold pulse amplitude (voltage) relatively constant, altering output intensity by changing the pulse duration and repetition rates of the e-stimulus. Other devices alter output intensity by increasing pulse amplitude and keeping pulse duration and frequency relatively constant, depending on the electrode-skin load. When skin resistance is low, pulse amplitude is decreased; whereas when skin resistance is high, pulse amplitude is increased. The high, medium, and low variations that are generated at different levels by some collars appear to be achieved by altering pulse duration and repetition rates rather than involving changes affecting output amplitude.

Threshold Values

Prior exposure to ES exerts a number of modulatory influences over electrocutaneous thresholds, with experienced human subjects tolerating at least twice the electrical intensity tolerated by naive subjects (Kaczmarek et al., 1991). Although long-duration ES results in a reduction in cutaneous impedance, it is also associated with stimulus fatigue and a reduced sensitivity to the e-stimulus (Tursky et al., 1970). Consequently, low-level continuous stimulation used in the context of attention training may help to elevate reactive thresholds, thereby reducing the risk that medium-level ES will evoke adverse arousal. The presentation of brief nonpainful prepulses of ES also serves to elevate pain thresholds. Studies with human subjects have shown that presenting a 0.5-second prepulse of ES 40 to 60 msec before a stronger ES serves to reduce pain thresholds significantly (Blumenthal et al., 2001). In persons with low-pain thresholds, 40-msec prepulses of current set to match perceptual threshold levels resulted in a 54% reduction in perceived pain. Presenting a vibratory stimulus to dogs just in advance of the electrical event (60 to 300 msec) appears to help reduce startle arousal while at the same time facilitating the integration of the event as an informative signal via sensorimotor gating processes. Another useful technique for reducing the risk of reactive responses in dogs with low thresholds is to introduce ES gradually in combination with a continuous vibratory stimulus overlapping the e-stimulus.

Surprisingly little data have been reported about dogs with respect to electrical threshold values. What little is known suggests that the thresholds for shock produced by high-voltage generators (approximately 500 to 600 V at 60 Hz) do not significantly differ between puppies and adult dogs (Lessac and Solomon, 1969). The minimum electrical intensity required to evoke a leg flexion for both puppies and dogs was found to be around 0.80 mA (range, 0.50 to 1.25 mA). The yelp response in both young and adult dogs was evoked at approximately 2.80 mA (range, 2.0 to 3.0 mA). Brush (1957) found that the efficiency of avoidance learning increases with intensities up to 4.8 mA, with latencies to escape appearing to increase at intensity levels above 5.0 mA. The maximum electrical shock delivered to the feet without inducing tetany has been determined to be around 10.0 to 12.5 mA (Solomon and Wynne, 1953). These specifications are not of much relevance with respect to e-collars, however, since significantly more electrical amplitude is needed to reach the detection threshold in the case of narrow-diameter electrode devices than is required by the larger electrodes and grids used in the experimental setting. At 500 V, a sustained current of 6.0 to 8.0 mA passed through a narrow electrode, as used in e-collars, barely reaches detection thresholds; however, the same current applied through a 2-inch-diameter electrode produces extreme discomfort. Conversely, directing the lowest detectable current produced by an e-collar through a 2-inch electrode results in a highly aversive event.

Standardization and Safety Considerations

Although many advances in collar design and quality have been made over the past several years, there is a significant lack of product standardization. The quality of electronic training collars varies among manufacturers, but most provide the means to adjust the collar to deliver stimulation at low and medium levels, producing a tickling or tingling effect, as well as high level electrical stimulation (HLES) capable of producing significant pain and distress in most dogs. High-quality collars produce a smooth stimulus effect, whereas cheap and poorly designed devices tend to produce a rough and unpleasant sensation, even at low levels, making them inappropriate for cynopraxic training purposes. Unfortunately, many devices produce a high-end shock that *far* exceeds what is needed by the average dog and owner. Although an occasional dog may need the higher levels of stimulation, such devices should be made available only through special order. Alternatively, an electronic key or code might be inserted into the circuit of such devices that would keep the high-end off, at least until the user found a real need for it and requested the code from the manufacturer. Such owners could be given appropriate counseling and referrals to trainers for further advice and instruction on how and when to use HLES. The ability to switch from low, medium, and high scales would provide the user with a greater range of output levels to meet specific needs and reduce the risk of accidental painful shock.

The high-end output of certain contemporary devices suggests the need for an optional safety device to prevent ES from occurring above a certain level and to prevent activation by unauthorized users (e.g., children). Accidental stimulation at high levels can produce significant distress and emotional harm to a dog. There is also a need for a product that would enable trainers to shape the e-stimulus according to specific needs. Devices that would enable professional users to set pulse amplitude, durations, and frequency (waveforms) as well as to control the duration of momentary stimulation and pulse-burst patterns would be highly desirable in the context of behavior-therapy applications. An external electrode interface might be designed to capture and condition collar output in various ways to make it safer and more compatible with low-level electrical training procedures. Meanwhile, the effective electrical output of an e-collar can be easily stepped down by placing an appropriate voltage divider (resistor) or miniature potentiometer between the electrodes. The lower the resistance is, the more voltage is shunted away from the skin. By carefully selecting a resistor with the correct ohm value, the entire output range of the collar can be adjusted down to low levels of ES, converting the strongest e-collar into a "tickle collar." The resistor wires should be appropriately sealed with nonconducting paint or sheathing. (*Note:* Users should check with the manufacturer for specific instructions and safety guidelines pertinent to such product modifications.)

SUBJECTIVE FACTORS AND ELECTRICAL STIMULATION

Electricity is a basic force of nature and life itself, with electrical currents streaming along the double-helical strands of DNA (Boon and Barton, 2002) and mediating every sensory transmission and action of the body. Nerve cells communicate with one another through the exchange of minute electrical charges, thereby producing sensory feelings of pleasure and pain and all forms of neural activity and bodily movement from the most primitive reflex to complex thought processes and motor skills. Millions upon millions of electrical signals travel through the body unnoticed while serving critical biological and behavioral functions. Given the ubiquity of electricity, it seems odd that dogs and most other mammals have not evolved sensory receptors specifically dedicated to sensing electrical stimuli.

While a true RMS multimeter or an oscilloscope can give trainers useful technical information, the direct experience of the e-stimulus translates the quantitative specifications into a qualitative and subjective appreciation for the event. Knowing the electrical dynamics of the e-stimulus is helpful for many reasons, but nothing can replace the feel or subjective index of stimulus quality and magnitude—the most sensitive way to evaluate the e-stimulus is to feel it. The subjective experience of electricity arises from the activation of cutaneous mechanoceptors. When touch receptors are activated by noxious stimulation or injury, electrical impulses communicate to the brain that damage or a threat of physical injury has occurred. Although the e-stimulus used in dog training does not produce any physical damage to the skin or underlying tissue, its presentation produces an illusion of noxious stimulation by activating mechanoceptors transmitting tactile sensations along myelinated A-delta and A-beta fibers (Sang et al., 2003). At low-intensity levels, low-threshold myelinated A-delta fibers transmit tapping, tickling, tingling, twitching sensations, whereas, at medium levels, high-threshold A-beta fibers are triggered evoking sharp pricking and jabbing sensations. Higher levels of ES may activate high-threshold cutaneous and muscular C-fiber nociceptors and mechanoceptors associated with a burning sensation. The throbbing and burning aftersensations of painful trauma are transmitted by high-threshold unmyelinated C-fibers occurring as the result of physical injury. Although no actual injury occurs, the reflexive actions elicited by aversive ES and the instrumental behavior emitted by dogs at such times are similar in many respects to responses occurring when physical pain is actually experienced (e.g., inhibitory startle and escape).

The advantage of ES is that it can be presented in highly controlled (intensity, duration, and density) and timely doses, producing corresponding levels of behavioral arousal, ranging from increased alertness and searching activity to intense startle and frantic escape efforts. Essentially, ES appears to confuse local mechanoceptors and nociceptors, causing the organism to respond as though a significant contact threat was present requiring immediate attention and escape. The e-stimulus is a purely subjective and psychological event. Tortora (1982) nicely states the aversive illusion produced by LLES:

> Safe electrical stimulation utilizes your dog's senses and causes your dog to respond as if there is physical damage, when in reality no damage is occurring. There is no better way to cause safe, timely, controllable short-term discomfort. (11)

Radio-controlled electronic training techniques can be divided into three general categories, depending on the behavioral objective and level of stimulation:

Low-level ES (LLES): escape/avoidance (negative reinforcement) and safety training
Medium-level ES (MLES): inhibitory training (punishment and negative reinforcement)
High-level ES (HLES): rapid suppression and aversive counterconditioning.

At low levels, the e-stimulus is annoying and disruptive; at medium levels, it is startling and inhibitory; and, at high levels, it can evoke significant pain and emotional distress. Although collar-produced shock can produce acute pain, the painful event does not and cannot produce physical injury. Pain is the subjective experience associated with somatic irritations and traumatic injury (e.g., stinging, throbbing, aching, or burning sensations). The experience of electrical pain is highly variable and not dependent on the activation

of nociceptors specific to electricity; in fact, the mammalian somatosensory system appears to lack receptors specifically dedicated to electrical stimuli. Significant individual differences exist with respect to the dog's tolerance for electrical pain. In addition to the dog's temperament and relative threshold sensitivities to aversive stimulation, the subjective experience of pain is modulated by a number of variables, including stress, fear, frustration, and anger. Further, pain thresholds can be significantly elevated by the elicitation of incompatible emotional and motivational states associated with olfaction, food, sex, massage, affection, and the effect of person. On a neurophysiological level, the pain associated with strong ES is modulated to some extent by the secretion of opioid substances in the brainstem that interact with nociceptive signals (Johnson, 1998).

Although electronic training devices can produce significant pain and distress, the subjective effects of low to medium ES do not warrant the term *pain*, as defined by the International Association for the Study of Pain (IASP) (Merskey and Bogduk, 1994). The IASP defines pain as "An unpleasant sensory and emotional experience associated with actual or potential tissue damage, or described in terms of such damage" (210). The standard set by the IASP clearly makes a distinction between stimuli producing momentary discomfort, but which are physiologically harmless, and states of pain resulting from actions leading to or having the capacity to produce injury: "Experiences which resemble pain but are not unpleasant, e.g., pricking, should not be called pain" (IASP, 2003). These distinctions appear to exclude the low-level to medium-level e-stimuli that produce a pricking sensation from being referred to as pain. As such, pain is subjective and depends on the evocation of an emotional state evidencing significant discomfort and distress.

Further, the physiologically harmless ES produced by e-collars should not be lumped with ordinary household electrical shock because the former has no potential for injuring tissue whereas the latter can produce physical injury, including severe burns. As such, the e-stimulus is not a priori a painful event and can be applied to the skin without producing any pain whatsoever. The most interesting and useful applications of the e-collar involve stimulation levels at just above threshold levels—tickles, tingles, and twitches. Electrical stimulation producing pricking sensations is also used without generating significant pain or distress. In fact, the vast majority of training objectives using ES involve low and medium levels. HLES is reserved for aversive counterconditioning, often delivered in the form of extremely brief momentary pulses and used for such things as snake proofing and the suppression of predatory behavior.

Though dogs may find ES alarming at low levels and startling at medium-intensity levels, these stimulation levels are far less aversive or intrusive than many conventional corrections delivered by slip, prong, or halter collars. Even when ES is delivered at moderately high levels, the subjective sensation of momentary stimulation approximates the feeling of a standard-sized rubber band stretched 5 or 6 inches away from the skin and released sharply on the wrist. Repeated ES delivered to the human hand at various levels used for training purposes produces no redness and minimal lingering sensations of discomfort. Comparable stimulation with a rubber band results in significant irritation and redness, and aching persists. Traditional training collars and tools produce an aversive effect by various means, such as abruptly compressing or jabbing the neck (slip and prong collars), clamping around the muzzle and twisting the head and neck (halter collars), or sharply striking the dog's body (e.g., throw objects). All of these techniques are relatively safe and humane when used properly but could damage the throat or neck if misused or abused. Electronic stimulation, on the other hand, is distinguished by being relatively harmless with respect to producing physical damage to a dog's skin or body. Furthermore, since mechanical techniques work by forcefully stimulating mechanoceptors and nociceptors, such tools may cause local irritation or muscle strain. Unlike the aversive effect of ES, which rapidly dissipates after being discontinued, forceful stimulation of skin and muscle tissue

can result in a chain of biochemical events that may cause sustained throbbing, local irritation, or bruising.

Anyone who has ever witnessed a dog experiencing acute (real) pain knows that they yelp repeatedly and show other autonomic and behavioral signs of sustained and unmistakable agony. The response dogs typically show in response to low to medium ES cannot be construed as pain. Dunbar (2000), during a panel discussion on dog-training equipment at the Tuft's Expo, acknowledged the capacity of "electronic stimulation collars" to produce a harmless and effective stimulus for training dogs, suggesting that such devices offer unique alternative for humane punishment:

> When you see an electronic stimulation collar working, then we need a different word for it, it's a "tickling collar" is what it is. And, you know, go to the companies; ask them, "Do you have anything that tickles me?" Put it on your hand, zap it out; so, I guarantee that we will have dog-friendly e-collars and autoshaping devices that do loads. They will be distracting dogs in all sorts of ways: with wisps of smells, uh, sounds that we can't hear, and maybe little tickles on the skin, and what have you. Then I think that the dog training area will start to come together, because you now have a greater choice of the punishments that you can choose on. And now, there is literally no need ever, ever to shock a dog. There, there's no need for it. No one can convince me of that. Why? Because we have the alternative, it's high tech, yeah, but it doesn't hurt. (transcribed from audio recording)

Just as dropping a bowling ball on one's foot will certainly produce a significantly different effect than that produced by a falling tennis ball, ES produces variable subjective and physiological effects, depending on the intensity of the stimulation used. To speak about the behavioral and emotional effects of electricity in general and biased ways is counterproductive. The objective effects of ES range from below-threshold to tetanizing and life-threatening shock. When referring to ES, an effort should be made to specify the sort of ES being discussed. Several basic categories are hereby proposed to guide future discussions:

Below threshold of perception
Mild tingling and attention (stimulus recognition)
Annoyance or tickling stimulation
Prickly startle reaction
Discomfort, distress, and escape arousal
Extreme pain and distress

STRESS, DISTRESS, AND POTENTIAL ADVERSE SIDE EFFECTS OF ELECTRICAL STIMULATION

Biological Stress and Psychological Distress

Learning is always distressful to some extent, with anxiety and frustration representing important incentives motivating adjustment, just as biological adaptation and the maintenance of stability in change (*allostasis*) are vitally dependent on a dog's ability to generate a stress response. Although stress and distress are not the same thing, some authors appear to treat these phenomena as though they were the same (see Schilder and Van der Borg, 2004). Just as physical exercise produces biological stress while building muscle mass and endurance, short-term stress in the context of training is not necessarily without robust long-term benefits. Psychological distress (anxiety, frustration, and startle) per se is not necessarily an impediment to learning, nor does it necessarily represent a threat to a dog's welfare (i.e., a state conducive to and promoting an adaptive coping style in response to an environmental challenge or threats). Distress is first and foremost a healthy response to an environmental challenge requiring an unaccustomed adjustment. Stress and distress only become problematic when they occur under social or environmental circumstances that prevent a dog from coping (adjusting or adapting) effectively—conditions that may result in various behavioral and biological disturbances as indexed, for example, by allostatic load and overload (Wingfield, 2003).

Dogs exhibit considerable variation in their response to ES. In addition to the electrical characteristics of the e-stimulus event,

various behavioral and psychological influences exert significant modulatory effects on a dog's response to ES. Prominent among these influences are habituation, sensitization, and opponent processes (relief/relaxation). The genetic heterogeneity and variation, even among dogs of the same breed, confer upon them a highly variable capacity for coping with aversive stimulation. Vincent and Michell (1996) found, within a population of 227 trainee guide dogs, that 96 (42.3%) were stress prone, a propensity that correlated with a trend toward higher blood pressure and heart rate. Dogs exhibiting a heightened vulnerability to stress will likely respond to shock in a more reactive and stressful way than will dogs less prone to stress.

When coping with a threat or challenge, a dog may show variable signs of anxiety or frustration but become problematically distressed only if the situation proves uncontrollable, whereupon anxiety (the situation lacks predictability) may grow into fear or frustration (the situation lacks controllability) may escalate into anger or aggression. While mobilizing the flight-fight system (FSS), the sympathoadrenal-medullary system (SAM) helps to promote a state of arousal and bodily readiness to react to a situation perceived as dangerous and uncontrollable. A slower opponent regulatory system, the hypothalamic-pituitary-adrenal (HPA) axis, is brought into play by the action of corticotropin-releasing factor (CRF) on the pituitary, stimulating the release of adrenocorticotropic hormone (ACTH) into the bloodstream. ACTH acts on the adrenal cortex to stimulate the release of glucocorticoid hormones (e.g., cortisol), which perform a number of adaptive biological functions within the body and brain. As cortisol enters the brain, it counteracts the reactive emergency state of arousal and begins to restore balance by exerting a general calming effect, including a negative-feedback control over the release of CRF that in turn inhibits the release of ACTH, which in turn decreases the secretion of cortisol, as things are gradually normalized. With respect to the use of aversives in dog training, the dog appears to have evolved antistress and antinociceptive capabilities that enable it to cope with such demands, perhaps mediated by a specialized oxytocinergic-opioid network (Panksepp et al., 1997; Uvnäs-Moberg, 1998) that enables it to cope (flirt and forbear) with significant psychological distress without prompting the activation of the SAM and HPA systems, provided that the distressing event is perceived by the dog as controllable. Dess and colleagues (1983) performed a series of experiments to evaluate the effects of event predictability and controllability versus event unpredictability and uncontrollability on plasma cortisol levels in dogs exposed to shock (7 mA for up to 15 seconds and 5 mA for up to 5 seconds). The dogs were divided into several groups, some of which could escape the stimulation, whereas others received shock regardless of what they did to escape from it. The researchers found that dogs that could control the occurrence of shock by escape exhibited a significantly attenuated cortisol response than did dogs having no control over the shock stimulus.

Among dogs, controllable aversive events may generate signs of temporary distress and precursor submission behaviors, but it is highly unlikely that such events rise to the sort of biological challenge or threat that might pose a significant threat to a dog's welfare or quality of life. Submissive precursor behaviors mediated by the corticobulbar social engagement system (Porges, 2001) are frequently mistaken for fear and evidence of stress. By carefully drawing lines between biological stress, quantified by changes in the release of adrenal steroids, and psychological distress, as indicated by autonomic changes (e.g., heart rate and HRV), one might avoid some of the confusion. Having a set of behavioral markers that might be used to assess biological stress would also be convenient, but until such behavioral markers have been properly validated, the use of ambiguous behavioral signs and ambivalent behaviors to index stress is fraught with the risk of subjectivism (see *Electronic Training and Working Dogs: A Shocking Study*). Beerda and colleagues (2000) have warned that ambiguous "stress behaviors" (e.g., subtle postural changes, oral displacement activities, paw lifting, yawning,

and so forth) may lead to false interpretations, unless the behaviors can be closely tied to physiological markers of stress (e.g., cortisol). Salivary samples can be obtained within 30 seconds or so (Kobelt et al., 2003), making such minimally intrusive sampling convenient for verifying the presence of stress. Without physiological markers, the attribution of stress to ambiguous behaviors is unwarranted and interpreting them as indicators of stress lacks scientific support. Changes in cortisol appear to be useful for detecting long-term adverse effects associated with shock in training (Stichnoth, 2002) and may be revealing even in the absence of overt behavioral signs of stress (Vincent and Michell, 1992).

Stress, Traumatic Avoidance, and Laboratory Conditioning with Shock

Evidence for individual differences affecting the way dogs cope with the most severe and debilitating electrical shock has been reported by several researchers. Perhaps the most extreme of these studies was performed by Houser and Paré (1974), who subjected two dogs to a daily regimen of electrical conditioning for 6 months. The dogs were restrained in a Pavlovian hammock, with electrodes delivering a 0.5-second 4.0-mA shock every 20 seconds to a hind leg. Each daily session lasted 3 hours. The dog could avoid the shock and postpone it for 20 seconds, provided it performed at least one key-pressing response during the 20-second period. During the last 2 months of the study, a classical conditioning contingency was superimposed on the Sidman avoidance schedule just described, thereby significantly increasing stress. Every day for 2 months the dogs received seven unavoidable 8-mA shocks lasting 0.5 seconds that were preceded by a 3-minute conditioned stimulus (light). Bear in mind that the dogs had to keep track of the temporal avoidance contingency simultaneously while bracing for the repeated presentation of unavoidable shock. Aside from demonstrating that human ingenuity for cruelty knows no bounds, the study showed that dogs possess a profound adaptive capacity for coping with the most assaultive and stressful circumstances. A dog's capacity to endure such laboratory conditioning is strongly dependent on individual differences, and the two dogs showed very different patterns of heart rate and cortisol release during the *300* hours of data collection.

Among psychological influences, the amount of control that a dog has over the aversive event directly affects the amount of fear and stress that it will likely experience when exposed to ES. For example, inescapable painful or traumatic shock may produce temporary and perhaps permanent debilitating effects on a dog's ability to cope competently with aversive situations, as well as stimulate a variety of stress-related physiological changes. However, generalizing to the notion that ES is debilitating per se is not justified by the relevant scientific literature. Under laboratory conditioning, dogs have demonstrated extraordinary capacities for coping with severe shock and other forms of traumatizing treatment (Solomon and Wynne, 1953; Kamin, 1954). A worker in Pavlov's laboratory trained a dog to salivate and to show negligible signs of defensive behavior or cardiovascular distress by pairing increasing levels of shock with food, gradually reaching levels of intensity sufficient to burn the skin, emphasizing the extraordinary adaptability that dogs exhibit with respect to electrical shock arranged to predict appetitive gratification:

> The conditioned food reflex was elaborated not from an indifferent agent but from a destructive one evoking an inborn defensive reflex. The skin was irritated by an electric current and at the same time the dog was fed, although at first the feeding had to be forced. A weak current was applied which was later increased to the maximum. The experiment ended thus: with the strongest current, as well as with burning and mechanical destruction of the skin, there could be provoked only the food reaction (the corresponding motor reaction and the salivary secretion) and there was no trace of any interference by the defensive reaction, there were no changes in breathing or heart beat, characteristic of this last reaction. (Pavlov, 1928:341)

The critical issue at stake appears to be the degree of perceived control that the dog has

over the aversive event. In the case of classical conditioning where food is associated with shock, the dog may perceive the shock as a controllable event contingent upon it waiting for some brief period after which the shock ends (safety) and food appears (comfort). The loss of control over aversive stimulation appears to increase the risk of inducing problematic cognitive, emotional, and behavioral effects. Littman and colleagues (1964) exposed rats of different ages to five sessions (each at 1 mA for 3 minutes) of continuous inescapable shock and found that shock thresholds and latencies for escape were significantly increased when traumatized rats were tested 1 day later. The adverse effects of uncontrollable trauma were still evident after 2 months.

When Seligman and Maier (1967) exposed dogs to escapable and inescapable shock to test various hypotheses regarding the effects of event controllability and uncontrollability on avoidance learning, they found that adverse cognitive and emotional interference effects and learned helplessness were primarily exhibited by dogs that lacked control over shock, whereas dogs with control over shock were less disturbed by the experience. A yoked design resulted in both groups of dogs receiving identical stimulation, except that the dogs under the escapable shock condition could terminate shock by pressing a panel located next to the head, whereas the dogs in the inescapable group had no control over the shock event. The dogs were restrained in a Pavlovian hammock with holes cut out for their legs, which were immobilized by cords lashed above the feet and tied to the floor. The only difference between the two groups was that dogs in the escapable group could terminate shock by pushing a panel located next to the head. The inescapable group received 64 shocks (6.0 mA), at 5 seconds each, delivered to the pads of their hind feet. During subsequent escape testing, both groups were exposed to 10 trials in which a 10-second conditioned stimulus was presented (a dimmed light), followed by 50 seconds of "severe pulsating shock" (1969:322). The intertrial interval varied from 60 to 120 seconds.

Approximately two-thirds of the dogs (N = 82) previously exposed to inescapable shock showed evidence of impairment in their ability to initiate escape behavior. Dogs that failed to jump over the barrier could be taught to overcome the interference effects of inescapable shock by being repeatedly pulled over the barrier by leash, gradually learning (some requiring 50 trials) to hop over it with the slightest tug and finally do so on their own (Seligman et al., 1968). If the dogs were allowed to rest for 48 hours prior to escape testing, these dramatic interference effects were not observed despite repeated exposure to inescapable shock (Overmier and Seligman, 1967). However, if the inescapable exposure was repeated, more durable interference effects were observed. Seligman and Groves (1970) showed that dogs with a variegated history of prior exposure to aversive stimulation had a greater resistance to the adverse effects of inescapable shock, requiring four blocks of 64 trials in which 5-second shocks were given on each trial for a total of 1280 seconds of exposure to shock in order to establish learned-helplessness effects. In contrast, cage-reared dogs showed a greater susceptibility to escape impairments, requiring two blocks of 64 trials in order to show enduring learned-helplessness effects—lasting at least a week. Caged dogs may receive insufficient opportunities to acquire coping skills, making them more vulnerable to the adverse effects of uncontrollable aversive stimulation. Lessac and Solomon (1969) found that severe isolation lasting for 1 year resulted in escape/avoidance behavior resembling learned helplessness—deficits that were prevented by electrical escape/avoidance training at week 12.

Electrical Stimulation Controllability and Safety

A large body of scientific evidence supports the notion that opponent poststimulation relief and relaxation is an important motivational aspect of escape/avoidance learning. The immediate effect of ES termination is emotional relief, which is subsequently followed by opponent-relaxation effects that develop more sluggishly and automatically over the next 2 to 3 minutes (Denny, 1991). As a result, the cessation of a controllable e-stimulus or its avoidance appears to promote hedonic emotional changes conducive to reward and safety (Denny, 1971). Further, conditioned stimuli associated with shock (S1) or the absence of shock (S2) have been shown to promote differential behavioral changes consistent with the safety hypothesis (Rescorla and LoLordo, 1965) (see *Safety Signal Hypothesis* in Volume 1, Chapter 8). While performing a Sidman avoidance task, dogs increased avoidance responding while in the presence of the excitatory S1, whereas they decreased avoidance responding when the inhibitory S2 was presented. Using a paradigm of classical conditioning similar to that employed by Rescorla and LoLordo, Billman and Randall (1980) confirmed that discriminated excitatory (paired with shock, S1) and inhibitory (not paired with shock, S2) conditioned stimuli also exert a differential effect on cardiovascular activity consistent with preparatory aversive arousal/threat and relaxation/safety effects, respectively. The signaled cessation of shock and partial reinforcement in dogs has also been shown to produce conditioned changes in heart rate consistent with the safety hypothesis (Fitzgerald, 1966; Royer, 1969). Finally, basic learning research with rodents (Galizio, 1999) appears to support the notion that stimuli predicting safety from shock (S2) acquire persistent reward properties that continue after extinction of the avoidance response has occurred. Poststimulation relief and relaxation has been successfully used to treat avoidance-motivated aggression in dogs (Tortora, 1983) and other refractory canine behavior problems (e.g., aggression toward strangers and other dogs) (Schwizgebel, 1992). In combination, the foregoing laboratory work supports the notion that safety in association with the successful escape/avoidance of aversive stimulation may augment the value of social rewards (e.g., petting and praise) used by the trainer to support cooperation and obedience to command. Properly performed electronic training promotes a confidence-building pattern of escape to safety that can be highly beneficial and useful in the context of canine behavior therapy

(see *Escape to Safety versus Escape from Danger* in Chapter 8)

ELECTRICAL STIMULATION TECHNOLOGY

Electrical stimulation has been used in various ways to influence motivation and behavior. In medicine, ES is used to aid in the control of heart problems, ranging from defibrillators resuscitating a lost heartbeat to pacemakers helping to maintain the heart's rhythm. Intracranial electrodes implanted in various parts of the dog's brain have been used to monitor and modify brain electrical activity and behavior (Himwich et al., 1965; Wagner et al., 1967). Vagal nerve stimulators have been successfully implanted and used to control seizure activity in dogs not responsive to anticonvulsant medication (Munana et al., 2002). Theoretically, certain intractable aggression problems or compulsive disorders associated with sympathovagal dysregulation or temporal seizure activity might benefit from vagal nerve stimulation (VNS), but to my knowledge such devices have not been evaluated for the control of serious canine behavior problems.

The use of ES on the skin has several applications in medicine. ES has been successfully used in acupuncture, as well as other applications for the control of pain, such as transcutaneous electrical nerve stimulation (TENS). Medical stimulators have also been developed to improve muscle tone via high-voltage constant-current stimulation. Several groups of bioelectrical engineers have been working for many years on sensory-substitution applications using electrocutaneous stimulation (ECS) and vibrocutaneous stimulation. These devices are aimed at assisting blind or deaf users or those needing to use prostheses (Kaczmarek et al., 1991). The modern e-collar has benefited significantly from these research and development advances in ECS technology. Perhaps the most common and controversial scientific use of ES has been in the contexts of the learning laboratory (Solomon and Wynne, 1953), aversion therapy (McGuire and Vallance, 1964), and behavior-modification programs

(Lovaas et al., 1965; Lovaas and Simmons, 1969). Researchers investigating fear and pain have also made considerable use of ECS (Tursky, 1973). In combination, many hundreds of studies have been dedicated to the sensory, autonomic, emotional, and behavioral effects of ES for motivating and controlling behavior (Campbell and Masterson, 1969), making ES the most carefully and exhaustively studied aversive stimulus available for use by dog trainers. An early radio-controlled device designed for laboratory conditioning with dogs used a harness-and-collar arrangement. The collar produced a 30-mA current (1000-V peak amplitude output) delivered through electrodes positioned on the dorsal surface of the dog's neck (Caldwell and Judy, 1970). One of the earliest radio-controlled devices explicitly designed for dog-training purposes appeared in the 1950s (Cameron and Hopkins, 1955). The radio-controlled receiver delivered a high-voltage, low-amperage current of electrical charge to the shoulders of the dog via electrodes fastened to a harness. The device produced one level of stimulation and was designed primarily to punish undesirable behavior.

Numerous electronic training aids have been developed in recent years incorporating a mild electrical or spray stimulus (e.g., aerosol citronella) to modify dog behavior. These devices can be divided into two general categories, depending on whether they are activated by a trainer controlling a radio transmitter or directly activated by the dog's behavior. Radio-controlled electronic devices are used to deliver various signals (e.g., tones, clicks, or vibrations) and aversive stimulation via a receiver attached to the dog's collar. Activation of the collar is controlled by a hand-held transmitter that provides the trainer with precise control over the presentation of both conditioned and unconditioned aversive stimuli at a distance. In addition, some collar systems include a reward tone or click that can be paired with successful escape/avoidance or the presentation of appetitive-positive or social-positive reinforcement (e.g., food or petting). Most current products permit the user to adjust the level of stimulation from a nearly imperceptible level or annoying tingle or tickle to a strongly aversive prickly twitching sensation.

Behavior-activated electronic training collars are most commonly used in applications involving outdoor containment and the control of excessive barking. Unlike radio-controlled electronic training aids, behavior-activated collars are not dependent on the presence of a human operator. In the case of containment systems, both conditioned (warning tone) and unconditioned (electrical or spray) stimulation are delivered automatically as the dog approaches an underground wire that encircles the property. The wire boundary forms a closed loop with a circuit box that transmits a radio signal to the receiver collar worn by the dog. Whenever the dog approaches within a certain distance (approximately 2 to 10 feet) of the boundary line (warning-signal field), a tone stimulus is activated that is immediately discontinued if the dog backs away; however, if the dog encroaches further into the warning field, an aversive electrical or spray stimulus is delivered. In the case of bark-activated e-collars, a microphone or a vibration sensor that makes contact with the dog's neck closes a circuit causing the collar to deliver a brief e-stimulus. Another device that has become popular with some trainers and behaviorists in recent years uses aerosol citronella sprayed from a collar. When activated by barking, the solenoid valve releases an aerosol spray directed up toward the dog's head. Unfortunately, the velocity of spray flow and the intensity of the odorant delivered cannot be adjusted to meet specific training needs. The device does, however, allow the user to deliver a short or long spray stimulus.

Many other electronic devices are in use to control dog behavior. These gadgets include electronic systems designed to protect specific areas of the house against intrusion or destructiveness. One device, used to protect furniture and other surfaces in the home, delivers static shock via an electrified mat. Other devices depend on the generation of loud audible and ultrasonic sounds to deter various actions. Some devices emit a loud high-pitched tone that is activated by motion, body heat, or vibration. After a variable period (ranging from 2 to 20 seconds), the sound stimulus shuts off and resets. Although loud auditory stimulation appears to work well on certain problems, ultrasonic devices do not appear to be as efficacious (Blackshaw et al., 1990). In comparison to electrotactile stimulation, loud sounds appear to be significantly less aversive (Campbell and Bloom, 1965).

Radio-controlled Electrical Stimulation

Over the past decade or so, electronic training has become increasingly popular among dog trainers for establishing increased control and reliability when a dog is off leash and for treating a variety of behavior problems. The wide acceptance of electronic tools by the dog-training community has been in part the result of significant design improvements in the size, adjustability, reliability, and safety of e-collars. Electronic devices are also becoming increasingly affordable. The e-collar's ability to deliver a consistent and precise ES at a distance makes the device extremely attractive and useful. Recently, relatively inexpensive collars have come to the market that are small, lightweight, and loaded with sophisticated features, including the ability to increase or decrease the level of stimulation from the transmitter instantly and in real time by turning a dial. This feature enables a trainer to accurately match the stimulation level to an individual dog's sensitivity and temperament. These electronic training collars deliver a relatively consistent and measured level of aversive stimulation, ranging from a tickle, tingle, twitch, or prickly twinge to a highly aversive electrical event that produces significant discomfort and startle but without risk of producing physical injury or pain. These devices also feature the ability to deliver a continuous stimulus lasting as long as the button is held down or until the receiver unit automatically shuts off and resets after approximately 8 to 12 seconds. Alternatively, a stimulus lasting a fraction of a second can be selected for the delivery of precise stimulation and prompting effects similar to that produced by leash checks. These various operational features satisfy the technical requirements for effective punishment and negative reinforcement, and give the trainer fingertip control over the timing, intensity, and duration of aversive stimulation. In addition to the delivery of a controlled e-stimulus, various tone and vibratory stimuli can be delivered in close pre-event and postevent association with ES, so that conditioned positive and negative reinforcers, punishers, and other signals (e.g., safety signals) can be developed and used to facilitate electronic training objectives. In combination, these various features help to minimize the amount of aversive ES needed to reach training objectives while maximizing a trainer's creative control over the delivery, intensity, and duration of aversive stimulation.

The effective use of ES requires significant skill and understanding of the training process. Ideally, such devices should be used only in the context of supervised training and behavior modification. Once a foundation of reward-based training is in place incorporating positive reinforcement, structured play, and various conventional directive efforts, remote electronic enhancement can be employed to achieve improved control at a distance (Tortora, 1982). Electronic training is also used to establish basic control that is not otherwise efficiently obtained by reward-based techniques alone. Once the training objectives are achieved via electronic procedures, positive reinforcement is used to maintain and generalize the behavior. Combining escape/avoidance training with positive reinforcement appears to optimize conditioning effects. For example, Franchina (1969) found that trained behavior is enhanced by exposing animals to a contingency in which target responses are followed by both shock offset and the presentation of a food reward. In the case of animals where the food reward was omitted but the shock-escape contingency held constant, the performance of animals declined below levels attained by the use of negative reinforcement alone. These findings stress the importance of combining both positive- reinforcement and negative-reinforcement procedures to optimize performance reliability. Despite a significant potential for misuse and abuse, electronic training tools provide significant advantages for skilled users (Table 9.1).

Electronic training is efficacious and warranted in situations where enhanced remote control of a dog is needed or when problem-solving objectives demand accurate, timely,

TABLE 9.1. Advantages of electronic devices for delivering aversive stimulation (ES, electrical stimulation)

ES is the most thoroughly studied aversive used in animal behavior and learning research.

ES at the levels used in dog training is virtually harmless, giving no evidence of lasting pain, tissue damage, or psychological trauma.

ES has many aversive control applications, ranging from escape/avoidance training (negative reinforcement) and suppression (positive punishment) to aversive counterconditioning.

ES intensity can be adjusted from very low and barely perceptible stimulation up to startling and highly aversive levels, thereby accurately matching a dog's specific needs and temperament.

ES duration can be precisely regulated, ranging from a fraction of a second to several seconds long.

ES can be delivered instantaneously at various distances from a dog.

ES can be delivered without the owner being present or being directly associated with the owner as its cause.

ES training appears to depend more on startle and annoyance than pain.

ES training techniques are highly compatible with instrumental training procedures (e.g., clicker training), enhancing performance, reliability, and assisting in problem-solving activities.

ES training techniques facilitate safe and reliable off-leash control and recall training.

ES training aids are relatively easy to use.

and remote aversive stimulation. Although radio-controlled e-collars are inappropriate for use as the initial or primary means for establishing basic obedience control, no comparable techniques or tools currently available can match the efficacy and safety of the e-collar for establishing safe and reliable off-leash control. In any case, humane electronic training procedures employ a minimal level of aversive stimulation to achieve behavioral objectives. Most dogs are highly responsive to ES set at levels that are barely perceptible to human touch. For the vast majority of training objectives, stimulation never exceeds a painless tingling or occasional twitching or pricking level. When properly used, electronic stimulation produces rapid and steady avoidance learning or, when applied at higher levels of stimulation as a punitive stimulus, suppression is often immediate and lasting. If minimizing the intensity, duration, and frequency of aversive stimulation during training is recognized as a significant factor in the definition of humane dog training, the radio-controlled e-collar must then be ranked as one of the most humane dog-training tools currently available.

Although most obedience-training objectives can be adequately achieved using a combination of reward-based methods and directive techniques, such approaches may not be sufficient to achieve effective control over high-spirited dogs under circumstances of increased motivation or distraction. Maintaining control under such circumstances may be especially problematic with adult dogs that have learned to evade the owner or run out of control when let off leash outdoors. Further, some dog owners may simply lack the physical strength and coordination to effectively use a leash and collar, long line, or throw tools. For example, elderly dog owners may be challenged beyond their means when faced with the behavioral excesses of an overly active dog. For such owners, leash and collar or halter restraint may not provide adequate means of control. Furthermore, despite the most conscientious reward-based training efforts, such training may not adequately curb canine appetites and excesses to a point of ensuring safe interaction with a fragile or physically disabled handler. Under such cir-

cumstances, electronic training aids may prove extremely useful and beneficial. Properly introduced, surprisingly low levels of ES can cause otherwise inattentive and uncooperative dogs to learn rapidly to comply with owner demands and directives that previously went unheeded. Basic control elements such as sit, down, stay, and come can be quickly enhanced and made more reliable by brief exposure to escape/avoidance training involving LLES. A combined approach incorporating both positive and negative reinforcement optimizes training efforts (see *Behavioral Equilibrium*). Optimization results in a rapid increase in performance reliability and fluency over a wide range of motivational and environmental conditions.

First and foremost, electronic training provides efficient means to enhance attention and impulse control under adverse environmental and motivational conditions requiring close timing of aversive stimulation, especially when a dog is off leash. The e-collar can be effectively used to induce a dog to perform more reliably under challenging situations in which it is most likely to hesitate, refuse, or disobey by engaging in behavior incompatible with training objectives. Obviously, securing a dog's attention provides a powerful means for initiating impulse-control training. In combination with attention training, training efforts that focus on relevant intentional movements that anticipate the loss of impulse control help to facilitate more reliable behavioral control. Establishing control over orienting behavior and intentional movements requires a high degree of precision. If a dog is kept in close proximity on leash or otherwise restricted, various nonaversive tools and techniques may suffice; however, with the dog at some distance away, operating under the influence of natural environments and contingencies of reinforcement, nothing provides the required control and fine-tuning more efficaciously than an e-collar. Most dogs can be trained effectively without electronic enhancement, but in cases in which dogs exhibit dangerous behavior that risks injury to itself or others, intervention with electronic training is definitely a viable and humane alternative to traditional punishment techniques.

As is discussed in the section *Electrical Stimulation and Aggression*, electronic training and enhancement of basic-training modules and routines may play a valuable therapeutic role in counteracting established patterns of inappropriate and reactive behavior occurring under aversive or threatening situations. Highly structured and systematic training using ES may help to enhance a dog's social competence and confidence by teaching it that it can control (avoid or escape) aversive events by means of cooperative behavior, thereby potentially reducing the likelihood of maladaptive aggression or panic responses when confronted with adversity. Of course, using electrical training techniques to control potentially aggressive dogs requires that trainers possess significant knowledge and experience with such dogs and a working understanding of the benefits and hazards of electrical training. Inappropriately painful or poorly timed stimulation may make such problems worse or elicit an aggressive response (Polsky, 2000). Radio-controlled ES has the advantage of minimizing the need for direct manual control of an aggressive dog—a valuable asset in the case of dogs prone to attack when touched or handled.

BEHAVIOR-ACTIVATED ELECTRONIC TRAINING

Citronella-spray Collars

Bark-activated citronella collars appear to be effective for controlling certain barking problems (Wells, 2001) but are not necessarily less aversive to dogs than are electronic counterparts. One study comparing the punitive effects of a citronella collar with an electrical device reported that the citronella treatment was more effective than shock in suppressing nuisance barking in dogs (Juarbe-Diaz and Houpt, 1996). The authors found that 89% of the owners using the citronella collar to control excessive barking reported satisfactory results, whereas 44% of owners using an e-collar reported satisfactory results. Unfortunately, the study was limited to nine dogs, and the authors may have been biased with respect to citronella devices (Wells, 2001)—a bias that one of the authors appears to

acknowledge in another context (Juarbe-Diaz, 1997). Given the acuity of a dog's olfactory sensibilities, it is not surprising that a potent aerosol odorant sprayed near a dog's nose and mouth would be aversive. What is surprising, however, is that the citronella device outperformed the electronic one—a finding that one should view with some skepticism, at least until a larger controlled study is performed and the findings confirmed. Although the citronella odor may be annoying to dogs, bark-activated spray devices appear to depend primarily on the effects of startle, with the odor of dilute citronella playing a secondary role. Citronella scent delivered without spray does not appear to suppress barking, but the scent may become an inhibitory stimulus as the result of aversive conditioning.

Recent studies seem to indicate that the citronella scent may not play a significant role in the inhibition of barking. Beaudet (2001) found that both scented and unscented spray collars worked about equally well to suppress barking, with 85% of owners reporting satisfaction with the citronella-scented stimulus versus 80% satisfaction with the unscented stimulus (N = 33). Similarly, Moffat and Landsberg (2001) have shown that unscented spray collars can produce a significant reduction in barking, comparable to that produced by citronella-scented collars (78% improved or controlled with citronella collars versus 57% improved or controlled with unscented collars; N = 36). The hiss produced by spray collars may be preferentially processed by the amygdala, eliciting unconditioned fear and startle. In addition, the amygdala is a primary destination of olfactory inputs, preparing and enabling a conditioned aversive association between a novel odor and startle to develop rapidly.

Bark-activated citronella collars produce approximately 15 to 25 gradually diminishing spray bursts until the spray reservoir is depleted—an operational limitation that habitual barkers may learn to exploit. Given the tendency of dogs to habituate to odors and noises, it is reasonable to assume that repeated bursts of citronella spray may progressively produce less of an effect on dogs. The effect of habituation may be significantly more troublesome in situations where a dog is left alone and exposed to a high level of bark-evoking stimulation. Along these lines, Wells (2001) has reported that a significant amount of habituation does occur in response to repeated spray stimulation. Her study indicates that, after producing a pronounced initial reduction in barking, dogs gradually habituated to the spray event—an effect that continued during the 3-week treatment program. Interestingly, she found that intermittent treatment (dogs wearing the collar every other day) produced a more lasting suppressive effect over nuisance barking than did the continuous treatment program. Both the continuous and intermittent treatment groups were exposed to bark-provoking stimulation for 30 minutes a day. In addition to a rapidly depleted spray reservoir, a problematic feature of citronella devices is microphone activation. Ambient noises, including the barking of nearby dogs, may activate the devise, thus exposing the dog to inappropriate and non-contingent punishment—apparently a fairly common complaint (Juarbe-Diaz and Houpt, 1996). Also, under outdoor conditions, the spray may be affected by wind and other influences, perhaps making it less effective for such use. Finally, citronella spray as an olfactory deterrent may be inappropriate for dogs used for tracking, search and rescue, or other activities requiring sharp olfactory abilities, since repeated exposure may potentially blunt olfactory acuity. A major advantage of the citronella-type collar is that it does not depend on prong-to-skin contact to deliver stimulation, thereby avoiding unnecessary irritation and discomfort to dogs with sensitive skin.

Electrical Bark Collars

The sustained noise generated by multiple dogs barking in kennel situations commonly exceeds 100 decibels (dB) and often reaches levels as high 125 dB—a range that can damage both human and canine hearing (Sales et al., 1997). The noise associated with excessive barking can hurt ears, and it can harm neighbor relations and lead to legal consequences involving citations, fines, and eviction notices. These pressures can cause a dog owner to take extreme measures, such as relinquishing the dog, resorting to severe punishment, or employing inappropriate restraint procedures. Most dogs can rapidly learn to inhibit excessive barking after the contingent delivery of a brief e-stimulus presented in close association with the barking action each time that a dogs barks (Arguello, 1986). Bark-activated collars can be adjusted to match a dog's temperament and specific behavioral needs. Some devices provide a brief obligatory intertrial interval, during which barking or yelping does not activate the collar. One device also keeps count of the stimulations delivered, providing a useful source of data. A voice-activated recorder can also be used to keep track of barking activity. Unfortunately, not all bark-activated collars perform reliably, and only the highest-quality collars should be selected for use in the context of behavior therapy. Although some collars are designed to be relatively insensitive to nearby loud noises (e.g., other dogs barking) and impact vibrations, certain cheap collars sold in pet stores are activated by being bumped or when scraped when the dog lies down or moves about. This defect can be especially problematic and harmful with dogs confined to crates. Some of these problems can be prevented by encasing the collar in a thin protective foam sheath or by covering it with a bandana worn by the dog. Proper control of excessive barking depends on an accurate and detailed evaluation of underlying causes. In addition to performing behavioral assessment, the trainer should explore minimally aversive behavior-control techniques and reward-based strategies before opting to use bark-activated ES (see *Barking* in Chapter 5). The introduction of a bark collar should not be decided casually and never without giving serious thought to potential side effects that might result from bark-activated ES. Certain behavior problems that present with excessive barking, such as separation distress and panic (see *Electrical Stimulation and Excessive Barking*), may be exacerbated by aversive electrical procedures.

Ideally, whenever behavior-activated electronic devices are used in the context of behavior therapy, preliminary radio-controlled training incorporating LLES should be performed with the goal of training the dog to *perceive* that it has control over the occurrence of the ES. Preliminary training should begin with the enhancement and refinement of various basic modules and routines, especially attention and orienting responses, sit, stay, back and wait, slack-leash walking, and recall training. In addition, barking behavior should be brought under stimulus control, whereby the dog learns to bark on command and to stop barking on command. Stimulus control is established via reward-based discrimination learning. Training a dog to bark on command appears to increase its ability to autoregulate bark-related arousal and impulses without becoming overly inhibited. Once basic stimulus control over the bark response is established, a vibratory stimulus is used in conjunction with a stop-bark command, followed by LLES alone or LLES embedded in a brief continuous vibratory stimulus overlapping undesirable or off-cue barking behavior. As the barking activity ceases, the stimulation should also immediately stop, followed by social and appetitive rewards. On every occasion in which the dog barks inappropriately, the e-stimulus is delivered along a staggered intensity gradient until a level is reached that instantly suppresses the bark response and results in sustained bark avoidance, thereby approximating the level of stimulation needed by the bark-activated collar to maintain the bark inhibition. The goal is to establish a level of ES sufficient to inhibit barking but without causing the dog undue discomfort or distress. Before transitioning to a bark-activated collar, transfer training and tests are performed with the dog left in various bark-stimulating situations while wearing a radio-controlled collar. Many potential problems are avoided by slowly introducing ES via radio-controlled training before advancing to the bark-activated stimulator.

Electronic Containment Systems

The most common use of behavior-activated electronic devices involves ES to train dogs to stay within the confines of a property boundary. The exact number of electronic boundary systems in current use is not known, but one large company alone has reported installing some 500,000 units from 1982 to 1997 (Polsky, 2000). Some electronic boundary systems use a relatively strong e-stimulus that may cause some dogs to experience significant pain, fear, and distress. Dogs inappropriately exposed to boundary ES may show intense fear and avoidance of the yard, especially when a young dog has been denied access to the yard for play and training prior to the event. Prior safe exposure to the yard appears to promote latent inhibition and conditioned associations incompatible with fear (comfort and safety). The first experience of some dogs to being walked on leash by a stranger is one in which they are pulled into the boundary field and forced to experience intense ES by a containment-system salesperson or installer. As a result of such exposure, such dogs may show strong generalized anxiety or reactive behavior whenever they are put on leash, along with a lasting wariness or autoprotective behavior toward strangers encountered near the boundary, especially those that might reach for or attempt to restrain the dog. In cases where stimulation occurs while the dog is in the presence of two persons, one familiar and one unfamiliar, the event shows an associative affinity for the unfamiliar person, even though the dog might actually be in a slightly closer proximity to the more familiar person at the moment of stimulation. The resulting social fear response toward the unfamiliar person may be highly durable and resistant to extinction and counterconditioning efforts. Adventitious ES occurring in association with safe activities, such as play or tagging along with children, can exert a profound loss of trust and security that may compromise a dog's ability to feel safe or to relax when engaged in those activities. Dogs exhibiting problematic temperament traits (e.g., excessive fearfulness or aggressiveness) should not (or only cautiously) be contained electronically, because in some dogs ES may elicit global panic reactions or an increased risk of directing aggressive behavior toward persons or animals entering the property. However, even dogs without an established history of aggressive behavior or fearfulness, *may*, under certain circumstances, become aggressively aroused when electrically stimulated (Polsky, 1998 and 2000). Obviously, particular caution should be used when employing such devices indoors, where there exists an increased likelihood of stimulation in close proximity to people. To reduce the stress associated with electronic containment, the fenced area should be large enough to allow the dog to move about freely without fear of triggering ES.

Preliminary enhancement of basic modules and routines with a radio-controlled collar is useful and avoids many of the present pitfalls associated with boundary training. Such training instills positive prediction-control expectancies and establishing operations conducive to a competent escape-to-safety pattern of proactive adjustment to ES. After a basic introduction to attention, stay, back and wait, halt-stay, and recall training, boundary training is introduced using these basic modules, as needed. Eventually, the boundary collar can be fastened in combination with the radio-controlled collar in order to establish appropriate conditioned escape/avoidance responses, beginning with LLES and then gradually introducing additional distractions and increasing intensity as required to maintain and enhance the avoidance response. The idea is to train the dog to perceive the LLES as a controllable event (e-stimulus) or cue (e-signal) predictive of safety, provided that it turn or back away in response to the warning signal. Initially, the dog is kept on a long line so that any hesitation or contrary response can be immediately countered with appropriate prompting or redirection. As training progresses, failure to turn or back or turn away is followed by an appropriately intense event to establish reliable deterrence. Throughout the process, the trainer should provide constructive support and offer the dog a haven of safety and play as it learns to respond to boundary warning tone as an avoidance signal. In addition to learning that the boundary ES is controllable, the dog must be given sufficient exposure to play and rewarding activities in the yard to make it a viable escape-to-safety destination. In addition to learning the boundary rule, various important secondary inhibitory lessons (e.g., all-stop, stop-change,

and go/no go) and enhanced impulse control can be acquired in the context of boundary training, thereby further maximizing the potential add-on benefits that might be obtained through the process.

Puppies at 16 to 20 weeks that are destined to undergo inhibitory boundary conditioning probably stand to benefit most from the gradual introduction of controllable ES via preliminary radio-controlled training using LLES. During preliminary training, the trainer can get an accurate idea of the amount of ES needed to establish reliable behavior-activated boundary control. In addition to the benefits of a radio-controlled introductory phase, emotional distress associated with boundary training can be reduced significantly by incrementally introducing the deterrent level of ES through steps of appropriate exposure and training. If the containment system lacks sufficient adjustability to match the output level of the e-collar to the particular needs of the dog, a set of insulated resistors or an adjustable potentiometer might be used as a voltage divider to achieve the desired adjustability. Any modifications of this nature to an e-collar device should be performed under the advisement of an electrical technician and only after consulting with the manufacturer for any potential incompatibilities. Finally, unless extraordinary circumstances warrant otherwise, electronic boundary training in earnest should not be commenced until the puppy is 6 months of age.

Although electronic containment systems are effective when properly installed and maintained, whenever possible a physical fence is preferable to an electronic one for confining dogs. In addition to keeping the dog in the yard, a physical fence keeps other dogs and people out. With dogs that jump over or dig under fencing, an electronic fence can be installed to discourage such escape behavior. To be effective, e-collars must be snugly fitted to ensure that both electrodes make contact with the dog's skin. This operational feature can be a source of significant discomfort, especially if the collar is kept on a dog for long periods. After prolonged and continuous wear, the skin may become irritated or experience significant tissue damage (contact necrosis) (Polsky, 1994). Another problem becomes evident only after a dog escapes from the yard and attempts to get back inside, whereupon it is stimulated and caused to flee the property. In neighborhoods where many of the same electronic containment systems are installed, the roaming dog may be repeatedly stimulated, perhaps causing it to seek safety in the worst possible place: the middle of the road! Hopefully, manufacturers will design systems in the future that allow the dog to reenter the yard and devise safeguards against extraneous stimulation by other containment systems. In addition, a telephone paging system that automatically calls and warns the owner, or triggers an alarm within the house, whenever the dog escapes the yard would be a valuable enhancement of such systems. Given the risks of escaping from the yard and the potential danger posed by other dogs freely entering the property, containment systems should include video surveillance for observing the goings-on in the yard. The cable feed could be put into the ground at the same time the containment system is installed. There is an obvious marketing angle here that might be of interest to the containment-system distributors, whereby the combination of containment and surveillance arguably provides a combination of enhanced home security and safety benefits. Such video capability would also offer an enhanced means for keeping a closer eye on children playing in the yard. A miniaturized rf-video camera and microphone built into the collar itself would also be of immense utility. Finally, video surveillance is an extremely useful means for studying dog behavior as well as addressing a variety of common outdoor behavior problems with the aid of radio-controlled spray or ES. Inexpensive two-way radios often have a variety of tones and voice-transmission capabilities that can provide a flexible communication interface when the receiver is placed at a fixed location such as near a door or when it is attached to the dog's collar.

Dogs that repeatedly run through electronic boundaries are a potential threat to themselves and to the public safety. There are several causes associated with the failure of such containment systems:

> Damage to the boundary wire
> Inoperative transmitter or receiving collar
> Worn-out batteries
> Improper fitting of the collar
> Improper training

Of this group, the leading cause of failure appears to stem from improper training. In one case, an owner deliberately encouraged a dog to run across the boundary field by calling and cajoling it from the other side, with the dog held on leash by another family member. The dog eventually pulled into the field and reached the owner, whereupon it was pulled back through the field and into the yard as punishment. The dog subsequently exhibited pronounced submission behavior (crawling on her belly, rolling over, and hunching up tightly) when approached by anyone coming into the yard. The dog also showed increased submissive-type urination when greeting visitors at the door. In another case, a dog learned to run through the field after children were instructed to run back and forth across the boundary, with the goal of proofing the inhibition. Other dogs inappropriately exposed to boundary training while off leash have succeeded in escaping from a yard after taking several e-stimulations while running wildly around the yard in a panic, until they finally dash headlong through the field. Many have learned to run through the field while pursuing another dog or while chasing wildlife off the property. One dog was strongly tempted by the lure of livestock kept by a neighbor. The dog would periodically break through the boundary to harass the animals, after which he would return home and wait for the owner to turn off the system so that he could get back inside the yard. In some cases, dogs sharing a residence may follow one another through the boundary. In one instance, a male and female pair occasionally escaped from the yard to jolly about in the neighborhood. On one of these occasions, the family was devastated when they learned that both the dogs had been killed while attempting to cross a four-lane highway near the home. Other sorts of problems periodically involve more idiosyncratic behaviors and causes. In one of these exceptional cases, a dog developed an odd habit resembling learned helplessness, whereby he would stand in the stimulation field shaking stoically and unable to back away or to move forward through the boundary without the help of a family member who had to physically pull the dog back out of the field. This particular dog apparently experienced the e-stimulus around its neck as an inescapable event. Another dog learned to habitually run through the boundary after she had been equipped with a bark-activated collar. Prior to this change, the dog had never broken through the boundary and had learned to closely hug the warning field, from where it persistently barked at other dogs and passersby. Once equipped with the bark collar, the dog began to run out of the yard whenever the collar was activated, perhaps confusing the bark-activated ES as an uncontrollable stimulus coming from the containment system. After a while, the barking behavior stopped, but the dog continued to run through the boundary, even though she received a strong e-stimulus on each occasion.

Dogs that habitually run through the warning and stimulation field appear to have learned an escape/avoidance strategy that is incompatible with containment. Since the act of running over the line ultimately terminates stimulation, the sequence undergoes significant reinforcement every time the dog succeeds. The situation is compounded if the dog attempts to return to the safety of the yard, since the collar is activated a second time. Instead of backing away from the field in response to the warning signal, these dogs acquire an opposite habit whereby they attempt to charge through the field as quickly as possible. In cases where an intractable escape habit has been well established and retraining has failed to improve a dog's response, a special procedure may be useful. A 30- to 50-foot nylon rope is secured to some stationary object and attached to the dog. The stationary line should be set up near locations where the dog has habitually escaped. The rope should be arranged to give the dog enough room to activate the warning field, but prevent the dog from going beyond it.

During such training, a radio-controlled collar is used in combination with the containment collar to enable the trainer to apply sufficient ES to deter inappropriate escape. At such times, the stationary line can be used to pull the dog out of the warning field, if necessary. As a result of the foregoing procedure, the inappropriate escape response is thwarted, making retreat into the safety of the yard the only escape option available. Once it is evident that the dog has learned the appropriate avoidance response, various proofing procedures should be performed to further reduce any risk that the dog will charge through the boundary in the future. Dogs that continue to run off the property despite such additional training and deterrence efforts are not good candidates for such confinement.

The use of electronic containment systems for indoor behavior control and restriction should be seriously reexamined with regard to behavioral and social considerations. Although one practitioner has suggested that an indoor ES delivered by such systems can be useful as a means to "protect children from pets and help orchestrate space sharing by pets" (Overall, 1997:288), electrical boundary training indoors can produce significant fear and consequently risks generating reactive behavior in association with approach-avoidance conflict and anxiety, especially around locations where the collar has been activated in the past while the dog was approaching, following, or playing with a family member or another companion animal sharing the household. Defining a property boundary by means of ES seems to be of a radically different nature than training a dog to avoid following family members within the context of the home. Further, given the possibility that boundary-activated devices may elicit aggression in some emotionally reactive and predisposed dogs (Polsky, 2000), the use of indoor electrical barriers to control the movements of dogs likely to show an escalation of aggression in response to ES should be avoided. Indoor electronic containment might be considered in some situations involving dogs that exhibit persistent house-training problems or destructive behaviors, but only after conventional training efforts have been attempted and failed to train the dog to stay out of forbidden parts of the house, and then only when gates or doors are not practical as the primary means of confinement. Indoor electronic containment may be useful for the control of some problems involving cat chasing and harassment; however, with highly motivated or aggressive dogs, electronic fencing does not provide a fail-safe barrier and should not be used to contain dogs with a history of attacking cats. Finally, properly performed electrical training minimizes associative linkages between the aversive event and the trainer, while encouraging the dog to seek comfort and safety from the owner in association with postevent relief, relaxation, and various rewards.

Caution: The quality of radio-controlled training collars and containment systems varies greatly, requiring that prospective users research the available products to ensure that the system selected is reliable, effective, and humane. Malfunctions resulting in the delivery of uncontrolled ES are uncommon; nonetheless, and despite numerous improvements over the years, no electronic device is entirely fail-safe. Further, not all radio-controlled and behavior-activated electronic training devices provide the same level of safe operation and adjustable stimulation. The quality and "feel" of ES vary among the devices available, with the best products producing a pulse that minimizes pricking and stinging effects. Professional use of such products demands careful attention to the functional fitness and humaneness of the electronic training aids selected. A number of manufacturers have emerged as leaders in the field of electronic training, and professional trainer/behaviorists are well advised to use only those products that offer the highest standards of operational reliability and incorporate low-level stimulation. Selecting from systems that feature rechargeable batteries in both the transmitter and the receiver unit—ultimately a wise selection criterion given the cost of replacement batteries for such devices—significantly narrows the field of possible collars from which to choose. Electronic training devices that produce excessively painful or traumatic shock should be avoided, as should techniques calling for such stimulation.

BASIC TRAINING AND ENHANCEMENT

Electronic training is most effective when it is used to enhance basic modules and routines previously shaped by means of conventional reward-based training. Ideally, the trainer performs introductory electrical training and gradually transfers control of the transmitter to the owner as a basic understanding of the process developed. Most dogs show little or no emotional reactivity or signs of distress to LLES. Although they may find the stimulus annoying, they are not usually frightened by it. Initially, some dogs may exhibit very minor and transient signs of alarm in response to LLES—signs that rapidly habituate and give way to increasing confidence and relaxation as they learn to control the electrical event. Although the vast majority of dogs appear to be highly receptive and responsive to electronic training, some may exhibit an adverse response to ES. Dogs that show signs of reactive aggression, fear, persistent anxiety, insecurity, or depression in response to ES are not good candidates for such training. Also, dogs exposed previously to electronic containment training may exhibit signs of hypersensitization and problematic escape and avoidance behavior in response to LLES. Aside from brief phantom biting and mouthing movements in the direction of the collar, the author has never observed a dog react aggressively toward a person or another dog in response to radio-controlled ES. However, reactive aggression has been reported in association with electronic containment systems (Polsky, 2000). Also, Beaudet (2001) mentions a Jack Russell terrier that appeared to become "mad" when sprayed by a bark-activated citronella collar, causing it to bark more when corrected by the device. Although reactive aggression appears to be relatively rare, such undesirable behavior should be considered a risk in dogs showing unstable temperaments or a standing history of aggressive behavior, where ES is delivered while the dog is in close proximity (particularly while making physical contact) with a person or another dog.

For dogs showing insecure behavior in response to LLES, electronic training can be introduced in combination with vibrotactile stimulation and target-arc training. A vibration stimulus is paired with an established target-arc stimulus in order to facilitate a safe preemptive bias toward the stimulus while habituating inappropriate aversive responses to the stimulation. The lowest level of ES is gradually introduced by embedding it within the vibration stimulus, thereby amplifying the orienting response, which is followed by a click and a flick of the right hand. Such dogs are given basic radio-controlled training that shadows previous reward-based training, especially orienting and recall modules and routines, until the dog shows a highly competent and confident response to conditioned signals and LLES. Successful responses are bridged and rewarded with food and other rewards presented on a schedule conducive to positive prediction error (surprise). Signs of fearful behavior are interrupted at the earliest point by evoking a target-arc response, followed by an orienting "Good!" (or a click), hand flick, and reward. The evocation of strong escape/avoidance behavior should be avoided, but such behavior that does occur should be blocked with a leash or long line worn by the dog at all times during the initial stages of training. At such times, the dog is turned around (with the long line if necessary), whereupon "Relax" is spoken just as the e-stimulus is turned off. The most common cause of excessive reactivity is sensitization resulting from previous traumatic exposure to electronic training or exposure to sensitizing aversive events (e.g., bark-activated and boundary-activated collars). Electronic training procedures using HLES should be performed under the supervision of experienced trainers who are knowledgeable concerning the benefits and potential risks associated with safety training.

Attention Training

Most problems necessitating electronic intervention stem from attention and impulse-control deficiencies. Electronic enhancement of attention and orienting behavior is introduced in the context of moderate environmental distraction with the dog on a leash or a long line. A continuous low-level pulse is delivered that is sufficient to get the distracted dog's attention but without evoking startle or evidence of distress. The attention-controlling effect of ES is attained in many dogs at very low levels of stimulation, often imperceptible to human touch; however, since dogs differ with respect to their sensitivity to ES, some may require a significantly stronger level to motivate an attentional response, especially when acting under the influence of strong distractions. Whatever the case, it is critical that ES levels be precisely calculated and controlled to match an individual dog's specific needs, circumstances at the time of stimulation, and the training objectives. Consequently, only electronic training collars that deliver a finely adjustable and reliable e-stimulus, ideally in combination with vibrotactile capability, should be used for such training purposes. As the e-stimulus is delivered, a smooching, squeaker, or whistle sound is made to attract the dog's attention. If the dog fails to orient toward the trainer as the ES continues, it is prompted with the long line to turn its head. As the dog turns, conditioned negative reinforcement (S^{r-}) (voice, click, or tone) is timed and presented to occur just before the e-stimulus is discontinued (Figure 9.1). The S^{r-} identifies the specific behavior that turns off the e-stimulus (escape phase), and, when presented in association with the controlling discriminative stimulus, the S^{r-} signifies that the response successfully avoided the aversive event. In the latter case, the S^{r-} not only serves to reinforce the avoidance response, but its presentation predicts safety from aversive stimulation. Several layers of reward are associated with the successful control of aversive motivational incentives.

Since the termination or reduction of aversive stimulation is perceived as a rewarding event, actions and stimuli paired with the discontinuation of ES gradually acquire reward value of a positive nature—that is, the dog will work to produce them—helping to explain the power of conditioned negative reinforcement to support avoidance learning. In addition, successful escape promotes rewarding associations with social and contextual stimuli paired with successful escape-to-safety behavior, and such stimuli (conditioned safety signals) acquire potent motivational significance for the dog (e.g., praise). As opposed to escape-from-fear associations, associations acquired during escape to safety may possess significant reward value that can be used in a variety of training situations (e.g., praise supporting the maintenance of obedience to command) and behavior-therapy contexts, but may be especially useful in the context of facilitating social attachment and confidence. The most significant source of reward for dogs that is obtained in the context of electronic training is mediated by the successful control of the aversive event. Perceiving that the e-stimulus is controllable by purposive efforts is not only a profound source of reward mediated by enhanced comfort and safety, but such learning contributes to the integration of an adaptive coping style via the organization of control-expectancy modules (prediction-control expectancies, calibrated establishing operations, and specific actions or sequences). When an aversive event is successfully terminated, reduced, postponed, or avoided in accordance with a rule or set of prediction-control expectancies, the dog acquires an increased sense of confidence or power over the threatening event. Repeated successful control over aversive events promotes competence, confidence, and a high-power control style conducive to elation, contentment, and well-being.

With the dog orienting toward the trainer, it is induced to come with affectionate encouragement and rewarded in ways conducive to promoting a sense of safety. If the dog attempts to turn away from the trainer instead, the LLES is applied and sustained until the dog turns back again. Once more, as the dog turns its head, S^{r-} (voice, click, or tone) is delivered just before stimulation is discontinued. After brief intertrial delays, similar trials are repeated until the dog rapidly turns its attention toward the trainer as soon as the e-stimulus is delivered. This escape phase of training is followed by an avoidance phase in which the dog's name is spoken just before the smooching or squeaker sound is made to intensify the orienting response. If the dog fails to orient, the e-stimulus is applied at a slightly higher level and immediately removed just as the dog turns toward the trainer. If the dog responds to its name alone, the reward bridge ("Good") is delivered just as it turns toward the trainer.

RECALL ENHANCEMENT

Recall enhancement is easily integrated with attention-control training by saying "Come" just as the dog steps in the direction of the trainer. On every occasion in which the dog successfully comes, it should be enthusiastically praised, rewarded, and released following the various procedures described in Chapter 1. Compelling a dog to come via ES is usually unnecessary and should be avoided unless special circumstances warrant such training. In some cases, prompting (repeated momentary pulsing) with LLES may be necessary to compel a highly resistant dog to come; however, most dogs learn to come reliably with positive reinforcement alone, especially after electronic training is used to enhance attention and impulse control. During the early phases of recall and attention-control training, there is a strong tendency for inexperienced trainers to point or poke the handheld transmitter at the dog as they deliver stimulation. This is not necessary and may actually cause the dog to become overly aware of the trainer as the source of stimulation and adversely affect its response to electronic training. The dog does not need to know where the stimulation is originating in order for it to be effective. As a general rule, it is best not to move or show the dog the transmitter. This precaution helps to minimize the risk that the dog might associate the movement of the hand with the e-stimulus. This is especially critical in situations where the trainer is in full view of the dog. Stimulation should prompt the dog to seek security by making contact or by cooperating with the trainer's instruction. Throughout the electronic training process, the trainer's role is that of constructive guide and source of support and security. As a

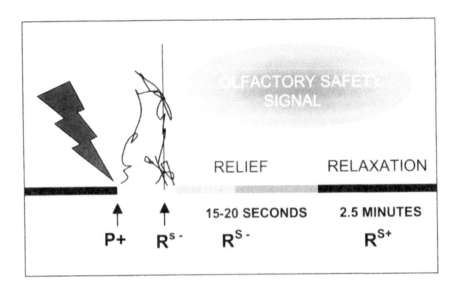

FIG. 9.1 The conditioned negative reinforcer R^{r-} immediately precedes the termination of the e-stimulus (P+), followed by opponent relief and relaxation (safety), providing both positive (R^{S+}) and negative (R^{S-})reinforcing effects. An olfactory stimulus presented to overlap with the postevent opponent relief and relaxation effects may gradually acquire conditioned associations capable of producing feelings of safety.

result, properly employed electrical training may significantly enhance a dog's connection and willingness to cooperate with the trainer.

Enhancing the Freeze Response

Training a dog to freeze on command dramatically enhances impulse control and recall reliability. The following procedure assumes that the dog has received long-line training as discussed in Chapter 1 and has been exposed to preliminary recall enhancement with LLES. With the dog on a long line and bolting toward some distraction, the command "Stay" is spoken in an abrupt and assertive tone just in advance of a brief pulse of high-end MLES. As the dog stops, the trainer quickly moves to the dog's position or calls it to "Come," whereupon the response is appropriately reinforced with sustained petting and food. An intertrial period of 2 1/2 to 3 minutes is provided to give the dog time to benefit fully from the ensuing postaversive relief and relaxation response. During this relief/relaxation period, various reward-based training and play activities are used to enhance the dog's confidence in the trainer as

a source of safety and nurturance. The foregoing procedure is repeated under increasingly difficult and distracting circumstances until the dog learns reliably to freeze in response to the "Stay" command without ES. With each level of mastery, the dog is trained to freeze, stay, and to come when called. Recall is highly prepared under such circumstances, with the dog seeking the safety of close contact with the trainer. After the dog comes to a halt, its name is called. If the dog turns, a reward bridge is presented (e.g., "Good" or click), and the dog is called to "Come." As the dog reaches the trainer, it is appropriately rewarded with appetitive-positive and social-positive reinforcement. If the dog fails to orient (as may occur under the influence of a strongly distracting stimulus), a whistle or squeaker is presented and, if necessary, LLES is delivered together with directive prompting with the a long line. If the dog begins to come, but then turns away toward the distraction, a stronger level of LLES is delivered to secure control and turn the dog's attention away from the distraction. In cases involving dogs with particularly strong motivational interests in some activity or object in the environment, higher levels of aversive ES may be needed to counteract the attraction. In general, establishing strong impulse control by conditioning a reliable freeze response is a necessary preliminary to obtaining a consistent and reliable recall sequence. After exposure to the stronger e-stimulus used in freeze training, a dog's response to LLES may undergo sensitization, perhaps allowing the trainer to use even lower levels of ES in the future.

Wait and Back

A useful way to enhance impulse control is to apply brief low-level stimulation during the wait and back exercises at the door when leaving the house for a walk. Preliminary training of the wait exercise teaches the dog to respond to the opening of the door by backing away ("Back") and waiting ("Wait") to be released ("Okay"). If the dog lunges ahead before being released, LLES is applied and repeatedly pulsed until the dog backs away from the doorway. The dog quickly learns that it can control stimulation and escape or avoid it by backing away or waiting in response to the door opening or by responding to the vocal signals "Back" and "Wait." Training a dog to wait and to back away from the door is a useful preliminary to enhancing slack-leash and controlled-walking behavior.

Walking on a Slack Leash

Excessive pulling on leash is a common complaint of dog owners. Although pulling can be controlled with traditional methods or halter restraint, such methods for some owners may be impractical or unsuccessful. Conventional halter training is particularly problematic because, when the halter is removed and the dog walked on a flat or slip collar, the pulling behavior may immediately recover despite conscientious positive reinforcement of more acceptable walking behavior while on the halter. Dogs exhibiting persistent habits of lunging or bolting at people, vehicles, or other animals show a pronounced and lasting benefit from even a very brief exposure to electronic training while on leash. The simplest approach is to directly link the presentation of low stimulation at the earliest moment in the pulling sequence and discontinue stimulation at the instant the dog backs off the leash. Surprisingly, most dogs with only modest preliminary training can learn not to pull, requiring only a few low-level stimulations (barely perceptible or imperceptible to human touch). Another method that is highly compatible with slack-leash techniques (see Chapter 1) is to pair momentary stimulation at a higher level with the spring release of slack or just after saying "Easy." An alternative method involves turning away from the pulling dog and applying stimulation just as the leash slack is dropped. By responding in a timely way to these cues, the dog can avoid ES. Once the dog is walking without pulling, appropriate rewards are used to strengthen more focused slack-lease walking, including periodic quick-sit/stay and instant-down/stay exercises.

Enhancing Emergency Exercises: Quick-sit and Instant-down

In the context of problem solving, electronic training is sometimes used to enhance emergency exercises that a dog has already learned (e.g., quick-sit, instant-down, and stay) through positive-reinforcement procedures. Also, in some situations, it may be necessary to improve the speed or reliability of the quick-sit or instant-down, especially when a high degree of impulse control is needed to maintain control in the presence of disruptive environmental distractions or adverse motivational arousal. Using ES to enhance behavioral control assumes as a starting point that the dog possesses a working understanding of the response being strengthened. For example, in the case of the quick-sit, the dog should demonstrate a viable sit response acquired through positive reinforcement and directive training. Again, the basic procedure is carried out with the e-collar set at the lowest level needed to evoke an orienting response and mild annoyance but without causing evidence of startle or discomfort. During the escape phase, ES is presented just before delivery of hand and vocal signals, which provide the dog with previously acquired information that it can use to escape, that is, control the e-stimulus. Just as the dog begins to sit, the S^r is presented and LLES is immediately discontinued, followed by vocal encouragement and the delivery of various other rewards as the dog completes the action. This procedure is repeated until the dog responds without hesitation and rapidly sits, indicating that it has learned that sitting turns off ES. If the dog has trouble sitting in the presence of ES, the response is induced by appropriate leash prompting or physical manipulation. The avoidance phase is a critical step in which the dog learns that hand and vocal signals can be used to avoid turning on ES in the first place, while setting the occasion for the subsequent delivery of positive reinforcement. During the avoidance phase, the dog's name is spoken to obtain its attention just before the command "Sit" is given in a normal tone followed by the hand signal—a delayed prompt. As the dog sits, appropriate positive reinforcement is delivered; however, if the dog fails to sit, the e-stimulus is applied together with leash prompting and physical manipulation sufficient to induce the dog to sit. If the dog successfully avoids the e-stimulus by sitting in response to the vocal and hand signals alone, the reward bridge ("Good" or click) is presented, followed by positive reinforcement. At the conclusion of each exercise or sequence of exercises, the dog is released with an "Okay" and hand clap.

In addition to strengthening the sit response with negative reinforcement, electrical training can be effectively used to enhance sit-stay reliability. This is a significant shift in emphasis. Instead of strengthening an active response through escape-to-safety training, the goal is to inhibit some action, improve impulse control, and increase the duration of the selected response. The stay exercise is carried out at both the sit-front position and the starting position at the trainer's side, as well as practiced under various naturalistic situations. Electrical stimulation should be delivered together with the command "Stay" at the earliest sign of movement indicating an intention to break the sit-stay position. If necessary, the dog is prompted by leash or physically guided

back into the sit position. An important aspect of effective stay training is to emphasize the duration of the response and the release. In fact, in an important sense, stay behavior is most effectively trained by conceiving it as a antecedent waiting period or contingency in anticipation of a response leading to reward. As such, the release signal "Okay" or the opportunity to perform some other response is integrated with the stay behavior. The release from the stay contingency is explicitly trained with reward, just as any other control module. In basic training, control modules (e.g., sit, down, and stand) are treated as default stay exercises; that is, the dog should learn to remain in the position until it is explicitly released with an "Okay" or another command. Gradually, the dog is exposed to progressively more distracting and difficult situations until the quick-sit and stay response is reliable and steady.

Training dogs to drop instantly on command and to stay there is a very useful exercise for highly active, impulsive, and otherwise difficult-to-control dogs. Although the vast majority of dogs can learn to perform the necessary sequence of behaviors without the use of electronic techniques, some highly intrusive, impulsive, and oppositional dogs may resist conventional training efforts. Such dogs often rapidly benefit from electronic enhancement training of the emergency instant-down and stay response. The instant-down is particularly useful for owner's who lack sufficient physical strength or motor ability to otherwise control such dogs. Preliminary training should include intensive reward-based conditioning and shaping efforts and conventional inhibitory training. In advance of electronic enhancement, the dog should exhibit a well-developed understanding of the instant-down and down-stay behavior. Electrical enhancement of the down response is carried out with the dog in both the sit and the stand positions, with the trainer stepping on a slack leash as LLES is delivered, followed by the appropriate vocal and hand signal. If the dog fails to lie down, momentary pulsing of LLES together with appropriate leash prompting or physical assistance should be applied. Once the dog learns to escape the e-stimulus by quickly lying down, the vocal and hand prompts are given before stimulation. If the dog responds appropriately, the reward bridge is presented at the moment in which the dog begins to lie down, followed by petting, food, and other rewards as the response is completed. Evidence of strong resistance to lying down in the presence of ES usually indicates that additional preliminary reward-based training is needed. The instant-down and stay exercise is practiced in a way similar to the procedure described for the quick-sit and stay. If the dog attempts to get up, ES, coupled with necessary leash prompting, is delivered at the earliest signs of movement and continued until the dog lies back down, whereupon ES is immediately discontinued and followed by appropriate bridging and positive reinforcement. At the conclusion of the instant-down and stay exercise, the dog is released with "Okay" and a hand clap. As with the quick-sit and stay, the instant-down and stay is practiced under varying conditions, lengths of time, distances, and distractions, thereby improving its usefulness and reliability for emergency control purposes.

BEHAVIORAL EQUILIBRIUM

Any highly motivational training technique may produce behavioral imbalances. As a result, certain classes of highly reinforced behavior may gradually dominate a dog's repertoire to such an extent that the expression of other behavior may be significantly impeded or blocked. For example, in reward-based training, a dog may tend to stay excessively close to its trainer in an effort to maximize its chances of getting food, gradually making it more difficult to shape exercises that either require it to move away from the trainer or to stay away at some distance. Other reinforcement-related imbalances may take the form of anticipatory behavior. For example, dogs that have been repeatedly called after a brief sit-stay may learn to anticipate the recall signal and come without waiting as required. In this case, the recall response is stronger than the stay response, reflecting an imbalance of readiness to perform the one response at the expense of the other. Simply returning to the

dog occasionally and rewarding it for staying can help to offset the anticipatory imbalance and restore equilibrium (see Tortora, 1983).

Electronic devices are frequently used to discourage undesirable behavior via punishment. As a result, the dog gradually learns to regard the e-stimulus as an inhibitory signal, causing it to freeze when the collar is activated. This would be a highly undesirable outcome if one wished to negatively reinforce a behavior requiring the dog to move toward or away from the trainer. Ideally, the dog should learn to increasingly respond to ES as an e-signal anticipating safety and reward rather than an aversive event compelling escape. Other problems may emerge if the device is used exclusively to reinforce a fixed sequence of exercises negatively, such as sit and down, always sequencing them in the same order. Numerous other potential imbalances may emerge during training, some beneficial and others detrimental to training objectives. The single most important consideration to keep in mind to avoid problematic imbalances is to engender in the dog a confident attitude with respect to its ability to predict and control significant events, whether attractive or aversive. Dogs that habitually fail to exercise control over significant outcomes, particularly aversive ones, may develop a pattern of inflexible and ritualistic behaviors to cope with difficult situations. Even though such rituals are ineffective as means to control attractive and aversive events, they may serve to reduce distressing arousal (e.g., escalating anxiety and frustration) associated with behavioral incompetence. Behaviorally incompetent and insecure dogs tend to prefer familiar activities that minimize the risk of failure, even though they produce a low rate of reinforcement, whereas competent and confident dogs are more willing to engage in risk-taking activities and experimentation (actions with uncertain outcomes) to produce an optimal range and quantity of reward and safety. Perhaps the best general strategy to ensure beneficial balance is to encourage the dog to engage in behavioral experimentation that involves a balance of both attractive and aversive events arranged to occur with sufficient difficulty to increase the dog's functional competence and confidence.

PUNISHMENT AND AVERSIVE COUNTERCONDITIONING

Radio-controlled e-collars are commonly used to punish (suppress) unwanted behavior. Since the intent of punishment is to produce rapid and complete suppression of the target behavior, the process typically involves significantly higher levels of stimulation than used to shape behavior with negative reinforcement. As a result, the levels of ES used for punishment purposes pose significantly more risks and potential problems than those associated with LLES. The more aversive the stimulation, the more accurate and precise the stimulation needs to be in order to avoid problems. Consequently, HLES is typically delivered in the form of a brief pulses lasting a fraction of second. Only e-collars incorporating a momentary function that prevents overexposure to HLES should be used to deliver such stimulation.

In contrast to LLES, HLES is prone to produce a number of undesirable side effects that require a great deal of care and expertise to prevent or manage. HLES can produce significant pain, fear, and distress, aversive arousal that may persist in some dogs by becoming associatively linked with the context or neutral stimuli present during inappropriate or lengthy HLES. Instead of promoting escape/avoidance behavior with negative reinforcement, HLES risks indiscriminately producing fear of the place or things present at the moment of stimulation, causing the dog to acquire a lasting aversion toward them, even though they might be entirely irrelevant to the actual cause of stimulation. Further, rather than learning to emit behavior instrumental to escape or avoid the stimulation, the dog may simply learn to be afraid of it. The intense emotional arousal elicited by HLES may impede efficient learning or evoke undesirable reactive behavior, even aggression, in some predisposed dogs. Fearful or aggressive behaviors immediately preceding the cessation of aversive stimulation may undergo significant negative reinforcement. Consequently, a major concern associated with punitive procedures is the risk of generating and reinforcing highly undesirable behavior in place of the target behavior being punished. For example, punishing a dog with HLES when it jumps up on guests may cause it to avoid entering the foyer or, perhaps, depending on the dog's temperament and propensity for such behavior, elicit intense fear or aggression toward the visitor at the moment in which stimulation is delivered. Dogs that succeed in running through an electrical boundary may inadvertently learn to avoid ES by running through the field in the future. Such dogs may subsequently run through the boundary as quickly as possible when threatened by the warning tone rather than simply backing away from it.

Aversive counterconditioning is most often used to counter or offset the appeal of intrinsically reinforcing activities. These techniques are most often used to control activities or appetites that might threaten dogs with injury or death. The intent of such training is to instill a lasting aversion toward some object or place. For example, many dogs are fascinated and beguiled by the sound made by rattlesnakes. By applying an intense ES as the dog approaches a rattling snake, it learns, often after a single trial, to avoid such sounds and creatures. In aversive counterconditioning, an attractive stimulus is paired with a strongly aversive one. The goal is to reduce the appetitive value of the stimulus for the dog. Punishment, on the other hand, is primarily focused on reducing the frequency or strength of some instrumental behavior. A common problem involves dogs that persistently chase cars or bicyclists. Because cars and bikes are common things, causing a dog to become overly fearful and avoidant toward such things would not be desirable. Instead, the goal is to suppress the chase response itself by means of aversive stimulation. Successful suppression appears to combine both behavioral avoidance and object-place aversion, with the associated object-place serving as a discriminative stimulus signaling avoidance.

ELECTRONIC TRAINING AND PROBLEM SOLVING

Electronic collars have been recommended and shown effective for the rapid suppression of numerous behavior problems, including chasing after a variety of objects and other animals, territorial aggression, excessive barking, stealing and destroying household items, pica, coprophagia, aggressive-intent (lunging) behavior toward other dogs, compulsive behaviors (e.g., tail chasing), fence jumping and other boundary-escape behaviors, and refractory mouthing and biting in puppies (Polsky, 1994). Hart and Hart (1985) have described e-collars as an effective way to remotely punish misbehavior in dogs. Aside from the advantage of remote application, e-collars enable trainers to deliver a highly controlled stimulus, at variable intensities, with a degree of accuracy and consistency that is not available by any other means.

Electrical Stimulation and Excessive Barking

Although many authorities deem the use of bark-activated collars inappropriate for controlling nuisance barking at separation, such devices appear to exert a significant suppressive effect over separation-related barking behavior. In addition to producing a sharp reduction of barking at separation, many owners and trainers have noted a significant calming effect associated with the use of such collars. A survey of dog owners that used e-collars found that many owners noted that their dogs were calmer and "more settled" after its use. Those owners that used a bark-activated collar noted universally a calming effect (Coleman and Murray, 2000). A disturbing finding detected by this survey was that among the 30 respondents, only one dog was regularly permitted in the house. Aside from suggesting that excessive barking and roaming problems may be causally related to rigid exclusion of the dog from the household, it emphasizes the importance of preliminary behavioral counseling that focuses on quality-of-life causes that might underlie the etiology of such problems. Without identifying and modifying such contributing causes, reliance on punitive measures (electronic or otherwise) is a highly problematic and ill-advised strategy of behavior control. Beaudet (2001) has suggested that the use of bark-acti-

vated spray collars is an effective adjunct to control territorial and protective barking as well as barking associated with separation anxiety, fear, or compulsive etiologies. This is a somewhat unexpected benefit, especially if one considers separation distress to be an anxiety-based problem. Given such an emotional etiology, one would predict that startle should exacerbate the problem barking—not reduce it. How can this apparent paradox be resolved? First, obviously, not all separation-related barking is exclusively caused by anxiety, and this could account for many instances of improved behavior (see *Separation Distress and Coactive Influences* in Volume 2, Chapter 4). But, even in cases of separation distress where anxiety clearly appears to play a role, a significant number of dogs appear to improve rapidly after exposure to electronic training when an electrical or spray stimulus is used. In the case of ES, a plausible way to interpret these observations is in terms of relief/relaxation and emotional opponent processing that ensue after shock is terminated. According to opponent-process theory, aversive stimulation evokes slave affects of opposite hedonic valence (Solomon and Corbit, 1974). After repeated exposure to aversive stimulation, the slave or b-processes become progressively robust, pronounced, and sustained (see *Opponent-process Theory and Separation Distress* in Volume 2, Chapter 4). These opponent b-processes include the confluent evocation of relief and relaxation. Denny (1971), who has thoroughly studied this phenomenon in the laboratory (see *Safety Signal Hypothesis* in Volume 1, Chapter 8), has found that relief rapidly displaces fear shortly after the termination of shock and continues to build in strength for 10 to 15 seconds into the post-shock period. This relief response is primarily autonomic in nature and gradually followed by a more generalized relaxation response. Paradoxically, so long as aversive stimulation is brief, escapable, and spaced in time, the net result predicted by opponent-process theory and the safety-signal hypothesis is progressive relaxation—not increased anxiety. In the case of separation-related barking, added beneficial effects may accrue as the dog learns to avoid stimulation by not barking. Theoretically, each time the impulse to bark is inhibited, thereby avoiding stimulation, the dog may experience repeated and deepening episodes of relief, relaxation, and enhanced confidence. If this theoretical assessment is accurate, the overall emotional effect of such training is progressively to generate a very significant internal counterconditioning influence, perhaps of sufficient magnitude to offset anxious arousal during periods of separation. Additional benefits could be obtained by presenting a continuous olfactory safety signal timed to coincide with the onset of relief following ES and continuing for 3 minutes, thereby overlapping both the relief and the relaxation stages of the opponent process. A bark-activated collar could be designed and programmed to perform this task. In addition, the collar could periodically deliver the odorant in small, nonstartling amounts at variable times so long as barking has been absent during the period immediately preceding the odor's presentation. The use of an intermittent olfactory safety signal would serve to calm and reassure the dog while simultaneously reinforcing quiet behavior.

Whether one chooses to use a bark-activated spray collar or an e-collar, such devices must be used with great care with dogs exhibiting separation distress with coactive anxiety or panic symptoms. Bark-activated collars work because they produce a strong inhibitory effect over barking, but, in some dogs, instead of calming them as previously suggested, such devices may evoke increased excitability, distress, or even global panic. One illustrative case involves a female Brittany spaniel that was 11 years old when her owner moved into an exclusive high-rise condominium and had gone back to work after a long hiatus between jobs. The dog's reaction to this change in routine was to bark continuously and to eliminate whenever the owner left her alone. According to the owner, both of these problems arose only after the change in home and routine. The dog's incessant barking led to a flurry of nasty complaints by her new neighbors. The owner consulted a veterinarian (her brother) who recommended that she use a crate and a bark-activated e-col-

lar. Rather absentmindedly, she put the collar on the dog and left her alone in the crate for the day. She later confessed that she had rushed out of the apartment to avoid hearing the dog yelp when the collar went off. When the owner returned home, she discovered to her horror that the dog had broken out of the crate. The dog's efforts to escape from the crate had resulted in severe lacerations of her feet and caused her to break off several teeth. The dog was covered in urine, feces, and blood—materials that were tracked and smeared into carpets and furniture. This is a rather exceptional case, but it does underscore the potential dangers involved when using crates or antibark devices to control separation problems. Such tools should be recommended with great care and their use avoided in the case of highly unstable and reactive dogs.

Electrical Stimulation and Refractory Compulsive Behavior

Refractory compulsive behaviors are a source of considerable distress for many dogs and owners. In addition to evidencing psychological stress, such problems often result in physical injuries to dogs. Compulsive habits may persist despite intensive behavior-modification efforts, prompting the use of various means of physical restraint and medical interventions involving psychotropic drugs. Excessive self-directed licking may result in acral lick dermatitis (ALD) (see *Excessive Licking* in Chapter 5), which is often associated with dermal hyperplasia and ulcerated lesions developing on affected areas, especially the carpus and tarsus joints. ALD may resist treatment efforts unless the dog's licking activity can be prevented. Prevention measures often include the use of Elizabethan-type collars, bandages, or various repellents applied to the affected area. Some of the treatments may cause the dog significant discomfort (e.g., glucocorticoids injected directly into the lesion) and require repeated administration. Although various pharmacological agents (e.g., clomipramine and fluoxetine) may significantly attenuate the habit, the benefits of such medications to control excessive licking depend on the sustained use of the drugs, with the unwanted behavior often recurring when the medication is discontinued. Not only are the long-term side effects of prolonged psychotropic medication unknown in dogs, such medications are relatively expensive and may represent a significant strain on the household budget of many dog owners.

Eckstein and Hart (1996) performed a study to evaluate the use of radio-controlled ES to suppress excessive licking associated with ALD. The five dogs selected for the study were equipped with an e-collar (Tri-Tronics), providing the delivery of three momentary stimulations (3.3, 13.2, and 59.0 msec). Owners were instructed to use the minimum duration of stimulation needed to interrupt licking behavior. For all dogs, the medium duration (13.2 msec) was sufficient to inhibit licking. Initially, the owner delivered the stimulation while hidden from the dog's view, but, as the training progressed, ES was delivered in different contexts, including at times when the dog was in the owner's presence. Between training sessions, dogs were required to wear Elizabethan collars, at least until licking had been absent or rare for 6 hours or more. On average, licking was suppressed in four of the five dogs after a mean of 11.8 electrical events delivered over 12 to 50 days. The suppressive effect of the protocol was highly durable, and relapse was quickly resolved with a brief period of remedial training. The variable length of time required to obtain full suppression may have been due to differences in the amount of time owners devoted to the training program.

Considering the extremely rapid and lasting benefits derived from a dozen or so brief pulses of momentary ES, the procedure described by Eckstein and Hart would seem to represent an important advance in the humane treatment of such problems. A significant advantage of the procedure is its simplicity—a factor that recommends its use by average dog owners. Interestingly, though, Hewson and Luescher (1996) have criticized the method as being too difficult for the average owner to follow because "the technique was used according to a particular protocol, something most owners cannot do" (156).

Oddly, they then go on to recommend an arguably more complicated protocol requiring that the owner train the dog to perform some response that is incompatible with licking. When licking occurs, the owner is instructed to distract (startle) the dog from the activity by blowing on a duck call or shrill whistle, whereupon it is cued to perform the incompatible response. This general procedure is repeated every time the dog licks during the 6-week treatment program. In addition, the authors recommend that the owner never "rebuke or punish" the dog since such treatment might worsen the problem, but offer no concrete evidence supporting their rationale or data demonstrating the effectiveness of their treatment protocol. Eckstein and Hart preemptively respond to potential "humane" criticisms, writing,

> The use of electronic shock collars may be questioned by some animal handlers; however, compared with the discomfort of intralesional injections, prolonged use of Elizabethan collar, or both, a limited number of momentary shocks should be considered a humane alternative. (1996:226)

Employing ES in the treatment of ALD should include a preliminary veterinary examination and appropriate treatment of any active lesions. The trainer should attempt to identify and remove sources of behavioral stress adversely impacting the compulsive habit. The long-term benefit of electrical conditioning for the control of ALD is enhanced by the incorporation of various enrichment and training programs. In addition to daily exercise and social activities involving play and compliance training, various counterconditioning efforts involving the use of food and massage should be employed. If an e-collar is selected to help control excessive licking, the dog should be first properly introduced to it in the context of safety training. *Safety training* involves a strategy designed to enhance a dog's control over aversive events while simultaneously exploiting the inherent relief/relaxation effects associated with the successful escape and avoidance learning. The dog learns that ES is controllable and safe by the trainer introducing it at low levels—those just sufficient to reinforce previously conditioned orienting and basic obedience exercises (e.g., sit and stay). Such preliminary training helps to reduce the risk of inducing undesirable fear or stress in association with aversive training.

Using ES to train a dog not to lick should consist of three phases: escape, avoidance, and reinforcement of an alternative behavior. During the escape phase, LLES is applied to interrupt licking. The moment the dog stops licking, a conditioned negative reinforcer (e.g., "Good" or click) is presented and the e-stimulus is immediately turned off and the vocal signal "Relax" is delivered. The avoidance phase of training involves the presentation of a vocal avoidance signal (e.g., "Stop") just before the e-stimulus is activated. By responding immediately to the avoidance signal, the dog can avoid the presentation of the e-stimulus. With the cessation of licking, the dog is tossed a treat or toy, thereby further reinforcing the response and providing the dog an alternative outlet for oral activity.

Once the dog learns that it can escape or avoid the e-stimulus, a more aversive event can be introduced with the goal of further suppressing the compulsive ritual. Now, if the dog fails to respond immediately to the avoidance cue "Stop," a momentary stimulus consisting of a stronger intensity is delivered, depending on the dog's sensitivity to ES. During this phase of training, a dilute odor and repellent taste can be applied sparingly to the area with a cotton squab, thereby providing an additional reminder not to lick the area. As the result of aversive ES, significant emotional relief typically follows within 3 to 5 seconds, with opponent relaxation building after another 2 to 3 minutes. During the relaxation phase, a safety odor (e.g., citrus scent or dilute lavender) can be presented together with a toy and reassuring affection. The idea is to associate the odor with relaxation while redirecting the licking activity away from the dog's body toward a toy. This procedure is repeated as necessary. The e-stimulus involved need not be too intense, but it should be strong enough to suppress the licking behavior rapidly (see Eckstein and Hart, 1996). Although the initial sensitizing exposure should be moderately strong, subsequent

stimulations can be milder, with the voice reprimand "Stop" often being sufficient. For optimal effectiveness, the e-stimulus should be paired with the earliest intentional movements anticipating a licking episode. A radio-controlled spray device (with or without odorant) might also be useful for such purposes. To guard against excessive contextualization, the dog should be observed in various situations and ES appropriately applied, as needed. Finally, it is particularly important to observe and apply ES with the owner both in and out of the dog's view. A remote wireless camera can be very effective for such purposes. Between sessions, the dog should wear an Elizabethan collar until it is evident that the licking compulsion has abated. In all cases, daily basic training should be performed together with exercise, play, massage, and other quality-of-life enhancements, as appropriate. In addition to providing an effective alternative for refractory ALD, electrical training is a viable adjunctive treatment procedure for the control of a variety of other compulsive habits requiring immediate interruption and precise timing of aversive stimulation (e.g., tail chasing and whirling).

Electrical Stimulation and Aggression

The value of electronic training for the control of aggressive behavior has been known for many years, but procedures incorporating ES remain a lightning rod for controversy. A common and erroneous allegation suggests that ES elicits aggression in dogs or makes aggressive dogs more aggressive. While it is certainly possible that exposure to a highly aversive and uncontrollable e-stimulus may elicit aggressive panic and phantom snapping in some reactive dogs, ES delivered in measured and controllable doses can be effectively used to enhance behavioral control in dogs prone to show aggression in response to direct control or restraint techniques. LLES has been recommended as an adjunct to other behavior-therapy efforts for the control of noncompliant behavior associated with dominance aggression (Borchelt and Voith, 1996). Of course, ES is used only for dogs not likely to escalate aggression in response to such stimulation. ES can be particularly useful in the treatment of location- and object-guarding behavior, providing a highly effective way to compel the dog to relinquish control over some location or object while channeling incompatible safety-seeking behavior toward the trainer. The power of ES to control aggression is probably the result of the dog learning that compliance and cooperation are more effective than aggressive threats and biting as a means of controlling such events. The net result is twofold: (1) a rapid disconfirmation of established prediction-control expectancies and establishing operations mediating aggressive threats and attacks, and (2) the establishment and subsequent confirmation of alternative prediction-control expectancies and establishing operations that promote social behavior incompatible with aggression.

When properly introduced and applied, ES does not typically cause dogs to escalate aggressive behavior, but generally exerts an opposite inhibitory effect. If delivered well in advance of the flash point of no return (see *Proactive versus Preemptive Processing and Cynopraxis* in Chapter 8), the most common effect of contingent ES is to trigger behavioral inhibition and deescalate aggressive arousal. In the context of a comprehensive cynopraxic therapy program, most dogs showing mild to moderate aggression problems appear to become increasingly pacified, relaxed, and cooperative as the result of exposure to radio-controlled training, provided that the preliminary reward-based training and enhancement procedures, as described previously, are carried out by a competent and skilled cynopraxic trainer. In particular, radio-controlled ES or vibrotactile stimulation can be highly effective for the control of intraspecific aggression—especially aggression between dogs sharing the same household. When brief LLES/MLES or vibratory stimulation is applied in a timely manner, such that an incipient threat sequence or juncture responsive to de-escalation is overlapped by the contingent presentation and cessation of ES, the stimulated dog usually shows a pattern of phasic inhibition and attenuation of aggressive arousal, followed by a heightened responsiveness to vocal

command and trainer control efforts. In the context of escalating interdog tensions, ES may cause the provocative dog to emit postural and intentional changes that the target dog may interpret as signifying cutoff or submission, causing both dogs to adopt a motivational shift incompatible with fighting. Many target dogs exhibit an unsettled appearance after observing the unexpected and rapid shift in intent and behavior shown by the stimulated provocator, and appear to be surprised and concerned about the unknown cause of the change. In addition to helping to defuse aggressive tensions between the dogs, the motivational shift (establishing operation) evoked at such times is conducive to the integration of alternative behavior previously acquired in the context of reward-based training. Finally, radio-controlled ES enables a trainer to manage proxemic distances and dynamics between potential adversaries while minimizing the risk of producing adverse interference effects that might otherwise occur as the result of direct interactive control efforts.

Undoubtedly, aversive stimulation can cause certain dogs exhibiting a reactive coping style to respond with fear and escape behavior or even to show autoprotective aggression, especially when escape is barred and the stimulation is perceived as otherwise uncontrollable or extraordinary in terms of threat magnitude. However, under structured and controllable circumstances, ES may also be used to temporarily attenuate or even permanently suppress aggression in dogs (Tortora, 1983). When confronted with an aversive social event, a dog is prone to exhibit a combination of two general coping patterns or *styles*, depending on the severity of the event and the degree of control it perceives to have over the event. Threatening aversive events perceived as lacking controllability tend to preferentially activate the flight-fight system (FFS) and prompt reactive adjustments, whereas safe aversive events perceived as predictable and controllable tend to facilitate adjustments in accord with acquired prediction-control expectancies and calibrated establishing operations, thereby promoting competent and confident adjustments. In safe aversive events, the positive hedonic processing and rewards associated with repeated escape to safety appears to antagonize and countercondition elicited fear stimulated by the event, thereby gradually reducing reactive escape-from-fear adjustments. That aversive events exert variable effects on dogs is consistent with the presence of individual temperament differences and differentiating learning experiences affecting the way dogs cope with and perceive aversive social challenges and threats. Whereas social challenges and threats perceived as such may invigorate aggressive behavior in dogs operating in accord with a reactive coping style, social challenges and threats perceived as safe and controllable tend to promote adjustments conducive to appeasement and reconciliation.

Obviously, significant conflict is apt to occur if the trainer is viewed by the dog as both the source of aversive stimulation and the provider of guidance and safety. Consequently, efficient safety training depends on the dog not linking the e-stimulus with the trainer. When stimulated, the dog should learn to look to the trainer for help while learning to escape and avoid the e-stimulus. In an important sense, the trainer should be perceived as a source of safe guidance to the dog, providing commands, hand signals, conditioned reinforcers, and leash prompts while helping the dog to escape and avoid the aversive event while learning to obtain safety and the comfort of various other rewards controlled by the trainer (e.g., play, massage, petting, and food). Consequently, in addition to reducing aggressive behavior and promoting prosocial behavior, radio-controlled training may enhance attachment dynamics and communication between the trainer and the dog. Finally, insofar as the dog perceives the trainer as a source of safety (relief and relaxation), the trainer may also acquire potent and lasting reward properties (see *Electrical Stimulation and Harm to the Handler-Dog Bond*).

Many types of canine aggression have been described and categorized according to the eliciting situation or motivational states presumed to mediate the threat of attack (see *A Nomenclature of Aggressive Behavior* in Volume 2, Chapter 6). Tortora (1983) has subsumed

several common types of aggressive behavior under the functional category of avoidance learning, suggesting that aggression is often learned as a means to control aversive social situations (see *Avoidance Learning and Aggression* in Volume 2, Chapter 6). According to Tortora's hypothesis, aggression toward people is learned via escape/avoidance (negative reinforcement) conditioning involving stressful or threatening situations. By training a dog to escape or avoid aversive or threatening stimulation with cooperative behavior, avoidance-motivated aggression is gradually replaced with a repertoire of behaviors that are incompatible with reactive opposition and aggression. Learning to successfully escape or avoid aversive stimulation promotes the development of expectancies of safety, further enhancing the dog's ability to cope with adverse social interaction in a more confident and prosocial way.

To achieve this change, Tortora devised a controversial program for rehabilitating aggressive dogs. The protocol focused on training dogs to perform 15 basic obedience exercises (AKC-CDX). The initial training process involved object and interactive play and force training. Training progressed from a continuous schedule of reinforcement, where every correct response was rewarded with play, to an intermittent schedule [variable ratio (VR) 5 and, eventually, VR 15]. Once the 15 exercises selected were under basic control, training with ES commenced. During the training process, the selected exercises were shaped through progressive stages to meet demanding performance criteria. In addition to training on the kennel grounds, the dogs were conditioned to respond reliably under a variety of circumstances:

Sidewalks with pedestrians and traffic
Busy shopping malls
A local shelter with many barking dogs
Household-type environments
A classroom with 20 to 60 students

Escape training was initiated with LLES just sufficient to get the dog's attention but not eliciting fearful behavior. The level of ES was progressively increased during training, until the dogs could tolerate and perform under HLES. As the dogs emitted the appropriate escape response, a safety signal consisting of a tone was immediately presented as the e-stimulus was turned off. The arrangement was designed to establish a conditioned association between the tone and poststimulation relief and relaxation. Poststimulation relief and relaxation serve to positively reinforce escape/avoidance behavior, as well as evoke a state of emotional arousal incompatible with fear. Conditioned stimuli repeatedly paired with the onset of relief and relaxation can gradually acquire the ability independently to elicit similar states of arousal and be employed to countercondition fear. Denny (1983), commenting on Tortora's study, summarized the significance of relief and relaxation in the process of safety training:

> Relief is conceived of as a short latency, autonomic event that lasts only 15 to 20 sec. Relaxation, on the other hand, seems to be a long latency, striate muscle event that requires at least a 2.5-min nonshock period to be effective. Both relaxation and relief are assumed to be effective in making the stimuli associated with a nonshock period positive, or safe, during the acquisition of avoidance and in providing the responses that can compete with fear and help mediate its extinction. According the theory, both relief and relaxation occur automatically with the extended removed of an aversive or well-conditioned aversive stimulus. Nothing else is required. (215)

In addition to establishing a safety signal, a warning vibrotactile buzz (conditioned avoidance stimulus) was presented just after the command. The dogs learned that they could escape ES by quickly performing the required obedience response or what Tortora refers to as an *operand*. With the emission of the target response, the safety signal was delivered for 2 seconds. An avoidance procedure brought the obedience response under the stimulus control of a command. By responding in a timely and correct manner, a dog could avoid ES and produce the positive reinforcement via the safety signal and play. During the avoidance-training phase, progressive improvement was observed in the dogs' performance, even though ES was no longer delivered. Gradually, both the safety tone and periods of play

were placed on an intermittent schedule. As dogs reached this point in the training process, they were exposed to various stress and distraction tests designed to maximize the generalization and transfer of safety training. Dogs were tested for aggressive propensity "under maximally stressful and aggression-inducing circumstances, for example, while the animal was roughly handled and beaten about the body with a rolled-up newspaper or switch" (1983:188). During this phase of testing, failure to comply with obedience commands or the display of aggressive behavior was followed by the delivery of HLES (full intensity). This final stage or *normalization* also involved phasing out the e-collar and transferring the trained behavior to the dog's home environment.

Tortora treated 36 dogs with the foregoing protocol. The reported results are very impressive, with all treated dogs showing a "complete and permanent" cessation of aggressive behavior. Tortora observed a number of other benefits directly attributed to safety training:

> Produces highly durable and reliable compliance responding
> Reduces fear and other stress reactions
> Promotes an appearance of enhanced confidence in the dog

Tortora's work appears to reveal several significant factors in the acquisition and control of aggression in dogs, but the treatment program is rather extreme and may benefit from various refinements and modifications. The general protocol may be made more effective and usable by minimizing aversive stimulation while maximizing the use of positive reinforcement, play, and safety conditioning. The use of full-intensity HLES and other procedures involving provocative and aversive handling of dogs raises significant welfare concerns. Tortora does not demonstrate the necessity of such highly aversive and potentially traumatic experiences for effective safety training. Further, dogs selected for the study were exposed to the same general procedures irrespective of temperament and individual sensitivity differences. The treatment protocol was identical for different dog breeds exhibiting varying behavioral propensities (Saint Bernard, German shepherd, chow chow, Dalmatian, standard poodle, springer spaniel, and Kerry blue terrier, among others). Also, positive reinforcement was limited to the safety signal and an opportunity to play—an activity that is not equally rewarding for all dogs, especially those with a history of aggression. The schedule of intermittent positive reinforcement used to maintain the repertoire of obedience responses was extremely lean— probably unnecessarily so. Perhaps significant benefit and minimization of aversive stimulation could be achieved by presenting food and other rewards on a more dense frequency of reinforcement that incorporates positive prediction error.

Another potential improvement in the protocol would be the use of an olfactory safety signal in combination with or in place of an auditory one. In contrast to the 2-second safety tone paired with relief following the termination of aversive stimulation, an olfactory stimulus (e.g., dilute lavender or chamomile) can form an association with the more sluggishly recruited relaxation responses, as well. In addition, the incorporation of vocal praise and encouragement with petting and massage would provide another form of constructive safe stimulation to pair with relief, perhaps helping to enhance relaxation and establishing more positive associations with human contact. An advantage of conditioning voice and tactile stimuli as safety signals is the ease with which they can be generalized and transferred to everyday activities in a dog's home environment. The benefit of pairing a sustained olfactory stimulus or set of social stimuli with both relief and relaxation may be significant for the maximization of the benefits of safety training and the promotion of trust between the dog and the trainer. Denny (1983) notes, in his comments regarding Tortora's report, that conditioned safety effects are doubled when the safety stimulus is paired with both relief and relaxation. Given the central significance of the safety signal in the safety-training protocol outlined previously, it is odd that the e-collar is gradually faded out and eventually removed from a dog altogether as part of the final normalization phase of training. Removing the collar from the dog appears highly problematic, because the delivery of the safety signal depends on the collar to deliver the requisite conditioned tone. This loss of signaling capability seems inconsistent with the repeated emphasis and importance placed on the safety signal for reducing fear and aggression and its value as a source of positive reinforcement for compliant behavior. In contrast, olfactory, vocal, and tactile conditioned safety signals would avoid such difficulties, perhaps enhancing the process of generalization and transfer, as well. Despite the apparent effectiveness of safety training for the treatment of aggression in dogs, the protocol has attracted little interest and, to my knowledge, has not been experimentally replicated, although safety training using ES offers many potentially beneficial applications in canine behavior therapy.

Electrical Stimulation and Chasing Behavior

Another common application of ES in dog training is the control of chasing and predatory behavior. The radio-controlled and behavior-activated delivery of ES has been proven effective for suppressing predatory behavior in dogs, coyotes, and wolves (see *Electronic Training and Wildlife Conservation*). For example, Andelt and colleagues (1999) at the National Wildlife Research Center's Predator Research Facility (Logan, Utah) found that HLES rapidly suppressed coyote predatory behavior toward lambs. Even when ES was delivered during attack, the researchers reported immediate suppression and no evidence of escalation or increased aggressiveness. In Norway, Christiansen and colleagues (2001a) evaluated the use of remote electronic training for suppressing canine predatory behavior toward sheep. The study period was 2 years and involved 114 dogs, consisting of three breeds: Norwegian elkhounds (35), English setters (56), and hare-hunting dogs (23). The dogs were administered a 1-second pulse of ES when they approached within 1 to 2 meters of sheep confined to a pen. The researchers found that a lasting suppression of predatory behavior was produced by the protocol (Christiansen et al., 2001b). After a year, only one dog that received ES training continued to attack sheep. The effect showed significant generalization to ordinary circumstances, with approximately 75% of the owners of trained dogs reporting that their dogs no longer showed an interest in sheep. Similarly, Stichnoth (2002) has demonstrated that the chase and hunting behavior of beagles can be rapidly suppressed with the aid of radio-controlled ES, without producing evidence of cardiovascular distress or physiological stress. As an adjunct to reward-based training efforts, radio-controlled ES can also be used to rapidly and effectively suppress the chasing of cats and other animals by dogs. Despite ample evidence that ES works effectively to control chasing and predatory behavior, organizations such as the Companion Animal Behavior Therapy Study Group (CABTSG) continue to suggest otherwise, but without offering any substantive research to backup their emotional convictions and charges of harm and ineffectiveness (CABTSG, 2003). In addition, they suggest that other methods are currently available that have been proven to provide better control and management of such problems, but fail to identify a method or offer a single citation referring to the powerful methods of control in question. Instead, they vent an emotionally charged diatribe of speculation that is largely contradicted by the prior research previously discussed.

Several advantages are derived from the radio-controlled application of aversive stimulation for the control of behavior problems associated with chasing behavior: It provides an exact level of stimulation, can be precisely timed and delivered at a distance, and helps to generalize training to situations in which the owner is absent. With a proper foundation of positive training in place, radio-controlled electrical or spray (e.g., citronella spray) stimulation offers a highly effective means to inhibit the territorial chase response in resistant dogs. Although electronic training can effectively deter persistent chasing behavior in dogs, the use of spray stimulation or ES should be considered only after a careful assessment and pre-

liminary training have been carried out. Once preliminary training has been performed, electronic training can help to enhance the reliability of inhibitory control.

Initially, the dog is exposed to recall training on a long line, with electronic training introduced only after the dog attains 90% reliability. The dog should be trained to orient to its name and halt forward movement in response to the command "Stay" spoken assertively. The orienting response can be effectively conditioned with LLES, whereas the inhibitory halt response may require a higher level of momentary stimulation to reach reliability. Electronic training should be combined with a conditioned stimulus (e.g., whistle or throw rings). By blowing a whistle or tossing a set of throw rings close to the dog immediately before and contiguous with the electrical event, a strong inhibitory association can be rapidly established. After pairing the throw rings with the e-stimulus, the jingling sound will produce a strong inhibitory response, providing an effective means to generalize a conditioned suppressive effect. Prior to every ES event, the throw rings are flipped once in the hand. The rings should be thrown only if the dog ignores the warning and requires remote stimulation. The throw rings need not strike the dog, but should bounce near enough to produce an impression. During the early stages of electronic training, the dog should be kept on a long line to ensure that the appropriate response is given during ES and to prevent unanticipated problems.

ELECTRONIC TRAINING AND WILDLIFE CONSERVATION

In addition to select dog-training and behavior-therapy applications, electronic training devices may play a significant future role in the management of wildlife, particularly tracking and deterrence systems used to protect endangered species or livestock from predation. Several studies have used radio-controlled or behavior-activated collar systems for predator control. For example, conservationists working in California found that foxes living on San Clemente Island preyed on nestling loggerhead shrikes (*Lanius ludovi-*

cianus mearnsi), a severely endangered bird species living on the island. Wildlife biologists affiliated with the Institute for Wildlife Studies (2000) employed an ordinary electronic dog-containment system to deter fox predation on shrike nestlings. Whenever the collar-equipped foxes came too close to the shrike nests, an electrical shock was delivered, thereby protecting the nestling shrikes from harm and training the foxes to avoid the nests. The technique of electrical deterrence was studied as an alternative to lethal control that would have been otherwise necessary to protect the shrikes from further decimation.

A similar effort to develop a predator-deterrence system has been launched by the U.S. Fish and Wildlife Service (USFWS) and U.S. Department of Agriculture (USDA) Wildlife Services, with the cooperation and support of the University of Montana and prominent wildlife conservationist groups. The objective of the study, under the scientific direction of John Shivik (USDA Wildlife Services), is to explore the efficacy of aversive electrical conditioning to control undesirable predation by wolves. Wolves that prey on domestic animals are often killed when other means of control fail. Four wolves suspected of repeated attacks on cattle were captured north of Gardner, Montana. The controversial experiment consisted of fitting the three surviving wolves (one of them, an adult female, died while in captivity) with containment dog-training collars and penning them with a calf fitted with an approach-activated transmitter. When wolves wearing radio-controlled collars approached the calf too closely, a brief tone stimulus was followed by the delivery of an ES producing "discomfort but not pain" (Bangs, 2000c). Successful deterrence has been reported with coyotes fitted with e-collars. Attack-contingent ES quickly conditioned coyotes to avoid attacking lambs that were placed in their pens (Andelt et al., 1999). Treated coyotes were exposed to the highest level of stimulation produced by the Tri-Tronics Model 100 Lite (325 pulses/second of 600 to 640 V at about 32 mA). The coyotes rapidly acquired a lasting avoidance of sheep that continued for several months after treatment without intervening electrical reinforcement.

Besides investigating the efficacy of aversive control on livestock predation, the researchers hope to learn whether treated wolves will desist from predation on cattle once the wolves are released into the wild and transmit the aversion as a tradition to other wolves subsequently raised by the pack. According to Bangs, the Wolf Recovery Coordinator for the USFWS, researchers in the former USSR (Republic of Georgia) successfully conditioned wolves with dog collars to avoid livestock when released from captivity. In addition, future generations of wolves learned through cultural transmission from the behavior of conditioned wolves to avoid livestock as prey animals. Research with dogs has not produced very promising results in this regard (Christiansen et al., 2001c). Sheep-chasing dogs paired with sheep-avoidant dogs (previously exposed to ES) showed an initial reduction in chase incentive but over time exhibited an increasing tendency to chase and attack sheep independently.

In the ongoing wolf experiment, preliminary results suggest that wolves may rapidly acquire an aversion toward calves as the result of approach-activated ES (Bangs, 2000a). One wolf that approached a calf hide with a transmitter placed on it was apparently stimulated, because it jumped back from the hide and avoided contact with it in the future. Other pack members watching the stimulated wolf's reaction seemed to have also acquired an avoidance response by observation. None of the three wolves subsequently approached the calf hide after the frightening incident. Further, avoidance behavior toward the calf hide appears to have generalized to live calves, at least temporarily. Calves were repeatedly left alone with the wolves, with one young calf spending a night in the wolf pen without evidence of molestation. It remains uncertain whether the avoidance is the result of predatory inhibition resulting from nervousness associated with close confinement or the result of the single (known) exposure to ES. Whatever the cause, the inhibition was not permanent, since the wolf that had been previously stimulated did finally attack a calf. Unfortunately, the collar either malfunctioned or the electrodes failed to reach the skin through the wolf's thick fur. Subsequently, the collar was repositioned for better contact with the skin, evidently correcting the problem, since a November update (Bangs, 2000b) noted that the calf now could follow or chase the wolves around the pen, having apparently learned to use the power afforded by its collar transmitter.

The use of conventional containment-type collars for predator deterrence is thwarted by significant design and operational problems. The long-term use of collars delivering ES through metal electrodes making direct contact with the skin is prone to produce skin irritations, gradually resulting in necrotic lesions and infection. Another problem with such devices is the need to change or recharge batteries periodically—a problem that might be solved by incorporating a miniature solar-recharging system integrated into the strap of the collar. The problems associated with the electrode-skin interface might be addressed by a high-voltage collar with the ability to arc through the fur barrier or by an e-collar equipped with electrodes that are only momentarily brought into close contact with the skin through a servomechanism activated at the time of stimulation.

ELECTRICAL STIMULATION AND WORKING DOGS: A SHOCKING STUDY

Electrical stimulation is frequently used in the context of training working dogs, aiding the trainer in establishing reliable control over highly motivated and potentially dangerous behavior. Schilder and Van der Borg (2004) have published a report of disturbing findings regarding the short-term and long-term effects of shock used in the context of training working dogs that is destined to become a source of significant controversy. The authors arrived at their conclusions after observing several training sessions and analyzing video records of Dutch handlers preparing dogs for IPO [Internationale Prüfungs Ordnung (International Examination Rules)] certification. The authors report that they observed 32 dogs receiving 106 shocks delivered by a radio-controlled collar. In addition, they combined the results of comparisons between 31 German shepherd dogs divided into shocked and nonshock groups, with 16 dogs (14 males and 2 females) receiving shock and 15 (12 males and 3 females) not receiving shock during training. The main differences observed between dogs receiving ES and those receiving other forms of correction included an altered ear posture detected during obedience work and free walking, tongue flicking (appeasement licking) during protection work, and submissive pawing actions during obedience work.

Electrical Stimulation and Harm to the Handler-Dog Bond

According to the authors, even brief and infrequent shocks may be perceived as traumatic by dogs, causing them emotional harm and permanent social fear. The notion that Dutch working dogs might have become fearful of their handlers as the result of shocks received in training is reported as an obvious fact that is never actually tested, leaving it to the reader to accept the speculation "as fact" or not. In practice, dogs do not appear to link ES with the handler, especially persons with whom the dog is closely attached and familiar. In fact, the most interesting uses of the collar depend on this lack of aversive association, including lasting reward and opponent safety effects (Denny, 1991). Interestingly, the IPO system has devised a good behavioral test for detecting mishandling and abuse. Surely, if an IPO dog had developed a fear or aversion toward its handler as the result of electrical training, the following IPO Watchdog Test [WH (Wachhunde Certificate)] requirement would likely reveal it, causing a great many dogs to fail if they were treated as badly as alleged by the present report:

Devotion to the Handler (10 pts)

The dog is put on lead and handed over to a second person. The handler then proceeds toward a group of people who are standing about 80 paces away. The dog is allowed to watch the departure of his handler until the handler has gone about 30 paces of the distance. At this point, the dog is taken behind a wall or similar structure so that his handler is no longer visible to him.

> When the handler arrives at the group, he walks into the center of the group and stops. While he is in the group, the handler may not make himself noticeable to the dog across from him. The dog is released from the lead by the second person. The behavior of the dog, especially the use of the nose, is to be observed during this exercise. When the dog has found his handler, he is to be praised. (Frawley, 2003)

If the electrical and physical stimulation during protection work were truly traumatic and stressful, one would expect that the traumatized dog might be apt to flee at the first instant it got a chance. Further, one would expect that its willingness to bite and hold the sleeve ought to decrease in proportion to the amount of fear and pain it experienced (e.g., causing the dog to come off the sleeve too early or not to bite as hard) or that the dog might even show signs of avoidance and fear toward the agitator. However, no such loss of drive or performance is reported. In fact, Dutch dogs are renowned for their hardness, work enthusiasm, and acrobatic attacks—attributes that are opposite to what one would expect from training that was overly stressful. With increased biological stress, as in sickness, one would expect to observe a drive-reducing effect on aggression and a loss of voluntary initiative, whereas increased fear should tend to suppress behavior rather than enhance it. The absence of reduced drive or behavioral suppression with respect to critical activities associated with shock (e.g., bite work) makes one skeptical about the lasting adverse effects that the authors claim to document. Although they offer no substantive evidence of trauma or harm to the dogs, they provide loads of speculation, anecdotes, insinuations of gender and educational inadequacies, and derogatory comments regarding the motivation and competence of IPO trainers in its place.

Most scientific evidence supports the notion that the cessation of aversive ES in the context of escape/avoidance training is more likely to enhance social attraction, promote feelings of safety, and calm a dog rather than make a dog afraid or apprehensive. These secondary effects of shock termination and pain reduction have long been recognized to promote conditioned and unconditioned effects conducive to reward and safety (see *Electrical Stimulation Controllability and Safety*). Instead of instilling social aversion and anxiety as suggested by the authors, competent electronic training may actually promote social attachment, reward, and safety. With the behavior-contingent cessation or avoidance of ES, dogs experience immediate emotional relief that subsequently merges into a state of progressive relaxation incompatible with social aversion and fear—a sequence of opponent emotional effects contrary to those alleged to occur in the case of working dogs exposed to ES in the context of training.

The opponent effects of relief and relaxation on social behavior are exemplified in a series of controversial experiments that used shock to promote desirable social behavior in profoundly autistic children. Lovaas and colleagues (1965) at the University of California, Los Angeles, used ES and its contingent termination to facilitate the expression of increased approach and affectionate behavior based on the following hypothesis:

> Any stimulus which is associated with or discriminative of pain reduction acquires *positive* reinforcing (rewarding) properties, i.e., an organism will work to "obtain" stimuli which have been associated with pain reduction. The action of such stimuli is analogous to that of stimuli whose positive reinforcing properties derive from primary positive reinforcers. (99)

The first of these experiments involved placing a child with pervasive emotional and social deficits between two experimenters who faced each other from a distance of 3 feet. Whomever the child faced encouraged him to approach closer with outstretched and gesticulating arms, saying "Come on" as a painful electrical current was delivered to the child's bare feet via strips of metal tape applied to the floor. If the child hesitated longer than 3 seconds, he was pushed forward into the beckoning arms of the "saving" experimenter by the other "helping" experimenter located behind the child. As the child moved in the direction of the experimenter, the shock stimulus was immediately terminated. In addition to rewarding social behavior via an escape to safety, the shock stimulus was contingently applied to suppress tantrums and self-stimulatory behavior. According to the authors, the experiment was highly successful, with the children (identical 5-year-old twins) subsequently exhibiting improved alertness, increased social approach behavior, and more affectionate behavior to the experimenters—changes that lasted for 9 months without any additional aversive stimulation. The boys also exhibited a significant decrease in tantrum and self-stimulatory behavior stemming from the contingent application of shock, and this changed behavior continued for 11 months without additional training. In another experiment involving these same twins, a radio-controlled stimulator (Lee-Lectronic Trainer) was fastened to a belt and situated so that the electrodes made contact with the child's buttocks. Affectionate social contact (kissing and hugging) was encouraged by the experimenter, who faced the child and bowed in his direction, saying "Kiss me" or "Hug me." If the child, who was held fast at the waist, failed to kiss the experimenter or hug him, a medium-level shock was delivered via radio control. As the result of the foregoing procedure, the boys were rapidly trained to kiss or hug the experimenter on cue. In a third study again with these same twins, the researchers evaluated the effects of shock reduction and safety in terms of acquired reward properties associated with the experimenter. As the result of an association established between the experimenter, pain reduction, and successful escape to safety, the presence of the experimenter became a significant source of reward for the children, as quantified by lever-pressing behavior whereby the children were given brief contact with the experimenter contingent upon performance of the lever-pressing task. The authors conclude with the following remarks regarding the apparent beneficial effects of contingent shock escape/avoidance and pain reduction:

> It seems likely that the most therapeutic use of shock will not lie primarily in the suppression of specific responses or the shaping of behavior through escape-avoidance training. Rather, it would seem more efficient to use shock reduction as a way of establishing social reinforcers,

i.e., as a way of making adults meaningful in the sense of becoming rewarding to the child ... Once social stimuli acquire reinforcing properties, one of the basic conditions for the acquisition of social behaviors has been met. (108)

These theoretical and experimental findings have been repeatedly validated in the context of formal obedience training, where dogs initially showing profound social inhibitions and fears become increasingly affectionate, confident, flexible, interactive, and playful in association with directive training (see *Electrical Stimulation Controllability and Safety*). Despite a significant amount of aversive stimulation used in the context of traditional dog training, dogs exposed to such training typically acquire a heightened level of affection toward the trainer, who is usually treated as a social reward object. The petting and praise that are strongly emphasized in such systems of training mediate significant reward, perhaps as the result of a similar paradoxical effect in response to pain reduction and the successful escape/avoidance (safety) of aversive collar stimulation and physical force, paralleling the findings of Lovaas and colleagues.

Fisher (1955) exposed several groups of puppies to different rearing conditions consisting of variable amounts of environmental enrichment, social contact, punishment, isolation, and control over aversive events. From around week 3 to week 15, one group of puppies [enriched (E)] were given 30 minutes of daily exposure to various sources of environmental and social stimulation, receiving consistent friendly handling by the experimenter, and were never punished. Another group of puppies [ambivalent (A)] were given 30 minutes of similarly permissive and playful environmental and social stimulation followed by 30 minutes of repeated punishment, consisting primarily of manhandling and hitting with a switch. During the punishment period, whenever a puppy attempted to approach the experimenter or another puppy, it was punished. The puppy was also punished if it explored the test area or played in the experimenter's presence. When receiving physical punishment, the puppy could flee to the safety of a hiding place but was often removed from there and punished more. Electric shock (via a 50-V dry-cell battery regulated by potentiometer) was used to punish social approach behavior within a small inescapable compartment. The shock punishment was delivered to the puppies' feet under two conditions: (1) whenever two puppies approached each other within the compartment and (2) after a puppy approached an experimenter coaxing it from outside the compartment. Two other groups were kept isolated, except that one group of isolates [punished (P)] was also treated roughly and exposed to the daily punishment treatment as group A; the other group of isolates remained in their cages until final testing. During subsequent testing at weeks 12 and 13, four of the six puppies exposed to the pattern of indulgence and punishment appeared to view the experimenter as an enhanced source of reward and security, spending significantly more time in close proximity with the experimenter than did indulged puppies. However, two of the puppies exposed to the combined indulgence and punishment treatment showed a strong avoidance of the experimenter indicative of aversion, suggesting that individual differences of a genetic origin may affect the way dogs respond to such treatment (see Freedman, 1958). Interestingly, the indulged-punished group showed a significant reduction in general activity and exploratory behavior and reacted more intensely toward extraneous noises and movements than did the consistently indulged group, perhaps indicative of a lowered startle threshold toward novelty. As such, aversive procedures used in the training of working dogs may promote strong one-person bonds and facilitate a desire to please via an acquired perception of the trainer as enhanced source of social reward and an increased alertness and reactivity for novelty and change consistent with the necessary preemptive readiness and social wariness of working dogs toward strangers.

Ambiguous Social Behavior: A Sign of Stress or an Enhanced Readiness to Submit and Obey?

Instead of instilling social aversion and anxiety as suggested by the authors, the foregoing animal and human research supports the notion that competent electronic training appears to promote positive social attachment, safety, and reward effects that may be provided and amplified via affectionate petting and reassuring praise. The preponderance of scientific evidence suggests that ES escape/avoidance and pain reduction should promote long-term effects that are incompatible with fear and stress, making the trainer an object of significant extrinsic reward that actually enhances the dog's welfare via an improved capacity for social coping, learning, and adaptation. Evidently, many of the shocks delivered by the handlers were far from traumatic experiences for the dogs, since the authors had to double-check with them to confirm the actual number of shocks received by the dogs. The following passage makes clear that the handlers probably used shock in a measured and contingent way that provided the dogs with significant behavioral control:

> The durations of most reactions to shocks were immeasurably short, possibly due to the fact that dogs were asked to obey some command or take some action immediately afterwards. (321)

From the foregoing description, it appears that ES was applied in a manner that met controllability standards, further making the attribution of stress and welfare harm resulting from electronic training seem more like an unfounded accusation than a scientific conclusion. Assuming that the handlers used both momentary and continuous levels of stimulation, the evidence also suggests that the dogs did not respond to longer durations of shock as being particularly painful; that is, the initial "immeasurably" brief reactions appear to indicate startle, a psychological response, but not reactive sequelae indicative of traumatic pain. In any case, for most dogs, the apparent enjoyment derived from the protection-training process itself far exceeds the periodic penalties that occur while learning how to play the "attack game" in accord with appropriate rules. Furthermore, once critical limits and fair-play rules are set via inhibitory conditioning (e.g., all-stop, stop-change, and go/no go), the social and play rewards associated with the activity itself should exert potent counterconditioning effects, thereby further reducing any secondary aversive emotional conditioning effects arising from inhibitory conditioning with shock. These various bits of circumstantial evidence conflict with the allegations that shock, as used by IPO trainers, promotes social fear, stress, and represents a serious threat of harm to the long-term welfare of trained dogs.

The ambiguous social behaviors that the authors represent as markers of fear and stress have been previously investigated and interpreted differently elsewhere (Beera et al., 1998). In that work, distinctions are drawn between behavioral indicators of fear, stress, and submission evoked by a moderately strong shock in comparison to other sources of startling stimulation. The researchers found that a robust cortisol release was produced by nonsocial fear-eliciting stimuli (e.g., electrical shock and blast of a nautical horn), however, provocative handling and startle (e.g., repeated physical restraint and opening an umbrella) in a social context produced negligible cortisol secretion. Significantly with respect to the behavioral correlations of the present study, they learned that nonsocial aversive stimulation, such as shock, produced a relative absence of oral behaviors (e.g., lip licking and tongue flicking). These previous findings suggest that activation of the HPA system occurs predominantly in response to nonsocial aversive events, whereas aversive stimulation occurring in a social context tends to produce precursor submission behaviors (intention movements) with a relative absence of concomitant biological stress. These findings are consistent with a motivational partition between stressful fear elicited by nonsocial aversive stimuli and submission behaviors evoked by social challenges and threats (startle), perhaps via a modulating effect of person. Whereas the increased oral behaviors and postural changes shown by laboratory dogs were previously interpreted as signifying an increased readiness to submit, these same behaviors now, as exhibited by working dogs toward their handlers, are characterized in an entirely different light, with the present authors now arguing that such

oral behaviors and changes in posture and gesture implicate fear and aversion toward the handler as the result of receiving shock in the handler's presence.

A substantial body of prior research has also shown that the critical factor affecting adverse stress and welfare parameters is the relative control that the dog has over the delivery of appetitive and aversive events. Despite this prior work regarding the important linkage established between event uncontrollability and stress, no effort was made by the authors of the present report to sort out the effects of controllable versus uncontrollable ES. Nevertheless, the dogs in the present study appear to adequately learn to control the electrical event, and since there is no significant evidence reported that suggests that the dogs suffered a loss of biological fitness or physical or mental harm due to ES, there is little justification for the use of the term "stress" to describe the present findings, especially so since prior evidence shows that contingent and controllable ES delivered by a radio-controlled collar in the context of dog training produces negligible immediate or lasting biological stress per cardiovascular and HPA-axis markers (Stichnoth, 2002).

If one defines *welfare* as "The state of an individual as regards its attempts to cope with its environment" (Broom and Johnson, 1993:1978), one might even argue that contingent ES probably exerts a long-term beneficial influence on the dog's welfare insofar as it enhances its efforts to acquire an adaptive coping style. Finally, if the behavioral differences attributed to shock in the handler's presence are interpreted in a manner consistent with the observations of Beerda and colleagues (1998), one arrives at an entirely different set of implications. Instead of indicating the presence of stress and fear, the slight lowering of posture, oral behaviors, and increased paw lifting are now viewed as precursor submission behaviors expressed in the context of coping successfully with an aversive social event. Consequently, if one accepts the behavioral changes described by the authors at face value, all that one might fairly conclude is that ES, in the context of obedience and bite work, generally establishes effective inhibitory control over target behaviors (e.g., bite release) while enhancing the dog's readiness to defer to handler command and control, as indicated by the presence of increased precursor submission behaviors.

In conclusion, contingent ES at the levels normally used in competent dog training is not intrinsically stressful or a threat to a dog's welfare and may be highly beneficial to the extent that it promotes adaptive behavioral change and improved coping skills (see *Stress, Distress, and Potential Adverse Side Effects of Electrical Stimulation*).

Is Physical Traumatization and Manhandling Really Better Than Shock?

The authors appear comfortable with the idea that "beatings and other harsh punishments, such as kicks or choke collar corrections" are somehow preferable to shock, since dogs exposed to such treatment do not show presumptive behavioral signs of stress and lasting fear that they claim occur from brief and contingent ES. Regardless of how one feels about the use of dogs for police and military work or dog training in general, implying that beating or kicking a dog is in some way preferable to brief ES is simply wrongheaded and makes no sense from a training or welfare perspective. Further, placing a slip-collar or prong-collar correction in the same category as beating or kicking a dog reflects a profound lack of knowledge and appreciation of the training process and how such devices are used to achieve training objectives. Many dog trainers on both sides of the e-collar controversy have struggled for decades to refine the training process into the humane and sophisticated art that it has become today, only to have it mandated that manhandling and brutalization are not a significant threat to a dog's welfare. There is no need for complicated statistics to demonstrate adequately that harshly striking a dog can exert potent and lasting adverse social and emotional effects that significantly impair its capacity to function and cope effectively, as amply demonstrated by Solomon and colleagues (1968). Abusive hitting and manhandling can also exert variable long-term developmental impairments of social behavior

dependent on individual differences and rearing histories (Fisher, 1955; Freedman, 1958).

Construing that physical abuse might be less of a threat to the welfare of working dogs than is a brief dose of harmless ES is simply bewildering and impossible to take seriously. The notion that dogs might be better off getting choked, beaten, and kicked rather than receiving contingent ES makes absolutely no sense and is contradicted by common practical experience. In dog training, not only is the e-stimulus precisely defined in terms of duration and intensity, it can be delivered and stopped with precision, with very little generalization (if any) to the handler, producing minimal signs of discomfort or subsequent distress to the dog and no sign of physical trauma. ES has the added benefit of hundreds of experimental learning studies involving dogs and other species, providing a comprehensive knowledge base for its use as a training tool. In addition to the slip, prong, and halter collars, a wide range of electronic training devices are recognized by the *Professional Standards for Dog Trainers* (Delta Society, 2001) as effective and humane tools of the trade. Along with radio-controlled electrical and spray collars, bark-activated and containment devices are included in the standard and treated as professional equipment for the control and improvement of dog behavior.

Methodological Concerns and Recommendations

Methodological aspects of the present contribution to the dog welfare literature are disturbing and deserving of further attention. The first of these concerns is the woeful lack of appropriate controls to limit experimenter bias and assumptions concerning the use of aversives in dog training. Neither of the authors openly acknowledge a prejudice or bias for or against electronic training, but the authors clearly bring to the study some established negative beliefs about the subject matter, as evident in the first line of the introduction, where electronic training is lumped together with beatings and other means that cause "wounds, pain and mental harm" (320) to dogs. Later in the text, they also link "choke collar corrections" with kicking, beating, and other "harsh punishments" (332), raising further concerns about the authors' knowledge and understanding of the dog-training process and the tools used by practical dog trainers. Schilder has previously urged that the *only* legitimate use of an e-collar is for suppressing predatory behavior (sheep killing) (*Applied Ethology Listserve*, September 20, 1996, 07:27:00.30), making the conclusions and recommendations of the present study appear somewhat like a foregone conclusion.

Despite the presence of obvious negative convictions toward dog training in general and electronic training in particular, the researchers took no measures to blind themselves to experimental and control groups, raising reasonable concerns about experimenter bias entering into the data collection process and post hoc treatments, which should necessarily be regarded as tainted and suspect. Further, the experimenters interacted with the trainers in ways that may have influenced them, thereby raising the possibility that a subtle element of participant bias had been introduced into the study. For example, to establish an accurate frequency of shock, they asked trainers how many times they had shocked their dogs. Aside from potentially making the handlers self-conscious about the number of shocks they delivered or, perhaps, causing them to increase or decrease the frequency of stimulation, such questioning may have caused some of them to deliver stronger levels of stimulation than might ordinarily be used in order to make the effects of shock more apparent to the observers. Several other potential participant bias effects might have easily slipped into the experiment as a consequence of handler interrogations regarding the frequency of the independent variable.

Although one might seriously doubt that any group of self-respecting trainers will ever again make themselves available for such a study, one possible way to perform blind and fair studies would be to have all the dogs wear an e-collar or a dummy collar. In addition, the experimenters might remain behind a blind while team assistants make video recordings of relevant training activities for later analysis. Once the training session is over, subsequent observations might then be made without the observers knowing which dogs were exposed to the independent variable. The experimenters manipulating and performing post hoc analyses of the collected data might only be permitted to see tapes and coded information in which the actual moment of stimulation is blocked from view, and an equal amount of video block is yoked to control dogs not receiving stimulation, thereby providing further precautions against bias. If a significant effect consistent with the hypothesis exists, the researchers should be able to identify it through observational and statistical means alone without knowing which dogs actually received the shocks. If correlations between particular behaviors and biological stress are of interest, in addition to observational data, relevant biological data should be collected at critical times before, during, and after the training session. In addition to obtaining salivary samples, temperature and real-time heart-rate measurements should be taken. By collecting various biological data before the e-collar is worn, while it is worn, and after it is removed, potentially significant within-subject effects might be identified and linked to associative learning resulting from ES. With a baseline of such relevant information, meaningful correlations between behavioral signs and biological stress might then be possible to establish. In the absence of biological markers, the attribution of significance to ambiguous or ambivalent behaviors presumed to index harmful stress struggles for footing at every step before collapsing, as it were, for lack of evidence.

Despite numerous variables affecting the quality, quantity, and subjective experience and potential harm of the e-stimulus, the authors make no effort to collect relevant data concerning the intensity or duration of the shock used by the handlers—variables that would significantly enrich the statistical analysis. The independent variable (ES) is treated as a constant of several thousand volts—a relatively meaningless open-circuit measure of electrical potential that is equivalent to the shock produced after scuffing one's feet on a carpet. In general, they treat shock as though any amount were bad, analogous to asserting that the toxic effect of taking one capsule of phenobarbital is equivalent to taking a full bottle. They repeatedly emphasize that such devices produce stress, but provide no evidence that ES in the context of dog training overtaxes biobehavioral control systems or harms a dog's biological fitness in any way, making the use of the term "stress" seem unwarranted (Broom and Johnson, 1993). The data in the present study are derived from a mean of three shocks of an unknown duration and intensity. To extract the subtle causal relations that the authors attribute to ES from such limited exposure to a vaguely defined electrical event seems a daunting challenge further complicating the process of sorting out cause-and-effect relations between shock and the specific changes in behavior that are attributed to it. Given the demonstrated fortitude and resilience of dogs to hundreds of repeated shocks under laboratory conditions and protocols resembling torture (see *Stress, Traumatic Avoidance, and Laboratory Conditioning with Shock*), it is highly suspicious indeed that working dogs, bred for hardness and drive, would fall victim to lasting harm as the result of receiving three or so shocks during training. If true as reported, the real news in this study is not the effects of ES, but the constitutional weakness of Dutch working dogs. How dogs cope with ES and other forms of aversive stimulation is largely determined by individual differences of a genetic nature and the relative controllability of the events (Corson et al., 1973) (see *Electrical Stimulation Controllability and Safety*).

The authors suggest that a goal of their study was to determine the short-term and long-term effects of shocks, yet they fail to provide any data relevant to the determination of long-term effects. The short-term differences between the two groups in the present study were derived from averaged scores obtained by one-zero sampling at various times relative to some significant interactive event between the dog and handler (e.g., at 1 minute into free walking, they assessed tail, body, and ear positions; and, during obedience exercises, tail and ear positions were graded 3 seconds after the command; whereas other behaviors were graded 10 seconds after

the command) and context. One might wonder what the results would have looked like if the sampling occurred after 2 minutes of free walking rather than 1 minute. Also, what would the results look like if a 3-second delay were used to sample target behaviors after the command in the aforementioned situations. For example, dogs stimulated 2 minutes prior to the observation window will likely show very different behavior from dogs stimulated 30 minutes prior to observation.

The small sample size, lack of controls for the effects of age (Beerda et al., 2000), interindividual differences and polymorphisms (Van der Berg et al., 2003), individual variations affecting stress proneness (see Vincent and Michell, 1996), and possible prior exposure to electrical training make the comparisons between shocked and nonshocked dogs statistically weak. Although the authors made some effort to match the shocked and nonshocked groups roughly in terms of breed and sex, controlling for the effects of age was completely neglected. This is not a minor point, because Beerda and colleagues (2000) had previously shown that socially ambiguous (nonspecific) displacement behaviors (e.g., increased licking) are strongly correlated with the dog's age. Despite an intimate familiarity with these earlier findings, the authors provide no information concerning the age of the dogs and apparently made no effort to control for this potentially significant source of error. The authors treat the presence of ambiguous social behaviors as an established behavioral index of stress, but, in fact, no such validated stress index exists.

The inventory of behaviors that the authors have identified in the present report as indicators of fear and stress have not been disambiguated under natural conditions, nor have they proven to be very reliable as markers of stress in the context of laboratory investigation. Ogburn and colleagues (1998) found that dogs wearing halters that clamp around the nose showed marked postural and behavioral differences (e.g., lowered head and ears back) indicative of fear and subordination in comparison to dogs wearing flat collars, who appeared more excited and difficult to control. Dogs restrained by halters also engaged in significantly more biting at and fighting against the leash and exhibited a higher level of pawing. While wearing a halter, dogs appeared to avoid looking at the handler during obedience training, suggesting an adverse motivational effect on social engagement not present in the case of dogs wearing a strap collar. Despite these relatively robust postural and behavior changes indicative of distress, physiological testing for sympathetic arousal and markers of stress showed no significant difference between dogs wearing halters and dogs wearing flat collars. The tests performed included measurement of blood pressure and heart rate, respiration rates, and pupillary dilation, as well as ACTH and cortisol levels. These prior findings significantly conflict with the notion that such behaviors are markers of stress that represent a serious threat to a dog's welfare. Further, Beerda and colleagues (2000) have explicitly warned against the use nonspecific displacement behaviors for indexing stress. This previous work acknowledged a danger of misinterpretation when one draws conclusions regarding stress from the presence of ambiguous social behaviors, giving rise to a curious violation of the law of noncontradiction: "Because stress behavior is rather variable and often nonspecific to stress, it is readily misinterpreted" (60). The foregoing is a muddled proposition. A collection or set of behaviors cannot be logically classified as simultaneously belonging to and not belonging to the defining category or class. Insofar as *stress* is not functionally present in some instance of behavior, that particular instance is not an example of *stress behavior* but a behavior with functional characteristics exemplifying another class. The hypothetical set consisting of behaviors classified as *nonspecific* to stress with respect to the class of behaviors such that stress is a defining characteristic would necessarily be an empty one. Although a behavior may belong to more than one class or category, insofar as it possesses complex functional or descriptive characteristics appropriate to the inclusion and exclusion criteria of each classification (e.g., both offensive and defensive aggression are types of aggressive behavior), claiming that the behavior in question is nonspecific (that is, it simultaneously

belongs and yet does not belong to one or the other category) would necessitate a third category (e.g., panic aggression). Finally, there are experimentally established ways for developing behavioral and physiological indices of stress, fear, and pain (see Broom and Johnson, 1993) that should be performed and rigorously validated before they are experimentally applied and used to justify a call for intrusive legislation. Traumatized puppies and dogs appear to show lowered startle thresholds and intensified startle responses, making tests evaluating prestimulation and poststimulation startle parameters a potentially useful index for evaluating the short-term effects of fear. Startle tests might also provide useful means for evaluating long-term fear effects in combination with physiological indicators of an impaired capacity to cope adaptively.

To increase the likelihood of extracting viable correlations from their data, the authors excluded behaviors that occurred in less than 50% of the dogs. While such a method might help to increase the likelihood of getting results, such post hoc manipulations also significantly reduce statistical power. Further, how can one be sure that this selection process is performed in evenhandedly? One obvious problem with the procedure is that certain traits that may have contributed to the selection of those dogs receiving electronic training might be confounded with the behavioral effects of ES. As a result, those common predisposing traits and behaviors exhibited by dogs receiving electronic training might be statistically amplified and mistakenly identified as representing between-group differences resulting from ES. For purposes of controlling these confounding variables, a baseline of within-subject data sets for the dogs receiving ES would need to be assembled prior to the exposure. A within-subject design (each dog serving as its own control) might help to avoid many of the aforementioned pitfalls. Such within-subject data collected for the experimental and control groups might be subsequently used to make more reliable between-subject comparisons between shocked and nonshocked dogs than allowed by the Schilder and Van der Borg design.

Alternatively, a larger sample might help to reduce some of the confounding effects resulting from individual differences and other uncontrolled sources of error.

The performance of multiple between-group comparisons in the absence of appropriate corrections for type 1 error is another troubling feature of the study. Type 1 error occurs when a statistically significant result is obtained due to chance. Repeated tests and comparisons can artificially cause the probability (p) value of some results to reach significance, just as flipping a coin enough times will eventually produce three heads in row. Consequently, to control the error rate associated with multiple comparisons, appropriate statistical precautions are taken, including the use of corrective procedures to avoid false positives. Without such corrections, there is a risk of turning up apparently significant results that do not actually exist. The more that statistical data are churned by multiple tests and comparisons, the greater is the risk that spurious results will be mistaken as significant differences. Despite an obvious potential for error favorable to their central hypothesis, the authors nevertheless rejected the need for a correction method because such treatment would likely cause much of what they held significant to vanish. The Bonferroni method was explicitly rejected, and the authors opted to publish their results in an uncorrected form to preserve the appearance of credible significance. Experimental findings that lack sufficient statistical strength to withstand appropriate corrections to prevent false positives are viewed with justifiable suspicion.

Implications

The authors grant that only small behavioral differences between the shocked and non-shocked dogs were found, yet they show little restraint or reserve in the way they interpret and amplify the significance of these slight differences with anecdotes and speculation. Even the title betrays a misleading implication with respect to the study's significance since the study design a priori lacks the capacity to make any meaningful determina-

tions about the effects of shock received during training on the long-term welfare of dogs. Of course, the authors acknowledge that long-term harm cannot be extrapolated from their findings but then go on anyhow to assert that such significance nevertheless somehow does exist: "We have not proved that the long-term welfare of the shocked dogs is hampered, but we have made clear that it is under serious threat" (332). It is bewildering to consider how one might justify the claim that a causal relation exists, such that P gives rise to a serious threat of harm to Q, without first demonstrating that P can actually harm Q—otherwise the assertion that P represents a serious threat of harm to Q does not make any sense. On the other hand, though, if one already knows that P represents an increased risk of harm to Q, how can one state that a causal relation of harm between P and Q has not been established, such that given the occurrence of P then Q is threatened with future harm. Lastly, if, as established by the first part of the authors' foregoing statement, the long-term welfare of a dog after exposure to shock is regarded as undetermined, then P could just as easily have a long-term beneficial effect on Q or possibly exert no measurable effect at all with respect to harm or benefit to Q. Since a causal relation has not been established between an exposure to shock and long-term adverse effects, one can only conclude that biased assumptions and beliefs led the authors to the speculation that shock is stressful and represents a serious threat to a dog's welfare. Even allowing that brief shock might momentarily produce changes in behavior consistent with pain and fear, obviously a specter of *post hoc ergo propter hoc* ("after this therefore because of this") looms over the speculation that the transitory effects of ES might represent a serious threat to a dog's long-term welfare—speculation that has no legitimate place in a scientific work of this nature. Finally, in the absence of consistent operational (descriptive and functional) definitions of stress and welfare, applied impartially, these notions will rapidly degenerate into shifting (and therefore increasingly meaningless) concepts of convenience for those wishing to impose their personal beliefs and preferences on others with respect to animal care and training.

Many of the negative statements and claims made by the authors conflict with prior evidence that they neglect to consider, stating that "no systematic investigations regarding possible long-term effects of the use of the collar have been published" (320). In fact, the available prior work provides behavioral and biological evidence that contradicts the allegation that contingent shock delivered by a radio-controlled collar is likely to promote long-term harm to a dog's welfare. Stichnoth (2002), for example, concluded, "If the dog is able to foresee and avoid the shock due to direct association with an object nearly no increase of salivary cortisol can be measured during the shock test and no increase four weeks later" (182). A similar lack of long-term adverse side effects has been reported in shock used to suppress predatory behavior (Christiansen et al., 2001a and b) and to control avoidance-motivated aggression (Tortora, 1982). Consequently, the authors of the present report have not proven that ES in the context of dog training poses a serious threat or any other harmful influence with respect to a dog's immediate or future fitness or adaptability (welfare). The assertion that shock used in the context of dog training poses a serious threat to a dog's welfare should be considered unfounded, at least until significant contrary evidence is made available.

Arndt and Bartko (2003) explore some of the ethical implications of intentionally failing to take appropriate measures to prevent false positives when performing behavioral studies involving multiple tests and comparisons:

> Since an underestimation of Type I error rates can lead to false impressions and treatment practices, this issue is of serious concern. While it may be comforting to speculate that follow-up studies will fail to replicate the spurious finding—hence eventually set the record straight—this attitude is becoming an increasingly shallow reassurance. All too often the popular press takes note of positive findings and reports them. Once the results are touted in the news, the public's knowledge about them is seldom corrected since follow-up negative studies are not deemed newsworthy. This not

only is misleading it also unfavorably affects scientific credibility. Furthermore, the rapidity of information transfer effectively removes the "waiting period" safeguards that science once enjoyed. In times past, there was a slow, cautious progression from when scientific results appeared in journals to when the findings surfaced in popular practice. Given rapid publication, electronic publishing, and the Internet, this safeguard is vanishing.

The obvious dangers underscored by the foregoing passage are not without relevance to animal welfare research. Already in February 2003, results prefiguring the findings of the present study (published in March 2004) were presented before the British Parliament, representing the lone bit of scientific evidence given in support of banning the manufacture, sale, and use of electronic training collars in England:

> A Dutch study by Dr. Joanna Van Der Borg compared dogs trained using electric shock collars with dogs trained using more conventional methods. The shocked dogs showed persistent and long-term behaviour differences that indicated that they were under stress and in fear. (Rendel, 2003:column 870)

It is noteworthy that these claims attributed to the present study (or a related study not cited by the authors) include the assertion that "persistent and long-term behaviour differences" were found to result from the use of ES in dog training—a conclusion that might also be easily taken away from the study by uncritical readers. The danger should be obvious. An opinion, even an erroneous and unfounded one, cloaked under the authority of science carries great potential power to influence public opinion and policy-making decisions. Unfortunately, even after a flawed study is debunked, many diehards will continue to embrace and defend it, making it the meme of the day. Slowly by repetition and political pressure, such "snark bait" may even worm its way into the law, thereby violating the rights of everyone compelled to obey it.

Arbitrarily restricting the manufacture, sale, and use of e-collars or any other training tool recognized by the dog-training profession as standard equipment (see Delta Society, 2001) may violate federal antitrust laws that guard against unfair infringements on free trade. In any case, such restrictions will not stop abusive behavior. Instead of making a beneficial change in the lives of Dutch working dogs, the most likely long-term consequence of the present effort to ban electronic training devices, should the efforts of Schilder and Van der Borg succeed, will be to increase the practical trainer's reliance on less efficient and potentially more harmful physical procedures, as needed to establish safe control over the working dogs' aggressive propensities and enthusiasm. Only education can hope to improve the way people interact with animals, but the power of education is based on the credibility and quality of the information provided and the integrity of the educator imparting it. Further, the arbitration of controversial welfare issues depends on a balance of science and ethics tempered by common sense and kindness. The key role of science in this process will only succeed to the extent that the scientist is recognized and trusted by all parties as a fair and objective arbiter, free of anthropomorphic emotionalism, private prejudice, malice, and legislative agendas. Legislation and policy changes that adversely impact established professional activities or infringe upon free trade are costly to society and represent a significant hardship to individuals and industries that are forced to bear the brunt of the burden. These sacrifices are part of social progress and human betterment, but they are costs that are onerous and hard to bear when the research used to achieve those ends is flawed. Every time a study published in a peer-reviewed journal contains unproven speculation that harms the interests of a particular group or product with misinformation, no matter how heartfelt the underlying sentiment, the whole scientific community will continue to suffer from the repercussions of mistrust long after the study is forgotten.

Electronic Training Collars in Perspective

Although generally reliable, effective, and humane, electronic training aids have attracted considerable criticism in recent years. Much of the criticism is based on incomplete, biased, or faulty information about the nature of ES and the techniques used to deliver it. Many of the critics of electrical training are strikingly ignorant regarding the use and effect of such tools, viewing them as draconian punishment devices causing significant pain and distress to dogs. Modern electronic training can produce consistent low-level ES or vibrotactile stimulation that causes very little discomfort. Technically, the electrical output of modern e-collars is similar in principle to the ES produced by medical devices used to treat pain. The devices are generally easy to use and perform reliably and very effectively as a minimally aversive means for establishing escape/avoidance control through negative reinforcement. Leading manufacturers of such devices strive to produce radio-controlled training devices that operate effectively at low levels of ES—starting at levels that are barely perceptible to human touch. As the result of sophisticated design and circuitry advances, modern e-collars cannot burn or otherwise damage skin tissue, except as might occur as the result of electrode irritation. Klein (2000) performed a series of tests on various collars in which the electrodes were placed on porcine skin preparations. The highest electrical currents produced by the collars tested were repeatedly applied to the skin for 5 minutes, under both dry and wet conditions. The tests showed conclusively that the electrical current produced by the e-collars tested does not cause burns of any kind. Contemporary devices do not produce significant heat on the skin, even after prolonged and repeated stimulation at the highest levels. Various soft and pliable electrode materials have been developed in recent years that will hopefully help solve skin irritation problems in the future. Disposable conducting rubber or siliconlike caps placed over metal electrodes would potentially help to solve some of these problems.

Despite the relatively harmless and innocuous character of the stimulation delivered by modern electrical training devices, some veterinarians, behaviorists, and animal welfare authorities have alleged that such devices hurt dogs (Frank, 1999), burn the skin (Seksel,

1999), and promote harm to the human-dog bond and welfare of the dog (Schilder and Van der Borg, 2004). Many anti-e-collar campaigns have centered around misinformation supported by veterinary misdiagnoses regarding the capacity of e-collars to produce burns. At least one person has been unfairly prosecuted and convicted on cruelty charges stemming from accusations that a bark-activated collar she used severely burned her dog's neck (Wellington, 1999). In some quarters, there is considerable pressure under way to make the case that e-collars are cruel (Kisko, 2003), with some organizations virtually pleading for anecdotes and hearsay with which to build a case in lieu of a genuine body of scientific evidence. The following, presented before the British Parliament, is an example of the sort of disinformation that governing bodies are spoon fed with the explicit purpose of biasing their decisions and promoting restrictive legislation:

> Other cases include those of dogs that have been brought to vets with severe neck burns. Of course, it is always claimed that such injuries are the result of a malfunction of the collar rather than deliberate mistreatment. One inevitable cause of malfunction is that the electrical properties of an animal's neck are affected by how wet it is. (Rendel, 2003:column 870)

With respect to the first point, to my knowledge no recognized authority has claimed that skin irritation and lesions are the result of burns caused by a malfunction of a collar stimulator. The assertion that electrode lesions are caused by a collar malfunction is a strawdog argument with no substantive evidence to support it. In fact, no one has ever proven that even the slightest burn can be produced by one of these devices. Of course, a simple series of experiments on an anesthetized dog would rapidly put the matter to rest, perhaps helping to prevent future misinformation, false charges of cruelty, and legal wrangling, such as recently occurred in the Australian federal courts. In that situation, statements made by a senior Australian Royal Society for the Prevention of Cruelty to Animals (RSPCA) inspector asserting that e-collars produced electrical shocks sufficient to cause severe burns prompted an e-collar distributor

and a manufacturer to file suit seeking damages and to set the public record straight. The judge decided the case on the merits of testimony given by an electrical engineer retained by the respondents. The expert stated that although the open circuit electrical potential of the collar in question was indeed 2705 V, the actual voltage driving electrical current at the electrode-skin interface was estimated to be on the order of 2 V! As a result, the judge found that the public statements asserting that e-collars inflicted a 3000-V shock were, "in every sense, misleading or deceptive" (Federal Court of Australia, 2002), and decided in favor of the complainants and awarded the e-collar company $100,000 in damages. As previously discussed (see *Electrical Potential, Current, and Power*), the open-circuit voltage produced by these devices is rather meaningless for estimating the size and potential for harm delivered to a dog. The judge in making his ruling found that e-collars are incapable of producing burns (Brine, 2002).

To some extent, the apparent confusion regarding electronic training is due to a lack of working knowledge and experience with electronic training tools. Many critics appear to lump together all forms of ES, regardless of intensity, under the same rubric of an imminent potential for harm and malfeasance. This unscientific and irresponsible practice blurs significant distinctions between the effects of the radio-controlled ES produced by modern e-collars and the effects of traumatic electrical shock, as historically used in the laboratory to induce learned helplessness and traumatic behavioral adjustments, namely, shock capable of doing great physical and psychological harm. It is of utmost importance when discussing shock and ES to specify with some precision the level of stimulation to which one is referring. As noted previously, ES that is virtually imperceptible to human touch can be extremely effective for some dog-training purposes, just as HLES that produces localized and physically harmless pain can be effectively used to rapidly deter highly motivated and undesirable behavior. Electricity, like gravity, has varying degrees of intensity and potential to do biological harm. By way of illustration, consider the very different effects resulting from the action of dropping a bowling ball on one's foot versus the effects caused by dropping a tennis ball instead. Although gravity mediates both of these actions, the pain and physical damage caused by the bowling ball would obviously be significantly greater than the effects produced by the tennis ball. Although electrical current delivered at high amperage can be life-threatening or produce significant burns, the ES levels most commonly used in dog training are extremely low, often being barely perceptible or producing a mild tingling or pricking sensation to human touch. A dog's experience is probably more akin to an annoying tingle (low level) or startling twitch (moderate level) sensation—not painful shock. Of course, at higher levels, the electrical output of such collars can be both painful and startling, but such stimulation is infrequently used in the context of electronic training.

Modern techniques and devices incorporating LLES are distinguished by the capacity to produce a graded and relatively harmless level of stimulation. Breland-Bailey (1998) has stressed that ES is highly controllable and can be precisely adjusted to meet exacting specifications. She argues that the controllability of ES recommends its use as a laboratory tool as well as a practical means for decreasing undesirable behavior:

> A. The amount of shock can be precisely determined and measured. It can likewise be precisely controlled so as to avoid physical damage and evaluate the amounts needed to achieve certain behavioral effects.
> B. This means that a shock need not be the same as hitting a fly with a cement block. It can be as strong or as weak as desired. Some ES can be so weak as to resemble only a slight tingling. Indeed, some human observers even report a mild, pleasant effect.

She then goes on to describe how such stimulation has been used to control self-injurious behavior in autistic and retarded children:

> This kind of electrical stimulation has sometimes been used in controlling self-destructive behavior in autistic and retarded children. It is not so much a punishment for such behavior,

because the "shock" is so mild, as it is an alerting of the child that he is beginning to emit such behavior. If he then stops, his subsequent response can lead to positive reinforcement.

This description precisely captures how ES is most effectively applied in dog training.

Although uncontrollable shock and pain may produce significant stress and fear that can interfere with effective learning, the low to medium levels of ES most often used in the context of electronic training produce minimal distress and typically result in very effective, efficient, and lasting behavioral change. Dogs receiving such training usually exhibit very little distress or confusion; to the contrary, most dogs show signs of enhanced relaxation, confidence, and playfulness subsequent to electronic training. This practical observation is supported by many laboratory studies that have shown how escapable ES is followed by opponent emotional relief and relaxation—safety (Denny, 1971 and 1976). Many authors have emphasized the role of pathological anxiety and stress in the etiology of compulsive self-directed licking, but none have actually quantified the alleged presence of anxiety or demonstrated evidence of elevated cortisol secretion or other physiological markers of stress in dogs showing compulsive behavior. Assuming that anxiety and stress are significant factors in the etiology of such problems, and granting for the moment that ES is fear-eliciting and stressful for dogs, one would expect that such stimulation should increase licking behavior. However, as discussed previously, Eckstein and Hart (1996) found that remote ES reduced psychogenic licking significantly in several dogs, with no significant adverse side effects. Similar benefits of radio-controlled and behavior-activated ES have been found in treatment of aggressive behavior and separation-related excesses (see *Separation-related Problems and Punishment* in Chapter 4). Electrical stimulation in the treatment of behavior problems requires that the cynopraxic trainer/therapist possess appropriate technical knowledge and skills together with a sensitive appreciation for potential adverse side effects.

Electronic training has many potential applications in the context of behavior therapy that remain unexplored, largely because of prejudice, misunderstanding of the process, and an exaggeration of the risks posed by electronic behavior therapy and training. An area of considerable interest for future practical application and research is the use of remote-controlled LLES, scentless spray, and vibrotactile stimulation in the context of puppy training, especially with highly impulsive and reactive young dogs showing excessive mouthing, biting, chasing behavior, aggressive tendencies, or social deficits not adequately responsive to food-based conditioning, play training, and conventional directive efforts alone. Although Polsky (1994) has suggested that ES might be used as a stand-alone modality for inhibiting "incessant" mouthing and biting in puppies, such training would be best applied in the context of appropriate reward-based efforts aimed at integrating excessive competitive behavior into an appropriate play outlet. Electronic training collars used for such purposes should be fitted with appropriate amplitude control (e.g., a voltage divider) to ensure that the ES delivered does not exceed a mild, attention-controlling level (tickle/tingle), even when delivered at the highest level. Early preliminary exposure to LLES may prove highly beneficial for hunting and working dogs, especially when electronic training is likely to figure prominently in adult training activities and fieldwork. The goal of early electronic training is to establish a positive bias toward ES as a controllable deterrent introduced within the context of reward-based training and play.

Aside from an incomplete understanding of the training process and lack of familiarity with electronic training devices, some of the irrational criticisms of ES may stem from phobic emotional and cognitive elaborations. For most people, the first experience they have with electricity is painful shock. Electricity is a common household hazard that parents repeatedly warn or punish young children about not approaching in order to instill fear and avoidance. Consequently, as the result of direct fear-eliciting experiences and fear-instilling parental warnings of the potential harm of electricity, most people are inculcated with a powerful aversion toward ES. The inculcation of negative associations with electricity is further magnified by the extreme images of electroshock therapy and electrocution that further bias people against the biological and psychological effects of ES. Other lasting fallout may stem from the use of electrified floors, belts with studs for the remote delivery of shock to buttocks, and the use of cattle prods to control the self-injurious behavior of institutionalized autistic and retarded children (see Lovaas et al., 1965; Lovaas and Simmons, 1969). In one of these studies (Lovaas and Simmons, 1969), children that banged their heads against walls, struck themselves, or bit into their skin were exposed to a brief (1 second) aversive shock delivered by a battery-powered "inductorium"—a cattle prod. The image of severely retarded children being repeatedly shocked with a cattle prod makes one cringe—the more so when the procedures are described in the emotionless and sterile language of a behaviorist. The emotional controversy provoked by the use of shock to control child behavior may have negatively biased the public's perception regarding the humaneness of ES for training purposes, whether for the control of children or dogs.

FUTURE PROSPECTS AND TRENDS

When properly understood and employed, ES can be effectively used to modify dog behavior without eliciting significant stress or fear. Given the potential benefits of LLES for dog behavior control and the relatively harmless and innocuous nature of LLES, it is nothing short of appalling that so many respected authorities, who otherwise show evidence of intellectual integrity and scientific restraint, have chosen to condemn electronic devices, based on personal prejudice and the hearsay opinions of others. Some outspoken critics appear to lose all perspective and semblance of reasonableness when it comes to electrical training aids, accepting and perpetuating patently emotional and misleading arguments as matters of fact. Individuals who otherwise may strive to shape their opinions and attitudes in concordance with verifiable empirical evidence betray their lax commitment to sci-entific method when they pronounce sweep-ing and unsubstantiated generalizations denouncing electronic training aids as inhu-mane tools that are used to abuse dogs. The same persons who reject LLES may embrace without question the use of highly intrusive restraint tools (e.g., halters and muzzles) or blast dogs at close quarters with compressed-air nautical horns without blinking. Consider-ing the widespread incidence of dog behavior problems and the questionable efficacy of many current treatment strategies, one would expect greater open-mindedness with respect to tools (electronic and otherwise) that might offer significant and unexpected therapeutic benefits.

The manufacture and distribution of elec-tronic training devices have become big busi-ness. Worldwide sales of e-collars for the year 1999 reportedly topped 3,000,000 units in that year alone (Holliday, 2000). Probably many more are sold today, with tens of mil-lions of these devices in current use. In the United States, in particular, a growing num-ber of professional dog trainers and dog behavior consultants have integrated elec-tronic devices into their reward-based training and therapy programs as adjunct tools. Numerous public seminars and workshops are now dedicated entirely to providing the dog-owning public with detailed instruction on how to use electronic training devices effec-tively to promote desirable behavior and deter undesirable behavior. If a threat of harm existed at a population level, as alleged by critics, one would expect that many more dogs would have behavior problems and phys-ical injuries stemming from the use of such devices, including various behavioral com-plaints involving fear and stress-related distur-bances directly tied to electronic training. In fact, adjustment problems resulting from such devices are extremely rare and, in any case, most frequently found in association with behavior-activated systems, not radio-con-trolled devices. With respect to harm resulting from remote e-collars, to my knowledge there are no scientific reports that provide any proof of actual harm. Polsky (2000) has iden-tified a possible risk of pain-elicited aggression

with containment systems, but otherwise such devices appear to be relatively innocuous in comparison to other factors contributing to the development of behavior problems. There is currently no substantive evidence justifying claims of harm produced by electronic train-ing devices, but there is significant evidence of benefit derived from the proper use of such devices for the control of undesirable dog behavior. Consequently, Scott-Park's (2002) suggestion that "there is little data available to prove either their misuse or positive applica-tions" is only half right; in fact, as discussed throughout this chapter, there is substantial evidence of benefit in a variety of professional dog-training and wildlife applications. With respect to unsupervised owner use of such devices, one preliminary survey of dog owners in Australia indicates only minor adverse effects, primarily related to electrode irrita-tions to the skin, with 97% of the respon-dents indicating that they were either satisfied or "more than satisfied." Among those respondents indicating that they were more than satisfied, 70% reported that they were "very satisfied" or "absolutely delighted" (Coleman and Murray, 2000).

Although the design and safety of elec-tronic training aids have progressed signifi-cantly over the years, much still remains to be done to improve the effectiveness and humaneness of these various products (e.g., standardization of the electrical output of col-lars). Perhaps the most important area needful of attention is user education. Average dog owners typically lack the necessary training skills and appropriate behavioral knowledge to use remote e-collars effectively and safely to train their dogs. Manufacturers of such devices should make a dedicated effort to develop educational materials and programs, such as videos, interactive CDs, and instruc-tional manuals, providing step-by-step instruction on the operation and use of the devices. Whenever possible, however, inexpe-rienced dog owners should be encouraged to receive hands-on instruction from skilled trainers and other professionals experienced in e-collar use. Providing instructional seminars to retailers, trainers, veterinarians, breeders, and other dog-related professionals would be a helpful means to disseminate pertinent information widely. Many e-collars are sold over the counter to dog owners with little by way of instruction on how to use them properly to train dogs or control a dog's undesirable behavior. The humane use of electronic training equipment depends on an educated end user; oddly enough, though, few manufactures have come to grips with their responsibility in this regard and, along with pet-supply retailers, appear content with the status quo and the short-term profits derived from the sale of these products to a relatively ignorant dog-owning public—a state of affairs that is difficult to fathom when one considers the high stakes. Eventually, this strategy may prove foolhardy, perhaps leading concerned individuals and organizations critical of such devices to seek legislative action to restrict their sale and use by the public, altogether.

As with any training device or technique capable of producing significant discomfort to dogs, trainers have an obligation to use the least intrusive and aversive means necessary to achieve necessary behavioral change. In addition to eschewing techniques that produce unnecessary distress and pain, trainers should be guided by an overarching spirit of kindness and respect for dogs. Despite such problems and limitations, little doubt exists that electronics in one form or another will significantly influence the future of dog training and dog behavior therapy. Further, as more trainers and behaviorists discover the usefulness of LLES, novel applications and advances for the use of radio-controlled and behavior-activated devices will certainly develop. The potential of training systems incorporating LLES and positive reinforcement to enrich the lives of companion dogs and improve their behavior will be limited only by the creative imagination of progressive trainers and the ingenuity of bioelectrical engineers to make such devices as painless as possible.

REFERENCES

Andelt WF, Phillips RL, Gruver KS, and Guthrie JW (1999). Coyote predation on domestic sheep deterred with electronic dog-training collar. *Wildl Soc Bull*, 27:12–18.

Arguello S (1986). Behavioral debarking: Regression and Resolution. *Anim Behav Consult Newsl*, 3(1).

Arndt S and Bartko JJ (2003). Why you need to correct for multiple tests. Part 2: The solutions. *Psychiatry Research/Statistical Tutorials: Statistics for Readers and Writers*. http://sarndt.psychiatry.uiowa.edu/Webpage/methresources/StatTutorials.html.

Bangs E (2000a). Status of gray wolf recovery (9/22–10/6). US Fish and Wildlife Service, Mountain-Prairie Region. http://www.r6.fws.gov/wolf/wk10062000.htm.

Bangs E (2000b). Status of gray wolf recovery (11/06–11/10). US Fish and Wildlife Service, Mountain-Prairie Region. http://www.r6.fws.gov/wolf/wk11102000.htm.

Bangs E (2000c). Wolf/livestock aversive conditioning: Letter to Andrea Lococo. US Fish and Wildlife Service, Mountain-Prairie Region. http://www.r6.fws.gov/wolf/lococo.htm,

Beaudet R (2001). Comparing the effectiveness of citronella with unscented odours in the anti-barking spray collar. In KL Overall, DS Mills, SF Heath, and D Horowitz (Eds), *Proceedings of the Third International Congress on Veterinary Behavioural Medicine*, Vancouver, BC, August 7–8.

Beerda B, Schilder MBH, Van Hooff JARAM, et al. (1998). Behavioural, saliva cortisol and heart rate responses to different types of stimuli in dogs. *Appl Anim Behav Sci*, 58:365–381.

Beerda B, Schilder MBH, Van Hooff JARAM, et al. (2000). Behavioral and hormonal indicators of enduring environmental stress in dogs. *Anim Welfare*, 9:49–62.

Billman GE and Dujardin JP (1990). Dynamic changes in cardiac vagal tone as measured by time-series analysis. *Am J Physiol*, 258:896–902.

Billman GE and Randall DC (1980). Classic aversive conditioning of coronary blood flow in mongrel dogs. *Pavlovian J Biol Sci*, 15:93–101.

Blackshaw JK, Cook GE, Harding P, et al. (1990). Aversive responses of dogs to ultrasonic, sonic and flashing light units. *Appl Anim Behav Sci*, 25:1–8.

Blumenthal TD, Burnett TT, and Swerdlow CD (2001). Prepulses reduce the pain of cutaneous electrical shocks. *Psychosomatic Med*, 63:273–281.

Boon EM and Barton JK (2002). Charge transport in DNA. *Curr Opin Struct Biol*, 12:320-329.

Borchelt PL and Voith VL (1996). Dominance aggression in dogs. In VL Voith and PL Borchelt (Eds), *Readings in Companion Animal Behavior*. Trenton, NJ: Veterinary Learning Systems.

Boyce WT, Essex MJ, Alkon A, et al. (2002). Temperament, tympanum, and temperature: Four provisional studies of the biobehavioral correlates of tympanic membrane temperature asymmetries. *Child Dev*, 73:718–733.

Brace CL (1962). Physique, physiology, and behavior: An attempt to analyze a part of their roles in the canine biogram [PhD dissertation: Introduction and Summary]. Boston: Harvard University.

Breland-Bailey M (1998). Electric shock as a form of aversive stimulation (punishment). *Anim Trainer's Forum Newsl* (SIG Association for Behavior Analysis), Winter.

Brine K (2002). RSPCA to pay $100,000 for defaming dog-collar firm. *Canberra Times*, July 20. http://canberra.yourguide.com.au/detail.asp?class=News&story_id=165679&subclass=national&m=7&y=2002.

Broom DM and Johnson KG (1993). *Stress and Animal Welfare*. London: Chapman and Hall.

Brush FR (1957). The effects of shock intensity on the acquisition and extinction of an avoidance response in dogs. *J Comp Physiol Psychol*, 50:547–552.

CABTSG (Companion Animal Behavior Therapy Study Group) (2002). Electronic training devices: A behavioral perspective. *J Small Anim Pract*, 44:95–96.

Caldwell WM and Judy AB (1970). A radiotelemetry stimulator for conditioning of large animals. *Psychophysiology*, 7:499–502.

Cameron RC and Hopkins JW (1955). Radio controlled electric cutaneous signal type animal obedience device. United States Patent Office, patent 2,800,104.

Campbell BA and Bloom JM (1965). Relative aversiveness of noise and shock. *J Comp Physiol Psychol*, 60:440–442.

Campbell BA and Masterson FA (1969). Psychophysics of punishment. In BA Campbell and FA Masterson (Eds), *Punishment and Aversive Behavior*. New York: Appleton-Century-Crofts.

Cattell RB and Korth B (1973). The isolation of temperament dimensions in dogs. *Behav Biol*, 9:15–30.

Chesney CJ (1995). Measurement of skin hydration in normal dogs and in dogs with atopy or a scaling dermatosis. *J Small Anim Pract*, 36:305–309.

Christiansen FO, Bakken M, and Braastad BO (2001a). Behavioral changes and aversive conditioning in hunting dogs by the second-year confrontation with domestic sheep. *Appl Anim Behav Sci*, 72:131–143.

Christiansen FO, Bakken M, and Braastad BO (2001b). Behavioral differences between three breed groups of hunting dogs confronted with domestic sheep. *Appl Anim Behav Sci*, 72:115–129.

Christiansen FO, Bakken M, and Braastad BO (2001c). Social facilitation of predatory, sheep-chasing behaviour in Norwegian elkhounds, grey. *Appl Anim Behav Sci*, 72:105–114.

Clark GI (1994). The relationship between emotionality and temperament in young puppies [PhD Dissertation]. Fort Collins, CO: Colorado State University.

Coleman T and Murray R (2000). Collar mounted electronic devices for behaviour modification in dogs. Urban Animal Management Conference Proceedings, Hobart, Australia. http://www.ava.com.au/content/confer/uam/proc00/murray.htm.

Corson SA, O'Leary Corson E, Kirilcuk B, et al. (1973). Differential effects of amphetamines on clinically relevant dog models of hyperkinesis and stereotypy: Relevance to Huntington's chorea. In A Barbeau, TN Chase, and GW Paulson (Eds), *Advances in Neurology*, Vol 1. New York: Raven.

Delta Society (2001). *Professional Standards for the Dog Trainers: Effective, Humane Principles*. Renton, WA: Delta Society. http://www.deltasociety.org/standards/standards.htm.

Denny RM (1971). Relaxation theory and experiments. In R Brush (Ed), *Aversive Conditioning and Learning*. New York: Academic.

Denny MR (1976). Post-aversive relief and relaxation and their implications for behavior therapy. *J Behav Ther Exp Psychiatry*, 7:315–321.

Denny MR (1983). Safety catch in behavior therapy: Comments on "Safety training: The elimination of avoidance-motivated aggression in dogs." *J Exp Psychol*, 112:215–217.

Denny MR (1991). Relaxation/relief: The effect of removing, postponing, or terminating aversive stimuli. In MR Denny (Ed), *Fear, avoidance, and phobias: A fundamental analysis*. Hillsdale, NJ: Erlbaum.

Dess NK, Linwick D, Patterson J, et al. (1983). Immediate and proactive effects of controllability and predictability on plasma cortisol responses to shock in dogs. *Behav Neurosci*, 97:1005–1016.

Diorio D, Viau V, and Meaney MJ (1993). The role of the medial prefrontal cortex (cingulate gyrus) in the regulation of hypothalamic-pituitary-adrenal responses to stress. *J Neurosci*, 13:3839–3847.

Dix GI (1991). Investigation of sonic invisible boundaries unit. New Zealand Department of Scientific and Industrial Research, report ECAEO0521.

Dunbar I (2000). Dog-training equipment: Panel discussion [Tape R4637]. In *Tufts Animal Expo*, Boston, October 10–13.

Dykman RA and Gantt WH (1997). Experimental psychogenic hypertension: Blood pressure changes conditioned to painful stimuli (schizokinesis). *Integr Physiol Behav Sci.* 32:272–287. (Originally published by the *Bulletin of the Johns Hopkins Hospital*, Aug 1960, Vol 107.)

Eckstein RA and Hart BL (1996). Treatment of acral lick dermatitis by behavior modification using electronic stimulation. *J Am Anim Hosp Assoc*, 32:225–229.

Endo Y and Shiraki K (2000). Behavior and body temperature in rats following chronic foot shock or psychological stress exposure. *Physiol Behav*, 71:263–268.

Fisher AE (1955). The effects of early differential treatment on the social and exploratory behavior of puppies [PhD dissertation]. State College: Pennsylvania State University.

Fitzgerald RD (1966). Some effects of partial reinforcement with shock on classically conditioned heart-rate in dogs. *Am J Psychol*, 79:242–249.

Fonberg E, Kostarczyk E, and Prechtl J (1981). Training of instrumental responses in dogs socially reinforced by humans. *Pavlovian J Biol Sci*, 16:183–193.

Forbes TW and Bernstein AL (1935). The standardization of sixty-cycle electric shock for practical use in psychological experimentation. *J Gen Psychol*, 12:436–442.

Fox MW (1978). *The Dog: Its Domestication and Behavior*. Malabar, FL: Krieger.

Franchina JJ. (1969). Effects of food reward and frustrative nonreward during escape training. *Psychon Sci*, 14:95–96.

Frank D (1999). Electronic collars "hurt" [Letter]. *Aust Vet J*, 77:408–409.

Frawley E (2003). Watchdog test. http://www.leerburg.com/wh.htm#gr.

Freedman DG (1958). Constitutional and environmental interactions in rearing of four breeds of dogs. *Science*, 127:585–586.

Fu QL, Shen YQ, Gao MX, et al. (2003). Brain interleukin asymmetries and paw preference in mice. *Neuroscience*, 116:639–647.

Galizio M (1999). Extinction of responding maintained by timeout from avoidance. *J Exp Anal Behav*, 71:1–11.

Gantt WH, Newton JE, Royer FL, Stephens JH (1966). Effect of person. *Cond Reflex*, 1:146–160.

Godsil BP, Quinn JJ, and Fanselow MS (2000). Body temperature as a conditional response measure for Pavlovian fear conditioning. *Learn Mem*, 7:353–356.

Greenblatt DJ and Tursky B (1969). Local vascular and impedance changes induced by electric shock. *Am J Physiol*, 216:712–718.

Groenink L, Van der Gugten J, Zethof T, et al. (1994). Stress-induced hyperthermia in mice: Hormonal correlates. *Physiol Behav*, 56:747–749.

Harmon-Jones E (2003). Anger and the behavioral approach system. *Pers Individ Differ*, 35:995–1005.

Harmon-Jones E and Sigelman J (2001). State anger and prefrontal brain activity: Evidence that insult-related relative left-prefrontal activation is associated with experienced anger and aggression. *J Pers Soc Psychol*, 80:797–803.

Hart BL and Hart LA (1985). *Canine and Feline Behavioral Therapy*. Philadelphia: Lea and Febiger.

Hewson CJ and Luescher UA (1996). Compulsive disorder in dogs. In VL Voith and PL Borchelt (Eds), *Readings in Companion Animal Behavior*. Philadelphia: Veterinary Learning Systems.

Himwich WA, Knapp FM, and Steiner WG (1965). Electrical activity of the dog's brain: Telemetry and direct wire recording. *Prog Brain Res*, 16:301–317.

Holiday JA (2000). Letters to the Editor. *Aust Vet J*, 78:133–134.

Hopkins WD and Fowler LA (1998). Lateralized changes in tympanic membrane temperature in relation to different cognitive tasks in chimpanzees (*Pan troglodytes*). *Behav Neurosci*, 112:83–88.

Houser VP and Paré WP (1974). Long-term conditioned fear modification in the dog as measured by changes in urinary 11-hdyrocorticosteroids, heart rate, and behavior. *Pavlovian J Biol Sci*, 9:85–96.

Institute for Wildlife Studies (2000). Island fox conservation. http://www.iws.org/island_fox_conservation.htm.

Johnson LR (1998). *Essential Medical Physiology*, 2nd Ed. Philadelphia: Lippincott-Raven.

Juarbe-Diaz S (1997). Assessment and treatment of excessive barking in the domestic dog. *Vet Clin North Am Prog Companion Anim Behav*, 27:497–514.

Juarbe-Diaz SV and Houpt KA (1996). Comparison of two antibarking collars for treatment of nuisance barking. *J Am Anim Hosp Assoc*, 32:231–235.

Juhasz C, Behen ME, Muzik O, et al. (2001). Bilateral medial prefrontal and temporal neocortical hypometabolism in children with epilepsy and aggression. *Epilepsia*, 42:991–1001.

Kaczmarek KA, Webster JG, Bach-y-Rita P, and Tompkins WJ (1991). Electrotactile and vibrotactile displays for sensory substitution systems. *IEEE Trans Biomed Eng*, 38:1–16.

Kamarck T and Jennings JR (1991). Biobehavioral factors in sudden cardiac death. *Psychol Bull*, 109:42–75.

Kaplan F, Oudeyer PY, Kubinyi E, and Miklósi A (2002). Robotic clicker training. *Robotics Autonomous Syst*, 38:197–206.

King T, Hemsworth PH, and Coleman GJ (2003). Fear of novel and startling stimuli in domestic dogs. *Appl Anim Behav Sci*, 82:45–64.

Kisko C (2003). Animals (Electric Shock Collars) Bill. *Vet Rec*, 153:475–476.

Klein D (2000). Electronic stimulus devices: Basics, effects, and potential dangers with regard to their use in training dogs [Dipl. Ing. Dieter Klein, Orthopaedische Universitaetsklinik, Funktionsbereich Bewegungsanalytik]. Muenster, Germany.

Klimenko LL (2001). Dynamics of parameters of the energy metabolism in cerebral hemispheres in late ontogenesis in rats [Abstract]. *Izv Akad Nauk Ser Biol*, March–April:213–219.

Koolhaas JM, Meerlo P, De Boer SF et al. (1997). The temporal dynamics of the stress response. *Neurosci Biobehav Rev*, 21:775–782.

Kouwenhoven WB and Milnor WR (1958). The effects of high-voltage, low-capacitance electrical discharges in the dog. *IRE Trans Med Electronics*, 9:41–45.

Kovach JA, Nearing BD, and Verrier RL (2001). Angerlike behavioral state potentiates myocardial ischemia-induced T-wave alternans in canines. *J Am Coll Cardiol*, 37:1719–1725.

Lessac MS and Solomon RL (1969). Effects of early isolation on the later adaptive behavior of beagles: A methodological demonstration. *Dev Psychol*, 1:14–25.

Little CJ, Julu PO, Hansen S, and Reid SW (1999). Real-time measurement of cardiac vagal tone in conscious dogs. *Am J Physiol*, 276:758–765.

Littman RA, Stevens DA, and Whittier JL (1964). Previous shock experience and response threshold to shock. *Can J Psychol*, 18:93-100.

Lovaas OI and Simmons JQ (1969). Manipulation of self-destruction in three retarded children. *J Appl Behav Anal*, 2:143–157.

Lovaas OI, Schaeffer B, and Simmons JQ (1965). Building social behavior in autistic behavior in autistic children by use of electric shock. *J Exp Res Pers*, 1:99–109.

Maier SF, Anderson C, Lieberman DA (1972). Influence of control of shock on subsequent shock-elicited aggression. *J Comp Physiol Psychol*, 81:94–100.

McGuire and Vallance (1964). Aversion therapy by electric shock: A simple technique. *Br Med J*, 1:151–153.

Meerlo P, De Boer SF, Koolhaas JM, et al. (1996). Changes in daily rhythms of body temperature and activity after a single social defeat in rats. *Physiol Behav*, 59:735–739.

Meerlo P, Sgoifo A, De Boer SF, and Koolhaas JM (1999). Long-lasting consequences of a social conflict in rats: Behavior during the interaction predicts subsequent changes in daily rhythms of heart rate, temperature, and activity. *Behav Neurosci*, 113: 1283–1290.

Merskey H and Bogduk N (1994). *Classification of Chronic Pain: Descriptions of Chronic Pain Syndromes and Definitions of Pain Terms*. Seattle, WA: IASP. See http://www.iasp-pain.org/terms-p.html.

Moffat K and Landsberg G (2001). Effectiveness and comparison of both a citronella and scentless spray bark collar for the control of barking in a veterinary hospital setting. *Newsl Am Vet Soc Anim Behav*, 23(2/3):6–7.

Munana KR, Vitek SM, Tarver WB, et al. (2002). Use of vagal nerve stimulation as a treatment for refractory epilepsy in dogs. *JAVMA*, 221:977–983.

Neveu PJ and Moya S (1997). In the mouse, the corticoid stress response depends on lateralization. *Brain Res*, 749:344–346.

Neveu PJ, Bluthe RM, Liege S, et al. (1998). Interleukin-1-induced sickness behavior depends on behavioral lateralization in mice. *Physiol Behav*, 63:587–590.

Niwano S, Kitano Y, Moriguchi M, et al. (2001). Leakage of energy to the body surface during defibrillation shock by an implantable cardioverter-defibrillator (ICD) system: Experimental evaluation during defibrillation shocks through the right ventricular lead and the subcutaneous active-can in canines. *Jpn Circ J*, 65:219–225.

Ogburn P, Crouse S, Martin F, and Houpt K (1998). Comparison of behavioral and physiological responses of dogs wearing two different types of collars. *Appl Anim Behav Sci*, 61:133–142.

Overall K (1997). *Clinical Behavioral Medicine for Small Animals*. St. Louis: CV Mosby.

Overmier JB and Seligman MEP (1967). Effects of inescapable shock upon subsequent escape and avoidance responding. *J Comp Physiol Psychol*, 63:28–33.

Pagani M, Lombardi F, Guzzetti S, et al. (1986). Power spectral analysis of heart rate and arterial pressure variabilities as a marker of sympatho-vagal interaction in man and conscious dog. *Circ Res*, 59:178–193.

Palazzolo JA, Estafanous FG, and Murray PA (1998). Entropy measures of heart rate variation in conscious dogs. *Am J Physiol*, 274:1099–1105.

Panksepp J, Nelson E, and Bekkedal (1997). Brain systems for the mediation of social separation-distress and social-reward: Evolutionary antecedents and neuropeptide intermediaries. *Ann NY Acad Sci*, 807:78–100.

Parr LA and Hopkins WD (2000). Brain temperature asymmetries and emotional perception in chimpanzees, *Pan troglodytes*. *Physiol Behav*, 71:363–371.

Pavlov IP (1928). *Lectures on Conditioned Reinforcement*, Vol 1. WH Gantt (Trans). New York: International.

Poletto CJ and Van Doren CL (1999). A high voltage, constant current stimulator for electrocutaneous stimulation through small electrodes. *IEEE Trans Biomed Eng*, 46:929–936.

Polsky RH (1994). Electronic shock collars: Are they worth the risk? *J Am Anim Hosp Assoc*, 30:463–468.

Polsky RH (1998). Shock collars and aggression in dogs. *Anim Behav Consult Newsl*, 15(2).

Polsky RH (2000). Can aggression in dogs be elicited through the use of electronic pet containment systems? *J Appl Anim Welfare Sci*, 3:345–357.

Porges SW (2001). The polyvagal theory: Phylogenetic substrates of a social nervous system. *Int J Psychophysiol*, 42:123–146.

Preobrazhenskaia LA (2000). Functional asymmetry of the neocortex electrical activity during food conditioning in dogs [Abstract]. *Zh Vyssh Nerv Deyat Im I P Pavlova*, 50:434–446.

Price KP and Tursky B (1975). The effect of varying stimulus parameters on judgments of nociceptive electrical stimulation. *Psychophysiology*, 12:663–666.

Quaranta A, Siniscalchi M, Frate A, and Vallortigara G (2004). Paw preference in dogs: Relations between lateralised behaviour and immunity. *Behav Brain Res*, 153:521-523.

Raine A, Buchsbaum M, and LaCasse (1997). Brain abnormalities in murderers indicated by positron emission tomography. *Biol Psychiatry*, 42:495–508.

Raine A, Meloy JR, Bihrle S, et al. (1998). Reduced prefrontal and increased subcortical brain functioning assessed using positron emission tomography in predatory and affective murderers. *Behav Sci Law*, 16:319–332.

Rendel D (2003). Bill to ban the manufacture, sale or use of collars which administer electric shocks to animals. UK Parliament, February 12, 2003:column 870. http://www.parliament.the-stationery office.co.uk/pa/cm200203/cmhansrd/vo030212 /debtext/30212-04.htm.

Reese WG, Newton JE, Angel C (1982). Induced immobility in nervous and normal Pointer dogs. *J Nerv Ment Dis*, 170:605–613.

Rescorla RA and LoLordo (1965). Inhibition of Avoidance Behavior. *J Comp Physiol Psychol*, 59:406–412.

Richter CP (1957). On the phenomenon of sudden death in animals and man. *Psychosom Med*, 19:191–198.

Rosell J, Colominas J, Riu P, et al. (1988). Skin impedance from 1 Hz to 1 MHz. *IEEE Trans Biomed Eng*, 35:649–651.

Royce JR (1955). A factorial study of emotionality in the dog. *Psychol Monogr Gen Appl*, 69: 1–27.

Royer FL (1969). Uncertainty of reinforcement consequences in Pavlovian conditioning of dogs. *Psychol Rep*, 24:147–152.

Sales G, Hubrecht R, Peyvandi A, et al. (1997). Noise in dog kennelling: Is barking a welfare problem for dogs? *Appl Anim Behav Sci*, 52:321–329.

Sang CN, Max MB, and Gracely RH (2003). Stability and reliability of detection thresholds for human A-Beta and A-delta sensory afferents determined by cutaneous electrical stimulation. *J Pain Symptom Manage*, 25:64–73.

Schilder MBH and Van der Borg JAM (2004). Training dogs with help of the shock collar: Short and long term behavioural effects. *Appl Anim Behav Sci*, 85:319–334.

Schwizgebel D (1992). Safety training: A complex procedure in the behavior therapy in dogs. *Kleintierpraxis*, 37:241–253.

Scott JP and Fuller JL (1965). *Genetics and the Social Behavior of the Dog*. Chicago: University of Chicago Press.

Scott-Park F (2002). BSAVA's position on electronic training devices for dogs and cats. *J Small Anim Pract*, 43:567.

Seksel K (1999). Comments on collars policy: No. *Aust Vet J*, 77:78.

Seligman MEP (1975). *Helplessness: On Depression, Development and Death*. San Francisco: Freeman.

Seligman MEP and Groves D (1970). Non-transient learned helplessness. *Psychonom Sci*, 19:191–192.

Seligman MEP and Maier SF (1967). Failure to escape traumatic shock. *J Exp Psychol*, 74:1–9.

Seligman MEP, Maier SF, and Geer JH (1968). Alleviation of learned helplessness in the dog. *J Abnorm Psychol*, 73:256–262.

Sgoifo A, De Boer SF, Buwalda B, et al. (1998). Vulnerability to arrhythmias during social stress in rats with different sympathovagal balance. *Am J Physiol*, 275:460–466.

Sgoifo A, Koolhaas JM, Musso E, and De Boer SF (1999). Different sympathovagal modulation of heart rate during social and nonsocial stress episodes in wild-type rats. *Physiol Behav*, 67:733–738.

Sgoifo A, Pozzato C, Costoli T, et al. (2001). Cardiac autonomic responses to intermittent social conflict in rats. *Physiol Behav*, 73:343–349.

Shevelev IA, Tsykalov EN, Budko KP, et al. (1986). Movement of temperature waves across the cerebral cortex of the white rat [Abstract]. *Neirofiziologiia*, 18:340–346.

Simonov PV, Rusalova MN, Preobrazhenskaia LA, and Vanetsian GL (1995). The novelty factor and asymmetry in brain activity. *Zh Vyssh Nerv Deyat Im I P Pavlova*, 45:13–17.

Solomon RL and Corbit JD (1974). An opponent-process theory of motivation. I. Temporal dynamics of affect. *Psychol Rev*, 81:119–145.

Solomon RL and Wynne LC (1953). Traumatic avoidance learning: Acquisition in normal dogs. *Psychol Monogr*, 67:1–19.

Solomon RL, Turner LH, and Lessac MS (1968). Some effects of delay of punishment on resistance to temptation in dogs. *J Pers Soc Psychol*, 8:233–238.

Stichnoth J (2002). Stress reactions of dogs due to the use of electronic shock collars [PhD dissertation]. Hanover: Hanover Veterinary University.

Sullivan RM and Gratton A (1999). Lateralized effects of medial prefrontal cortex lesions on neuroendocrine and autonomic stress responses in rats. *J Neurosci*, 19:2834–2840.

Tan U (1987). Paw preferences in dogs. *Int J Neurosci*, 32:825–829.

Tan U and Caliskan S (1987a). Allometry and asymmetry in the dog brain: The right hemisphere is heavier regardless of paw preference. *Int J Neurosci*, 35:189–194.

Tan U and Caliskan S (1987b). Asymmetries in the cerebral dimensions and fissures of the dog. *Int J Neurosci*, 32:943–952.

Tham I (2002). What your dog is really thinking. MSNBC, May 10. http://stacks.msnbc.com/news/750404.asp#BODY.

Thayer JF and Lane RD (2000). A model of neurovisceral integration in emotion regulation and dysregulation. *J Affect Disord*, 61:201–216.

Tomaz C, Verburg MS, Boere V, et al. (2003). Evidence of hemispheric specialization in marmosets (*Callithrix penicillata*) using tympanic membrane thermometry. *Braz J Med Biol Res*, 36:913–918.

Tortora DF (1982). *Understanding Electronic Dog Training*. Tucson, AZ: Tri-Tronics.

Tortora DF (1983). Safety training: The elimination of avoidance-motivated aggression in dog. *J Exp Psychol*, 112:176–214.

Tursky B (1973). Physical, physiological, and psychological factors that affect pain reaction to electric shock. *Psychophysiology*, 11:95–112.

Tursky B, Greenblatt D, and O'Connell D (1970). Electrocutaneous threshold changes produced by electric shock. *Psychophysiology*, 7:490–498.

Uvnäs-Moberg K (1998). Oxytocin may mediate the benefits of positive social interaction and emotions. *Psychoneuroendocrinology*, 23:819–835.

Van den Berg L, Schilder MB, and Knol BW (2003). Behavior genetics of canine aggression: Behavioral phenotyping of golden retrievers by means of an aggression test. *Behav Genet*, 33:469–483.

Verrier RL and Dickerson LW (1991). Autonomic nervous system and coronary blood flow changes related to emotional activation and sleep. *Circulation*, 83(Suppl 4):81–89.

Vincent IC and Michell AR (1992). Comparison of cortisol concentrations in saliva and plasma of dogs. *Res Vet Sci*, 53:342-345.

Vincent IC and Leahy RA (1997). Real-time non-invasive measurement of heart rate in working dogs: A technique with potential applications in the objective assessment of welfare problems. *Vet J*, 153:179–184.

Vincent IC and Michell AR (1996). Relationship between blood pressure and stress-prone temperament in dogs. *Physiol Behav*, 60:135–138.

Visser EK, Van Reenen CG, Van der Werf JT, et al. (2002). Heart rate and heart rate variability during a novel object test and a handling test in young horses. *Physiol Behav*, 76:289–296.

Wagner AR, Thomas E, and Norton T (1967). Conditioning with electrical stimulation of motor cortex: Evidence of a possible source of motivation. *J Comp Physiol Psychol*, 64:191–199.

Wellington B (1999). RSPCA: Collar charges [Letter]. *Aust Vet J*, 77:618.

Wells DL (2001). The effectiveness of a citronella spray collar in reducing certain forms of barking in dogs. *Appl Anim Behav Sci*, 73:299–309.

Wells DL (2003). Lateralised behaviour in the domestic dog, *Canis familiaris*. *Behav Processes*, 61:27–35.

Williams NG and Borchelt PL (2002). Full body restraint as a treatment for dogs with defensive aggressive behavior. In *Abstracts for the Interdisciplinary Forum for Applied Animal Behavior Meeting*, Tampa, FL, March 1–3.

Williams NG, Borchelt PL, Sollers III JJ, et al. (2003). Ambulatory monitoring of cardiovascular responses during behavioral modification of an aggressive dog. *Biomed Sci Instrum*, 39:214–219.

Wingfield JC (2003). Control of behavioural strategies for capricious environments. *Anim Behav*, 66:807–816.

Wittling W and Pfluger M (1990). Neuroendocrine hemisphere asymmetries: Salivary cortisol secretion during lateralized viewing of emotion-related and neutral films. *Brain Cogn*, 14:243–265.

Wittling W (1990). Psychophysiological correlates of human brain asymmetry: Blood pressure changes during lateralized presentation of an emotionally laden film. *Neuropsychologia*, 28:457–470.

Wittling W, Block A, Genzel S, Schweiger E (1998a). Hemisphere asymmetry in parasympathetic control of the heart. *Neuropsychologia*. 36:461–468.

Wittling W, Block A, Schweiger E, and Genzel S (1998b). Hemisphere asymmetry in sympathetic control of the human myocardium. *Brain Cogn*, 38:17–35.

10

Cynopraxis: Theory, Philosophy, and Ethics

Attention, Model/Rival Learning, and
   Mirror Neurons

PART 1: TRAINING THEORY

WHAT IS CYNOPRAXIS?

The term *cynopraxis* combines the Greek roots
cyno (*kunos*) or "dog" and praxis (*prassein*),
meaning "to do" or doings with the dog. In
accordance with Aristotle's use of the term,
the notion of praxis consists of goal-directed
action performed in accordance with three
criteria: the action is voluntary, regulated by
informed and rational choice, and performed
as an end in itself (Irwin, 1985). More specifically, these *doings* refer to the collective
exchanges and transactions between the
trainer, dog, and family aimed at promoting
interactive harmony, mutual appreciation, and
an improved life experience with the dog.
Cynopraxis is a pragmatic process constrained
to the complementary goals of enhancing the
human-dog bond while improving the dog's
quality of life.

CYNOPRAXIC TRAINING THEORY

A successful training theory should possess a
number of defining characteristics. The theory should be based on a limited number of
processes, explain a wide range of related
behavioral phenomena, and generate predictions that are testable by direct observation
and experimentation. First and foremost,
however, a training theory must successfully
account for behavioral organization that
simultaneously results in order and increasing
variability as the result of experience. In addition, the value of such a theory depends significantly on how well its postulates and predictions connect with the factual and
theoretical accounts of related disciplines,
especially those already possessing a high
degree of scientific veracity and maturity. As a
result of such cross-discipline linkages, the
explanatory significance of the theory is made
more general, convincing, and useful. In particular, a training theory should be consistent
with the experimentally established findings
of formal learning theory and neurobiology,
especially those findings that pertain to the
organizing processes that contribute to the
learning process. Finally, a cynopraxic training theory must satisfy a set of special
requirements peculiar to the cynopraxic
process itself to provide an explanatory
account for the ability of cynopraxic procedures to facilitate competent social skills and
change conducive to mutual appreciation,
interactive harmony, and affectionate playfulness. A training theory need not be infallible,
but theoretical conjecture and speculation
should take a form that admits to the possibility of experimental falsifiability. Cynopraxic training theory appears to meet these
basic requirements as well as possessing interesting implications for understanding human
behavior and learning. An introductory orientation of the theory is provided in *A Brief
Critique of Traditional Learning Theory* in Volume 1, Chapter 7.

BASIC POSTULATES, UNITS, PROCESSES, AND MECHANISMS

Cynopraxic training theory argues that
instrumental behavior cannot be studied in
isolation from affects, incentives, expectancies, and establishing operations, without
losing its functional integrity and significance. On a very basic level, behavior is
rewarded or punished as the result of its ability to predict and control the occurrence of

significant motivational events (see *Tolman's Expectancy Theory* in Volume 1, Chapter 7). Reward occurs when an action successfully controls the occurrence of an anticipated resource or threat, whereas punishment occurs when such control efforts fail. According to this viewpoint, successful actions serve to confirm prediction-control expectancies, whereas failed efforts disconfirm them. The success and failure of purposive action result in the evocation of emotional state changes that exert significant modulatory (excitatory and inhibitory) changes on behavior; contrary to the law of effect, however, these state changes affecting arousal, alertness, and action readiness are consequent to the effects of reward and punishment and are not themselves the cause of reward and punishment. Successful control is associated with surprise and increased excitability when the outcomes are better than expected, on the one hand, or comfort and safety and increased calming when the outcome is just as expected. By contrast, failure occurs when purposive action results in worse-than-expected outcomes. Failure is associated with disappointment and conflict between excitation and inhibition (distress) or *loss of comfort*, on the one hand, and increased apprehensiveness of danger and an aversion to risk, heightened vigilance, and a heightened action readiness to flee or hide in response to a *risk to safety*. Accordingly, the emotional effects or *affects* associated with adaptive learning are consequent to the confirmation or disconfirmation of prediction-control expectancies.

Thus, learning by reward and punishment is not simply a matter of confirming or disconfirming expectancies but proceeds in accordance with cognitive, emotional, and behavioral adjustments to discrepancies or *prediction errors* between what a dog expects to occur and what actually occurs as the result of its control efforts. According to this hypothesis, an important aspect of learning is the acquisition of reliable predictive information (knowledge) by testing prediction-control *hypotheses* (Tolman and Brunswik, 1935). Dickinson (1980) nicely summarizes the importance of prediction error and uncertainty for adaptive learning:

It could be argued that there is something intuitively implausible about the central idea of Mackintosh's theory [see Mackintosh, 1975], the idea that animals learn about an event to the extent that it has been a reliable and good predictor in the past. Certainly an animal should control its behaviour on the basis of the information provided by such reliable predictors. It is far less clear, however, that the learning capacity of an animal should be largely devoted to processing events which in the animal's recent history have been constituents of stable relationships. Rather one might expect the animal to devote most of its processing capacity to analyzing events whose predictive significance is uncertain in an attempt to discover relationships involving these events. (153)

Cynopraxic training theory postulates two primary units of behavioral organization: the control module and the adaptive modal strategy. The *control module* consists of prediction-control expectancy, emotional establishing operation, and a goal-directed action. Prediction-control expectancies and calibrated establishing operations operate through the agency of flexible and purposive actions. When control modules are being integrated, positive and negative error signals encode changes to predictive expectancies and establishing operations that refine future control incentives and efforts. Prediction error also promotes excitatory and inhibitory motivational changes in the directions of increased or decreased approach or increased or decreased withdrawal. The emotional effects of reward (positive prediction error) mobilize active modal strategies (e.g., searching, exploring, and risk taking) whereas affects associated with punishment (negative prediction error) mobilize passive modal strategies (e.g., hesitating, ritualizing, and risk avoiding). Active modal strategies mobilized by the affective responses to positive error signals serve to orient a dog toward the source of reward to prolong contact with the location in order to derive information relevant to the control module. Passive modal strategies mobilized in response to negative prediction error serve to orient a dog away from the source of punishment or to hesitate before acting, again with the purpose of obtaining information relevant to error signals.

Adaptive modal strategies consist of both active and passive aspects mobilized in response to positive and negative prediction error in order to maximize resource benefits against costs and to manage competently the risk associated with unexpected windfalls and setbacks. In combination, control modules and adaptive modal strategies enhance a dog's ability to cope with the uncertainty of unexpected change by orienting and prolonging contact with valuable resources, as well as startling events, while extracting information to improve future control efforts. Many confident dogs engaged in an activity interrupted by a sudden startle will jump back to a safe distance (escape-to-safety response) from where they will often immediately return to the spot and cautiously investigate it to obtain information about the unexpected event. Such dogs respond to startle as an impetus to curiosity and increased exploratory activity, which is a pattern that they also show in response to novelty and attractive surprise.

PREDICTION ERROR AND ADAPTATION

Reward and punishment depend on the relative success or failure of instrumental efforts to anticipate and control motivationally significant events. Consequently, aversive and attractive motivational events share a common function of enhancing canine adaptability and security (comfort and safety) by promoting control incentives and goal-directed efforts, with aversive control efforts aimed at seeking and obtaining safety (relief and relaxation) and attractive control efforts aimed at seeking and obtaining appetitive and tactile gratification (comfort and calming). As such, reward-based training incorporates both aversive and attractive incentives presented and withdrawn in highly predictable and controllable ways. Just as stimuli paired with actions that anticipate the successful control of appetitive events are valenced with attractive significance, so are stimuli paired with actions anticipating the successful avoidance of aversive events (Dinsmoor, 2001); that is, they are both represented as reward signals. In an important sense, competent dog training is

reward based regardless of the hedonic valence of the antecedent and consequent motivational stimuli used to activate control incentives and to facilitate behavioral change and control. A balance of controllable attractive and aversive contingencies in the context of social exchange promotes learning conducive to the integration of secure place and social attachments.

Prediction error results in significant alterations affecting social expectancies and mood. The direction of these changes depends on the relative proportion of surprising versus disappointing outcomes produced by control efforts. Dogs producing proportionately more surprises (positive prediction errors) than disappointments (negative prediction errors) tend toward elated mood and a positivity bias—changes reflected in a high level of optimism, confidence, relaxation, and persistence at tasks setting the occasion for prediction errors. Dogs operating under a positivity bias expect to produce positive prediction errors (reward). On the other hand, dogs producing proportionately more disappointment than surprise associated with social exchange tend to show dysthymic mood, irritability, and a negativity bias, as indicated by increased insecurity, anxiety and frustration, and a lack of persistence at tasks setting the occasion for positive prediction errors—dogs affected by a negativity bias expect to produce negative prediction errors (punishment) and conflict when they interact with people.

When properly performed, cynopraxic training provides a foundation of orderly interaction between the owner and the dog that can rapidly enhance mood and alter expectancy bias in the direction of increased optimism. The facilitation of an elated mood and an optimistic expectancy bias provides a valuable preliminary foundation for the implementation of more specific behavior-therapy procedures. In addition to improving an owner's ability to control and manage the dog, the highly predictable and controllable nature of training events helps to improve the dog's attention and impulse-control abilities—executive functions that are centrally involved in the organization of competent behavior.

Behavior resulting in a high degree of verification is relatively free of conflict and stress but lacks the excitement and surprise associated with the production of positive prediction errors. The safe and comfortable (but boring) status quo consisting of highly verified control modules are often put aside by dogs, at least momentarily, for the sake of exploring and experimenting, perhaps in search of unforeseen ways to exploit some resource more thoroughly, possibly discovering new solutions to old problems or taking risks with potentially dangerous situations, all in order to obtain the surprise and delight of producing positive prediction errors (cortical rewards). Reward resulting from better-than-expected outcomes helps to optimize prediction-control efforts. Contingencies of positive prediction error that are associated with adventure and discovery produce powerful incentives, sufficient to risk life and limb. Rather than resting content and enjoying the gratification of reliable and safe contingencies, cortical reward and punishment promote incentives to explore and take risks (active modal strategies), or to wait and minimize risks (passive modal strategies) if risk taking is unlikely to pay off.

Actions resulting in cortical reward cannot continue to produce reward by simply repeatedly producing the same rewarding outcome. Paradoxically, the more effective a response becomes, the less it can produce reward. This notion of reward conflicts substantially with the traditional formulation of the law of effect. In contrast to conventional assumptions, a central function of cortical reward according to cynopraxic training theory is to confirm the prediction-control expectancy while simultaneously producing surprise conducive to the mobilization of active modal strategies (e.g., increased seeking, searching, exploring, and experimenting). These observations point to another corollary of the prediction-error hypothesis: formally speaking, behavior cannot be certain to produce cortical reward; it can only increase the probability that a change will occur to produce surprise or relief. The most effective behaviors for this purpose are adaptive modal strategies, that is, a combination of active and passive modal strategies consisting of searching, exploring, risk taking, hesitating, waiting, and ritualizing. The aleatory nature of prediction error marks behavior in search of reward with a characteristic quality of hopefulness. Hope is the condition of behaving in accordance with uncertain, albeit expected, contingencies of reward (surprise), with hope occasionally being dashed by disappointment (see Mowrer, 1960).

Consequently, the surprise of cortical reward increases alertness and exploratory activity while orienting attention toward the windfall. As a result, the cortical reward does not simply increase the future probability of the reward-producing response but also serves to increase the probability of discovering information relevant to the optimization of the action. In addition to active modal strategies, passive modal strategies (e.g., waiting, begging, and ritualizing) are employed to decrease the likelihood of producing negative prediction errors. Passive modal strategies are especially likely to occur under conditions in which active strategies are more likely to produce negative prediction error than positive prediction error. The evolutionary provision of motivational incentives to activate environmental exploration and experimentation as well as to support waiting and ritualizing under adverse environmental conditions is consistent with the behavioral flexibility needed to optimize adaptability and survival fitness.

Learning by means of knowledge derived from experience and prediction error organizes behavior into a base of highly effective and reliable instrumental responses, routines, and patterns conducive to comfort and safety (order), while at the same time increasing exploration, experimentation, and risk-taking behavior (variability), thus optimizing a dog's ability to engage in competent exchanges with the environment. The advent of behavioral organization shaped by positive prediction error and negative prediction error heralds a sophisticated evolutionary advance that succeeds in organizing behavior toward increasing order while at the same time facilitating behavioral variability.

ADAPTATION, PREDICTION ERROR, AND DISTRESS

According to cynopraxic training theory, adaptive adjustments are organized to cope with the conflict and distress associated with error signals produced in association with the control of attractive and aversive motivational events. Control incentives operate in close association with prediction-control expectancies, calibrated emotional establishing operations, and goal-directed actions to prepare and enable a dog to obtain the full value of anticipated outcomes while managing risk and avoiding harm. The function of control incentives is to establish the value of available outcomes and thereby adjust effort to appropriate motivational levels, to increase or decrease a dog's tolerance for distress (frustration and anxiety), and to determine the amount of risk taking that the reward is worth.

Learning by reward and punishment depends on prediction-control expectancies functioning in close coordination with emotional establishing operations and abolishing operations (see *Instrumental Control Modules and Modal Strategies* in Chapter 1). Calibrated emotional establishing operations serve to modulate (excite or inhibit) control incentives in accordance with prediction error and a variety of cross-associative linkages between the event, action, and the hedonic value of the resulting exchange or *transaction*. These predictive relations are subject to constant revision and refinement in response to positive and negative error signals. The emotional establishing operation consists of specific motivational state changes that undergo continuous refinement in conjunction with the revision of prediction-control expectancies in response to prediction-error signals generated by goal-directed actions. In contrast, abolishing operations oppose the emotional and motivational effects of emotional establishing operations (e.g., fear and hunger) through the active inhibition of the motivational state evoked. According to this hypothesis, the inhibitory effects of abolishing operations serve to counter the emotional excitatory effects of establishing operations, but abolishing operations do not generate new motivational states incompatible with the discon-firmed expectancy. The pure inhibitory functions of abolishing operations point to an origin within the executive prefrontal cortex. For example, in response to an emotional establishing operation mediating fear or appetence, the abolishing operation actively inhibits fear and hunger but without replacing it with feelings of safety and comfort (satiation). The incompatible states of safety and comfort are mediated by emergent alternative emotional establishing operations developing in association with the integration of modified prediction-control expectancies.

The reward and punishment of control modules require that a dog be actively engaged in expectant efforts to control some significant attractive or aversive event. Significant events that simply happen to a dog out of the blue may produce temporary or even permanent conditioned excitatory or inhibitory effects on reactive modal behavior but not necessarily alter the control module. The organization of prediction-control expectancies requires the presence of antecedent signals to activate control incentives and preparatory emotional establishing operations in anticipation of the event in order to engage in efforts to control it. Without predictive signals to activate appropriate prediction-control expectancies and emotional establishing operations to guide changes of behavior at the critical moment, the dog may continue to repeat the same behavior over and over again, as Guthrie (1935) relates in a pertinent story that illustrates this aspect of expectancy learning:

> My own view of the way in which unpleasant or unsatisfactory consequences of action affect learning might be further illustrated by a minor incident in the routine of a certain psychologist. He rented an apartment for the summer with a garage which had a large swinging door. From the top of the door hung a heavy chain. Opening the door hurriedly the first morning the chain swung about slowly and struck a blow on the side of the subject's head, a distinctly painful and "unsatisfactory" event. But this continued to happen each morning for some two weeks. Why the long delay in learning to stand aside?
>
> The answer, I believe, is that the act of opening the door was performed while looking

at the exterior of the door. The chain struck after the door had opened and the scene changed. Dodging was not conditioned on the sight of the door because a sight of the door had not accompanied flinching from the blow. The flinching movement which occurred as the rear of the car came into view was too late. Only after the bruised ear became a chronic reminder and the incident had been talked about and finally had been told to a visitor on the way to the garage, did caution show itself in time. (1935:159)

To intensify attention and to activate control incentives, many dog-training techniques involve the use of attractive or aversive events presented independently of a dog's ability to control them. As the result of such stimulation, attention is intensified and behavior activated into reactive seeking or fleeing modes. When such events are deliberately presented for the purpose of interrupting ongoing behavior, they are referred to as *diverters* (attractive events) and *disrupters* (aversive events) (see *Diverters and Disrupters* in Volume 1, Chapter 7). Diverters and disrupters are often linked to appetitive or emotional establishing operations and used as occasion-setting events to activate control modules incompatible with the interrupted target activity.

COMPARATOR PROCESSING, ALLOSTASIS, AND ADAPTIVE OPTIMIZATION

Adaptive behavior is organized to cope proactively with the uncertainty of change. Anticipated outcomes are rarely exactly as expected but are sometimes slightly or far worse than expected, sometimes partly expected and partly unexpected, sometimes slightly or far better than expected, and sometimes more or less as expected. The sum effect of these outcomes is varied still further by diverse motivational states coincident with the outcomes produced. According to cynopraxic theory, predictive relations and transactions that produce positive and negative prediction errors are part of a reality-constructing process. The comparator processing of prediction error is hypothesized to represent an evolutionary opening out of neuroregulatory systems origi-

nally dedicated to track energy gains and losses maintaining physiological balance and homeostasis. The behavioral system includes a capacity to respond to error as alarm and warning signals triggering preparatory responses in anticipation of physical and psychological stressors as well as reward signals in anticipation of relief and comfort. Experiences of autonomic arousal triggered by emotional distress (frustration and anxiety), passive modal strategies organized to reduce loss and risk, and somatic reward (feelings of comfort and safety or security) are closely coordinated with energy conservation and homeostasis. Whereas homeostasis is concerned with the maintenance of physiological conditions within narrow ranges of deviation, allostasis mediates adaptive fitness by means of predictive relations shaped to maintain "stability through change" (Sterling and Eyer, 1988), a concept posited as an important evolutionary development in the way biological systems cope with change in the process of optimizing adaptability.

Adjustments to positive and negative prediction error enables dogs to optimize the extraction of useful predictive relations and patterns while limiting risks incurred as the result opening and exploring new things and places. The resulting *opening out* of experience is comfortable and safe (zona securitas) but sufficiently aleatory and dynamic (zona optimus) to maintain a feed-forward momentum, thus offsetting the adverse effects of internalizing (axipetal) and externalizing (axifugal) load. *Load* refers to a loss of adaptability stemming from a binding up biobehavioral energy into entropic activities that impair a dog's ability to initiate flexible control efforts in accord with prediction-control expectancies and calibrated emotional establishing operations (see *Big Bangs and Black Holes: Extraversion, Introversion, and Disorganizing Load*). Specifically, adaptability refers to the ability of dogs to integrate an expansive coping style (freedom) in the process of developing competent skills and the confidence to use them (power).

Feed-forward comparator processing links many different neural systems together into brainwide attunement networks and nodes that resonate in response to prediction error and confirmation signals to organize adjustments relevant to adaptive needs (Simonov, 1994). The resulting organization is sufficiently complex and orderly to support energy homeostasis, while sufficiently uncertain and varied to enable dogs to cope flexibly with novelty and unexpected change by means of versatile control modules and adaptive modal strategies conducive to allostasis. A complex network of interconnective nodes links the orbital and medial prefrontal cortex (PFC) to the hypothalamus (Öngür et al., 1998), the head ganglion of the autonomic nervous system, which performs numerous integrative functions associated with autonomic attunement, appetitive and defensive motivation, reproduction, and energy homeostasis. In addition to hypothalamic projections, networks comprising the orbital-medial PFC have strong interconnectivities with the basolateral amygdala, basal ganglia, superior colliculus, hippocampus, the ventral tegmental area, the periaqueductal gray, and brainstem vagal system. Multiple levels of comparator processing work in unison to decipher patterns of significance (reward value) adhering to prediction error and to integrate the information obtained into an expanding interactive space opened and exploited in the process of optimizing adaptive skills. Such a layered comparator processing system is consistent with the notion of a behavioral guidance system comprised of cortical-autonomic attunement nodes that assign motivational significance (arousal, incentive, and hedonic value) to attractive and aversive events, select appropriate goal-directed actions, and mobilize adaptive modal strategies in response to error signals. Thus, sensory input processed for error and significance by frontal and limbic networks is projected to the hypothalamus to modulate complex neuroendocrine and autonomic effector systems. These reciprocal pathways between the cortex, limbic areas, and the hypothalamus give rise to a subjective awareness of emotion and motivational state changes via humoral, visceromotor, and afferent vagal feedback from the body (see Nauta, 1971).

The evolution of the neocortical mantle was probably related to adaptations necessitated by the added metabolic demands of thermoregulation. The increased metabolic costs of sustaining temperature homeostasis were met by a matching increase in the early mammal's ability to procure food and other basic survival resources via predictive information and environmental maps organized by the cortex. Interesting, within the developing embryo, the first part of the neocortex to develop is localized around the mouth, with the remaining development of different cortical areas concentrically building out from this core area (Allman, 2000). An increased capacity for organizing behavior in accord with prediction-control expectancies and calibrated establishing operations is hypothesized to be the result of a revolutionary shift from reactive adjustments to internal and external demands to a more flexible and proactive pattern of *adaptive optimization*. This shift toward the organization of behavior in accordance with prediction error and an increased awareness of internal emotional states is likely a result of evolutionary changes to the mammalian brain organized to cope with the complex demands of social life and the extended care of offspring. Awareness of one's emotional state of arousal is a necessary precondition for the hesitation and proactive adjustments needed to avoid conflict, enabling dogs to wait and delay or to select alternative courses of action. Choosing among alternative courses of action probably traces its origins to a habitual pattern of hesitating and refraining to act immediately in anticipation of social exchange, thereby giving rise to an ability to consider and rehearse various control options in advance of initiating action based on the option that *feels* best (more likely to succeed or safer). The ability to hesitate and choose or wait provides dogs with a strong element of voluntary control over social exchange. By means of *feel*-forward comparator processing, emotional establishing operations are calibrated to meet the anticipated needs of ongoing goal-directed projects and ventures based on affective adjustments to prediction-control expectancies and action-mediated prediction error.

The process is analogous to the operation of a radio. A radio is designed to detect and decode subtle patterns of information encoded into electromagnetic signals that are transmitted at the speed of light through the atmosphere, picked up, separated, and conducted through various feed-forward circuits in the process of decoding, converting, and amplifying electromagnetic information into acoustical signals delivered at a rate and strength to enable the listener to experience a coherent and realistic pattern of acoustical stimulation represented to awareness as crystal clear music. A major difference between a radio system and the adaptive brain system is related to the processing of prediction error. Everything governing the operation of the radio is highly predictable and closed. A radio cannot improve over time but merely wears out. The canine brain is designed to improve senso-effector capacities over time by means of adaptive adjustments in response to prediction error. Accordingly, prediction-error signals are converted into energy/information values (energy gains and losses) and uploaded into feed-forward comparator processors that amplify the energy/error signal, converting it into feed-forward predictive relations having information and hedonic value. These energy/information values are selectively amplified while their significance is being determined and thus reach various cognitive (orienting and attending), emotional (arousal, incentive, and valence), and behavior (action mode) threshold values.

Control efforts result in a transfer of energy, the result of which is to open space and to optimize energy gains and losses via the organization of predictive relations. According to this general hypothesis, the moment-to-moment predictive relations that guide goal-directed efforts result in either better-than-expected or worse-than-expected outcomes (i.e., energy gains and losses relative to energy expenditures). These energy gains and losses are scaled and converted into changes of affective awareness and arousal having motivational relevance for ongoing control efforts. Consequently, the discovery of motivationally significant events while engaged in exploratory exchanges with the environment results in incentive (need) and hedonic (like and dislike) changes that increase autonomic arousal and invigorate attention (awareness) commensurate to energy gains or losses calculated to have resulted from the transaction.

Actions are not dissociable from feed-forward comparator processing but are the voluntary and goal-directed manifestations of such processing; that is, adaptive behavior is a complex energy/information exchange system that includes information collecting, processing, and testing functions. Technically, actions are not separate from experience but exist to mediate experience to acquire knowledge. *Experience* is understood as an active process of signification mediated by behavioral experiment, as in sense of the Latin, *experientia*, "knowledge gained by trial and test." Actions can shape objects but cannot be shaped into objects. Behavior is an activity in constant change, and only a dead dog "behaves" like an object. As such, behavior lacks an objective nature except as regards the history of effects that it leaves on objects. Behavior can produce knowledge by virtue of exchanges with objects (culture) but cannot be known itself accept as a subjective experience of hedonic value, referred to as *appreciation*. During social exchange, the partner's behavior is the object of esthetic and empathetic appreciation. Learning in accord with the formation of prediction-control expectancies is conducive to the development of increasing social awareness, appreciation, and competence.

Behavior consists of exchanges and transactions with the environment that open and extend fields of predictive relations into the uncertainty of change by collecting, processing, testing error signals. Thus, goal-directed actions are integrated into a stabilizing matrix of prediction-control expectancies and emotional establishing operations or control modules. The feed-forward comparator processing and amplification of error signals as experiential information mediating adjustment is conserved across distant phyla, ranging from conditioned reflexive adjustments to conscious awareness. The nature of such processing is limited by the complexity of the organism's nervous system. With every level of comparator processing, the significance of the error signal is extracted and amplified. During highly significant events, the error signal attains affective significance by its representation to awareness as an experience possessing hedonic value. The comparator process involves a complex interactive system of brainwide networks that cooperatively convert and amplify prediction error into significance, with experiential events of significant value attaining to subjective awareness after reaching threshold values prompting attentive interest or concern. Accordingly, habituated stimuli do not attract attention or evoke emotional arousal rising to awareness because they fail to rise above the preattentive sensory threshold of significance. Dishabituated stimuli are represented to experience as significant events by attaining to the threshold value of error signals prompting attention and interest.

The theory postulates that all categories of experience, including sensation, perception, cognition, emotion, and action, are the result of feed-forward comparator processing that extracts, amplifies, and interprets the value and significance of error signals. Error signals reaching preattentive thresholds (saccades) precede sensory and perceptual thresholds (orienting), sensory and perceptual thresholds precede cognitive thresholds (attention), and thresholds of cognitive significance precede affective thresholds attributing hedonic value (conscious awareness and appreciation). Thus, feed-forward comparator processors and dedicated algorithms convert sensory and cognitive values into affective or hedonic values (likes and dislikes) that in turn vector control incentives (needs) on objects of interest or concern with an intent to control them. The attainment of esthetic and empathetic appreciation represents the highest level of comparator refinement and amplification of error signals reaching thresholds of conscious awareness.

The organization of different predictive relations into a unified system entails that some common scalable and interchangeable factor or constant hold between them. The energy gains and losses resulting from social transaction may be scaled, encoded, and invested with value, as information, emotion (incentive and distress), and hedonics (energy gains and losses experienced as pleasure or displeasure). Accordingly, positive prediction error yielding surprise and elation (energy gain) results in an enhanced state of awareness, whereas outcomes that merely match expectancies are encoded to yield feelings of comfort and safety. As such, both attractive and aversive events have allostatic and autonomic value insofar as they evoke arousal/alertness and activate comfort- or safety-seeking action modes. This hypothesis suggests that sensory and emotional experiences are differentiated in terms of the neural energy expended to represent them as subjective experiences, with excitatory events appearing to require a greater expenditure of energy to represent than inhibitory ones. Whereas excitatory events carry an attractive or aversive valence that generates an increased vigilance and readiness to act, inhibitory events conduce a state of autonomic de-arousal (Collet et al., 1999). Finally, there is an optimal level of attractive or aversive arousal that promotes adjustment and reward, stimulation under or over which evokes irrelevant or conflictive responses (Hebb, 1955).

SOMATIC VERSUS CORTICAL REWARD, PROJECTS AND VENTURES, AND POWER INCENTIVES

The integration of prediction-control expectancies, calibrated emotional establishing operations, and actions into control modules gives dogs a significant degree of choice in defining and pursuing goal-directed objectives, referred to as *projects* (riskless) and *ventures* (risky). Although adaptive behavior is responsive to the motivational influences of emotional command systems, according to cynopraxic training theory, autonomic arousal and modal activity evoked by conditioned and unconditioned attractive and aversive motivational stimuli do not directly regulate behavior by means of reinforcement and punishment, but instead motivational events generate control incentives (e.g., hunger, thirst, fear, anger, and loneliness) and distress (frustration and anxiety) in association with excitatory and inhibitory state changes that alter alertness and action readiness.

Technically, reward and punishment refers to the relative success or failure of goal-directed projects or ventures to control significant motivational events. Control efforts that match expected outcomes confirm or *reinforce* the control module. Although such matches or somatic rewards may verify control modules, gratify control incentives, promote relaxation, and generate security (comfort and safety), they do not add anything new to a dog's ability to predict or control the event; that is, they do not reduce uncertainty adhering to change. Since the verified action is asymptotic in its capacity to produce reward, verification establishes an increasingly stable plateau of order (see *Reinforcement and the Notion of Probability* in Volume 1, Chapter 7). Verifying events serve to gratify dogs motivationally and to maintain the status quo—a condition of no change and no need to change. Under highly verified and regimented environmental conditions, learning may be significantly impeded by a lack of sufficient prediction error to produce cortical reward. The reduction in reward under such circumstances may produce various deleterious and damaging behavioral effects paradoxically despite a high degree of order and adequate basic resources and safety from danger. For example, a dog may engage in risky sensation-seeking behavior to raise the intensity and variety of stimulation to obtain positive affects from social exchange.

Whereas the confirmation of a control module results in reinforcement (verification), the disconfirmation of a control module results in its rapid or gradual extinction. *Rapid extinction* occurs as the result of the signaled discontinuation of the instrumental control contingency, with the previously rewarded behavior now failing to control the aversive or attractive motivational stimulus. In contrast, *gradual extinction* occurs as the result of an unsignaled discontinuation of the control contingency such that a significant amount of uncertainty remains regarding the status of the contingency. In addition to disappointment and discomfort, the gradual extinction of a control module produces sig-

nificant anxiety and frustration associated with uncertainty. Avoidance learning is particularly problematic in this regard. An unsignaled discontinuation of an avoidance contingency gives a dog little information about the necessity of the avoidance response. Since the dog cannot know whether the avoidance response is necessary without testing the contingency by withholding the avoidance response, it may continue to perform the response long after it is unnecessary to do so. Consequently, in order to learn the status of the avoidance contingency requires that the dog take risks and test it periodically by withholding the avoidance response or forgetting to respond. In highly aversive or traumatic events, the risks are so great that dogs may persist in the avoidance response indefinitely rather than test the contingency, obtaining significant reward from the safety produced by the strategy. The major difference between rapid and gradual confirmation and disconfirmation of learned behavior is the relative degree of certainty that the dog possesses regarding the status of the control contingency.

Many common behavior problems stem from inconsistent efforts to disconfirm and extinguish social control modules and routines operating in association with intrusive modal strategies (e.g., begging and attention seeking), thereby producing significant positive prediction error and reward when the dog unexpectedly succeeds in compelling the interactive partner to yield more than he or she may wish to give, a disruptive source of reward that serves to increase intrusive limit testing, demanding behavior, and social risk taking. Consequently, the gradual disconfirmation of control modules and routines may provide a problematic backdrop for inadvertent reward, invigorate undesirable modal strategies, generate significant anxiety and frustration associated interactive conflict, and support vicious-circle behavior (i.e., increasing persistence associated with escalating punitive efforts). As a result of these problems, rapid disconfirmation via the signaled discontinuation of the control contingency is usually preferred to gradual extinction, not simply because it is faster acting (a criterion that is not always consistent with long-term interests), but because it minimizes the risks and side effects associated with inconsistent extinction efforts. Although the disconfirmed instrumental control module is taken out of service, it is not unlearned or removed from storage, and it remains available for future use should it be needed. Alternative control modules are generally trained to replace undesirable behaviors associated with problematic or excessive modal behavior (e.g., attention seeking and begging). In an important sense, cooperation is simply attention-seeking and begging routines refined by training and established rules or control contingencies that set limits on the opportunity to gain the social and appetitive rewards sought by the dog.

When purposive control efforts produce better-than-expected or worse-than-expected outcomes, feed-forward comparator neural processors detect the mismatch and extract energy/information from the error signal. In contrast to the calming and relatively neutral emotional effects of somatic reward, the comparator processing of positive prediction error yields state changes that range from elevated interest and concern to power elation and emotional relief. As the error signal rises to the significance of hedonic value and *cortical reward*, it is encoded into comparator network nodes and engrams that inform prediction-control expectancies and calibrated establishing operations. The revision and optimization of the control module are associated with increased alertness and attention, vectoring reward value on the action and context producing the surprising event while activating adaptive modal strategies.

Neuringer (1969), for example, demonstrated that pigeons and rats would engage in key pecking and lever-pressing actions to earn food, even though the same food was made freely available to them within the experimental chamber (see *Contrafreeloading* in Volume 1, Chapter 5). These findings are consistent with the notion that successful control efforts are valenced with positive hedonic value and that the organization of adaptive behavior by reward does not depend on the satisfaction of needs or the escape/avoidance of danger but instead depends on a hedonic factor derived

from the successful control of significant events: "Responding for food, like play and exploring, appears to be a natural part of the behavior of animals and does not necessarily depend upon any prior motivating operation....the present findings suggest that animals often emit instrumental responses which reduce no biological need and abolish no threat" (401). According to cynopraxic training theory, exchanges yielding positive hedonic value serve to promote active modal strategies (exploring and experimenting), whereas outcomes or exchanges yielding negative hedonic value and increased risk promote passive modal strategies (e.g., hesitating and ritualizing). The differentiation of adaptive modal activity into active and passive strategies in response to positive and negative prediction error promotes behavioral variability, thereby improving a dog's ability to exploit unexpected windfalls while exercising appropriate caution and restraint.

From the perspective of adaptive optimization, reward (power/energy gain) and punishment (power/energy loss or risk) are both viewed as having positive significance insofar as they contribute information that refines a dog's prediction-control efforts. The essential difference between them from an experiential viewpoint is subjective; that is, reward is experienced as a gain having positive hedonic value (pleasure and power elation), whereas punishment is experienced as a loss or risk having a negative hedonic value (displeasure and power deflation). Actions that succeed in establishing effective control over a significant resource acquire positive hedonic value, whereas actions that fail acquire negative hedonic value. A principle difference between the occurrence of unexpected attractive motivational stimuli and cortical rewards yielding hedonic value is *power*. Attractive and novel events that merely happen to a dog may yield significant changes that affect arousal and modal behavior but not yield significant hedonic value. In the absence of purposeful control efforts guided by expectancies and establishing operations, such events will tickle the appetite with desire but not satisfy it. Thus, impulsive and hyperactive dogs are driven to seek novelty and reward relentlessly and recklessly but cannot be satisfied so long as their control efforts are performed independently of control modules and power incentives. Such intrusive and exploitive dogs (unstable extraverts) epitomize behavioral powerlessness. In contrast, cortical reward and power elation are the result of occasions that anticipate opportunity and the successful optimization of control modules organized to exploit it.

The combined cognitive and hedonic effects of reward and punishment are reflected in autonomic changes affecting mood (lasting tonic effects) and feelings (transient or phasic emotional effects) conducive to selective attention, impulse control, attachments, and power. *Power* is defined as the acquisition of competent social and motor skills and the confidence to use those skills to optimize control over significant attractive and aversive events. As such, power conduces a state of optimism and increased action readiness (voluntary initiative) to practice and develop adaptive skills. Power is tempered by timing (hesitation and delay) and expansion into novel domains through skilful exploration, experimentation, and discovery aimed at maximizing the success of control efforts while minimizing risks and losses. Power is embedded in timely events that open space and invigorate emergent freedom incentives.

The cynopraxic training process enables the human-dog dyad to pursue an enhanced life experience by organizing social exchanges that mediate mutual appreciation and interactive harmony. Interactive harmony depends on the mutual acquisition of power by social partners to engage in social exchanges free of stressful conflict dynamics. Under the combined influence of power and freedom incentives, competent social exchange systematically increases the complexity and hedonic quality of proxemic relations while expanding the range of interactive relations into the living space by means of increasing cooperation and compromise.

EXPECTANCIES, EMOTION, AND STRESS

The ability to regulate emotion adaptively depends on the coordinated refinement of prediction-control expectancies and calibrated emotional establishing operations. The discovery of a discrepancy or mismatch between what a dog anticipates and what actually occurs as the result of its action is adaptogenic; that is, both surprise and disappointment prompt adaptive change (see *Autonomic Nervous System-mediated Concomitants of Fear* in Volume 1, Chapter 3). Control modules resulting in worse-than-expected or less-than-expected outcomes (negative prediction error) produce anxiety or frustration in proportion to the degree of the detected discrepancy, whereas better-than-expected outcomes (positive prediction error) produce surprise and power elation. The adaptive anxiety and frustration associated with negative prediction error exert varying levels of inhibitory or excitatory emotional change that mobilize behavioral adjustments via the activation of the behavioral inhibition system (BIS) or the behavioral approach system (BAS). As the match is secured, the evoked frustration and anxiety are reduced in association with relaxation and feelings of comfort and safety. According to this hypothesis, comfort and safety result from adjustments that reduce frustration and anxiety by producing *as expected* outcomes, that is, outcomes that match or verify prediction-control expectancies. Rewards producing comfort and safety promote security and a calming effect in association with passive coping strategies (e.g., hesitating, waiting, and watching) and the avoidance of punishment (i.e., the loss of comfort or safety). The calming effect associated with enhanced comfort and safety appears to be mediated by the parasympathetic branch of the autonomic nervous system (ANS), suggesting the term *somatic reward*. In an important sense, somatic reward serves to mediate adjustments conducive to both behavioral and biological adaptation (homeostasis) via the reduction of error signals generating frustration and anxiety.

The reward associated with positive prediction error mobilizes intrinsically rewarding active modal strategies (e.g., seeking, hunting, and exploring), increased excitement and alertness, and elated mood via the activation of dopaminergic mesocorticolimbic reward pathways. The surprise associated with better-than-expected outcomes mediates adaptive optimization (order with variety) and is referred to as *cortical reward*, emphasizing its executive organizing, exciting, and mood-enhancing effects. Learning is stressful but less so to the extent that adjustments are gradual and voluntary, based on reliable prediction-control expectancies, and organized in a social environment (home) generally perceived as safe and supportive. The ability to competently organize behavioral output toward the optimization of somatic and cortical rewards while avoiding punishment (loss of comfort and safety) is referred to as an *adaptive coping style*. Dogs showing adaptive coping behavior efficiently select control modules, monitor and assess outcomes, and make appropriate adjustments in accordance with prediction-error discrepancies.

When an established social expectancy is disconfirmed in a dramatic, threatening, and uncontrollable way (loss of trust), a dog's behavior may rapidly fall under the influence of stressogenic emergency arousal (fear or anger) and the activation of species-typical autoprotective coping strategies. Whether the dog confronts the threat, backs down, attacks, or runs away depends on the nature of the provocation, the size of the perceived discrepancy and amount of threatened loss or harm, the strength of elicited aversive arousal (anger or pain), the quality and strength of affiliative buffers (effect of person), protective quality-of-life (QOL) factors, behavioral thresholds controlling flight-or-fight behavior, acquired ability to regulate emotion, outcomes of past agonistic encounters, and so forth. In general, the way dogs respond to social threats and challenges can be divided into five types depending on reactive thresholds (see *Behavioral Thresholds and Aggression* in Volume 2, Chapter 8). Most dogs will cower to the ground and become immobile (high-flight and high-fight thresholds—type 1), others may attempt to run away (low-flight and high-fight threshold—type 2), some may stand their ground and confront the challenge but not attack unless provoked (high-flight and medium-fight threshold—type 3), some may attack without hesitation (high-flight and low-fight threshold—type 4), and a few may respond with panic and rage (low-flight and low-fight threshold—type 5). If a dog's efforts to escape are thwarted, an attack threshold may be rapidly reached, and under the influence of escalating fear and anger, a panicked attack with rage may follow. A dog that is prepared to confront a challenge or threat may hold ground but rapidly attack if reached for or grabbed, and escalate the attack in accordance with the perceived degree of threat. As the result of such agonistic encounters, reactive thresholds may be significantly altered, and the dog may become more reactive under similar future circumstances. Also, after experiencing a disconfirmatory mismatch between expected outcomes and actual outcomes, a dog may exhibit an increased dependence on direct sensory input for assessing the situation, appearing to lose its trust in expectancies for assessing social safety (see *Practical Example* in Volume 1, Chapter 7).

AUTONOMIC AROUSAL, DRIVE, AND ACTION MODES

At a basic level, acting in accord with modal drive is intrinsically gratifying, whether it results in approach and seeking or withdrawal and avoiding behavior; however, thwarting drive behavior is intrinsically annoying regardless of its motivational direction. For example, preventing a dog's flight to safety while operating under the aversive arousal of a threat will likely increase the direction and pressure (control incentives) of its escape efforts with frustration (annoyance). In contrast, behavioral exchanges that result in an unexpected opening to safety while under the added aversive arousal of annoyance may produce a pleasurable surprise consisting of elated relief and an emergent state of relaxation that yields feelings of safety. The reward associated with successful escape to safety promotes the integration of prediction-control expectancies, emotional establishing operations, and avoidance behaviors that lead to safety when exposed to similar future threats and circumstances. Likewise, preventing a hungry dog from taking food placed within its reach is annoying, whereas allowing it to approach and eat the food is satisfying. Forbidding a dog to approach and eat appears to increase appetitive drive and control incentives via the aversive motivational effects of annoyance (frustration) under the modulatory influence of risk monitoring and anxiety. As the result of increased modal activity and mobilization of control incentives, those behavioral efforts that facilitate access to the food will be strengthened by reward, especially so in the case of novel solutions that the dog discovers as the result of experimenting or struggling under the pressure of distress.

Although the various action modes, drive, and emotional command systems are functionally partitioned, they are not entirely insulated and appear to exert a variety of excitatory and inhibitory influences on one another (see *Emotional Command Systems and Drive Theory* in Chapter 6). In contrast to the relatively strict segregation of quiet and affective attack modes, seeking and fighting modes do not appear to be strictly incompatible (see *Intraspecific State and Trait Aggression* in Chapter 8), whereas social and appetitive seeking and flight modes do show evidence of reciprocal inhibition, as evidenced by the psychogenic anorexia induced by social anxiety. In addition to diagnostic significance, the foregoing observations are of considerable relevance with respect to the benefits and drawback of appetitive counterconditioning as a therapeutic tool for reducing the reactive arousal anticipating certain forms of extrafamilial aggression. Behavioral treatment programs that exclusively rely on appetitive counterconditioning may reduce social anxiety (defense drive) without significantly reducing social anger (fight drive). For example, a mature watchdog when threatening a visitor fully expects that the target will retreat or that the target will fight back. At such times, the dog is attuned with autonomic arousal to engage the visitor in combat—not to make nice—so the presentation of food at such times is entirely out of context. With encouragement, some of these dogs will happily take food from the stranger but still remain in a reactive state of suspicion and suspense. The persistent wariness and readiness of such dogs to attack is only

natural when one considers the circumstances and that only a few moments before they were engaged in behavior that established an adversarial relation with the visitor. Actually, the food-giving behavior of the visitor might be interpreted by the dog as a ruse to cause it to lower its guard, thereby making it vulnerable to a surprise attack. As the dog takes food, anxious arousal associated with defensive flight modes may be attenuated, allowing the visitor even to pet the dog without reducing the risk of an attack. The instant the visitor stops feeding or petting the dog or engages in overt actions (stands up) perceived as a threat, the change may trigger a strong catastrophic escalation of aggressive arousal.

When under the heightened arousal of drive compatible with the activation of seeking and prey-catching activities, the opportunity to chase a deer is intrinsically energizing and gratifying for a dog whether the chase succeeds or not, whereas compelling a dog to abstain from chasing a deer is intrinsically annoying. In addition, even though restraint is annoying, it will not help to reduce the future strength of the deer-chasing action mode. Accordingly, mere annoyance is not synonymous with punishment. Annoyance actually may significantly augment arousal and drive while generating more of the predatory action mode by virtue of agitation effects on drive. For example, the use of passive leash restraint (horizontal hanging) to block impulsive control efforts (e.g., seeking, chasing, and fighting) appears to escalate drive significantly by invigorating sympathetic arousal and energizing action modes. The action mode selected is determined by the combined pressure and direction of the motivational event, so that attractive events evoke comfort-seeking incentives and serve to activate approach modes, whereas aversive events are valenced to evoke withdrawal and safety-seeking action modes (escape to safety). A dog may shift from one mode into another under the combined influence of distress (frustration and anxiety) and increased aversive stimulation, thereby recruiting more energetic arousal and effort (escape from danger) with the goal of overcoming the interference blocking the dog's access or ability to produce a situational change promising to confer comfort or safety.

Efforts aimed at thwarting motivated behavior without first causing a dog to disengage impulsive control efforts are generally unsuccessful. The amplified energetic state changes produced by holding the dog back on leash, for example, are encoded into emotional establishing operations signaling the dog to try harder, thereby increasing the strength of seeking and fighting modes and causing the dog to escalate its efforts when faced with similar circumstances in the future, making the impulsive pattern dominant over other coping options. Forcing a dog to stop an attack risks fanning the fierceness of the attack, just as blocking a dog's escape efforts may cause it to abruptly transition out of the flight mode into a fight mode. Finally, withdrawing social stimulation while a dog is in social drive is intrinsically annoying, whereas providing social attention at such times promotes social attraction and attachment. These are but a few of many linkages between modal activity, autonomic arousal, and drive that impact significantly the efficacy of behavior therapy.

The emotional effects of reward and punishment are closely integrated with the activation and deactivation of relevant drive modes. In addition to the differential effects of attractive and aversive arousal, as reflected in active and passive modal strategies, drive activity can be excited or inhibited by natural triggers or by classically conditioned stimuli. Also, drives can be modulated or interrupted by deliberately educing other drives. Drive deficits and excesses can be manipulated toward equilibrium by educing compatible (excitatory) and incompatible (inhibitory) state changes via the activation of relevant emotional command systems. Teasers are arousal-enhancing tools that are used to tune and boost activity or to attract a dog's attention with repeated lip smacking, clapping, changes of pace, crouching, and sundry other gestures. Drive eduction is often performed by means of diverters and disrupters (generic establishing operations) used to interrupt or balance drive-related activities. A cautionary note here is that stressing excessive reliance on training

methods that reduce drive activity by educing incompatible drive (e.g., educing fear to decrease appetitive seeking) may introduce imbalance and destabilize the emotional command system, especially if such stimulation is applied severely or unpredictably or in the absence of stabilizing reward-based training efforts.

Drive and emotional command systems combine to give control incentives direction, pressure, continuity, and momentum, but only actions integrated into control modules are amenable to the effects of reward and punishment. However, reward appears to be more directly related to the hedonic value attributed to transactions rather than the gratification or drive reduction obtained by eating (Young, 1955) or escaping to safety. The actual eating of food and the escape to safety might mediate modal alterations and state changes (relaxation), but such consummatory effects alone may not mediate reward effects. For example, an anticipated food reward that is *bigger* but less savory than expected might actually be represented as a disappointment, whereas a food reward that matches expectations may prevent extinction but fail to support additional learning. Thus, reward appears to be more directly related to the hedonic value of the outcome (Young, 1959) and its capacity to optimize goal-directed efforts than its ability to satisfy a need. Consequently, increasing appetitive drive by food or social deprivation is not typically a very useful way to augment counterconditioning or instrumental control efforts. Alternatively, instead of increasing need (incentive value), a far more valuable effect can be achieved by increasing the hedonic value of the reward (i.e., by use of a more savory food item) or by switching to a different type of reward (novelty) to increase the enjoyment value of the reward object. The manipulation of hedonic value and novelty provides a powerful means to enhance reward value and increase the therapeutic value of food rewards (Zernicki, 1968).

Crespi (1942) showed that the reward value of food can be increased or decreased by changing its size during a post-training test phase relative to the size of the reward used in the training phase. Initially, Crespi trained three groups of rats to run to a goal box where they received 1, 16, or 256 pellets, respectively. These groups were subsequently tested and compared for motivational differences by giving each of them 16 pellets and then measuring running speed. The experimenter found that rats trained with 16 pellets showed no change in running speed, whereas those that had been originally trained with 1 pellet showed a significant increase (elation effect) in running speed, and those trained with 256 pellets showed a significant decrease (depression effect) in running speed. These findings are consistent with the expectancy hypothesis, whereby a bigger-than-expected outcome (positive prediction error) generates surprise and elation, thereby increasing the hedonic value of the food reward, whereas a smaller-than-expected outcome (negative prediction error) produces disappointment and depression, thereby decreasing the reward's hedonic value.

Actions operating under the guidance of prediction-control expectancies and calibrated emotional establishing operations (control module) are refined or *optimized* by social and environmental transactions that yield surprise or disappointment. Further, the hedonic value of any given transaction is determined by the difference between the gain anticipated from the energy invested in the action and the actual gain produced, less the energetic costs and risks incurred by pursuing the project or venture. Energy is invested in behavioral projects and ventures with an expectation of a profit. Consequently, the optimization of control modules is closely coordinated with an *unconscious* process organized to maximize energy gains while minimizing energy losses and reducing risk. Energy gains and losses are encoded into conscious awareness as pleasurable or displeasurable alterations commensurate to the positive or negative hedonic value of the outcome. Energy gains and losses (i.e., physiological state changes) are scaled or translated into affective state changes that rise to the level of awareness by the amplification error signals provided by feed-forward comparator processing networks that simultaneously construct an experiential engram that

informs and modifies the control module. According to this hypothesis, the energy gains and losses inferred from positive and negative prediction error are represented to awareness as affective changes having hedonic significance. These affective changes rise to awareness as substrate neurophysiological alterations are integrated into synaptic elaborations or attunement nodes and nodal networks that alter synaptic sensitivity and mediate long-term reverberation and resonance effects affecting mood and action readiness. The composite synaptic activity of attunement nodes and nodal networks, and corresponding effects on mood and a dog's readiness to initiate voluntary action, are hypothesized to vary depending on the proportion of transactions perceived as resulting in energy gains (positive hedonic value) or losses (negative hedonic value).

The ability of an attractive or aversive motivational incentive to promote instrumental learning depends on its ability to generate sufficient emotional arousal to mobilize an appropriate control module without being so strong that it triggers reactive adjustments. The generation of emotional arousal via the presentation of attractive (appetitive and social) and aversive stimuli varies greatly among dogs. These breed and individual differences reflect the combined influence of genetic predisposition and prior experience on social approach-withdrawal thresholds (social temperament dimensions), coping styles, transient motivational states (e.g., isolation and hunger), survival-mode activity, and autonomic attunement. Dogs combining low-approach and high-withdrawal thresholds consistent with *extraversion* are more likely to persist in conflictive social exchange under the influence of escalating autonomic arousal yielding frustration, whereas dogs expressing high-approach thresholds and low-withdrawal thresholds consistent with introversion are more likely to withdraw from social conflict under the influence escalating arousal yielding anxiety. These tendencies to persist or withdraw in response to conflict exert potent organizing effects on social behavior, mood, and coping styles.

The preference shown by extraverts for signals of reward, novelty, and risk taking predisposes them to acquire proactive skills that tend to individuate leader personality traits and roles in association with confidence/playfulness (strong power/freedom incentives), whereas the preference of introverts for signals of loss and risk (harm avoidance) inclines them to express follower and dependency relations in association with greater social insecurity/submissiveness (strong comfort/safety incentives). Ultimately, since most dogs possess both extraverted and introverted traits, the coping styles, social roles, and personality characteristics that they express are highly flexible and tend to shift toward a centrist position under the influence of an adaptive coping style and constructive attunement dynamics. Under the influence of a reactive coping style and misattunement, though, extraversion and introversion become increasing unstable and extreme, with unstable extraverts becoming increasingly exploitive, intrusive, and impulsive, and unstable introverts becoming increasing cautious, withdrawn, and reactive.

PLAY AND DRIVE

Play possesses unique qualities and capacities to mediate rewarding exchange via the activation of a wide assortment of drive-related behaviors educed and liberated from functional significance, including sundry sex-related exploratory activities, seeking and exploratory behavior (object play), social exchanges (flirting, i.e., playful fleeing and fighting), and prey-predator interactions (stalking, chasing, body blocking, and grabbing). Play engenders a sense of empowering confidence that imbues the nervous system and body with a tonic balance of vigor and euphoric feelings of well-being or joy. Play is suspected to promote significant adaptogenic influences over critical neuropeptide and neurotransmitter systems that mediate autonomic attunement and antistress functions (see *Play and Autonomic Attunement* in Chapter 8).

As a specialized modal activity, play allows dogs to access various drive and motor programs and arousal systems but without activating the emotional command and hypothalamic effector systems that normally motivate

these drives in earnest. The sum of the foregoing characteristics and neurobiological evidence suggests that play is probably integrated into a far-reaching network of neuronal pathways and attunement nodes that are orchestrated at an executive level (Vanderschuren et al., 1997). A reasonable candidate site of executive control is the dorsolateral PFC, a cortical area that appears to mediate the organization of proactive coping strategies in response to conflict. Some interesting work with juvenile rats has found that 30 minutes of rough-and-tumble play elevates brain-derived neurotrophic factor (BDNF) transcription in the dorsolateral frontal cortex and the amygdala (Gordon et al., 2003). This finding supports the idea that repeated play bouts may exert profound neurodevelopmental effects on executive function and lasting epigenetic influences on a dog's ability to cope with conflict (see *Cortical and Subcortical Comparator Functions and Adaptation*).

A prefrontal localization is consistent with the diverse anticonflict and attunement capacities that play appears to coordinate via an active appreciation of the attentional and emotional state of the play partner (see Horowitz, 2002). To sustain playful interaction, dogs must learn to limit exploitive excesses and to avoid causing play partners pain or fear. These various demands encourage dogs to play fairly and to reciprocally adjust to the play partner's needs, thereby promoting empathy for the sake of harmonious exchange. The distinctive reward features of play probably depend on play partners possessing the ability to regulate play exchanges in accord with a principle of fairness (see *Fair Play, Emergent Social Codes, and Cynopraxis* in Chapter 8). The autonomic and behavioral flexibility of play is likely to contribute an increased confidence and tolerance for unexpected social events. Play arousal is antagonistic to most aversive emotional states, providing a natural antidote against social anxiety, irritability/intolerance, and depression. During cynopraxic training, control modules and routines are brought under the modal control of play incentives. The harmony and fluid rhythms of play exchange are consistent with the integration of autonomic attunement nodes that promote increasing attraction, attachment, and confidence as social familiarity and play skills develop. Play behavior appears to attune people and dogs to sustained cooperative exchange. The invigorated mutual attention and social engagement, harmonious modal shifting, choreographed proxemics, and mutual appreciation and joy give play exchanges an interactive form and beauty.

FAIR PLAY AND THE GOLDEN RULE

There is an inherent unfairness in the relative freedom of a trainer and a dog to initiate purposive exchanges and to control the dispensation of rewards—a disparity that requires a novel cynopraxic solution whereby the trainer's advantage is subordinated to the adaptive interests of the dog. Cynopraxic bond and life-experience imperatives are achieved in various ways, but ultimately all training and therapy activities are subordinated to enhancing a dog's ability to engage others in competent social exchange conducive to affection, play, and trust. People and dogs naturally derive significant hedonic value from play and tend to form lasting attachments as the result of social exchanges that entice and sustain playful interaction. Play is incompatible with social aversion, mistrust, and QOL deficiencies, while helping to promote social competence, confidence, and trust; in short, play is the expressive actualization of power. Play activities help to shape optimistic expectancies and improve a dog's ability to cope proactively with social uncertainty. In situations where playfulness is lacking, cynopraxic counseling and therapy efforts are energetically focused on enlivening playful dynamics between the family and the dog, placing the highest priority on enabling the family and the dog to engage in safe play. Working under the assumption that the most important reason to keep dogs is to enjoy their companionship, cynopraxic therapy and training canalize affectionate playfulness toward the attainment of interactive harmony, mutual appreciation, and joy. Regardless of a trainer's orientation, the training process is only truly humane and meaningful to the extent that it succeeds in establishing an affectionate and playful coexistence.

The prohibitions against competitive play that are frequently espoused in the popular dog literature are tailor-made to promote problems. The notion that play (e.g., tug games and roughhousing) promotes aggression is extremely misleading and destructive. In fact, play appears to enhance a dog's ability to cope proactively with conflict situations and unexpected changes that might otherwise result in more serious reactive contests. Players take and give advantage to optimize the reward intrinsic to play. To sustain such play activities, they must be sensitive to one another's needs and play fairly. In the process, dogs learn the *golden rule*: do as one wishes done in return. The leader is not distinguished by possessive irritability and a short-fuse temper that flares into rage at any provocation. A leader's status is measured by the amount of power and freedom he or she has to integrate playful exchanges with others—a prerequisite for integrating cohort relationships, guiding cooperative projects, and performing successful courtship rituals.

Dogs with good play skills exemplify the golden rule in the active and careful way they avoid violating the social code around the rights of first possession, apparently with some expectation that other dogs do the same in turn (see *Fair Play, Emergent Social Codes, and Cynopraxis* in Chapter 8). The code is respected regardless of the other dog's ability or willingness to defend the object in its possession. Leader-type dogs will even refuse direct countermands prompting them to take objects in violation of the code. When in possession of a valued object, however, these same dogs defend the code by a variety of strategies, often by stiffening over the object, which is an action that might also be interpreted in terms of the golden algorithm; that is, the stiffening may be intended to cause the other to hesitate or stop. If necessary, an expression of default dominance consisting of a startling growl-bark or fang whack may be used to defend the code, often followed by the dog shifting away with the object or taking it off to another location. Of course, such dogs can deliver a vigorous defense against persistent intruders, if need be. A similar pattern of code-regulated behavior and default dominance may be shown around food and other highly valued resources, thereby exercising significant control over conflict-related tensions. The increased willingness of dogs to share valued objects and toys with people probably stems from the greater likelihood of people giving things to the dogs. Again, following the golden rule, giving to a dog is reciprocated by increased tolerance and capacity for sharing by the dog, perhaps fostering human-dog codes and attunement dynamics around shared comfort objects and resources that reduce the risk of conflict. In contrast, people that do not give but instead take, deprive, restrain, and threaten dogs may mobilize a pattern of exploitive and autoprotective dynamics in those dogs. The golden rule provides a useful social algorithm for guiding exchanges conducive to sharing, attuning dogs toward fair exchange and helping to decipher intent guiding canine social behavior.

For the average dog, the benefits of play for mediating social harmony and mutual enjoyment far outweigh any risks incurred by the activity. The common dire warnings and prohibitions against inhibitory training, tug games, and other social play activities often have the effect of *self-fulfilling prophecies*. By following the prohibitions against play, the very problems that an owner sought to avoid are actually facilitated. Many new dog owners hoping to calm an excitable puppy or reduce excessive mouthing or biting fall headlong for this idea. These sorts of arbitrary rules and prohibitions usually need to be imposed on other family members with considerable pressure, since the style of interaction required of them will likely feel stymied and unnatural, perhaps causing them to gradually withdraw their interest from the newcomer altogether. The loss of playful exchange is a tremendous sacrifice for everyone. Puppies and dogs appear to be attuned to play as a way to enjoy and become familiar with people and other dogs. The failure to engage in social play essentially denies a dog access to the interaction needed to integrate the relations required to become a full member of the household.

Note: The normal partition preventing play fighting and competition, roughhousing, and tug games from escalating into aggression in earnest may breakdown in certain dogs, especially certain fighting and guard-type breeds. Such dogs may be preemptively biased to respond to increased competitive arousal and excitement by shifting from a play mode into an attack mode. These dogs can be extremely dangerous for naive people to handle. In addition, nervous and reactive dogs can be dangerous when efforts are made to provoke them into play.

NEURAL COMPARATOR SYSTEMS

Preattentive Sensory Processing

Adaptive orienting behavior is mediated by spontaneous and search eye movements in response to auditory and visual stimuli. Spontaneous saccadic eye movements turn the visual apparatus toward the source of stimulus change in anticipation of an orienting response. These reflexive eye movements help to maintain a audiovisual interface with the immediate surroundings, enabling dogs to represent and map significant changes taking place in the immediate surroundings. Saccadic eye movements are associated with the target-arc response that precedes an orienting response. The target-arc response and saccadic eye movements are functionally associated with a complex network of interconnections between the PFC, superior colliculus (SC), limbic system, and brainstem. The encoding and representation of multimodal input into oculocentric sensory maps at the level of the SC has many implications for understanding how rapid adjustments to sudden change and novelty are perceived and integrated into adaptive and reactive preparatory adjustments. In addition to providing an audiovisual spatial representation mapping encoded sensory input, the SC via interconnectivity with cortical and limbic processing is intimately involved in expectant and preemptive processing of an emotional nature that affects how novelty and change are interpreted. The detection and processing of change having potential significance appears to be mediated by preattentive interconnectivity between the SC, amygdala, PFC, basal ganglia, and brainstem, which rapidly process incoming sensory information. As a result, sensory processing may acquire a preemptive significance or lack thereof depending on a dog's history of exposure to aversive and attractive motivational events (Carretie et al., 2001; Ikeda and Hikosaka, 2003). As such, the emotional significance of reward and punishment appears to have a far-reaching influence on the preattentive and preemptive organization of perception, cognition, mood, and modal activity. For example, reward-mediated interconnectivity between the SC, PFC, and basal ganglia appears to bias orienting responses in a positive direction, whereas aversive emotional experiences activating preattentive networks between the SC, PFC, amygdala appears to promote a negativity bias (anticipatory anxiety) toward novelty and unexpected events (uncertainty). In addition, the SC may encode template information relevant to the detection of species-typical threats and has direct access to defensive centers organized at the level of the central nucleus of the amygdala, hypothalamus, periaqueductal gray (PAG), and basal ganglia that generates automatic and rapid-onset fear modules at the earliest stage of sensory processing and gating (see Öhman and Mineka, 2001).

The relative ability of an unexpected event to produce an orienting response depends on its conspicuousness, its phylogenetic significance, or its relevance to an ongoing project or venture. The detection of an inconsistency or mismatch in the flow of sensory data is cross-associated with the concurrent sensory input from other modalities contributing to the content of sensory maps represented at the level of the SC (e.g., sight, hearing, touch, and balance). The coordinated processing of preattentive sensory information deemed significant is tagged with hedonic value, resulting in appropriate emotional and autonomic arousal to promote attentional focus or intensification, as needed to guide adaptive actions. On the other hand, sensory events that are sufficiently conspicuous or salient to prompt

an orienting response but lack relevance with respect to control incentives are gradually gated out by habituation and ignored by means of active inhibition associated with selective attention. In addition, the repeated exposure to a highly salient stimulus that attracts attention but without significant consequence will cause the stimulus to merge gradually into the background and prevent future associations from forming via latent inhibition (Dess and Overmier, 1989). Latent inhibition appears to cause dogs to actively ignore the event via inhibitory processing at the level of the PFC and SC, a stimulus biasing influence in the direction of irrelevance that must be unlearned for it to form significating associations that are relevant to a dog's control interests. If such a stimulus is repeatedly paired with some significant future event, it will gradually acquire prediction-control significance; however, the associative link between the two events may be more readily dissolved if the contingency between the events is discontinued than would be the case if the stimulus had never been previously presented independently of significance. Similarly, stimuli acquiring attractive or aversive significance resist change or conversion in the direction of an opposite hedonic valence or accepting new associative linkages with events of contrary motivational significance. Conditioned aversive and attractive stimuli acquired in association with first impressions at an early age may leave relatively permanent positive or negative biases that can be rapidly reinstated and guide behavioral output despite intensive counterconditioning or extinction efforts. Exposure and habituation to a broad assortment of uneventful environmental stimuli may reduce the risk of undesirable positive and negative biases that contribute to inappropriate appetites and aversive reactivity later in life via the shielding effects of latent inhibition.

Detecting and Processing Prediction Error

Neurobiological research indicates that reward, motivation, and mood are strongly modulated by mesolimbic and mesocortical dopamine (DA) activity. Dopamine neurons located in the ventral tegmental area (VTA) show an increased firing rate when putative rewards occur unexpectedly or when such events exceed a dog's expectations. In contrast, DA neuron activity remains unchanged when an anticipated event matches a dog's expectations; when an anticipated event is less than expected or omitted, however, the firing rate is decreased (Schultz, 1998; Schultz and Dickinson, 2000). The VTA projects to the nucleus accumbens and forms a network of connectivity with the PFC, the amygdala, and various subcortical networks that perform comparator and valuative functions that enable dogs to interpret the motivational significance of novel and anticipated events and to adjust behavior accordingly, with cholinergic neurotransmission likely playing a prominent modulatory role (see Miranda et al., 2000; Giovannini et al., 2001; Kobayashi and Isa, 2002; McIntyre et al., 2003; Wu et al., 2004). The expectancy-comparator model proposes that prediction-control expectancies, calibrated establishing operations, and goal-directed actions are organized into control-expectancy modules and adaptive modal strategies. Control-expectancy modules and modal strategies are shaped by positive and negative prediction error into adaptive adjustments with the goal of optimizing instrumental control over significant motivational events (see *Prediction and Control Expectancies* in Chapter 1).

In the case of classical conditioning, when prediction mismatches occur, error signals mediate the recalibration of emotional establishing operations by selectively exciting or inhibiting relevant emotional command systems (valuative modulation), thereby increasing or decreasing motivational incentives and adjusting arousal to match the behavioral needs of the situation. Hypothetically, when control-expectancy mismatches occur, error signals are relayed along comparator loops and interconnecting pathways that mediate valuative changes coordinated with the recalibration of emotional establishing operations, thereby refining the control-expectancy module and modulating state arousal and action readiness to reflect the new information.

Prominent neural substrates and circuits hypothesized to perform this information-integrating process include plastic networks between the following:

Basolateral amygdala: a central hub coordinating the evaluation and attribution of emotional significance to novel and conditioned attractive and aversive motivational stimuli

Bed nucleus of the stria terminalis (BSNT): an extension of amygdala playing an important role in the mediation of seeking incentives, emotion, and vigilance

Ventral tegmental area (VTA): the source of the mesocortical DA pathway projecting to the PFC and activated by the central amygdala in response to psychological stressors

Nucleus accumbens: the mesolimbic DA reward area that plays a significant role in the coordination of incentive and hedonic value attributed to the gain and loss of reward objects

Pedunculopontine tegmental nucleus (PPTN): the origin of cholinergic neurons responsive to prediction error/novelty and serving to modulate mesolimbic DA neurons mediating reward

Superior colliculus (SC): organizes multimodal sensory maps of the surroundings and orienting response

Lateral hypothalamus: contains hypocretin/orexin cells that promote arousal and alertness via complex interactions with cortical and limbic reward networks, autonomic effector systems, and feed-forward programming of serotonin and norepinephrine release associated with waking states

Basal forebrain: the origin of cholinergic networks modulating awareness and attentional response, hesitation, and increased exploratory activity in response to novelty and surprise

The PFC and the anterior cingulate area coordinate activity in these various limbic and subcortical systems while promoting selective attention and impulse control and organizing flexible control-expectancy modules and routines (see Schoenbaum and Setlow, 2001; Cardinal et al., 2002).

Attention, Impulse Control, and Processing Prediction Error

The executive selective attention and impulse-control functions of the PFC are largely dedicated to inhibition, but the PFC also mediates excitatory processing related to cortical reward via glutaminergic pathways, including excitatory input from the amygdala, information relevant to conditioned reinforcement in association with the control of aversive and attractive motivational incentives. Prefrontal and amygdalar-glutaminergic pathways also project to the nucleus accumbens and the VTA, areas of the brain that are strongly involved in mediation of reward (see *Prediction and Control Expectancies* in Chapter 1). Among the inhibitory effects of the PFC, the gating out of irrelevant or insignificant stimuli, as described in the previous section, are critical functions necessary to promote selective attention. In addition to selective attention, the PFC narrows response possibilities down to a single best bet based on ongoing control incentives, prediction-control expectancies, and emotional establishing operations. The PFC inhibits actions that are unlikely to succeed and disinhibits actions that are more likely to succeed, while contributing to the activation of active modal strategies via the surprise associated with outcomes. As such, the PFC appears to modulate behavioral output and emotional arousal through the exertion of tonic inhibition and phasic inhibition or disinhibition and the excitatory influence of reward. When instrumental behavior results in outcomes that are better than expected, the mismatch or *positive prediction error* results in phasic disinhibition and elation via excitatory inputs and outputs to reward centers. Conversely, if the behavior produces outcomes worse than expected, the mismatch or *negative prediction error* results in phasic inhibition and disappointment. When functioning under optimal conditions, tonic disinhibition promotes calming and mood states conducive to comfort and safety via the cumulative effects of somatic reward, whereas

phasic disinhibition and excitation result in cortical reward and increased exploratory activity and inquisitiveness (active modal strategies), and phasic and tonic inhibition results in hesitation and delay (passive modal strategies). Under adverse conditions, excessive cortical inhibition may cause numerous disturbances of affect, motivation, and attention (hypervigilance) associated with inescapable loss and risk—disturbances that affect voluntary initiative. Disturbances affecting excitatory prefrontal reward systems or loss of appropriate inhibitory and disinhibitory modulation of reward-related behavior may play a significant role in the expression of exploitive novelty-seeking behavior and impulsivity, on the one hand, or incompetent power-seeking behavior, on the other (Van Erp and Miczek, 2000).

An important goal of cynopraxic therapy is to restore functional executive capacity to selective attention and impulse-control functions and to enliven spontaneity and playfulness—the result of a harmonious balance of somatic reward and cortical reward. A foundation of inhibitory control afforded by basic training provides an indispensable anchor for controlling reactive adjustments via the modulatory effects of prediction-control expectancies and provides reactive dogs with the autoregulation necessary to integrate an adaptive coping style and a repertoire of effective behavior. Establishing a reliable repertoire of basic modules and routines (e.g., formal heeling and automatic sit, controlled walking and quick sit, slack-leash walking, and reliable sit-stay and down-stay) is of tremendous value, both as a platform for behavior modification and for the intrinsic calming effects and enhanced social attraction that such training produces.

Cortical and Subcortical Comparator Functions and Adaptation

The selective attention and impulse control mediated and refined by goal-oriented prediction-control expectancies and emotional establishing operations are organized at the level of the PFC; in particular, orbital and medial PFC networks appear to play a crucial role in governing control-expectancy modules and modulating shifts in attention and motivational direction (Öngür and Price, 2000), as needed to maintain purposive focus and to optimize control efforts (see *Cortical and Subcortical Comparator Functions and Adaptation*). Cortical reward and elation induced by the detection of positive prediction error serve to mobilize active modal strategies vectored on the search for additional opportunity. Reward arousal appears to be constrained by opponent processing, whereby the energy used to represent and experience reward is countered by an opposing *antireward* that restores homeostasis. Conflict monitoring and the detection of negative prediction error also set limits on reward-seeking activities. The anterior cingulate cortex (ACC) is hypothesized to play a key role in the monitoring and encoding of error signals (conflict) occurring in the context of instrumental projects and ventures. Conflict monitoring may be an important way for dogs to obtain control-relevant information not otherwise available. The detection of negative prediction error by the ACC results in motor inhibition and increased activity at the level of the dorsolateral PFC (DLPFC), where refinements to the control module may be integrated (MacDonald et al., 2000; Kerns et al., 2004). Consequently, in addition to monitoring control expectancies for action error or conflict, the ACC probably plays a central role in the mediation of passive modal strategies organized to minimize risk and loss (i.e., calculated hesitation, ritualization, and avoidance).

The conflict-monitoring and inhibitory functions performed by the ACC appear to divert executive attention to error (Luks et al., 2002), perhaps with the goal of "training" the executive PFC, as the egocentric object of emotional pain and distress, to avoid future similar adjustments to conflict. Conflict avoidance is likely a central contribution of the PFC to the integration of an adaptive coping style. In addition, the DLPFC appears to mediate an active interface that anticipates interactive conflict and selects response options that serve to resolve conflict proactively (Badre and Wagner, 2004). With the integration of reliable control modules, ACC

error and conflict signals should decrease as executive attention and impulse-control capacities become increasingly competent (see Milham et al., 2003). In contrast to the proactive skills exhibited by dogs operating in accord with an adaptive coping style, reactive dogs treat attractive and aversive motivational stimuli in a highly impulsive manner. The pattern of reactive behavior shown by such dogs depends on their individual differences and specific motivational incentives, variably involving intrusive exploitation, despotic control efforts, social avoidance, or reactive inhibition (helplessness). These cognitive and behavioral changes are consistent with the nervous, exploitative, and autoprotective behaviors shown as the result of a *reactive coping style*.

The ACC is also a locus of interest with respect to the etiology of compulsive behaviors (Ursu et al., 2003; Van Veen and Carter, 2002). Whereas the PFC appears normally to integrate response error and conflict-related information in the process of modifying the control module, in the case of compulsive behavior the diversion of attentional resources for conflict monitoring may become dysfunctional, operating with a high degree of autonomy from the executive refinement of control modules. The increased conflict monitoring and behavioral inhibition mediated by the ACC may impair a dog's ability to vary behavior in response to executive adjustment signals. Whereas increased ACC activity appears to promote compulsive behavior, decreased ACC activity may facilitate impulsive behavior and inappropriate explosive adjustments in response to threats or challenges perceived to lack controllability. The ACC is also nicely positioned to monitor subcortical emotional signals arising in association with conflict (i.e., anxiety, frustration, resentment, worry, and despair) and increased autonomic arousal (Eisenberger et al., 2003). As such, the ACC appears to play a prominent role in the mediation of the reactive coping style emerging within the introversion dimension associated with persistent social ambivalence and entrapment dynamics. In contrast to the central role of the ACC for monitoring and coping with social conflict and aversive state changes (emotional pain) mediated by autonomic state changes (Thayer and Lane, 2000), the DLPFC appears to actively counteract and prevent aversive state changes associated with social ambivalence and distress (Badre and Wagner, 2004) by heading off conflict by means of fair exchange, compromise, and cooperation. Decreased activity in the PFC may significantly impair a dog's capacity to maintain the flexible interface of autonomic attunement needed to regulate preparatory arousal in support of nonconflictive exchange.

PHYLOGENETIC SURVIVAL MODES

According to cynopraxic theory, the cognitive and motivational changes occurring in response to conditions of plenty (favorable) and activity success versus conditions of adversity (unfavorable) and activity failure appear to mediate the expression of different phylogenetic survival modes (PSMs). In general, favorable conditions promote a coordinated *modal phase shift* consisting of cognitive and motivational changes conducive to social extraversion, power, expansion, elation, and well-being, whereas unfavorable conditions result in a coordinated cognitive and motivational shift in an opposite direction conducive to social withdrawal, inhibition and passivity, anxiety, irritability, intolerance, and autoprotective reactivity. Adaptation to persistent stressors may alter a dog's ability to shift flexibly in or out of modes. An inability to produce modal shifts conducive to autonomic attunement may occur as the result of the accumulated physiological and state changes or *allostatic load* acquired in the process of coping with chronic stressors that gradually impede rather than support adaptation (see *Survival Modes and Allostasis* in Chapter 8).

Survival Modes and Adaptation

PSMs exert overarching influences on the emergence of adaptive and maladaptive behavior by shifting motivational pressures, preferences, and priorities. Evidence for the existence of a switch activating PSMs in response to changing environmental conditions and metabolic pressures has been observed in the sedentary and nomadic behavior of male nonterritorial tree lizards (Knapp et al., 2003). Unlike aggressive counterparts who remain true to a territory, nonterritorial males are variably site-faithful or nomadic rovers, depending on environmental conditions. During harsh years of reduced rainfall the nonterritorial males tend to rove, whereas during more favorable years of increased rainfall they tend to stay put. Both male territorial and nonterritorial tree lizards show increased corticosterone levels during harsh years, but only nonterritorial males exhibit reduced testosterone levels. These two behavioral phenotypes appear to be differentiated by a polymorphism that includes a stress-sensitive switch that toggles on PSMs that affect aggression levels, territoriality, and reproductive tactics. During unfavorable years, elevated corticosterone levels and reduced testosterone appear to combine to toggle on a dispersal mode facilitating nomadic roving. However, during more favorable years in which corticosterone levels are low and testosterone high, the modal switch toggles on a sedentary mode conducive to site-faithful behavior.

Among laboratory rodents, the loss of control associated with restraint stress (defeat) or exposure to situations perceived as unfamiliar has been shown to affect agonistic and affiliative thresholds differentially in male and female rats. Female rats exposed to a single 30-minute period of restraint stress show little change in aggressive behavior when tested 24 hours later (Albonetti and Farabollini, 1995). However, if this same strain is exposed to novelty or novelty with restraint stress, the rats show significant change in both agonistic and affiliative behavior. Exposure to novelty alone appears to reduce agonistic behavior selectively while leaving affiliative behavior and allogrooming unaffected, whereas novelty plus restraint simultaneously increases both social agonism and affiliative behavior. The simultaneous activation of both agonistic and affiliative modes may reflect a general increase in autonomic arousal resulting in increased behavioral output in an effort to cope with changing (novel) social and environmental circumstances, improving the rat's ability to compete, on the one hand, and to engage in conciliatory behaviors, on the other. Interestingly, a factor analysis revealed that exposure to novelty alone not only decreased the frequency of aggressive behavior but also modified the way it was organized. Whereas controls showed two distinct factors partitioning offensive and defensive aggression, the rats exposed to novelty showed only one factor, suggesting that reactive thresholds controlling active and passive defensive reactions had been significantly altered by exposure to the treatment, perhaps enabling stressed rats to cope more effectively with environmental uncertainty.

Evidence consistent with survival-mode hypothesis has been reported in dogs and monkeys (see *Diet Change and the Integrate-or-Disperse Hypothesis* in Chapter 7). In the case of dogs, upgrading to a high-quality diet containing increased levels of fat and protein may either have a calming effect or increase reactivity toward novelty, depending on the presence or absence of social enrichment. Hennessy and colleagues (2002) found that dogs fed enhanced diets showed fewer signs of reactive arousal in response to novelty and startle, but only if they also received supplemental social interaction and training. Dogs receiving the fat- and protein-enhanced diet without social enrichment showed an opposite trend toward increased signs of anxious arousal. Two other groups of dogs were fed a diet containing significantly less fat and protein with and without social enrichment. In contrast to the beneficial effects of increased social interaction and training in the case of dogs fed the enhanced diet, dogs fed the diet containing less fat and protein showed more signs of anxious arousal in comparison to dogs not receiving social enrichment. Among cynomolgus macaques, Kaplan and colleagues (1996) showed that monkeys fed a high-fat diet were less aggressive and showed more affiliative behavior than monkeys fed a low-fat diet—changes linked to reduced serotonin turnover (Kaplan et al., 1994) (see *Fat, Cholesterol, Fatty Acids, and Impulsive Aggression* in Chapter 7).

Survival Modes, Neuropeptides, and Heterochrony

A comparison of genes expressed in the brain tissue of wolves, coyotes, and dogs has revealed that the most substantial genetic differences between domestic dogs and related wild canids are localized within the canine hypothalamus, with a high proportion of hypothalamic genes having been downregulated (Saetre et al., 2004). The study also found that gene expression in the frontal lobes reflected anticipated evolutionary distances, with dogs and wolves showing a closer genetic relatedness than exhibited by the coyotes to either. The third area examined, the amygdala, also showed some interspecific genetic variation, but clearly the hypothalamus appears to have undergone the most significant evolutionary remodeling as the result of domestication. In addition, several peptide systems have undergone significant change, including neuropeptide Y (NPY) and calcitonin-related polypeptide B, both playing important roles in energy homeostasis and appetitive behavior. NPY neurons are localized in the arcuate nucleus of the hypothalamus from where NPY fibers project widely to different areas of the brain. The hypothalamus regulates basic biological (e.g., energy homeostasis) and motivational functions and plays a key role in the coordinated release of numerous bioregulatory peptides in response to adaptive pressures. These ancient peptide systems bridge the brain-body gap, playing profoundly influential roles in the physiological processes associated with metabolism, thermogenesis and thermal regulation, visceral functions, growth, and reproductive activities.

In comparison to wolves and coyotes, dogs show a downregulation of the neuropeptide in the hypothalamus and an upregulation of NPY receptors expressed in the amygdala. NPY receptors in the basolateral nucleus of the amygdala appear to exert potent anxiolytic and antistress effects by dampening the activity of co-localized corticotropin-releasing factor (CRF) receptors (Sajdk et al., 2004). NPY has also been shown to regulate the release of oxytocin and vasopressin by the posterior pituitary (Sheikh et al., 1998), as well as exert modulatory effects on hypothalamic-pituitary-adrenal (HPA) activity in dogs (Inoue et al., 1989; Miura et al., 1992). During sympathetic arousal, NPY release appears to mediate a pronounced inhibition of vagal tone by binding to acetylcholine receptors expressed on parasympathetic nerve endings (Rios et al., 1996). In addition to modulating stress reactions, NPY interacts with orexin to promote feeding behavior. Orexin is a neuropeptide believed to play a prominent role in energy homeostasis and alertness. Low levels of circulating leptin, a peptide produced by adipose cells that monitor energy reserves, stimulate NPY neurons to increase feeding behavior (Jéquier, 2002), while at the same time resetting the hypothalamic-pituitary-thyroid (HPT) axis in the direction of energy conservation and hypothyroidism (Fekete et al., 2001 and 2002). Circulating leptin levels vary in response to fasting and dietary state. Whereas NPY neurons are inhibited by high levels of circulating leptin, orexin neurons originating in the lateral hypothalamus project dense fibers to the arcuate nucleus that may stimulate NPY neurons to increase food intake independently of leptin signaling (Willie et al., 2001), perhaps suggesting a role of hedonic value dissociated from appetitive drive need.

The lateral hypothalamus receives strong projections from the orbitofrontal cortex (OFC), a prefrontal area believed to attribute hedonic value to food rewards (Rolls, 2000) and tactile stimulation. In addition to connectivity with the alertness-promoting cholinergic neurons of the basal forebrain, the lateral hypothalamus projects to the ventrolateral periaqueductal gray (vlPAG) (Öngür and Price, 2000), where it drives parasympathetic adjustments. The effector capacity of orexin and the wide distribution and interconnectivity of orexin receptors in key areas of the brain associated with reward, alertness, and energy homoeostasis (see Willie et al., 2001) suggest that the neuropeptide may play a pivotal role in scaling prediction error in terms of energy gain or loss as well as modulating arousal shifts in response to novelty and the subjective experience of reward. For example, orexin cells stimulate the dorsal raphe nucleus and the locus coeruleus via a feed-forward mechanism involving glutamatergic interneurons modulating the release of both serotonin (5-hydroxytryptamine or 5-HT) and norepinephrine (NE), which, in turn, exert an inhibitory feedback effect over orexin neurons (Li et al., 2002). The interconnectivity between the lateral hypothalamus and the orbitofrontal cortex and reward systems is consistent with the possibility that orexin stimulation of NPY neurons may play a role in sustaining modal seeking activity in response to goal-directed appetitive transactions yielding hedonic value.

The interconnectivity between the OFC, the lateral hypothalamus, and the vlPAG is also interesting with respect to canine narcolepsy, a disorder caused by a mutation of the hypocretin (orexin) receptor 2 gene (Lin et al., 1999). When excited by food or play, narcoleptic dogs are prone to cataleptic attacks stemming from deficit orexin neurotransmission (Fujiki et al., 2002). A network between the lateral hypothalamus, the dorsal raphe nucleus, and vlPAG may play a prominent role in this disorder, especially since the activation of the vlPAG results in tonic immobilization.

The upregulation of NPY receptors in the amygdala and the downregulation of the hypothalamus, as indicated by the finding of Saetre and colleagues (2004), are compatible with a reduced vulnerability for reactive arousal in response to social stressors, a functional change consistent with the differentiation of enhanced abilities to cope with stressful conflict situations. According to this hypothesis, corticohypothalamic nodes and networks interact reciprocally with various hypothalamic effector neurons to modulate allostatic drive and motivational state changes via direct enervation of sympathetic and parasympathetic ganglia as well as by releasing numerous peripheral hormones and neuroendocrine substances within the brain to coordinate metabolic changes conducive to attunement and energy homeostasis. In the wake of increasingly complex social relations and extended care/attachment relations associated with domestication, cortical executive networks appear to have evolved enhanced capacities to integrate sensory and motor functions with hypothalamic effector systems to regulate drive functions in the direction of increasing sociability and tameness, bringing autonomic and metabolic processes under the enhanced efficiency and unification of centralized prediction-control mechanisms, enabling dogs to respond proactively in anticipation of events and thereby promoting adaptive optimization through social exchange.

In addition to reducing the excitability of hypothalamic effector neurons mediating flight-or-fight reactions, the reduction in predatory behavior by genetic alterations in limbic and hypothalamic nuclei governing prey-seeking drives (see Arons and Shoemaker, 1992) would have likely freed up enormous energy reserves, normally dedicated to the pursuit of predatory priorities, that perhaps turned to the pursuit of social and object play as a compensatory outlet or cooperative hunting for sport. Selection pressures for reduced predatory behavior and increased playfulness would probably have been a high priority with respect to adaptations enabling early dogs to interact safely with children. Similarly, the sexual pair bonding and extended parental behavior that wolves show toward their offspring are reduced in most dogs. Instead, dogs appear to sublimate pair bonding and parental caregiving into what Perin (1981) has described as "superabundant love," combining the sociosexual drives of the wolf mother and father into the playful affection and innocent attentiveness that transforms dogs into supernormal attachment objects (see *Supernormal Attachment Hypothesis* in Volume 2, Chapter 4). The various autonomic and interactive dimensions opened by the downregulation of hypothalamic effector systems mediating predatory and reactive behavior infuse the human-dog relationship with extraordinary capacity for social complexity and adaptability. The downregulation of hypothalamic effector mechanisms mediating flight-or-fight reactions in response to social approach should reduce the flight distance while simultaneously increasing social attraction, thereby elevating fear and aggression thresholds while lowering approach/exploratory thresholds. These

behavioral changes are consistent with improved capacities for social engagement, increased tolerance for novelty, and reduced stress reactivity.

Physiological and behavioral support for this hypothesis has been reported among silver foxes selected for reduced fear and aggression toward humans. Foxes showing tameability and increased exploratory behavior have a significant reduction in plasma cortisol levels in comparison to reactive farm-bred counterparts (Trut, 2001). In additon to decreased HPA-axis tone, foxes selected for increased tameability show higher 5-HT levels in the midbrain and hypothalamus (Popova et al., 1991), suggesting that increased 5-HT levels may play a role in the inhibition of defensive behavior. Problematically, with respect to applying the fox model of domestication to dogs, the cortisol levels of wolf pups and adults do not vary appreciably from the baseline cortisol levels of dogs (Seal et al., 1975 and 1987). Further, among free-living wolves, there is no detectable correlation between cortisol levels and high rates of aggression and agonistic exchange (Sands and Creel, 2004). These findings appear at odds with those reported previously by McLeod and colleagues (1996), who described a significant correlation between glucocorticoid levels and rates of aggressive exchange between wolves. Sands and Creel suggest that a significant factor that may explain the heightened stress reactivity shown by captive wolves is related to the vulnerability of subordinates to unavoidable and severe attacks that are more common among captive wolf populations than among free-living groups. Finally, cortisol levels do not significantly differ between reactive and nonreactive dogs, until these two types of responders are exposed to fear-eliciting events and situations (Hydbring-Sandberg et al., 2004).

Other authors have emphasized the importance of the HPT axis and the hypothalamic-pituitary-gonadal (HPG) axis as playing a critical role in regulating developmental and physiological rates modulating neuronal excitation and inhibition. The extensive experimental work by Anderson (1941) and James (1941) was largely dedicated to investigating the effects of thyroid hormone on the differentiation of behavioral and morphological types among dogs. They argued that temperament dimensions affecting relative excitability and adaptability might be driven by metabolic differences stemming from the level or quality of thyroid or pituitary secretion. They believed, for example, that the physical form, excitability, high activity levels, and alert typology of German shepherds was probably a reflection of an increased responsiveness to thyroid activity, whereas the physical morphology and behavior of basset hounds reflected a slowing physiological rate and reduced responsiveness and ability to acquire conditioned reflexes. To compare the effects of thyroid on behavior and development, numerous classical conditioning experiments were performed on German shepherd and basset hound crosses. The researchers found that they could alter the relative excitability of these intermediate types toward the hyperexcitability of German shepherds by altering thyroid and epinephrine levels, whereas ablation of the thyroid glands, gonads, and adrenal glands resulted in changes in the direction of the inhibited phenotype. These findings are consistent with heterochrony mediating the differentiation of breeds, whereby certain canine developmental rates are accelerated, resulting in peromorphosis (the German shepherd typology), whereas others are slowed down and result in paedomorphosis (the basset hound typology).

Dogs do appear to express individual differences with respect to the production and utilization of thyroid hormone. For example, a comparison of five breeds (beagle, sheltie, cocker spaniel, wirehaired fox terrier, and the basenji) showed that the basenji uses thyroxin at a higher rate than European breeds (Nunez et al., 1970). Whereas the basenji showed a mean thyroidal half-life of 3.3 days, dogs of a European ancestry showed a mean thyroidal half-life of 7 to 10 days. The monoestrous basenji is adapted to an equatorial environment and exhibits an annual breeding cycle timed to occur with the decreasing daylight that occurs around September or October (Scott et al., 1959), whereas the wolf is adapted to temperate climates and programmed to initiate reproductive activity as daylight increases in January or February. Nunez and colleagues speculate that the changes to the reproductive cycles of the basenji may be the result of a genetic alteration in thyroid functions. Among wolves, the reproductive cycle reportedly varies with latitude, occurring earlier in the year at lower latitudes (Seal et al., 1987). Interestingly, Cape hunting dogs shift the timing of reproductive cycles a full 6 months when moved from Southern Africa to Ireland (reported by Seal et al., 1987). In contrast to the basenji, the reproductive cycle of European breeds appears to operate in relative independence to seasonal light periods and the endocrine control mediated by the pineal gland. Dogs that are housed together with other dogs or that come into contact with wolves reportedly show evidence of synchronizing their estrus cycles with the estrus cycles of other females (Harrington and Asa, 2003); further, dogs are kept in close proximity with wolves appear to show evidence of increased reproductive photoperiodicity, coming into estrus in January–February and then again in August–September (Kreeger, 2003).

Hiestand (1989) has speculated that the previously discussed research of James and Anderson suggests the possibility that the neoteny hypothesized to distinguish dogs from wolves (see *Paedomorphosis* in Volume 1, Chapter 1) may be due to genetic alterations affecting the sensitivity of different dog breeds to the effects thyroid hormones—speculation consistent with the notion that early domestication may have resulted in significant changes affecting the pulsatile release and turnover of thyroid (Crockford, 2002). The pulsatile secretion of thyroid-releasing hormone (TRH) by the hypothalamus acts on the anterior pituitary to produce thyroid-stimulating hormone (TSH) and the release of thyroid into the bloodstream (Kooistra et al., 2000). Given the negative-feedback effects of circulating thyroid hormones on TRH and TSH activity, increased episodic production of TRH would likely promote hypothyroidism and elevated prolactin levels (Kaufman et al., 1985), a change in thyroid function consistent with the neoteny hypothesis.

However, somewhat problematic for the neoteny hypothesis are the results of chemistry studies of blood taken from wild-caught wolf pups (4 to 7 months) indicating that young wolves show a tendency toward lower thyroid (T4) concentrations in comparison to dogs (beagles) (Seal et al., 1975). Similar trends toward hypothyroidism have been shown in adult wolves. The thyroid levels of wolves undergo seasonal changes, with thyroxin (T4) levels increasing in the winter and decreasing in the summer (Seal et al., 1987).

Dogs appear to express varying degrees and types of developmental rate changes consistent with dissociated heterochrony. According to this hypothesis, dog breeds are not more or less neotenous but rather show evidence of selective developmental changes that delay (paedomorphosis) or accelerate (peromorphosis) the organization of various behavioral and physiological systems. Alterations in thyroid activity at different prenatal and postnatal periods may yield altered sensitivities to thyroid and mediate functional and morphological changes to the canine phenotype.

Strong evidence indicates that developmental changes in thyroid levels regulate the timing of the metamorphosis of tadpoles into frogs (Bentley, 1976). Evidence of similar thyroid-mediated effects on developmental rates among mammals is less secure, but some well-controlled investigations do indicate that the timing of developmental markers is altered in response to treatments that increase or decrease thyroid activity during prenatal and postnatal development. Maternal thyroid has been demonstrated to alter the expression of the neuroendocrine-specific protein (NSP) and a gene encoding the Oct-1 transcription factor in the cortex and limbic system of the rat brain (Dowling et al., 2000). NSP is believed to play a critical role in the differentiation of neuronal tissue via the modulatory influence of thyroid hormone. Animals exposed to increased fetal thyroid show lasting focal changes in NSP expression in the hippocampus that is enhanced by adult hypothyroidism, whereas Oct-1 expression in the cortex and hippocampus is suppressed in adulthood. Even relatively slight changes in maternal thyroid

levels can lead to lasting changes affecting neural development and learning abilities (Colburn, 2004).

In addition to prenatal effects, neonatal hypothyroidism has been shown to exert profound ontogenetic effects over the regulation of genes that program the development of the brain and sensory abilities, including neuronal differentiation, cell migration, synaptogenesis, dendritic structure, and myelination. Thyroid hormone (T3) or triiodothyronine is instrumentally involved in the postnatal organization of 5-HT neural pathways that regulate the stress management system (see *Antistress Neurobiology, Maternal Care, and Coping Style in Chapter 8*). Alterations of thyroid activity can exert lasting impairments affecting the animal's ability to learn and to adapt (see Thompson and Potter, 2000). Recently, Yilmazer-Hanke and colleagues (2004) have shown that the induction of neonatal hyperthyroidism hastens the opening of eyes as well as producing morphological changes consistent with peromorphism (e.g., snout elongation). In addition, transient hyperthyroidism produced several key changes affecting amygdalar activity that continued into adulthood, including a reduction of CRF neurons in the central nucleus of the amygdala and an increase of NPY neurons in the basolateral complex, while increasing the density of tyrosine-hydrolase-positive fibers (indicative of DA transmission). These various amygdalar changes were found to exert various anti-anxiety effects consistent with increased adaptability and tameness. The presence of increased DA activity suggests that part of these changes might be due to sensitization of DA neurons in the VTA, a connection that may play a pivotal role in the process of attributing and updating the hedonic value of motivational stimuli (Baxter and Murray, 2002).

Developmentally, foxes selected for tameness show a steady trend toward increasing exploratory activity and fearlessness in response to novelty, whereas farm-bred foxes become increasingly fearful and inhibited in response to novelty (Belyaev et al., 1984/85). The eyes of tameable fox pups are completely opened sooner than are those of reactive farm-bred counterparts. Also, foxes selected for tameness show a slightly earlier orienting response to sound. These changes accelerating the opening of the eyes and tendencies toward increased exploratory activity are consistent with the aforementioned effects produced by the administration of thyroid on developmental rates in rats (see Brosvic et al., 2002). Whether these alterations in timing affecting the emergence of fear-related behavior and sensory development among foxes selected for tameness is due to maternal thyroid changes is currently unknown, but the findings do raise a number of interesting questions for future research.

A dissociated heterochrony appears to affect the timing of sensory development and the eruption of teeth among coyotes, wolves, and dogs. Snow (1967), for example, found that coyotes opened their eyes, on average, at day 14, but the milk teeth of coyote pups can already be felt at day 10, 10 days before the canine incisors of dogs can be felt through the gums (Scott and Fuller, 1965). Mech (1970) observed that the front teeth of two wolf pups he raised emerged at day 15, whereas the eyes began to open at day 12 and were wide open by day 15. The developmental dissociation between the eruption of teeth and the opening of eyes in coyotes, wolves, and dogs is consistent with paedomorphosis affecting dentition but not sensory development, with the eyes of dogs opening, on average (with significant breed variation), around day 13 (Scott and Fuller, 1965). The early emergence of reproductive behavior among dogs may reflect an acceleration of developmental rates consistent with peromorphosis, whereas the extended playfulness of dogs may represent a change consistent with a paedomorphic delay affecting social and emotional development.

Since thyroid activity is sensitive to external temperature, with cold temperatures causing an elevation of circulating thyroid (Seal et al., 1987), wolf mothers gestating under cold climate conditions ought to produce more circulating thyroid hormone than mothers gestating under warmer conditions. Given the high degree of fetal responsiveness to maternal thyroid levels, it is reasonable to expect differences resulting from winter gestation and that these differences might affect the

adaptability of offspring, with adults showing an increased sensitivity to thyroid levels, causing them to tend toward seasonal hypothyroidism. Hypothyroidism during summer months might enable wolves to conserve and store energy reserves in the form of fat, whereas hyperthyroidism in the winter would enable them to use these fat reserves to maintain thermal homeostasis.

These changes fit nicely with the genetic alterations of the amygdala and hypothalamus identified by Saetre and colleagues (2004) and the thyroid hypotheses posited by Hiestand (1989) and by Crockford (2002). Reduced hypothalamic NPY activity might result in periodic shifts toward hyperthyroidism coincident with critical prenatal and postnatal developmental periods that might result in adult changes inclining toward hypothyroidism via neural sensitization and enhanced negative feedback regulating thyroid release. These alterations in thyroid activity might also reduce the number of CRF neurons in the central nucleus (thereby reducing HPA-axis reactivity) while supporting connectivity between NPY interneurons in the basolateral complex with mesolimbic and orbitofrontal reward circuits projecting to the lateral hypothalamus, completing a feedforward loop involving orexin-mediated excitatory effects on NPY activity. According to this hypothesis, orexin neurons in the lateral hypothalamus may play a prominent role in the modulation of NPY neurons in the process of mediating hedonic value and a heightened state of alertness, action readiness, and increased exploratory activity, as discussed previously in this section. In addition, a network of neural activity of this sort is consistent with enhanced antistress capabilities, increased sociability, and adaptive optimization.

Survival Modes, Control Incentives, and Reward

The relatively small social and dietary QOL enhancements needed to mobilize mode changes suggest the involvement of conditioned associations, perhaps involving NPY regulated release of arginine vasopressin

(AVP) and oxytocin (Sheikh et al., 1998). Among rats, for example, food deprivation results in a persistent state of biological distress that elevates AVP activity, promotes adrenal hypertrophy, and mediates a twofold increase in NE turnover in brainstem (El Fazaa et al., 2000). Food- and water-deprived rats also show elevated glucocorticoid levels and a potentiated increase in catecholamine release in response to acute immobilization (Kiss et al., 1994). In contrast, the closely related neuropeptide, oxytocin, plays many complementary antistress and antiaggression roles by way of linkages among sucking, ingestion, tactile stimulation, social affiliation, and autonomic attunement antagonistic to the stress-mediating effects of AVP. These oxytocin effects are consistent with an important role in the activation of the social engagement system (SES) and the integration of secure attachments. AVP and oxytocin appear to modulate thresholds regulating autonomic tone and a dog's ability to obtain hedonic value from social, appetitive, and tactile exchanges while organizing an adaptive coping style (Ostrowski, 1998).

AVP is hypothesized to play a role in mediation of state changes underlying nervous attachments, irritability, and repulsion consistent with the loner-dispersal mode, whereas oxytocin promotes changes consistent with secure attachments, including the calming, comfort and safety, and pleasure derived from eating, petting, and warmth. According to this hypothesis, oxytocin may increase neural activity in pathways conducive to social engagement by lowering the excitation thresholds of neurons and circuits mediating increased parasympathetic tone and attributing positive hedonic value (attraction and calming) to social attention, appetitive rewards, and tactile stimulation. In contrast, AVP may route neural activity consistent with the loner-dispersal mode by lowering excitation threshold of neurons and circuits mediating sympathetic arousal and attributing negative hedonic value (aversion and agitation) to social attention, appetitive rewards, and tactile stimulation, thereby increasing social irritability, intolerance, and autoprotective behavior. Neuropeptide-mediated alterations of neu-

ronal responsiveness to the hedonic value of social stimuli would serve a potentially beneficial function by limiting attachment behaviors to appropriate social partners. Consistent with such social functions, oxytocin and AVP play complex roles in the establishment of durable social memories (e.g., kin recognition) and affiliative bonds, as well as mediate potent states of social aversion and aggression toward unfamiliar conspecific intruders.

Although the survival mode is immensely influential, it does not dictate the behavior expressed by a dog but rather serves to modify behavior by altering the incentive and hedonic value of social exchange. According to the integrate-or-disperse hypothesis, the hedonic value of social exchange may shift depending on the survival-mode active at the time (see *Diet Change and the Integrate-or-Disperse Hypothesis* in Chapter 7). In particular, the hypothesis predicts that QOL enhancements in the absence of increased affiliative exchange promote anxiety and insecure attachments. A further prediction asserts that QOL diminishments made while increasing social interaction tend to promote dispersive tensions, which, if blocked, generate social ambivalence and entrapment dynamics. Consequently, persistent exposure to inescapable social situations that provide poor QOL resources (entrapment) but nevertheless make high demands on a dog for social contact, may amplify dispersive tensions and promote antipredatory and autoprotective adjustments in response to ambiguous signals. Accordingly, QOL changes may generate significant motivational changes promoting social integration or dispersion, depending on the availability of adaptive social options consonant with the activated survival mode.

The quality of social or place attachments exerts an immense effect on the hedonic value of transactions resulting in social and appetitive reward. For example, under circumstances perceived as secure, the contingent delivery of social attention, tactile stimulation, and play may produce positive hedonic value and state changes conducive to social attraction and integration. In contrast, under the influence of circumstances perceived as insecure or unsafe, the same social exchange will produce aversive state changes conducive to reactive adjustments and social dispersion. The reward value of affectionate petting and hugging will greatly vary, depending on the survival mode active at the time of receiving it and the quality of attachment between the dog and the person giving it. Whereas petting and hugging or playful teasing may yield a high degree of positive hedonic value (e.g., calming and enjoyment) for a dog operating under the influence of autonomic attunement and secure attachments (social integration mode), the autonomic state changes and physiological alterations of neuronal substrates and target organs mediating the loner-dispersal mode may cause such playful and affectionate actions to yield a negative hedonic value (e.g., resentment and irritability), especially in the presence of a QOL diminishment.

Survival Modes, Energy Homeostasis, and Stress

During stressful arousal in anticipation of increased energy demands, complex physiological changes are orchestrated to protect or restore energy homeostasis. Thus, neuropeptide signals (principally CRF and AVP) converging on the pituitary modulate the release of adrenocorticotropic hormone (ACTH) into the bloodstream. ACTH stimulates the adrenal cortex to release glucocorticoids, thus activating numerous metabolic, anti-inflammatory, and cognitive-emotional changes conducive to adaptation and energy homeostasis. The size of this adaptation and denouement phase (allostasis) is followed by several key changes affecting flight-or-fight thresholds. The activation of the HPA axis and the release of adrenal glucocorticoids into the bloodstream promotes a state of positive energy balance (excess), whereas the activation of the HPT axis in response to severe stressors produces an energy deficit by increasing the metabolic rate (Horvath et al., 2004).

In addition to the varied caloric requirements needed by working dogs to maintain energy homeostasis, genetic peculiarities may influence a dog's capacity to anticipate and efficiently supply the changing energy requirements needed by the brain and body to sup-

port goal-directed behavior. The recent finding that a structure of genetic relatedness between different dog breeds collects principally around four clusters of genomic variation (Parker et al., 2004) raises the possibility that individuals belonging to these different genetic groups may express digestive and metabolic variations that require different nutritional support to achieve energy homeostasis. For example, Frank (1987) has reported preliminary evidence suggesting that Northern breeds (e.g., the malamute) may possess more efficient metabolic capacities than other dog breeds or wolves. The metabolic and nutritional requirements of breeds specialized for sprint racing and long-distance racing varies significantly. Whereas sled dogs appear to perform best when fed diets containing high fat (50%) and high protein (30%), greyhounds appear to perform best when fed diets containing more moderate levels of fat and protein (Hill, 1998). The groupings identified by Parker and colleagues may provide a valuable frame of reference for investigating nutritional differences and, if necessary, formulating canine diets compatible with the specific needs identified. According to this hypothesis, diverse breeds, such as the Bernese mountain dog, greyhound, and the Shiba Inu, have probably evolved very different nutritional requirements and metabolic capacities due to local customs and food availability. A mismatch between a dog's diet and its breed-specific and individual differences affecting metabolism may result in compensatory appetitive and motor efforts to achieve the requisite state of balance and metabolic repose.

A failure to achieve a state of metabolic comfort and energy homeostasis may mobilize disorganized striving and increased catecholamine activity via the activation of sympathetic-adrenomedullary (SAM) system. Whereas epinephrine appears to play a prominent role by mobilizing a rapid state of generalized arousal and increased glucose metabolism (McGuinness et al., 1997), NE appears to mediate lipid metabolism in preparation for sustained physical exertion (Connolly et al., 1991). In addition to promoting rapid preparatory thermogenic and visceral changes serving to prime and mobilize the emergency system into a state of heightened arousal and readiness, the SAM system exerts excitatory cardiovascular and muscle-tone changes inclining dogs toward confrontation or retreat (see *Periaqueductal Gray and Autoprotective Adjustments to Social Stressors*). Verrier and Dickerson (1991) found that NE predominates the catecholamine flow evoked by anger in dogs. Among cats, different catecholamine proportions emerge, depending on the nature of psychological stressors presented (Stoddard et al., 1987). Among dogs, NE released at $ß_1$-adrenergic receptors appears to play a prominent role in mobilizing cardiovascular changes associated with acute anger states, with cardioselective $ß_1$-adrenergic antagonist, metoprolol-blunting T-wave alternans (TWA), a heart beat pattern reflecting cardiac instability that is evoked by anger and stress, not a secondary instability resulting from an elevated heart rate. This research suggests the possibility that TWA, perhaps in conjunction with heart-rate variability tests, may provide a useful marker for evaluating sympathovagal tone and canine aggressive propensities in response to anger-evoking stimulation (see *Heart-rate Variability* in Chapter 9). Interestingly, sympathectomized dogs (Brouha et al., 1936; Brouha and Nowak, 1939) or dogs under the influence of strong ß-adrenergic blockade (Roossien et al., 2000) show evidence of parasympathetic-driven cardiac accelerator effects conducted by vagal receptors, perhaps mediated by the combined action of acetylcholine and vasoactive intestinal peptide (VIP) (Roossien et al., 2000). Brouha and colleagues (1936) include a photograph of two dogs straining on leashes to fight, even though the sympathetic pathways of both dogs had been surgically disrupted. Despite severe sympathetic impairments, the dogs appeared to show normal running, jumping, playing, and active and passive defensive reactions, suggesting that sympathetic arousal systems are integrated into voluntary behavior at another level of neural organization.

Dogs cope with exchanges perceived as challenges or threats by increasing arousal, vigilance, and readiness—changes that are mediated by cortical and limbic signal converging on the hypothalamus. The activation of emotional systems involved in coping with psychological stressors and demands causes numerous endocrine changes that shift the body into a catabolic state in anticipation of energy outflow. As conflict is resolved, these catabolic processes are substituted by increased anabolic activity organized to conserve and restore energy reserves and to mediate energy conservation, bodily repair, and healing. By means of prior exchanges with others and the environment, predictive information is acquired that enables dogs to match adaptive control efforts with the energy resources needed to succeed. Under conditions of chronic interactive conflict, a state of persistent heightened arousal and *vigilance* (anxiety) may result in a chronic state of physiological stress affecting a dog's ability to competently utilize, produce, and conserve metabolic resources in a manner that promotes energy homeostasis and heath. In addition to the adverse stress effects of persistent anxiety, appetitive frustration promoting heightened arousal and *action readiness* may exert damaging effects on the body and behavior. For example, extinction procedures have been shown to increase HPA-axis activity. Several studies investigating the physiological effects of extinction have shown that rats and monkeys experience a significant rise in glucocorticoid release when exposed to appetitive extinction procedures. Although an increased frequency of reward results in a decrease of glucocorticoid activity during the acquisition phase of training, rewards that fall short of expectations result in increased glucocorticoid activity (Lyons et al., 2000), suggesting that circuits regulating the HPA axis are sensitive to positive and negative prediction error signals. During the extinction phase of a control module, the magnitude of change in HPA-axis activity is proportional to the value of the rewards obtained during the acquisition phase of training (Kawasaki and Iwasaki,1997). The increased active modal activity that often occurs during the initial extinction phase appears to be corticosterone-mediated, with adrenalectomy abolishing the extinction burst in rats (Thomas and Papini, 2001).

Circulating glucocorticoids enter the brain and interact there with mesolimbic dopamine pathways, perhaps playing a facilitative role in the process of extinction by mediating the expression of active modal strategies in response to surprising nonreward, to borrow Papini's term (Papini, 2003). Instrumental extinction is an active learning process, whereby the animal preserves the general structure and sequential organization of a previously effective action pattern, while exploring and experimenting with the changed situation in an effort to reestablish and optimize effective control (see Neuringer et al., 2001). Whereas the acute activation of the HPA system in response to the temporary loss of control over a previously controllable attractive or aversive event may augment adaptive capacities, chronic exposure to distressing frustration and anxiety in association with uncontrollable motivational events appears to gradually diminish the dog's ability to experience reward and to integrate an adaptive coping style. The net result of chronic stress is a reduction of purposive reward-seeking activity in combination with mood changes conducive to social withdrawal, anxiety, irritability, and incompetence. The widely held assumption that the activation of the HPA-axis is indicative of adverse stress is obviously flawed. The foregoing findings suggest that cortisol measures may not be a very useful stand-alone indicator of the dog's welfare status. In fact, a robust adrenal release of cortisol in response to the disconfirmation of expectant prediction-control efforts appears to actually facilitate behavioral changes conducive to adaptive optimization. Actually, one might better argue that diminished HPA-axis activity in response to the repeated disconfirmation of a previously reliable control module would be more indicative of disruptive stress and allostatic load than adaptive stability.

Dog breeds and individuals show significant differences in their ability to cope and adjust to adverse environmental circumstances. Hydbring-Sandberg and colleagues (2004) have reported that dogs showing low-auditory startle thresholds in response to gunshots exhibit a robust cortisol and progesterone response not shown by dogs exhibiting high-startle thresholds. The same loud-noise stimulation has little effect on the release of cortisol and progesterone in the latter, less sensitive group. Interestingly, the experimenters found that baseline measures (e.g., heart rate, hematocrit values, cortisol, progesterone, endorphin, and vasopressin) taken from fearful and fearless dogs did not significantly differ. The relative dependence of stress-related adjustments on the vagaries of individual difference raises significant questions concerning the objectivity of assumptions and generalization regarding the intrinsic stress potential of different classes of sensory stimuli. The blast of a shotgun for a hunting dog signals a very different chain of associative events than the blast produced by a firecracker thrown into the backyard. Similarly, careening down a snow-covered mountain on long fiberglass runners fastened to the feet would represent a robust and terrifying experience for a nonskier but be a source of pleasurable exhilaration for an expert skier. The key differences between stressors and nonstressors revolve around relative predictability, controllability, and familiarity, on the one hand, and the possession of appropriate skills and the confidence needed to use them effectively, on the other. The study draws into serious doubt the value of psychological stress studies that fail to separate dogs into test groups based on behavioral thresholds and temperament types.

GENETIC INFLUENCES ON ADAPTIVE AND REACTIVE COPING STYLES

Dopamine Regulatory Polymorphisms and Reactive Behavioral Phenotypes

Complex interactions between hereditary influences and experience influence how dogs cope with adversity (loss of control). The way a dog responds to novelty and unexpected events appears to exert a profound stabilizing or destabilizing influence on its temperament and coping style. There are four general ways in which the dog responds to novelty and strangeness: fearlessly, conflictively, aggressively, and fearfully. A possible genetic factor affecting how dogs respond to novelty and unfamiliar persons or other dogs may be traceable to polymorphisms regulating the expression of DA receptors, especially D_2 and D_4 subtypes (see *Neural and Physiological Substrates* in Volume 2, Chapter 5). Mice lacking the D_4-receptor gene show a significant reduction of exploratory behavior and increased approach-avoidance conflict toward novel objects in comparison to wild mice (Dulawa et al., 1999). The functional significance of D_4-receptor polymorphisms on temperament in humans is currently controversial and clouded with contradictory findings (Kluger et al., 2002). Whether D_4 polymorphisms adversely affect canine adaptive behavior is unknown, but some intriguing evidence is highly suggestive with regards to the possibility of such an effect. Niimi and colleagues (1999) have reported significant differences in the distribution of D_4 alleles in the genomes of the golden retriever and the Shiba inus. They have cautiously suggested that these genetic variations may contribute to some of the temperament differences exhibited by these two breeds. For example, the long D allele prominent in the Shiba inu may contribute to the breed's reputed territoriality and propensity for reactive excitability toward other dogs. The Shiba also appears to express variant D_4 alleles not found in the genome of other dog breeds thus far studied (e.g., beagle, sheltie, golden retriever) (Niimi et al., 2001), consistent with the breed's ancient origins and relatively close genetic relationship with the wolf (see Parker et al., 2004).

Another line of relevant research in dogs has investigated polymorphisms affecting the gene responsible for the production of catechol-O-methyltransferase (COMT) (Masuda 2004), an enzyme that metabolizes dopamine and norepinephrine (Tunbridge, 2004). The polymorphisms affecting the canine COMT gene are similar to those that have been identified in humans, suggesting that COMT may play a role in the elaboration of dopamine-related predispositions underlying certain adjustment problems. Tunbridge and colleagues (2004) have reported that the inhibition of COMT release at the level of the prefrontal cortex serves to enhance attention functions by increasing dopamine availability. Interestingly, the effects of COMT are only evident under conditions of increased arousal

when increased prefrontal dopamine activity appears to facilitate flexible attention shifting. These findings are consistent with the hypothesis that polymorphisms affecting the COMT gene may contribute to selective attention and impulse control deficits associated with impulsive aggression. Too little or too much dopamine release in the PFC at times of increased arousal appear to be conducive to impulsive and reactive adjustments. These findings suggest the possibility that polymorphisms affecting the dopamine transporter gene might also contribute an adverse predisposing influence affecting the functional competency of executive functions.

Breed and Individual Difference and Reactive/Impulsive Behavior

Breed and individual differences affecting excitability, emotional reactivity (anger and fear thresholds), and cognitive organization (attention and impulse control) exert significant influences on how dogs cope with the conflictive exchange and emotional tensions generated by social ambivalence and entrapment (James, 1939; Sgoifo et al., 1996). Van Der Velden and colleagues (1976) described a pattern of impulsive CDA exhibited by a population of Bernese Mountain dogs in the Netherlands. Of 800 questionnaires sent to owners, 404 were returned and analyzed. The researchers found that not less than 20% of the owners reported that their dog had attacked family members intermittently with "blind aggressiveness" (404). The dogs that had threatened owners or delivered attacks were most often males (76%), whereas females were over represented in the group showing shyness and "unbalanced" temperaments only when away from their home territory. The attacks exhibited by the affected dogs were episodic and out of character with otherwise friendly behavior. Some of the dogs appeared insecure (shy and nervous) while others were reported to exhibit hypersexual behavior. The provoking stimulus was frequently a command or prohibition, even when given in a friendly and nonthreatening way. Some of the dogs responded to the least amount of restraint or force with "real panic"

(404). Often the owner was unable to identify an evoking stimulus triggering the attack. Dogs showing this behavior were reported as shy or avoidant as puppies, especially with respect to strangers. As puppies and adults, the dogs showed a "clear lack of communication" (404). The owners described a rutilant glow in the dog's eyes immediately before the attack took place. Attacks were directed against family members in circumstances consistent with a dominance-aggression interpretation. Interestingly, when rehomed aggressors only began to attack family members again after they had established social attachments with them. Since the attacks were described as resembling impulsive fits or seizures, a series of neurological tests [kindling and electroencephalogram (EEG)] were performed to exclude epilepsy. In addition, necropsies and microscopic examination of the brain tissue from 8 dogs found no evidence of pathology. Intracranial EEG recordings of 7 dogs presenting varying signs of reactivity, including a history of attack behavior, were taken by inserting electrodes bilaterally into the temporal and orbitofrontal cortex, the amygdala, and the hippocampus. The testing failed to reveal evidence of epileptic-like spontaneous activity. The authors stress the likely role of genetic factors in the etiology of the impulsive aggression exhibited by these dogs.

Other breeds, notably the cocker spaniel and English springer spaniel, have also attracted clinical and scientific interest stemming from similar presenting signs, often collectively described as dominance-related. Mugford (1984) found that English cocker spaniel dogs (N=50) with aggression problems, showed a highly uniform pattern of attacks directed exclusively against family members in association with moodiness and the defense of bones, food, and defended areas (e.g., under furniture). Aggressive propensities appeared to decrease when the dogs were in less familial surroundings. Male dogs delivered most attacks (68%), with males also showing more severe aggression than females. The eyes of attacking dogs changed color and the attack worsened as the result of physical punishment. Most dogs appeared confused and contrite after the attack. Mugford's data suggests that a linkage between temperament and coat color may exist in the English cocker spaniel, since 74% of the aggressors were red or golden in color, 20% were black, 6% were designated as other (e.g., parti-colored); a relationship later confirmed by Podberscek and Serpell (1996). The apparent reduced incidence of aggression in parti-colored English cocker spaniels is consistent with data collect by Belyaev and colleagues (Trut, 1999). Belyaev's group found that piebald pelage is highly correlated with tameness in foxes (see *The Silver Fox: A Possible Model of Domestication* in Volume 1, Chapter 1).

A similar pattern of dominance-like behavior has been reported to occur disproportionately among English springer spaniels. According to Reisner (1996), the English springer spaniel is the breed presenting most frequently for treatment of dominance-aggression problems. The results of a large questionnaire survey involving 1,053 springer owners (53.1%) indicate that 26.4% reported that their dog had bitten someone, which was often a family member or a person familiar to the dog (65.2%) (Reisner, 1996). Reisner reports that nearly half (48.4%) of these domestic aggressors had growled, snapped, or bitten in situations associated with dominance. In a sample of 53 cases involving springer spaniels diagnosed as dominance-related aggression, males presented twice as often as females (Reisner, 1993). Again, attacks were most common around food and prized objects, with dogs also showing aggression in response to punishment or when disturbed while resting or sleeping. Interestingly, with respect to a possible genetic defect, a statistic analysis of pedigree data revealed that a particular kennel and sire was highly associated with dogs showing the aggressive trait (p=0.002) (Reisner, 1996), suggesting the possibility of a popular sire effect (see *Prospects for the Future* in Volume 1, Chapter 1). The results of a similarly large survey of English cocker spaniel owners also found evidence of a combined genetic and behavioral influence, but then conclude that domestic attacks occurring suddenly and without apparent provocation are not of some separate category (Podberscek and Serpell, 1996), but are "clearly associated with other symptoms of dominance-type aggression" (87) and therefore should be interpreted in terms of social dominance incentives. In addition to intrafamilial aggression, the authors found that a large percentage of the dogs showed extrafamiliar aggression, threatening or attacking persons visiting the home or strangers away from home. Allen and colleagues (1974) have described a sibling group of Alaskan malamutes that showed severe fighting and predatory behavior that support the notion that individual constitutional influences may strongly affect breed propensities toward intraspecific trait and predatory aggression, since other sled dogs raised under similar circumstances did not show the sort of extreme aggression exhibited by these dogs. After bilateral mechanical disruption and aspirative ablation of the prefrontal cortex, several of the dogs showed a pronounced reduction of fighting and killing behavior, without impairing their drive to pull a sled. In contrast, many of the family dogs presenting with domestic aggression problems showed improvement while in the laboratory, but little of this change transfered to the home, consistent with a complex etiology involving both genetic vulnerability and additive experiential influences.

NEUROBIOLOGY AND LOSS OF ADAPTABILITY

Neuopeptides, Monoamines, Impulsivity, and the Dissolution of the Bond

Aggression is of particular interest from a theoretical cynopraxic standpoint insofar as it represents the castastrophic dissolution of the social bond and thus mirrors in reverse significant factors influencing the bonding process. Social interaction perceived as ambiguous, uncertain, or uncontrollable (i.e. portending a potential loss or risk) may acutely activate NE and DA pathways in the process of enhancing vigilance (NE) and readiness (DA) to cope with the challenge or threat. The arousal mediating impulsive CDA probably originates at a preattentive level that reaches a catastrophic point of no return while the dog is preoccupied with conflict monitoring, suggesting that the diversion of attentional resources away from executive prefrontal functions to cope with social conflict may play a critical role in the mediation of impulsive aggression (see *Cortical and Subcortical Comparator Functions and Adaptation*). The risk of catastrophic impulsivity and aggression is particularly high in the case of ambiguous (uncertain) social signals or social demands forcing the dog to make conflict-laden choices between unacceptable alternatives. According to this hypothesis, chronic social ambivalence and entrapment diverts attentional resources away from executive functions (selective attention and impulse control) to conflict monitoring, a process that disrupts the dog's ability to competently regulate emotion, integrate an adaptive coping style, and to competently inhibit or disinhibit aggressive impulses.

Although a causal linkage between frontal serotonergic activity and aggression in dogs has not been definitively established, speculation implicating 5-HT in the etiology of aggression has long circulated in the applied and veterinary literature. However, most of this speculation has focused on the aggression-facilitating effects of 5-HT deficiencies. The present hypothesis suggests that both deficiencies and excesses of prefrontal 5-HT and DA may promote impulsivity (Dalley et al., 2002) and aggressive behavior (see De Boer et al., 2003). Depending on the specific receptor subtype, 5-HT appears to exert variable inhibitory and disinhibitory neuromodulatory effects over motivated behavior. On the one hand, psychological stressors may alter 5-HT function by various mechanisms. The adverse effects of altered 5-HT activity may be further amplified or attenuated by changes to the 5-HT transporter. For example, the principle antianxiety and antiaggression benefits of serotonergic medications is probably mediated by the inhibition of 5-HT transporters, thus enhancing the neurotransmitter's capacity to linger longer in the synaptic cleft and to modulate other neurotransmitters and neuropeptides conducive to relaxation, social attraction, and an adaptive coping style. In contrast, however, under the influence of excessive 5-HT activity, some 5-HT receptors may mediate problematical inhibitory or disinhibitory influences over impulsive and reactive behavior via disruptive interaction with glutaminergic, dopaminergic, and GABAergic pathways. Depending on the type and chronicity of the stressors involved, stress-mediated deficiencies or excesses of 5-HT and DA may perturb selective attention, impulse control, and mood. According to this hypothesis, chronic stress results in disturbances affecting 5-HT modulatory function, while disrupting the integrative functions of DA, thereby impairing the dog's ability to organize control modules in a proactive and competent fashion. Effective cognitive processing and emotional regulation requires a precise balance of inhibitory, disinhibitory, and excitatory neuromodulation, that is, autonomic attunement and allostasis.

Oxytocin- and AVP-containing neurons express a variety of 5-HT receptor subtypes that promote a diversifying function on arousal and behavior (see *Oxytocin, Arginine Vasopressin, and Autonomic Attunement* in Chapter 8) via the release of oxytocin and AVP in response to stress. Both oxytocin and AVP neurons express $5HT_{2A/C}$ receptors, but only oxytocin neurons express $5\text{-}HT_{1A/B}$ receptors (Jorgensen et al., 2002). $5\text{-}HT_{1A}$ receptors may exert a major modulatory effect over the antianxiety and antiaggression effects mediated by oxytocin. $5\text{-}HT_2$, $5\text{-}HT_4$, and $5HT_7$ receptors appear to play prominent roles in AVP-mediated behavioral and physiological effects (Jorgensen et al., 2003a). Also, circulating cortisol entering the brain appears to selectively inhibit AVP and CRF release but spares oxytocin, leaving it unchanged (Papanek and Raff, 1994), suggesting that central oxytocin may perform a post-stress calming effect, consistent with an amnestic reconciliation function. Petting the stressed dog may facilitate this calming forgetfulness and facilitate social attraction by augmenting the release of central oxytocin. The oxytocin stimulating effects of petting and praise (vocal petting) appear to mediate the cumulative bond-enhancing and calming effects of basic training (see *Neuropeptides and Social Behav-*

ior in Chapter 4 and *Oxytocin-opioidergic Hypothesis* in Chapter 6).

During episodes of acute stress AVP appears to augment the CRF-mediated release of adrenocorticotropic hormone (ACTH) (Klingbeil et al., 1988). Keck and colleagues (2002) found that an AVP receptor antagonist blocks the stimulatory effect of CRF on ACTH release in high-anxiety rats, supporting the hypothesis that AVP plays a mediational role in the expression of individual differences in response to acute psychological stressors. Although acute stress facilitates the production of both AVP and CRF, chronic stress exerts a differential upregulating effect on AVP while downregulating CRF activity (Ma and Lightman, 1998). As a result of exposure to chronic restraint stress, both CRF and glucocorticoid activity are reduced over time, whereas AVP gene expression is increased. The $5HT_{2A}$ receptor is known to control the release of AVP at the paraventricular nucleus (Ramage, 2001; Jorgensen et al., 2003b) and to modulate NE release by the locus coeruleus (Millan, 2003), while NE regulates the release of CRF (Itoi et al., 1999), which in turn modulates the release of 5-HT via the dorsal raphe nucleus (Thomas, et al., 2003) (see *Septal Distress, Relief, and Panic*). The notion that glucocorticoid activity decreases over time while AVP levels increase draws into question the value of cortisol levels as an objective index for assessing the welfare implications of chronic stressors, suggesting that AVP levels and AVP-related indicators such as antidiuresis, thermogenesis (elevated body temperature), cardiovascular changes as reflected in heart rate, heart rate variability (HRV), and blood pressure, and other compensatory behavioral and physiological adjustments (e.g., persistent hyperpnea), might represent more useful endophenotypic markers of allostatic load resulting from chronic stress than isolated cortisol levels (see *Restraint, Unavoidable Aversive Stimulation, and Stress*). The foregoing findings suggest that exposure to chronic psychological stress (social ambivalence and entrapment) may promote either allostatic hyperdrive (high cortisol) or hypodrive (low cortisol) depending on the neural systems activated and the nature of the stress. Whereas acute stressors activate reactive adjustments in association with allostatic hyperdrive and *hypercortisolism*, exposure to chronic stress and allostatic hypodrive in association with increased NE and AVP activity may switch on a PSM conducive to impulsivity.

Social exchanges posing difficult to discriminate options or ambiguity are a source of significant distress for dogs operating under the influence of entrapment and social ambivalence. The diversion of attention to monitor conflict may drain the executive resources needed to process and select behavioral options. With the reduction of executive capacities to maintain selective attention, the nodal regulation of sympathetic arousal may be disrupted, threatened with dissolution, and loss of impulse control. The resulting state of reactive readiness and vigilance may rapidly saturate available inhibitory networks and flood the dog with emotional pain and anger. Thus, impulsive CDA appears to involve the breakdown of the autonomic attunement and mutual awareness that emerges in response to social exchanges that mediate the friendly familiarity, belongingness, and the caring protectiveness of secure attachments. If the owner at such times would merely withdraw from the dog, the sequence of events might be averted, allowing dysregulated arousal to subside and the threat to pass. However, if the dog is further aroused by encroachment and nervous ambiguity or worse yet physical punishment it appears to enter a momentary state of utter incompetence and confusion or lapse of awareness as a catastrophic flash point of no return is reached. Hoaken and colleagues (2003), referring to disturbances of impulse control in human aggressors, nicely state the situation with respect to impulsive CDA, as well:

> Aggression is a primal social response option, a simple response option to an exceedingly rich and complex mélange of contextual cues. It may be that individuals with poor ECF (executive cognitive functioning), demonstrating poor social information processing skills and an inability to cope with overwhelming response options, fail to access more socially appropriate options and make default aggressive responses to provocative situations. (28)

Stress, 5-HT$_{2A}$ Receptor Upregulation, and Aggression

Recent developments in neurobiological research are making significant progress with respect to getting a handle on the neural disturbances contributing to the development of impulsive CDA. For example, a neuroimaging study performed by Peremans and colleagues (2003ab) suggests a possible link between impulsive aggression and an imbalance of central serotonin activity. The researchers found that dogs with a history of serious aggression problems show evidence of increased 5-HT$_{2A}$ receptor binding potential in frontal cortex. No significant differences were found in the receptor binding characteristics of aggressive and nonaggressive dog with respect to 5-HT$_{2A}$ receptor expression in subcortical areas. Nor were there significant differences between aggressive and non-aggressive dogs in terms of regional cerebral blood flow. The aggressive dogs studied were referred for imaging by behavioral consultants and all of the dogs had been diagnosed with "dominance aggression." Precisely why aggressive dogs show increased cortical 5-HT$_{2A}$ receptor binding potential is unknown, but at first glance, given the common assumption that "dominance aggression" is due to a lack of synaptic 5-HT, one might be tempted to interpret the increased binding potential as an adaptive upregulation of receptor activity in response to decreased 5-HT (Walsh and Dinan, 2001). The upregulation hypothesis is problematical since the 5-HT$_{2A}$ receptor does not appear to upregulate in response to reduced synaptic 5-HT (Peremans et al., 2003b). Although chronic exposure to decreased 5-HT release might result in alterations affecting 5-HT$_{2A}$ receptor sensitivity and numerous other changes influencing 5-HT function, decreased 5-HT levels alone might not account for the receptor binding changes found in aggressive dogs. Another possible explanation for the increased binding index exhibited by such dogs is prior exposure to antidepressant medications commonly used to treat canine aggression problems. Chronic fluoxetine treatment in rats has been shown to significantly increase the density of 5-HT uptake sites and to upregulate the expression of 5-HT$_2$ receptors in the frontalparietal cortex by 31-38% (Hrdina and Vu, 1993). However, none of the dogs enrolled in the present study had ever received psychotropic drugs, modified diets, or behavioral therapy prior to the imaging study (Peremans, personal communication, 2003), thus excluding a drug effect as a possible explanation. The lack of differences between aggressive and nonaggressive dog pertaining to cerebral blood flow is a bit surprising and might represent an artifactual peculiarity of the study design, which required that the dogs be anesthetized for brain imaging.

Early developmental stress may exert influential effects on the organization of reactive thresholds. Prenatal stress has been shown to promote widespread changes affecting the organization of most major neurotransmitter systems so far studied (see *Ontogeny, Coping, and Social Behavior*). In addition to the impact of elevated maternal glucocorticoids reaching the fetal brain, perinatal gonadal hormones may alter the expression of serotonergic pathways in the young dog that may affect the adult dog's vulnerability to psychological stress. Early social stressors have been implicated in numerous neurophysiological changes relevant to attachment problems and aggression, including the upregulation of the 5-HT_{2A} receptor. For example, rats given corticosterone or ATCH for 10 days show a significant increase of 5-HT_{2A} receptor binding potential in the frontal cortex (Takao et al., 1995; Takao et al., 1997; Kuroda et al., 1992). Also, cortisol has been shown to increase the expression of 5-HT transporter sites in vitro (Tafet et al., 2001), raising the possibility that increased glucocorticoid levels resulting from chronic stress might increase the re-uptake efficiency of serotonergic terminals, causing 5-HT to be rapidly cleared from the synaptic cleft. Such an enhancement of 5-HT transport could result in the premature termination of 5-HT-mediated neural transmission. Under a highly motivated state, rapid clearance of 5-HT could result in muddled judgment, behavioral dysregulation, and the catastrophic sequencing and loss of control associated with impulsive aggression.

In addition to stress-related endocrine changes, sex steroids also appear to exert an upregulating effect on 5-HT_{2A} receptors in frontal and cingulate cortical areas of rats (Sumner and Fink, 1998). Male rats show a greater concentration of 5-HT_{2A}-receptor activity in the ventromedial hypothalamus, a gender dimorphism that is eliminated by castration (Zhang et al., 1999). The ventromedial hypothalamus is associated with the expression of affective aggression [see *Neurobiology of Aggression (Hypothalamus)* in Volume 1, Chapter 3]. Isolation rearing can also enhance 5-HT_{2A} receptor binding and increase aggressive behavior (Sakaue et al., 2002), conversely, enhanced 5-HT_{1A} receptor activity appears to exert an antiaggression influence. Similarly, among cats the 5-HT_{1A} receptor appears to mediate an inhibitory effect over affective aggression, whereas the 5-HT_2 receptor may facilitate it (Gregg and Siegel, 2001). 5-HT_{1A} agonists exert potent inhibitory effects on 5-HT_{2A}-mediated behavior as well as downregulating the 5-HT_{2A} receptor (Eison and Mullins, 1996). 5-HT_{1B} agonists have also been shown to exert a potent inhibitory effect on aggression between rats facilitated by frustration and social instigation (de Almeida and Miczek, 2002). Interestingly, a prominent effect of 5-HT_1 receptors is to exert an inhibitory autoreceptor effect over the release 5-HT, with 5-HT_1 agonists reducing synaptic 5-HT availability.

Panic, Separation Distress, and Aggression

Increased dopamine (DA) activity stimulated by apomorphine has been shown to upregulate the 5-HT_{2A} receptor as well as to facilitate the expression of impulsive behavior, including aggression in predisposed animals (Matto et al., 1999), however, increased 5-HT_{2A} activity does not appear to alter the latency or intensity of apomorphine-mediated aggressive behavior, at least among rats (Skrebuhhova-Malmros et al., 2000). Aggression mediated by dopaminergic pathways may either be facilitated or inhibited by 5-HT_2 receptor activity depending on the cortical or subcortical site and the receptor subtype involved. For example, the 5-HT_{2A} receptor appears to mediate a phasic disinhibitory influence (i.e., lifts tonic inhibition) over cortical DA release in response to anticipated social stressors, while 5-HT$_{2C}$ receptors appear to exert a tonic inhibitory effect (Gobert and Millan, 1999). At the level of the ventral tegmental area (VTA), 5-HT$_{2C}$ appears to promote phasic and tonic inhibitory influences over the release of DA (Di Matteo et al., 2002), whereas the 5-HT$_{2A}$ receptor mediates a phasic disinhibitory influence over DA release. Prefrontal regulatory influences over mesolimbic reward circuits is also mediated by the modulatory effects of 5-HT on excitatory glutaminergic pathways projecting to the VTA and the nucleus accumbens (Charney, 2004). In addition to receiving glutaminergic input from the amygdala, the thalamus also communicates with the mPFC via a glutaminergic circuit (Martin-Ruiz et al., 2001)—a circuit that might produce significant disruption of executive function and perceptual disturbance in cases where 1A- and 2A-receptor activity is in a state of flux or imbalance. Elevated DA activity, increased 5-HT$_{2A}$ receptor binding potential, and disturbances affecting 5-HT or DA clearance within the PFC may combine to produce devastating cognitive disturbances. Hallucinogens (e.g., LSD) exhibit a high affinity for the 5-HT$_{2A}$-receptor subtype, suggesting the possibility that some impulsive attacks may be associated with perceptual confusion or hallucination.

Prefrontal 5-HT and DA systems undergo alteration as the result of aggressive interaction. Van Erp and Miczek (2000), for example, have shown that episodic fighting between rats produces a potent effect on prefrontal DA and 5-HT balance, resulting in a sustained 120% increase of DA and an 80% decrease of 5-HT turnover in the mPFC. In a parallel study performed in the same laboratory, found that repeated aggressive encounters between rats resulted in conditioned changes in heart rate and the release of DA and 5-HT in anticipation of a fight (Ferrari et al., 2003). In this study, aggressive rats were brought together to fight on 10 consecutive days at precisely the same time. On day 11 the scheduled fight was cancelled and various real-time measurements were taken to assess 5-HT and DA activity. During the hour

immediately before the usual fight time, the rats showed a conditioned increase of heart rate and a potent efflux of accumbal DA. The 5-HT levels of experienced rats stayed relatively constant throughout, until approximately several minutes before the normally scheduled fight, whereupon 5-HT levels dipped and decreased by 30-35% over the next hour or so before slowly returning to baseline levels. During the first fight encounter, in contrast, 5-HT levels showed a slight dip during the fight period itself and remained relatively steady for 30 minutes, during which time DA levels increased with the onset of the fight and continued to increase over the course of the same 30-minute period. The subsequent increase of DA appeared to shadow a decrease of 5-HT levels, suggesting that 5-HT may exert an inhibitory effect on DA activity, perhaps via the action of the 5-HT$_{1A}$ autoreceptor. Taken together these findings suggest that DA establishes a motivational readiness to fight, whereas 5-HT may either inhibit or disinhibit aggressive behavior, thereby forbidding or permitting aggression but without directly affecting the motivational state. Surprisingly, in contrast to the conditioned changes in DA and 5-HT levels, the rats that fought showed only a slight increase of anticipation-related heart rate change in comparison to control mice that had not fought.

The feed-forward or proactive nature of preparatory aggressive arousal is also true for the way dogs cope with social stressors, explaining why the same aversive event might activate the HPA system or not depending on the degree of control or *power* (competence and confidence) that the dog perceives it has over the event. The foregoing findings support the idea that aggressive exchanges are under the regulatory influence of feed-forward conditioning effects. The evident adjustment and coordination of DA and 5-HT activity in anticipation of events, including the preparation of physiological states required to enable the animal to cope effectively with impending motivational demands strongly supports the notion that aggressive behavior can be regulated by control expectancies and emotional establishing operations integrated in the process of establishing an adaptive coping style. Psychological stressors perceived as uncontrollable challenges or threats exert a disorganizing effect (reactive coping style), whereas the same aversive motivation stimuli, when perceived as predictable and controllable, generate an organizing effect on behavior (adaptive coping style) precisely because adaptation is organizational and designed to learn and cope proactively with motivational challenges and threats rather than to merely react to them. These observations support the hypothesis that reward and punishment in association with positive and negative prediction error is critically dependent on the nucleus accumbens and its interconnectivity with the orbitofrontal cortex, amygdala, and VTA, neural processing networks that regulate the expression of motivated behavior in accord with proactive prediction-control expectancies and calibrated establishing operations.

Septal Distress, Relief, and Panic

The septum pellucidum is a limbic structure believed to perform a number of important functions in learning and the regulation of endocrine activity and emotion by virtue of its close relationship with the hippocampus and interconnectivity with the amygdala, the hypothalamus, the cingulate cortex, and the PAG. Reciprocal communication between the septum and the hippocampus occur via cholinergic tracts, with septal signals providing a pacemaker effect on hippocampal theta rhythms as well as serving to switch the hippocampus from an information processing mode to information collecting mode (Ikonen, 2001). The septum plays an important role in the process of forming expectancies about the timing and contingency of unconditioned stimuli (Garcia and Jaffard, 1996). Under the influence of aversive arousal septal stimulation appears to produce reward (relief), whereas under nonthreatening circumstances septal stimulation is hedonically neutral (Grauer and Thomas, 1982), suggesting that the septal-hippocampal connectivity may mediate passive avoidance, anxiety, and relief, whereas the central amygdala and the

BNST are involved in the elaboration of fear and active avoidance. Medial septal lesions appear to significantly impair an animal's ability to respond adaptively to signals of punishment and nonreward (Gray, 1971). Impaired animals show deficits with respect to the inhibition of an activity once it has started, despite the presence of clear signals of punishment and nonreward. Unable to respond to stop signals, septal-impaired animals may nevertheless remain acutely aware that they are threatened by an impending loss or risk resulting from their failure to stop.

In response to emotional alarm or uncertainty, the central amygdala may activate anxiety-mediating excitatory pathways that reach the lateral septum via the paraventricular nucleus (PVN) and the BNST (Nail-Boucherie et al., 1998). Also, efferent AVP fibers project from the medial amygdala to the ventral hippocampus as well as the lateral septum directly and via the BNST (Caffe et al., 1987), suggesting that CRF and AVP (see DeVries et al. 1983) may synergistically interact in the lateral septum to mediate anxiety- and distress-related behavior. Interestingly, Thomas and colleagues (2003) have shown that CRF exerts a regulatory effect at the level of dorsal raphe nucleus over the release of 5-HT in the lateral septum, with low levels of CRF reducing septal 5-HT release and high levels of CRF increasing septal 5-HT release. This pattern of connectivity may promote a durable state of aversive arousal and punishment-resistant vigilance in response to a variety of acute psychological stressors requiring caution and persistence but not escalating into a state of reactive fear or anger. Significantly, paroxetine exerts an inhibitory effect over the release of 5-HT via the 5-HT$_{1B}$ autoreceptor, an effect that takes place most prominently in the ventral hippocampus (Gardier et al., 2003). 5-HT also appears to modulate cholinergic transmission via postsynaptic 5-HT$_{1B}$ receptors expressed on the terminals of cholinergic neurons within the hippocampus. Fish and colleagues (2000) have shown that 5-HT$_{1B}$ agonists mediate a suppressive effect over mouse distress vocalization to maternal separation (Fish et al., 2000), suggesting a possible mechanism for the beneficial effects of paroxetine for the control of separation distress and panic. Consistent with this hypothesis, nicotine, a cholinergic agonist, has also been shown to decrease separation distress vocalizations in chicks, whereas the antimuscarinic scopolamine increases distress vocalizations (Sahley et al., 1983). Further, the electrical stimulation of the ventral septum produces a high level of separation-distress vocalizations, as does stimulating the BNST (Panksepp, 1998). Recently, Degroot and colleagues (2004) have reported that the septal-hippocampal system plays a prominent role in the modulation of different anxiety states via glutaminergic, GABAergic, and cholinergic pathways. Finally, GABAergic plasticity at the level of the septum determines how animals cope with inescapable stressors, with the stress-mediated downregulation of septal $GABA_B$ receptors appearing to exert a protective influence against learned helplessness (Kram et al., 2000). In addition to the panic occurring in association with separation distress, the lateral septum and BNST may also play a role in mediating the panic associated with certain forms of aggression expressed in association with a reactive coping style (see Koolhaas et al., 1998).

The panic and persistence associated with separation distress is consistent with what one would expect to occur in association with faulty septal-hippocampal processing, whereby the dog appears to become "obsessively" fixated on an expectation of impending relief, despite foreknowing (signals of nonreward) that the owner will not likely come home any time soon, consistent with impairments affecting passive avoidance learning. The precise etiology of such problems is unknown, however, it is reasonable to suggest that social ambivalence and entrapment occurring in association with insecure or nervous attachments may promote complex disturbances disrupting glutaminergic, GABAergic, opioidergic, or cholinergic transmission and that these dynamics might produce a detrimental imbalance at the level of the septum and other limbic areas conducive to separation distress. The involvement of these systems in the mediation of separation distress may help to explain why people often

increase their consumption alchohol, sugar, sweet and fatty dairy products (e.g., ice cream), and tobacco at times involving social loss and separation. The consumption of sugar, for example, may produce a self-medicating effect via a glucose-mediated reduction of opioid restraint over cholingergic activity, whereas nicotine consumption may alter activity in cholinergic-dopaminergic pathways. Ragozzino and colleagues (1992) found that passive avoidance was impaired when morphine was injected into the medial septum, whereas the administration of glucose reversed the deficit. Under the influence of an insecure attachment heightened oxytocin activity may mediate a sensitization to opioid and DA activity, making the dog vulnerable to opiate-like addiction and withdrawal symptoms when the insecure social attachment object maintaining DA, opioid, and oxytocin levels is withdrawn. Interestingly, clomipramine, a drug commonly used to treat separation-related problems, reduces central opioid levels, down regulates opioid-binding sites, and attenuates morphine-induced analgesia. In addition, among humans, clomipramine has been shown to increase oxytocin and to decrease CRF levels in the cerebral spinal fluid (CSF) (McDougle et al., 1999), perhaps contributing to the stabilizing effect that the medication appears to exert over canine separation distress.

The finding that glucose interacts with opioids in a function-restoring fashion, suggests that at least in some cases of separation distress, a sugar pill may be more than just a placebo. Also, given the apparent attenuating effects of nicotine on separation distress, it would be interesting to learn whether there is any discernable relationship between cigarette smoking in households with dogs and the risk of separation-related problems. Whether feeding the dog sweet-flavored treats or giving it toys that have been coated with a sweet solution would have any benefit on separation-related problems is unknown but such research may be interesting to pursue, since the dog definitely has a sweet tooth (Ferrell, 1984). Among human infants undergoing painful medical procedures, sucrose and non-sucrose sweeteners have been shown to diminish signs of pain for up to 5 minutes, with peak effects observed at 2 minutes after ingestion (Blass and Shah, 1995). These findings suggest the obvious possibility that similar benefits might be obtained in the case of puppies and dogs receiving vaccination shots or undergoing painful grooming procedures (e.g. cleaning ears). In addition to analgesic effects, among rat pups that have been separated from their mother, ingestion of sucrose also produces a calming effect in the distressed infant (Blass et al., 1987). Milk also appears to produce similar effects among infant rats (Blass and Fitzgerald, 1988), apparently not as result of lactose (Blass and Shide, 1994), but perhaps due to the casomorphine contained in milk casein or as the result of milk fat. The calming effect of sucrose on separation distress is robust, reducing distress vocalizations by 50% (Blass and Shide, 1994). Interestingly, with respect to the cholinergic-opioid hypothesis outlined above, the analgesic effect of sweet substances appears to be mediated by nicotinic cholinergic receptors (Irusta et al., 2001). Casual observations by the author indicate that small amounts of whipped cream or soft cheese delivered from a pressurized can do seem to mediate a transient comforting effect. The use of food items may provide benefits in the case of puppies that are overly resentful or reactive to routine veterinary or grooming procedures. In any case, given the reports from human and animal studies of an analgesic effect, some investigation is warranted to explore whether food items such as whipped cream or soft cheese might be useful for reducing the discomfort and fear associated with veterinary examinations and treatments. The first visit is the most critical since those impressions are extremely durable. Using a combination of food, odors, petting/massage, and toys might help to reduce the risk of the dog forming lasting aversive associations linked to veterinary visits, while at the same time promoting positive expectations.

Periaqueductal Gray and Autoprotective Adjustments to Social Stressors

Social disengagement, confrontation, and aversive communication systems appear to converge subcortically at the level of the PAG (periaqueductal gray) (Keay and Bandler, 2001). The PAG projects to the nucleus ambiguous (Farkas et al., 1997) where it may increase heart rate and blood pressure and participate in the expression of threat displays (e.g. direct stare, snarling, ears forward, and growling) (lateral PAG) or decrease heart rate and blood pressure and contribute to the expression of defeat and appeasement displays (e.g., averted eye contact, head down, ears pinned back, and yelping) (ventrolateral PAG). Active and passive coping reactions in response to threats are under the regulatory influence of both cortical and limbic pathways (e.g., amygdala, hippocampus, and hypothalamus) (see *Stress-related Potentiation of the Flight-Fight System* in Chapter 6). These reactions include emotional vocalizations expressing distress, discomfort, and alarm/threats, social communication that appears to be mediated by the PAG and vocal-motor nuclei located in the brainstem. The strong connectivity between the prefrontal cortex and the PAG emphasizes the role of psychological stressors (e.g., violations of prediction-control expectancies) on the development of fear and aggression problems. PAG flight-or-fight adjustments appear to be under the modulatory control of reciprocal inhibition, that is, when PAG flight networks are activated PAG fight programs may be actively restrained while a converse effect appears to occur when the fight network is activated (Jansen et al., 1998). The rostral aspects of the dorsolateral (dlPAG) and lateral (lPAG) columns of the PAG mediate confrontational threat and attack (anger) (fight system), while the caudal aspect of the dlPAG and lPAG mediate the mobilization of defensive escape (fear) (flight system). The rostral portion of the lPAG receives ascending somatosensory input originating from the face and forelimbs, whereas the caudal portion of the lPAG receives afferent input from the lower portion of the body. This organization of somatosensory organization suggests that frontal threats are more likely to evoke anger and offensive aggression than threats coming from behind, which are more likely to evoke fear and defensive adjustments. The ventrolateral PAG (vlPAG) mediates opioid-mediated analgesia, bradycardia and hypotension, and tonic immobilization, suggesting that the vlPAG plays a role in facilitating the aggression-suppressing effects of repeated social defeat (Depaulis et al., 1994).

When the dog is challenged or threatened in a serious way a pathway linking the medial amygdala, the bed nucleus of the stria terminalis (BNST) (an area that may promote intensified vigilance at such times), and the medial hypothalamus may be activated to mobilize an avalanche of neurophysiological activity at the level of the PAG that might promote catastrophic autoprotective adjustments. Both the rostral and caudal aspects of the lPAG and the dlPAG produce tachycardia and hypertension but do so in association with different patterns of vasodilation and vasoconstriction. Defensive arousal associated with the caudal lPAG results in a diversion of blood from the head and viscera to the skeletal muscle. In contrast, offensive arousal associated with the rostral dlPAG result in an increased heart rate and blood pressure associated with a diversion of blood from the skeletal muscles and viscera to the head via increased extracranial blood flow. The vasodilation and increased blood flow associated with dlPAG offensive arousal may explain the reddish glow that dogs show immediately before launching into an attack. Unlike the lPAG, the dlPAG column receives no significant spinal, trigeminal, or medullary inputs, but is strongly enervated by descending inputs from the right mPFC. These mPFC efferent pathways also target the anterior and ventromedial hypothalamus, a pattern of connectivity that suggests that the mPFC in coordination with the hypothalamus serves to modulate the expression of aggression and escape behavior (Keay and Bandler, 2001). The lPAG receives strong cortical enervation from the cingulate area (An et al., 1998), perhaps mediating aversive state arousal and behavioral activation associated with the detection of social conflict and loss. Kyuhou and Gemba (1998) found that the area of the guinea pig PAG that evokes separation-distress vocalizations, receives "massive input" from the ACC, lending support to a possible

linkage between separation distress/panic and the PAG.

PART 2: BONDING THEORY

ONTOGENY, COPING, AND SOCIAL BEHAVIOR

The disorganizing influence of runaway allostatic load and the integration of maladaptive behavioral phenotypes may be initiated or prefigured early in a dog's ontogeny. Dogs exposed to adverse prenatal and postnatal stress, perinatal trauma, or maternal maltreatment may show a more dramatic and exaggerated allostatic response and tendency to integrate adaptation-impairing load in response to stressors than dogs exposed to more favorable ontogenetic programming early in life. The type, amount, and timing of early stress may profoundly affect the expression and functionality of PSMs and the ability of a dog to adjust in a functionally coordinated way. Developmental programming and insults that cause modal disturbances affecting sensorimotor processing (preattentive and preemptive arousal) and various motivational and motor systems integrating drive and behavioral output may impair a dog's ability to achieve coherent and stable adjustments.

In addition to psychological stressors, damage associated with infectious disease and environmental toxins have been implicated in etiology of adult and childhood behavioral disorders. Mothers exposed to viral infections early in the gestation period may transmit pathological antibodies or cytokines across the placenta that produce lasting harmful effects. Rat mothers, for example, infected with influenza virus during day 9 of gestation showed alterations in exploratory activity, including increased aversion toward novelty together with deficits affecting prepulse inhibition in response to auditory startle (Shi et al., 2003). Brown and colleagues (2004) have reported that babies born to mothers exposed to influenza during the first trimester showed a sevenfold increase in risk for developing schizophrenia in adulthood. Since the influenza virus only rarely crosses the placenta, the researchers implicate maternal immunoglobulin G antibodies activating fetal brain antigens or a virus-induced excess of maternal cytokines. Infant exposure to environmental toxins has been implicated in the expression of a wide spectrum of behavioral disorders, including attention-deficit hyperactivity disorder, retardation, and autism (Zoeller et al., 2002; Colburn, 2004). The effects of thyroid are pervasive and time dependent, affecting the organization of neural tissue and connectivity via myelination and synaptogenesis. Thyroid plays a significant role in the organization of the glucocorticoid, cholinergic, and serotonergic systems and the structural development of the cortex, basal forebrain, cerebellum, hypothalamus, and hippocampus (Meaney et al., 2000; Thompson and Potter, 2000; Smith et al., 2002; Zoeller et al., 2002). The prenatal role of thyroid in the development of neuronal systems mediating the organization of social coping styles emphasizes the importance of fetal thyroid balance. Exposure to a variety of common medications and cytokine-producing vaccinations during the first trimester of gestation may exert far-reaching effects on a progeny's behavioral adaptability in adulthood (see *Antistress Neurobiology, Maternal Care, and Coping Style* in Chapter 8 and *Immune Stress and Cytokines* in Chapter 6).

Although PSMs and the various interconnected modal networks and motor programs subserving their development and expression may remain relatively quiescent and unintrusive under the influence of minimal change and stress, dormant dysfunctional modes may be activated later in life under the influence of psychological stressors or in association with epigenetic shifts heralding major developmental transitions (e.g., puberty and adulthood). These late epigenetic elaborations and patches may be particularly vulnerable to disorganization and instability. Under the influence of aberrant polymorphisms or stressors, problematic PSMs may integrate at an age-inappropriate time and thereafter exert adverse epigenetic changes to modal drive networks and emotional command systems. For example, paedomorphic behavioral phenotypes may be the result of such developmental delays and shifts in organization serving to prolong youthful sociability and playfulness, with many dogs appearing to operate under a predominant play drive. Late developmental epigenetic elaborations or patches that add on to or activate modal networks and motor programs organized early in life but left in a dormant state (e.g., the gender dimorphic effects of perinatal sex hormones) are prone to mobilize instability and allostatic load when mediating disruptive social dynamics associated with social ambivalence and entrapment. Accordingly, dormant dysfunctional PSMs activated while adult sociosexual phenotypes are being elaborated may be particularly sensitive to conflictive social dynamics, dispersive tensions, and show an increased vulnerability for the expression of reactive and impulsive behavior.

The dysfunctional mode and subservient modal networks may become progressively autonomous and disruptive while degrading or abolishing executive control and fostering a reactive coping style associated with accumulating allostatic load, ambivalence, and entrapment. Under the influence of social and environmental stressors perceived as inescapable (entrapment), a dog may attempt to adjust by retracting the SES while disengaging executive attentional resources, giving rise to dispersive tensions (e.g., resentment, irritability, and intolerance) and autoprotective dynamics, on the one hand, and mediating persistent anxiety, autonomic deregulation, and impairment of the dog's ability to cancel/inhibit or activate/disinhibit autonomic and emotional processing appropriately in coordination with purposive drive and functionally appropriate behavior (see *Breed and Individual Difference* and *Reactive/Impulsive Behavior*).

Prenatal Stress: Born to Flee or to Bite?

The enduring developmental effects of prenatal stress have been traced to various changes in all major neurotransmitter systems (Weinstock, 1997). In addition to altering NE and serotonin (5-HT) activity, prenatal stress reduces DA turnover in the nucleus accumbens while increasing DA turnover in the PFC. Chronically elevated DA activity in the PFC may disrupt executive attention and impulse-control functions (see *Startle and Fear Circuits* in Chapter 3), whereas a reduction in DA turnover in the mesolimbic system may diminish an animal's ability to produce reward and mobilize reward-dependent active modal strategies (e.g., exploratory behavior and social engagement). In fact, animals exposed to prenatal stress have been shown to exhibit a diminished responsiveness to reward (Matthews et al., 1996; Matthews and Robbins, 2003). The intrinsic reward that mediates play appears to depend on a balance of DA and opioid activity, whereas acetylcholine and NE appear to be involved in the cognitive, exploratory, attentional, and arousal aspects of play behavior (Vanderschuren et al., 1997; Panksepp, 1998).

Developmental perturbations of the DA reward system would likely disrupt a young dog's ability to refine control modules, thereby adversely influencing its ability to integrate adaptive behavior. Such prenatal disturbances affecting reward processing suggest an explanation for the *reward resistance* exhibited by some dogs to behavior-therapy procedures dependent on the conditioning of reward signals. The tendency of unstable introverts to show a heightened sensitivity to signals of punishment and a reduced responsiveness to signals of reward is consistent with a prenatal origin of such temperament differences as well as the anxious/irritable dysthymia exhibited by such dogs. In addition to an increased sensitivity to stimuli producing anxiety and a blunted responsiveness to reward, prenatal exposure to maternal anxiety and anger may program neurobiological changes that might confer an increased risk for developing behavior problems associated with anger and impulsivity in adulthood. For example, babies born to high-anxiety, angry, and depressed mothers show parallel biochemistry profiles (low DA and 5-HT levels), decreased vagal tone, and right hemisphere electroencephalographic asymmetry (Field et al., 2003), perhaps predisposing them to integrate similar mood and behavioral propensities.

Postnatal Handling: Protective and Destructive Influences

Postnatal stimulation may accentuate, diminish, or reverse the adverse effects of prenatal stress. Whereas long periods of separation from the mother can result in HPA-axis disturbances in adult rats, briefer periods of separation tend to produce a moderating effect on emotional reactivity and HPA-axis activity. Adverse maternal separation stress produces a downregulation of glucocorticoid-binding sites in the hippocampus, as well as increases hypothalamic CRF mRNA expression. This combination of neural changes may result in an adult animal that is stress prone, showing a greater vulnerability to the adverse effects of chronic environmental and psychological stressors via impaired hippocampal negative-feedback control over CRF release and increased CRF activity. Although the stress-mediated facilitation of CRF gene expression exerts highly durable and perhaps irreversible changes on the CRF system, the brain shows remarkable capabilities to make compensatory adjustments. For example, among rats exposed to harmful maternal separation, social and environmental enrichment procedures ameliorate the adverse effects of early stress on HPA-axis activity and fearful responses to psychological stressors (Francis et al., 2002).

The critical factor affecting the long-term effects of early stress probably depends on the quality of maternal care received by an infant. Several studies have shown that it is not the *stress* produced by separating an infant from its mother or exposure to environmental insults, but rather the benefits are due to subsequent changes in the mother's caregiving behavior when the infant is returned to the nest (see *Antistress Neurobiology, Maternal Care, and Coping Style* in Chapter 8). Maternal caregiving behavior appears to be invigorated by the pup's absence from the nest and upon reunion the separated infant becomes the object of intensified exploratory interest, licking, and other maternal contact behaviors. Among rats, adoptive mothers are typically more attentive to adopted pups and tend to give them more grooming and licking than provided by natural mothers. Maccari and colleagues (1995) have shown that the increased care provided by adoptive mothers appears to reverse the adverse behavioral effects of prenatal stress on HPA-axis activity.

An infant's ability to cope with stress in adulthood appears to be mediated by an anti-stress system that is integrated by the central release of oxytocin in response to maternal licking and other caregiving activities. Repetitive stroking and other forms of stimulation similar in effect to maternal care and grooming have been shown to induce oxytocin release and to exert a protective influence or to reverse the effects of prenatal stress on developmental disorders in adult animals (Weinstock, 2002) (see *Handling and Gentling* in Chapter 4). The obvious implication of these various findings is that the amount and quality of maternal attention and care received by the infant exert a significant programming effect on adult coping styles (see *Ontogeny and Reactive Behavior* in Chapter 8).

Ontogeny, Olfactory Cortex, Attunement Nodes, Engrams, and Networks

During the first 2 weeks of life, a puppy is adapted to an off-line state dedicated primarily to nursing and sleeping (Fox and Stanton, 1967) adjusting as needed to internal and external stressors by means of an array of sensorimotor reflexes. Sensory inputs are reduced to a minimum with the eyes and ears remaining closed, but as these sensory channels open between weeks 2 and 3, respectively, a dog becomes increasingly active and interactive. By the time a dog reaches week 3, it already shows a strong preference for the smell of kin bedding (Mekosh-Rosenbaum et al., 1994) consistent with the existence of a motivated preference and attachment. At weeks 4 1/2 to 5 1/2 (Hepper, 1986), they orient, presumably using both auditory and visual channels (although auditory information may play a subordinate role), and ambulate into the proximity of familiar siblings and avoid other puppies of a similar age, breed, and sex. The olfactory memories and preferences integrated during this time appear to degrade with respect to the recognition of separated siblings but remains intact with respect to the reciprocal recognition shown mothers and offspring after 2 years of separation (Hepper, 1994). In addition to confirming these earlier studies, Gillis and colleagues (1999) have demon-strated that dogs not only recognize their mother but also recognize the scent of the breeder well into adulthood and probably for much of their lives (Appel et al., 1999).

With the onset of the socialization period at week 3, a rapid integration of corticohypothalamic networks and exchange-mediated autonomic attunement nodes emerges to regulate drive and emotion and to guide sympathovagal tone toward a state of balance conducive to alertness and social engagement (see *Socialization: Learning to Relate and Communicate* in Volume 1, Chapter 2). During these early weeks, social expectancies, autonomic attunement, and play facilitate increased social attraction and awareness. A puppy's ability to learn appears to reach a high level by weeks 7 and 8, abilities that may already start declining after week 16 (see *Learning and Trainability* in Volume 1, Chapter 2).

Weaning and Parent-Offspring Conflict

According to an influential theory of parental investment (PI) proposed by Trivers (1972), both parents invest in the care of offspring, but the PI of males is typically much less than that of females. In some species, such as dogs, the male PI consists only of donating sperm, whereas other mammalian males contribute more equitable investments to the care of the young. The amount of PI given by the mother and father appears to exert a profound influence on the reproductive relationship, the social organization of the group, and the quality of interaction among members of the group. Besides nurturance, a significant part of PI involves protection. Among wolves, mothers and fathers share a major investment in the care and protection of the young (Mech, 2000). They form lasting pair bonds, show evidence of a division of labor, and organize relatively stable family groups. The mother wolf suckles and cares for the young and protects the denning area, whereas the father appears to play a greater role in the defense of the home territory while provisioning the mother and young with food. In contrast, males in animal societies where they contribute minimal PI to their offspring may nevertheless contribute strongly to the gene pool to the extent that they can compete successfully with other males seeking females to fertilize. In such animal groups, intermale competition may be more prominent, necessitating a variety of biological (e.g., endocrine control of agonistic thresholds) and social adaptations (e.g., dominance hierarchies) to moderate competitive tensions.

The weaning process exhibited by wolf mothers appears to be relatively peaceful, at least when adequate amounts of alternative food are available to feed the young. Packard and colleagues (1992) observed only one occasion prior to week 7 in which the mother terminated a nursing bout by muzzling a pup. From week 6 onward, however, they observed a trend toward more frequent mother-initiated terminations of nursing bouts and infant-directed agonism, culminating in weeks 8 and 9, when the mother terminates 80% of the nursing bouts by agonistic means. The use of muzzling to control nursing activity was usually associated with signs of discomfort on the mother's part (wincing). The wincing action itself acquired the ability to interrupt nursing. After the mother winced or muzzled them, the pups stopped nursing and did not persist.

Under domestic conditions, the mother and the breeder contribute the primary sources of PI in the care of puppies. In addition to giving the mother emotional support, the breeder assists the dam by feeding the puppies solid food or by confining the puppies or by helping the mother stay out of the offsprings' reach, perhaps by providing a ledge or other place for the mother to retreat. In the early stages of nursing, the mother appears to derive considerable gratification from the contact with her offspring (Korda, 1974), initiating nursing bouts and spending large amounts of time caring for them (Rheingold, 1963). Licking bouts are most frequent and lengthy during the first 2 weeks postpartum. As the mother's willingness to nurse declines toward week 4, there is an increase in offspring-initiated approaches and nursing bouts, which may rapidly exceed the mother's optimum PI and require the breeder's intervention to control. In addition to the food given to the puppies by the breeder, some

canine mothers may regurgitate. Regurgitation serves to transition the puppy from the ingestion of the preferred mother's milk to the search for solid food (James, 1960; Malm, 1995). Martins (1949) observed that the appearance of regurgitation is closely associated with the decline in lactation and continues only a few days after weaning is complete, whereas Korda (1974) found that regurgitation routinely continued long after puppies were able to eat solid food—conflicting findings that suggest the existence of a high degree of individual variability affecting the habit. Domestic male dogs can be induced to regurgitate in response to et-epimeletic displays if they are confined in close proximity with puppies (Korda, 1974), but the tendency to provision food to offspring appears to be generally atrophied in male dogs. Feral male dogs may stay with the mother, sleep nearby, and even play with the puppies but do not provide the young with food (Macdonald and Carr, 1995). This lack of PI by male dogs is a peculiarity of domestication and in sharp contrast to the behavior of wild canids.

During weaning, the competent mother appears to calm the puppy with affectionate tactile stimulation, complementing the more energetic, playful, and competitive exchanges among littermates. Gently muzzled puppies may be transitioned to receive a sustained licking or nibbling bout, maternal activities that they appear to enjoy by rolling on their side or back, laying still, and often closing their eyes. Puppies may show signs of growing sibling agonism during this period of transition, but they rarely attempt to provoke such interaction with the mother. Often by means of the mildest assertions of maternal force, a puppy defers or walks away—a response that may be followed by the mother going to the puppy and intermittently mouthing or licking around the scruff of the neck. The mother appears to actively mediate a reconciliation process with the discouraged youngster. Contingent assertions of power, affectionate reconciliation, and periodic absences serve to reduce undesirable behavior while at the same time stimulating emotional establishing operations that prime conflict-resolving adjustments and compromise. The assertion of maternal power mediates various passive modal activities (e.g., hesitating, waiting, and submissive ritualizing) that are valuable for promoting impulse control and cooperative behavior.

The conflictive dynamics of exchange between the mother and puppy appear to promote an emergent coping style consistent with many of Trivers' predictions regarding parent-offspring conflict (Trivers, 1974) (see *Parent-Offspring Conflict and Interactive Conflict* in Chapter 8). The puppy's efforts to get care in excess of the mother's parental investment, while avoiding punishment (e.g., loss of care and risk of physical restraint), provides a framework of positive and negative incentives that may point to the origin of propensities toward interactive conflict and exploitive exchange, on the one hand, or interactive harmony and fair exchange, on the other.

Mothers pushed beyond the limits of their PI may become increasingly reactive and abusive toward their young (see *Maternal Mistreatment* in Chapter 8). In a study by Scott and Fuller (1965), canine mothers and offspring were kept together until week 10 under relatively austere conditions of close confinement. This rearing practice may have been highly stressful for both mothers and offspring, perhaps accentuating the effects of prenatal stress on the emotional reactivity of the puppies and explaining the high level of agitation and aggression exhibited by mothers toward offspring (Rheingold, 1963). On the other hand, removing puppies too early from the mother may result in lasting impairments diminishing the offsprings' ability to achieve autonomic balance.

In any case, disruptive influences stemming from maternal mistreatment may exert profound and lasting adverse effects on a dog's ability to cope adaptively with complex social demands. However, the same flexibility that makes a puppy vulnerable to destructive influences also makes it highly resilient and responsive to protective influences, perhaps helping to explain the apparent lack of significant maternal effects shown by German shepherd dogs in a recent study performed by Strandberg and colleagues (2004). Whereas exposure to inescapable aversive stimulation shortly after weaning profoundly disturbs adult escape behavior, exposure to controllable aversive events early in life appears to have an immunizing effect against the adverse effects of inescapable aversive events in adulthood (Hannum et al., 1976). How a puppy is treated in the home ultimately seals its fate by either accentuating problematic aspects of developmental programming or by providing it with social and environmental conditions that promote compensatory adjustments conducive to an adaptive coping style and allostasis—*stability through change.*

ATTUNEMENT, ATTACHMENT, AND THE HUMAN-DOG BOND

According to the affect-attunement hypothesis, dogs and people relate by feeling their way through exchanges and by shifting arousal and output to match the emotional intensity, duration, and shape of the partner's reciprocating actions. The mutual appreciation or sharing of attention, intention, and affective states is marked by the emergence of an interactive attentional nexus and an allocentric relational space within which human and canine partners build complex predictive relations that serve to synchronize arousal and affective states. From a foundation of care relations mediating autonomic attunement, the dog shows an increasing appetite for socially mediated and shared experiences with others. When facing problems or circumstances evincing difficulty or uncertainty, dogs, like infants studied by Stern (1985), may look toward the social partner for "affective content, essentially to see what they should feel, to get a second appraisal to help resolve their uncertainty" (132). The dog's ability to grab and steer the human partner's attention to the location of out-of-reach toys or food reflects a capacity for relating to the other allocentrically, indicating the operation of a cognitive functions that enable the dog to appreciate the perspective of the partner relative to objects of interest to the dog. Affect attunement is commonplace in the interaction between people and dogs (Finck, 1993), especially in the context of caregiving and play exchanges. Affect attunement occurs when a partner's actions convey the feelings of a shared affective state, and it serves to focus attention on the "quality of feeling" that underlies expressive behavior: "Imitation renders form; attunement renders feeling" (Stern 1985:142).

Affect attunement gives social interaction a quality of sharing an experience and existence that stands outside of oneself. The personal nature of attachment entails that social transactions be tagged with unique social and contextual identifiers. Only exchanges with a specific individual can be encoded and stored in that person's social account, so to speak. Attunement imbues attachment relations with an implication of *responsibility* to the other, as one might feel responsible for how the dog feels and then adjust exchanges to compensate, as needed, to produce affective shifts conducive to a more desirable state, that is, to protect and care for it. As such, the affective changes associated with attunement dynamics that promote social and place attachments have the ontic property of belonging to the other who has an *identity*. To attach is to belong and incur an obligation to care for and to protect the interests of the attachment partner (loyalty). These attachment and attunement dynamics set the framework for many of the benefits of dog ownership as well as potential adjustment problems. Interestingly, when reminiscing over a previous family dog, many dog owners are apt to tell stories that illustrate the belongingness qualities of the attachment by referring to extraordinary caregiving behavior, fidelity, and heroic stories involving the protection of children.

As the result of the autonomic and affective attunement associated with the integration of secure attachments, a bond of belongingness is formed that links the dog and family together to *share* a secure living space held in a common trust (see *Social Spaces, Frames, and Zones* in Chapter 8). Secure social and place attachments shape a dog's identity into one who belongs as an object of care and protection. Social exchanges operating under the modulation of competent attunement serve to anticipate and match autonomic arousal to prediction-control expectancies,

calibrated emotional establishing operations, and goal-directed actions (control modules) that enable dogs to accumulate hedonic value in support of optimistic mood, social attraction, cooperation, play, and the integration of an adaptive coping style.

OPPORTUNITY WITH LIMIT

Attaining cynopraxic objectives depends on decisive action at the right time (*kairos*). In dog training, the coordination, selection, and timing of social exchanges are critical for success. The notion of kairos goes to the inner nature of such intuitive action and timely exchange. The word *kairos* was used in a variety of ways by ancient Greeks to describe timely action or opportunity. White (1987) suggests that the term was used to refer to the brief moment allowed for a weaver to pass a thread through a gap opened momentarily in the warp of a cloth being woven. In the *Odyssey*, Homer combines this early meaning of kairos with a manipulation of time used by Penelope to postpone the time agreed by her to decide and choose among the suitors. Penelope promised the suitors that as soon as she had finished a shroud that she was weaving for Odysseus' father that she would choose a new husband. But the promise was only a ruse to gain time, since at night she undid the work she accomplished during the day. A symbolic implication of her trick is that placing a thread through the kairos advanced time and pulling the thread out again held time back, at least with respect to the timing of the moment for her decision. Eventually, her subterfuge was discovered and the suitors demanded that she now decide and choose. Here, a second meaning of kairos enters the story, bringing the separated husband and wife closer together and setting the occasion for a decisive event. Instead of acquiescing to the suitors' demand, Penelope devised a contest for them to decide the matter of her hand. The challenge required that the winner string Odysseus' horned bow and then shoot an arrow through the hub of 12 axes aligned in a row. Like the passage of a thread through the warp of a cloth, the passage of an arrow through the opening of the hub of axes aligned in a row is also referred to as kairos (White, 1987), thus linking the two meanings in the critical moment when Odysseus, disguised as a beggar, takes the bow in hand and asserts his status and real identity as husband by stringing the bow and sending the arrow through the kairos. Unbeknownst to her at the time, Penelope's stalling had set the occasion of the contest in synchrony with the return of Odysseus and all that would follow. Having revealed his identity as husband, Odysseus is now united with Telemachus, as father and son, to take the moment of surprise to mete out justice upon the corrupt band of suitors who had invaded his home.

These two meanings of kairos derived from weaving and archery combine a balance of feminine and masculine energy (work or effort) to effect change and restore order and stability to a state of disorder by means of timely action. Thus, the ideal cynopraxic trainer combines the steady patience and intuitive vision of the weaver, on the one hand, and the mental steadiness and strength of the archer, on the other, to act decisively at the best opportunity. The opportune moment is not found by means of spontaneous opportunity-taking efforts, but by acting in accord with limit, by setting the stage, and by letting the opportune moment happen, as exemplified by Penelope's strategic stalling and the circumstances of the contest that she set for the suitors that enabled Odysseus to reclaim his identity heroically as husband and father.

Hitting and Missing the Mark

Social interaction is significantly complicated by the mutual control that social partners have over the moment of exchange and the circumstances surrounding exchange. As a result, social exchange is vulnerable to *tricks* of timing and other efforts used by interacting partners to make exchanges happen in ways that allow them to take an advantage or to engage in preemptive social strategies aimed at protecting themselves against the loss and risk associated with exploitive interaction. The

result of such interactive subterfuge is mistrust and misattunement, that is, putting the other out of step by concealment and deception, much as Penelope manipulated the exploitive and obtrusive suitors by her clever ruse. The process of adaptive optimization depends on the reciprocal give and take of opportune moments for attaining reward while staying within fair-play limits to keep the exchange going and thus opening a *social space* of interactive possibility expanding under the pressure of complementary power and freedom incentives. Symbolically, the forces at both ends of the bow must be applied in equal measure to send the arrow straight to the mark. For social exchanges to resonate autonomic nodes conducive to attunement and interactive harmony, they need to be perceived as fair and rewarding. Just as the archer must master the art of letting the bowstring jump with a surprise from the fingers, there is a surprise element that enables social exchanges to *hit the mark* (tychon); that is, social exchanges need to be made at a propitious moment with an element of surprise to arouse interest and to promote learning.

The social skills and confidence acquired in resolving interactive conflict naturally involve attunement dynamics compatible with mutual appreciation and interactive harmony. With improving social skills and confidence, a dog is empowered to pursue a wider range of cooperative projects with its owner in pursuit of freedom incentives. Social exchanges that hit the mark promote enhanced awareness (attentive mindfulness), secure attachments, mutual appreciation, and interactive harmony. Exchanges that miss the mark (hamartia) promote an imbalance of *opportunity without limit* that generates increasing disorder and impulsivity (big-bang effect), whereas exchanges promoting an imbalance of *limit without opportunity* are prone to mediate behavioral reactivity and rigid inhibition (black-hole effect). A persistent failure to engage in fair exchange elevates social distress and promotes conflict monitoring, incompetence, instability, and a state of persistent autonomic misattunement. The resultant reactive coping style is hypothesized to underlie a wide gamut of social adjustment problems.

BIG BANGS AND BLACK HOLES: EXTRAVERSION, INTROVERSION, AND DISORGANIZING LOAD

Behavioral adjustments may either hit the mark or miss it. One performing actions that hit the mark depends on experience to learn the most opportune moments (occasion-setting criteria) to act and what to expect as the result of actions, and to tune energy expenditures and preparatory arousal to act in accord with those expectancies. Behavioral adjustments are said to *hit the mark* when expectancies, preparatory arousal, and action modes promote social exchanges conducive to reward, autonomic attunement, secure attachments, and an adaptive coping style. On the other hand, a failure to attune arousal and action readiness in accord with reliable predictive information, causing a dog to motivationally overshoot or undershoot the mark or miss the right opportunities to act, promotes behavioral adjustments that *miss the mark*. Social exchanges that consistently overshoot the mark because of a lack of predictive modulation regulating excitatory arousal and action readiness tend to promote an externalizing (approach) imbalance in the direction of hyperactivity, novelty seeking, and exploitive social interaction. At the other extreme, dogs lacking predictive modulation over inhibitory processes may miss the mark by consistently undershooting the mark because of an internalizing imbalance in the direction of behavioral inhibition, social avoidance, and withdrawal. These inhibited types show caution in response to novelty and an active intolerance for situations that require risk taking. Behavioral adjustments that persistently undershoot or overshoot the mark promote autonomic misattunement and insecure or nervous attachments associated with a reactive coping style.

Theoretically, the viability of an adaptive behavioral system is determined by its potential for correspondence, complexity, and flexibility; that is, its ability to achieve a balance between order and variety while constructing a coherent reality organized to cope with uncertainty and change. Behavior-organizing constraints that limit opportunity and variety are hypothesized to result in a loss of adaptive capacity or *adaptability*. A preoccupation with the familiar and the safe renders a dog vulnerable to the pull of axipetal load. Conversely, systems that fail to limit variety and opportunity tend to become increasing energetic, expansive, and disorderly, showing a preoccupation with novelty and stimulus change (uncertainty) under the push of axifugal load. Where axipetal load is associated with excessive energy loss (drain), axifugal load is associated with excessive energy gain (strain). The drain and strain of load impairs a dog's ability to construct a viable *umwelt* and cope proactively with change. These opposite forms of instability represent the extreme ends of allostatic load, whereby energy is tied up in processes that prevent the dog from organizing predictive relations and change conducive to stability.

Axipetal load mediating unstable introversion (high-approach/low-withdrawal thresholds) appears to reduce prediction error gradually to a negative significance—a negativity bias that degrades a dog's ability to cope with loss and risk proactively. These extreme features of unstable introversion roughly correspond to what Pavlov referred to as the *melancholic* (m) type. An m-type dog treats novel and unexpected change as inherently threatening. As a result, the ability of affected dogs to encode and invest novel social exchange with hedonic value is significantly curtailed. Such dogs only slowly habituate to social novelty and tend toward social inhibition and withdrawal. The effect of internalizing load is akin to an affective black hole, where social space is narrowed and closed under the influence of increasing passive modal activity. Instead of searching for reward opportunities, unstable introverts turn attentional resources toward a heighten vigilance for signals of loss and risk in association with an active disinterest in exploratory activity. The adaptive strength of negative prediction error to conserve energy and to limit loss and risk becomes a significant hindrance when isolated from the balancing influence of cortical reward and active modal activity. As a result, affected dogs may become increasingly preoccupied with conflict monitoring, compulsive rituals, and autoprotective concerns (see *Attention, Dopamine, and Reward* in Chapter 5).

By contrast, unstable extraverts appear to operate under an opposite bias toward novelty and stimulus change. These dogs, corresponding to Pavlov's *choleric* (c) type, tend to treat stimulus change and novelty as intrinsically rewarding, regardless of predictive significance causing them to rapidly accumulate energy gains that produce a state of externalizing load analogous to the big bang, whereby an enormous amount of energy is expended in the vain pursuit of reward signals. Axifugal load accelerates feed-forward processing in the direction of extraversion (low-approach/high-withdrawal thresholds), simultaneously flattening and stretching out space and reducing prediction error to a positive significance. The stretching out of axifugal social space is correlated with a decline in awareness and attentional tone, behavioral disorganization, and dispersive independence (autonomy). The novelty-seeking efforts of c-type dogs are driven by arousal and energy expenditures that have little apparent relevance for the maintenance of homeostasis and security (comfort and safety). In addition, they are unable to engage in fair exchange or to show affect-attunement behaviors. Although they are intensely aroused by the pursuit of novelty and stimulus change, the hedonic significance of their actions does not rise to the level of awareness, and consequently they fail to encode awareness-dependent expectancies and engrams. Affected dogs treat everyone they encounter with the same energetic and exploitive enthusiasm, making few distinctions with respect to the way they engage insiders and outsiders.

A balance of opportunity with limit is crucial for managing information entropies in the direction of adaptive optimization. Goal-directed actions may successfully open the zona securitas but become increasingly rigid with order if not opened to sufficient opportunity. This pattern of progressive deteriora-tion of adaptability is countered by means of utilizing the "noise" (prediction error) associated with the opening of the zona optimus consisting of modal adjustments to positive prediction error (cortical reward). Adaptive coping skills and the confidence to use them under varying circumstances are integrated by means of positive and negative prediction error in association with emergent power and freedom incentives. The strategy promotes competent skills (power) and freedom incentives sufficient to open and share social spaces consistent with the integration of secure attachments and adaptive optimization.

Autonomic attunement nodes activated around points of conflict alter thresholds controlling approach and withdrawal behavior and thus play a significant role in adjusting arousal and social exchange toward the *central field* (i.e., the point of balance between extraversion and introversion) and the opening of the zona securitas (somatic reward promoting comfort and safety) and zona optimus (cortical reward promoting hedonic value and elation). The adaptive optimization that normally occurs as the result of social exchange regulated by reliable expectancies is largely disrupted by a reactive coping style. Instead of organizing competent exchanges conducive to mutual appreciation, fairness, and interactive harmony, the social styles of c-type and m-type dogs tend to become increasingly impulsive and reactive incompetent. Finally, whereas dogs integrating an adaptive coping style are relaxed and ready in anticipation of rewarding social exchange, impulsive/reactive dogs respond to impending social exchange with preparatory anxious or frustrative arousal in anticipation of interactive conflict, thus mediating a heighten readiness to flee, exploit, or confront in response to social stimuli.

According to cynopraxic theory, both m types and c types are extremes that result from a failure to acquire the necessary autoregulation and awareness needed to integrate an adaptive coping style. Most dogs are distributed along the extraversion-introversion continuum by virtue of attachment and attunement dynamics (relative social attraction and aversion), their history of socialization and training efforts, their acquired capacities to cope with interactive conflict, and their ability to process somatic and cortical reward competently. Although some individual dogs may closely resemble the extreme m and c types, the vast majority of dogs, under the stabilizing influence of an adaptive coping style and exchanges conducive to mutual reward (e.g., comfort, safety, and surprise) and attunement, integrate a phenotypic balance of extraversion (E) and introversion (I), showing behavior roughly corresponding to Pavlov's *sanguine* (s) types (stable extravert) and *phlegmatic* (p) types (stable introvert). The stable introvert and extravert operate under the influence of activity success within the central field organized around a sanguine-phlegmatic axis. The major difference between s types and p types is their respective sensitivity to signals predicting reward and punishment. Whereas s-type dogs are more sensitive to positive prediction error (better-than-expected outcomes) and cortical reward mediating active modal strategies (testing, searching, and exploring), p-type dogs show a greater sensitivity for negative prediction error (worse-than-expected outcomes) and somatic reward (comfort and safety) mediating passive modal strategies (hesitating, waiting, and ritualizing) aimed at securing comfort and safety while minimizing loss and risk.

In contrast, under the destabilizing influence of misattunement and interactive conflict (e.g., loss, risk, and disappointment), extraverts and introverts integrate reactive coping styles to accumulate destabilizing axifugal and axipetal load, roughly corresponding to Pavlov's c type (unstable extravert) and m type (unstable introvert)—behavioral tendencies conferring an increased vulnerability to impulsive and reactive disturbances, respectively (see *Experimental Neurosis* in Volume 1, Chapter 9). A third temperament variation combines features of both m and c types, referred to as a *nervous* (n) type. An n-type dog shows low reactive thresholds, making it prone to panic and helplessness associated with chronic insolvable conflict. N-type disturbances are characterized by conflict intolerance, compulsivity, and panic occurring under the influence of a *dysfunctional bias*

toward change that cause affected dogs to persistently attribute danger and uncontrollability to significant events, even though the events are benign and highly amenable to proactive control efforts. N-type disturbances combine m-type and c-type characteristics along with persistent mood changes combining high levels of toxic anxiety and frustration (dysthymia).

Dogs showing n-type disturbance appear to cope with change through the distortion of a dysfunctional bias of danger and powerlessness that causes them to believe that whatever they do will have little effect on what ultimately happens. In situations involving choices between highly motivated alternatives (flight-or-fight conflict), such dogs are prone to panic (low reactive thresholds) or fall into a state of helpless resignation. Genetic predisposition, prenatal and postnatal stress, abusive rearing practices, and highly emotional social interaction lacking predictability and controllability may contribute to the expression of n-type disturbances. Paradoxically, highly ordered environments and social exchange that encourage excessive dependency and insecure social and place attachments may also impair a dog's ability to cope adaptively with the uncertainty of social and environmental change, contributing to a perception of change as being intolerably risky, unpredictable, and uncontrollable (see *Defining Insolvable Conflict* in Volume 1, Chapter 9). As a result, socially sheltered dogs may prefer insular conditions (e.g., they may "like" crate confinement) and seem most satisfied with rigid and monotonous routines.

The anxious–state arousal of dogs showing n-type disturbances appears to be of a different qualitative order than the stimulus-oriented anticipatory anxiety and bias for signals of punishment shown by m-type dogs or the action readiness and bias for signals of reward shown by c-type dogs. The persistent and conflict-reactive anxiety and anger-reactive responses to frustration associated with n-type dysfunction promote catastrophic conflict, with the affected dog appearing to lose consciousness. The panic behavior characteristic of n-type dogs depends on the predisposing influence of reactive thresholds controlling the escalating activation of fear and anger. Dogs expressing low flight (fear bias) and low fight (anger bias) thresholds are prone to reactive panic in response to social exchanges perceived as posing an uncontrollable danger. Such dogs may show highly inappropriate and incompetent behavior in response to benign social stressors or impediments to freedom. N-type dogs sometimes show an anomalous intolerance for tactile stimulation, reacting to gentle handling and petting with panic-driven paroxysmal attacks.

Reactive emotional adjustments to change (e.g., depression, anxiety, worry, and panic) are prone to develop under social and environmental conditions perceived by a dog as unsafe and inescapable. According to this hypothesis, the impulsive and exploitive tendencies of the c type, on the one hand, and the anxious withdraw tendencies of the m type, on the other, are the default coping strategies of dogs exposed to situations perceived as uncontrollable, unsafe, annoying, and/or inescapable. The terms *social ambivalence* and *entrapment* are used to refer to these general social and environmental influences promoting a reactive coping style. Finally, stable and unstable orientations to reward (extraversion) and punishment (introversion) may originate in organizational processes first appearing in association with the parent-offspring conflict.

COPING WITH CONFLICT

Household social interaction, in all its nuances and refinements, is the result of human and canine adaptations to the competition and possessiveness arising from interactive conflict. Conflict sets the stage for the emergence of both reactive and proactive adjustments, depending on the abilities of the owner and the dog to prevent or avoid conflict when opening and sharing a *social space* (see *Social Spaces, Frames, and Zones* in Chapter 8). Although a dog's control interests are mostly confined to the pursuit of attractive motivational stimuli under a freedom incentive, an owner's control incentives are more often informed by power incentives. The owner may experience a strong sense of failure

and inadequacy when unable to limit the dog's undesirable behavior. The loss of control experienced by the owner may heighten aversive feelings of anger and resentment toward the dog while mediating a state of misattunement, marginalization, entrapment, and social ambivalence. Many owners are under the persuasion of bad advice that a dog's conflictive efforts are motivated by a dominance incentive, causing the owner to engage the dog in exchanges that perpetuate and worsen the problems, rather than restoring social attraction and trust.

By necessity, while in pursuit of motivational interests, the dog is forced to negotiate around the owner's interference and control efforts. The attunement and social skills acquired when integrating an adaptive coping style serve to reduce conflict, whereas a chronic history of coercion, exploitation, frustration, loss, risk, and discomfort is likely to attune the dog and its owner to anticipatory expectancies that virtually ensure conflictive exchanges whenever they interact. The anticipation and preparation for conflictive exchange can be turned around and harnessed to cynopraxic objectives by integrating social exchanges with the dog that disconfirms the conflict expectancy. Instead of evoking unfair and conflictive exchanges where reward for one depends on loss or risk for the other, cynopraxic training focuses on restructuring and attuning social exchange toward mutual reward, cooperation, and trust. Social exchanges that satisfy the owner's social control needs (power incentives) while simultaneously gratifying canine seeking needs (freedom incentives) provide a basic structure that enables people and dogs to engage in mutually rewarding social activity.

Social interaction perceived as uncontrollable, unsafe, or biologically unfavorable may promote social and cognitive (attentional) disengagement, lower reactive flight-or-fight thresholds, and cause the dog to become increasingly irritable, intolerant, and reactive to social interference via the activation of a loner-dispersal survival mode. Chronic exposure to an impoverished or threatening social or living space in association with the dispersive tensions generated by an involuntary subordination strategy (ISS) may gradually exhaust a dog's stress-regulating abilities and sharpen household tensions. The degradation of interactive relations as the result of unresolved conflict may gradually result in exchanges unable to support secure attachments. As a result, the dog may become increasingly reactive toward ambiguous and relatively benign social signals as the emotional regulation afforded by attunement is lost in association with encroaching estrangement and mistrust.

The establishment of organized household relations is rarely achieved without significant interactive conflict along the way. Depending on how interactive conflict is managed, a dog may either adopt a voluntary subordination strategy (VSS) or an ISS (see *Interactive Conflict, Stress, and Social Dominance* in Chapter 7). Psychologically, a dog is organized to predict and control (i.e., manage) social events to exploit them for advantage. Excesses and deficits associated with such management interests are tempered by a sense of fairness, playfulness, and a love of social companionship with people. Under the benign influences of social leadership and the nurturance of a friendly VSS, interactive conflict and reactive tensions are gradually superseded by social attraction, mutual appreciation, and interactive harmony. Social and autonomic attunement serve to align and coordinate the cognitive and emotional processing needed by a dog to pursue its private interests competently while preventing, limiting, or resolving interactive conflict, as needed to consolidate social relations. Dogs adopting a VSS tend to become increasingly relaxed and confident while organizing an adaptive coping style and integrating secure social and place attachments. The pursuit of private interest becomes a public or household concern when it gives rise to competition and possessiveness aimed at *getting* and *keeping* some valued resource at an expense or harm to others sharing the home.

To achieve a state of relative harmony and peaceful coexistence, a dog must be compliant to owner control efforts, but the owner must in turn be able to compromise and to share the living space with the dog (see *Unilateral, Bilateral, and Pluralistic Relations* in Chapter 8). Most puppies and dogs come into the home as default subordinates but lack knowledge of the specific rules for sharing in household activities and resources. Subsequent interactive conflict results when the puppy or dog attempts to engage in reward-seeking activity in ways that conflict with owner power incentives. A puppy is best introduced into the home by means of identifying points of conflict and converting them into points of mutual reward and interactive harmony. Interactive compliance training (ICT) plays a critical role in facilitating social adjustments conducive to a VSS by means of conflict-resolving interactions. ICT serves to consolidate and refine the owner's control interests while the dog learns how to control valued resources and activities without engaging in disruptive competition. These rules are taught in process of integrating flexible *ascendant* and *descendant* relations based on a principle of fairness and pluralism, whereby sharing the living space is at the owner's consent and ability to assert veto power and *default dominance*, if necessary.

In the process of cynopraxic training, the owner and the dog shift from a reactive orientation fueling interactive conflict to a proactive orientation or *adaptive coping style* by means of social exchanges that optimize fair exchange and mutual reward, enhance the dog's ability to pursue power and freedom incentives in the absence of reactive arousal and interference, and integrate secure social and place attachments. Cynopraxic training theory postulates the following working hypotheses and claims regarding the integration of an adaptive coping style:

1. The loss and risk resulting from interactive conflict are experienced as emotional distress (anxiety and frustration) that preemptively conditions social approach with a negative efficacy bias (low-power orientation) in anticipation of conflictive exchange.
2. Emotional distress provides an aversive incentive conducive to the integration of proactive adjustments organized to prevent or avoid conflict.
3. The integration of prediction-control expectancies and calibrated emotional establishing operations organized in accord with fair exchange and reward promotes mutual attunement, causing

social approach to become increasingly relaxed and expectant of friendly exchange under the preemptive influence of a positive efficacy bias (high-power orientation).

4. Attunement coordinates energy-state changes via calibrated establishing operations and control expectancies to promote mutual reward and fair exchanges incompatible with conflict.

5. Chronic interactive conflict results in mutual powerlessness, entrapment dynamics, social ambivalence, and the activation of autoprotective modes, whereas conflict resolution promotes mutual empowerment, freedom, and secure attachments promoting mutual comfort and safety, mutual appreciation, and playfulness.

6. Cynopraxic training converts the energy diverted into conflictive exchange and resulting in homeostatic distress (energy loss) and turns it toward energy-conserving exchanges organized to resolve or prevent conflict in process of producing energy gains and homeostatic balance.

7. Exchanges yielding transactions producing energy gains are hypothesized to encode attunement via the calibration of emotional establishing operations. The preattentive comparator processing of energy gains scaled to hedonic value gives rise to a heightened state of awareness of pleasure. As such, the hedonic value attributed to energy gains and losses is an interpretive function or algorithm converting energy gains derived from better-than-expected outcomes into experiences and memories having the significance of pleasure (positive hedonic value), whereas the energy losses representing worse-than-expected outcomes are encoded into experiences having the significance of displeasure (negative hedonic value).

8. The energy gains obtained as the result of preventing and avoiding interactive conflict provide the trainer and the dog with the enhanced awareness and capacity to encode the significance of social exchange as experiences and memories needed to foster the social skills,

autonomic attunement, and confidence (power) to engage in mutually rewarding cooperative projects and ventures. The power derived from the energy gains stemming from the resolution of conflict is integrated into predictive relations that open social space under the expansive dynamics of a freedom incentive. In contrast, the power lost due to energy losses stemming from interactive conflict results in the contraction of predictive relations, the closure of social space, and the accumulation of axipetal and axifugal load collecting in the opposite directions of unstable introversion and extraversion.

9. The effective resolution of conflict depends on the initiative and leadership abilities of the trainer to organize and guide mutually rewarding exchanges based on a principle of fairness (the golden rule), compromise, and cooperation around situations previously generating conflict.

10. Learning to prevent and resolve conflict results in mutual empowerment and liberation, with the dog and the trainer integrating the skills and the confidence needed to obtain mutual reward in the context of fair exchange and cooperation, as exemplified in play.

11. The translation of conserved energy into positive mood, mutual attunement, and stable predictive relations serves to promote social attraction and to open a social space within which people and dogs integrate secure social and place attachments.

12. Power and freedom incentives are most fully expressed in the form of affectionate play.

13. An attentional nexus conducts exchanges between the trainer and dog around points of common interest in the process of activating the SES and mediating autonomic attunement. The autonomic attunement and social awareness resulting from the activation of the SES simultaneously serve to disengage disruptive autonomic arousal driving conflictive control incentive and vectors, thereby enabling the trainer to turn his or her attention on the dog (and vice versa) as an object of affectionate appreciation and play.

14. With the emergence of power and freedom incentives focused on the mutual integration of social skills and confidence to avoid conflict, a principle of fairness and social codes naturally emerges to facilitate social exchange and attunement dynamics incompatible with conflict.

15. The mutual reward mediated by fair exchange serves to promote attunement, heightened awareness, and the joy arising from mutual appreciation and interactive harmony, as exemplified in affectionate play.

Under the influence of social ambivalence and entrapment, dogs appear to cope by withdrawing from the insecure/nervous attachment object, on the one hand, and by increasing their dependency on locations having conditioned associations with security (comfort and safety), on the other. Building social tensions (e.g., anxiety, frustration, irritability, and intolerance), impulsivity, lowered reactive thresholds (e.g., fear, anger, and panic), a preemptive negativity bias causing dogs to anticipate conflict with the approach of the owner, and the breakdown of social communication set the stage for reactive and impulsive autoprotective behavior. In addition to the retraction of the SES, a key factor in this process of estrangement and marginalization appears to involve the diversion of attentional resources to conflict monitoring, and *tuning out* the ambivalent attachment object. According to cynopraxic training theory, attention and impulse control are intimately interconnected and interdependent upon each other.

The disengagement of attentional resources combines synergistically with social withdrawal to imperil dogs with autonomic dysregulation and vulnerability for impulsive and reactive adjustments. These hallmarks of a nervous attachment make it difficult for dogs to experience coherent feelings of social security and belongingness in the home. The pervasive cognitive and emotional perturbations of chronic interactive conflict substantially disrupt a dog's ability to selectively attend to and decode the transactional significance of social exchanges with family members and to cope proactively with the most

ordinary and benign social stressors. The ensuing dispersive tensions and marginalization may mediate an untenable insider-outsider orientation between the dog and the family members. In essence, the dog appears to undergo a process of estrangement and dissociation that gradually causes it to experience family members as "super pals" (tuning in) or as strangers and threats (tuning out), making them fit targets for impulsive attacks. If left untreated, such dogs not dispersed by rehoming or relinquishment, much as a captive wolf, unable to freely disperse or integrate is badgered and finally killed, may face a predicament of intensified social ambivalence, entrapment, and punishment, until at last the intolerable situation is disposed of by means of veterinary proxy.

RESTRAINT, UNAVOIDABLE AVERSIVE STIMULATION, AND STRESS

Most dogs express flexible antistress and antiaggression capability but not in equal measure, with some breeds, on average, showing a greater proclivity toward reactive behavior than others (Malhut, 1958). Also, there is tremendous variation among individuals within the same breed that affects fearful behavior. In addition to differences affecting reactive thresholds in response to innocuous novel stimuli, Malhut found that breed-related differences affected the sort of coping style exhibited by the dogs. Corson and O'Leary Corson (1976) have also reported significant individual variation in the way dogs cope with isolation, physical restraint, and unavoidable electrical stimulation. Certain dogs—notably those belonging to herding, spaniel, and terrier breeds—show an ensemble of reactive behavioral and physiological changes when exposed to psychological stressors. These reactive dogs, which the researchers refer to as *antidiuretic* or low-adaptation types, exhibit a persistent pattern of increased metabolic activity and autonomic activation—physiological changes that typically occur in association with the sympathetic arousal and muscular exertion used to fight off or escape from a serious threat or challenge. In contrast to the reactive pattern exhibited by antidiuretic low-adaptation dogs, other dogs showed a more passive coping style in response to unavoidable aversive stimulation and restraint. Many of these high-adaptation or *diuretic* types showed a transient antidiuretic response that diminished after several sessions of conditioning, whereas other dogs (most notably beagles and other hounds) showed little sign of disturbance in response to the stressors.

The antidiuretic stress response is hypothesized to be the result of an emotional conflict consisting of a strong incentive to escape coupled with an inability to break free of the Pavlovian-restraint apparatus. The ensuing conflict, escalating anxiety, frustration, and defensive arousal may result in elevated body temperature and various compensatory thermoregulatory activities aimed at restoring thermal homeostasis, including hyperpnea (panting), elevated heart rate, increased respiration, profuse salivation, high levels of plasma AVP (antidiuretic hormone), and reduced urine production (Corson and O'Leary Corson, 1969):

> In spite of the inability of the antidiuretic dogs to engage in fighting or to escape, the physiologic reactions of these animals appear to be those associated with severe muscular effort. We postulated that these dogs pant in order to dissipate the extra heat production associated with anticipatory responses to muscular effort. The excessive salivation serves to provide the water required for evaporative cooling during the hyperpnea. The antidiuresis serves the purpose of conserving water by the kidneys so as to make the water available for the increased secretion of saliva. (155)

The researchers found that after an avoidance contingency was introduced that allowed the dogs to avoid the electrical stimulus, many of the reactive antidiuretic dogs showed a marked shift toward normalization of autonomic tone and balance, but some of the dogs failed to adapt despite the most thorough training efforts (Corson et al., 1973). Among these nonresponders, a subgroup of antidiuretic dogs persistently reacted to restraint in the Pavlovian stand, with some chewing through harnesses and cables in their frenzied efforts to escape. The emotional effects of restraint were especially pronounced when the experimenter left the room, which suggests that the experimenter's presence exercised a significant stabilizing effect. The reactive behavior in response to restraint described by Corson and colleagues as hyperkinetic is reminiscent of a dog described by Pavlov that showed a similar pattern of reactivity and profuse salivation when restrained. Pavlov attributed the persistent autonomic reactivity shown by the dog to a thwarted *freedom reflex* (Pavlov, 1928) (see *Liddell: The Cornell Experiments* in Chapter 9, Volume 1). The descriptions by Pavlov of the dogs behavior seem consistent with the classical signs of separation distress/panic, representing the earliest known description of such disorder in dogs:

> One of our many dogs, used during the past year for the study of acquired, or conditioned, salivary reflexes exhibited especial characteristics. This animal when first used by us for experimentation gave, when placed on the stand, in distinction from all other dogs, a spontaneous and constant secretion of saliva during an entire month. This, of course, rendered it unsuitable for our experiments. This secretion of saliva is as we know from previous observations, dependent upon a general excitation of the animal, and is usually accompanied by dyspnea. Such excitation of the dog is evidently analogous to the state of excitation in the man, where it is manifested, however, by sweating instead of salivation. A short period of such excitation is seen in many of our dogs during the first experiments with them, and especially among the untamed and wilder of them. On the contrary, though, the dog in question was very tame and quickly became friendly with us all. That made it even more strange that for a month the excitation in the experimental stand did not diminish to any degree....The spontaneous salivary secretion continued, and gradually increased with each experimental séance. Also the animal constantly moved, struggling in every possible way in the stand, scratching the floor, and pulling and biting at the frame, etc. (283)

Months of intensive counterconditioning failed to calm the dog and hypersalivation increased over time. Only after 4 1/2 months of isolation in a separate cage did the dog finally stabilize and become amenable to handling and experimentation. Interestingly, in a language reminiscent of Nietzsche's "instinct for freedom" and slave morality, Pavlov contrasts the "reflex to freedom" with a "reflex of slavish submission," thereby placing the etiology of such behavior into the context of social imperatives and dialectics consistent with the interactive dynamics believed to contribute to the expression of nervous and insecure place/social attachments. Freedom of movement is a precondition for a dog to act effectively in accord with control and power incentives. As such, the loss of freedom associated with excessive crate confinement results in a significant loss of reward, as it forcibly separates the dog from the means needed to produce reward via the control of attractive and aversive motivational incentives. As a result of the combination of social isolation and loss of freedom imposed by confinement, the dog may experience a persistent state of internal conflict combining heightened anxious arousal and frustration.

The potent effects of crate confinement on the inhibition of urine production may stem, in part, from the release of AVP triggered by restraint and isolation of crate confinement. Corson (1966) reported that dogs living in small cages were prone to develop various nervous behaviors, including antidiuresis, reduced appetitive drive (e.g., anorexia and adipsia), and avoidance of social novelty (e.g., running away from strangers). QOL enhancements, which included housing the dog in a room and providing it with daily walks, helped to eliminate these aberrant behaviors. Social abuse, isolation, and restraint stress may underlie some of the persistent learning deficits exhibited by dogs exposed to excessive isolation and crate confinement. For example, increased opioid activity resulting from aversive interaction and chronic restraint stress may impair memory and associative learning capacities (Westbrook et al., 1997; McNally and Westbrook, 2003; McNally et al., 2004). Also, chronic stress causes glucocorticoid-mediated disturbances in cortical and mesolimbic DA reward pathways, and degrades cholinergic hippocampal circuits that preferentially mediate spatial and contextual learning.

These various stress-related changes in combination with autonomic imbalance and a concomitant rise in CRF, AVP, and NE may help to explain the crate-dependent aggression exhibited by some dogs. When restrained, crate-conditioned triggers may mobilize autonomic state changes and phase shifts in the direction of autoprotective action modes. When removed from the crate, these dogs appear to shift rapidly out of the dysregulated state into a state of excited arousal facilitating exploitive and impulsive exchanges but do not show any evidence of hostility. A similar pattern of arousal and dysregulation is predictably exhibited by some dogs while on leash, causing them to show an escalating state of aggressive arousal toward other dogs until they are released, whereupon they may rapidly (but not always) shift into a state of autonomic regulation conducive to exploitive and intrusive play.

A linkage with social isolation in the development of aggression has been frequently observed in the laboratory. Lagerspetz and Lagerspetz (1971), for example, found that mice selected for aggressiveness and nonaggressiveness for 19 generations showed significant variability with respect to learning aggression and their ability to cope with isolation stress. In one experiment, male mice were taken from these two groups at weaning and housed for several months in small groups. At month 8, mice selected for aggressiveness were housed in separate cages and tested on a weekly basis for 2 months. When tested at 8 months (prior to the first week of isolation), well-socialized aggressive mice showed no aggression when put in a novel cage with a nonaggressive mouse. After only 1 week of isolation, however, these same mice showed a rapid increase in aggressive reactivity that remained at a high level during the 8-week testing period. Even mice selected for nonaggressiveness showed increased aggression after 2 weeks of isolation. The authors emphasize the importance of social punishment as the decisive factor limiting aggressive impulsivity. As the result of retaliation and defeat consequent to aggressive actions, socialized mice appear to learn how to regulate their agonistic impulses. In the absence of punitive social feedback, the predisposition toward aggression is heightened, a finding also reported among Hereford bulls (see *Play, Social Engagement, and Fair Play* in Chapter 8).

Paradoxically, after months of crate confinement, the crate may become a potent source of autonomic regulation promoting relaxation and sleep. Many dogs show a strong preference for sleeping in the crate and, if denied access to this "safe haven," often show signs of heightened autonomic distress and an inability to relax until they are put in their "den." Such dogs frequently show unproductive exploratory pacing, persistent panting, increased gut motility, and other signs indicative of autonomic dysregulation— all while the owner is nearby. When given access to their crate, these dogs immediately regain their composure, perhaps as the result of place attachments and security that they associate with the location. The behavior of these dogs is consistent with the distress behavior exhibited by dependent and insecure dogs when left alone. These sorts of observations have convinced many advocates of long-term cage and crate confinement that dogs really like being crated day and night—a bizarre belief that is used with great effectiveness on the low-power owner in order to help assuage guilt and rationalize excessive confinement of the dog. That a dog should prefer a state of social and physical privation and loss of freedom to the security and enjoyment of close company with family members is more rightly interpreted as evidence of social pathology than a healthy preference. The bond and QOL deficiencies evident in such a "preference" for social isolation and loss is antithetical to the goals of cynopraxic training and therapy (see *Mechanical Suppression of Behavior*).

ATTENTIONAL NEXUS, ALLOCENTRISM, AND ATTUNEMENT

The opening of an attentional nexus implies an appreciation of the other's viewpoint, that is, an allocentric orientation. The integration of an allocentric perspective translates the human umwelt into messages sensible to the canine umwelt and vice versa. Attunement is consequent to affective inferences (anthropomorphism) and attributions concerning the nature of the dog's doings. In fact, anthropomorphism plays a prominent role in the process of constructing a viable interface of affectionate and flexible exchange between people and dogs. These anthropic attributions and valuations provide a profoundly rich and complex cultural backdrop from which to receive and transmit affective information. Attunement dynamics are integrated at an early age, beginning with the undifferentiated approach behavior of neonatal puppies in search of contact comfort, appetitive gratification, and thermoregulation from the mother. These early protobehaviors are gradually incorporated in complex rituals used by dogs to negotiate conflict and allelomimetic behaviors. Among puppies, social facilitation invigorates the coordinated pursuit of common interests, at least until the activity threatens to escalate into conflictive exchange, whereupon social inhibition is evoked (Scott and McCray, 1967). These early attunement dynamics serve to promote social enthusiasm while curbing motivational momentum that might lead to overt antagonism.

ATTENTIONAL NEXUS, SOCIAL COMMUNICATION, AND CONTROL

Domestication has significantly improved the dog's capacity to cope with stress and social uncertainty via the evolution of antistress and antiaggression capacities, enhanced attention and impulse-control abilities, exchange-mediated autonomic attunement, and the integration of a sophisticated SES consolidating these various changes (see Porges, 2003). As a result, the dog's ability to explore and rapidly establish social relations under a positive expectancy of reward is generally ascendant to negative expectancies and the social aversion associated with dispersion and entrapment dynamics. Dogs appear to respond to the presence of a person as an intrinsically rewarding object, with social contact possessing both incentive significance and hedonic value. For many dogs, petting is not only calmative but is also restorative in nature (see

Affection and Friendship in Volume 1, Chapter 10). The mere presence of a person nearby activates antistress capacities that enhance a dog's ability to cope with pain and stress. In addition to generally enjoying human social contact, dogs have evolved a proactive sociability that enables them to smooth over social tensions with conciliatory exchanges before they escalate into conflict. In short, dogs are developmentally organized to attune and commune with people. Along with these various changes affecting canine sociability and emotional adaptability, dogs appear to have acquired complementary sensory and cognitive capabilities that enable them to socially engage and communicate with people and to follow human instruction (Warden and Warner, 1928; Szetei et al., 2003).

Some authors have emphasized that the dog's enhanced abilities to initiate communicative interaction with people is due to an enhanced capacity for social gazing (Miklosi et al., 2003), perhaps augmenting the dog's abilities to decipher the significance of human social signals (see Hare et al., 2002). McGreevy and colleagues (2004) report that brachiocephalic breeds tend to concentrate receptor ganglion cells around the central area, in contrast to dogs with elongated muzzles that tend to express a visual streak (see *Orienting, Preattentive Sensory Processing, and Visual Acuity* in Chapter 8). Consistent with the aforementioned social-gaze hypothesis, these authors speculate that a genetic trend toward a frontal placement of the eyes and shortening of the muzzle might have developed as the result of selection pressures favoring visual capacities that enabled dogs to focus on the human face.

Relevantly, Viranyi and colleagues (2004) have observed that canine begging behavior is preferentially directed toward an attentive person rather than a person looking away from the dog. The authors suggest that such preferences might reflect an appreciation of human attentional cues insofar as they help to improve the success of instrumental food-sharing projects. The authors also found that a dog's ability to perform a basic obedience exercise ("Down") in response to a recorded command varied depending on whether the owner was out of sight, faced the dog, turned away, or faced another person while giving the command. The best performance was obtained when the owner gave commands while facing the dog, followed by commands given as the owner turned his or her head away from both the dog and person. The dog showed an equal disruption of performance when the owner was out of sight as when facing a nearby person. The authors interpret these findings as evidence of special attention-dependent capabilities. However, since most dogs can be trained to lie down rapidly and consistently in each of the previously mentioned stimulus and contextual conditions, and given the limited controls used in the experiment, it would seem extremely difficult to sort out what is attributable to the effects of owner-training skills versus the effects of special cognitive abilities expressed by dogs as a group. Although some acquired skills appear to depend on the help of directional cues for a dog to perform well, others do not. Warden and Warner (1928) explored many of these problems in the case of the dog named Fellow, finding that tasks such as sitting and lying down on command were not appreciably affected by changes in attentional focus or directional cueing, whereas routines that required the dog to move toward places or to select objects were much more dependent on attentional and directional cueing (see *Nora, Roger, and Fellow: Extraordinary Dogs* in Volume 1, Chapter 4).

Several authors have hypothesized that dogs have acquired, as the result of domestication, unique capacities for interpreting and responding to human directional cues. The dog's ability to translate directional information derived from gross and subtle pointing and indicating movements is well developed (Hare and Tomasello, 1999), seeming to surpass the abilities of chimpanzees and wolves (Hare et al., 2002). Although dogs are undoubtedly responsive to human deictic (pointing) signals, nonverbal directive signals, and social gaze, capabilities that trainers have fostered for centuries, it is not clear that this capacity is the result of special cognitive adaptations. To take an extreme example, unstable pointer dogs would likely show significantly less responsiveness to directional gaze and pointing cues than would stable counterparts, not because pointers lack such ability but because preemptive reactions toward humans prevent them from showing that they have it. The ability of such dogs to use directional signals in appropriate ways only becomes fully evident when training them to hunt, as demonstrated by McBryde and Murphree (1974). In addition to training, the participation of an eager and playful pointer appeared to prime and attune an unstable pointer with arousal and direction that helped to break the spell of cataplexy. Once in their umwelt, the unstable pointers rapidly learned to show and respond to pointing signals:

> The performances of both nervous and normal dogs were quite comparable on an overall basis. The nervous dogs scored about as well throughout and just as well as the normal subjects on their last two trials which were intended to evaluate each dog's final abilities after rehabilitation. On an individual basis some of the nervous dogs did better than the normal controls. (81)

Despite significant changes away from the laboratory, their confident and human-friendly behavior did not generalize back to the laboratory, where they rapidly reverted to the same unstable and nervous behavior shown before field training. Apparently, in the absence of natural stimuli promoting drive arousal conducive to hunting activity (prey-seeking action modes and modal strategies), these dogs get *stuck*. The disorder does not appear to be primarily caused by fear or an aversion to novelty, since nervous dogs rapidly lost most of their timidity and could tolerate close human contact and the blast of a shotgun while hunting. Instead, these dogs appear to be affected by an overspecialization of function genetically encoded around hunting. Perhaps more fundamental, though, is the presence of a genetic defect affecting parasympathetic braking and accelerator functions. The ability to attenuate and accelerate arousal competently while remaining in a parasympathetic mode of activation may be an important aspect of domestication and herald the emergence of the canine SES (Porges, 2003).

Thus, individual differences affecting the dog's arousability and sociability (approach and withdrawal thresholds), motivational interest (incentive and hedonic value) in the reward object, susceptibility to conflict and distress during testing (anxiety and frustration thresholds), age, and relative social dependency (see Topál et al., 1997) would likely generate significant variability into any cognitive test relying on social and motivational variables not equally distributed among experimental subjects. These various influences represent additive confounds that have long been recognized as obstacles to the scientific investigation of animal cognition and continue to plague it with ambiguity.

To take an experimental example of the sort of risks involved in cognitive theorizing, Triana and Pasnak (1981) tested 32 cats and 23 dogs in eight standardized object-permanence tasks using a soft toy as the objects. Although dogs and cats completed some of the tasks, they consistently failed (with the exception of one dog) to solve the invisible displacement tasks. In a second experiment, two additional naive dogs and three cats were tested, but this time the researchers used savory treats and chunks of hamburger as rewards. Under the influence of enhanced motivation, the two dogs and three cats completed all eight of the tasks in a "logical manner." Now, if one took the results of the first test as a true estimate of canine and feline cognitive abilities, the interpretation would be consistent with the results of the experiment but wrong with respect to the dog's actual object-permanence abilities. Further, the second experiment might be erroneously interpreted as evidence of extraordinary cognitive skills, but neither experiment actually says much about cognition per se and instead underscores the reality that cognition and motivation are not easily dissociable, especially when the one variable is manipulated to test the other. Consequently, object-permanence tests employing such things as rubber toys may not measure the extent of cognitive capabilities as much as they measure a dog's motivational interest in getting the object concealed and their willingness to invest the attentional resources and energy needed to encode a working memory of it.

Pointing at a container concealing a treat is not a neutral deictic signal but may also carry the added significance of a command; that is, the directional cue may signify a demand "Go there"—not merely indicating where the food is (i.e., a "There it is" signal) but carrying the added implication of a dominance imperative. Further, standing behind and pointing directly over an object may not necessarily be interpreted by the dog as a "Here it is" signal or a "Go there" signal but rather may project a "This is mine" significance. Accordingly, standing over and pointing at an object while repeatedly glancing from it to a dog should cause many dogs to withdraw from the object. In fact, many dogs can be caused to avoid forbidden objects merely by alternating glances toward the dog and back again while intently staring and pointing at the object. The effect can be very strong and appears to accumulate over repeated trials and may be augmented with auditory orienting signals. With regard to such dogs, learning to approach and take objects that are pointed at from above may be contraprepared. Dogs rarely, if ever, relinquish food to other dogs by dropping it and then glancing at the other dog and staring at the object to indicate that the other dog should take it. Such social signals when they do occur more likely carry an opposite significance, that is, represent a dare or challenge. Typically, when dogs give up objects, they indicate this intent by moving away from them. They are not particularly well adapted to engage actively in showing behavior with conspecifics when it comes to highly valued objects. The "Go there" imperative should also be subject to the influence of individual differences. In all of these cases, extraverts (with low-approach/high-withdrawal thresholds) should outperform the introvert (with high-approach/low-withdrawal thresholds).

The finding by Hare and colleagues (2002) that puppies perform the object-choice task fairly well from the start and that the "skill" does not appear to be much affected by rearing or social exposure to people seems inconsistent with the findings of other authors (see Soproni et al., 2001). The lack of effect resulting from rearing and social experience is especially puzzling given the findings reported by Topál and colleagues (1997), who found a strong correlation between the number of glances toward the owner, social dependency, and reduced prob-

lem-solving efficiency. Of course, one way to explain Hare and colleagues' findings is the possibility that the learning needed to decipher the significance of directional cues is epigenetically articulated into puppy behavior at an early age. The notion that complex social skills might emerge in the context of early ontogeny should not come as any surprise, nor should its significance be downplayed.

The social-cognition hypothesis faces other more formidable problems when the results are judged in the light of prior experimental work performed in Konorski's laboratory. In a series of delayed-response experiments performed by Lawicka (1959), dogs were taught a 3-choice response that depended on the directional information provided by a 3-second orienting signal, a buzzer emanating from one of the different locations. After a variable duration delay, with or without intervening distractions (e.g., feeding the dog or taking the dog from the room), the dogs were released to choose. Dogs readily learned to make the correct location-choice responses, despite distractions, long delays, and even after falling asleep. In one dog, delays of over 18 minutes proved of little difficulty, with the dog making no errors in 7 trials (see Lawicka, 1959:202). Thus, the dogs did not depend on body orientation, but appeared rely on an oculocentric map to orient toward the signalled location.

Lawicka's findings suggests that the distance between the boxes from where the buzzer emanated appeared to enhance the integration of predictive information into the canine localizing map. When the boxes were widely spaced apart (e.g., over 12 feet) the dogs perform the location-choice task after long delays with few errors, whereas when the boxes are placed close together the delay abilities of the dog are "drastically reduced." These observations are extremely interesting since they appear to suggest that delayed response capabilities are partially dependent on the spatial distribution of reference points scaled to coordinate action to locate stationary objects concealed at some distance away, perhaps revealing significant features of the canine umwelt. One might expect that moving objects, including those in slow motion, would not yield lasting memory traces of a location but might yield predictions concerning the future location of the object based on a trajectory, speed, and prominent terrain markers. Accordingly, allowing the dog to briefly (2 seconds) observe another dog walk by in front of the house before closing the door and taking it to another room for a brief delay, reveals that the dog immediately angles off in the direction last observed, even though, in fact, the dog was immediately turned about and walked in a opposite direction after the door was shut.

Lawicka and Konorski (1959) observed that prefrontal dogs treated directional cues much like a pointer orients and freezes its focus and posture in the direction of the cued location, thereby depending on proprioceptive and vestibular signals to hold on point. Since the arrangement could not exclude the possibility that the dog was relying on bodily signals when orienting and making location-choice responses, the researchers discounted the value of such responses with respect to cognitive function, referring to them as "pseudo-delayed." In addition, Konorski and Lawicka (1964) found that dogs suffering prefrontal lesions are still able to correctly follow directional signals, so long as the signals were closely tied to the object's location and that the dog was released during or shortly after the directional cue was discontinued. Now, if dogs with massive prefrontal lesions can "solve" such problems by remaining physically oriented on the location during the delay period, it makes it difficult to assume that the performance is strictly speaking of a cognitive nature. These findings are bad news for the social-cognition hypothesis. If a dog without a functional prefrontal cortex can perform the requisite orienting and approach response, then the social-cognitive hypothesis is falsified, that is, the action might not depend on cognitive ability at all.

In order to overcome these confounding influences, delayed-response procedures can be designed with built-in interference effects that filter out positional information, e.g., the dog is turned around, distracted with food or petting, and even momentarily taken away from the starting point before being released again to choose. Interesting work performed by Nippack and colleagues (2003) appears to have avoid many of these obvious experimental pitfalls while exploring the effect of delay on latency and response accuracy.

SENSITIVITY TO HUMAN ATTENTIONAL STATES

One might expect that under circumstances in which deictic signals result in interference or exploitation by an observer that a dog might employ gaze amd directional cues to turn the other's attention away from the location or object of interest. The results of a study by Call and colleagues (2003) might be interpreted as evidence of tactical behavior organized to evade interference by adjusting risky ventures to changes in human orientation, proximity, and attention. In their study, dogs were exposed to training in which a piece of food was placed on the floor, whereupon the experimenter looked at the dog and said "Aus!" (Out!), followed by a second event in which the dog's name was called and followed by "Aus!" again. The dogs were subsequently exposed to a series of test trials that continued until the dog either took the food or 3 minutes had elapsed. If the dog took the food without permission, it was not punished, nor was it rewarded if it refrained from taking the food. As such, the procedure appears to asymmetrically favor approach over avoidance, since dogs that took the forbidden food were merely ignored, just as those that obeyed the prohibition were ignored. With only one exception, all of the dogs took the food at least once, and some of them took food on several occasions while they were watched. However, watched dogs generally avoided the forbidden food but readily took the food if released to do so or when left alone with it. In a follow-up experiment, the dogs appeared to be aware of the attentional state of the experimenter based on the orientation of the experimenter's direction of gaze. When the experimenter faced the dog with closed eyes, the dog tended to respond to the frontal orientation as it did when the experimenter's back was turned to the dog. These findings suggest the possibility that dogs might know when they are being carefully observed. When closely watched, the dogs broke the prohibition against taking the food much less frequently, engaged in more indirect approaches to the forbidden item, and appeared less relaxed (i.e., sat more often and laid down less often) during the test trial. The indirect approach might have enabled the dogs to keep an eye on the experimenter while nearing the object or taking a more advantageous position from where to approach the food item.

A remarkable aspect of the experiment by Call and colleagues is the degree of appetitive suppression achieved by virtue of two vocal warnings, essentially events that emphatically served to draw the dogs attention to the food in association with a social startle/threat implication. One possible explanation for the extraordinary control exerted by vocal reprimands may stem from the unfamiliarity of the testing situation and the person delivering the threat. Another possible factor might be traced to prior inhibitory training. Some of the dogs may have received aversive inhibitory training that conditioned them to refuse food not given to them by the owner (e.g., poison proofing). Poison-proofed dogs usually show a strong avoidance and rejection of illicit food that they might find or have offered to them by strangers. In contrast, the dogs in the test group eventually took food when released or when left alone, strongly suggesting that they were not behaving under the influence of situational anxiety or aversive inhibition. Apparently, the experimenter remained neutral whether a dog ate the food or not. From a behavioral aspect, the effect of such a procedure would be far from neutral. In fact, such a strategy should have resulted in a significant differentiating effect with respect to dogs that ate and those that were inhibited. Dogs that ate the food in the presence of the neutral experimenter should have been doubly gratified by the disconfirmation of the avoidance contingency and by the successful control established over the food item without cost or interference. Learning theory predicts that such rewarding outcomes should reduce inhibition and conflict in dogs about taking food in comparison to dogs that continued to avoid the food.

Appetitive Suppression, Social Attraction, and the Attribution of Intention

Matters are further complicated by the fact that dogs tend to cope with social inhibitory conditioning in ways that are highly variable and strongly influenced by constitutional differences and prior rearing practices (Freedman, 1958). Freedman studied the ontogeny of these effects in several breeds. Puppies selected from these breeds were divided into two groups: one group had been reared with disciplinary handling and the other reared with social indulgence. At week 8, disciplined and indulged puppies received several days of inhibitory training during which they received swats on their rumps together with loud vocal reprimands whenever they ate meat from a bowl that was located in the middle of a room. The aversive contingency exerted a differentiating effect on social and appetitive approach behavior that was correlated strongly with the rearing breed of the puppy and only partially with rearing history.

After the experimenter left the room, basenjis, which showed a strong environmental and novelty orientation, tended to eat from the bowl straightaway, whether they had been punished or indulged, whereas shelties, which showed a strong social avoidance, consistently avoided the food during the full 8 days of testing, regardless of their rearing history. In contrast to the social aloofness of the basenjis and the social avoidance of the shelties, the beagles and wirehaired fox terriers showed a high level of attraction and interest in the experimenter. Depending on their previous rearing history, these breeds also differentiated into separate groups after punishment training. Indulged puppies showed a greater amount of avoidance toward the meat than did puppies that received disciplinary treatment prior to punishment. Of particular interest with respect to the long-term effects of such treatment, indulged beagle puppies receiving punishment training at week 8 showed evidence of delayed changes in social behavior consistent with a loss of trust and safety stemming from the earlier punitive experience. During follow-up tests from weeks 11 to 15, these indulged-punished beagle puppies became wary when approached by handlers and increasingly difficult to catch—behavior that sharply contrasted with their earlier sociable attitude and behavior. The so-called second fear period may actually be related to the retraction of residual social attraction or its loss as the result of interactive conflict, releasing conditioned social fear acquired earlier in life.

Freedman's findings indicate that early rearing practices and individual differences can strongly influence how dogs respond to appetitive inhibitory training. The individual differences associated with appetitive inhibitions would seem to represent a significant confounding influence for cognitive studies such as the one performed by Call and colleagues. According to Freedman's work, some dogs should simply avoid food in the presence of the experimenter, whereas others should simply ignore the warning and take the food at the first opportunity. Dogs most likely to differentiate behavior in response to reprimands would need to have a high level of social attraction.

Another problematic influence is prior safe or unsafe exposure to food. Under normal household conditions, dogs frequently find bits of food fallen to the floor, which they are usually permitted to eat without consequence. Most dogs are also accustomed to obtaining food as rewards from their owners or to obtaining it by searching countertops and trash bins—efforts that are intermittently successful and may persist despite the use of contingent and belated punitive efforts. Dogs regularly receive small portions of food as rewards consequent to the performance of obedience tasks. Food is also sometimes used to relax anxious dogs via its calming effects on aversive emotion and arousal. The idea here is that preexposure to food would likely build a significant level of prior conditioning and bias that should impede or facilitate the acquisition of inhibitory conditioning (see *Stimulus Factors Affecting Conditioned-stimulus Acquisition and Maintenance* in Volume 1, Chapter 6). Further, there might be an intrinsic contrapreparedness associated with learning to avoid appetitive objects via aversive threats. Rats, for example, exposed to brief foot shock and other aversives (e.g., ammonia, mustard,

or quinine) as they approached a highly preferred food item (an Oreo cookie), or as they ate the cookie, continued to show a persistent appetite for the object. In contrast, rats exposed to nausea-producing lithium chloride acquired a rapid and cross-contextual aversion toward the cookie, perhaps indicating a certain degree of independence between cutaneous and alimentary defense systems. When subsequently tested, the shocked rats showed only momentary hesitation before eating the cookie in the training cage where the shock took place but showed no hesitation before eating the cookie while in the home cage or when tested in a novel cage (see *Prepared Connections: Taste Aversion* in Volume 1, Chapter 5).

Despite biological contrapreparedness, lasting food inhibitions can be established rapidly with severe physical or electrical punishment but not without risking neurotogenic elaborations. Lichtenstein (1950) demonstrated that appetitive behavior could be fully suppressed by the delivery of one to three electrical shocks (2 seconds of 85-volt AC each), if the aversive events were timed to overlap the act of eating, whereas significantly more repetitions of shock stimulation (23 to 29 shocks) were required if it was delivered immediately before the presentation of food (see *Lichtenstein's Experiments* in Volume 1, Chapter 9), again raising additional questions about the size, durability, and ease with which Call and colleagues were able to establish a stable inhibition of appetitive behavior.

Chairs and Minds: On Knowing What a Dog Knows About Attentional States

A more serious set of problems for Call's attentional state hypothesis is posed by the findings reported by Solomon and colleagues (1968). The experimenters were interested in the delay of punishment effects on the highly motivated appetitive behavior of starving dogs. During the training phase of the experiment, the dogs were deprived of normal rations and caused to lose more than 20% of their normal body weight. They were presented with two food bowls, one containing 20 grams (approximately a tablespoon and a half) of dry food and the other containing 200 grams (less than a cup) of horse meat. The food bowls were arranged so that they were within the reach of the experimenter, who sat in a nearby chair armed with a tightly rolled-up newspaper in hand. If the dogs limited their interest to the dry food, which they were permitted to eat, they were ignored without consequence; if the dogs ate the meat, however, they were hit sharply across the nose with the newspaper. Some of the dogs were swatted just before they touched the forbidden food, whereas others were punished after a 5- or 15-second (s) delay, during which they were allowed to eat. Dogs showed a spectrum of intense fearful behaviors and sustained food aversion differentiated in various ways depending on the timing of punishment. Approach toward the forbidden food item was suppressed rapidly in all three groups of dogs, requiring as few as three or four hard swats.

After the training phase, the dogs were given several daily 1-hour feedings to allow them to regain the weight they had lost. At the end of this period, the dogs were deprived of all food for 2 days. During the testing phase, all food was obtained during "temptation tests," which consisted of dry kibble and a bowl of horse meat. The experimenters found that dogs were so intimidated by the treatment that they would starve themselves, on average, for 16.3 days (no delay), 9.7 days (5-s delay), and 1.5 days (15-s delay) rather than eat the preferred meat, even though the experimenter was out of the room and the punishment contingency had been discontinued.

An interesting aspect of this disturbing study is the finding that the dogs showed opposite patterns of social behavior, depending on whether punishment was immediate or delayed. The no-delay group, upon entering the experimental room, skulked around with the head and tail down and staying as far away from the experimenter and the forbidden food as possible. In contrast, the delay groups entered the experimental room with an appearance of immense excitement, tail wagging, and jumping up on the experimenter. As they approached the food and took a few bites, their behavior dramatically changed: with their tail drooping down, they would slink behind the experimenter's chair or circle the room, go to a wall, and then crawl on their belly to the experimenter, whereupon they would wag their tail, furtively take some more food, and retreat again. During the test phase, when the dogs were left alone they behaved as though the experimenter was still present. Even though they were free to eat the meat, they could not initially do so. In the case of no-delay dogs, the taboo broke down very slowly, but when they finally began to eat the meat they did so in an uninhibited fashion, wagging their tail and not showing any sign of anxiety. In contrast, when the delay dogs finished eating the dry food, they would often put their paws on the experimenter's chair or go behind it from where they would wag their tail when they looked in the direction of the empty chair. The dogs appeared to treat the chair in ways that mirrored the behavior they showed when the experimenter was in the room. For these dogs, the taboo against eating the meat broke down much more rapidly, but they never lost their apprehensiveness while eating and remained anxious after eating.

The findings reported by Solomon and colleagues are at significant odds with the attentional state hypothesis. The 18 dogs in this experiment appeared unable to differentiate the relative degree of threat posed by the presence or absence of the experimenter. In fact, in the case of those dogs punished after a brief delay, they continued to treat the experimenter with animated excitement at the beginning of each session, only showing evidence of fear after they had taken some food. The trigger stimulus of anxious arousal relative to the experimenter was elicited by the act of taking food, not by the presence of the experimenter. During the test phase, the delay dogs were observed to approach the chair and behave as though the experimenter was still present. Of course, a chair does not possess an attentional state, but the dogs nevertheless showed behavior toward the chair and surroundings as though it did. The authors interpreted this social behavior in vacuum as an expression of *conscience*.

Whether the previously described experiment performed by Solomon and colleagues would qualify as such falsification is not clear, but it does raise a number of questions about how dogs perceive and use human attentional states. The questions raised here need to be answered by means of clever experimental designs that can unambiguously rule out lower levels of organization (e.g., stimulus and context learning). The accumulated data of 100 studies performed to prove some inductive belief or generality are vulnerable to upset based on a single well-designed experiment demonstrating an irrefutable counterexample. The use of vocal threats or physical punishment to test cognitive capacities seems particularly onerous, clumsy, and inappropriate to the task, especially insofar they are likely to impact a dog on numerous levels, making it difficult to disambiguate a canine orientation to attentional states and a complex chain of conditioned responses associated with the object and surroundings.

A problematic aspect of Solomon and colleagues' method deserves mention, to wit: how was the experimenter able to swat dogs belonging to the 15-s-delay group while they were still eating. Considering that these dogs were starved, one would expect that several of them (at least) should have been able to bolt down 200 grams of meat in less than 15 s and thereby beat the punishment contingency. Frankly, the notion that a starving dog would take 15 s to eat less than a cup of meat seems inconceivable.

COMPLEX SOCIAL BEHAVIOR AND MODEL/RIVAL LEARNING

Dogs appear to be highly sensitive to social modeling and training effects that occur in the context of exchanges between two human demonstrators—a trainer and a model/rival—interacting with an attractive object in the dog's presence. The method of model/rival (M/R) training has been most thoroughly investigated in the context of training parrots (see Todt, 1975; Pepperberg et al., 1999; Pepperberg, 2002). Todt's work with parrots is organized around the incentive value of attention directed toward a familiar and previously cooperative person who has ceased to be so and made to become a *rival* for the attention of a second person who remains a cooperative *partner* to the bird. In this paradigm of instruction, the rival's vocal expressions prompt close attention and interest by the partner (trainer), thereby modeling vocal behavior relevant to attracting attention and interest from the cooperative partner. Whether the incentive governing the acquisition of vocal behavior is related to reward associated with social attention or merely the result of focusing the bird's attention on the rival's behavior is unclear, but Todt notes that, while the birds learned words from the rival, they tended to use words to communicate with partner/trainer.

A study by McKinley and Young (2003) purports to compare the relative efficacy of a modified M/R method with shaping for training a vocally discriminated selection-and-retrieval task. The authors suggest that both methods perform about equally well. However, since the design is not adequately controlled for making comparative assessments (e.g., all of the dogs had been previously trained to retrieve), it is difficult to say what the study results actually measure. From the brevity of the training used to reach criteria levels and the weight of other evidence provided, the comparable performance of the dogs tested was probably the result of transient motivational changes, classical conditioning, and prior training to retrieve, rather than reflecting effects specifically due to instrumental or M/R training. Another possibility is that the results reflect a prepared ability to rapidly associate word meanings with the act of retrieving objects via a process akin to *fast mapping* (Kaminski et al., 2004). At a minimum, such experiments require that baseline data be obtained to assess prior learning and skills that might confound the behavioral change that one wishes to use as a comparison to measure the relative effects of the independent variables. Since such baseline data were not collected, it is impossible to determine from their data whether any significant effect on retrieve behavior occurred as the result of either of the training procedures. Further, the experimenters moved immediately from the training procedure to the test trial, suggesting that the comparable effects of the two methods may have been due to arousal and motivational changes (establishing operations) activated by the target object that in turn served to recruit previously learned retrieval responses.

Preliminary Experiments and Observations

Preliminary results of a series of experiments performed to explore possible effects of a modified M/R method indicate that dogs may be more sensitive and responsive to social learning via observation than previously suspected. These experiments appear to reveal a form of rapid complex social learning in dogs that was not previously described in the scientific literature. The experiments indicate that dogs may rapidly acquire and integrate the attunement dynamics of two persons making exchanges involving an object valued by the dogs.

The procedure consists of an observing dog, a partner/trainer (P/T), a model/rival (M/R), and an object of significant interest (OSI) to the dog. The M/R plays a combined role of stimulating rivalry for the trainer's attention while attuning and modeling behavior in response to the P/T's signals, prompts, and rewards. The experiments were performed in a home environment and involved two familiar demonstrators, who sat on the floor facing each other approximately 3 feet apart. The dog, a 2-year-old, male, Belgian Malinois, was signaled by the P/T to lie down and to stay at approximately 6 feet away from the P/T and the M/R. The dog showed a strong interest in both objects used in experiments 1 and 2.

Experiment 1

The first experiment (1A) involved the dog observing the demonstrators interacting with a favorite toy (a ball). In the first interaction, a brief fuss was made over the ball while the demonstrators tugged back and forth on it. The P/T finally pulled the ball forcefully away from the M/R, and then, after a brief

pause, the ball was put on the floor approximately 2 feet away from an identical ball. The dog was released and observed. A second experiment (1B), employing an identical arrangement, was performed immediately after experiment 1A. This time, though, the demonstrators interacted more quietly and cooperatively, with the P/T now giving the M/R the ball with "Take it," saying "Good," and then asking the M/R to give the ball back with "Out." As the M/R handed the ball back, the P/T said "Good" and immediately thereafter gave the object back again in a friendly way, saying "Take it" and "Good" as the M/R took the ball again. This pattern was repeated two or three times before the ball was placed on the floor in the manner previously described.

The results of these experiments were extremely surprising. Observing human interaction with the ball beforehand exerted a pronounced affect on the dog's subsequent response to the object. In the case of experiment 1A, the dog went directly to the ball, rapidly picked it up, became unusually possessive over it, and made vigorous efforts to evade being caught when the P/T tried to take the ball. This behavior was in striking contrast to the dog's ordinary willingness to give and release toys. Equally striking and remarkable was the dog's change and demeanor following experiment 1B. After observing the demonstrators interact in a more friendly and cooperative way with the item, the dog went to the ball, picked it up in a much more relaxed manner, went to the P/T, and allowed him to take it away. Extraordinarily, these dramatic changes in complex social behavior were produced within the context of a 10-minute period.

Experiment 2

Several days later, the same dog was observed under a similar basic arrangement, but this time another toy (e.g., a stuffed animal) was used and the P/T and M/R staged another set of exchanges for the dog to observe. In the first of these experiments (2A), the P/T showed the object to the M/R, sharply said "Leave it," and made a slapping action toward the M/R's hand. This procedure was repeated two or three times. After a brief delay, the toy was put on the floor and the dog released. In the second experiment (2B), the P/T presented the toy to the P/T, saying "Take it," and then "Good" as the M/R took the object. After a moment, the P/T, saying "Give," asked nicely for the object, whereupon the M/R handed the toy back and P/T said "Good." This friendly exchange was repeated two or three times, before the object is placed on the floor and the dog released.

Again, quite unexpectedly and surprisingly, the dog's behavior toward the toy changed rapidly in directions consistent with the way in which the P/T and M/R interacted with the object beforehand. In the case of experiment 2A, the dog, normally highly object driven and enthusiastic, only slowly and tentatively approached the object, then hesitated, and turned away without picking it up. Instead of taking the object, the dog went to the M/R, as though to check on her, while appearing to ignore and avoid the P/T. By contrast, after observing the cooperative interaction between the P/T and the M/R staged in experiment 2B, the dog went directly to the toy, picked it up, and took it to the P/T.

Social Cognition, Scripts, and Modal Styles

The clarity, contextual appropriateness, and rapidity of the complex behavioral adjustments shown by the dog in response to observing social exchanges between the P/T and M/R were truly extraordinary, going well beyond what one might expect from the low estimations normally attributed to observational learning in dogs (see *Social Learning* in Volume 1, Chapter 7). The dog seemed to grasp accurately the social significance of the interaction between the P/T and the M/R and to adjust its behavior immediately toward the object and the demonstrators accordingly, as though he had directly experienced the stimulation firsthand. These remarkable changes in behavior, occurring in response to staged demonstrations, suggest that the model/rival procedure may offer a powerful tool for studying developmental processes,

affect-attunement dynamics, and canine proxemics (see *Model/Rival Theory, Fair Play, and Sibling Hierarchy* in Chapter 8), as well as suggest a variety of behavior therapy and training applications. For example, in addition to an apparent value for developing object preferences and avoidance, dogs exhibiting possessive or overt guarding behavior might be helped to interact in a more friendly and cooperative manner by observing a trainer and model/rival exchanging positive vocal signals and gestures signifying safety and comfort around trigger objects. In addition, it may have value in the context of reducing impulse-control deficiencies by demonstrating to the dog more calm and cooperative exchanges organized around desirable objects. The apparent attunement and social scripting fostered by M/R method may help to explain certain social excesses associated with hyperactivity. For example, in situations where children routinely roughhouse around objects of interest to a dog, M/R learning effects may strongly affect the dog's behavior toward the children and the objects.

The robust and remarkable effects produced by the M/R method is deserving of experimental scrutiny. The apparent sensitivity that dogs exhibit for attunement information derived from social demonstration suggests that such learning may play a significant role in behavioral organization. The arrangement does not exclude the possibility that the dog might be responding to conditioned or unconditioned stimuli that generate preparatory arousal and subsequent expressive behavior similar to the rival's modeled behavior. Of course, such preparatory influences would not necessarily be incompatible with the possibility that such interaction might also exert cognitive organizing effects. Further, even if the effects are restricted to the transmission of attunement effects, such capacities for behavior-therapy purposes are not insignificant. The dramatic and rather precise nature of the behavioral output associated with M/R demonstrations is consistent with the possibility that M/R learning might involve processes that conduce attunement and encode modal scripts or styles of exchange with the object mirroring the model/rival's behavior. This hypothesis is consistent with the tendency of some young dogs to adopt various modal styles and nuances of behavior shown by other dogs perceived as possessing effective leadership qualities (perceived high power). Model/rival learning appears to enable observing dogs to mirror the affect and actions observed between the M/R and the P/T. Structuring behavior in accord with attunement scripts observed taking place between the M/R and P/T would allow dogs to integrate rapidly into social activities. Such abilities might be particularly active in the modal behavior and styles of playful newcomers and young animals seeking acceptance into an established social group. The capacity to exhibit behavior that "feels" like the style of others may cause group members to perceive the newcomer as being familiar and to more readily accept and integrate the *poser* into the group.

Attention, Model/Rival Learning, and Mirror Neurons

The ability of dogs to *style* behavior in conformity with the attunement dynamics observed between demonstrators would suggest the involvement of a complex computational apparatus for extracting socially significant information and making accurate affective inferences about its significance. One line of neurobiological research in monkeys has shown that the ventral premotor cortex encodes a mirror representation of the actions made by others of a form similar to the representation made when the animal makes the action itself (Umilta et al., 2001; Ferrari et al., 2003). In addition to actions seen, these mirror neurons represent what is heard in association with actions but remain inactive to other sounds (Kohler et al., 2002). Mirror neurons appear to provide the animal the ability to discriminate action based on auditory, visual, and motor information (Keysers et al., 2003). These findings suggest the possibility that these mirror neurons may be part of a larger network comprising a neural matching/comparator system that would enable social animals to rehearse the form or script of social behavior observed in the behavior of others

before acting on it. Thus, the encoding of a mirror representation at the stage of premotor processing may be "transformed into potential actions in the mirror system such that the perception-action link related to action representation is activated already during observation" (Nishitani and Hari, 2000:918). The ability of parrots to acquire and express complex vocal sounds based on hearing in the context of model/rival enactments may be facilitated by a similar process of mirror representation whereby complex vocal sounds are encoded by auditory mirror neurons and subsequently decoded by motor programs controlling vocal behavior.

The observed action represented as potential action by mirror neurons may be attributed with affective significance by cortical and limbic processing before being expressed as an action attuned to the social circumstance. Unlike parrots with their imitative behavior, dogs may be more inclined to recast the potential action represented by mirror neurons by turning attention toward the quality of feeling informing the observed exchange. According to this hypothesis, dogs are more interested in the affective significance of the M/R demonstrations than in imitating the specific form. These sorts of prepared social learning capacities may be particularly important to domestic dogs, whose social acceptance depends on their ability to attune and commune with family members. The genetically augmented play capacities of dogs may include an automatic representational framework for decoding and attributing affective significance to potential actions, enabling dogs to transition from the external form of playful exchanges to a subjective experience of shared internal feelings (joy) arising in the process of mediating attunement and secure attachments.

PART 3: ETHICS AND PHILOSOPHY

CYNOPRAXIS AND ETHICS

A Delta Society publication aspiring to set professional standards for dog trainers lists three primary ethical criteria that the authors believe qualify a procedure as humane:

"Humane dog trainers use and advocate methods that rely on: eliciting and reinforcing desired behaviors, inhibiting and discouraging unwanted or potentially dangerous behaviors, minimizing the use of aversives while doing either of the above" (Delta Society, 2001:2). Defining ethical behavior exclusively in terms of technical means irrespective of aims is inherently circular and limited with respect to ethical practices.

Ends

Without defining the aims of training, such rather tinny behavioristic criteria as set by the Delta Society are virtually meaningless with respect to humane-practice criteria. Numerous questionable training activities might be construed as ethical and humane practices merely because they are performed in adherence to these sorts of standards. The second criterion violates the dead-dog rule and the third criterion neglects to consider the adverse impact of overly intrusive methods (see *Hydran-Protean Side Effects, the Dead-dog Rule, and the LIMA Principle*). According to these recommendations, putting a dog in a crate and training by means of a tedious autoshaping program would be considered ethical and humane, even though a human is never involved in the training process. Evaluating the ethical and humane use of means in the absence of appropriate consideration of the ends to which they are applied is logically flawed and produces many absurd implications. For example, dogs trained by the Russians during World War II were desensitized and conditioned with food rewards until they either ran between the treads of an approaching tank or ran alongside it, whereupon an ordinance strapped to their bodies was detonated. Since antitank dogs were trained by "eliciting and reinforcing desired behaviors," applying the aforementioned criteria suggest that training of antitank dogs was ethical and humane.

The criteria listed for identifying behaviors to be reinforced or "inhibited" are strictly limited to anthropic interests; that is, those canine activities that the trainer finds desirable or undesirable without reference to the dog's needs and QOL. Canine adjustment problems cannot be effectively treated without normalizing the social and environmental circumstances producing the objectionable behavior. Merely reinforcing or punishing what one likes and dislikes is not likely to prove very beneficial in the long run.

These concerns emphasize the profound influence that training objectives have on matters pertaining to ethical standards. A ruthless person may use kindness and gifts in order to deceive and gain the confidence of others, with the goal of eventually harming or taking advantage of them in some way. Such manipulation is obviously unethical and can hardly be considered humane. In a poignant way, Bertrand Russell (1997) has stressed the potential risks associated with the formation of faulty expectations based on an assumed uniformity between means and ends:

> Domestic animals expect food when they see the person who feeds them. We know that all these rather crude expectations of uniformity are liable to be misleading. The man who has fed the chicken every day throughout its life at last wrings its neck instead, showing that more refined views as to the uniformity of nature would have been useful to the chicken. (63)

Russell's chicken, like the Russian antitank dogs, was duped by a faulty extrapolation from means to ends.

Under natural conditions, animals change their behavior in order to improve their ability to control environmental resources and events that contribute to their survival and well-being. Accordingly, instrumental behavior is strengthened when it succeeds in enhancing an animal's ability to predict and control the occurrence of some significant event and weakened when it fails. Dog training is based on a contrivance that exploits canine learning to shape and control an artificial repertoire of behaviors patterned toward some training objective that may or may not be in a dog's best interest. In the context of training, reward and punishment are arbitrarily arranged to occur in accord with the trainer's plans to render the dog's behavior more predictable and controllable. The dog's ability to predict and control these events is preempted by rules established by the trainer in advance; that is, the game is rigged to allow only those changes in the dog's behavior that suit the trainer's purposes.

Just as a dog's behavior is shaped by its ability to control attractive and aversive events arranged by a trainer, the trainer's behavior is subject to modification by the relative success or failure of training exchanges to meet objectives. Efforts that successfully increase control over a dog's behavior are strengthened, whereas efforts that fail to increase control are weakened. As such, practical dog training is inherently reward based insofar as contingencies are arranged to enable dogs to gain control over motivational events by means of signaled actions consistent with the training objective. Only an irrational trainer would set up contingencies that were deliberately arranged to make a dog fail. The most unethical and punishment-based training does not stem from the use or nonuse of aversive motivational stimuli but rather from incompetence. Incompetent trainers may lack the basic know-how and skill to use basic procedures humanely or to organize the contingencies and steps of a training plan. As a result of an inconsistent or incoherent organization of training events, dogs may be unable to control significant attractive and aversive motivational stimuli, thus resulting in persistent punishment, distress, and an adverse overall impact on their ability to cope.

Competent dog training is intrinsically rewarding and bond enhancing, whereas incompetent training is intrinsically punishing and bond degrading. The enhanced control resulting from successful training yields an enhanced capacity for the partnership to produce mutually rewarding exchanges that enable the partners to enjoy each other while adjusting and learning about each other. Conversely, social exchanges that result in a loss of mutual control tend to promote increased punitive interaction and conflict. The interactive conflict stemming from incompetent exchanges contributes to an increased reliance on excessive confinement and isolation, emphasis on passive head and jaw restraint, and needless distress.

The practical ends of dog training have significant welfare implications, especially for dogs trained to perform services that are inherently aversive and require significant compulsion to achieve. One cannot disclose the nature of one's training objectives to a dog in advance, nor can it appreciate intuitively the significance of its training. To some extent, the dog's innocence and ignorance with respect to the end task renders the ethical dilemma somewhat less consequential than if the dog was deliberately kept in the dark by deception and omission regarding ultimate aims and purposes. However, to the extent that the dog is an object of care, its innocence about such matters obligates the trainer, as a *humane* being, to consider thoughtfully the ethical implications of training procedures and the practical purposes for which the dog is trained. Training goals that are ultimately enslaving or harmful to a dog are inherently unethical and cruel, regardless of the means used to attain them.

One hypothetical test that can serve as a general guideline for making decisions about practical use is to ask oneself whether the dog, given a choice, would likely select the career being chosen for it. The notion that a dog might truly love to work is not far-fetched, since selective breeding has produced a staggering array of canine skills integrated with ready-made motivational systems that make their performance intrinsically rewarding. Breeding biologically prepares dogs with drives and functional capacities that are uniquely compatible with certain practical tasks while being inimical to others. Dogs are born with a set of innate threshold values predisposing them toward certain traits and action modes. These predispositions point toward activities that a dog seeks and is gratified to perform. These various preferred activities represent a core focus of competency that a dog is naturally inclined to integrate skills around. Discovering a dog's core competency and building on those interests and incentives is an important aspect of both cynopraxic and practical dog training. Integrating skills relevant to a dog's core competency serves to activate power and freedom incentives, which are typically expressed in playful activities of various kinds. The availability of these playful activities can be budgeted and made to overlap with the performance of related practical activities of significant value to the trainer but of no particular significance to the dog, except insofar as resonating with core interests and affording an opportunity to play or the possibility to obtain other rewards. When training working dogs, the competent trainer discovers, stimulates, refines, and sublimates various innate appetites and propensities (drives) conducive to the performance of useful services in accordance with the accepted cultural and functional expectations of the breed.

Just as a competent craftsperson would not use a screwdriver in place of chisel or a wood saw to cut metal pipe, a competent trainer would not train a beagle to hunt grouse or train a Brittany spaniel to hunt rabbit. In essence, the practical trainer's work is to actualize an innate potential present in the dog for some useful activity. As a result of such training, a convergence human and canine interests dovetails, with the dog obtaining significant gratification and playful stimulation as the result of performing some valuable practical activity, thereby satisfying both the trainer's objectives and the dog's interest in play and companionship. Dogs successful in such work have an increased likelihood of being bred and thereby perpetuating the genes responsible for their responsiveness to training.

The foregoing represents the ideal circumstances surrounding the training of working dogs, whether they are used for military scouting and reconnaissance, drug and explosive detection, search and rescue, hunting, herding, and so forth—dogs work to play. Some training objectives, however, require that dogs perform work for which they are neither biologically prepared nor from which they can obtain play gratification. Training dogs for such purposes requires the implementation of means other than play to shape and render reliable the requisite repertoire of trained behavior needed to perform the service. Typically, such dogs are systematically manipulated by social encouragement together with the presentation and withdrawal of attractive and aversive motivational stimuli in the process of compelling adjustments compatible with the training objective

that they would otherwise not perform. These issues raise difficult ethical questions, requiring that one weigh the cost of such training and service to the dog versus the potential social benefits that the service provides for the end client. If the social value of the service is minimal or harmful to society, it is easy to conclude that such training is inappropriate. It is sobering, though, to consider the previously mentioned Russian antitank dogs in the context of a social cost-benefit assessment. From the perspective of the Russian military and a great many Russian people faced with a mortal threat, such an end use of dogs was probably considered a tremendous social good. Indeed, the use of such dogs may have saved Russian lives, but the notion of training dogs to become living bombs is abhorrent, just as making prostitutes of adolescent children for the sake of espionage is abhorrent. In both instances, the violations of innocence and trust make such uses intrinsically inhumane. This example underscores the danger of ethical judgments weighted in the direction of social cost-benefit assessments and social consensus without appropriate consideration having been given to the cost and harm to the dog.

The line becomes even more blurred in the case of some canine services that provide a significant amount of social benefit, such as those performed by assistance and guide dogs, but involve the training of unprepared action sequences. As noted previously, in addition to reward-based training efforts, such practical training activities often require a significant amount of inhibitory training and compulsion. Unlike working dogs in which the end use is compatible with breed-typical appetites and drives, some service applications are intrinsically foreign to dogs (see Serpell et al., 2000). Dogs that perform such services do so as the result of intensive training that gradually shapes a repertoire of behaviors having little intrinsic reward value for the dogs themselves but possessing immense comfort and reward value for persons needing such assistance. Although the close interaction and companionship provided by the client-caregiver provide the dog some compensation, nevertheless such dogs would also benefit from special compensatory stimulation consistent with their breed-typical play and work interests when not performing services, including appropriate opportunities to play and exercise—activities that the client-caregiver may not always be able to provide the dog. Perhaps what is needed is a national volunteer-type organization that would provide *assistance* to these dogs and their owners in the form of play and other outdoor activities not otherwise available to them.

There is nothing intrinsically incompatible between cynopraxic priorities and work, provided that the training process is competent and consists of bond-enhancing exchanges that improve a dog's QOL. These cynopraxic priorities stress that the working dog *team* is the result of a mutual process of adaptation conducive to belongingness, playfulness, and trust. Even relatively unnatural skills, if trained in a competent manner and gradually brought under the motivational influence of power and freedom incentives, can become the source of significant pleasure for a dog to perform.

Although practical dog training can involve behavioral objectives that are exploitive or inimical to a dog's well-being, many practical uses of dogs can be achieved in a manner that does not run afoul of cynopraxic bond and life-experience imperatives. Some authors have argued that working dogs, in principle, cannot be effective workers while living in a home as companions, suggesting that selective breeding for traits that make them good working dogs bars them from making good household companions. These sorts of general hypotheses conflict with numerous counterexamples indicating that working dogs can, and do, enjoy the QOL benefits of companionship and still remain effective workers (see Kiley-Worthington, 1990). Finck (1993), who studied the affect attunement between children and dogs, found that working and hunting dogs were generally highly receptive to a child's attunement efforts, which is consistent with the enhanced abilities of such dogs to follow human instruction.

Breeding that would so alter behavioral thresholds in ways that preemptively excluded a dog from household companionship would

likely also significantly impair the dog's capacity to perform most types of cooperative work. The notion that canine traits conducive to work are incompatible with domestic life is unfounded and contradicted by common experience, since thousands of police dogs have demonstrated that they can be both good workers and welcome household companions. Many police departments in the United States use dogs that work and then go home with the officer/handler as companions. Police dogs share the risk of a dangerous job and are entrusted to make safe contact with the general public. Why, then, should they be denied the familiar surroundings of the home after their duty shift is over? How might the isolation and confinement of overnight and weekend stays in a kennel help such dogs in their work? Dogs are first and foremost companions who are also helpers, and specialized uses of canine labor that preemptively exclude them from living in a home or deny them the benefits of human companionship so that they can be made into cheap and useful "tools" raise a number of significant welfare concerns.

Means

The purposes and ultimate goals of training obviously affect the ethical assessment of the means. With the broader picture of ends in place, a more sensible discussion of means is possible. First and foremost, procedural means are employed to produce some series of immediate effects toward the realization of an ultimate goal or objective. In dog training, these means consist of a variety of manipulations involving the differential application and removal of attractive and aversive stimuli with the intent of altering a dog's behavior in some way. The ethical implications of means depend on a number of competing considerations. There is a widely held belief that attractive stimuli are of a more humane and ethical nature than aversive ones. Of course, both people and dogs share a preference for pleasure over pain; however, the ultimate significance of attractive and aversive stimuli depends not only on their momentary hedonic and emotional effects but also to a significant extent on ultimate ends and the aggregate effects that such events have on the human-dog relationship and the dog's QOL. The experience of brief discomfort in exchange for the acquisition of long term safety from pain or injury, together with increased opportunities for pleasure and liberty, unquestionably warrants the limited use of such stimulation, especially if other means are not available for producing a similar effect in a timely manner. However, using only mildly aversive or annoying procedures might be considered inhumane in situations where nothing of lasting benefit is achieved.

Motivational stimuli consist of hedonic (likes and dislikes) and incentive (needs) values. Seeking pleasure, comfort, and safety, on the one hand, and avoiding pain, loss, and risk, on the other, are strong motivational incentives regulating both human and dog behavior. Such events also exert influential excitatory (arousal) and inhibitory (calming) autonomic effects. Training consists of the response-contingent application of both attractive and aversive events in order to change a dog's behavior in some specific or general way. Applying aversive stimulation excessively, incompetently, or unnecessarily represents prima facie abusive treatment. Although the arbitrary and incompetent use of attractive and pleasurable events does not invite similar criticism, it too can be highly abusive and destructive. Since attractive incentives can be used to deceive or to obtain ends harmful to a dog or fail to obtain beneficial ends, a reliance on nonaversive procedures may be unethical in cases where the training objectives are contrary to the dog's best interests or when they result in harm to the dog that could have been averted by the use of a more effective but aversive procedure. Conversely, aversive procedures that cause significant discomfort but act as a means to some beneficial end (e.g., prevent the dog from running into the street) may confer a positive moral value to the procedure insofar as it is efficacious and achieves, on the whole, an ultimate good that could not have been achieved by nonaversive efforts alone.

When considered independently of ends, attractive events and aversive events are morally indeterminate, although the former is hedonically preferable to the latter. Consequently, on balance, if some behavioral objective is equally obtainable by attractive or aversive means, then the trainer, with due respect for the dog's preference for pleasure, is ethically bound to use attractive means rather than aversive ones. On the other hand, if some behavioral objective promising benefit to the dog is obtainable only by aversive means, then the trainer, with due consideration for the dog's well-being, is ethically obligated to use the least aversive procedure necessary. However, on the whole, the competence and confidence needed to integrate an adaptive coping style depend on a balance of reward derived from the successful control of both attractive and aversive motivational stimuli. To conceive of attractive stimuli as being intrinsically good and beneficial to a dog's welfare and aversive stimuli as being intrinsically bad and inimical to a dog's welfare is the brew of fanatics, not the fruit of science or a sincere concern for the dog's welfare. From the perspective of cynopraxic theory, punishment, especially those efforts that thwart or attempt to suppress a dog's control efforts by incompetent interference or excessive confinement or restraint, is a far more significant and serious threat to canine welfare than is the balanced use of aversive motivational stimuli in the context of reward-based training.

In practice, the decisions regarding the use of valenced motivational stimuli involve a variety of practical and ethical considerations. At minimum, for attractive and aversive events to be used humanely, the trainer must possess sufficient skill to apply them effectively for the purpose of attaining well-defined target objectives (competency factor) and possess a reasonable idea of the immediate and remote consequences of the events used, including a realistic appreciation of potential side effects. In addition to general training and behavioral knowledge, the trainer must also possess significant experience with dogs of different breeds and temperament types at various ages—factors that strongly influence the selection and appropriateness of training procedures.

OWNER CONTROL STYLES AND WELFARE AGENDAS

Hiby and colleagues (2004) have collected and analyzed questionnaire data ostensibly relevant to owner control and disciplinary styles, however, the interpretation and conclusions they present of their findings appears to belie a negative bias and agenda against the use of aversive motivational stimuli in dog training. Among these findings, they found that dogs receiving high obedience ratings from their owners were rewarded more often than counterparts receiving low obedience ratings. This finding suggests a rather obvious and straightforward implication: owners are more likely to reward obedient behavior than they are to reward disobedient behavior. That low obedience ratings were associated with a higher frequency of punishment suggests a similarly obvious implication: dog owners tend to punish disobedient behaviors and refrain from rewarding them, at least not intentionally. The authors also found a strong correlation between punishment and the relative incidence of behavior problems. That the greatest number of problem behaviors were reported by owners using the most punishment or those combining punishment and reward, yields an obvious corollary of the foregoing, just as commonsense might predict, namely, owners of problem dogs are more likely to react with punishment or a combination of aversive and attractive means in an effort to control behavior problems. In contrast, dogs showing the least number of problems would naturally tend to receive more rewarding interaction—again an obvious finding, after all what would lead a sane person to shout or cause discomfort to their dog if it were not in reaction to some undesirable behavior.

The authors also found that dogs that walked obediently on leash were more likely to be praised by their owners than dogs that pulled, a finding that suggests that obedient dogs may have received some prior inhibitory training, perhaps combining leash jerking

with praise, such as a method popularized in England by Woodhouse and widely practiced in one form or another in the United States. Praise and petting in the context of inhibitory training may serve to support consequent autonomic attunement and safety. Once limits are set on pulling, reward-based exchanges can, indeed, help to maintain obedient walking habits; however, praise-alone would hardly be an adequate incentive to prevent or stop pulling by normal dogs. The notion that average dogs might be trained by their owners to walk "at heel" in public by using a praise-alone technique is highly improbable. Practical experience dictates that a combination of techniques incorporating both attractive and aversive motivational incentives fitted to the individual dog's needs works best for controlling leash-pulling excesses and other behavioral complaints resulting from the incessant canine appetite for drive-activating stimulation and novelty that most dogs show when outdoors.

The authors appear to assume that the increased reward received by obedient and well-adjusted dogs carries the necessary implication that well behaved dogs are made that way by means of reward-alone methods—an approach that they claim was practiced by an astonishing 20% of their owner respondents. They also report that nearly 10% of dog owners used a punishment-only method of control. Logically, it is difficult to consider how reward-only or punishment-only training might be implemented, since by definition the contingent withdraw or withholding of an attractive event is punishing, just as the contingent withdraw or omission of an aversive event is rewarding. How an owner might be able to carry on everyday exchanges with the dog that only resulted in reward or punishment is hard to imagine. In general, the findings reported by Hiby and colleagues point to the obvious conclusion that highly excitable, impulsive, and disobedient dogs are more likely to receive more punishment than dogs considered by their owners to be relatively calm, well-behaved, and obedient to command—dogs that are more likely to become the object of affectionate appreciation. Here is the real welfare implication of their study, viz., problem dogs are at greater risk of becoming the object of owner frustration, anger, and abuse.

Most dishearteningly, however, after acknowledging that their findings lacked causal significance (i.e., correlations of this sort do not prove cause-effect relationships), the authors nevertheless go ahead and treat them as though they were causally significant, concluding that reward-only methods represent "a more effective and 'welfare-compatible' alternative to punishment for the average dog owner" (2004:68). Instead of considering the most obvious and plausible implications of their findings, the authors draw upon a far less plausible generalization in order to promote what appears to be for them a foregone conclusion: aversives are *bad* for dogs and *good* owners and trainers should not use them. The authors appear to be so swayed by their heartfelt convictions and morality-speak regarding the "welfare-incompatible" implications of aversive training techniques that they entirely neglect to consider the most reasonable alternative hypothesis, namely, that aversive control efforts might actually offer significant welfare-compatible benefits. The oblique tone and pejorative commentary contained in this study also warrants mention. Not only is such diatribe demeaning with respect to the trainer's art and tradition, the particulars of the commentary are generally in conflict with a large body of practical and scientific evidence indicating that aversive motivational incentives can be effectively used in the context of reward-based training to enhance the human-dog bond and improve the dog's QOL.

The question is not whether aversives should or should not be used in the context of reward-based training; aversives *are* an integral aspect of competent dog training and aversive procedures will surely remain an instrumental and standard part of the dog trainer's practice (see Delta Society, 2002). What is more likely to change in a beneficial way is the relative reward-to-punishment ratio, the severity, and the frequency with which aversive procedures are used—a fairly constant trend that is evident in the tradition of dog training as well as in contemporary

improvements and progress in training methodology and skills. The debate would be far more constructive if it focused on how such procedures might be most effectively and efficiently used to minimize adverse side effects while maximizing potential welfare benefits in the context of reward-based training. The humane use of dog training methods depends on trainer competency, which, in turn, depends on suitable experience and reliable scientific information—not the imposition of moralistic agendas opposed *on principle* to the use of aversive procedures in dog training.

ANTHROPIC DOMINANCE IDEATION, PERCEIVED POWER, AND CONTROL STYLES

Bugental and colleagues (1993) have studied the dominance dynamics between caregivers and children. This work provides a number of useful insights into dominance and its destructive influences on dependent familial relationships. The attribution of dominance to children (and dogs) appears to be the expression of an insecure cognitive bias affecting an individual's perception of the power dynamics between themselves and dependent others. The power ideation and narrative used by persons with low perceived power are often employed to rationalize the abusive behavior-control tactics that such low-power persons are prone to employ in order to control dependents. Low-power parents interpret challenging behavior as being determined predominantly by causes under the child's control (e.g., stubborn or dominant attitude) rather than being the result of causes under proactive parental control. The researchers found that, while observing child behavior perceived as challenging, low-power parents filter and interpret what they see in terms of threatening implications. The reactive bias shown by such parents is indexed by changes in autonomic activity consistent with defensive arousal and a vulnerability to form nervous/insecure attachments. In contrast, high-power parents perceive the causes of challenging behavior to be predominantly under proactive control and remain in a state of autonomic balance while viewing challenging child behavior—a profile consistent with a capacity for autonomic attunement and the formation of secure attachments.

In addition to autonomic differences indicative of a reactive coping style and defensiveness, low-power parents show significant changes affecting dominance ideation when operating under the influence of cognitive load. Under cognitive load, low-power parents tend to exaggerate the power disparity between themselves and their children, tending to rank the child as being more dominant, and justifying deprivational, emotional, and physical abuses toward the child as *self-defense*. However, when these same low-power parents are not under the pressure of cognitive load, they appear to adopt an opposite attitude and estimation of social power relative to the child, tending to rank themselves as possessing more power than the child. These power-dominance vacillations inject a disruptive dynamic of ambivalence that increases the risk of gratuitous retaliation against the child (Bugental et al., 1997). Similar power dynamics appear to filter the way low-power owners and behavior modifiers interpret challenging dog behavior.

Whereas low-power behavior modifiers dwell on causes beyond their control, high-power behavior modifiers focus their attention and training efforts on matters that are within their reach and ability to change. The prominent findings of Bugental's research can be summarized and extended to behavior modifiers, as follows:

1. Low-power behavior modifiers are more likely to indiscriminately interpret challenging or oppositional behavior as a power contest beyond the reach of proactive behavioral interventions.
2. Low-power behavior modifiers are more likely to engage in highly intrusive or aversive deprivational, emotional, or physical practices.
3. Low-power behavior modifiers are more likely to interpret challenging and oppositional behavior in terms of malevolent social power intentions.
4. Low-power behavior modifiers unsure of their authority and power to control a dog

in proactive ways are more likely to resort to coercive emotional tactics, abusive force, or deprivational strategies.

5. Low-power behavior modifiers tend to justify highly intrusive and aversive training activities by appealing to self-defense and public safety.
6. Low-power behavior modifiers are more likely to interpret and respond to the uncertainty of ambiguous situations as threats, causing them to respond with inconsistent and reactive punishment.

Recurrent cycles of passive resentment followed by reactive and abusive power assertions appear to activate social ambivalence and entrapment dynamics, perhaps inoculating the dog with anxiety, irritability, and social withdrawal (dispersive tensions) or activating incompetent and reactive autoprotective strategies for coping with the low-power owner's inconsistent behavior and uncontrollable mistreatment. Exposure to cyclical patterns of passive resentment and arbitrary social and emotional deprivation, excessive confinement and restriction, and uncontrollable physical punishment may infuse social interaction between the dog and offending family members with a high degree of conflict, uncertainty, and mutual mistrust (distrust), perhaps causing the children and the dog alike to adopt preemptive and autoprotective strategies for coping with the reactive power shifts governing the low-power owner's control efforts. Alpert and colleagues (2003) found that children of parents diagnosed with depression (low-power state) and comorbid anger attacks were more vulnerable to develop post-traumatic stress disorder (PTSD) or increased aggressive behavior than were children of parents diagnosed with depression without comorbid anger attacks. These patterns of increased autoprotective behavior of children appear to parallel the reactive coping styles shown by dogs exposed to a history of maltreatment and abuse by low-power owners. The same research group also found that children of parents with early-onset depression were more vulnerable to develop a variety of psychological and social disturbances (e.g., delinquency and aggression) than were children of parents with late-onset depression

(Petersen et al., 2003). These psychiatric findings suggest a possible linkage between dog owners affected by depression (low-power state) with anger and an increased risk of reactive/impulsive aggression and other challenging behavior problems in dogs—a hypothesis that might be used to test and falsify the antipredator/autoprotective account.

Low-power individuals appear to be prone to behave in ambiguous or impetuous ways toward the dog or send social messages having passive-aggressive implications that may contribute to social ambivalence and reactive adjustments. A dog owner that abruptly grabs a sleeping dog around its head to give it a firm kiss on the mouth is not performing an act of loving appreciation, but is tempting fate with arrogance standing on the shoulders of ignorance. The evident abandonment of common sense at such times is the sort of thoughtless and inconsiderate action that has frequently resulted in devastating bites. As demonstrated in the case of children (Bugental et al., 1999b), dogs also appear to *tune out* ambiguous social signaling. Unfortunately, in human-dog interactions, the disengagement of social and attentional resources in response to ambiguous social interaction may trigger autonomic arousal, executive, and physiological functions coordinated and attuned by selective and sustained attention.

The finding that persons prone to low-power estimations are vulnerable to distort and shift their perception of relative control depending on cognitive load appears to question the validity of questionnaires and self-reports for estimating the efficacy of aggression-treatment programs. Low-power owners, depending on the quality of emotional support provided during counseling, may subsequently judge their personal power over the dog in a highly inflated or deflated way. Consequently, the estimates of behavioral improvement that such owners may attribute to medications or behavioral treatments may be confounded with changes in their dominance ideation and perception of control rather than effects specific to the intervention, which may not actually exist (false positives) or may exist but are not recognized (false negatives). The work by Bugental and colleagues has obvious implications with respect to providing a theoretical framework for studying the effects of owner control styles on the differentiation of adaptive and reactive coping styles. Study of owner control styles would be relevant to cynopraxic theories of social aggression and separation distress, and might also have general implications for understanding how proactive and reactive behavior is shaped. In addition to needing a questionnaire validated for the detection and assessment of low-power and high-power dog owners, such research would likely benefit from a design in which between-group comparisons could be made of dogs meeting the criteria of stable versus unstable extraversion. A similar sequestering of dogs according to criterion of stable and unstable introversion might also be performed. How stable and unstable extraverts and introverts progress under the influence of owners with high-power or low-power control styles may reveal interesting relationships between the stable-to-unstable continuum and the owner's control style. The study might be revealing with respect to dynamics mediating adaptive and reactive coping styles and factors contributing to the integration of secure and insecure attachments. Topál and colleagues (1997), for example, have found that the problem-solving ability of dogs is inversely related to the strength of the dog's attachment to the owner (i.e., problem-solving abilities decrease as attachment measures increase), which is consistent with the notion that dogs with insecure attachments would be more vulnerable to interactive conflict and a reactive coping style. Finally, such research might be readily performed in the context of an animal shelter with the human questionnaire and canine personality testing performed as a routine part of the adoption process.

POWER-DOMINANCE IDEATION AND TREATMENT PROTOCOLS

The power-dominance motivation attributed to canine domestic aggression is widely accepted as a leading cause of intrafamilial aggression. Appeal to social rank as a cause of aggression is a central theme guiding much of the applied and popular dog behavior literature, with most authors rehashing the narrative account or tweaking it to justify their particular dominance-oriented treatment program. However, instead of helping family members to understand the causes of dog aggression, such emphasis on dominance and rank may serve only to perpetuate a malevolent interpretation of canine intent and purposiveness that places undue and inappropriate focus on causes that are predominantly beyond an owner's control and rarely significant for the treatment of domestic aggression problems. Instead of interpreting the etiology of intrafamilial aggression problems and their treatment in terms of adversarial hierarchical dynamics, counseling and training activities are better served by focusing on the antecedent events and establishing operations specific to interactive exchanges triggering reactive behavior, insofar as these behavioral elements are accessible and subject to change by means of social exchange.

The dominance narrative not only has obscured the causes of aggression problems but has also resulted in a considerable amount of conceptual confusion that continues paralyze research, concealing far more than it reveals by way of a simplistic explanation regarding the causes of aggression. The anthropic dominance bias frames an excessively myopic and simplistic perspective on canine social behavior, giving rise to circular diagnostic labels and treatment rationales based on the dominance narrative. The effects of this misconception are not just of theoretical interest, because the dominance narrative and unfounded assumptions arising from it are used to justify a variety of highly intrusive and aversive practices in the name of rational therapy. The dominance narrative frames autoprotective and challenging dog behavior in a manner that contributes to the use of abusive emotional deprivation, aversive physical control and restraint tactics, and unproven pharmacological and surgical procedures. A leading cause of ineffectual management and treatment is the habitual targeting coercive tactics at quashing the "dominant" dog's attitude or perception of rank. The default use of drugs to treat such problems is especially

problematic because it appears to shift the domain of causation from the dog's attitude to its physiology—a domain of causality that is sufficiently vague for both the owner and the behavior modifier to promote magical thinking about the efficacy of such treatments.

Although some dogs with severe aggression problems may be victims of inadequate socialization and training, their care and training are frequently not that much different from the way many millions of other dogs are treated that do not develop aggression problems. Given the notable lack of (1) formalized-threat sequencing, (2) the severity of attacks, (3) the explosive and situational inappropriateness of attacks, (4) the benign nature of the provoking challenges or threats, and (5) the general incompetence exhibited by the aggressor and the victim, diagnosing such attacks as "dominance aggression" seems akin to pounding a square peg into a round hole and calling it a perfect fit. Most dogs with serious aggression problems do not appear to have been victimized by physical punishment. Instead, aggression seems to emerge under the influence of a genetic predisposition and the incubation of nervous or insecure attachments, interactive conflict and tensions, entrapment dynamics and social ambivalence, adverse dietary and environmental conditions, inadequate exercise and play, excessive confinement and restraint (isolation), suboptimal attention and tactile stimulation, autonomic dysregulation, or the absence of appropriate training and play. In short, as the result of an emergent reactive coping style, selective attention and impulse-control capacities may be degraded and impaired, causing the dog to become increasingly inattentive, uncooperative, aloof, or impulsive—attributes often claimed to be evidence of dominance problems.

These various issues stress the danger inherent to approaches that take anthropic ideas and symbols such as *dominance* and reify them into substantive causes or proximate relations in order to rationalize intrusive and aversive behavior-change procedures that ironically are not too dissimilar from the *real* causes of aggression. A substantive body of human research indicates that perceived power and dominance ideation promotes a number of cognitive and behavioral effects on how parents, teachers, and caregivers cope and respond to the challenging behavior of vulnerable dependents (Bugental et al., 1993, 1997, and 1999a), findings that are directly relevant to how family members and professionals cope with the management and treatment of problem canine behavior. The designation of low perceived power or high perceived power is based on the relative importance that owners place on accessible and controllable behavioral causes versus causes that are predominantly under a child's control or causes that are perceived as being uncontrollable by both a dog and its owner (e.g., disease model). For example, the attribution of stubbornness as a cause of uncooperative behavior is an indicator of low perceived power, since the lack of cooperation is perceived predominantly as being under the control and intent of a stubborn dog or child. Similarly, consultants and trainers operating under the influence of a low-perceived-power construct may attribute a dominant attitude and other highly speculative causes to explain the etiology of aggression and challenging behavior. The tendency to attribute attitudinal causes associated with the dominance ideation may be linked with excessively intrusive or aversive training strategies or reliance on unproven nutritional or psychopharmacological protocols.

Low-power owners (like low-power parents with regard to their children) tend to explain their dog's misbehavior in terms of causes that lie outside of their control or understanding. The low-power behavior modifier may perpetuate this perception by searching for causes of the problem in the dog's attitude or distant history that resonate with the anthropic dominance myth. From the very outset of such therapy relationships, the dog's behavior may be framed in terms of power-ascendant motives and a preoccupation with finding ways to leverage power and control over it. Instead of highlighting how social ambivalence and inconsistent control efforts may have contributed to the problem, the counselor may assign an attitudinal cause to behavior and give the owner a diagnostic label with which to justify abusive deprivational and emotional treatment procedures that resonate with and confirm the owner's powerlessness. Unfortunately, by locating the causes of aggression in a dominant attitude or perception of rank, the trainer/consultant may only succeed in strengthening the owner's private distortions and belief, thereby perpetuating problematic power-dominance dynamics. The seeking and getting of a diagnostic label may tap a primitive urge to possess a magical name, causing a low-power owners or supplicant to seek out the wisdom of a low-power behavioral hierophant, hoping for a revelation, a magical name, a vision of the future, a potion, or a set of rituals with which to placate the mysterious forces causing the dog to misbehave. With the possession of a name, the low-power owner may feel empowered by virtue of the arcane scientific authority and significance attributed to it. Obviously, the practice of diagnostic labeling is extremely problematic, and especially so when the name shifts from a merely descriptive significance to causal significance; that is, the diagnostic label is no longer used to specify a collection of symptoms but now implies explanatory power to identify a physiological or phylogenetic cause. The interpretations used by low-power behavior modifiers are often little more than descriptive platitudes and elaborate myths that lack coherent causal significance. Unfortunately, the nominal fallacy (i.e., confusing naming with explaining) is widely committed in the context of treating canine adjustment problems.

The autoprotective perspective is more parsimonious and consistent with the collection of known facts than is the dominance account (see *Antipredatory Strategy and Autoprotection versus Dominance* in Chapter 8). Although an oversimplification itself, the antipredator hypothesis is a much less harmful over simplification than is the dominance myth. The antipredator model puts the owner in an instrumental role, thereby correctly emphasizing that human-dog interaction and, in particular, human action, rather than malevolent canine intent and power-dominance motivations, are the primary causes to blame (if any) for domestic aggression; dogs, like most prey animals, rarely go out of their way to instigate aggressive contests, at least not without significant agitation and due cause for such anomalous behavior. In general, dogs are not in need of therapy to modify a distorted "perception of rank," but the dog and its owner may need to learn how to build relations conducive to cooperative exchanges and autonomic attunement while integrating secure social and place attachments. Like a dog living under social ambivalence and dispersive tensions, an abused child may also adopt an antipredatory orientation toward the parent and acquire the habits of a frightened prey animal but secretly harbor or surreptitiously act out fantasies of cruelty on the dog. As the child enters into power relations with other children and the family dog, the parent's predatory model may become apparent in the child's abusive and ambiguous relations with the dog, perhaps causing him or her to become increasingly exploitive and intrusive toward the dog while extracting pleasure from its distress and victimization. Children that treat dogs abusively and communicate ambiguous affection and play signals might, therefore, reflect some of the same dynamics expressed in the reactive behavior of the dog. The child and the dog may mirror and express similarly reactive behaviors, ambivalence, and impulsivity flowing from exposure to the same parental emotional or physical abuse.

The relationship formed between the owner and the behavior modifier appears to exert a profound influence on the owner's perception of control, depending on the nature of the causes (accessible versus inaccessible) attributed to the problem, and the treatment strategy selected to resolve it. The typical treatment strategy adopted is based on either a proactive open-stance orientation directed toward accessible causes or a reactive closed-stance orientation directed toward inaccessible causes (i.e., relatively uncontrollable or unknown). A major ethical and welfare consideration recommending the autoprotective account of canine domestic aggression is that it avoids evoking anthropic dominance ideation and the biased framing of

challenging dog behavior in terms that encourage the use of abusive or ineffectual treatment programs aimed at coercing a change in the dog's "dominant" attitude or perception of rank. The dominance narrative is widely associated with the use of abusive emotional deprivation, traumatizing physical punishment and restraint tactics, and unproven pharmacological interventions.

The cynopraxic approach emphasizes counseling and therapy aimed at facilitating improved attention and impulse control, integrating affectionate and playful relations, supporting autoinitiated behavior and emotional autoregulation, and promoting a gratifying life experience—changes that naturally reduce the risk of domestic aggression. An important goal of cynopraxic counseling and therapy is to empower the owner with basic skills and dog sense to promote a fair balance of control and appreciation of the dog's needs, while improving the dog's ability to engage in interactive prosocial exchanges rather than resorting to reactive antisocial behavior. In particular, play represents a potent tool for adjusting the social imbalance contributing to impulsivity and reactive behavior. Comprehensive cynopraxic training and behavior-therapy efforts serve to promote changes that facilitate a functional equilibrium at virtually every level of behavioral organization. These social changes are brought about by the integration of secure attachments and an enhanced QOL that benefits both the dog and the family members.

PROBLEMATIC TRENDS AND OBSTACLES TO ADAPTIVE COPING AND ATTUNEMENT

In addition to avoiding training procedures that are needlessly aversive, cynopraxic trainers avoid procedures that intrude excessively upon a dog's freedom incentive (see *Hydran-Protean Side Effects, the Dead-dog Rule, and the LIMA Principle*). Training efforts that inappropriately restrict a dog's ability to initiate goal-directed behavior not only adversely impact the dog's QOL but often do so without contributing any real therapeutic benefit. For example, inappropriate restraint or isolation, pointless deprivation procedures, intrusive rules of interaction, and tedious extinction and training rituals may be of little positive benefit with respect to training goals but impose time-consuming hardships on the owner, impede the bonding processes, and impair the dog's ability to adjust, perhaps making the problem worse. Although highly intrusive procedures do not generate physical pain, they can produce significant *emotional pain* and distress while augmenting interactive conflict.

Pharmacological Control of Behavior

In recent years, the introduction of a medical model of dog behavior has led some practitioners to treat adjustment problems as mental disorders having physical causes and often to emphasize the role of disease as the underlying cause of behavior problems (Mills, 2003). Although the medical model is not entirely without merit, as some valid parallels exist between certain psychiatric disorders and canine behavior disorders and undoubtedly some behavior disturbances are the result of disease, overly speculative assumptions, problematic diagnostic labels, and an excessive reliance on psychotropic drugs based on rationale borrowed from human psychiatry serve only to compound the current puzzlement regarding the etiology and functional significance of canine adjustment problems. In addition to emphasizing disease etiologies and the importance of drugs to treat behavior problems, many practitioners who stress the medical model claim special authority pertaining to matters of diagnosis whereby the "physical" causes of the problem are purportedly identified, usually by means of speculative inferences from emotional and behavioral signs. These putative but unproven physical causes are then targeted with various medications believed to mediate a resolution of the problem. Unfortunately, the various inclusion and exclusion criteria used to make behavioral diagnoses and related drug-treatment decisions tend to cause referring professionals and owners to defer treatment until the canine adjustment problem reaches a form that threatens the dog with relinquishment or

euthanasia, rather than initiate behavioral treatment at the first sign of a problem. The pharmacological approach resonates with the low-power owner's basic assumptions, placing the causes of the dog's adjustment problems beyond the scope of conventional training and socialization efforts. The adjustment problem is encapsulated within an involuntary subdomain of physiology that places it outside of the dog's voluntary control and prevents its resolution without the help of drugs. In contrast, the cynopraxic approach views the physical changes to brain that mediate disturbance as the result of the accumulative effect of conflictive social exchanges and reactive adjustments in response to environments chronically lacking sufficient predictability and controllability to promote an adaptive coping style. Conversely, by changing interactive habits of social exchange to promote interactive harmony in combination with appropriate QOL changes that support the dog's needs, the physiological causes of disturbance are replaced by physiological changes conducive to adaptive optimization and social adjustment.

Although drugs are potentially useful in some refractory cases, the current state of the art remains investigational, and the ultimate benefits of drug therapy are uncertain, especially with respect to the control of domestic aggression problems (see *Pharmacological Control of Aggression* in Chapter 6). Even in the realm of human psychiatry, the efficacy of the most commonly prescribed mood-altering drugs used to treat anxiety and depression disorders has been questioned. Kirsch and colleagues (2002; see also Kirsch and Sapirstein, 1998), for example, who performed an extensive meta-analysis of treatment data submitted to the U.S. Food and Drug Administration (FDA) between 1987 and 1999, found that 80% of the clinical response of humans to six commonly prescribed antidepressants was duplicated in placebo control groups, suggesting that the selective serotonin reuptake inhibitors (SSRIs) tested may have little clinical effect separable from that of placebo. A remarkable neuroimaging study of human patients treated for depression has shown that placebo responders and fluoxetine responders show similar changes in glucose metabolism in specific cortical and limbic areas, concluding that the "administration of placebo is not absence of treatment, just an absence of active medication" (Mayberg et al., 2002). In addition, the study revealed that the two groups responded differently to fluoxetine, with the drug producing specific changes in the hippocampus and brainstem of fluoxetine responders after 1 week of therapy that predicted a long-term response to the medication. Responders also showed a switch effect in response to drug therapy that resulted in an initial elevation of posterior cingulate metabolic activity followed by a decrease and then a gradual increase over the 6-week period of therapy—a pattern of change not exhibited by placebo responders. These distinct metabolic changes that differentiate responders from nonresponders suggest that tympanic temperature fluctuations might be present among dogs that could be tracked to help identify serotonergic responders from nonresponders (see *Functional Lateralization and Tympanic Temperature* in Chapter 9).

Although the FDA appears to enforce strict standards of efficacy to gain approval on certain classes of drugs, there appears to be a troubling double standard with respect to others, perhaps including the level of stringency applied to psychotropic drugs such as SSRIs. However, the most egregious and disturbing example of a double standard used to evaluate drug efficacy is the special and protected status afforded to homeopathic substances, described by one FDA representative as "kinder, gentler medicine" (Stehlin, 1996). Incredibly, homeopathic remedies are approved as drugs without meeting the rigorous standards of proven efficacy set for other drugs issued FDA approval. A meta-analysis of 89 studies using homeopathic substances to treat various medical conditions concluded, "Our study has no major implications for clinical practice because we found little evidence of effectiveness of any single homoeopathic approach on any single clinical condition" (Linde et al., 1997:840).

With regard to serotonergic antidepressants and dog behavior problems, even when apparently efficacious in the short term, aggression-controlling medications are unlikely to succeed in the long term without the support of complementary behavior therapy. The therapeutic use of social placebo is acknowledged as a valuable tool in the cynopraxic treatment of behavior problems (see *Social Placebo* in Volume 2, Chapter 10), but the administration of costly psychotropic drugs that exert potential health-threatening side effects for the sake of questionable benefits that do not rise above placebo alone raises serious ethical and welfare concerns. In any case, no drug or combination of drugs currently available can provide the sweeping range of dramatic and subtle balancing and integrative effects that are mediated by cynopraxic training and play therapy (see *Modulatory and Unifying Effects of Play* in Chapter 6). Comprehensive cynopraxic training and therapy efforts promote changes that facilitate a functional equilibrium at virtually every level of neural organization. Cynopraxic therapy is based on the assumption that social exchange promoting adjustments conducive to an adaptive coping style and secure attachments serve simultaneously to mediate physical alterations of the neuronal substrates mediating social ambivalence and reactive behavior. In particular, play therapy represents a potent tool for adjusting autonomic imbalance and reducing the allostatic load perturbing the complex feed-forward trafficking of neuronal networks that contribute to the etiology of adjustment problems (see *Cynopraxis: Allostasis, Adaptability, and Health*).

When drugs are used to manage intractable behavior problems, the goal should be to alleviate allostatic load and to promote neurobiological changes conducive to social affiliation and playfulness. Pharmacological efforts used merely to suppress undesirable behavior seem wrongheaded, violate the dead-dog rule, and are intrinsically problematic with respect to the basic bond and QOL tenets of cynopraxis. Dogs that engage in autoprotective behavior usually do so out of emotional extremis associated with chronic stress and allostatic load. Using behavior modification, restraint and isolation, emotional deprivation, or drugs to suppress undesirable behavior, without alleviating the underlying social and environmental causes hindering a dog's ability to cope adaptively, violates basic welfare principles (Broom and Johnson, 1993).

Mechanical Suppression of Behavior

The restrictive loss of freedom imposed by excessive crate confinement is especially prone to cause harm in cases where the procedure is used in the absence of constructive training efforts; that is, where crate confinement is made into a way of life or a *steel straitjacket* for the purpose of preventing some undesirable behavior by mechanically suppressing all behavior. The word *crate* carries the implication of a temporary container used for the purpose of stowing an animal away, whereas the word *cage* has the added onus of being a permanent place of restrictive confinement used to control an animal's behavior, particularly an animal regarded as dangerous and untrustworthy. A cage serves to isolate and restrain an animal in a way that makes it constantly available for various exploitive purposes that are generally performed against its will, such as a spectacle for public viewing in zoos, for entertainment on a stage, or as an object of scientific investigation. Whereas a dangerous wild animal might be briefly crated for transport or medical treatment, its permanent place of confinement and isolation from other animals and people is a cage. In contrast, domestic animals are *housed* in pens, coops, stalls, and so forth, depending on the needs of the species and the uses made of the animal. In the case of dogs, long-term confinement generally involves the use of a kennel and adjoining run appropriate to the dog's size, an arrangement that gives the dog access to both indoor and outdoor environs to rest or move about freely and to eliminate away from its sleeping and eating areas. When a dog must be kenneled on a long-term basis, at a minimum the arrangement should include the company of another dog, preferably of a similar size, friendly disposition, and a compatible same or opposite sex companion. In designing and managing environments used for animal confinement, appropriate consideration should be given to making the living space compatible with species-typical social predilections and group-organizing tendencies. Of critical importance for the housing of dogs is the provision of adequate opportunities to engage in pack-coordinated activities, which require access to large open areas for social interaction. In the case of a dog living in a home, putting the dog in the backyard alone is inadequate with respect to social needs—space alone does not confer significant benefit. Social activity needs are nicely satisfied within in the home by the combination of daily training, tug-and-retrieve play, and neighborhood walks.

Many advocates of long-term crate confinement claim that dogs are phylogenetically preadapted to live in a crate. These conclusions are based on various fallacious assumptions derived from inappropriate comparisons with the use of dens by wild canids and feral dogs. In reality, a crate has far more in common with a trap (or grave) than it does with a den. Further, a den actually has far more in common with a home, the natural environment of a dog, providing access to communal indoor and outdoor living spaces via a two-way door. An obvious distinction between a den and a crate is physical entrapment, isolation, and inescapability. While the den provides the mother with the seclusion and security that she needs to deliver and care for her young, it does not restrict her freedom of movement, as the crate does. Instead of providing a safe environ for her young, the crate serves the express purpose of separating the dog from social attachment objects. Further, instead of promoting comfort and safety, the inescapable exclusion imposed by crate confinement appears to confer an increased vulnerability for disruptive emotional arousal and insecure place attachments. Most puppies and dogs show a high degree of aversive arousal when first exposed to crate confinement, which is consistent with the foregoing comparison. After learning that the crate is inescapable, however, dogs appear to treat the crate in a paradoxical manner analogous to persons affected by the Stockholm syndrome (Ochberg and Soskis, 1982); that is, they appear to form strong attachments with the crate, which becomes the place they identify as home.

The primary motivation governing the use of crates is similar to the reason certain wild animals are isolated in cages; viz., a dog's freedom is perceived as representing some sort of threat or risk, usually in association with destructive habits or elimination problems. The daily ritual of cajoling and luring the dog into the crate may also gradually result in the dog acquiring a growing mistrust toward the owner, as reflected in its refusal to cooperate in other ways not directly related to confinement. The widespread practice of routinely caging a dog at night and then again during the day for periods totaling 16 to 18 hours (or more) is an extremely problematic practice that should not be condoned or encouraged, because it probably underlies the development of many adjustment problems, including aggression.

For many pet trainers, pet-trade breeders, and like-minded veterinarians, caging is frequently promoted as a humane alternative to more time-consuming and skill-intensive training efforts. Although crate confinement can be a useful asset when integrated into a competent training program, to expose a dog repeatedly to 16 to 18 hours of daily caging makes no sense. The fact that a dog can survive many months of such solitary confinement in a space barely big enough for it to turn around is testament to its flexibility. In addition to crate confinement, various devices are used to supplement intrusive control efforts, such as muzzles used to restrict barking, thereby extending mechanical control over the dog's vocal behavior while it is in the cage. In other cases, owners use various behavior-activated collars designed to deliver a deterrent spray or electrical charge to control undesirable behavior while the dog is inside the crate. To restrain compensatory excitability and impulsivity, some ill-informed advisers might further recommend that the owner stop all play activities, especially tugging and roughhousing. To complete the picture, the owner may be sold on homeopathic remedies and vitamin supplements, fragrant odors and pheromones, or flower essence drops put in the dog's water to help reduce its stress!

Cynopraxis: Allostasis, Adaptability, and Health

At every step in a dog's ontogeny, predictive relations are refined and integrated into a base of genetic and experiential *prior knowledge*. These predictive relations are organized to promote stability through change, referred to as *allostasis* (Sterling, 2004). Allostatic adjustments enable dogs to anticipate and avoid future risks to stability, thus enhancing adaptive efficiency by responding to predictive signals. The genes that regulate neuronal activity depend heavily on experience for the information needed to maintain the brain's functional stability and capacity for coping proactively with change. The feed-forward unfolding of genetic information via experience-dependent gene activation and suppression is consistent with the notion that regulatory genes are responsive to positive and negative prediction-error signals. Consequently, causing neuronal activity to increase or decrease results in the production of structural proteins and enzymes, and thereby alters the neurophysiology in the process of mediating allostasis (Sterling and Eyer, 1988). Thus, the process of emergent individuation is seamlessly interwoven into a multitude of neurobiological changes that mediate cognitive, motivational, and behavioral adjustments. During such accommodation and allostatic change, the activation of neural protein synthesis and synapse building serves to integrate predictive information into the physical substance of the organism, leading to far-reaching benefits or harm influencing not only behavioral adaptation but also biological adaptation. By such means, *knowledge* acquired by experience is directly integrated into the neurobiological phenotype from where it exerts numerous adaptive and maladaptive effects on the developing organism (Kolb and Whishaw, 1998).

Acute stress is triggered in response to the detection of discrepant events that exceed the normal *safe* range of accustomed variability in combination with a perception of uncontrollability; that is, stress is a biological response to the violation of expectancy or a failure to establish predictive control over significant motivation events. Such events elicit intense state arousal, active vigilance, and increased action readiness in anticipation of reactive emergency or defensive adjustments. Thus, chronic and uncontrollable challenges (loss of comfort), threats (loss of safety), and unconditioned aversive events mismatching prediction-control expectancies promote stress and allostatic load that adversely affect a dog's adaptability. Chronic exposure to aversive conflict situations perceived as uncontrollable tends to become increasingly problematic when they are also inescapable. Allostatic load associated with social ambivalence and entrapment is hypothesized to orchestrate widespread neuronal changes and emotional disturbances that adversely affect selective attention and impulse control.

Under social and environmental circumstances where a balance of predictive exchange is lacking, the ensuing instability and allostatic load make the work of adaptation increasingly costly. A failure to integrate a mutually satisfying household relationship based on predictable and controllable relations is not only disruptive at the level of social exchange—the consequences of such influences impact at various levels of a dog's biology and may gradually impair its capacity to adapt. According to cynopraxic theory, many maladies affecting canine health and well-being are traceable to dis-ease associated with chronic interactive conflict and compensatory allostatic load adversely impacting critical biological systems necessary to sustain health and survival fitness (see *Immune Stress and Cytokines* in Chapter 6 and *Stress, Thyroid Deficiency, Hypocortisolism, and Aggression* in Chapter 8). As such, cynopraxic therapy serves to promote both behavioral and biological stability by mediating changes that reduce interactive conflict and promote mutual appreciation and interactive harmony while enhancing the human-dog bond and improving the dog's QOL. The capacity of cynopraxic therapy to promote beneficial changes depends on the integration predictive control relations mediated by social exchange and transactions governed by a principle of fairness promoting mutual reward, cooperation, and affectionate playfulness between interactive partners around points of common interest and potential conflict.

HYDRAN-PROTEAN SIDE EFFECTS, THE DEAD-DOG RULE, AND THE LIMA PRINCIPLE

Aversive procedures are legitimate and valuable tools for controlling undesirable behavior, but such techniques can be rapidly debauched into a form that substantially complicates matters. Technically, punishment results when established control expectancies are disconfirmed, for example, when the trainer discontinues an attractive or aversive contingency. Punishment occurs when the dog recognizes that some previously successful action no longer controls the occurrence of some attractive or aversive event. Severe and sustained aversive stimulations in the absence of options to escape (e.g., beating) are of no use in dog training and for whatever reasons such nasty actions are performed they are likely to foster a far worse problem.

Just as chopping off the mythical Hydra's head only caused her to sprout more monstrous and threatening replacements growing out of the severed stump, the use of inappropriate physical punishment, restraint, and manhandling may only serve to stimulate autoprotective behavior and initiate various unanticipated vicious-circle effects. In such cases, the escalation of conflict and aversive arousal evoked by severe physical punishment may cause difficult behaviors to transform into even worse forms, especially in cases where the root causes of the problem are left unresolved. Homer's story of Proteus illustrates other aspects of potential harm wrought by inappropriate punishment and interactive conflict. For ancient seekers wishing to foresee the future, the water divinity had to be seized and held tightly as he morphed through a frightful array of threatening forms, until he finally gave in and returned to his normal form to give prophecy. The myth has obvious positive implications related to the constructive use of response prevention and blocking techniques, but more importantly with respect to the present topic, the myth resonates symbolically with the adverse effects of interactive struggles and tensions around points of conflict where the future is left uncertain until the conflict is resolved. Actions that emerge in the context of persistent conflictive exchange are often highly reactive and pose many significant training challenges and risks. Further, as a result of a history of contentious interaction, dogs and people may gradually lose their capacity for mutual attraction and tolerance, becoming increasingly ambivalent, intolerant of uncertainty, and reactive toward the ordinary losses and risks associated with social exchange. Instead of engaging in friendly cooperation, the owner and dog may engage one another as adversaries in the process of morphing a veritable pantheon of adjustment problems out of the toxic conflict dynamics that bind them together.

All variation in canine social behavior develops in the context of coping styles emerging in various ways around interactive conflict. As such, the intersection of human and canine control vectors define the field of interactive possibility. Only by working through conflict by holding protean advantage-seeking efforts at bay and by opening a space of fair exchange and mutual appreciation around conflict situations can the other be perceived as a cooperator rather than a dominator or exploiter. With the restoration of *normal exchange*, the unifying relations and governance needed to promote an adaptive coping style can be pursued as a harmonious social space is extended over the field of conflict situations.

Despite obvious limitations and risks, aversive procedures are a necessary aspect of dog training and behavior-problem solving that cannot be neglected or substituted for (e.g., by drugs) when competent inhibitory control over highly motivated behavior is being established. These procedures are of great value in the context of basic training, the treatment of adjustment problems, and the integration of secure attachments. To maximize the benefits and to minimize the adverse effects of training procedures that compel dogs to act or not act in particular ways, two general guidelines appear to be useful: the least intrusive and minimally aversive (LIMA) principle and the dead-dog rule. The LIMA principle addresses the excesses and abuses that might arise when aversive or intrusive dog-training procedures are implemented. As such, it applies to both positive and negative punishment, and covers procedures that generate states of emotional

pain and deprivation (e.g., long-term cold shouldering, crate confinement/isolation, and various restraint techniques). The LIMA principle entails that trainers use the least intrusive and minimally aversive technique likely to succeed in achieving a training objective with minimal risk of producing adverse side effects. Essentially, the LIMA principle is a competency criterion, since only competent trainers possessing the necessary know-how can make the required assessments and have the skills needed to ensure that the least intrusive and aversive procedure is in fact used. To speak of the effective and humane use of dog-training procedures in the absence of competency criterion borders on the ridiculous. Accordingly, incompetent uses of attractive and aversive motivational stimuli to modify dog behavior are liable to produce harmful effects that violate the dog's interests and breech the trust of the responsible dog owners seeking help.

A second general guideline that promotes the effective use of training procedures is the dead-dog rule, which recommends that training criteria and objectives be defined in terms that a dead dog cannot satisfy (see *Dead-dog Rule* in Volume 2, Chapter 2). In essence, the dead-dog rule is a complementary logic for framing the LIMA principle. By converting training goals into affirmative statements and identifying objectives that can be achieved only by a live dog, the resultant perspective is biased toward reward-based training efforts. For example, instead of training a dog not to bite (dead dogs do not bite), the dog is trained to be friendly and trusting, that is, to show affectionate, cooperative, and playful behavior incompatible with aggression— behavior that a dead dog cannot do. In the case of aversive motivational stimuli used in the context of aversive inhibitory control, the training objective is best described in terms of positive behavioral change that places the primary emphasis on escape-avoidance adjustments and the establishment of a *training space*, based on the acquisition of predictive information and a socially acceptable *escape-to-safety* response that result in reward. When properly performed, all training is reward based insofar as the dog learns how to control attractive and aversive events while negotiating conflict. In the context of reward-based training, the dead-dog rule and the LIMA principle provide general guidelines for the use of attractive and aversive motivational stimuli to modify dog behavior (see *Compliance* in Volume 2, Chapter 2). When aversive procedures are used, the trainer should possess an objective rationale and the skills necessary to implement the procedures safely and effectively. The suppression of behavior by means of inhibitory procedures is appropriate and useful when regulating behavior governed by an excitatory imbalance and impulsivity but only to the extent that it is performed in the context of coordinated reward-based activities aimed at filling the void.

Cynopraxic trainers acknowledge and respect the dog's preference for pleasure by advocating the use of procedures that utilize reward and minimize punishment. However, to train a dog to a reasonable degree of reliability, the use of both attractive and aversive motivational incentives is an inescapable fact of life. In an important sense, reward and punishment are not properties of motivational stimuli or evoked attractive or aversive states but rather flow from the dog's ability to produce outcomes that either meet or exceed prediction-control expectancies. Training is not about making dogs feel good or bad—rather it is about enabling them to adapt well.

REFERENCES

Albonetti ME and Farabollini F (1995). Effects of single restraint on the defensive behavior of male and female rats. *Physiol Behav*, 57:431–437.

Allen BD, Cummings JF, and De Lahunta A (1974). The effects of prefrontal lobotomy on aggressive behavior in dogs. *Cornell Vet*, 64:201-216.

Allman J (2000). *Evolving Brains*. New York: Scientific American Libraries.

Alpert JE, Petersen T, Roffi PA, et al. (2003). Behavioral and emotional disturbances in the offspring of depressed parents with anger attacks. *Psychother Psychosom*, 72:102–106.

An X, Bandler R, Ongur D, and Price JL (1998). Prefrontal cortical projections to longitudinal columns in the midbrain periaqueductal gray in macaque monkeys. *J Comp Neurol*, 401:455-479.

Anderson OD (1941). The role of the glands of internal secretion in the production of behavioral types in the dog based on a study of behavior by the conditioned reflex method. In CR Stockard (Ed), *The Genetic and Endocrine Basis for Differences in Form and Behavior as Elucidated by Studies of Contrasted Pure-line Dog Breeds and Their Hybrids* (American Anatomy Memoir 19). Philadelphia: Wistar Institute of Anatomy and Biology.

Appel J, Arms N, Horner R, and Carr WJ (1999). Long-term olfactory memory in companion dogs. Presented at the Annual Meeting of the Animal Behavior Society, Bucknell University, Lewisburg, PA, 27–30 June.

Arons CD and Shoemaker WJ (1992). The distribution of catecholamines and beta-endorphin in the brains of three behaviorally distinct breeds of dogs and their F_{1} hybrids. *Brain Res*, 594:31–39.

Badre D and Wagner AD (2004). Selection, integration, and conflict monitoring: Assessing the nature and generality of prefrontal cognitive control mechanisms. *Neuron*, 41:473–487.

Baxter MG and Murray EA (2002). The amygdala and reward. *Nat Rev Neurosci*, 3:563–572.

Belyaev DK, Plyusnina IZ, and Trut LN (1984/85). Domestication in the silver fox (*Vulpes vulpes*): Changes in physiological boundaries of the sensitive period of primary socialization. *Appl Anim Behav Sci*, 13:359–370.

Bentley PJ (1976). *Comparative Vertebrate Endocrinology*. New York: Cambridge University Press.

Blass EM and Fitzgerald E (1988). Milk-induced analgesia and comforting in 10-day-old rats: Opioid mediation. *Pharmacol Biochem Behav*, 29:9-13.

Blass E, Fitzgerald E, and Kehoe P (1987). Interactions between sucrose, pain and isolation distress. *Pharmacol Biochem Behav*, 26:483-489.

Blass EM and Shah A (1995). Pain-reducing properties of sucrose in human newborns. *Chem Sens*, 20:29-35.

Blass EM and Shide DJ (1994). Some comparisons among the calming and pain-relieving effects of sucrose, glucose, fructose and lactose in infant rats. *Chem Senses*, 19:239-249.

Brosvic GM, Taylor JN, and Dihoff RE (2002). Influences of early thyroid hormone manipulations: Delays in pup motor and exploratory behavior are evident in adult operant performance. *Physiol Behav*, 75:697–715.

Brouha L and Nowak SJG (1939). The role of the vagus in the cardiac-accelerator action of atropine in sympathectomized dogs. *J Physiol*, 95:439–453.

Brouha L, Cannon WB, Dill DB. (1936). The heart rate of the sympathectomized dog in rest and exercise. *J Physiol*, 87:345–359.

Brown AS, Begg MD, Gravenstein S, et al. (2004). Serologic evidence of prenatal influenza in the etiology of schizophrenia. *Arch Gen Psychiatry*, 61:774–780.

Bugental DB, Blue J, Cortez V, et al. (1993). Social cognitions as organizers of autonomic and affective responses to social challenge. *J Pers Soc Psychol*, 64:94–103.

Bugental DB, Lyon JE, Krantz J, and Cortez V (1997). Who's the boss? Differential accessibility of dominance ideation in parent-child relationships. *J Pers Soc Psychol*, 72:1297–1309.

Bugental DB, Lewis JC, Lin E, Lyon J, and Kopeikin H (1999a). In charge but not in control: The management of teaching relationships by adults with low perceived power. *Dev Psychol*, 35:1367–1378.

Bugental DB, Lyon JE, Lin EK, et al. (1999b). Children "tune out" in response to the ambiguous communication style of powerless adults. *Child Dev*, 70:214–230.

Caffe AR, Van Leeuwen FW, and Luiten PG (1987).Vasopressin cells in the medial amygdala of the rat project to the lateral septum and ventral hippocampus. *J Comp Neurol*, 261:237-252.

Call J, Bräuer J, Kaminski J, and Tomasello M (2002). Domestic dogs are sensitive to the attentional state of humans. *J Comp Psychol*, 117:257–263.

Cardinal RN, Parkinson JA, Hall J, and Everitt BJ (2002). Emotion and motivation: The role of the amygdala, ventral striatum, and prefrontal cortex. *Neurosci Biobehav Rev*, 26:321–352.

Carretie L, Martin-Loeches M, Hinojosa JA, and Mercado F (2001). Emotion and attention interaction studied through event-related potentials. *J Cogn Neurosci*, 13:1109–1128.

Charney DS (2004). Psychobiological mechanisms of resilience and vulnerability: Implications for successful adaptation to extreme stress. *Am J Psychiat*, 161:195-216.

Colborn T (2004). Neurodevelopment and endocrine disruption neurodevelopment and endocrine disruption. *Environ Health Perspect*, 112:944–948.

Collet C, Dittmar A, and Vernet-Maury F (1999). Programming or inhibiting action: Evidence for differential autonomic nervous system response patterns. *Int J Psychophysiol*, 32:261–276.

Connolly CC, Steiner KE, Stevenson RW, et al. (1991). Regulation of glucose metabolism by norepinephrine in conscious dogs. *Am J Physiol*, 261:764–772.

Corson SA (1966). Conditioning of water and electrolyte excretion. In R Levine (Ed), *Endocrines and the Central Nervous System*. Baltimore: Williams and Wilkins.

Corson SA and O'Leary Corson E (1969). The effects of psychotropic drugs on conditioning of water and electrolyte excretion: Experimental research and clinical implications. In A Pletscher, A Marino, and P Pinkerton (Eds), *Psychotropic Drugs in Internal Medicine: The Theoretic Experimental and Clinical Bases for a Rational Application of Psychopharmacotherapy in Internal Diseases*. Amsterdam: Excerpta Medica Foundation.

Corson SA and O'Leary Corson E (1976). Constitutional differences in physiologic adaptation to stress and distress. In G Serban (Ed), *Psychopathology of Human Adaptation*. New York: Plenum.

Corson SA, O'Leary Corson E, Kirilcuk B, et al. (1973). Differential effects of amphetamines on clinically relevant dog models of hyperkinesis and stereotypy: Relevance to Huntington's Chorea. In A Barbeau, TN Chase, and GW Paulson (Eds), *Advances in Neurology*, Vol 1. New York: Raven.

Crespi LP (1942). Quantitative variation of incentive and performance in the white rat. *Amer J Psychol*, 55:467-517.

Crockford SJ (2002). Animal domestication and heterochronic speciation: The role of thyroid hormone. In N Minugh-Purvis and K McNamara (Eds), *Human Evolution Through Developmental Change*. Baltimore: Johns Hopkins University Press.

Dalley JW, Theobald DE, Eagle DM, et al. (2002). Deficits in impulse control associated with tonically-elevated serotonergic function in rat prefrontal cortex. *Neuropsychopharmacology*, 26:716-728.

De Almeida RM and Miczek KA (2002). Aggression escalated by social instigation or by discontinuation of reinforcement ("frustration") in mice: Inhibition by anpirtoline: a $5-HT_{1B}$ receptor agonist. *Neuropsychopharmacology*, 27:171-181.

De Boer SF, Van der Vegt BJ, and Koolhaas JM (2003). Individual variation in aggression of feral rodent strains: A standard for the genetics of aggression and violence? *Behav Genet*, 33:485-501.

Degroot A and Treit D (2004). Anxiety is functionally segregated within the septo-hippocampal system. *Brain Res*, 1001:60-71.

Delta Society (2001). *Professional Standards for the Dog Trainers: Effective, Humane Principles*. Renton, WA: Delta Society. http://www.deltasociety.org/standards/standards.htm.

Depaulis A, Keay KA, and Bandler R (1994). Quiescence and hyperactivity evoked by activation of cell bodies in the ventrolateral midbrain periaqueductal gray of the rat. *Exp Brain Res*, 99:75-83.

Dess NK and Overmier JB (1989). Generalized learned irrelevance: Proactive effects on Pavlovian conditioning in dogs. *Learn Motiv*, 20:1–14.

Di Matteo V, Cacchio M, Di Giulio C, and Esposito E (2002). Role of serotonin (2C) receptors in the control of brain dopaminergic function. *Pharmacol Biochem Behav*, 71:727-734.

Dickinson A (1980). *Contemporary Animal Learning Theory*. Cambridge: Cambridge University Press.

Dinsmoor JA (2001). Stimuli inevitably generated by behavior that avoids electric shock are inherently reinforcing. *J Exp Anal Behav*, 75:311–333.

Dowling AL, Martz GU, Leonard JL, and Zoeller RT (2000). Acute changes in maternal thyroid hormone induce rapid and transient changes in gene expression in fetal rat brain. *J Neurosci*, 20:2255–2265.

Dulawa SC, Grandy DK, Low MJ, et al. (1999). Dopamine D4 receptor-knock-out mice exhibit reduced exploration of novel stimuli . *J Neurosci*, 19:9550-9556.

Eisenberger NI, Lieberman MD, and Williams KD (2003). Does rejection hurt? An fMRI study of social exclusion. *Science*, 302:290–292.

Eison AS and Mullins UL (1996). Regulation of central 5-HT$_{2A}$ receptors: a review of in vivo studies. *Behav Brain Res*, 73:177-181.

El Fazaa S, Gharbi N, Kamoun A, and Somody L (2000). Vasopressin and A1 noradrenaline turnover during food or water deprivation in the rat. *Comp Biochem Physiol [C]*, 126:129–137.

Farkas E, Jansen AS, and Loewy AD (1998). Periaqueductal gray matter input to cardiac-related sympathetic premotor neurons. *Brain Res*, 792:179-192.

Fekete C, Kelly J, Mihaly E, Sarkar S, et al. (2001). Neuropeptide Y has a central inhibitory action on the hypothalamic-pituitary-thyroid axis. *Endocrinology*, 142:2606–2613.

Fekete C, Sarkar S, Rand WM, et al. (2002). Neuropeptide Y1 and Y5 receptors mediate the effects of neuropeptide Y on the hypothalamic-pituitary-thyroid axis. *Endocrinology*, 143:4513–4519.

Ferrari PF, Gallese V, Rizzolatti G, and Fogassi L (2003). Mirror neurons responding to the observation of ingestive and communicative mouth actions in the monkey ventral premotor cortex. *Eur J Neurosci*, 17:1703–1714.

Ferrell F (1984). Preference for sugars and nonnutritve sweeteners in young beagles. *Neurosci Biobeh Rev*, 8:199-203.

Field T, Diego M, Hernandez-Reif M, et al. (2003). Pregnancy anxiety and comorbid depression and anger: Effects on the fetus and neonate. *Depress Anxiety*, 17:140–151.

Finck KS (1993). Children, their pet dogs, and affect attunement [PhD dissertation]. Garden City, NY: Institute of Advanced Psychological Studies, Adelphi University.

Fine AH (2000). The welfare of assistance and therapy animals: An ethical comment. In AH Fine (Ed), *Handbook on Animal-assisted Therapy: Theoretical Foundations and Guidelines for Practice*. New York: Academic.

Fish EW, Sekinda M, Ferrari PF, et al. (2000). Distress vocalizations in maternally separated mouse pups: modulation via 5-HT(1A), 5-HT(1B) and GABA(A) receptors. *Psychopharmacology*, 149:277-285.

Fox MW and Stanton G (1967). A developmental study of sleep and wakefulness in the dog. *J Small Anim Pract*, 8:605–611.

Frank M (1987). A pilot for the study of digestive and metabolic efficiency in wolves and dogs under conditions of unrestricted activity. In H Frank (Ed), *Man and Wolf: Advances, Issues, and Problems in Captive Wolf Research*. Dordrecht, The Netherlands: Dr W Junk.

Freedman DG, King JA, and Eliot O (1961). Critical period in the social development of dogs. *Science*, 133:1016–1017.

Fujiki N, Morris L, Mignot E, and Nishino S (2002). Analysis of onset location, laterality and propagation of cataplexy in canine narcolepsy. *Psychiatry Clin Neurosci*, 56:575–576.

Garcia R and Jaffard R (1996). Changes in synaptic excitability in the lateral septum associated with contextual and auditory fear conditioning in mice. *Eur J Neurosci*, 8:809-815.

Gardier AM, David DJ, Jego G, et al. (2003). Effects of chronic paroxetine treatment on dialysate serotonin in 5-HT1B receptor knockout mice. *J Neurochem*, 86:13-24.

Gillis C, Legarsky M, Lenker L, et al. (1999). Scent-mediated kin recognition and a similar type of long-term olfactory memory in domestic dogs (*Canis familiaris*). In RE Johnston, D Muller-Schwarze, and PW Sorensen (Eds), *Advances in Chemical Signals in Vertebrates*. New York: Plenum.

Giovannini MG, Rakovska A, Benton RS, et al. (2001). Effects of novelty and habituation on acetylcholine, GABA, and glutamate release from the frontal cortex and hippocampus of freely moving rats. *Neuroscience*, 106:43–53.

Gobert A and Millan MJ (1999). Serotonin (5-HT)2A receptor activation enhances dialysate levels of dopamine and noradrenaline, but not 5-HT, in the frontal cortex of freely-moving rats. *Neuropharmacology*, 38:315-317.

Gordon NS, Burke S, Akil H, et al. (2003). Socially-induced brain 'fertilization': Play promotes brain derived neurotrophic factor transcription in the amygdala and dorsolateral frontal cortex in juvenile rats. *Neurosci Lett*, 341:17–20.

Grauer E and Thomas E (1982). Conditioned suppression of medial forebrain bundle and septal intracranial self-stimulation in the rat: Evidence for a fear-relief mechanism of the septum. *J Comp Physiol Psychol*, 96:61-70.

Gray JA (1971). *The Psychology of Fear and Stress*. New York: McGraw-Hill Book Co.

Gregg TR and Siegel A (2001). Brain structures and neurotransmitters regulating aggression in cats: Implications for human aggression. *Prog Neuropsychopharmacol Biol Psychiatry*, 25:91–140.

Guthrie ER (1935). *The Psychology of Learning*. New York: Harper and Brothers.

Hannum RD, Rosellini RA and Seligman MEP (1976). Learned helplessness in the rat: Retention and immunization. *Dev Psychol*, 12:449–454.

Hare B and Tomasello M (1999). Domestic dogs use human and conspecific social cues to locate food. *J Comp Psychol*, 113:173–177.

Hare B, Brown M, Williamson C, and Tomasello M (2002). The domestication of social cognition in dogs. *Science*, 298:1634–1636.

Harrington FH and Asa CS (2003). Wolf communication. In LD Mech and L Boitani (Eds), *Wolves: Behavior, Ecology, and Conservation*. Chicago: University of Chicago Press.

Hebb DO (1955). Drives and the C.N.S. (conceptual nervous system). *Psychol Rev*, 62:243–254.

Hennessy MB, Voith VL, Travis L, et al. (2002). Exploring human interaction and diet effects on the behavior of dogs in public animal shelter. *J Appl Anim Welfare Sci*, 5:253–273.

Hepper PG (1986). Sibling recognition in the domestic dog. *Anim Behav*, 34:288–289.

Hepper PG (1994). Long-term retention of kinship recognition established during infancy in the domestic dog. *Behav Processes*, 33:3–15.

Hiby EF, Rooney NJ, and Bradshaw JWS (2003). Dog training methods: Their use, effectiveness and interaction with behaviour and welfare. *Anim Welfare*, 13: 63-69.

Hiestand NL (1989). A comparison of problem-solving and spatial orientation in the wolf (*Canis lupus*) and dog (*Canis familiaris*) [PhD dissertation]. Storrs: University of Connecticut.

Hill RC (1998). The nutritional requirements of exercising dogs. *J Nutr*, 128(Suppl 12):2686S–2690S.

Hoaken PNS, Shaughnessy VK, and Pihl RO (2003). Executive cognitive functioning and aggression: Is it an issue of impulsivity? *Aggress Behav*, 29:15-30.

Horowitz AC (2002). The behaviors of theories of mind, and a case study of dogs at play [PhD dissertation]. San Diego: University of California.

Horvath TL, Diano S, and Tschop M (2004). Brain circuits regulating energy homeostasis. *Neuroscientist*, 10:235–246.

Hydbring-Sandberg E, Von Walter LW, Hoglund K, et al. (2004). Physiological reactions to fear provocation in dogs. *J Endocrinol*, 180:439–448.

Ikeda T and Hikosaka O (2003). Reward-dependent gain and bias of visual responses in primate superior colliculus. *Neuron*, 14:693–700.

Ikonen S (2001), The role of the septohippocampal cholinergic system in cognitive functions [PhD dissertation]. Kuopio, Finland: University of Kuopio.

Inoue T, Inui A, Okita M, et al. (1989). Effect of neuropeptide Y on the hypothalamic-pituitary-adrenal axis in the dog. *Life Sci*, 44:1043–1051.

Irusta AE, Savoldi M, Kishi R, et al., (2001). Psychopharmacological evidences for the involvement of muscarinic and nicotinic cholinergic receptors on sweet substance-induced analgesia in *Rattus norvegicus*. *Neurosci Lett*, 305:115-118.

Irwin T (1985). *Aristotle: Nicomachean Ethics*. Indianapolis, IN: Hackett.

Itoi K, Helmreich DL, Lopez-Figueroa MO, and Watson SJ (1999). Differential regulation of corticotropin-releasing hormone and vasopressin gene transcription in the hypothalamus by norepinephrine. *J Neurosci*, 19:5464-5472.

James WT (1941). Morphological form and its relation to behavior: A study of the behavior of pure breed and hybrid dogs by conditioned salivary and motor reactions. In CR Stockard (Ed), *The Genetic and Endocrine Basis for Differences in Form and Behavior as Elucidated by Studies of Contrasted Pure-line Dog Breeds and Their Hybrids* (American Anatomy Memoir

19). Philadelphia: Wistar Institute of Anatomy and Biology.

James WT (1960). Observations of the regurgitant feeding reflex in the dog. *Psychol Rep*, 6:142.

Jansen AS, Farkas E, Mac Sams J, and Loewy AD (1998). Local connections between the columns of the periaqueductal gray matter: A case for intrinsic neuromodulation. *Brain Res*, 784:329-336.

Jéquier E (2002). Leptin signaling, adiposity, and energy balance. *Ann NY Acad Sci*, 967:379–388.

Jorgensen H, Knigge U, Kjaer A, and Warberg J (2002). Serotonergic involvement in stress-induced vasopressin and oxytocin secretion. *Eur J Endocrinol*, 147:815-824.

Jorgensen H, Kjaer A, Knigge U, et al (2003a). Serotonin stimulates hypothalamic mRNA expression and local release of neurohypophysial peptides. *J Neuroendocrinology*,15:564-571.

Jorgensen H, Riis M, Knigge U, et al. (2003b). Serotonin receptors involved in vasopressin and oxytocin secretion. *J Neuroendocrinol*,15:242-249.

Kaminski J, Call J, and Fischer J (2004). Word learning in a domestic dog: Evidence for "fast mapping." *Science*, 304:1682–1683.

Kaplan JR, Shively CA, Fontenot MB, et al. (1994). Demonstration of an association among dietary cholesterol, central serotonergic activity, and social behavior in monkeys. *Psychosom Med*, 56:479–484.

Kaplan JR, Fontenot MB, Manuck SB, and Muldoon MF (1996). Influence of dietary lipids on agonistic and affiliative behavior in *Macaca fascicularis*. *Am J Primatol*, 38:333–347.

Kaufman J, Olson PN, Reimers TJ, et al. (1985). Serum concentrations of thyroxine, 3,5,3'-triiodothyronine, thyrotropin, and prolactin in dogs before and after thyrotropin-releasing hormone administration. *Am J Vet Res*, 46:486–492.

Kawasaki K and Iwasaki T (1997). Corticosterone levels during extinction of runway response in rats. *Life Sci*, 61:1721–1728.

Keay KA and Bandler R (2001). Parallel circuits mediating distinct emotional coping reactions to different types of stress. *Neurosci Biobehav Rev*, 25:669-678.

Keck ME, Wigger A, Welt T, et al. (2002). Vasopressin mediates the response of the combined dexamethasone/CRH test in hyper-anxious rats: implications for pathogenesis of affective disorders. *Neuropsychopharmacology*, 26:94-105.

Kerns JG, Cohen JD, MacDonald III AW, et al. (2004). Anterior cingulate conflict monitoring and adjustments in control. *Science*, 303:1023–1026.

Keysers C, Kohler E, Umilta MA, et al. (2003). Audiovisual mirror neurons and action recognition. *Exp Brain Res*, 153:628–636.

Kiley-Worthington M (1990). *Animals in Circuses and Zoos: Chirons World?* Harlow, England: Aardvark.

Kirsch I and Sapirstein G (1998). Listening to Prozac but hearing placebo: A meta-analysis of antidepressant medication. *Prevention and Treatment*, 1. http://journals.apa.org/prevention/volume1/pre0010002a.html.

Kirsch I, Moore TJ, Scoboria A, and Nicholls SS (2002). The emperor's new drugs: An analysis of antidepressant medication data submitted to the U.S. Food and Drug Administration. *Prevention and Treatment*, 5. http://journals.apa.org/prevention/volume5/pre0050023a.html.

Kiss A, Jezova D, Aguilera G (1994). Activity of the hypothalamic pituitary adrenal axis and sympathoadrenal system during food and water deprivation in the rat. *Brain Res*, 663:84–92.

Klingbeil CK, Keil LC, Chang D, and Reid IA (1988). Effects of CRF and ANG II on ACTH and vasopressin release in conscious dogs. *Am J Physiol*, 255:46-53.

Kluger AN, Siegfried Z, and Ebstein RP (2002). A meta-analysis of the association between DRD4 polymorphism and novelty seeking. *Mol Psychiat*,7:712-717.

Knapp R, Hews DK, Thompson CW, et al. (2003). Environmental and endocrine correlates of tactic switching by nonterritorial male tree lizards (*Urosaurus ornatus*). *Horm Behav*, 43:83–92.

Kobayashi Y and Isa T (2002). Sensory-motor gating and cognitive control by the brainstem cholinergic system. *Neural Networks*, 15:731–741.

Kohler E, Keysers C, Umilta MA, et al. (2002). Hearing sounds, understanding actions: Action representation in mirror neurons. *Science*, 297:846–848.

Kolb B and Whishaw IQ (1998). Brain plasticity and behavior. *Annu Rev Psychol*, 49:43–64.

Konorski J and Lawicka W (1964). Analysis of errors by prefrontal animals on the delayed-response test. In J. M. Warren and K. Akert (Eds), *The Frontal Granular Cortex and Behavior*. New York: McGraw-Hill.

Kooistra HS, Diaz-Espineira M, Mol JA, et al. (2000). Secretion pattern of thyroid-stimulating hormone in dogs during euthyroidism and hypothyroidism. *Domest Anim Endocrinol*, 18:19–29.

Koolhaas JM, Everts H, De Ruiter AJ, et al. (1998). Coping with stress in rats and mice: differential peptidergic modulation of the amygdala-lateral septum complex. *Prog Brain Res*, 119:437-448.

Korda P (1974). Epimeletic (care-giving) vomiting in dogs: A study of the determinating factors. *Acta Neurobiol Exp (Warsz)*, 34:277–300.

Kovach JA, Nearing BD, and Verrier RL (2001). Angerlike behavioral state potentiates myocardial ischemia-induced T-wave alternans in canines. *J Am Coll Cardiol*, 37:171, 917-925.

Kram ML, Kramer GL, Steciuk M, et al. (2000). Effects of learned helplessness on brain GABA receptors. *Neurosci Res*, 38:193-198.

Kreeger TJ (2003). The internal wolf: Physiology, pathology, and pharmacology. In LD Mech and L Boitani (Eds), *Wolves: Behavior, Ecology, and Conservation*. Chicago: University of Chicago Press.

Kuroda Y, Mikuni M, Ogawa T, and Takahashi K (1992). Effect of ACTH, adrenalectomy and the combination treatment on the density of 5-HT_2 receptor binding sites in neocortex of rat forebrain and 5-HT_2 receptor-mediated wet-dog shake behaviors. *Psychopharmacology*, 108:27-32.

Kyuhou S and Gemba H (1998). Two vocalization-related subregions in the midbrain periaqueductal gray of the guinea pig. *Neuroreport*, 9:1607-1610.

Lagerspetz KMJ and Lagerspetz KYH (1971). Changes in the aggressiveness of mice resulting from selective breeding, learning and social isolation. *Scand J Psychol*, 12:241–248.

Lawicka W (1959). Physiological mechanism of delayed reactions. II. Delayed reactions in dogs and cats to directional stimuli. *Acta Biol Exp Vars*, 19:199-219.

Lawicka W and Konorski J (1959). Physiological mechanism of delayed reactions. III. The effects of prefrontal ablations on delayed reactions in dogs. *Acta Biol Exp Vars*, 19:221-231.

Li Y, Gao XB, Sakurai T, and Van den Pol AN (2002). Hypocretin/orexin excites hypocretin neurons via a local glutamate neuron: A potential mechanism for orchestrating the hypothalamic arousal system. *Neuron*, 36:1169–1181.

Lichtenstein PE (1950). Studies of anxiety. I. The production of a feeding inhibition in dogs. *J Comp Physiol Psychol*, 43:16–29.

Lin L, Faraco J, Li R, et al. (1999). The sleep disorder canine narcolepsy is caused by a mutation in the hypocretin (orexin) receptor 2 gene. *Cell*, 98:365–376.

Linde K, Clausius N, Ramirez G, et al. (1997). Are the clinical effects of homeopathy placebo effects? A meta-analysis of placebo-controlled trials. *Lancet*, 350:834–843.

Luks TL, Simpson GV, Feiwell RJ, and Miller WL (2002). Evidence for anterior cingulate cortex involvement in monitoring preparatory attentional set. *Neuroimage*, 17:792–802.

Lyons DM, Fong KD, Schrieken N, and Levine (2000). Frustrative nonreward and pituitary-adrenal activity in squirrel monkeys. *Physiol Behav*, 71:559–563.

Ma XM and Lightman SL (1998). The arginine vasopressin and corticotrophin-releasing hormone gene transcription responses to varied frequencies of repeated stress in rats. *J Physiol*, 510:605-614.

Maccari S, Piazza PV, Kabbaj M, et al. (1995). Adoption reverses the long-term impairment in glucocorticoid feedback induced by prenatal stress. *J Neurosci*, 15:110–116.

MacDonald III AW, Cohen JD, Stenger VA, and Carter CS (2000). Dissociating the role of the dorsolateral prefrontal and anterior cingulate cortex in cognitive control. *Science*, 288:1835–1838.

MacDonald DW and Carr GM (1995). Variation in dog society: Between resource dispersion and social flux. In J Serpell (Ed), *The Domestic Dog: Its Evolution, Behaviour, and Interaction with People*. New York: Cambridge University Press.

Mackintosh NJ (1975). A theory of attention: Variations in the associability of stimulus with reinforcement. *Psychol Rev*, 82:276–298.

Malm K (1995). Regurgitation in relation to weaning in the domestic dog: A questionnaire study. *Appl Anim Behav Sci*, 43:111–121.

Martin-Ruiz R, Puig MV, Celada P, et al. (2001). Control of serotonergic function in medial prefrontal cortex by serotonin-2A receptors through a glutamate-dependent mechanism. *J Neurosci*, 21:9856-9866.

Martins T (1949). Disgorging of food to the puppies by the lactating dog. *Physiol Zool*, 22:169–172.

Masuda K, Hashizume C, Kikusui T, Takeuchi Y (2004). Breed differences in genotype and allele frequency of catechol O-methyltransferase gene polymorphic regions in dogs. *J Vet Med Sci*, 66:183-187.

Matthews K and Robbins TW (2003). Early experience as a determinant of adult behavioural responses to reward: The effects of repeated maternal separation in the rat. *Neurosci Biobehav Rev*, 27:45–55.

Matthews K, Wilkinson LS, and Robbins TW (1996). Repeated maternal separation of preweanling rats attenuates behavioral responses to primary and conditioned incentives in adulthood. *Physiol Behav*, 59:99–107.

Matto V, Skrebuhhova T, and Allikmets L (1999). Apomorphine-induced upregulation of serotonin 5-HT$_{2A}$ receptors in male rats is independent from development of aggressive behaviour. *J Physiol Pharmacol*, 50:335-344.

Mayberg HS, Silva JA, Brannan SK, et al. (2002). The functional neuroanatomy of the placebo effect. *Am J Psychiatry*, 159:728–737.

McBryde WC and Murphree OD (1974). The rehabilitation of genetically nervous dogs. *Pavlov J Biol Sci* 9:76–84.

McDougle CJ, Barr LC, Goodman WK (1999). Possible role of neuropeptides in obsessive compulsive disorder. *Psychoneuroendocrinology*, 24:1-24.

McGreevy P, Grassi TD, and Harman AM (2004). A strong correlation exists between the distribution of retinal ganglion cells and nose length in the dog. *Brain Behav Evol*, 63:13–22.

McGuinness OP, Shau V, Benson EM, et al. (1997). Role of epinephrine and norepinephrine in the metabolic response to stress hormone infusion in the conscious dog. *Am J Physiol*, 273:E674–E681.

McIntyre CK, Marriott LK, and Gold PE (2003). Patterns of brain acetylcholine release predict individual differences in preferred learning strategies in rats. *Neurobiol Learn Memory*, 79:177–183.

McKinley S and Young RJ (2003). The efficacy of the model-rival method when compared with operant conditioning for training domestic dogs to perform a retrieval-selection task. *Appl Anim Behav Sci*, 81:357–365.

McLeod PJ, Moger WH, Ryon CJ, et al. (1996) The relation between urinary cortisol levels and social behaviour in captive timber wolves. *Can J Zool*, 74:209–216.

McNally GP and Westbrook RF (2003). Anterograde amnesia for Pavlovian fear conditioning and the role of one-trial overshadowing: Effects of preconditioning exposures to morphine in the rat. *J Exp Psychol [Anim Behav]*, 29:222–232.

McNally GP, Pigg M, and Weidemann G (2004). Blocking, unblocking, and overexpectation of fear: A role for opioid receptors in the regulation of Pavlovian association formation. *Behav Neurosci*, 118:111–120.

Meaney MJ, Diorio J, Francis D, et al. (2000). Postnatal handling increases the expression of cAMP-inducible transcription factors in the rat hippocampus: The effects of thyroid hormones and serotonin. *J Neurosci*, 20:3926–3935.

Mech LD (1970). *The Wolf: The Ecology and Behavior of an Endangered Species*. Minneapolis: University of Minnesota Press.

Mech LD (2000). Leadership in wolf, *Canis lupus*, packs. *Can Field Nat*, 114:259–263.

Miklosi A, Kubinyi E, Topal J, et al. (2003). A simple reason for a big difference: Wolves do not look back at humans, but dogs do. *Curr Biol*, 13:763–766.

Milham MP, Banich MT, Claus ED, and Cohen NJ (2003). Practice-related effects demonstrate complementary roles of anterior cingulate and prefrontal cortices in attentional control. *Neuroimage*, 18:483–493.

Millan MJ (2003). The neurobiology and control of anxious states. *Prog Neurobiol*, 70:83-244.

Mills DS (2003). Medical paradigms for the study of problem behaviour: A critical review. *Appl Anim Behav Sci*, 81:265–277.

Miranda MI, Ramirez-Lugo L, and Bermudez-Rattoni F (2000). Cortical cholinergic activity is related to the novelty of the stimulus. *Brain Res*, 882:230–235.

Miura M, Inui A, Teranishi A, et al. (1992). Structural requirements for the effects of neuropeptide Y on the hypothalamic-pituitary-adrenal axis in the dog. *Neuropeptides*, 23:15–18.

Moger WH, Ferns LE, Wright JR, et al. (1998). Elevated urinary cortisol in a timber wolf (*Canis lupus*): A result of social behaviour of adrenal pathology? *Can J Zool*, 76:1957–1959.

Mowrer OH (1960). *Learning Theory and Behavior*. New York: John Wiley and Sons.

Mugford RA (1984). Methods used to describe the normal and abnormal behaviour of the dog and cat. In RS Anderson (Ed), *Nutrition and Behavior in Dogs and Cats*. New York: Pergamon Press.

Nail-Boucherie K, Garcia R, and Jaffard R (1998). Influences of the bed nucleus of the stria terminalis and of the paraventricular nucleus of the hypothalamus on the excitability of hippocampal-lateral septal synapses in mice. *Neurosci Lett*. 246:112-116.

Nauta WJH (1971). The problem of the frontal lobe: A reinterpretation. *J Psychiatr Res*, 8:167–187.

Neuringer AJ (1969). Animals respond for food in the presence of free food. *Science*, 166:399–401.

Neuringer A, Kornell N, and Olufs M (2001). Stability and variability in extinction. *J Exp Psychol Anim Behav Process*, 27:79-94.

Niimi Y, Inoue-Murayama M, Kato K, Matsuura N, et al. (2001). Breed differences in allele frequency of the dopamine receptor D4 gene in dogs. *J Hered*, 92:433-436.

Niimi Y, Inoue-Murayama M, Murayama Y, et al. (1999). Allelic variation of the D4 dopamine receptor polymorphic region in two dog breeds, Golden retriever and Shiba. *J Vet Med Sci*, 61:1281-1286.

Nippak PM, Chan AD, Campbell Z, et al. (2003). Response latency in *Canis familiaris*: mental ability or mental strategy? *Behav Neurosci*, 117:1066-1075.

Nishitani N and Hari R (2000). Temporal dynamics of cortical representation for action. *Proc Natl Acad Sci USA*, 97:913–918.

Nunez EA, Becker DV, Furth ED, et al. (1970). Breed differences and similarities in thyroid function in purebred dogs. *Am J Physiol*, 218:1337–1341.

Ochberg FM and Soskis DA (1982). *Victims of Terrorism*. Boulder, CO: Westview.

Öhman A and Mineka S (2001). Fears, phobias, and preparedness: Toward an evolved module of fear and fear learning. *Psychol Rev*, 108:483–522.

Öngür D, An X, and Price JL (1998). Prefrontal cortical projections to the hypothalamus in macaque monkeys. *J Comp Neurol*, 401:480-505.

Öngür D and Price JL (2000). The organization of networks within the orbital and medial prefrontal cortex of rats, monkeys and humans. *Cereb Cortex*, 10:206–219.

Ostrowski NL (1998). Oxytocin receptor mRNA expression in rat brain: Implications for behavioral integration and reproductive success. *Psychoneuroendocrinology*, 23:989–1004.

Packard JM, Mech LD, and Ream RR (1992). Weaning in an arctic wolf pack: Behavioral mechanisms. *Can J Zool*, 70:1269–1275.

Panksepp J (1998). *Affective Neuroscience: The Foundations of Human and Animal Emotions*. New York: Oxford University Press.

Papanek PE and Raff H (1994). Physiological increases in cortisol inhibit basal vasopressin release in conscious dogs. *Am J Physiol*, 266:1744-1751.

Papini, MR (2003). Comparative psychology of surprising nonreward. *Brain Behav Evol*, 62:83-95.

Parker HG, Kim LV, Sutter NB, et al. (2004). Genetic structure of the purebred domestic dog. *Science*, 304:1160–1164.

Pepperberg IM (2002). In search of King Solomon's Ring: Cognitive and communicative studies of grey parrots (*Psittacus erithacus*). *Brain Behav Evol*, 59:54–67.

Pepperberg IM, Sandefer R, Noel D, and Ellsworth CP (2000). Vocal learning in the grey parrot (*Psittacus erithacus*): Effects of species identity and number of trainers. *J Comp Psychol*, 114:371–380.

Peremans K, Audenaert K, Coopman F, et al., (2003a). Regional binding index of the radiolabeled selective 5-HT$_{2A}$ antagonist 123I-5-I-R91150 in the normal canine brain imaged with single photon emission computed tomography. *Vet Radiol Ultrasound*, 44:344-351.

Peremans K, Audenaert K, Coopman F, et al. (2003b). Estimates of regional cerebral blood flow and 5-HT$_{2A}$ receptor density in impulsive, aggressive dogs with (99m)Tc-ECD and (123)I-5-I-R91150. *Eur J Nucl Med Mol Imaging*, 30:1538-1546.

Perin C (1981). Dogs as symbols in human development. In B Fogle (Ed), *Interrelations Between People and Pets*. Springfield, IL: Charles C Thomas.

Petersen TJ, Alpert JE, Papakostas GI, et al. (2003). Early-onset depression and the emotional and behavioral characteristics of offspring. *Depress Anxiety*, 18:104–108.

Podberscek AL and Serpell JA (1996). The English cocker spaniel: Preliminary findings on aggressive behavior. *Appl Anim Behav Sci*, 47:75-89.

Popova NK, Voitenko NN, Kulikov AV, and Avgustinovich DF (1991). Evidence for the involvement of central serotonin in mechanism of domestication of silver foxes. *Pharmacol Biochem Behav*, 40:751–756.

Porges SW (2003). The polyvagal theory: Phylogenetic contributions to social behavior. *Physiol Behav*, 79:503–513.

Ragozzino ME, Parker ME, and Gold PE (1992). Spontaneous alternation and inhibitory avoidance impairments with morphine injections into the medial septum. Attenuation by glucose administration. *Brain Res*, 597:241-249.

Ramage AG (2001). Central cardiovascular regulation and 5-hydroxytryptamine receptors. *Brain Res Bull*, 56:425-439.

Rheingold HL (1963). Maternal behavior in the dog. In HL Rheingold (Ed), *Maternal Behavior in Mammals*. New York: John Wiley and Sons.

Rios R, Stolfi A, Campbell PH, and Pickoff AS (1996). Postnatal development of the putative neuropeptide-Y-mediated sympathetic-parasympathetic autonomic interaction. *Cardiovasc Res*, 31:E96–E103.

Rolls ET (2000). The orbitofrontal cortex and reward. *Cereb Cortex*, 10:284–294.

Roossien A, Brunsting JR, Zaagsma J, et al. (2000). The vagal cardiac accelerator system in the reflex control of heart rate in conscious dogs. *Acta Physiol Scand*, 170:191–199.

Russell B (1997). *The Problems of Philosophy*. New York: Oxford University Press.

Saetre P, Lindberg J, Leonard JA, et al. (2004). From wild wolf to domestic dog: Gene expression changes in the brain. *Mol Brain Res*, 126:198–206.

Sahley TL, Panksepp J and Zolovick AJ (1981). Cholinergic modulation of separation distress in the domestic chick. *Eur J Pharmacol*, 72:261-264.

Sajdyk TJ, Schober DA, and Gehlert DR (2002). Neuropeptide Y receptor subtypes in the basolateral nucleus of the amygdala modulate anxiogenic responses in rats. *Neuropharmacology*, 43:1165–1172.

Sajdyk TJ, Shekhar A, and Gehlert DR (2004). Interactions between NPY and CRF in the amygdala to regulate emotionality. *Neuropeptides*, 38:225-234.

Sakaue M, Ago Y, Sowa C, et al. (2002). Modulation by 5-hT$_{2A}$ receptors of aggressive behavior in isolated mice. *Jpn J Pharmacol*, 89:89-92.

Sands J and Creel S (2004). Social dominance, aggression and faecal glucocorticoid levels in a wild population of wolves, *Canis lupus*. *Anim Behav*, 67:387–396.

Schoenbaum G and Setlow B (2001). Integrating orbitofrontal cortex into prefrontal theory: Common processing themes across species and subdivisions. *Learn Memory*, 8:134–147.

Schultz W (1998). Predictive reward signal of dopamine neurons. *J Neurophysiol*, 80:1–27.

Schultz W and Dickinson A (2000). Neuronal coding of prediction errors. *Annu Rev Neurosci*, 23:473–500.

Scott JP (1968). Evolution and domestication of the dog. In T Dobzhansky, MK Hecht, and WC Steere (Eds), *Evolutionary Biology*, Vol 2. New York: Appleton-Century-Crofts.

Scott JP and Fuller JL (1965). *Genetics and the Social Behavior of the Dog*. Chicago: University of Chicago Press.

Scott JP and McCray C (1967). Allelomimetic behavior in dogs: Negative effects of competition on social facilitation. *J Comp Physiol Psychol*, 63:316–319.

Scott JP, Fuller JL, and King JA (1959). The inheritance of annual seasonal breeding cycles in hybrid-basenji-cocker spaniel dogs. *J Hered*, 50:255–261.

Seal US, Mech DL, and Van Ballenberghe V (1975). Blood analyses of wolf pups and their ecological and metabolic interpretation. *J Mammal*, 56:64–75.

Seal US, Plotka ED, Mech DL, and Packark JM (1987). Seasonal metabolic and reproductive cycles in wolves. In H Frank (Ed), *Man and Wolf: Advances, Issues, and Problems in Captive Wolf Research*. Dordrecht, The Netherlands: Dr W Junk.

Serpell J, Coppinger R, and Fine AH (2000). The welfare of assistance and therapy animals: An ethical comment. In AH Fine (Ed), *Handbook on Animal-assisted Therapy: Theoretical Foundations and Guidelines for Practice*. New York: Academic.

Sheikh SP, Feldthus N, Orkild H, et al. (1998). Neuropeptide Y2 receptors on nerve endings from the rat neurohypophysis regulate vasopressin and oxytocin release. *Neuroscience*, 82:107–115.

Shi L, Fatemi SH, Sidwell RW, and Patterson PH (2003). Maternal influenza infection causes marked behavioral and pharmacological changes in the offspring. *J Neurosci*, 23:297–302.

Simonov PV (1994). Cortiohypothalamic relationships during the development and realization of the conditioned reflex. *Neurosci Behav Physiol*, 24:267–273.

Skrebuhhova-Malmros T, Pruus K, Rudissaar R, et al. (2000). The serotonin 5-HT(2A) receptor subtype does not mediate apomorphine-induced aggressive behaviour in male Wistar rats. *Pharmacol Biochem Behav*, 67:339-443.

Smith JW, Evans AT, Costal B, and Smyth JW (2002). Thyroid hormones, brain function and cognition: A brief review. *Neurosci Biobehav Rev*, 26:45–60.

Snow CJ (1967). Some observations on the behavioral and morphological development of coyote pups. *Am Zool*, 7:353–355.

Solomon RL, Turner LH, and Lessac MS (1968). Some effects of delay of punishment on resistance to temptation in dogs. *J Pers Soc Psychol*, 8:233–238.

Soproni K, Miklosi A, Topal J, and Csanyi V (2001). Comprehension of human communicative signs in pet dogs (*Canis familiaris*). *J Comp Psychol*, 115:122–126.

Stehlin I (1996). Homeopathy: Real Medicine or Empty Promises. Washington, DC: US Food and Drug Administration. http://www.fda.gov/fdac/features/096_home.html.

Sterling P (2004). Principles of allostasis: Optimal design, predictive regulation, pathophysiology, and rational therapeutics. In J Shulkin (Ed), *Allostasis, Homeostasis, and the Costs of Adaptation*. New York: Cambridge University Press.

Sterling P and Eyer J (1988). Allostasis: A new paradigm to explain arousal pathology. In S Fisher and J Reason (Eds), *Handbook of Life Stress, Cognition and Health*. New York: John Wiley and Sons.

Stern DN (1985). *The Interpersonal World of Infants: A View from Psychoanalysis and Developmental Psychology*. New York: Basic.

Stoddard SL, Bergdall VK, Conn PS, and Levin BE (1987). Increases in plasma catecholamines during naturally elicited defensive behavior in the cat. *J Auton Nerv Syst*, 19:189–197.

Strandberg E, Jacobsson J, and Saetre P (2004). Direct genetic, maternal and litter effects on behaviour in German shepherd dogs in Sweden. *Livestock Production Science* (article in press).

Sumner BE and Fink G (1998). Testosterone as well as estrogen increases serotonin2A receptor mRNA and binding site densities in the male rat brain. *Brain Res Mol Brain Res*, 59:205-214.

Szetei V, Miklosi, Topal, and Csanyi V (2003). When dogs seem to lose their nose: An investigation on the use of visual and olfactory cues in communicative context between dog and owner. *Appl Anim Behav Sci*, 83:141–152.

Tafet GE, Toister-Achituv M, and Shinitzky M (2001). Enhancement of serotonin uptake by cortisol: A possible link between stress and depression. *Cogn Affect Behav Neurosci*, 1:96-104.

Takao K, Nagatani T, Kitamura Y, and Yamawaki S (1997). Effects of corticosterone on 5-HT$_{1A}$ and 5-HT$_2$ receptor binding and on the receptor-mediated behavioral responses of rats. *Eur J Pharmacol*, 333:123-128.

Takao K, Nagatani T, Kitamura Y, et al. (1995). Chronic forced swim stress of rats increases frontal cortical 5-HT$_2$ receptors and the wet-dog shakes they mediate, but not frontal cortical beta-adrenoceptors. *Eur J Pharmacol*, 294:721-726.

Thayer JF and Lane RD (2000). A model of neurovisceral integration in emotion regulation and dysregulation. *J Affective Disord*, 61:201–216.

Thomas BL and Papini MR (2001) Adrenalectomy eliminates the extinction spike in autoshaping with rats. *Physiol Behav*, 72:543-547.

Thomas E, Pernar L, Lucki I, and Valentino RJ (2003). Corticotropin-releasing factor in the dorsal raphe nucleus regulates activity of lateral septal neurons. *Brain Res*, 960:201-208.

Thompson CC and Potter GB (2000). Thyroid hormone action in neural development. *Cereb Cortex*, 10:939–945.

Todt D (1975). Social learning of vocal patterns and modes of their applications in grey parrots. *Z Tierpsychol*, 39:178–188.

Tolman EC and Brunswik E (1935). The organism and the causal texture of the environment. *Psychol Rev*, 42:43–77.

Topál J, Miklósi A, and Csányi V (1997). Dog-human relationship affects problem solving behavior in the dog. *Anthrozoos*, 10:214–224.

Triana E and Pasnak R (1981). Object permanence in cats and dogs. *Anim Learn Behav*, 9:135–139.

Trivers RL (1972). Parental investment and sexual selection. In B Campbell (Ed), *Sexual Selection and the Descent of Man*. Chicago: Aldine.

Trivers RL (1974). Parent-offspring conflict. *Am Zool*, 14:249–264.

Trut LN (1999). Early canid domestication: The farm-fox experiment. *Amer Scient*, 87:160-169.

Trut LN (2001). Experimental studies of early canid domestication. In A Ruvinsky and J Sampson (Eds), *The Genetics of the Dog*. New York: CABI.

Tunbridge EM, Bannerman DM, Sharp T, and Harrison PJ (2004). Catechol-o-methyltransferase inhibition improves set-shifting performance and elevates stimulated dopamine release in the rat prefrontal cortex. *J Neurosci*, 24:5331-5335.

Umilta MA, Kohler E, Gallese V, et al. (2001). I know what you are doing: A neurophysiological study. *Neuron*, 3:155–165.

Ursu S, Stenger VA, Shear MK, et al. (2003). Overactive action monitoring in obsessive-compulsive disorder: Evidence from functional magnetic resonance imaging. *Psychol Sci*, 14:347–353.

Van Der Velden NA, De Weerdt CJ, Brooymans-Schallenberg, JHC, and Tielen AM (1976). An abnormal behavioral trait in Bernesse mountain dogs (Berner sennenhund). *Tijdschr Diergeneesk*, 101:403-407.

Van Erp AM and Miczek KA (2000). Aggressive behavior, increased accumbal dopamine, and decreased cortical serotonin in rats. *J Neurosci*, 20:9320–9325.

Van Veen V and Carter CS (2002). The anterior cingulate as a conflict monitor: fMRI and ERP studies. *Physiol Behav*, 77:477–482.

Vanderschuren LJ, Niesink RJ, and Van Ree JM (1997). The neurobiology of social play behavior in rats. *Neurosci Biobehav Rev*, 21:309–326.

Verrier RL and Dickerson LW (1991). Autonomic nervous system and coronary blood flow changes related to emotional activation and sleep. *Circulation*, 83(Suppl 4):81–89.

Viranyi Z, Topal J, Gacsi M, and Miklosi (2004). Dogs respond appropriately to cues of humans' attentional focus. *Behav Processes*, 66:161–172.

Walsh MT and Dinan TG (2001). Selective serotonin reuptake inhibitors and violence: a review of the available evidence. *Acta Psychiatr Scand*, 104:84-91.

Warden CJ and Warner LH (1928). The sensory capacity and intelligence of dogs, with a report on the ability of the noted dog "Fellow" to respond to verbal stimuli. *Q Rev Biol*, 3:1–28.

Weinstock M (1997). Does prenatal stress impair coping and regulation of hypothalamic-pituitary-adrenal axis? *Neurosci Biobehav Rev*, 21:1–10.

Weinstock M (2002). Can the behaviour abnormalities induced by gestational stress in rats be prevented or reversed? *Stress*, 5:167–176.

Westbrook RF, Good AJ, and Kiernan MJ (1997). Microinjection of morphine into the nucleus accumbens impairs contextual learning in rats. *Behav Neurosci*, 111:996–1013.

White EC (1987). *Kaironomia: On the will-to-invent*. Ithaca, NY: Cornell University Press.

Willie JT, Chemelli RM, Sinton CM, and Yanagisawa M (2001). To eat or to sleep? Orexin in the regulation of feeding and wakefulness. *Annu Rev Neurosci*, 24:429–458.

Wu M, Zaborszky L, Hajszan T, et al. (2004). Hypocretin/orexin innervation and excitation of identified septohippocampal cholinergic neurons. *J Neurosci*, 24:3527–3536.

Yilmazer-Hanke DM, Hantsch M, Hanke J, et al. (2004). Neonatal thyroxine treatment: changes in the number of corticotropin-releasing-factor (CRF) and neuropeptide Y (NPY) containing neurons and density of tyrosine hydroxylase positive fibers (TH) in the amygdala correlate with anxiety-related behavior of wistar rats. *Neuroscience*, 124:283-297.

Young PT (1955). The role of hedonic processes in motivation. In *Nebraska Symposium on Motivation*. Lincoln: University of Nebraska Press.

Young PT (1959). The role of affective processes in learning and motivation. *Psychol Rev*, 66:104–125.

Zernicki B (1968). Two cases of experimental neuroses in dogs cured by a temporay change of reinforcement. *Acta Biol Exp* (Warsaw), 28:213-216.

Zhang L, Ma W, Barker JL, and Rubinow DR (1999). Sex differences in expression of serotonin receptors (subtypes 1A and 2A) in rat brain: A possible role of testosterone. *Neuroscience*, 94:251-259.

Zoeller RT, Dowling ALS, Herzig CTA, et al. (2002). Thyroid hormone, brain development, and the environment environmental health perspectives. *Environ Health Perspect*, 110:355–361.

Appendix A

Sit-Stay Program

Modified Sit-Stay Instructions
Sit-Stay Tasks
Reference

MODIFIED SIT-STAY INSTRUCTIONS

Sit-stay training fosters competent skills for obtaining reward and avoiding its loss by training the dog to defer, wait, and relax in the process of seeking rewards. Sit-stay training is integrated with play, providing an additional source of reward and balance. In addition to affectionate petting and attention, sit-stay behavior is reinforced with food rewards of variable size, type, and frequency. The schedule and duration of stay periods also has a potentially rewarding effect on stay behavior. That is, once a standard expectancy is established, comparatively short stay periods may be conducive to reward via surprise. On the other hand, longer-than-usual stay periods may produce punitive effects that are inimical to sit-stay objectives. As a result, stay periods should only be gradually increased in duration and arranged to occur so that longer ones are followed by a series of shorter ones, play, or other sources of positive surprise (e.g., better-than-usual food rewards). Stay-training sessions are generally begun with short-stay periods, followed by a mix of variable duration periods in between, and finished with a long-stay period at the end. Each session is introduced and concluded with a period of play.

The initial lesson consists of training the dog to come to a closed hand after retrieving a ball or simply coming in the case of dogs showing little interest in ball play (see *Introductory Lessons* in Chapter 1). Just before the hand is opened, the bridge signal "Good" is spoken in a playful tone. The ball is taken

and tossed for the dog to retrieve. Dogs that are uninterested in fetching a ball are permitted to explore the training situation freely between trials. Additional trials are initiated by calling the dog's name and making a smooch or squeaker sound after the dog picks up the ball, thus evoking an orienting response. As the dog turns in the direction of the trainer, the trainer can deliver a click and then flick the right hand to the side. The vocal signal "Come" is spoken in a friendly and encouraging way, followed by the voice bridge "Good" and the delivery of the reward concealed in the right hand. After each exercise, the dog is encouraged to retrieve a ball or move away with the release signal "OK" and a clap or two.

Improved orienting behavior can be achieved by putting a squeaker bulb in the right hand (held by the last two fingers), and squeezing it just as the dog approaches the hand. The bridge "Good" is spoken just before the hand is opened. In addition, an odor (orange or orange-lemon mix) can be placed in the squeaker, thereby establishing a linkage between the odor, squeaker sound, and food. As the result of repeated associations between the squeaker and food, the squeak sound acquires an enhanced potential for evoking an orienting response. Bridging the occurrence of the orienting response with a click and treat can further improve attention control. Olfactory conditioning is included in sit-stay training in cases where a platform for counterconditioning and desensitization is being prepared (see *Systematic Desensitization* in Chapter 3 and *Olfactory Conditioning* in Chapter 6).

With the dog coming rapidly to the closed hand, the trainer encourages the dog to sit by moving a hand up and behind the dog's head, causing it to follow and sit. The sit response is

739

reinforced with the bridge "Good," which is timed to coincide with the earliest movement in the direction of sitting. The sit response should be well trained to a hand signal before a "Sit" signal is added as a cue or command. The easiest way for most dogs to learn how to sit on command is to pair the "Sit" signal with a hand signal. The vocal signal is only paired with the hand signal after the dog is sitting consistently in response to the hand movement. If the dog fails to sit in response to the vocal cue, the hand signal is used to prompt the response. The trainer should avoid repeating the "Sit" command, but instead should use the hand to lure the dog into position, if necessary. The dog should gradually learn to sit equally well to both vocal or hand signals, but normally the signals are presented together. Although physical prompting, fading, and shadowing procedures are ordinarily used to increase reliable stimulus control over sit-stay behavior, these techniques are generally avoided with the goal of training the dog to defer without resorting to force of any kind.

Each successful sit response is rewarded, and additional rewards are given to the dog after varying durations of waiting in the sit position. The duration component of stay training is accomplished in the context of shaping an attending response. With the dog sitting in front, the trainer makes a smooch or cluck-click sound to encourage the dog to look up at the trainer and then to make eye contact before saying "Good" or clicking and delivering a food reward and affectionate pet. During such training, the trainer should make a friendly face expressing pleasure at the dog's effort and keep the training session upbeat and fun spirited. Initially, the bridge is timed to occur immediately as the dog looks up, but gradually requires that the dog hold eye contact for 1 or 2 seconds. As the dog learns to look up into the trainer's eyes, its name is presented just in advance of the smooch or cluck-click sound, a prompt that is progressively delayed and gradually faded altogether, but reinstated as needed to capture the dog's wavering attention. After every trial of attention training, the dog is released with "OK" and a clap or two. If the dog breaks the stay

position, a brief unrestrained time-out (TO) or rest period of 15 seconds is initiated during which the dog's efforts to obtain food or attention are ignored. The dog is signaled by name to orient, to come, and to sit in accord with a previously mastered criterion that the dog is likely to perform successfully, even going back to conditioning the bridge signal, if necessary.

Distance is gradually introduced after a high degree of reliability is established over the duration element with the dog both in front and on the left side. With the dog looking up, the trainer presents the right hand, palm toward dog, and vocally praises the dog as it continues to stay in place, followed by a food reward and release. The vocal signal "Stay" is subsequently paired with the hand signal as the trainer takes a 1-foot step back, bridges the stay response, and quickly returns to the dog to reward it. This process is repeated a number of times with variable durations without releasing the dog. The dog is trained to expect additional rewards to follow rather then learning to get up in anticipation of being released. If the dog breaks without being released, a 15-second TO-rest period is initiated. Reliable stay at increasing durations and distances is achieved over several sessions. If at any point in the process the behavior breaks down, the trainer should go back to a previously successful step and continue from there. The duration of sit-stay sessions varies according to the dog's needs and motivation, but should be periodically interrupted with ball play or other play activities. Stay training can be repeated several times during the day in different locations around the house. Once a high degree of reliability is established over duration and distance control, an element of increasing difficulty and distraction can be added in accordance with sit-stay program criteria (see *Stay Training* in Chapter 1).

Dogs that repeatedly break the stay position may benefit from response blocking (e.g., active-control line) and vocal prompts ("Eh, eh"); however, stern reprimands, directive prompts, or forceful handling should be avoided. The goal is to train the dog to sit and stay to obtain attractive rewards and avoid their loss. When gentle vocal prompting is used, it should be applied to the earliest intentional movements rather than applied after a dog breaks. An active-control line can be effectively used to help prevent unnecessary errors by training a dog to first stand-stay and then returning to sit-stay training. If a dog breaks completely, a brief TO-rest period follows during which the dog is ignored. If the dog barks during sit-stay training, the barking response should be brought under stimulus control. Jumping up should be treated in a similar way (see instructions for bring barking and jumping up under stimulus control in *Hyperactivity and Social Excesses* in Chapter 5). Once under adequate stimulus control, the opportunity to bark or jump up can be used as a reward. In the case of highly disruptive behavior, the trainer can leave the training room with the dog left on the other side of the door with the leash pinched in the doorjamb. The time-out lasts for 30 seconds provided that the dog has not scratched or barked for at least 10 seconds.

Once the sit-stay is mastered, a similar pattern of control is established involving down-stay training. Whereas the sit-stay is practiced with the dog in front and at the left side, the down-stay is practiced exclusively with the dog at the left side. In addition to luring and shaping techniques as described in Chapter 1, the down module can be trained by using an attention-cuing procedure. In this case, the trainer establishes eye contact and then glances at a point just in front of the dog. A constant gaze is fixed on the spot as the trainer steadily points and then taps over it. If the dog fails to lie down, the trainer looks at the dog, establishes brief eye contact, and then glances back at the spot and repeats the pointing-tapping procedure. As the dog begins to lie down, the bridge "Good" is delivered, followed by a treat after the action is completed. Many dogs resistant to lying down by other methods are often surprisingly responsive to this technique. Alternatively, a small square of cotton adhesive tape or Band-Aid is scented and presented to the dog to sniff and paired with food several times. The scented Band-Aid is then taped to the floor. The same attention-cuing procedure as

described previously is used to train the dog to orient and sniff the scented tape and then to lie down. The scented tape can be gradually placed at greater distances from the dog. Again, the trainer makes eye contact with the dog, breaks it off to glance toward the scented tape, and then points at the spot. The dog is encouraged to go to the spot and sniff (click), wait there or lie down in response to a pointing-tapping action ("Good" and reward), and required to stay until it is released ("OK" and clap). In one variation, the pointing-down signal is gradually faded, and the dog learns to lie down in response to the scented tape alone. The scented tape can be affixed to a variety of objects that are left in plain view or hidden for the dog to find, perhaps becoming the basis of an interesting game for dogs possessing a proclivity for such activity. Procedural variations based on the spotting technique can be used in a variety of training applications requiring a precise search and down-stay component.

The various daily sit-stay skills listed in Figure A.1 represent a guide, not a rigid program. Instead of practicing all of the tasks listed for a particular day, trainers should limit practice activities to as many items as the dog can successfully learn and perform without becoming overly stressed. The goal of sit-stay training is to establish control while encouraging a set of positive secondary emotional associations with the training process, in particular imbuing the act of sitting and staying with feelings of to enhanced comfort, safety, and relaxation. In addition to benefits for dogs, reward-based sit-stay training can be helpful to owners by introducing the rudiments of training and opening up a new perspective on behavioral change and control. By avoiding coercive techniques, family members are obliged to learn more positive strategies and ways to affirmatively frame the dog's behavior (e.g., the dead-dog rule) and to use reward more effectively. While training the dog to sit and stay, a new level of appreciation for the dog's abilities and needs may be engendered. Finally, as the result of using a reward-based method, even briefly, owners may learn to think more clearly and rationally about the process of mediating behavioral

Dog's Name:		Date:
SIT-STAY TASKS		

PRELIMINARY SIT TRAINING	DIFFICULTY RANK 1–5	NO. TIMES REPEATED
The dog sits for a food reward		
The dog sits quietly for 5 seconds		
The dog sits quietly for 10 seconds		
The dog sits quietly for 15 seconds		
Day 1: The dog should		
Sit		
Sit for 5 seconds		
Sit for 5 seconds		
Sit for 10 seconds		
Sit for 5 seconds		
Sit for 10 seconds		
Sit while you take 1 step backward and forward		
Sit while you take 1 step sideways, to the right, and return		
Sit while you take 1 step sideways, 1 step to the left, and return		
Sit while you step back 3 steps and return		
Sit while you take 3 steps to the left and return		
Sit while you take 3 steps to the right and return		
Sit for 10 seconds		
Day 2: The dog should		
Sit		
Sit for 5 seconds		
Sit for 5 seconds		
Sit for 10 seconds		
Sit while you step back 3 steps and return		
Sit while you take 3 steps to the right and return		
Sit while you take 3 steps to the left and return		
Sit for 10 seconds		
Sit while you walk halfway around the dog		
Sit while you walk halfway around the dog in the opposite direction		
Sit while you take 5 steps back and return		
Sit while you walk around the dog		
Sit while you take 5 steps to the right and return		
Sit for 10 seconds		
Sit while you take 5 steps to the left and return		
Sit while you take 10 steps back and return		
Sit for 20 seconds		
Sit while you take 10 steps to the right and return		
Day 3: The dog should		
Sit for 5 seconds		

FIG. A.1. Sit-stay program. Modified from a client handout with permission by Victoria L. Voith (1979).

Sit for 10 seconds		
Sit for 20 seconds		
Sit for 10 seconds		
Sit while you walk halfway around the dog and return		
Sit while you take 5 steps back and return		
Sit for 5 seconds		
Sit while you walk halfway around the dog and return		
Sit while you take 10 steps backward and return		
Sit while you take 5 steps to the left and return		
Sit while you take 5 steps to the right and return		
Sit while you walk completely around the dog		
Sit while you run back 10 steps and return		
Sit while you take 10 steps to the right, walk briskly to an equidistance to the left, and return		
Sit while you do the above in the opposite direction		
Sit for 10 seconds		
Day 4: The dog should		
Sit for 5 seconds		
Sit while you walk around the dog		
Sit for 20 seconds		
Sit while you take 20 steps backward and return		
Sit for 20 seconds		
Sit while you take 10 steps briskly backward and then toward the dog		
Sit while you take 10 steps to the right, walk an equidistance to the dog's left, and return		
Sit while you do the above in the opposite direction		
Sit while you walk briskly around the dog twice		
Sit while you slowly walk out of the room and immediately return		
Sit while you leave the room for 5 seconds		
Sit while you walk around the dog 3 times		
Sit while you run 10 steps to the left of the dog and walk briskly back		
Sit for 30 seconds		
Sit while you leave the room for 5 seconds		
Sit while you leave the room for 10 seconds		
Sit for 10 seconds		
Day 5: The dog should		
Sit for 10 seconds		
Sit for 15 seconds		
Sit for 20 seconds		
Sit for 10 seconds		
Sit for 20 seconds		
Sit while you walk around the dog		
Sit while you briskly walk around the dog twice		
Sit while you walk back 10 steps briskly and return		
Sit while you run to the left 10 steps and return		
Sit while you run 10 steps to the right and return		

743

Sit for 20 seconds		
Sit for 5 seconds		
Sit while you walk around the dog		
Sit while you leave the room for 5 seconds and return		
Sit while you leave the room for 10 seconds and return		
Sit while you leave room for 5 seconds and then return and walk around the dog before rewarding the dog		
Sit while you walk around the dog twice		
Sit while you leave room for 10 seconds and, on returning, walk around the dog before rewarding the dog		
Sit for 20 seconds		
Sit for 5 seconds		
Day 6: The dog should		
Sit for 10 seconds		
Sit for 15 seconds		
Sit for 20 seconds		
Sit while you walk around the dog		
Sit while you run 10 feet to the left and return		
Sit while you run 10 feet to the right and return		
Sit for 20 seconds		
Sit while you leave the room for 10 seconds		
Sit while you leave the room for 20 seconds		
Sit while you walk around the dog		
Sit while you leave the room for 10 seconds and walk around dog when you return		
Sit while you leave the room for 15 seconds and circle the dog when you return		
Sit for 5 seconds		
Sit while you circle the dog twice		
Sit while you walk 15 feet to the left, run 15 feet past the dog to the right, and walk back		
Sit and repeat the above		
Sit while you do the above in the opposite direction		
Sit for 5 seconds		
Day 7: The dog should		
Sit for 5 seconds		
Sit for 10 seconds		
Sit for 5 seconds		
Sit while you step back from the dog, sit down, and return		
Sit while you step back 5 feet from dog, sit down for 5 seconds, and return		
Sit while you walk across the room, sit (on a chair) for 15 seconds, and return		
Sit for 5 seconds		
Sit while you walk briskly 20 feet to the right away from the dog and return		
Repeat the above to the left		
Sit for 5 seconds		
Sit for 30 seconds		
Sit while you walk around the dog twice		
Sit while you take 10 steps briskly backward and then toward		

the dog		
Sit for 10 seconds turned away from the dog		
Sit for 20 seconds		
Day 8: The dog should		
Sit for 5 seconds		
Sit for 10 seconds		
Sit for 20 seconds		
Sit while you leave the room for 10 seconds		
Sit while you leave the room for 15 seconds		
Sit for 5 seconds		
Sit for 30 seconds		
Sit for 10 seconds		
Sit while you run 15 feet to the left and then to the right and back		
Sit while you do the above in the opposite direction		
Sit for 10 seconds		
Sit while you walk 10 feet away, circle the dog, and walk back		
Sit while you repeat the above at a brisk walk		
Sit while you circle the dog at 10 feet at a brisk walk		
Sit while you circle the dog at a brisk walk twice		
Sit for 10 seconds		
Sit while you leave the room for 10 seconds		
Sit for 5 seconds		
Sit while you circle the dog at 10 feet away		
Sit for 30 seconds at 5 feet away		
Sit for 10 seconds while 5 feet behind the dog		
Day 9: The dog should		
Sit for 10 seconds		
Sit for 60 seconds		
Sit for 10 seconds		
Sit while you circle the dog		
Sit while you leave the room for 10 seconds		
Sit while you back up 10 feet, sit down for 15 seconds, and return		
Sit while you circle the dog at 10 feet at a run		
Sit while you circle the dog twice at a run		
Sit while you reach for your toes		
Sit while you touch your toes twice		
Sit while you walk 15 feet to the right and then left before returning		
Sit while you do above in the opposite direction		
Sit for 10 seconds		
Sit for 30 seconds while you sit 5–10 feet away		
Day 10: The dog should		
Sit for 5 seconds		
Sit while you back up 10 feet and circle the dog at a brisk walk		
Sit while you walk to a chair and sit down for 10 seconds		
Sit while you walk to a chair sit down for 20 seconds and return		
Sit while you walk 20 feet to the right and run past the dog to		

20 feet to the dog's left and walk back		
Sit while you do above in opposite direction		
Sit for 10 seconds and both of you sit for 60 seconds		
Sit while you walk to a chair, sit for 10 seconds, walk briskly to 10 feet past the dog, and return slowly		
Sit while you repeat above		
Sit while you repeat above at a jog		
Sit while you repeat above at a fast jog		
Sit for 10 seconds		

Observations:

change, thereby becoming less reliant on punishment and adopting a more constructive and balanced approach to their dog's training. As control over the sit-stay module is established, family members can be encouraged to integrate it into everyday activities possessing reward value for the dog.

Encouraging owners to keep a journal and other records associated with sit-stay training can help them to become more aware and objective with respect to their dog's behavior—changes of viewpoint that are particularly important in cases involving serious adjustment problems. The dog's response to sit-stay training and daily progress should be tracked by keeping a record of daily training activities. The relative difficulty of each sit-stay requirement is estimated by the owner in terms of a five-point scale between 1 (easy: almost without error) through 5 (difficult: dog made many mistakes). The owner should jot down each day of exercises on a separate sheet of paper, giving space for notes and detailed observations about the dog's response to sit-stay training. Later, the estimated relative difficulty is recorded on the master sheet, along with a letter grade (+A-, +B-, +C-) based on overall working attitude and the

number of times that the response had to be repeated to reach criteria. In addition to estimating the difficulty for the dog and performance grading, the time of day, situational variables (e.g., distractions), motivational state (e.g., before or after meals), adverse influences, positive secondary changes, and so forth should be noted. Owners should be encouraged to write down their concerns and successes, thereby helping them to think more clearly about the dog's response to training projects.

Note: The foregoing instructions are in large measure consistent with Voith's intent and include some specific items that she included in her original instruction sheets (Voith, 1979); however, the procedures deviate in several significant ways from her original instructions.

SIT-STAY SKILLS

See Figure A.1.

REFERENCE

Voith VL (1979). Sit-Stay Program. Modified from a client handout with permission by Victoria L. Voith.

Appendix B

Sit, Down, Stand, and Stay Practice Variations

<table>
<tr><td>Dog's Name:</td><td>Date:</td></tr>
</table>

SIT VARIATIONS

Exercises Session	1	2	3
Sit with hand signal only			
Sit with voice signal only			
Sit from stand position after 3-second stay			
Sit from down position after 5-second stay			
Quick-sit while controlled walking			
Sit after starting exercise and 10-second stay			
Sit with the trainer in front after making and holding eye contact for 2 seconds			
Sit after the dog moves from the trainer's left side to the front			
Sit with the trainer behind the dog after 3-second stay			
Sit with the dog to the right after 10 seconds			
Sit with the trainer crouching			
Sit with the trainer sitting on the ground			
Sit with the trainer lying on the ground			
Sit while the trainer walks by at 3 feet away			
Sit while the trainer walks 5 feet away			
Sit from a stand at a distance of 3 feet			
Sit from stand after interrupted auto sit			
Sit from down position at a distance 5 feet			
Sit from a separate room			
Sit while another dog walks by			
Sit before a ball is tossed			
Sit at 10 feet away before a ball is tossed			
Stay and sit after a ball is tossed; dog is then released to chase the ball			
Sit after the dog turns around and stays 5 seconds			
Sit after moving to the right			
Sit after moving to the left			
Sit before jumping through a hoop or over a hurdle			
Quick-sit in the presence of a strong distraction (e.g., a squirrel)			
Quick-sit before a ball is tossed			

Observations:

<table>
<tr><td>Dog's Name:</td><td>Date:</td></tr>
</table>

DOWN VARIATIONS

Exercises Session	1	2	3
Down from sit with hand signal only			
Down from sit voice signal only			
Down from starting position after 5-second stay			
Down from the stand after 10-second stay			
Down from sit in front after 15-second stay			
Down from sit with the trainer to the left			
Down from sit with the trainer behind			
Down from sit with the trainer turned away			
Down from sit with the trainer crouching			
Down from sit with the trainer sitting on the ground after 10-second stay			
Down from sit with the trainer lying on the ground after 5-second stay			
Down from stand with the dog in front			
Down from stand with the dog to the right			
Down from stand with trainer behind the dog			
Instant-down			
Down from sit at a distance of 3 feet			
Down from sit from a separate room			
Down from sit at a distance 5 feet after 15-second stay			
Down from sit as another dog walks by			
Down from stand while another dog walks by			
Down from sit before the dog is released to chase a ball			
Down from sit after a ball is tossed; the dog is then released to chase the ball			
Down at 10 feet away before a ball is tossed			
Down after turning around			
Down on recall			
Down from sit after moving to the left			
Down after jumping through a hoop or over a hurdle			
Down from sit while near traffic			
Instant-down while running along side the trainer			

Observations:

Left form:

Dog's Name: Date:

STAND VARIATIONS

Exercises Session	1	2	3
Stand with one step forward			
Stand with voice signal only			
Stand from the starting position after 5 seconds			
Stand from the down after 30 seconds			
Stand from sit with the dog in front after 10 seconds			
Stand from down after 45-second stay			
Stand from sit with the trainer behind the dog			
Stand from sit with the trainer turned away			
Stand from down with the trainer crouching			
Stand from sit with the trainer sitting on the ground			
Stand from sit with the trainer lying on the ground			
Stand from down with the trainer in front			
Stand from down with the trainer to the left			
Stand from down with the trainer behind			
Stand after instant-down			
Stand from down at a 5 feet away			
Stand from down as another dog walks by			
Stand from sit at a distance 5 feet near a busy corner			
Stand from down with hand signal at a distance of 10 feet after 30-second second stay			
Stand from sit while another dog walks by			
Stand from down at 5 feet away before the dog is released to chase a ball			
Stand from sit after a ball is tossed; the dog is then released to chase the ball			
Stand from down at 15 feet away before tossing a ball			
Stand and stay after turning around			
Stand from down after drop on recall			
Stand from sit after moving to the left			
Stand after quick-sit and 10-second stay			
Stand after instant-down and 30-second stay			
Walking stand-stay while alongside the trainer			

Observations:

Right form:

Dog's Name :   Date:

SIT, DOWN, AND STAND COMBINATIONS

Exercises Session	1	2	3
Stand and stay for 10 seconds			
Sit from stand with voice and hand signal			
Down from sit after 5-second stay			
Sit from down after 5-second stay			
Stand from sit after 5-second stay			
Stand stay for 10 seconds 5 feet away			
Sit-stay for 20 seconds 5 feet away			
Down-stay for 30 seconds 5 feet away			
Walking stand-stay and then facing the dog at 5 feet away for 10 seconds			
Sit from stand at 5 feet away			
Down from sit at 5 feet away			
Sit from down at 5 feet away			
Stand from sit at 5 feet away			
Starting exercise with auto sit from the left side			
Starting exercise with stand interruption			
Starting exercise to heeling w/o auto sit			
Starting exercise, auto sit, and stay for 30 seconds for recall, front sit, and finish to the left side			
Walking stand-stay to starting position and auto sit after 10-second stay			
Starting exercise to auto sit, sit-stay, and 10-second stay before down and sit from down at a distance 15 feet			
Sit-stay for 30 seconds at 20 feet to recall, sit-front, and finish to right side			
Starting exercise to auto sit, down, and stay for 1 minute at 15 feet away before returning and dog is released to fetch a ball			
Sit, down from sit, stand from sit, and stay for 20 seconds at 15 feet away			
Down from stand at 20 feet, followed by stand from down after 1-minute stay			
Walking stand-stay, sit, and down from 10 feet followed by 30 seconds			
Drop on recall, sit from down, and stand 30-second stand-stay followed by ball play			
1-minute sit-stay followed by ball play			
5-minute down-stay followed by recall and finish from 20 feet away			

Observations:

FIG. B.1. Practice variations: sit, down, and stand. These tasks are intended as a general guideline. They should be gradually mastered and practiced in progressively longer and more difficult sequences. Many of the tasks depend on a well-established stay response that has been made reliable by sit and down-stay training. Tasks practiced are checked off after every daily session.

	GOOD CONDITIONING	ATTENTION ORIENTING	COME SIT/FRONT	SIT AND STAY	DOWN AND STAY	STAND/SIT/DOWN CYCLE	COME SIT/FRONT FINISH	STARTING EXERCISE	CONTROLLED WALKING	QUICK/SIT	BALL PLAY
1											
2											
3											

Observations:

FIG. B.2. Basic training practice checklist.

Appendix C

Posture-facilitated Relaxation (PFR) Training

BASIC GUIDELINES AND PFR TECHNIQUES

PFR training can be beneficial for puppies and dogs exhibiting a variety of adjustment problems. Of course, special precautions must be taken in the case of potentially aggressive dogs. Before being exposed to PFR training, such dogs should receive appropriate attention and integrated compliance training, and preliminary graduated counterconditioning as needed to reduce excessive reactivity to touching and handling. Adult dogs should be cautiously introduced to the procedure and may require a muzzle if they show signs of aggressive reactivity. The trainer should always be aware of the potential risks involved and error on the side of safety when performing such procedures, especially in the case of physically powerful dogs with a history of aggressive behavior.

Environmental Considerations

1. PFR training is first introduced in familiar situations with few distractions, but as a dog's relaxation response improves, it can be per-formed under more distracting and potentially stressful conditions. In the case of dogs exhibiting separation-related problems, massage should be performed in the room where the dog is left alone.

2. PFR training should be performed at times of need for de-arousal and increased relaxation.

3. A blanket or rug can be spread out for the dog to lie down on during PFR training. The rug gradually acquires a calming effect by way of association with PFR training. The dog can be trained to go to the rug and stay there at times of increased arousal associated with social excesses. Finally, the rug can be used to generalize the effects of relaxation and desensitization from the massage situation to other places. Conditioned comfort rugs can play a useful role in various fear-reduction procedures (Hothersall and Tuber, 1979).

PFR Techniques

1. PFR training progresses through graded postures ranked in terms of relative relinquishment of control and postural potential for inducing relaxation. The stepwise resistance (muscular tensing) and letting go in response to physical prompting and blocking is an intrinsic part of the PFR training process (see *Posture-facilitated Relaxation* in Chapter 6), without which a rapid and deep relaxation response is not achieved.

- PFR training begins with a collar control, reassuring eye contact, and a soft smile (friendly face), followed by a series of physical prompts causing the dog to stand, sit, lie down, and roll over onto its side. In addition to being the most control-relinquishing posture, the recumbent posture is the one most conducive to the

751

induction of a deep relaxation response (Figure C.1).

- If the dog becomes overly aroused or resistant, the massage is limited to actions and postures that it tolerates best and then additional steps are gradually added as its ability to relax and cooperate improves.
- Transitions triggering resistance can be worked through by repeating the same prompt and control with vocal reassurance ("Relax") and additional massage, until the dog shows signs of increasing acceptance and relaxation.

2. Each posture is physically prompted and maintained with vocal prompting "Relax." Otherwise, talking to the dog is minimized, except as needed to provide occasional reassurance and comfort.

3. The dog is paced through the massage sequence according to its response to each step. With practice, the speed of induction improves, especially with the aid of an olfactory-signature stimulus. Some puppies and dogs appear to be more responsive to a rapid sequencing of postural shifts and faster massage activity, whereas others require slower steps and more sustained massage.

4. The best results are achieved by matching handling and massage activities to the dog's temperament and needs. Some dogs prefer firm handling and massage, whereas others require more sensitive and gentle handling and massage. Oppositional behavior should be managed patiently but firmly, constantly guiding the dog back to the posture and position required. Going back to a previously successful step in the PFR cycle can be helpful, thereby increasing the relaxation response before trying to move ahead again.

- Physical assertions of control and TO, though sometimes necessary and expedient, are always reserved for those situations where affectionate persuasion has failed and where alternative courses of action are judged inappropriate.
- PFR training may challenge the dog and momentarily raise competitive tensions, but it should never be deliberately provocative or adversarial or degrade into manhandling. Competitive tensions are gradually resolved via the counterconditioning effects of increasing relaxation and trust.

5. Each massage stroke should be performed with the intention of intensifying the relaxation response. Absentminded rubbing does not produce the same benefit as focused massage.

6. The rhythm of massage should be slow and steady, with the time spent on each stroke, and the interval between strokes kept approximately the same. As the dog's response to PFR training improves, the massage stroke can be varied as needed to intensify the relaxation effect.

7. PFR training should be performed with a high degree of order, consistency, and precision from session to session. Predictable massage actions, controls, and manipulations gradually promote a dog's feelings of enhanced comfort, safety, and relaxation (security).

8. During the massage, the trainer should focus on breathing and project from the belly to the hands a feeling of comfort and care.

9. After several massages in which a progressively enhanced relaxation response is achieved, an olfactory signature is introduced in the context of thermal touch and the induction of a deep relaxation response. Gradually, the olfactory signature is presented at progressively earlier points in the PFR sequence. Eventually, the scent is presented just before the PFR cycle is initiated, thereby forming a conditioned association with the initiation and induction of relaxation. When fully conditioned, the odor should help to facilitate the PFR-training process, as well as improve the dog's responsiveness to various behavior-therapy procedures. The conditioned odor appears to enhance the dog's receptivity to counterconditioning efforts by directly helping to restrain aversive arousal or by altering the dog's appraisal of stimulation occurring in the presence of the odor.

10. A record of the dog's response to various prompts and controls should be kept to track its progress. In addition to general impressions regarding the dog's relative resistance or compliance at various stages of the PFR cycle, ranked on a point scale from 1 (resists: struggles constantly) to 5 (compliant: fully cooperative), heart rate should be recorded. A resting heart rate should be measured before PFR training is initiated, recorded after the dog is prompted to stand, and meas-

	PROMPT / CONTROL	STRUGGLE / RESISTANCE	COMPLIANCE/ COOPERATION	HEART RATE	COMMENTS
1	Collar				
2	Stand				
3	Sit				
4	Down				
5	Lateral				
6	Olfactory Signature				
7	Petting				

Dog's Name: Date:

Session No.:

PFR TRAINING CHART

FIG. C.1. PFR techniques.

ured immediately after the petting period at the conclusion of the PFR cycle, either by counting beats with fingers pressed over the femoral artery for 15 seconds or by using an inexpensive radiotelemetry device (see *Devices Used to Monitor Autonomic and Stress-related Changes* in Chapter 9). Changes in heart rate provide an objective measure of change occurring as the result of PFR training over time.

PFR TRAINING INSTRUCTIONS
Collar Control

The collar control is secured by grasping the collar at approximately at 4 and 8 o'clock.

While holding the dog's head securely, the jaw muscles are rhythmically massaged with the thumbs moving in a circular direction, while the trainer maintains affectionate eye contact, saying "Relax" in a reassuring tone.

Stand Prompt and Control

Next, the collar is grasped by the right hand at about 9 o'clock while the left forearm goes under the dog's belly bringing it up and around to the front. The trainer is aligned perpendicularly with the dog forming a T shape—an ethologically significant orientation (Fox, 1971). As the dog is steadied in the standing position, the left hand moves to the back of the neck where a rhythmic massage is applied to the neck, withers, and shoulders. The pressure of the massage stroke varies according to the dog's response to the stimulation. Some dogs and puppies may find such handling provocative and may attempt to wiggle out of the position, movement that should be prevented by placing the left forearm under the belly and shifting the puppy back into proper alignment.

It is important to maintain the massage for at least 30 seconds. If the dog struggles or attempts to sit, the action is prevented, and the dog is prompted back into the stand position. As the dog settles, its heart rate should be measured at the femoral artery by counting the number of beats that occur during a 15-second period.

Sit Prompt and Control

Once the dog accepts the stand control and massage, the left hand moves slowly and rhythmically down the spine until reaching the hip bone. The massage stroke along the spine is performed with a slow inchworm action. The hand is then opened across the breadth of the hip. With the thumb and first two fingers placed into the slight depression just anterior to the iliac crest, a gentle pincer pressure is applied until the dog sits. As the dog sits, the trainer says "Relax" and extends the massage to include the shoulder and lumbar muscles. When the sit posture is prompted, some dogs and puppies may resist and attempt to escape by shifting out of position or turning and mouthing on the hand. If such struggling does occur, it should be discouraged and the puppy prompted to complete the action, perhaps by pushing forward from behind the stifle. Pushing down on the rump should be avoided. Although assertive control and prompting are sometimes necessary, especially during the first or second cycle of PFR training, it is far better to achieve each postural transition without evoking excessive opposition.

Down Prompt and Control

The left hand grasps the collar from behind the neck at a point slightly left to the midline with the left forearm laid along the dog's

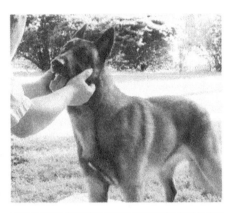

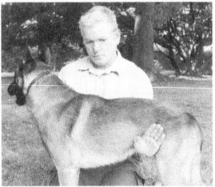

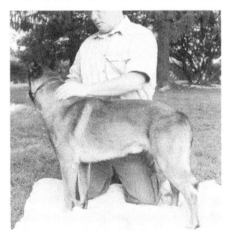

Fig. C.2.a. Stand prompt and control.

back. A steady downward pressure is applied as the right leg is grasped at the elbow and pulled forward as the dog is lowered down. When prompted into the down position, the dog's back should lean toward the handler. Once the dog settles into the down position, massage is applied over muscled areas of the shoulders, hips, and upper legs. The fingers of

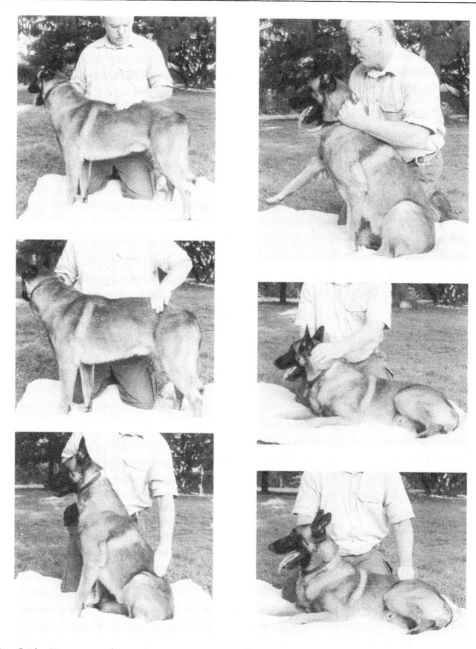

FIG. C.2.b. Sit prompt and control.

FIG. C.2.c. Down prompt and control.

the massage hand should be closed together and slightly cupped. The best all-purpose massage stroke is achieved by moving the fingers in a circular or spiraling movement over muscled areas. Carefully following and participating in the developing relaxation response help to guide the massage process intuitively. The trainer should focus on breathing in a rhythmic manner and actively feel the relaxing effects of the massage develop. When performed properly, massage benefits both the trainer and the dog.

Again, despite the most gentle and patient handling, some reactive puppies and dogs may respond aggressively to such manual control, perhaps necessitating more secure restraint (muzzling) or other emergency control measures (e.g., time-out). Limiting postural shifts to the stand and sit may be necessary in the beginning, at least until the dog learns to accept the massage and starts to relax, whereupon the down control can be attempted again.

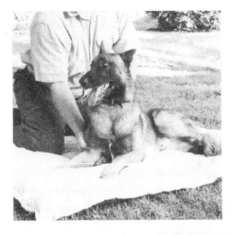

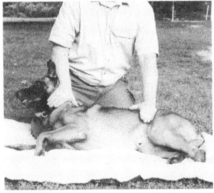

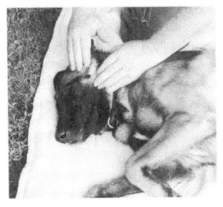

FIG. C.2.d. Lateral prompt and control.

Lateral Prompt and Control

Once the dog accepts and relaxes in the down position, it is rolled over onto its side. This maneuver is accomplished by placing the left hand on the lumbar muscle just in front of the hip. After pushing the dog's elbow under its body, the right hand is placed (knuckles up) over the neck so that the little finger is situated just behind the base of the jaw, whereupon the dog is rolled over onto its side. As the dog accepts the lateral control, the fingertips of the right hand are placed on the temporal muscle just in front of the ear while the fingertips of the left hand are placed on the masseter. A rhythmic massage is carried out with the fingers moving circularly in opposite directions. In addition to observing the dog's rate of breathing, the commissure of the eyelid should be monitored as an indicator of building relaxation. As the dog relaxes, the frequency of blinking decreases as the eye begins to close and finally shuts.

Ear, Jaw, and Lateral Massage

As the relaxation response deepens, the ear is taken by the thumb and index finger of the right hand and massaged. The thumb is then inserted gently into the ear canal and slowly moved outward to the tip of the ear. Most dogs and puppies appear to enjoy this very much and often exhibit a reflexive sigh as the thumb is moved about in the ear canal. This reflexive response, discovered in the context of PFR training and called the auricular relaxation reflex, usually precedes a deepening of the relaxation response. Next, the lower lip is massaged along the length of the jaw with tight spiraling movements. Attention is then turned to the upper shoulder and various muscles and joints of the foreleg. The front paws are carefully manipulated with each digit receiving focused massage. The massage is gradually moved over the rest of dog's body with focused massage applied to the lumbar area and hip, the hindquarters, the various joints, the tail, and the rear paws. In addition to the circular movement previously described, the heel of the hand is used to produce a simultaneous kneading effect, complementing the more focused movements of the fingertips. Lateral massage is limited to the left side of the dog's body.

Massage on the left side of the body produces a contralateral effect on the right hemisphere of the brain. The right somatosensory cortex plays a prominent role in social and emotional information processing (Adolphs, 2001). In addition, the right medial prefrontal cortex appears to be asymmetrically involved in the cortical integration of emotional and physiological responses to stressful arousal (Sullivan and Gratton, 1998). Massage-induced alterations of activity in the right cortex may promote positive social responsiveness as well as help to modulate emotional and physiological responses to restraint. Whether unilateral massage exerts a benefit via these cortical mechanisms is unknown, but unilateral massage does appear to perform better than bilateral massage for inducing a rapid and deep relaxation response.

Thermal Touch

As the relaxation response progresses and reaches a peak (as evidenced by decreased respiration rate, relaxed muscle tone, and lowered or closed eyelid position), the right index finger and forefingers are drawn together and placed on the temporal muscle mass located just in front of the ear. A gentle continuous pressure is applied for 10 to 15 seconds together with a steady care intention is focused on the dog. As a sensation of warmth develops between the fingertips and the point stimulated on the dog's head, the hand is slowly lifted away and centered approximately 2 to 3 inches above the dog's belly. From there, the hands are moved slowly over the dog's body, circulating a sensation of warmth in a manner resembling a slow movement through water.

Olfactory Signature

The last step in the massage is to link an olfactory stimulus or signature with the relaxation response. Normally, the odor of the owner's hand or other family members is presented as the olfactory signature. Alternatively, a dilute (1:30–50) odor (e.g., sandalwood, lavender, or chamomile) is presented during the thermal-touch procedure and the induction of a deep relaxation response. A scant drop of the dilute odor is rubbed into the hands. Alternatively, 2 or 3 drops of the odor

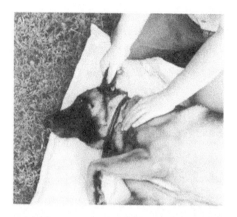

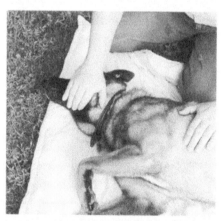

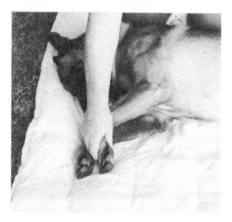

FIG. C.2.e. Ear, jaw, and lateral massage.

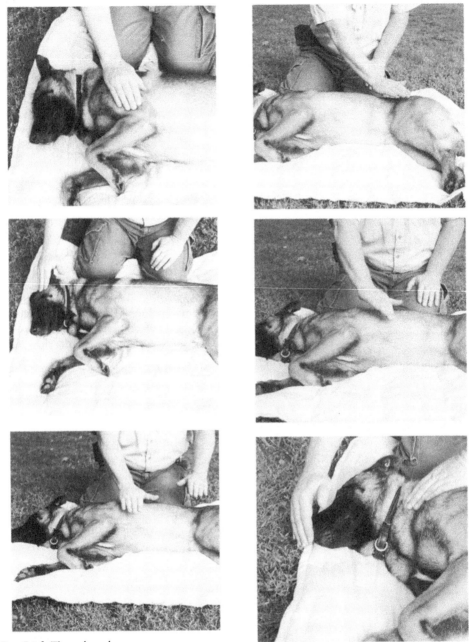

FIG. C.2.f. Thermal touch.

FIG. C.2.g. Olfactory signature.

are put on a tissue that is then folded several times into a small square that can be rubbed between the thumb and index finger to draw out the odor. Again, the hands are moved slowly above the dog's body without actually touching, but close enough for the heat and movement of the hands to be felt by the dog

as a thermal sensation. As the relaxation response deepens, the right hand is cupped gently around the dog's nose, stimulating a sniffing action and surprise. The surprise is of critical importance for forming a rapid and strong association between the state of deep

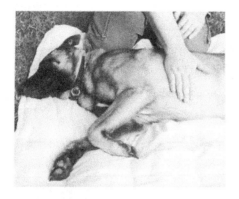

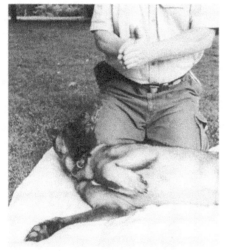

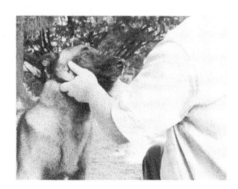

FIG. C.2.h. Transition petting and release.

relaxation (the physiological expression of acceptance and trust), the odor, and subsequent petting and release. Another method involves placing a small amount of the selected odor on the lips and blowing the scent slowly and unobtrusively over the dog's head from behind, just as an unscented hand is cupped over the dog's nose. The trainer should not blow sharply or directly into the dog's face and should sit upright and behind the dog when performing the procedure. Alternatively, a gentle smooch sound follows the scented breath and is timed to occur just as the unscented hand is placed in front of the dog's nose. The scented-breath technique is based on subtle associative linkages formed between the conditioned odor, surprise, and relaxation. Finally, in some olfactory-conditioning procedures, the odor is delivered from a squeaker bulb by slowly squeezing it and then releasing the slightly depressed bulb to produce a soft squeak.

Transitional Petting and Release

The dog is gradually transitioned out of the relaxation response with firm, long-stroke petting actions that consciously and deliberately follow the lay of coat over the head, neck, back, and chest. As the hindquarters are petted, the dog's heart rate should be measured again and recorded. At the conclusion of the petting phase, the trainer quietly says "OK" and gently claps a couple of times. As the dog stands up, the collar control is applied again with affectionate eye contact and vocal reassurance before the puppy or dog is released for play, training, or another cycle of PFR training. Note the more focused eye contact given by the dog in comparison to response exhibited with the collar control initiating the PFR cycle.

REFERENCES

Adolphs R (2001). The neurobiology of social cognition. *Curr Opinion Neurobiol*, 11:231–239.

Fox MW (1971). *Behaviour of Wolves, Dogs and Related Canids*. New York: Harper and Row.

Hothersall D and Tuber DS (1979). Fears in companion dogs: Characteristics and treatment. In JD Keehn (Ed), *Psychopathology in Animals: Research and Clinical Implications*. New York: Academic.

Sullivan RM and Gratton A (1998). Relationships between stress-induced increases in medial prefrontal cortical dopamine and plasma corticosterone levels in rats: Role of cerebral laterality. *Neuroscience*, 83:81–91.

Appendix D

Puppy Temperament Testing and Evaluation

Temperament Testing
Testing Procedures
    A. Social Attraction (Passive Handler)
    B. Social Attraction (Active Handler)
    C. Contact Tolerance
    D. Physical Controls
    E. Impulse Control (Possessiveness)
    F. Impulse Control (Delay of
       Gratification)
    G. Ball Play
    H. Rag Play
    I. Separation Reaction
    J. Reactivity and Problem Solving (Barrier
       Frustration)
    K. Startle Reflex
    L. Cognition (Expectancy)
    M. Cognition (Delayed Response)
    N. Social Cognition (Passive Direction)
    O. Social Cognition (Active Direction)
Significance and Interpretation
References

TEMPERAMENT TESTING

In Volume 2, much was left to the imagination with regard to the procedures used to perform puppy temperament tests (see *Puppy Temperament Testing and Evaluation* in Volume 2, Chapter 2). In addition to describing in detail how the various tests are performed, the potential significance of the information also remains to be discussed. The tests described below borrow from the basic research performed by Scott and Fuller (1965), the testing procedures used by the Bio Sensor Research Team (U.S. Army Super Dog Program), and testing recommendations suggested by Michael Fox (1972). Although temperament tests are not routinely performed, they can be used as an objective tool for eval-

uating a variety of social, emotional, cognitive, and motivational dimensions in puppies. For applied dog behaviorists needing a highly objective assessment tool for supplementing behavior questionnaires and other instruments (e.g., the Puppy Behavior Profile), such testing may be useful. Temperament tests may also be useful for research purposes, wherein an objective baseline of information is needed. For most practical training purposes, however, the Puppy Behavior Profile, along with interview information and direct observation, provides sufficient information to determine a puppy's training needs.

The Puppy Temperament Test may be most useful in the case of older puppies about whom little information is known. No test, no matter how comprehensive and detailed, can reveal every facet of a puppy's behavior or potential. In addition to specific tests, real-life observations of a puppy's behavior under various circumstances and stressors can be highly revealing and useful. Although an owner can play the role of handler in many of the tests, the administering trainer, especially in cases where special skills may be necessary to control the puppy properly, should perform the role of handler. The tests are designed for puppies from 10 to 20 weeks of age, but can be easily modified for use with younger and older dogs.

TESTING PROCEDURES

A. Social Attraction (Passive Handler)

Both the owner and the trainer can alternately play the role of handler. The scorer (owner) holds the puppy on a 6-foot leash as the handler moves to a spot approximately 20 feet away. After approximately 10 seconds, the handler calls the puppy's name and claps to get its attention and the scorer releases the puppy. If the puppy hesitates, it is encouraged vocally and the handler might crouch down, as well. As the puppy approaches, the handler should once again stand upright. After a brief moment of standing still, the handler should praise the puppy and toss a treat on the ground and pick up the leash. Further information can be obtained by reversing the roles of handler and scorer. Now, the trainer holds the puppy's leash as the owner walks away. The owner repeats the handler procedure in an identical manner. Differences in the puppy's behavior toward the trainer and the owner are noted.

B. Social Attraction (Active Handler)

Holding the end of a 6-foot leash, the handler steps away while calling the puppy's name. If the puppy hesitates, the handler (owner or trainer) calls the puppy's name again and slaps his or her thigh. If necessary, the leash can be dropped as the handler jogs away from the puppy while at the same time encouraging it to follow along with cajoling words and gestures. If the puppy forges into the leash, the handler should run along to keep up.

C. Contact Tolerance

Most puppies enjoy being petted and handled, but some are intolerant of tactile stimulation and may become agitated or overly aroused by taction. For highly reactive or excitable puppies, petting and handling should be limited to minimally provocative stimulation. In addition to petting the puppy's head, body, and tail, the handler should attempt to examine the puppy's mouth, ear's, and feet.

D. Physical Controls

These various controls are typically performed by the trainer, and the owner is later instructed on how to perform them in the context of posture-facilitated relaxation training. Care should be taken not to agitate the

puppy unnecessarily. During the performance of each control, the puppy is massaged and reassured. If the puppy becomes highly reactive and fails to calm in response to massage and vocal reassurance, the score for that control is noted and the physical control portion of the test concluded. At the beginning of the test, resting heart rate should be measured, followed by a second measure taken at the end. For specific instructions on prompting the controls, refer to Appendix C, *Posture-facilitated Relaxation (PFR) Training*.

E. Impulse Control (Possessiveness)

For the safety of children and others in the home, it may be helpful to determine the degree of risk that a puppy poses with respect to possessive aggression.

The trainer, taking care not to provoke the puppy unnecessarily, always performs this test with the puppy restrained on a leash. The beef bone or other desirable object used for this test should be tied to a piece of twine, allowing the trainer means to remove it safely from the puppy if the puppy becomes aggressively aroused. The puppy is left with the bone for 1 minute as the handler stands 10 feet away. As the handler approaches the puppy, the leash is picked up to restrain the puppy, if necessary, and the handler reaches toward the bone, just out of the puppy's reach. If the puppy growls or snaps, the attached twine is used to pull the bone away. In the case of a puppy that accepts close contact and petting while it chews on its prize, the trainer can attempt to take away the bone. If there is any doubt about the puppy's intention, the bone is removed by pulling the piece of twine, without applying a muzzle control. If the puppy releases the bone without objection, it is rewarded with a treat offered as trade and the opportunity to have the bone back again. In the case of threatening puppies or puppies appearing stiff with intense possessive interest, testing for bite propensity should be considered. In such cases, a piece of broomstick 1-foot long is covered on one end with an 8-inch square of cloth neatly wrapped around several layers of batting and secured with rubber bands at the base of the wad. The cloth and batting should be replaced after every use to minimize the presence of confounding odors. Alternatively, fingers of a glove can be filled with cotton balls and shaped into the form an approaching hand. The probe stick is passed under a jacket sleeve, with the padded end or glove protruding out. As the puppy is approached, the leash is secured and the probe stick is moved toward the bone, mimicking normal caution when doing so. If the puppy ignores the intrusion, it is petted, given a food reward, and left alone to enjoy the bone for an additional minute. If the puppy attacks the probe stick, the bone is snatched away and the puppy timed-out. This test is not designed for adult dogs, wherein more precautions and safeguards may be needed to ensure safety for the trainer and the dog. Although the test is useful for detecting possessive aggression tendencies, failure of the puppy to show such behavior should not be taken to imply that under some set of circumstances it may not exhibit aggression while in possession of some prized item.

F. Impulse Control (Delay of Gratification)

During this test, the handler (owner or trainer) requires that a puppy stand quietly before receiving a treat. If the puppy already knows how to sit, the handler vocally prompts the puppy to sit, but, additionally, requires that it hold the sit position as the treat is moved toward its mouth. The puppy is required to take the treat gently. By standing on the puppy's leash, jumping and lunging are thwarted.

G. Ball Play

A puppy's willingness to chase and retrieve a tennis ball is assessed by first briefly causing the puppy to mouth or tug it. Interest can also be enhanced by bouncing the ball against a wall a couple of times before throwing it. The ball is rolled approximately 15 feet away. If the puppy runs after it and picks it up, it is encouraged vocally and with smooching and clapping to return with it, whereupon the

puppy is rewarded with affection and tug before the ball is taken. The puppy is given three opportunities to fetch the ball and scored according to the best performance in terms of drive and cooperation, ideally chasing the ball enthusiastically and bringing it straight back without hesitation. In this test, the least favorable responses are to ignore the ball (deficient drive) or to run away with it (deficient cooperation), with the latter being preferable to the former. If the puppy fails to return or runs away with the ball, the handler should appropriately lure the puppy back or step on the leash or long line and take the ball away from the puppy. The puppy is returned to the original spot and allowed to mouth on the ball for a moment before the ball is thrown again. For smaller puppies, soft toys or smaller balls should be used.

H. Rag Play

A strip of cloth (e.g., burlap) is presented to the puppy and dangled or dragged back and forth for it to grab. If the puppy takes the rag, it is encouraged with praise to tug and hold on. Puppies are prompted to release the rag by offering them a treat. Another variation allows the puppy to keep the rag, and it is evaluated for its subsequent behavior. For example, the puppy runs off and shakes the rag, the puppy runs off and chews the rag, the puppy takes the rag and returns promptly to play more, or the puppy drops the rag. In addition, puppies are evaluated for their level of possessiveness when approached while in possession of the rag.

I. Separation Reaction

During the separation test, the puppy is usually placed into an unfamiliar room for 1 minute. A small room is ideal, but a larger room can also be used, as well. To prevent the puppy from wandering too much during isolation, it can be placed into a holding pen. A highly desirable treat or hollow rubber toy smeared inside with peanut butter is presented to the puppy. In the case of puppies showing a high level of separation reactivity, a piece of clothing with the owner's scent is left with puppy. A third variation involves evaluating the puppies response to a mirror secured to the back of the door.

J. Reactivity and Problem Solving (Barrier Frustration)

A wire-mesh barrier is set up by stretching out a hinged holding pen, forming a crescent or V shape. Stakes are placed in the ground to support the barrier so that it cannot be knocked down if the puppy runs into it or jumps against it. The puppy is placed in the middle of the convex side of the barrier while the handler (owner) stands about 5 feet away on the opposite side. The scorer holds the puppy by a leash as the handler drops several small treats into a bowl on the ground. The handler should move about 2 feet back from the bowl and call the puppy, as the scorer releases the leash. In addition to scoring the sort of behavior exhibited by the puppy, the length of time that it takes to get around the barrier should be noted. If the puppy fails to solve the problem within 1 minute, the handler goes around the barrier to join the puppy and then demonstrates to the puppy how to get around the barrier. The handler places another small treat in the bowl and steps back from the barrier. If the puppy still fails to get around the barrier, it is taken around by the scorer, whereupon the puppy is received with affection and permitted to eat the food in the bowl. In addition to the specific items on the score sheet, the scorer should note whether the puppy goes to the handler first or the food, improvement occurring as the result of demonstration, and unusual behaviors.

K. Startle Reflex

A relatively strange area is usually selected for this test. Normally, the handler is located about 3 to 5 feet behind the puppy, and a seven-penny shaker can is dropped to the floor from waist high. The distance and size of the shaker can are determined by the puppy's relative sensitivity to auditory startle. Startle tests are typically reserved for puppies over 12 weeks of age. Any modifications of the basic test format should be noted on the test form. Puppies showing extreme reactions

can be subsequently given a prepulse-inhibition test. In this case, the can is tapped with the flick of a finger as it is dropped. Any changes in the puppy's startle response are noted. After the startle event, the handler should encourage the puppy to come, receiving it with affection and petting, rewarding it with food, and tossing a ball. In addition to the auditory startle test, the puppy can be exposed to startle stimulation involving a visual component. For example, a spring-loaded umbrella can be opened at a perpendicular angle to the puppy from 6 to 8 feet away. Another variation involves dragging some novel rattling object (e.g., a toy wagon) near the puppy. Whenever possible bilateral tympanic temperature and heart rate measurements should be taken before and after exposure to novel and startling stimuli.

The following social cognition tests have been added to the original evaluation format:

L. Cognition (Expectancy)

The puppy is given 20 small treats from the right hand in the context of attention training (squeak, head turn, click). After a brief period, the handler presents a small biscuit held between the fingers of the left and right hands at approximately 12 to 16 inches from the puppy's nose. The hands are slowly separated so that the biscuit remains in the puppy's view, but is kept in the left hand. Since the puppy has learned to find the food treat in the right hand, it will tend to show a persistent tendency to follow the right hand, despite the presence of sensory information indicating an opposite fact (i.e., the treat is in the left hand) (see *Practical Example* in Volume 1, Chapter 7). The results (1 to 5) are measured by counting the number of trials the puppy requires to learn not to follow the right hand on two consecutive trials.

M. Cognition (Delayed Response)

The puppy is kept on leash at a doorway while the handler shows it a treat and places the treat in a small bowl situated behind one of three shoe boxes standing on their sides, thereby concealing the item from view. The boxes are placed 5 to 7 feet apart. The middle box never contains food. The puppy is given several practice trials allowing it to run to the box where the food is hidden after waiting 1, 3, 5, 10, 15 seconds. The practice is continued until the puppy is able to able to find the food without error. Next, after the food treat is concealed while the puppy looks on, the door is closed and opened again after an increasing period (1, 3, 5, 10, 15 seconds), whereupon the puppy is released to locate the food item. The puppy is given five progressively longer trials, provided that it goes to correct box each time; otherwise, it is required to repeat the step until it succeeds. The results are evaluated in terms of the longest delay in which the puppy performed correct choices after five trials (see *Learning and Trainability* in Volume 1, Chapter 2).

N. Social Cognition (Passive Direction)

The arrangement is the same as just described, except the food item is concealed after the door is closed. The handler remains standing behind the shoe box where the food item is hidden. The puppy is released after 10 seconds from behind the door. The results are evaluated in terms of the number of correct choices in five trials.

O. Social Cognition (Active Direction)

An identical arrangement as the foregoing is set up, except the handler stands or sits on a chair behind the middle box. The puppy is given 10 trials of increasing difficulty (ranked 1 to 5) with respect to handler directional cuing: the handler makes a tapping action toward the correct box, the handler reaches and points at the correct box, the handler orients and points toward the correct box, the handler repeatedly turns and glances toward the box, or the handler steadily stares at the correct box. The puppy is given 10 trials during which it is allowed to advance to the next step after a minimum of two successful choices. After two consecutive incorrect choices, the puppy is returned to a previously successful step. The results are evaluated in terms of the number errors and the ranked difficulty of directional cuing.

In addition to the specific tests just outlined, impressions are recorded about the puppy's response to familiar and unfamiliar situations and objects. General impressions of fearfulness, activity levels, and excitability should be recorded (e.g., high, moderate, or low). Any behavior observed during testing that may help clarify the direction and significance of the test results should be noted and given appropriate consideration. In some cases, it can be useful to repeat tests on a weekly basis to observe changes resulting from maturation or training.

SIGNIFICANCE AND INTERPRETATION

Several temperament tests have been devised and recommended to help place puppies in homes consistent with their behavioral needs (see *Temperament Testing* in Volume 1, Chapter 5). However, in recent years, the predictive value of such tests has fallen under significant doubt and controversy (see *Temperament Tests and Aggression* in Volume 2, Chapter 8). Although the results of such tests [e.g., restraining a puppy on its back, petting it along its topline, and lifting it off the ground (Campbell, 1972)] may be useful as general reactivity *indicators* (see Clark, 1994), they do not appear to be very useful as *predictors* or means for detecting stable *dominance* traits or propensity for dominance-related aggression (Beaudet, 1993).

The detection of stable traits and characteristics or interpreting the test scores as predictive indicators of adult behavior is not the primary purpose of the tests just described. The primary purpose of testing is to help define specific behavioral propensities and tendencies needful of training and therapy. Testing provides an objective picture of a puppy's behavioral potential (excesses and deficits) at the time of testing. In addition to identifying weaknesses needing attention, testing can also help to identify strengths to nurture and actualize further. Behavioral tendencies that persist despite dedicated training efforts and the influence of development may presage adult propensities.

Excesses associated with tests A and B are often misinterpreted as indicators of social dominance, appearing to confound oppositional behavior with playful competitiveness. Unfortunately, the mischaracterization of social exuberance as an oppositional threat is not just an innocuous error, but an evaluation that has resulted in significant misunderstanding and maltreatment of puppies in training. A host of manhandling techniques has been developed to "break" such puppies to make them more submissive—a sad situation because most of these puppies are already submissive and in search of leadership; that is, their behavior is actively submissive—not dominant. Although exceptions certainly exist, most often puppies that use threats and overt aggression toward people do so as the result of mishandling and a failure to establish more competent and cooperative means to negotiate interactive conflicts and tensions. Although puppies affected by oppositional problems may also exhibit intrusive excesses, for the most part low scores on these tests are indicative of excitability, social enthusiasm, confidence, and playful competitiveness; such puppies may be characterized as social extraverts. In the context of Pavlov's typology (see *Experimental Neurosis* in Volume 1, Chapter 9), such extraverted puppies correspond to the sanguine or s type: friendly, socially responsive, focused, energetic, and highly sensitive to the effects of reward and less responsive to the effects of punishment. Puppies with low scores (1 and 2) are socially (and usually physically) healthy and outgoing (stable extravert), but needful of social limits and compliance training. In addition, play training may be very beneficial as a means to redirect their competitive enthusiasm into more constructive and cooperative outlets. At the other extreme, puppies exhibiting high scores (4 and 5) may be affected by significant social tendencies associated with introversion. Such puppies may show a generalized lack of behavioral output (inhibited) and may be socially reserved, passive, adverse to play, and highly sensitive to the effects of punishment and less responsive to the effects of reward (Gray, 1991). Puppies scoring 3s on tests A and B show a healthy balance between extraverted and introverted influences and, depending on future developmental, socialization, and training influences,

may progressively move in the direction of increased introversion or extraversion (Figure D.1).

Under the influence of adverse developmental influences, extraverted puppies may become progressively unstable in the direction of Pavlov's choleric type (c type), being prone to show contact aversion (touch sensitivity and irritability), impulsive behavior, frustration and restraint intolerance, and nervous excitability. The c type is prone to panic-evoked aggression (rage) via the simultaneous and escalating arousal of fear and anger emotional systems. Unstable extraverts require highly structured reward-based training activities aimed at reducing interactive conflict and tension, together with management precautions designed to minimize provocative stimulation. The goal of training and management efforts is to reduce behavioral stress while increasing the dog's ability to gain a better state of security (comfort and safety) and trust. The c type tends to react to punishment rather than adjust to it, making physical punishment highly problematic in the case of such dogs. Mismanaged introverted puppies, on the other hand, may become progressively unstable and prone to develop melancholic tendencies (anxiety and depression) and behavior problems, e.g., social aversions, fears and phobias, and compulsive disorders. Whereas the c type tends to be affected by excessive excitability and impulsiveness (hyperactivity and stimulation seeking), the melancholic type(m type) tends to respond to the environment in a highly fearful, inhibited, or helpless manner. Under the influence of stability-enhancing training activities, introverted puppies can learn to cope more effectively with the environment and become progressively more confident and relaxed. In contrast, phlegmatic types (p types or stable introverts) tend to be passive, controlled, calm, and balanced with respect to their social and environmental interaction. Whereas s-type puppies may have trouble learning to wait and to delay gratification, such abilities come more naturally to p-type puppies. According to Pavlov (1994), all dogs can be grouped according to these four basic temperament types:

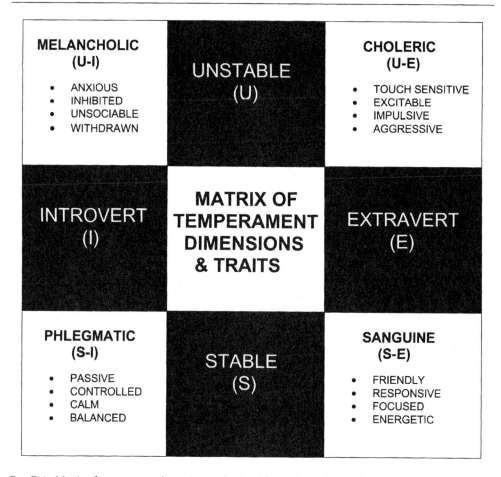

FIG. D.1. Matrix of temperament dimensions and traits. After Pavlov and Eysenck (see *Experimental Neurosis* in Volume 1, Chapter 9).

Thus all our animals are divided into four definite groups: two extreme groups of excitable and inhibitable animals [choleric and melancholic] and two central groups of balanced but different animals: some very quiet [phlegmatic] and others extraordinarily lively [sanguine]. We have to consider this a precise fact. (216)

Whereas tests A and B give some indication of a puppy's social development in terms of relative extraversion or introversion, subsequent tests may serve to detect specific stabilizing or destabilizing influences. For example, high scores (1 and 2) on test C may indicate heightened touch sensitivity and excitability consistent with Pavlov's c type, whereas low scores (4 and 5) may indicate some degree of insecurity or social aversion, indicators consistent with Pavlov's m type. Puppies scoring 3 exhibit a fairly balanced response to contact, consistent with p type (stable introvert). Stable extraverts (s types) also show strong playful responses (mouth, paw, and jump up) while being handled. The cause of their behavior is the result of playful enthusiasm and poorly defined social limits—not contact aversion or impulse dysregulation. Differentiating biting and other excesses due to contact aversion versus playful enthusiasm is facilitated by the control tests (D1–D5). During control tests, unstable extraverts (c types) may become progressively aroused and resistant despite vocal reassurance and massage. Stable extraverts (sanguine), on the other hand, are typically more receptive to the calming effects of reassurance and massage. C types may become reactive and aggressive when rolled on their side, whereas s types are more likely to accept such restraint without much resistance or struggle and rapidly calm down. S types are highly responsive to relaxation training, often falling rapidly into a deep relaxation response as massage proceeds. M types may struggle to get away or appear to resent physical restraint. P types typically show high scores (4 and 5) by passively accepting control and appearing to enjoy massage, but often enter into the relaxation response more slowly than s types.

Test E helps to differentiate these various temperament types further as well as providing an indicator of behavioral thresholds controlling aggression in response to appetitive loss or frustration (see *Anxiety, Frustration, and Aggression* in Volume 2, Chapter 8). Puppies getting low scores (1 and 2) in tests C and D1–5 that also show intense growling or snapping when approached while possessing a prized item may be at significant risk for serious problems unless significant and sustained behavioral efforts are undertaken. Well-socialized s and p types typically score 3 and 4 in the possessiveness test. M types may ignore the bone as the result of high levels of anxiety competing with appetitive arousal, a significant test for confirming such tendencies when other test scores appear to point in the direction instability (e.g., anxious, inhibited, unsociable, and withdrawn). Test F may have some value in detecting impulsive tendencies associated with hyperactivity, especially in the case of older puppies. Repeated jumping up and grabbing for the treat despite blocking (1), may reflect an inability to cope adaptively with frustration, a c-type trait. Stable extraverts (s type) tend to show high levels of excitement and enthusiasm but rapidly abandon impulsive efforts (2) to grab the treat and defer to physical restraint, whereas stable introverts (p type) show a more control and even appetitive response, together with a greater willingness to wait or sit when given a treat. In contrast, unstable introverts (m type) may refuse or avoid taking food.

Tests G and H can be particularly revealing. Puppies that show a natural aptitude for chasing and retrieving things are typically s types that are highly responsive to training for work and competition (see *Learning and Trainability* in Volume 1, Chapter 2). These tests can be further revealing by performing them under both familiar and unfamiliar circumstances. Choleric puppies may refuse to release the rag or stand guard over it with threats and snapping. P-type puppies may show a willingness to retrieve and tug, but typically lack real enthusiasm and sustained interest in the activity. M-type puppies may ignore the ball or halfheartedly chase it, but not pick it up or walk away after giving a brief chase. Unstable introverts (m type) may refuse to take a rag to play tug.

The separation-reaction test (I) helps to segregate excesses and deficits associated with attachment. Most puppies experience some degree of distress when separated in a strange situation. C-type puppies may exhibit sustained distress resulting from exaggerated reactions to loss and frustration. Such dogs may bark in a persistent and demanding way and scratch aggressively at doors. S-type puppies may also rebel at separation, but can be comforted with food or toys (e.g., peanut butter on the inside of a hollow rubber toy). While initially highly aroused, sanguine puppies may bark, but rapidly habituate to distress at separation and engage in diversionary activities. M-type puppies may be highly distressed at separation, reacting under the coactive influence of fear and anxiety, whereas p-type puppies may show a more restrained distress response when isolated for brief periods, but may become progressively distressed by longer separations. Whereas s types tend to bark more than whine, p types are more prone to whine than bark. Whereas s-type puppies appear to be responsive to the calming effects of food, p-type puppies appear to be more responsive to the presence of clothing and other items scented with the owner's odor.

The barrier test (J) is used to help evaluate a puppy's ability to cope with adverse emotional arousal (frustration) while solving a simple problem. Puppies that exhibit intense emotional reactivity and fail to solve the test within the allotted 1-minute period may be subject to significant stress. Again, the c type will tend to obtain low scores (1 and 2), whereas s and p types (exhibiting excitatory and inhibitory balance) will tend to obtain higher scores. M-type puppies may stay close to the scorer and not attempt to solve the problem. The barrier test may help to identify learning and impulse-control problems. By measuring the length of time it takes the puppy to get around the barrier, the degree of interference can be given an objective measure. The benefits of behavior-therapy efforts may be estimated by comparing barrier test scores over time. Additional information may be obtained in the case of puppies that initially struggle or fail, but learn how to get around the barrier more quickly by observing the handler demonstrating how to do it. Such responsiveness may point to enhanced social learning abilities and sensitivity to human sources of information used to solve problems (Pongrácz et al., 2001).

The way a puppy responds to startling events may strongly affect its ability to learn and perform under aversive situations. Whereas choleric puppies appear to be adversely influenced by frustration, melancholic puppies are typically more vulnerable to startling sounds or movements. During the auditory startle test, c-type puppies may bark at the handler or even run at and grab the shaker can. P-type puppies typically show some evidence of startle, but quickly recover without evidence of lingering fearful arousal. S-type puppies may show significant startle (3) and recover, although some sound-movement-sensitive types may exhibit significant fear with retreat from the situation. Such otherwise stable puppies should receive intensified desensitization and habituation efforts to elevate the relevant threshold. As one might predict, unstable introverts may be significantly affected by the startle test, typically receiving high scores (4 and 5). In addition, to behavioral measures of emotional reactivity, heart rates should be taken before and after startling stimulation. Poststimulation heart rates should be taken 10 to 15 seconds after the event and again after 1 minute. Active and fearless puppies exhibiting low standing heart rates may be prone to develop offensive aggression problems (see *Autonomic Arousal, Heart Rate, Aggression* in Chapter 6), especially if they exhibit threatening behavior during contact-tolerance tests, physical control tests, or impulse-control (possessiveness) tests

(see *Behavioral Thresholds and Aggression* in Volume 2, Chapter 8).

A prepulse-inhibition test may be useful in the case of puppies showing unusual responses to startle or other indicators of disorganizing reactivity. Normally, the presence of a comparatively weak stimulus presented just in advance of a startling acoustical stimulus serves to restrain the magnitude of the startle response. The absence of prepulse inhibition is a marker occurring in association with a variety of psychiatric disorders (Braff et al., 2001). Prepulse inhibition is conceptualized as performing a protective emotional function, on the one hand, and a cognitive processing function, on the other. With the occurrence of a startling (dangerous) event, it behooves the animal to stop what it is doing, collect as much relevant information as possible, and rapidly evaluate its significance. Without mechanisms such as prepulse inhibition, the animal may be emotionally overwhelmed by startling events and react blindly to them, perhaps endangering itself in the process. A lack of prepulse inhibition may reflect a gating deficiency affecting sensorimotor processing. Although published data are lacking in dogs, preliminary observations indicate that dogs generally exhibit a strong prepulse-inhibition effect. Future studies designed to evaluate prepulse inhibition in dogs exhibiting serious behavior problems may prove valuable in terms of understanding and treating certain severe canine behavioral disorders. In addition to providing an operational measure of cognitive function, such indicators may offer a neurological marker for confirming behavioral diagnostics and to evaluate treatment efficacy.

Delayed response testing provides another measure of cognitive function (Fox and Spencer, 1967). Delayed response and object permanence abilities operate under developmental constraints, with the dog's abilities appearing to improve with the maturation (Gagnon and Dore, 1994). Delayed response capacities depend on a complex coordination of emotional and cognitive functions that may be disrupted by stress and other disturbances affecting the frontal cortex and working memory (see *Cerebral Cortex* in Volume 1, Chapter 3). Deficiencies in delayed response capacity may help to more accurately characterize impulse-control problems, perhaps providing a baseline from which to objectively evaluate the benefits of training and behavior therapy. Another useful indicator of cognitive function is the puppy's ability to adjust expectancies in accordance with prediction discrepancies. Adjusting behavioral output to fit sensory input and outcomes associated with instrumental activity is an important aspect of adaptive learning. When events and outcomes occur on a regular basis, the formation of prediction and control expectancies may exert a dominant influence over choices, even in the face of contrary sensory information. On the other hand, a predominance of irregular events and outcomes lacking reliability and orderliness (or lacking the ability to detect and organize such reliability and order) may cause the dog to depend more on direct sensory information to make decisions, with heightened behavioral stress (anxiety and frustration), hypervigilance, and scanning. Test L evaluates a puppy's ability to form a simple predictive-control expectancy and the rapidity with which the expectancy is changed in response to contrary sensory information and the discontinuation of the expected outcome.

Dogs showing compulsive tendencies and therapy-resistant reactive adjustments in association with social anxiety and ambivalent behavior appear to show a strong tendency to perseverate on the right hand after learning to expect food from there. The unproductive choice may continue on for many trials, despite the presence of obvious sensory information to the contrary and growing signs of distress on the dog's part. Such behavior gives support to the notion that habit formation takes place at choice points with the choice itself signifying that the action has undergone reinforcement. It is only through the inhibitory action of attention and impulse control that intelligent hesitation enables the dog to process choice points proactively and to choose well. Thus, the perseveration revealed by this cognitive test may provide information useful for assessing the fitness of executive functions. In addition, the test may reveal the presence of interfering social anxiety and reactive arousal impairing the dog's ability to adjust its behavior to the change.

Dogs affected by this perseverant pattern may rapidly shift into a proactive selection mode when the test is performed by a family member or trusted person but may rapidly revert back to the previous pattern if startled or otherwise made uneasy.

The dog's ability to adapt to life with people is in large part mediated by social cognitive abilities. Normal puppies show an innate responsiveness to human directional cuing, especially pointing actions combined with gazing. The capacity of puppies to follow human pointing and gazing to find food and other attractive objects does not appear to depend on learning or developmental age, at least with respect to puppies 9 weeks of age or older (Hare et al., 2002). Interestingly, according to Hare and colleagues, the dog's ability to follow human pointing and gazing cues is superior to the abilities of the chimpanzee and the wolf to follow similar directional cues. The dog's ability to follow directional cues may be the result of linked social, emotional, and cognitive changes produced by domestication. According to Hare, the dog appears to have undergone a "process of phylogenetic enculturation" (1636) by which human and canine cognitive abilities have converged to make social bonding and cooperation possible. Tests M, N, and O provide useful information for assessing cognitive functions that may offer additional insight into the significance of other tests.

Deficits affecting a dog's ability to follow human directional cues or establish eye contact and sustained face gazing may reflect the presence of significant social anxiety and ambivalence, perhaps stemming from a persistent partial retraction of the social engagement system. In order to acquire social information of sufficient quality to promote autonomic attunement, the dog must orient and actively attend to the face in a relatively neutral and trusting way. Some dogs appear to show from an early age a tendency to treat eye contact and neutral facial expressions as threats. Some puppies may act on this negative bias by biting or snapping at the face instead of licking affectionately, which is the normal custom of most puppies. Even those puppies that are strongly motivated to compete and mouth on the hands will usually shift from biting to kissing when permitted to get close to the face. Even dogs expressing high-reactive thresholds may show such problems at an early causing them to gradually lose their capacity to connect in a rewarding way with people. Although such dogs are usually not at risk of developing aggression problems, they may become increasingly insular and hyperactive or withdrawn. Puppies showing any of these signs should receive intensive therapy aimed at promoting friendly eye contact and social gazing. Target-arc training and play therapy appears to be particularly useful in such cases as a means for invigorating the social engagement system (see *Attention and Play Therapy* in Chapter 8).

Temperament test scores may reveal significant information about how a puppy is emotionally and cognitively organized and prepared to respond to social and environmental stimulation. Four temperament types have been described and characterized in terms of functional behavioral and motivational systems (see *Emotional Command Systems and Drive Theory* in Chapter 6). These types are differentiated by the way they respond to various provocative situations and stimuli. Balanced responses are characteristic of stable extraverts (s type) and stable introverts (p type), whereas unbalanced responses are typical of unstable extraverts (c type) and unstable introverts (m type). While s and p types appear to function under the complementary and balancing influences of the behavioral approach system (BAS) and the behavioral inhibition system (BIS), the instability associated with c and m types appears to stem from heightened BIS sensitivity to signals of punishment (threat and loss) and a reactive affinity with the fight/flight system (FFS) (see *Prediction and Control Expectancies* in Chapter 1). The FFS mediates the expression of escape and attack in response to aversive stimulation and frustration (nonreward).

The BAS and BIS work in relative harmony to mediate adaptation, with the former doing the steering and the latter doing the braking. The FFS is an emergency system associated with the reactive expression of unconditioned fear and anger. S- and p-type puppies and dogs are differentiated by the amount of influence exerted by the BAS and

BIS. S types show an increased sensitivity to novelty and reward signals and operate under the dominant activating influence of the BAS (prone to approach), whereas p types are more sensitive to startle and reward signals associated with the avoidance of punishment and operate under the dominant inhibitory influence of the BIS (prone to hesitate). S and p types respond adaptively to signals of reward and loss of reward in the process of organizing behavior. S-type dogs tend to engage in modal strategies (searching, exploring, and competing) aimed at producing positive prediction error (surprise), whereas p-types tend to engage in modal strategies (e.g., hesitating, waiting, and deferring) aimed at avoiding negative prediction error (disappointment). In contrast, c and m types show a reactive sensitivity toward novelty and signals of punishment (risk and loss), predisposing them to reactive appetitive and emotional behavior resulting in opposite adaptations tending toward mania and exploitation, on the one hand, and anxious dysthymia and withdrawal, on the other. Further, whereas extreme c-types expressing low-aggression thresholds (trait aggression) are prone to respond in an invigorated fashion to signals of risk and loss under the influence frustration and anger (attack mode), m-types are prone to respond to risk and loss under the conflictive influence of anxiety or the invigoration of fear (escape mode), and may attack under the catastrophic influence of anger and fear (panic mode) if efforts to escape are blocked. Extreme c- and m-types appear to operate in close affinity with the FFS, recommending strongly against the use of punitive techniques in the control and management of puppies and dogs exhibiting such trait aggression or fear. C and m types require highly structured home environments and consistent reward-based training in order to stabilize them in the direction of the s and p type.

Temperament testing can be used most constructively in the context of assessing and guiding training and socialization activities. However, the results of such testing can easily produce significant potential harm when they are improperly generalized or used to forecast adult behavior. Although conventional temperament tests cannot reliably predict adult propensities, they may inadvertently influence the eventual development of such problems via social placebo and self-fulfilling prophecy effects (see *Social Placebo* in Volume 2, Chapter 10). With the recognition that temperament tests have limited predictive value, except in the most extreme and obvious cases, breeders and trainers using such instruments should take great care not to overly alarm or plant the seeds of doubt and worry when interpreting and discussing the results of puppy temperament testing. Telling a prospective owner that his or her puppy is dominant or aggressive may adversely influence the way the owner treats the puppy, perhaps setting into motion a chain of events that gradually shapes a relationship based on misunderstanding, mistrust, and misguided training activities—all stemming from the influence of a careless opinion. Instead of being used to prognosticate and label the puppy or dwell on its negative potential, the results should be used to help the owner understand the puppy's behavior and to guide socialization and training efforts toward the actualization of the puppy's positive potential.

References

Beaudet R (1993). Social dominance evaluation: Observations on Campbell's test. *Bull Vet Clin Ethol*, 1:23–29.

Braff L, Geyer MA, and Swerdlow NR (2001). Human studies of prepulse inhibition of startle: Normal subjects, patient groups, and pharmacological studies. *Psychopharmacology*, 156:234–258.

Campbell WE (1972). A behavior test for puppy selection. *Mod Vet Pract*, 12:29-33.

Clark GI (1994). The relationship between emotionality and temperament in young puppies [PhD dissertation]. Fort Collins: Colorado State University.

Fox MW (1972). *Understanding Your Dog*. New York: Coward, McCann and Geoghegan.

Fox MW and Spencer JW (1967). Development of the delayed response in the dog. *Anim Behav*, 15:162–168.

Gagnon S and Dore FY (1994). Cross-sectional study of object permanence in domestic puppies (*Canis familiaris*). *J Comp Psychol*, 108:220–232.

Gray JA (1991). The neuropsychology of temperament. In J Strelau and A Angleitner (Eds), *Explorations in Temperament: International Perspectives on Theory and Measurement*. London: Plenum.

Hare B, Brown M, Williamson C, and Tomasello M (2002). The domestication of social cognition in dogs. *Science*, 298:1634–1636.

Krauss JL (1976). The predictive value of a puppy test for determining future trainability for obedience work [PhD dissertation]. Cleveland, OH: Case Western Reserve University.

Pavlov IP (1994). *Psychopathology and Psychiatry*, G Windholz (Intro). New Brunswick, NJ: Transaction.

Pongrácz P, Miklósi A, Kubinyi E, et al. (2001). Social learning in dogs: The effect of a human demonstrator on the performance of dogs in a detour task. *Anim Behav*, 62:1109.

Scott JP and Fuller JL (1965). *Genetics and the Social Behavior of the Dog*. Chicago: University of Chicago Press.

Index